THE
CANADIAN
MEDICAL
ASSOCIATION

HOME MEDICAL
ENCYCLOPEDIA

A Dorling Kindersley book

Published in Canada in 1992 by
The Reader's Digest Association (Canada) Ltd.
215 Redfern Avenue
Westmount, Que. H3Z 2V9

Canadian edition
Copyright © 1992 Dorling Kindersley Limited, London

Based on *The British Medical Association Complete Family
Health Encyclopedia*
Copyright © 1990 Dorling Kindersley Limited, London

The Canadian Medical Association Home Medical Encyclopedia
provides information on a wide range of health and medical topics.
The encyclopedia is not a substitute for medical diagnosis,
however, and you are advised always to consult your physician for
specific information on personal health matters. The naming
of any organization, product, or alternative therapy in this
encyclopedia does not imply CMA endorsement; the omission
of any such names does not indicate CMA disapproval.

Canadian Cataloguing in Publication Data
Main entry under title:
The Canadian Medical Association home medical encyclopedia

1st Canadian ed.
Includes index.
ISBN 0-88850-186-2 (set)
ISBN 0-88850-184-6 (v. 1)
ISBN 0-88850-185-4 (v. 2)

    I. Medicine, Popular – Dictionaries. I. Morgan,
Peter, 1927 –   . II. Canadian Medical Association.
III. Reader's Digest Association (Canada). IV. Title:
Home medical encyclopedia.

RC81.A2C36 1991   610.3   C91-090378-6

Reader's Digest and the Pegasus colophon
are trademarks of The Reader's Digest Association, Inc.

Computerset by MFK Typesetting Limited, England
Reproduction by Mandarin Offset Limited, Hong Kong
Printed and bound in the U.S.A.

THE
CANADIAN
MEDICAL
ASSOCIATION

HOME MEDICAL
ENCYCLOPEDIA

VOLUME TWO · I – Z

MEDICAL EDITOR

Peter Morgan, M.D.

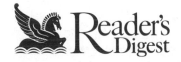

The Reader's Digest Association (Canada) Ltd.
Montreal

EMERGENCY FIRST AID TECHNIQUES

Use this quick-reference list to find illustrated first aid boxes containing step-by-step instructions for performing emergency techniques.

SYMPTOM CHARTS

Use this quick-reference list to find question-and-answer flow charts that indicate the possible causes and significance of many common symptoms.

CONTENTS

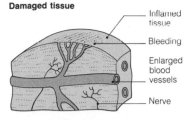

Damaged tissue
- Inflamed tissue
- Bleeding
- Enlarged blood vessels
- Nerve

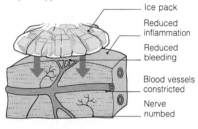

Ice pack application
- Ice pack
- Reduced inflammation
- Reduced bleeding
- Blood vessels constricted
- Nerve numbed

Use of an ice pack
Applying an ice pack to an area of damaged tissue helps relieve pain, reduce inflammation and tissue damage, and minimize bleeding and swelling.

Iatrogenic

A term meaning "physician produced" that can be applied to any medical condition, disease, or other adverse occurrence that results from medical treatment. The development of an iatrogenic condition does not necessarily imply a lack of care or knowledge on the part of the physician. Many common forms of treatment are seldom, if ever, entirely free of possible unwanted effects. The drowsiness produced by some antihistamine drugs is one example.

Ibuprofen

A *nonsteroidal anti-inflammatory drug* (NSAID) used as a painkiller in the treatment of headache, menstrual pain, and painful injury to soft tissues (such as muscles and ligaments). The anti-inflammatory effect of ibuprofen helps reduce the joint pain and stiffness that occurs in types of arthritis, such as *rheumatoid arthritis* and *osteoarthritis*.

Ibuprofen may cause abdominal pain, diarrhea, nausea, heartburn, and, rarely, dizziness. It may cause *peptic ulcer*, but is less likely to do so than some other NSAID.

Ice packs

Means of applying ice (in a towel or other material) to the skin to relieve pain, to stem bleeding, or to reduce inflammation. Cold causes the blood vessels to contract, thus reducing blood flow.

WHY IT IS DONE

Treatment with ice packs is used to relieve pain in a variety of disorders, including severe *headache*, *hemorrhoids* (piles), and pain in the throat after a *tonsillectomy*. Another common use is after sports injuries to minimize swelling, bruising, and further tissue damage. In the treatment of sports injuries, ice packs are usually used together with the application of a pressure bandage and the raising of the injured part. Ice packs may also be used to stop bleeding from small vessels, as in a nosebleed.

HOW IT IS DONE

Ice is wrapped in a wet cloth (to prevent it from "burning" the skin) and applied to the skin's surface. It is also possible to use special chemical packs that become very cold when they are shaken or struck.

Ichthyosis

A rare, inherited condition in which the skin is dry, thickened, scaly, and darker than normal due to an abnormality in the production of *keratin* (a protein that is the main component of skin). The name ichthyosis is taken from the Greek word "ichthus" (meaning fish); the condition is commonly called fish skin disease.

Ichthyosis usually appears at or shortly after birth and generally improves during childhood. The areas most commonly affected are the thighs, arms, and backs of the hands.

There is no special treatment, although lubricants and emulsifying ointments help the dryness and bath oils moisten the skin. Washing with soap makes ichthyosis worse and should be avoided. The condition improves in a warm, humid atmosphere.

Icterus

A term for *jaundice*.

Id

One of the three parts of the personality (together with the *ego* and *superego*) described by Sigmund Freud. The id is the primitive, unconscious store of energy from which come the instincts for food, love, sex, and other basic needs. The id seeks simply to gain pleasure and to avoid pain. (See also *Psychoanalytic theory*.)

Idiocy

An outdated term for the most severe degree of *mental retardation*.

Idiopathic

Of unknown cause. For example, epilepsy for which no specific cause can be found is referred to as idiopathic epilepsy. The word idiopathic comes from Greek "idios" meaning one's own and "pathos" meaning disease.

Idoxuridine

An *antiviral drug* used for the *topical* treatment of *herpes simplex* and *herpes zoster* infections. Idoxuridine may cause irritation of areas to which it is applied. Eye drops may cause photophobia (abnormal sensitivity to light) and blurred vision.

Ileitis, regional

An old name for *Crohn's disease*.

Ileostomy

An operation in which the *ileum* (lower part of the small intestine) is surgically severed and the end brought through an incision in the abdominal wall and formed into an artificial outlet to allow the discharge of feces into a lightweight bag attached to the skin. An ileostomy is usually permanent.

WHY IT IS DONE

A permanent ileostomy is usually performed for people with *ulcerative colitis* or *Crohn's disease* whose health, despite drug treatment, continues to deteriorate because of chronic inflammation of the colon. For these people, the only means of restoring health is to perform a *colectomy* (an operation to remove the colon and rectum) followed by an ileostomy.

Temporary ileostomy is sometimes required at the time of partial colectomy (removal of part of the colon) to allow the repair of the colon to heal before waste material passes through it. Temporary ileostomy may also be carried out as an emergency measure in a person who is very ill due to an obstruction high in the large intestine that is preventing the normal passage of feces. The ileostomy is made above the obstruction and, by allowing waste material to discharge, enables a patient to recover sufficiently to undergo a partial colectomy to remove the obstruction. Temporary ileostomies are closed when the rejoined colon has healed.

HOW IT IS DONE

When the whole of the colon and rectum has been removed, the cut end of the ileum is brought to the surface of the skin through an incision in the abdominal wall.

In the case of a temporary ileostomy, a loop of bowel is brought to the surface and opened so that waste material can pass through. The edges of this opening are then stitched to the skin at the edge of the abdominal incision to create a stoma (an artificial opening). The stoma is usually located on the patient's right side, about 5 cm below the natural waist and away from the hipbone.

POSTOPERATIVE CARE

For a few days, patients may need to be fed by *intravenous infusion*. After that, the intestine starts to function normally again; semiliquid waste is discharged through the stoma into a bag that is closely attached to the skin by adhesive seals.

During the convalescent period, patients with permanent ileostomies are given counseling to help them come to terms with an altered body image and the appearance of the stoma. They are also taught the practical aspects of stoma care. There is no muscle control over evacuation of body wastes through the stoma. These wastes are semiliquid and contain enzymes that can damage the skin around the stoma. For these reasons, it is usually necessary for the bag to be worn at all times. A member of the nursing staff (ideally a stoma-care nurse) teaches the patient how to empty, change, and dispose of the bag, and how to maintain a good seal between bag and body to protect the skin and prevent leaks.

Full recovery from the operation takes about six weeks, during which time patients should avoid vigorous physical activity.

OUTLOOK

The condition of patients who are given ileostomies after removal of a chronically inflamed colon usually improves dramatically. Because their ability to be active is enhanced, many of these people say they wish they had had the operation years earlier.

Following convalescence, patients should be able to return to their usual employment, life-style, and family and social activities. After an ileostomy it is necessary to drink increased

---

PROCEDURE FOR ILEOSTOMY

Two incisions are made in the abdominal wall (usually on the right side)—a small circular cut for the stoma (most often located about 5 cm below the waist and away from the hipbone and groin crease) and a vertical cut to give access to the intestine and *mesentery*.

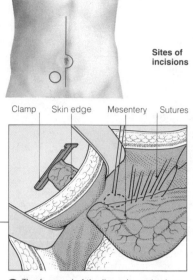

Sites of incisions

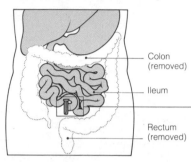

Colon (removed)

Ileum

Rectum (removed)

1 After removal of the colon, the cut end of the ileum is clamped and part of the mesentery is cut to free a short length of ileum for the stoma.

Clamp   Skin edge   Mesentery   Sutures

2 The free end of the ileum is pushed out through the circular incision in the abdomen; the mesentery is then stitched to the inner abdominal wall.

Clamp

Stoma

3 The main vertical incision is closed and the clamp is removed from the protruding end of the ileum (top) The end of the ileum is then turned back and attached to the abdomen with sutures (middle). When completed, this creates a small protruding stoma (bottom). A temporary ileostomy appliance is usually fitted immediately.

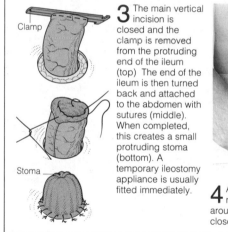

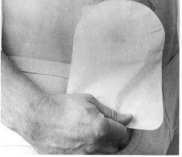

4 After the intestine begins to function normally, an ileostomy bag is fitted around the stoma. The bag is attached closely to the skin by adhesive seals.

---

amounts of water and to ensure that the intake of salt is adequate, thus compensating for the lack of a colon (the main functions of which are the absorption of water and salt). Apart from this recommendation, it is generally possible to eat a normal diet.

Only an occasional medical checkup is needed to make sure that the stoma is in good condition, although the physician should always be informed of any change in the function or appearance of the stoma. Occasionally, the channel of the stoma becomes narrowed or prolapses (protrudes too far from the abdomen), requiring surgical correction.

Various attempts have been made to devise ileostomies that require emptying only once or twice a day at fixed times and do not require an external appliance. These devices include internal reservoirs made from loops of small intestine, magnetic closures, and carbon filter systems for gas. However, none is consistently reliable; most patients are still offered a conventional ileostomy.

Ileum

The final, longest, and narrowest section of the small intestine. It is joined at its upper end to the *jejunum* and at its lower end to the large intestine.

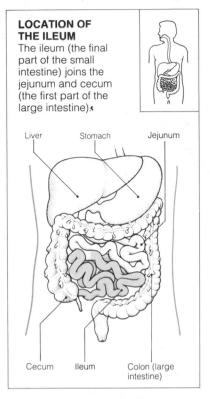

Liver   Stomach   Jejunum

Cecum   Ileum   Colon (large intestine)

The function of the ileum is to absorb nutrients from food that has been digested in the stomach and the first two sections of the small intestine. The millions of *villi* (finger-like projections) that line the ileum considerably increase its surface area and thus its powers of absorption.

DISORDERS
Occasionally, the ileum becomes obstructed—for example, by pushing through a weakness in the abdominal wall (see *Hernia*) or by becoming caught up with scar tissue following abdominal surgery (see *Adhesion*).

Other disorders of the ileum include *Meckel's diverticulum* (a pouch in the ileum wall that may become ulcerated) and diseases in which absorption of nutrients is impaired, such as *Crohn's disease, celiac disease,* tropical *sprue,* and *lymphoma.*

Ileus, paralytic
A failure, usually temporary, of the normal contractility of the muscles of the intestine. As a result, intestinal contents can no longer pass through the body and the intestine becomes obstructed. Paralytic ileus commonly follows abdominal surgery and may also be induced by severe abdominal injury, *peritonitis* (inflammation of the membrane lining the abdomen), internal bleeding, acute *pancreatitis* (inflammation of the pancreas), or interference with the blood or nerve supply to the intestine.

The symptoms of paralytic ileus include a distended (swollen) abdomen, vomiting, and failure to pass feces. The condition is usually successfully treated by sucking out the intestinal contents through a tube passed through the nose or mouth into the stomach or intestine and by maintaining body fluid levels by *intravenous infusion* (drip).

Illness
Perception by a person that he or she is not well. Illness is a subjective sensation and may have physical or psychological causes. Illness is also sometimes used as a synonym for disease or disorder.

Illusion
A distorted sensation. An illusion is based on misinterpretation of a real stimulus (for example, a pen is seen as a dagger, or the sound of a screeching brake is heard as a scream). An illusion is not the same as an *hallucination* in which a perception occurs without any stimulus.

Usually, illusions are brief and can be understood when explained. They may be due to tiredness or anxiety, to drugs of many sorts, or to certain forms of brain damage. *Delirium tremens* is a classic inducer of illusions.

Imaging techniques
Techniques that produce images of structures within the body that cannot otherwise be seen. Imaging techniques are an invaluable aid in diagnosing abnormalities and disease.

X RAYS
In 1895 the discovery of *X rays* revolutionized medical diagnosis by making it possible for the first time to visualize bone, organs, and other internal tissue without opening up the body. The rays are electromagnetic waves of short wavelength. Some are absorbed and others pass through tissues; the shadow that is cast is projected onto a fluorescent screen or a film.

CONTRAST MEDIA X-ray images of bones are distinct, but soft tissues show up less clearly. To overcome this, radiologists from the 1920s onward began using substances opaque to radiation as part of certain X-ray procedures. When such substances (known as contrast media) are introduced into internal organs, blood vessels, or ducts, they produce (on the X-ray screen or film) an outline of the cavities they fill.

A contrast medium can be introduced into the body in various ways. In *cholecystography* (carried out to examine the gallbladder and common bile duct) and in some *barium X-ray examinations* of the esophagus, the stomach, and the small bowel, the medium is swallowed in tablet or liquid form. In *bronchography* (used to diagnose various chest disorders) the contrast medium is introduced into the bronchi (airways) connecting the windpipe to the lungs. In *angiography* and *venography*, the contrast medium is injected into an artery or vein, respectively, to provide images of the blood vessels. In intravenous *urography*, the medium injected into a vein in the arm travels to the kidneys and urinary tract. In *ERCP* (by which the pancreatic duct and biliary system are examined), the medium is passed into the ducts by means of a catheter (tube) passed through a channel in an endoscope (a flexible viewing instrument).

SCANNING TECHNIQUES
Since the 1970s, many X-ray imaging techniques have been superseded by newer procedures that are simpler to perform and are safer and more comfortable for the patient. *Ultrasound scanning* consists of passing high-frequency sound waves through the body with a transducer placed against the skin. The waves are reflected to varying degrees by structures of different density, and the pattern of the echoes is electronically recorded on a screen. Ultrasound scanning is the first choice for diagnostic imaging of the gallbladder, female genital tract, and fetus. It also provides remarkably clear pictures of the kidney.

COMPUTERS Many scanning techniques use a computer to provide images. In *CT scanning* (computed tomography scanning), X rays are passed through the body at different angles. The computer produces cross-sectional images ("slices") of the tissues being examined. In *MRI* (magnetic resonance imaging), the patient is placed in a strong magnetic field and radiofrequency waves are passed through the body. A computer analyzes changes in the magnetic alignment of the hydrogen protons of the cells to give an image of the tissues.

CT scanning and MRI are particularly valuable in the diagnosis of brain disorders. So, too, is a more recent technique called *PET scanning* (positron emission tomography scanning),

I

IMAGING THE BODY

Over the past decade, many new methods of imaging the body have been developed. These new imaging techniques have made it possible to visualize internal structures in a variety of different ways. Today, in addition to conventional X rays (which show primarily bones), techniques such as CT scanning, radionuclide scanning, ultrasound scanning, MRI, and PET scanning are used to provide detailed diagnostic pictures of soft tissues and organs. The examples given here show some of the different ways in which the kidneys can be imaged.

X RAYS

Radiopaque contrast media may be utilized to give distinct X-ray images of soft tissues, as in intravenous urography, which is used to give clear images of the kidneys and urinary tract.

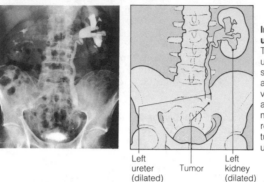

Left ureter (dilated) Tumor Left kidney (dilated)

Intravenous urogram
The intravenous urogram (far left) shows the left kidney and ureter, which are visible because they are filled with contrast medium that has been retained due to a tumor obstructing the ureter (see left).

SCANNING TECHNIQUES

Many new techniques have been developed for imaging the body, particularly the soft tissues. Some of these techniques, such as CT scanning, rely on computers to process the raw imaging data and produce the actual image. Others, such as ultrasound scanning and radionuclide scanning, can produce images without a computer, although one may be used for image enhancement.

Damaged left kidney

Normal right kidney

Radionuclide scanning
A radioactive substance is introduced into the body, and the radiation emitted is detected by a gamma camera, which converts it into an image. In the scan of the kidneys (left), the left one has taken up little of the radioactive substance (and thus appears faint), which indicates that it is damaged.

Ultrasound scanning

Ultra high-frequency sound waves reflected from tissues in the body are converted into an image by special electronic equipment. The scan (below left) shows a section through a diseased kidney; the inner tissues (calyx and pelvis) are greatly dilated and the outer cortex is abnormally thin (see diagram, below right).

Back   Thin cortex

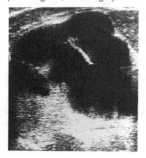

Renal calyx (dilated)   Renal pelvis (dilated)

CT scanning

A CT scanner produces cross-sectional images (slices) of the body. The CT scan (right) shows a greatly dilated right kidney (see diagram, below right).

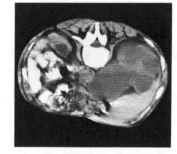

Back muscles

Tip of left kidney

Spine

Spinal cord

Right kidney (dilated)

Rib

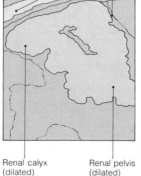

in which very short-lived radio-isotopes are introduced into tissues; the paths of gamma rays emitted are analyzed by a computer, giving information about brain function and structure.

In *radionuclide scanning*, a gamma camera records, and a computer transforms into images, radiation emitted from tissues into which a radioactive substance has been introduced. The computer may be used to obtain more information from the results.

Imipramine

A tricyclic *antidepressant drug*. Imipramine is most commonly used as a long-term treatment for *depression*, but may take up to six weeks to have a beneficial effect.

Possible adverse effects include excessive sweating, blurred vision, dry mouth, dizziness, constipation, nausea, and, in older men, difficulty passing urine. Overdose, particularly in a child, can be fatal.

Immersion foot

A type of *cold injury* occurring when the feet are wet and cold for a long time. It occurs in people who have been shipwrecked and in soldiers (in whom it is known as trench foot). Initially, the feet turn pale and have no detectable pulse; later, they become red, swollen, and painful, and have a strong pulse.

TREATMENT
If the feet are at the pale stage, they should be gradually and carefully rewarmed; overheating may lead to *gangrene* (tissue death). Conversely, if they are red and swollen, they should be gradually cooled. *Analgesic drugs* (painkillers) may be necessary.

If the condition is ignored and becomes severe, muscle weakness, skin ulcers, or gangrene may develop. Even with mild cases, the feet may be painful and sensitive to cold for several years afterward.

Immobility

Reduced physical activity and movement. Immobility is particularly harmful in the elderly because it causes muscle wasting and progressive loss of function.

CAUSES
Total immobility is rare; it occurs in coma, which is sometimes the result of *stroke*, *brain tumor*, or major *head injury*. *Catatonia* is associated with varying degrees of immobility.

Temporary loss of mobility, lasting a few days, occurs during recovery from any serious illness, such as a *myocardial infarction* (heart attack), or from a major surgical procedure.

Fractures in a lower limb may be treated by *traction*, which requires several weeks in bed, or by use of a *cast*, which also hinders mobility.

Loss of mobility may be caused by the symptoms of a specific medical disorder, such as *asthma* or *angina pectoris* (chest pain due to reduced blood supply to the heart muscle). Both these conditions may, in severe cases, be aggravated by exercise. *Arthritis* (inflammation of joints) limits mobility if the hips, knees, ankles, or feet are affected by pain and stiffness. Nervous system disorders that restrict mobility include *hemiplegia* (paralysis on one side of the body), *Parkinson's disease*, and *multiple sclerosis*.

A person may find it difficult to move around because of deteriorating eyesight; alternatively he or she may lack motivation due to *depression* or the effects of alcohol or other drugs (such as *tranquilizer drugs*).

COMPLICATIONS
Total immobility can cause *bedsores*, *pneumonia* due to the buildup of secretions in the lungs, or *contractures* (deformity caused by the shrinkage of tissue).

A common complication of partial immobility is *edema* (abnormal retention of fluid in body tissues), which causes swelling of the legs because the calf muscles are not pumping the fluid back to the heart via the circulation. Rarely, sluggish blood flow encourages formation of a *thrombus* (abnormal blood clot) in a leg vein.

Obesity is more likely to occur in people who do not exercise. Stiffness tends to develop in any joint that is not being used properly. Muscle wasting and *osteoporosis* (bone thinning) are common problems caused by immobility in the elderly.

TREATMENT
Regular *physiotherapy* and adequate nursing care are important for any person who is totally immobile. Frequent turning and the use of a special mattress and bed reduce the risk of bedsores. Stretching exercises may prevent contractures.

Early mobilization after serious illness or major surgery is usually encouraged to avoid the problems of prolonged bed rest. After a lower limb fracture, walking with the aid of crutches is started as soon as possible.

Aids for the disabled (see *Disability*) can increase mobility in people with leg weakness, stiffness, loss of

balance, or poor coordination. If a person is unable to walk despite assistance, exercises may be done in a chair or in bed to keep the muscles and joints in reasonable working order.

Immobilization

An orthopedic term for techniques used to prevent movement of joints or displacement of fractured bones so that the bones can unite properly. (See *Fracture*.)

Immune response

A defensive reaction of the body to invading microorganisms, cancer cells, transplanted tissue, and other substances or materials that are recognized as antigenic or "foreign" (that is, different from normal body components). The response consists of the production of substances called *antibodies* or *immunoglobulins*, sensitized cells called *lymphocytes*, and other substances and cells that act to destroy the antigenic material. (See also *Immune system*.)

Immune serum globulin

A preparation of *antibodies*, also known as immune globulin and gamma globulin, used to prevent and sometimes treat infectious diseases.

Mainly used to prevent viral hepatitis, immune serum globulin is also given to prevent infection in persons exposed to measles and rubella who previously had neither had these diseases nor been immunized against them. Immune serum globulin is also given to people with *immunodeficiency disorders*.

HOW IT WORKS
Immune serum globulin provides immunity to a range of common infectious diseases. It works by passing on antibodies obtained from the blood of large numbers of people who have previously been exposed to these diseases and thus have developed antibodies to them.

Immune serum globulin may cause rash, fever, and pain and tenderness at the injection site.

Immune system

A collection of cells and proteins that works to protect the body from potentially harmful, infectious microorganisms (microscopic life-forms), such as bacteria, viruses, and fungi. The immune system also plays a role in the control of *cancer* and is responsible for the phenomena of *allergy*, *hypersensitivity*, and rejection problems after *transplant surgery*.

THE INNATE IMMUNE SYSTEM

Each of us has many inborn defenses against infection, including external barriers (below), the inflammatory response (right), and phagocyte action (below right). Others include substances called complement (which is activated by and attacks bacteria) and *interferon* (which has antiviral effects).

All these defenses are nonspecific and quick-acting. By contrast, the adaptive immune system (see overleaf) mounts specific attacks against particular microbes. These cells are most effective on second exposure to the organisms.

The two parts of the immune system work together; antibodies produced by the adaptive immune system assist phagocyte action.

THE INFLAMMATORY RESPONSE

If microbes break through the body's outermost barriers, inflammation is the second line of defense. Chemicals (such as histamine) are released, prompting the effects shown below, including the attraction of phagocytes to the microbes. The symptoms of inflammation are redness, pain, swelling, and heat.

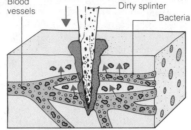

Following tissue injury (here caused by a splinter) and entry of bacteria or other microbes, blood vessels in the area widen and there is increased leakage of fluid from the blood into the tissues. This allows easier access for immune system components that fight the invaders, including phagocytes and soluble factors (such as the group of substances known as complement).

Physical and chemical barriers

These barriers, summarized below, provide the first line of defense against harmful microbes (bacteria, viruses, and fungi).

Eyes
Tears produced by the lacrimal apparatus help wash away microorganisms; tears contain an enzyme (lysozyme) that can destroy bacteria.

Mouth
Lysozyme present in saliva. destroys bacteria.

Breast-feeding
Antibodies (proteins with a protective role) formed by the mother against certain microbes are transferred to the baby in breast milk. This action provides some extra immunity until the baby can form his or her own specific antibodies.

Nose
Hairs in the nose help prevent entry of microorganisms on dust particles. This process is assisted by the sneeze reflex

Respiratory tract
Mucus secreted by cells lining the throat, windpipe, and bronchi traps microbes, which are then swept away by cilia (hairs on cells in the lining) or engulfed by phagocytes (types of white cells). The cough reflex also helps to expel microbes.

Stomach and intestines
Stomach acid destroys the vast majority of microorganisms. The intestines contain harmless bacteria (commensals) that compete with and control the harmful organisms.

Genitourinary system
The vagina and urethra also contain commensals and are protected by mucus.

Skin
Intact skin provides an effective barrier against most microbes. The sebaceous glands secrete chemicals that are highly toxic to many bacteria.

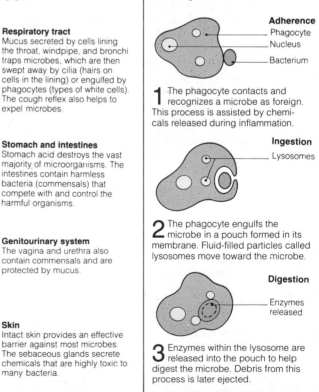

ACTION OF PHAGOCYTES
These white blood cells are attracted to infection sites, where they engulf and digest microorganisms and debris.

Adherence
- Phagocyte
- Nucleus
- Bacterium

1 The phagocyte contacts and recognizes a microbe as foreign. This process is assisted by chemicals released during inflammation.

Ingestion
- Lysosomes

2 The phagocyte engulfs the microbe in a pouch formed in its membrane. Fluid-filled particles called lysosomes move toward the microbe.

Digestion
- Enzymes released

3 Enzymes within the lysosome are released into the pouch to help digest the microbe. Debris from this process is later ejected.

Some of the main components of the body's immune system are described in the illustrated boxes on pages 570 and 572.

A newborn child is, to some extent, protected against infection by innate immunity. This consists of physical barriers, such as the skin; substances present in the mouth, urinary tract, or on the eye surface that destroy microorganisms; and *antibodies* or *immunoglobulins* (protective proteins) that have been passed to the child from the mother (including those received in breast milk).

Innate immunity cannot guard against all disease-causing organisms. As the child grows, he or she encounters organisms that overcome the innate defenses and thus cause disease. The second line of immune defense, called the adaptive immune system, then comes into play. As the name implies, this system adapts its response specifically to fight each invading organism. In addition, it retains a memory of the invader so that defenses can be rallied instantly in the future. The person is then said to have acquired immunity to the infection. If the same microorganisms invade again, they are quickly recognized and dealt with (which explains why it is rare for diseases such as measles and diphtheria to affect the same person twice).

The acquisition of immunity in response to an infection can take a few days or weeks to develop; in the interim, a child or adult can become very ill or even die. In the past, many did die. Today, our chance of surviving, recovering, or totally avoiding infectious diseases is much improved, partly as a result of better general health and nutrition (which bolsters the immune system) and partly through vaccination—artificial *immunization* against specific microorganisms.

INNATE IMMUNITY

The skin provides an impenetrable barrier to the vast majority of infectious agents, most of which can gain entry only via the mucous membranes (i.e., the lining of the mouth, throat, eyes, intestines, vagina, or urinary tract). These areas are protected by the movement of mucus and other fluids (such as tears) and the presence of enzymes (such as lysozyme) that destroy bacteria. If microorganisms penetrate the outer layer of the skin or a mucous membrane, they soon encounter white blood cells called phagocytes (literally, "devouring cells"), which attempt to destroy them, and other types of white cells, such as natural cell-killing (cytotoxic) cells. Microorganisms may also meet naturally produced substances (such as *interferon*) or a group of blood proteins called the complement system, which act to destroy the invading microorganisms.

ADAPTIVE IMMUNITY

The adaptive part of the immune system is extremely complex and only partly understood. Its function is to produce specific defenses against a vast range of different invading organisms or tumor cells. Broadly, however, it first must recognize part of an invading organism or tumor cell as an *antigen* (a protein that is foreign or different from any natural body protein).

A response (either humoral or cellular) is then mounted against the antigen. The humoral response consists of the production of soluble proteins, called antibodies or immunoglobulins, manufactured by cells called B-lymphocytes. Cellular responses center on the activities of cells called T-lymphocytes.

HUMORAL IMMUNITY This type of immunity is particularly important in the defense against bacteria. After a complex recognition process, certain B-lymphocytes are stimulated to multiply. These cells then begin to produce vast numbers of antibodies that are able to bind to the antigens. Once this binding process has taken place, the organisms bearing the antigens are easy prey to phagocytic ("cell-devouring") white cells. Binding of antibody and antigen may also activate the complement system, which increases the efficiency with which phagocytes engulf and destroy the invading organisms.

CELLULAR IMMUNITY This is particularly important in the defense against viruses, some types of parasites that hide within cells, and, possibly, cancer cells. The T-lymphocytes at the center of cellular immunity are of two types, called helper cells and killer cells. The helper cells play a role in the recognition of antigens. Along with various other functions, they activate the killer cells.

Killer lymphocytes lock onto cells that have been invaded by viruses or other parasites which have left recognizable antigens on the cell surfaces. The killers then destroy these parasitized cells. They may act in a similar way against tumor cells and against cells in transplanted tissue.

The memory of the immune system (which provides acquired immunity to certain diseases) relies on the long-term survival of lymphocytes that were activated or sensitized to antigens when these antigens were first encountered.

IMMUNE SYSTEM DISORDERS

The immune system is an essential asset for the protection of the body from infectious agents and probably cancer. In *immunodeficiency disorders*, suppression of the immune system occurs either as a result of an inherited disorder or after infection with certain viruses, including *HIV*, the virus that causes *AIDS*.

In another group of disorders, known as *autoimmune disorders*, the immune system misidentifies the body's own proteins as antigens and mounts an immunological attack against them.

Other disorders occur when the immune system mounts an inappropriate response to what are usually innocuous antigens, such as pollen, causing *hypersensitivity* or *allergy*.

IMMUNOSUPPRESSIVE THERAPY

In certain circumstances, such as after tissue transplants and in people with an autoimmune disorder, it is advantageous to suppress the immune system (especially its adaptive part) through use of *immunosuppressant drugs*. This prevents rejection of the donor organ by lymphocytes and other cells that recognize proteins in the transplanted tissue as antigens.

Immunity

A state of protection against a disease or diseases through the activities of the *immune system*. Innate immunity is present from birth and is the first line of defense against the majority of infectious agents. Acquired immunity is the second line of defense. It develops either through exposure to invading microorganisms (after they have broken through the innate immune defenses) or through *immunization*.

Immunization

The process of inducing *immunity* as a preventive measure against certain infectious diseases. The incidence of a number of diseases (e.g., *diphtheria*, *poliomyelitis*) has declined dramatically since the introduction of effective immunization programs; one disease (*smallpox*) has been eradicated.

Due to the persistent efforts of physicians, public health authorities, and with the support of legislation, the great majority of children in

THE ADAPTIVE IMMUNE SYSTEM

This system is based on cells called lymphocytes. It has two parts. Humoral immunity relies on the production, by B-lymphocytes, of antibodies, which circulate and attack specific microbes. In cellular immunity, cells called T-lymphocytes are activated and attack specific microbes or abnormal cells (such as virally infected or tumor cells)

HUMORAL IMMUNITY

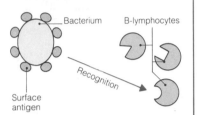

1 A humoral response is started when an antigen (foreign protein)—here on the surface of a bacterium—activates one type of B-lymphocyte.

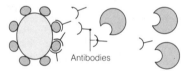

2 The particular type of B-lymphocyte multiplies, forming cells called plasma cells, which make antibodies designed specifically to attack the bacterium.

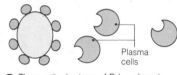

3 After a few days, the antibodies are released and travel to, and attach to, the antigen. This triggers more reactions, which ultimately destroy the bacterium.

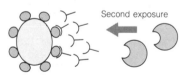

4 Some B-lymphocytes remain in the body as memory cells; if the bacterium enters the body again, they rapidly produce antibodies to halt the infection.

CELLULAR IMMUNITY

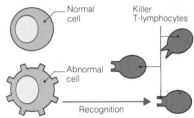

1 An antigen, here on the surface of an abnormal cell (such as a virus-infected or tumor cell), is identified by, and activates, specific killer (cytotoxic) T-lymphocytes.

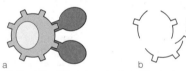

2 With the assistance of helper T cells (another type of T-lymphocyte), the killer T-lymphocytes begin to multiply.

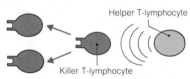

3 The killer T-lymphocytes travel to, and attach to, the abnormal cells (a), leading to their destruction (b). The T-lymphocytes survive and may go on to kill more targets.

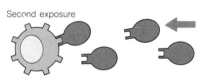

4 Some of the killer T-lymphocytes remain as memory cells, and quickly attack abnormal cells should they reappear (e.g., after reinfection with a virus).

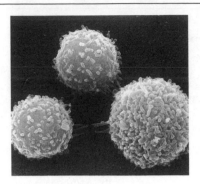

Lymphocyte
Lymphocytes are found in the blood and lymphoid organs (lymph nodes, spleen, and thymus). The two main types—B- and T-lymphocytes—have different functions but look similar under the microscope.

AIDS AND CELLULAR IMMUNITY

HIV—the AIDS virus—disrupts the cellular part of the adaptive immune system.

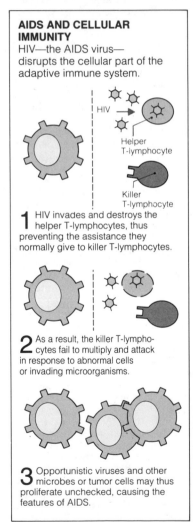

1 HIV invades and destroys the helper T-lymphocytes, thus preventing the assistance they normally give to killer T-lymphocytes.

2 As a result, the killer T-lymphocytes fail to multiply and attack in response to abnormal cells or invading microorganisms.

3 Opportunistic viruses and other microbes or tumor cells may thus proliferate unchecked, causing the features of AIDS.

EXAMPLES OF INFECTIOUS ORGANISMS COMBATED

Humoral immunity particularly important against:	Cell-mediated immunity particularly important against:
Some viruses (e.g., measles)	Many viruses (e.g., herpes simplex)
Many bacteria (e.g., cholera)	Some bacteria (e.g., tuberculosis)
Some parasites (e.g., malaria)	Some fungi (e.g., candidiasis)

TYPES OF IMMUNIZATION

There are two main types. In passive immunization, antibodies (protective proteins) are injected and provide immediate, but short-lived, protection against specific disease-causing bacteria, viruses, or toxins. Active immunization primes the body to make its own antibodies against such microorganisms and confers longer-lasting immunity.

PASSIVE IMMUNIZATION

1 Blood is taken from a person or, rarely, an animal previously exposed to a specific microorganism. The blood contains antibodies against that organism.

Antibodies

2 An extract of the blood containing the antibodies (called immune serum or antiserum) is injected into the person to be protected.

Serum

Bloodstream

3 The antibodies help destroy the microorganism if it is present in the blood or enters it over the following few weeks.

Microorganism

ACTIVE IMMUNIZATION

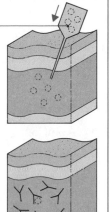

Vaccine

1 The person to be protected is inoculated with a killed or modified microorganism (vaccine) that does not cause disease.

2 The immune system is provoked to make antibodies against the modified microorganism; it also retains a "memory" of the organism.

Antibodies

3 If the real microorganism then enters the blood, antibodies are produced in large numbers to halt the infection.

Disease-causing microorganism

Canada is currently immunized; as a result, not only diphtheria and polio but also *measles* and *pertussis* have become rare. However, to keep the incidence of these diseases low, routine immunization must continue. If a large proportion of the population is not immunized, there is always risk of a new epidemic.

IMMUNIZATION AND VACCINATION

Immunization may be active or passive (see table below). The terms vaccination and active immunization are used interchangeably.

WHO SHOULD BE IMMUNIZED

Some types of immunization, such as immunization against polio, against measles, mumps and rubella, and against diphtheria, pertussis, and *tetanus* (see *DPT vaccination*), are aimed at the general population, primarily at young children. Others are intended for specific people, such as those exposed to dangerous infections during local outbreaks or those who are at risk of contracting unusual infections through occupational exposure (e.g., laboratory workers or veterinary surgeons).

Immunization before foreign travel may be necessary for entry into certain countries (today, this usually applies only to immunization against *yellow fever*) and to protect the traveler against infection. The traveler should determine a few months before departure which immunizations are necessary or recommended.

The accompanying table gives details of a typical immunization schedule during childhood. (See also *Travel immunization*.)

HOW IMMUNIZATION IS DONE

Most immunizations are given by injection, usually into the tissues under the skin or into the muscle of the upper arm. If the injection contains a large volume of fluid, it may be given in the buttock. Polio vaccine is given orally.

ADVERSE REACTIONS

There are usually no after effects following immunization. Some vaccines cause pain and swelling at the injection site and may produce a slight fever, a feeling of irritability and malaise, or flulike symptoms. Young children who develop fever after being immunized should be given *acetaminophen*. Some vaccines, such as the measles vaccine, may produce a mild form of the disease.

In very rare cases, severe reactions (such as seizures) occur following immunization. This has led to controversy about the advisability of some types of vaccination, notably against pertussis. However, for most people, the risks of vaccination are much smaller than the risks of damage from the disease.

Although most modern vaccines provide a reliable method of preventing disease, they do not all provide complete protection. *Cholera* and *typhoid fever* vaccinations, in particular, give only partial protection, so other precautions (principally food and water hygiene) must be observed during travel to areas where there is a risk of these diseases.

WHO SHOULD NOT BE IMMUNIZED

Immunization should not be given to any person who suffers from an *im-*

TYPICAL CHILDHOOD IMMUNIZATION SCHEDULE

Age	Disease	
3 months	Diphtheria, pertussis (whooping cough), tetanus*	Poliomyelitis†
5 months	Diphtheria, pertussis, tetanus*	Poliomyelitis†
9 months	Diphtheria, pertussis, tetanus*	Poliomyelitis†
15 months	Measles, mumps, rubella (German measles)*	
4 to 5 years	Diphtheria, tetanus*	Poliomyelitis†
	*Combined injection	†Oral

munodeficiency disorder or widespread cancer. Any person who is taking corticosteroid drugs or who has previously had a severe reaction to the same vaccine should not be vaccinated. Some vaccines (e.g., for typhoid and yellow fever) should not be given to very young children. Vaccination should be delayed if a person has a fever or infection. A number of vaccines should not be given during pregnancy because of the risk to the fetus.

Immunoassay

A group of laboratory techniques that includes ELISA (enzyme-linked immunosorbent assay) and radioimmunoassay. Both are used in the diagnosis of infectious diseases; variants of radioimmunoassay, such as the radioallergosorbent test (RAST) and the radioimmunosorbent test (RIST), are also used in the diagnosis of allergies and in the measurement of concentrations of hormones in the blood.

ELISA and radioimmunoassay can both determine the presence or absence in a person's blood of a specific protein—such as an antigen (a protein on the surface of a microorganism or an allergen), a specific antibody (a protein formed by the body's immune system to protect against a particular type of microorganism or allergen), or other protein, such as a hormone.

The principle underlying these techniques is that, for any specific antibody, there is a specific antigen. If molecules of these two proteins come in close contact, they will bind strongly to each other. Any specific antibody will bind only to its own antigen, and vice versa.

HOW IT IS DONE

First, the surface of a plate or the inside of a test tube is prepared with a covering of the specific protein (antigen or antibody) that will bind to the antibody or antigen whose presence in the blood is to be tested. For example, in the ELISA test for antibody to HIV (the virus responsible for AIDS), the inside of a test tube is lined with small amounts of antigen from HIV virus.

This surface is then exposed to plasma of the blood; if the antibody (or antigen) under test is present, it will stick strongly to the surface. The surface is then washed and a chemical added that will bind to the bound protein. This chemical is itself linked either to an enzyme called peroxidase (in the ELISA test) or to a radioactive isotope (in radioimmunoassay).

Any excess chemical is washed away, and, if the antibody or antigen was present, either peroxidase or radioactivity is left on the surface. Peroxidase can be detected by adding another chemical that changes color in its presence; radioactivity can be measured by a gamma counter.

The RIST differs from other types of radioimmunoassay in that the blood serum containing the substance being tested is first mixed with a solution containing the same substance, which has been radioactively labeled. The radioactive and the test versions compete to bind to the test plate. The result is that, after washing, the less radioactivity found on the test plate, the more test substance must have been present in the blood serum.

Immunodeficiency disorders

Disorders in which there is a failure of the immune system's defenses to fight infection and tumors. Immunodeficiency may be the result of an inherited or a congenital defect that interferes with the normal development of the immune system, or may be the result of acquired disease that damages the system's function. The result, in either case, is the appearance of persistent or recurrent infection by organisms that would not ordinarily cause disease, poor response to customarily effective treatment, incomplete recovery from illness, and an undue susceptibility to certain forms of cancer.

The infections seen in people with immunodeficiency disorders are sometimes called opportunistic infections because the microorganisms take advantage of the person's lowered defenses. Such infections include pneumonia caused by PNEUMOCYSTIS CARINII, widespread herpes simplex infections, and many fungal infections.

INHERITED IMMUNODEFICIENCY

The adaptive part of the immune system (which mounts specific defenses against particular microorganisms or tumor cells) has two major prongs. One of these, the humoral system, relies on the production of antibodies (or immunoglobulins) by B-lymphocytes. The other prong is called the cellular system and relies on the activity of T-lymphocytes. Congenital or inherited deficiencies can occur in either of these systems.

Deficiencies of the humoral system include hypogammaglobulinemia (in which the production of one or more types of immunoglobulin is interfered with) and agammaglobulinemia

(in which there is an almost complete absence of B-lymphocytes and immunoglobulins). The most common type of hypogammaglobulinemia affects about one person in 600 and usually causes no symptoms or may cause no more than repeated mild attacks of respiratory infection. Agammaglobulinemia is a rare, grave condition that often has a fatal outcome in infancy or childhood.

Congenital deficiencies of T-lymphocytes may lead to problems such as persistent and widespread candidiasis (thrush) affecting the skin, mouth, throat, and vagina. Problems of this type are caused by inability of the immune system to fight fungi.

A combined deficiency of both prongs of the immune system, called severe combined immunodeficiency (SCID), is also known. Affected infants usually die in the first year of life.

ACQUIRED IMMUNODEFICIENCY

Acquired deficiency of the immune system may result either from disease processes or from damage to the immune system as a result of its suppression by drugs.

Diseases that cause immunodeficiency include infection with HIV (human immunodeficiency virus), which leads to AIDS (acquired immune deficiency syndrome). Severe malnutrition, especially if there is protein deficiency, and many cancers can also cause immunodeficiency.

Deliberate suppression of the immune system with immunosuppressant drugs and corticosteroid drugs is usually carried out as part of the treatment of autoimmune disorders and after transplant surgery to minimize the risk of organ rejection.

IMMUNODEFICIENCY IN THE ELDERLY

A degree of immunodeficiency arises simply as a consequence of age. The thymus, which plays an important part in the production of T-lymphocytes, reaches peak size in puberty and steadily shrinks thereafter. This results in a decline in the number and activity of T-lymphocytes with age; there is also a decline in the numbers of B-lymphocytes.

Immunoglobulin

A type of protein found in the blood and in tissue fluids, also known as an antibody. Immunoglobulins are produced by cells of the immune system called B-lymphocytes. Their function is to bind to substances in the body that are recognized as foreign antigens (often proteins on the surface of bacteria and viruses). This binding is a crucial event in the destruction of the microorganisms that bear the antigens.

Immunoglobulins also play a central role in *allergies* and *hypersensitivity* reactions. In this case they bind to antigens that are not necessarily a threat to health, which may provoke an inflammatory reaction.

There are five classes of immunoglobulin; of these, immunoglobulin G (IgG) is the major immunoglobulin in human blood. The IgG molecule consists of two parts, one of which binds to an antigen; the other binds to other cells of the immune system. These other cells are principally white cells called phagocytes, which then engulf the microorganisms bearing the antigen.

The antigen-binding site of the IgG molecule is variable in its structure, the different versions of the molecule being capable of binding to an almost infinite number of antigens.

Immunoglobulins can be extracted from the blood of recovering patients and used for passive *immunization* against certain infectious diseases.

Immunoglobulin injection

Administration of preparations of *immunoglobulins* (*antibodies*) to prevent or sometimes treat infectious diseases. Such preparations are also known as immune globulin or gamma-globulin.

The main use of immunoglobulin injections is in the prevention of viral *hepatitis* (e.g., before traveling to a country where the disease is common). They are also given to prevent *measles* and *rubella* in people who are exposed to these infections and are not already immune to them from previous infection or *immunization*.

Immunoglobulin injections are also given to people with *immunodeficiency disorders* (impaired natural defenses).

HOW IT WORKS
Immunoglobulin injections provide immunity to a range of common infectious diseases. They work by passing on antibodies obtained from the blood of large numbers of people who have previously been exposed to these diseases and thus have developed antibodies to them.

POSSIBLE ADVERSE EFFECTS
Immunoglobulin injections may cause rash, fever, and pain and tenderness at the injection site.

Immunology
The discipline concerned with the *immune system*. Immunologists study the functioning of the immune system

and investigate and treat disorders of the immune system, including *allergies*, *autoimmune disorders*, and *immunodeficiency disorders* such as *AIDS*.

Specialists in immunology are also concerned with finding ways in which the immune system can be stimulated to provide immunity (principally through the use of *vaccines*).

Immunologists also play an important part in *transplant surgery*, looking preoperatively for a good immunological match between recipient and donor organ, and suppressing the recipient's immune system after transplantation to minimize the chances of organ rejection.

Immunostimulant drugs
A group of drugs that increase the efficiency of the body's *immune system* (natural defenses against infection and abnormal cells). Immunostimulant drugs include *vaccines* (see *Immunization*), and *interferon* and interleukin-2, which are used to treat viral infections and types of cancer.

Immunostimulant *adjuvant drugs* enhance the ability of a vaccine to stimulate the immune system and are added to the vaccine for this reason. Aluminium phosphate, for example, increases the effectiveness of the *tetanus* vaccine.

Immunosuppressant drugs

COMMON DRUGS
Corticosteroid drugs *Prednisolone Prednisone*
Cytotoxic drugs *Azathioprine Chlorambucil* *Cyclophosphamide Methotrexate*
Others *Cyclosporine*

A group of drugs that reduce the activity of the body's *immune system* (natural defenses). Immunosuppressant drugs are prescribed after *transplant surgery* to prevent the rejection of foreign tissues. They are also given to halt the progress of *autoimmune disorders* (in which the body's immune system attacks its own tissues) when other treatments are ineffective. They are unable, however, to restore tissue that has already been damaged.

Immunosuppressant drugs work by suppressing the production and activity of *lymphocytes*, a type of white blood cell that plays an important part in fighting infection and in eliminating abnormal cells that may form a malignant tumor.

POSSIBLE ADVERSE EFFECTS
Apart from the individual effects of each type, these drugs increase the risk of infection and of the development of certain cancers.

Immunotherapy
Stimulation of the *immune system* as a treatment for *cancer*. Immunotherapy as a cancer treatment is still largely experimental, but it may prove a useful adjunct to other therapies, such as the use of *anticancer drugs*, in the treatment of *leukemia*, *lymphoma*, and some other cancers. (The term immunotherapy is also sometimes used to describe *hyposensitization* treatment.)

TYPES
One type of immunotherapy used in the treatment of cancer relies on the use of *immunostimulant drugs*, substances that cause general stimulation of the immune system. Another technique is to inoculate the patient with tumor cells or cellular extracts, rendered harmless by irradiation, which have been taken from another person suffering from the same disease. The patient's immune system then produces its own *antibodies*, which attack the tumor cells.

Alternatively, a patient can be given antibodies from another person with the same type of tumor. More recently, monoclonal antibodies (see *Antibody, monoclonal*) directed against tumors have been produced artificially by *genetic engineering*. *Interferon* or chemical poisons can be linked to these antibodies to increase their ability to destroy tumor cells.

LIMITATIONS
One drawback to the administration of some of these anticancer treatments is that they, too, may be recognized as foreign by the person's immune system, causing either allergic reactions (such as serum sickness) or new antibody production, which interferes with anticancer activity.

Impaction, dental
Failure of a tooth to emerge completely from the gum at its normal time of eruption. An impacted tooth remains either fully or partly embedded in bone or soft tissue.

Dental impaction may occur because overcrowding (see *Overcrowding, dental*) leaves little room for the teeth that erupt last (the wisdom teeth and upper canines). Impaction may also occur when a tooth grows in the wrong direction, causing its eruption to be blocked by dense bone.

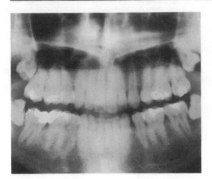

Impacted wisdom teeth
This X ray shows impacted wisdom teeth lying horizontally in the lower jaw. The impacted teeth are wedged against the adjacent molars and are not able to erupt normally.

IMPACTED WISDOM TEETH
These are common, but usually cause no trouble unless they partially penetrate the gum, leaving a flap of tissue over most of the crown. *Plaque*, bacteria, and food debris then collect between the tooth and the gum, which often becomes inflamed and painful. There may also be swollen *lymph nodes* in the upper neck and difficulty opening the mouth.

Rinsing the area with warm salt water and taking *analgesic drugs* (painkillers) may relieve symptoms but, if infection is present, *antibiotic drugs* are required. A dentist may decide that the tooth requires extraction to prevent more trouble.

IMPACTED UPPER CANINES
These teeth play a much more important part than do wisdom teeth in biting and chewing. If the upper canines are impacted, they are not usually removed, but instead are moved into the correct position by means of an *orthodontic appliance*.

Impetigo
A highly contagious skin infection, common in children, that usually occurs around the nose and mouth.

CAUSES AND INCIDENCE
Impetigo is caused by bacteria entering the skin through a broken area, such as a cut, *cold sore*, or an area affected by *eczema*. The infection occurs more often in warm weather. Impetigo was once extremely common, but occurs less frequently now because of improved standards of personal hygiene. Small epidemics occasionally occur in schools.

SYMPTOMS AND SIGNS
The skin reddens and small, fluid-filled blisters appear on the surface. The blisters tend to burst, leaving moist, weeping areas underneath; the released fluid dries to leave honey-colored crusts on the skin. The infected area may spread at the edges or another patch may develop nearby. In severe cases there may be swelling of the *lymph nodes* in the face or neck; accompanied by fever. Rarely, complications such as *septicemia* (blood poisoning) or *glomerulonephritis* (a type of kidney inflammation) develop.

TREATMENT
Because impetigo spreads rapidly, it is advisable to consult a physician. *Antibiotic drugs* in tablet or ointment form usually clear up the problem in about five days. Any loose crusts should be gently washed off with soap and water and the area dabbed dry.

To prevent transmission of the infection, pillowcases, towels, and facecloths should not be shared and should be boiled after use. Children should not touch affected skin and should stay away from school until the infection clears.

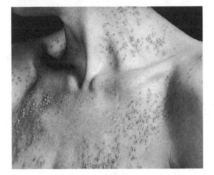

The appearance of impetigo
Fluid-filled blisters appear on the skin (in this case, on the neck and chest). The blisters often burst, releasing fluid that dries to leave pale brown crusts.

Implant
Any material, natural or artificial, inserted into the body for medical purposes (see box, facing page).

Implantation, egg
Attachment of a fertilized *ovum* (egg) to the wall of the *uterus*. Implantation occurs about six days after *fertilization*, when the blastocyst (early form of embryo) comes into contact with the wall of the uterus. As the cells of the developing *embryo* continue to divide, the outer cell layer penetrates the lining of the uterus to obtain oxygen and nutrients from the mother's blood; later, this layer develops into the *placenta*.

The embryo usually implants in the upper part of the uterus; if it implants low down near the cervix, *placenta previa* may develop. Rarely, implantation occurs in a fallopian tube, resulting in an *ectopic pregnancy*.

Implants, dental
Posts surgically embedded in the jaw for the attachment of a dental prosthesis (a type of false teeth). Titanium or synthetic materials may be used for the implants.

Implants are useful for people who have lost all their teeth and either are unable to tolerate a traditional *denture* or have lost so much tooth-bearing tissue through injury or disease that a denture would not be stable.

Fitting a dental implant is performed in stages, usually under local anesthesia. First, holes are drilled in the jaw and posts are inserted into them. Several months later, attachments that protrude above the gum are screwed into the posts. A few weeks later, a prosthesis is fitted.

Impotence
The inability to achieve or maintain an *erection*. Impotence is the most common male sexual disorder, affecting most men at some time in their lives.

CAUSES
In most cases, impotence is caused by psychological factors, which may be temporary (e.g., when caused by fatigue or stress) or long-standing (e.g., when caused by feelings of anxiety and guilt that originated in childhood). Impotence may also be a symptom of severe *depression*.

Approximately 10 percent of impotence is caused by a physical disorder (e.g., *diabetes mellitus* or a disorder of the *endocrine system*) or by a neurological disorder (e.g., damage to the *spinal cord* or an *alcohol-related disorder*). Impotence may be caused by taking various drugs—particularly *antidepressant drugs*, *antipsychotic drugs*, *antihypertensive drugs*, and *diuretic drugs*. Impotence is more common as men get older, possibly because of altered circulation or, very occasionally, lowered levels of the male sex hormone *testosterone*.

DIAGNOSIS AND TREATMENT
Tests may be performed to eliminate the possibility of any physical disorder. A change in medication may sometimes be advised to see whether impotence is affected.

If a physical cause is found, treatment will be given if possible. *Penile implants* help some men whose impo-

TYPES OF IMPLANTS

Implants may be inserted into various parts of the body. They can be used to replace a diseased structure, to improve appearance, to maintain proper functioning of an internal organ, to treat certain disorders, or to deliver drugs or hormones.

Hormonal
Some hormonal drugs (such as estradiol and progesterone) can be placed in implants that are inserted under the skin to release the drug slowly over time. There were no hormonal implants being sold or manufactured in Canada when this book was being prepared.

Breast
Implants can be used to restore breast shape after mastectomy (breast removal) for cancer or to increase breast size for cosmetic purposes (augmentation mammoplasty).

Therapeutic
Radioactive materials in sealed containers can be inserted into tissue to treat malignant tumors, for example, a cancer of the cervix.

Eye
An implant can be used to replace the lens of the eye after cataract removal, or the entire eyeball if it requires removal because of injury or disease.

Face
Pieces of bone taken from another part of the body, or shaped pieces of silicone, can be implanted on the face to make a receding chin more prominent or to improve the contour at a fracture site.

Heart
Cardiac pacemakers (battery-powered electronic devices connected by wires to the heart muscle) can be implanted in the chest to regulate the heartbeat; diseased heart valves may be replaced with artificial or natural substitutes.

Joints
Diseased joints can be replaced with artificial substitutes to help restore full function. The elbow, the hip, the knee, the finger joints, and the shoulder can all now be treated in this way.

Artery
Diseased sections of artery, such as the lower aorta and upper iliac arteries (shown here), can be replaced or bypassed with artificial tubular materials made from woven or knitted synthetic fibers.

tence is caused by disease. Injections of certain *vasodilator drugs*, especially papaverine, may be prescribed in some cases. An attempt will be made to treat depression or *alcohol dependence* if appropriate.

If the cause of impotence is psychological, *counseling* or *sex therapy* (preferably together with the person's partner) may be recommended. Such treatment is successful in more than half the cases of long-term impotence of psychological origin.

Impression, dental
A mold taken of the *teeth, gums,* and sometimes the *palate.* A quick-setting material, such as alginate or a rubber compound, is placed in a shaped tray that is eased over the area of which a replica is to be made and left in position until the material has set. After the mold has been removed, plaster of Paris is poured into it to obtain a model of the area. This is then used as a base on which to build a *denture, bridge,* or dental *inlay.*

Impressions are also used in *orthodontics* to study the position of the teeth and the structure of the mouth, and to make *orthodontic appliances* to correct irregularities.

Impulse control disorders
A group of psychiatric disorders characterized by the inability to resist an impulse or temptation to do something that ultimately proves harmful to oneself. The group includes pathological *gambling, kleptomania, pyromania,* and *explosive disorders.*

Incest
Sexual intercourse between close relatives. Incest is usually considered to include intercourse with a parent, a son or daughter, a brother or sister, an uncle or aunt, a nephew or niece, a grandparent or grandchild. However, the definition of what constitutes incest differs between cultures.

Incest is illegal or taboo in most societies and against the teaching of many religions. This almost universal prohibition is probably based on a perceived higher risk of congenital abnormality due to inbreeding.

The actual prevalence of incest is unknown. Research suggests that as many as 5 to 10 percent of women have had sexual contact with a father, brother, or other male relative, and that 1 to 2 percent of men have had sexual contact with a male or a female relative.

The existence of *child abuse* involving incest is now well recognized, and support for victims of this crime is increasingly available from telephone helplines; self-help groups; pediatric, psychiatric, and social services; and the courts. The child may be moved to safety, or the molester may be removed from the home.

Incidence
One of the two principal measures (the other is *prevalence*) of how common a disease is in a defined population. The incidence of a disease is the number of new cases that occur during a given period (e.g., 17 new cases per 100,000 people per year). Prevalence is the total number of cases of a disease in existence at any one time; it includes both new and old cases. Thus, in 100,000 people, there may be an incidence of, say, 400 cases of a specific type of cancer per year, but a prevalence of 4,000 cases, because the disease lasts an average of 10 years before being cured or causing death.

Incidence is most useful in expressing the frequency of a disease that has a definite or sudden onset, such as an infectious disease, most cancers, or stroke. (See table, p. 578.)

INCIDENCE OF VARIOUS CONDITIONS IN CANADA

Incidence (new cases per 100,000 population per year)	Categorization	Examples
More than 10,000	Extremely common	Common cold
1,000 to 10,000	Very common	Sexually transmitted diseases (all types)
100 to 1,000	Common	Myocardial infarction Stroke
20 to 100	Fairly common	Breast cancer Cancer of colon Symptomatic kidney stones Leukemia Lung cancer
5 to 20	Uncommon	Ovarian cancer Tuberculosis
0.5 to 5	Rare	Anorexia nervosa Hepatitis B Hodgkin's disease Meningococcal meningitis Motoneuron disease Syphilis
0.005 to 0.5	Very rare	Diphtheria Poliomyelitis Acute rheumatic fever Typhoid fever
Less than 0.005	Extremely rare	Botulism Histoplasmosis Rabies

Incision

A cut made into the tissues of the body by a scalpel (surgical knife). Most incisions are made to gain access to tissue inside the body (usually to repair or remove a diseased organ) or to relieve pressure (e.g., from pus in an abscess). Standard incision sites for abdominal surgery are shown in the illustrated box, facing page.

Incisor

One of the eight front teeth (four in the upper jaw and four in the lower) used for incising (cutting through) solid forms of food. (See *Teeth*.)

Incontinence, fecal

Inability to retain *feces* in the *rectum*. A common cause of fecal incontinence, especially in the elderly and in toilet-trained children, is *fecal impaction*, which is often itself caused by long-standing *constipation*. The feces lodged in the rectum irritate and inflame its lining and, as a result, fecal fluid and small pieces of feces are passed involuntarily. Temporary loss of continence may occur at any age in cases of severe *diarrhea*, when the need to evacuate the bowel becomes too great to withstand.

Less common causes include injury to the anal muscles (as may occur, for example, during childbirth or surgery), *paraplegia* (paralysis of the legs and lower trunk), *mental retardation*, and *dementia*.

TREATMENT
If the underlying cause of fecal impaction is constipation, recurrence may be prevented by a high-fiber diet. Suppositories containing *glycerol* or *laxative drugs* may be recommended. Fecal incontinence in people with dementia or a nerve disorder may be avoided by regular use of enemas or suppositories to empty the rectum.

Incontinence, urinary

Uncontrollable, involuntary passing of *urine*, often due to injury or disease of the *urinary tract*. Urinary incontinence often affects the elderly because the efficiency of the sphincter muscles surrounding the *urethra* declines with age. Women are affected more often than men.

TYPES AND SYMPTOMS

STRESS INCONTINENCE This refers to the involuntary escape of a small amount of urine when a person coughs, laughs, picks up a heavy package, or moves excessively (such as during athletic activity). Stress incontinence is common in women, particularly after childbirth, when the urethral sphincter muscles are stretched.

URGE INCONTINENCE In this type, an urgent desire to pass urine is accompanied by inability to control the bladder as it contracts involuntarily. Urge incontinence may occur when walking or sitting, but is frequently triggered by a sudden change in position. Once urination starts, it continues until the bladder is empty.

TOTAL INCONTINENCE This is a complete lack of bladder control resulting from the total absence of sphincter activity. In rare cases, total incontinence occurs because the urine bypasses the sphincter, as may occur in a person with a vesicovaginal fistula (a hole between the bladder and vagina) or an ectopic ureter (in which the ureter enters the urethra rather than the bladder).

OVERFLOW INCONTINENCE This occurs in chronic *urinary retention*, a condition in which the sufferer is unable to empty the bladder normally, often because of an obstruction such as an enlarged *prostate gland*. The bladder is always full, leading to constant dribbling of the overflow of urine. Relief of the obstruction will restore continence.

CAUSES
Incontinence may be caused by localized disorders of the urinary tract (including infections, bladder stones, or tumors) or by *prolapse* of the uterus or vagina. Incontinence due to lack of control by the brain commonly occurs in the young (see *Enuresis*), the elderly, and those with mental impairment. Damage to the brain or spinal cord by injury or disease also affects bladder control, as do stress, anger, and anxiety.

Weak pelvic muscles, a fractured pelvis, or cancer of the prostate can cause incontinence. *Irritable bladder*, in which the bladder muscle contracts intermittently, raises the pressure in the bladder to push some urine out of the urethra; this causes an intense desire to pass urine.

ABDOMINAL INCISIONS

Surgery is frequently performed on the abdomen. Standard incision sites provide access to the diseased portion with minimum weakening of the abdominal wall. The most commonly used of these standard incision sites are shown in the diagram below.

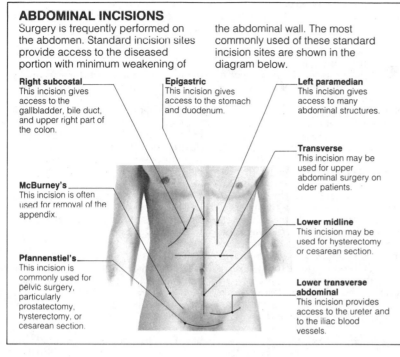

Right subcostal
This incision gives access to the gallbladder, bile duct, and upper right part of the colon.

Epigastric
This incision gives access to the stomach and duodenum.

Left paramedian
This incision gives access to many abdominal structures.

Transverse
This incision may be used for upper abdominal surgery on older patients.

McBurney's
This incision is often used for removal of the appendix.

Lower midline
This incision may be used for hysterectomy or cesarean section.

Pfannenstiel's
This incision is commonly used for pelvic surgery, particularly prostatectomy, hysterectomy, or cesarean section.

Lower transverse abdominal
This incision provides access to the ureter and to the iliac blood vessels.

DIAGNOSIS
Urinalysis (examination of the urine) is performed to eliminate the possibility of infection, inflammation, *diabetes mellitus*, or protein loss. *Ultrasound scanning*, intravenous *urography* (X rays of the kidney and ureters after injection of a radiopaque substance), and X rays taken while the patient is passing urine (see *cystourethrography, micturating*) are used to investigate the possibility of an obstruction. *Cystometry* (measurement of pressure within the bladder) can determine if the bladder is functioning normally or if there is any abnormality of the nerves supplying the bladder. *Cystoscopy* (examination of the urethra and bladder through a viewing instrument) is performed to look for the presence of bladder stones, tumors, or cysts.

TREATMENT
If weak pelvic muscles are causing stress incontinence, *pelvic floor exercises* may help to restore sphincter function. Sometimes, an operation is performed to tighten or lengthen the urethra. In severe cases, an inflatable artificial sphincter may be placed around the urethra; when urination is required, a trigger is pressed to deflate the mechanism in order to allow urine to flow.

Anticholinergic drugs are sometimes used to relax the bladder muscle if irritable bladder is the cause.

If, despite treatment, normal bladder function cannot be restored, special incontinence pants (with an internal pad to absorb the urine) can alleviate discomfort. Men can wear a penile sheath leading into a tube connected to a portable urine bag. Some people can avoid incontinence by self-catheterization (see *Catheterization, urinary*) four or five times a day to empty the bladder.

If these measures are unsuccessful and the condition is severe, a *urinary diversion* operation to bypass the bladder may be necessary.

Incoordination
Loss of the ability to produce smooth, harmonious muscular movements, leading to clumsiness and unsteady balance. Incoordination can also mean the failure of a group of organs to work together successfully. (See also *Ataxia*.)

Incubation period
The time during which any *infectious disease* develops, from the point when the infecting organism enters the body until the appearance of symptoms. Different infections have characteristic incubation periods—for example, 14 to 21 days for chickenpox and seven to 14 days for measles. The incubation period for cholera may be as short as several hours.

Incubator
A transparent plastic container in which oxygen, temperature, and humidity levels are controlled to provide premature or sick infants with ideal conditions for survival. An incubator also provides some protection from airborne infection.

Incubators have portholes to allow handling of the baby and smaller holes through which monitoring cables and intravenous and respiratory tubing can pass.

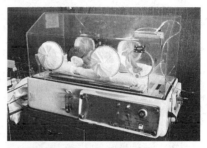

Premature infant in an incubator
Portholes make it possible to handle the infant without disturbing the special conditions provided by the incubator.

Indian medicine
In contrast to Chinese medicine, traditional Indian medicine was based on empirical observation and practice rather than on philosophy. The earliest Indian literature, the Vedas, which date from about 1500 B.C., contains details of numerous disorders and their treatments. Ayurvedism, as Vedic medicine is known, was based largely on herbal treatment, although early Vedic physicians also used simple surgical techniques and invented artificial limbs and eyes.

The Vedic era ended in about 800 B.C., but the medical traditions of ayurvedism survived and were further developed (especially the surgical aspect) under the Brahmins, the caste of wise men. As a result, by about 500 A.D., Indian medicine had become a scientifically based system with a wide range of surgical techniques (such as operations for cataracts and kidney stones) along with the herbal tradition. The Brahmins, however, cloaked their medical knowledge in theology and superstition and traditional Indian medicine stagnated. Today, most Indian medicine follows Western practices.

Indigestion
A common term covering a variety of symptoms brought on by eating, including *heartburn, abdominal pain,*

nausea, and *flatulence* (excessive wind in the stomach or intestine, causing belching or discomfort). The medical term for indigestion is dyspepsia.

Indigestion refers to discomfort in the upper abdomen, often brought on by eating too much, by eating too quickly, or by eating very rich, spicy, or fatty foods. Nervous indigestion is a common effect of stress. Occasionally, persistent or recurrent indigestion is associated with a *peptic ulcer, gallstones,* or *esophagitis* (inflammation of the esophagus).

TREATMENT
Self-help treatment includes avoiding foods and situations that bring on symptoms and eating regularly three or four times a day, without rushing. Taking *antacid drugs* or drinking milk may make symptoms subside.

Anyone who takes antacid drugs regularly should see a physician so that the underlying cause of the problem can be investigated. If abdominal pain persists for more than six hours, or if there are other symptoms, such as prolonged vomiting, vomiting blood (which may appear brown), passing very dark or black feces, or feeling weak or faint, a physician should be consulted immediately.

Indomethacin
A *nonsteroidal anti-inflammatory drug* (NSAID) used to relieve pain, stiffness, and inflammation in disorders such as *osteoarthritis, rheumatoid arthritis, gout, ankylosing spondylitis,* and *tendinitis.* Indomethacin is also prescribed to relieve pain caused by injury to soft tissues, such as muscles and ligaments.

Treatment with indomethacin may cause abdominal pain, nausea, heartburn, headache, dizziness, and an increased risk of *peptic ulcer.*

Induction of labor
Use of artificial means to initiate the process of *childbirth.* Labor is induced if the health of the mother or baby would be endangered by allowing the pregnancy to continue. If the pregnancy is not at full term, the risks of induction are weighed against the risks of *prematurity.*

WHY IT IS DONE
The commonest reason for inducing labor is that the pregnancy has continued past the estimated delivery date, which increases the chance of maternal and fetal complications occurring during childbirth. Most obstetricians induce labor if delivery is more than two weeks overdue.

Labor may be induced early if the mother is suffering from *preeclampsia,* or if she has chronic *hypertension.* Labor may also be induced if there is Rh incompatibility between the mother and baby (because of the risk of *hemolytic disease of the newborn*) or if there are indications of *intrauterine growth retardation.*

HOW IT IS DONE
The most common technique of inducing labor is to rupture the membrane around the baby to release some of the amniotic fluid. This is sometimes sufficient to start labor. If not, vaginal suppositories containing a *prostaglandin drug* (which stimulates the uterus to contract) may be inserted high in the vagina. Alternatively, an intravenous infusion of *oxytocin* (a hormone that stimulates the uterus to contract) may be used. Careful monitoring of the condition of both mother and baby is important during an induced labor. If attempts to induce labor are unsuccessful, the baby may be delivered by *cesarean section.*

Industrial diseases
Disorders related to the workplace. (See *Occupational disease and injury.*)

Infant
A term usually applied to a baby up to the age of 12 months.

Infantile spasms
A rare type of recurrent seizure, also called progressive myoclonic encephalopathy or salaam attacks, that affects babies. Infantile spasms occur most commonly between the ages of 4 and 9 months.

The condition is a form of *epilepsy.* In a seizure, the baby's head suddenly falls forward, the body stiffens, and the limbs bend. Following this, the arms and hands extend and move out. There may be several hundred such spasms per day, each lasting a few seconds and sometimes preceded by a cry. In most cases the seizures are a sign of brain damage and affected babies grow up with severe *mental retardation.*

Infant mortality
The number of infants who die during the first year of life per 1,000 live births. About two thirds of all infant deaths occur during the neonatal period (the first month of life). Most of those who die are very premature (i.e., all babies born before the 30th week of pregnancy) or have severe *birth defects.*

Infant mortality varies greatly among different countries and among different racial and social groups. A low infant mortality rate reflects good maternal nutrition, good medical and social conditions throughout pregnancy, and good care for the infant after birth. Since 1921, when national records were first kept, the infant mortality rate in Canada, as in all developed countries, has dropped remarkably. In 1921 it was 102.1 deaths per 1,000 live births; by 1956 it had dropped to 31.9, and it now is below eight per 1,000. It is still considerably higher in such disadvantaged groups as the very poor and native peoples. Rates for male babies are about 20 percent higher than those for female babies.

Infarction
Death of an area of tissue caused by *ischemia* (lack of blood supply). Common examples include *myocardial infarction* (heart attack) and pulmonary infarction, which is lung damage caused by a *pulmonary embolism* (a blood clot that has moved into a vessel in the lung and is obstructing the flow of blood). (See also *Necrosis.*)

Infection
 The establishment of a colony of disease-causing microorganisms (such as bacteria, viruses, or fungi) in the body. The organisms actively reproduce and cause disease directly by damage to cells or indirectly by toxins they release. Infection normally provokes a response from the *immune system,* which accounts for many of the features of the infection.

Toxic symptoms, such as fever, weakness, and aching joints, are expressions of *infectious disease.* In such cases, the microorganisms are often spread throughout the body (this is called "systemic" infection). Infection may also be localized within a particular tissue or area, often through spread of organisms from parts of the body where they are harmless to parts where they are harmful (e.g., through leakage from the intestines into the abdomen to cause *peritonitis*).

Entry of microorganisms from soil into wounds or during surgical procedures is another common cause of localized infection. Infection of internal body cavities was once the major risk to the patient. Antiseptic surgical techniques have largely eliminated this problem.

AVOIDANCE

Localized infections (as opposed to infectious diseases) can be avoided by standard hygienic measures, such as keeping the hands clean, not picking at blemishes, washing and covering cuts and grazes, having wounds attended to by a physician, and seeking regular dental treatment.

SYMPTOMS

Localized infection is generally followed by *inflammation*, which increases the flow of blood to the infected area, bringing white blood cells and other components of the immune system. Symptoms and signs usually include pain, redness, swelling, formation of a pus-filled abscess at the site of infection, and sometimes a rise in temperature.

TREATMENT

Any suspected infection should be brought to the attention of a physician. Once the nature of the causative microorganism has been discovered, treatment of the condition consists of an *antibiotic drug* or other antimicrobial drug.

Infection, congenital

Any infection present at birth that was acquired by the infant either in the uterus or during passage through the birth canal.

INFECTIONS ACQUIRED IN THE UTERUS

Many viruses, bacteria, and other microorganisms can pass from the mother's blood through the placenta and into the circulation of the growing fetus. Particularly serious are organisms responsible for *rubella* (German measles), *syphilis*, and *toxoplasmosis*, and the *cytomegalovirus*. Any of these infections may cause *intrauterine growth retardation*. Further effects depend on the stage of pregnancy at which the infection was acquired. Thus, rubella occurring before 12 weeks may cause *deafness*, congenital *heart disease*, and eye disorders. Some infections in later pregnancy, particularly with a *herpes* virus, may also damage the fetus severely.

A woman who is infected with the HIV virus (responsible for *AIDS*) risks passing the infection onto her baby during pregnancy.

INFECTIONS ACQUIRED DURING BIRTH

These infections are almost always acquired from the mother's vaginal secretions or uterine fluid that has become infected with microorganisms. If the membranes rupture prematurely, the baby is at risk of infection from organisms ascending into the uterus from the birth canal.

Conditions acquired in this way include *conjunctivitis* (sometimes caused by infection with the organisms responsible for *gonorrhea*), *herpes* infection, a *chlamydial infection*, and infantile *diarrhea*. *Meningitis, hepatitis B, listeriosis, staphylococcal infections* and *streptococcal infections* may also be acquired in this way. Babies who inhale infected maternal secretions may develop *pneumonia*.

PREVENTION

The risk of a baby acquiring an infection in the uterus is minimized if its mother was immunized against rubella when she was a child and if, during the pregnancy, she has no sexually transmitted disease or receives prompt treatment for any such disease she contracts. If a woman has an active genital herpes infection close to the time of delivery, a *cesarean section* is usually performed, because infection of the newborn baby with herpes simplex virus is particularly serious and commonly fatal.

TREATMENT

If a baby is diagnosed as having an infection at birth, treatment against the infecting agent is started. Any growth retardation that has occurred due to infection in the uterus cannot usually be reversed. Some types of birth defects caused by infection (such as some types of heart defects) are treatable; others (such as congenital deafness) usually are not.

Infectious disease

Any illness caused by a specific microorganism.

INCIDENCE

Infectious diseases are a large and important group of conditions and, until recently, were the major cause of illness and death throughout the world. (In many developing countries, they remain a major cause of death.) Over the last century or so, this situation has changed in the more developed countries as a result of four important advances. First, better methods are employed for controlling the spread of disease organisms—including better sanitation, water purification, housing, pest control, and personal hygiene. Second, many effective *antibiotic drugs* and other antimicrobial drugs have been developed. Third, vaccines and other preparations have been developed to provide immunity to certain infectious diseases (see *Immunization*). Fourth, better general health and nutrition have bolstered immunity and improved survival.

In developed countries, such measures have brought about a dramatic decline in the incidence of some serious diseases (such as *poliomyelitis, diphtheria*, and *tuberculosis*) and the total eradication of *smallpox*. In poorer countries, however, infectious diseases remain a huge problem, for reasons that include lack of resources, ignorance, low standards of public and personal hygiene, the presence of insect transmitters of disease, and, perhaps most importantly, malnutrition. Diseases such as measles may have a mortality of 20 percent in malnourished children.

CAUSES

Disease-causing organisms fall into a number of well-defined groups. Among the most important are *viruses, bacteria*, and *fungi*, along with three smaller groups, the rickettsiae, chlamydiae, and mycoplasmas. All are relatively simple organisms that can readily multiply in a host's tissues when defenses are low. Other groups include the *protozoa* (single-celled animal parasites), *worms*, and *flukes*. These more complex parasites may spend only part of their lifes cycle in human tissues; the rest of their life is spent in another animal or in soil. Colonization by worms and flukes (along with external parasites, such as *scabies* and *lice*) may be referred to as an *infestation* rather than an infection. (See the tables beginning on page 583 for examples of transmission mechanisms of various diseases.)

AVOIDANCE

Serious infectious diseases can largely be avoided by measures such as immunization, good hygiene with respect to food and drink and washing the hands after using the toilet, avoiding contact with animal feces and secretions, and prudence in the choice of sexual partners (or precautions, such as the use of condoms). For travel outside North America, Northern Europe, Australia, and New Zealand, extra immunizations, and, in some cases, antimalarial tablets and protective measures against insects may be recommended by your travel agent and confirmed by your physician.

SYMPTOMS AND DIAGNOSIS

The symptoms of an infectious disease are caused in part by microorganisms damaging cells and tissues, releasing toxins, and drawing on their host's reserves of nutrients; symptoms are also caused by the efforts of the body's defenses (including the *immune system*) to destroy the micro-

HOW INFECTIOUS DISEASES ARE TRANSMITTED

In developed countries, infectious diseases are usually spread by sexual transmission, airborne transmission, blood-borne transmission, or direct skin contact. In poorer countries, insect-borne, food-borne, and water-borne infections are other important mechanisms of transmission. Certain infections can also pass from a pregnant woman's blood across the placenta into the blood of the fetus.

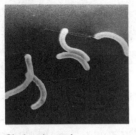

Cholera bacteria
The comma-shaped bacteria that cause the dangerous infectious disease cholera are spread by contamination of water.

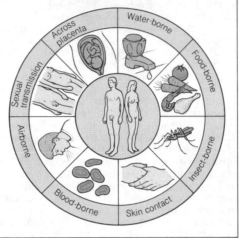

organisms. The outcome depends on whether the microorganisms or the defenses (sometimes aided by drug therapy) gain the upper hand. The strength of a person's immune system, which reflects his or her general health, strongly influences this outcome.

Fever is a feature in many infectious diseases; symptoms generally are related to the system or organ attacked—for example, cough, diarrhea, or skin rash.

Apart from diseases in which the symptoms and signs are usually easily recognizable (such as *chickenpox*), diagnosis relies on identifying the causative microorganism. Testing may be by microscopic examination of a specimen of infected tissue or body fluid, by *culture* techniques, or by detecting *antibodies* (proteins manufactured by the body to defend against a particular organism) in the blood (see *Serology*).

A particular problem with infectious diseases is that there is always a time gap (known as the incubation period) between the entry of the microorganisms into the body and the first appearance of symptoms. The incubation period may last from a few hours to several years; during this time, the infected person is likely to pass the microorganism to other people. Furthermore, symptoms may never develop in some infected people, but these people nevertheless continue to carry the disease organisms and unwittingly spread them to others.

As a result, an epidemic can be well established before it is recognized and before control measures are introduced. This can be particularly devastating when the disease is a new one and has a long incubation period and a high mortality (*AIDS* is a classic example).

TREATMENT
The mainstay of treatment is the use of antibiotic and other antimicrobial drugs. Drug treatment must be carefully selected by means of culturing and identifying the causative microorganisms because certain microorganisms are susceptible only to certain drugs. For many viruses, no effective *antiviral drug* is available and treatment relies on supportive measures, such as reducing temperature, maintaining food and fluid intake, etc.

OUTLOOK
Although great strides have been made in the fight against infectious diseases, many problems remain, even in developed countries. The spread of certain diseases (such as sexually transmitted infections) is difficult to control except by modifying human behavior. For many infections, no effective vaccine has been developed. The majority of viral diseases cannot be effectively combatted with drugs, and some bacteria have developed *resistance* to the drugs available. When a new infectious disease appears, it may be years before an effective vaccine or drug treatment can be devised. In the meantime, large numbers of people may die (once again, AIDS provides the most recent example.)

Infectious mononucleosis
See *Mononucleosis, infectious*.

Inferiority complex
A neurotic state of mind that develops because of repeated hurts or failures in the past. Inferiority complex arises from a conflict between the positive wish to be recognized as someone worthwhile and the haunting fear of frustration and failure. Attempts to compensate for the sense of worthlessness may take the form of aggression and violence, or of overzealous involvement in activities. (See also *Superiority complex*.)

Infertility
The inability to produce offspring. Conception depends on the production of healthy sperm by the man, healthy eggs by the woman, and *sexual intercourse* so that the sperm reach the woman's *fallopian tubes*. There must be no mechanical obstruction to prevent the sperm from reaching the egg, and the sperm must be able to fertilize the egg when they meet (see *Fertilization*). Next, the fertilized egg must be capable of implantation in the uterus (see *Implantation, egg*). Finally, the developing embryo must be healthy and its hormonal environment must be adequate for further development so that the pregnancy can continue to full term. Infertility may result from a disturbance of any of these factors.

INCIDENCE
As many as one in six couples requires help from a specialist. Infertility increases with age; the older a couple is when trying to conceive, the more difficult it may be.

CAUSES
About 30 percent of infertility cases are due to factors that affect the man, another 30 percent to factors that affect the woman. In 40 percent of cases, infertility is due to both partners.

MALE INFERTILITY The major cause of male infertility is failure to produce enough healthy sperm. *Azoospermia* (in which there is no sperm) and *oligospermia* (in which few sperm are produced) both cause infertility.

In some cases the sperm are malformed or their lifespan after ejaculation is too short for them to travel far enough to reach the egg. Defects in the sperm may be due to a blockage of the spermatic tubes or to damage to the spermatic ducts, usually due to a *sexually transmitted disease*, such as *gonorrhea*. A *varicocele* (varicose veins in the scrotum) may also be a factor. Abnormal development of the testes due to an endocrine disorder (see *Hypogonadism*) or damage to the testes by *orchitis* (inflammation of the testes) may also cause defective sperm. Toxins, cigarettes, or drugs can lower the sperm count. Infertility may also be caused by a failure to deliver the sperm into the vagina, as occurs in *impotence* or in disorders affecting ejaculation (see *Ejaculation, disorders of*).

SOME IMPORTANT INFECTIOUS DISEASES

VIRAL INFECTIONS

Infective agent	Transmission	Incubation period	Symptoms	Treatment
AIDS virus infection				
Human immuno-deficiency virus (HIV)	Sexual contact; sharing hypodermic needles; mother to child; infusion of infected blood products before May 1985	Variable, usually several years	Fever; weight loss; fatigue; diarrhea; swollen lymph nodes; shortness of breath	Treatment of complicating infections; zidovudine can prolong life expectancy
Chickenpox				
Varicella-zoster virus (herpes zoster virus)	Airborne droplets; direct contact	11 to 21 days	Slight fever; malaise; characteristic rash	Relief of symptoms; acyclovir beneficial in adults
Common cold				
Numerous rhino-viruses; corona-viruses	Airborne droplets; hand-to-hand contact	1 to 3 days	Sneezing; chills; muscle aches; runny nose; cough	Relief of symptoms
Hepatitis, viral				
Hepatitis virus types A and B; others	Infected food or water (type A); sexual contact; blood-borne transmission; sharing hypodermic needles (type B)	3 to 6 weeks (type A); a few weeks to several months (type B)	Influenzalike illness; jaundice; many people are asymptomatic	Relief of symptoms; interferon may be beneficial in some cases
Influenza				
Influenza viruses types A, B, or C	Airborne droplets	1 to 3 days	Fever; chills; aches; headache; sore throat; cough; runny nose	Relief of symptoms; fluids
Measles				
Measles virus (a paramyxovirus)	Airborne droplets	7 to 14 days	Fever; coldlike symptoms; characteristic rash; conjunctivitis	Relief of symptoms
Meningitis, viral				
Various viruses	Various methods, including via rodents	Variable	Fever; headache; drowsiness; confusion	Relief of symptoms; acyclovir in some cases
Mononucleosis, infectious				
Epstein-Barr virus	Possibly via saliva	1 to 6 weeks	Swollen glands; fever; sore throat; headache; malaise; lethargy	Relief of symptoms; rest; fluids
Poliomyelitis				
3 polioviruses	From feces to mouth via hands; airborne droplets	Minor illness—3 to 5 days. Major illness—7 to 14 days	Minor illness—sore throat; headache; vomiting. Major illness—fever; stiff neck and back; muscle aches; paralysis	Relief of symptoms
Rabies				
Rabies virus (a rhabdovirus)	Bite from infected animal	10 days to 8 months	Fever; general malaise; irrationality; throat spasms; hydrophobia	No effective treatment
Rubella				
Rubella virus	Airborne droplets; mother to child	2 to 3 weeks	Low fever; characteristic rash	Relief of symptoms

583

CHLAMYDIAL INFECTIONS

Infective agent	Transmission	Incubation period	Symptoms	Treatment
Nonspecific urethritis				
Chlamydia trachomatis	Sexual contact	1 to 4 weeks	Pain on passing urine; watery, mucus discharge	Antibiotics
Psittacosis				
Chlamydia psittaci	Inhalation of dust containing feces from infected birds	1 to 3 weeks	Flulike and feverish symptoms; shortness of breath	Antibiotics

RICKETTSIAL INFECTIONS

Infective agent	Transmission	Incubation period	Symptoms	Treatment
Q fever				
Coxiella burnetti	Inhalation of infected dust	7 to 14 days	Sudden onset of fever and sweating; cough; chest pains; headache	Antibiotics
Epidemic typhus				
Rickettsia prowazekii	Bite from infected body louse	About 7 days	Severe headache; high fever; muscle aches; weakness; rash	Antibiotics

BACTERIAL INFECTIONS

Infective agent	Transmission	Incubation period	Symptoms	Treatment
Gonorrhea				
Neisseria gonorrhoeae	Sexual contact; mother to baby	2 to 6 days	Pain on passing urine; discharge; pain in abdomen	Penicillin; ampicillin; other antibiotics for resistant forms
Meningitis, bacterial				
Neisseria meningitidis (meningococcus); *Streptococcus pneumoniae*; others	Mother to baby via vagina; infection reaching bloodstream from another organ	Less than 3 weeks, could be less than 24 hours	High fever; stiff neck; nausea; confusion	Antibiotic treatment
Pertussis (whooping cough)				
Bordetella pertussis	Airborne droplets	1 to 2 weeks	Runny nose and moderate fever; slight cough leading to characteristic cough spasms	Erythromycin in early stage; small children may require hospital admission
Pneumonia				
Streptococcus pneumoniae; *Legionella pneumophila*; others	Airborne droplets	1 to 3 weeks	Cough; fever; chest pain; shortness of breath	Antibiotics
Tuberculosis				
Mycobacterium tuberculosis	Airborne transmission; cow's milk	Several weeks to several years	Malaise; weight loss; cough; shortness of breath; chest pain	Various antibiotics; possibly surgery
Typhoid fever				
Salmonella typh	Food or water contaminated with infected feces	1 to 2 weeks, sometimes longer	Headache; lethargy, intestinal upsets; very high, prolonged fever	Several effective drugs, but fever takes a long time to control

FUNGAL INFECTIONS

Infective agent	Transmission	Incubation period	Symptoms	Treatment
Tinea				
Epidermophyton spp; *Microsporum* spp; *Trichophyton* spp	Direct contact with infected humans or animals	Variable	Itchy skin patches; patchy hair loss; cracking skin between toes	Antifungal drugs
Meningitis, fungal				
Cryptococcus neoformans	Inhalation of fungus from pigeon droppings	Unknown	Headache; stiff neck; photophobia	Antifungal drugs

PROTOZOAL INFECTIONS

Infective agent	Transmission	Incubation period	Symptoms	Treatment
Amebiasis				
Entamoeba histolytica	Food or water contaminated by feces	A few weeks to many years	Severe diarrhea	Antiprotozoal drug (e.g., metronidazole)
Giardiasis				
Giardia lamblia	Food or water contaminated by feces; sexual contact	3 to 40 days	Diarrhea; abdominal discomfort; bloating	Antiprotozoal drugs (e.g., metronidazole)
Malaria				
Plasmodium falciparum; *Plasmodium vivax*; others	Bite from infected mosquito	10 to 40 days	Chills; high fever; sweating; headache; fatigue	Various drugs (e.g., chloroquine)

In rare cases, there may be a chromosomal abnormality (such as *Klinefelter's syndrome*) or a genetic disease (such as *cystic fibrosis*) that causes infertility in men.

FEMALE INFERTILITY Anovulation (failure to ovulate) is the most common cause of female infertility. Failure to ovulate often occurs for no obvious reason. It can be caused by hormonal imbalance, stress, or a disorder of the *ovary*, such as a tumor or cyst.

Blocked fallopian tubes, which frequently occur after *pelvic inflammatory disease*, may prevent the sperm from reaching the egg. The woman may have one tube or no tubes because of a congenital defect or because they were removed surgically (e.g., because of an earlier *ectopic pregnancy*). Disorders of the uterus (such as *fibroids*) may cause infertility, as can *endometriosis*.

Infertility also occurs if the woman's cervical mucus provides a hostile environment to her partner's sperm by producing antibodies that kill or immobilize them.

Rarely, a chromosomal abnormality (such as *Turner's syndrome*) is the cause of a woman's infertility.

DIAGNOSIS
Tests for infertility are usually carried out if pregnancy has not resulted after a year of regular unprotected intercourse (about 90 percent of women trying to become pregnant do so within a year).

A physical examination of both the man and the woman will be performed to determine the general state of their health, and to eliminate untreated physical disorders that might be causing the infertility. The partners are interviewed, separately and together, regarding their sexual habits to determine if intercourse is taking place correctly for conception. If the cause of infertility remains undiagnosed after these examinations, additional tests may be performed (see box, p. 586).

TREATMENT
When no specific cause can be found, improving the general state of health may help. The physician may suggest changes in the patient's diet (e.g., reducing alcohol intake) and may suggest relaxation techniques and elimination of stress.

Treatment of male infertility is limited. Surgical reversal of vasectomy is possible in some cases. When azoospermia exists, the couple must usually accept their childless state or consider adoption or *artificial insemination* by donor. If the sperm count is low, artificial insemination by the husband may be tried, although its success rate varies. In cases due to a hormonal imbalance, drugs such as *clomiphene* or *gonadotropin hormone* therapy may prove useful.

For female infertility, failure to ovulate requires ovarian stimulation with a drug such as clomiphene, with or without a gonadotropin hormone. Microsurgery can sometimes repair damage to the fallopian tubes if it is not too severe. If surgery on the fallopian tubes is unsuccessful, *in vitro fertilization* is the only way that pregnancy may be possible. Uterine abnormalities or disorders, such as fibroids, may require treatment. If the cervical mucus has proved hostile, artificial insemination of the husband's semen directly into the cervix can prevent the sperm from coming into contact with the mucus.

Some cases of infertility, provided the woman has normal fallopian tubes, are treated by GIFT (gamete intra-fallopian transfer). In this technique, the ovaries are first stimulated by drugs. Then, by *laparoscopy* under general anesthesia, fluid is sucked out from the ovarian follicles through a needle and examined microscopically for eggs. The eggs are then replaced, together with a semen sample, in the fallopian tubes.

INVESTIGATING INFERTILITY

If no cause for infertility is found after a general checkup and/or a personal interview regarding sexual behavior, more specialized tests may be performed. Both partners may require testing because infertility can be attributed to one person, to both of them, or to mutual incompatibility.

CAUSES OF INFERTILITY

Conception is a complicated process; the organs involved can be affected in numerous ways, resulting in infertility. Some of the principal underlying causes of infertility—in men and women—are illustrated at right.

Vas deferens
Blockage or structural abnormality may impede passage of sperm.

Fallopian tubes
Blockage may prevent sperm from reaching egg; one or both tubes may be absent or damaged.

Penis
Failure to achieve or maintain erection; abnormality of ejaculation.

Ovaries
Eggs may fail to mature or may not be released.

Uterus
Abnormality or disorder may prevent implantation of fertilized egg.

Testes
Too few sperm produced; sperm are abnormally shaped, too short-lived, or have impaired motility.

Cervix
Cervical mucus may damage or destroy sperm.

FEMALE INFERTILITY

Investigations to discover the cause of a woman's infertility may include taking a menstrual history, a study of body temperature during the menstrual cycle (below), and/or blood and urine tests to discover whether ovulation is normal, hysterosalpingography (right), or laparoscopy (below right).

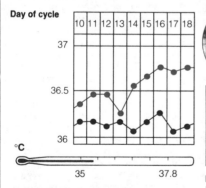

Day of cycle

°C

35   37.8

Body temperature and ovulation
Charting a woman's body temperature during her menstrual cycle can indicate abnormalities of ovulation. The chart above shows typical temperature fluctuations during a normal cycle (red line) and those associated with failure to ovulate (gray line).

Hysterosalpin-gography
This X-ray technique is used to visualize the uterus and/or fallopian tubes to determine whether or not there is any abnormality.

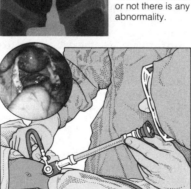

Laparoscopy
In this technique, a laparoscope (a type of viewing tube) is inserted through the abdominal wall to examine the woman's reproductive organs and determine whether an abnormality, such as a cyst or a tumor, is present. The laparoscope view (above) shows a tumor in the left ovary.

MALE INFERTILITY

The first test for investigating male infertility is semen analysis (below). If it reveals a low sperm count, more tests may be needed to investigate the underlying cause.

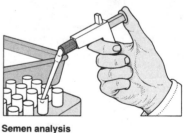

Semen analysis
Semen produced by masturbation is examined as soon as possible for the number, shape, and degree of motility of the sperm. A postcoital semen test may also be performed.

Abnormal sperm
The presence in the semen of large numbers of abnormally shaped sperm, such as the two-headed one (left), may reduce a man's fertility.

OUTLOOK

About half the couples professionally treated for infertility achieve a pregnancy. Each couple's chances depend on the cause of the infertility.

Infestation

 The presence of animal parasites (such as mites, ticks, or lice) in the skin or hair or of worms (such as tapeworms) inside the body.

Infibulation

A form of female circumcision in which the labia majora (the outer lips surrounding the vagina) are removed and the entrance to the vagina narrowed. See *Circumcision, female.*

Infiltrate

Accumulation of substances or cells within a tissue that are either not normally found in it or are usually present only in smaller amounts.

Infiltrate may refer to a drug (such as a local anesthetic) that has been injected into a tissue or to the buildup of a substance within an organ (such as of fat in the liver caused by excessive alcohol consumption).

Radiologists use the term to refer to the presence of abnormalities, such as the presence of a tumor or signs of pneumonia, on an X ray.

Inflammation

Redness, swelling, heat, and pain in a tissue due to chemical or physical injury, or to infection.

When body tissues are damaged, specialized *mast cells* release a chemical called *histamine* (other substances are also involved in the inflammatory response, but histamine is believed to be responsible for most of the effects). Histamine increases blood flow to the damaged tissue, which causes the redness and heat. It also makes the blood capillaries more leaky, resulting in fluid oozing out of them and into the tissues, which causes localized swelling. The pain of inflammation is due to stimulation of nerve endings by the inflammatory chemicals.

Inflammation is usually accompanied by an accumulation of white blood cells, which are attracted by the inflammatory chemicals. These white cells help destroy invading microorganisms and are involved in repairing the damaged tissue. Thus, inflammation is an essential part of the body's response to injury and infection.

If inflammation is inappropriate (as in *rheumatoid arthritis* and some other

autoimmune disorders), it may be suppressed by *corticosteroid drugs* or by *nonsteroidal anti-inflammatory drugs*.

Inflammatory bowel disease

A general term for chronic inflammatory disorders affecting the small and/or large intestine. The cause is unknown. Specific conditions are *Crohn's disease* and *ulcerative colitis*.

Influenza

A viral infection of the respiratory tract (air passages) that causes fever, headache, muscle ache, and weakness. Popularly known as "the flu," it is spread by virus-infected droplets coughed or sneezed into the air. Influenza usually occurs in small outbreaks or every few years in epidemics. Outbreaks tend to occur in winter; they spread particularly rapidly through schools and institutions for the elderly.

CAUSES

There are two main types of influenza virus, called A and B. Anyone who has been infected with a certain strain of the type A or B viruses acquires immunity to that strain. Both the A and B type viruses can alter to produce new strains that may be able to dodge or overcome immunity built up from a previous attack, thus leading to a new infection.

The type B virus is fairly stable, but it occasionally alters sufficiently to overcome resistance. The new strain often causes outbreaks of illness. The type A virus is more unstable; new strains arise constantly throughout the world. Among these strains are those that caused the influenza *pandemics* of this century, most notably Spanish flu in 1918, Asian flu in 1957, and Hong Kong flu in 1968.

The initial classic symptoms of flu (chills, fever, headache, cough, muscular aches, and fatigue) are brought on by both type A and type B influenza viruses. In general, type A is more debilitating than type B.

The general symptoms described are usually followed by a cough (often accompanied by chest pain), a sore throat, and a nasal congestion. Nausea or vomiting may occur in some cases of influenza but diarrhea is not characteristic of the disease. After two days, fever and other symptoms start to subside and, after five days, these symptoms have usually disappeared. Respiratory symptoms persist, however; the sufferer may feel weak and sometimes depressed. The illness usually clears up completely within

7 to 10 days. In rare cases, however, it takes a severe form, causing acute pneumonia that may be fatal within a day or two even in healthy young adults. The Spanish flu epidemic of 1918 killed millions of young adults in all countries of the world.

In children and adolescents treatment of influenza with acetylsalicylic acid has been associated with an increased risk of *Reye's syndrome*, a rare but serious illness involving the liver and brain. Fever caused by an influenza infection can cause febrile seizures in young children.

Secondary bacterial infection is common, particularly in the elderly and in those with lung or heart disease; it may cause fatal *pneumonia*.

PREVENTION

Anti-influenza vaccines, containing killed strains of types A and B viruses currently in circulation are available and have only a 70 percent success rate in preventing illness and even greater success in preventing serious complications or death due to influenza. Since the viruses are unstable and the immunity produced in response to influenza vaccine is short-lived, vaccination must be repeated each year just before the start of the influenza season. It is recommended that older people and anyone suffering from chronic respiratory or circulatory disease and people with immune system deficiencies and certain other chronic conditions, especially those living in institutions, be vaccinated each fall.

TREATMENT

In all but the mildest cases, a person with influenza should rest in bed in a warm, well-ventilated room. Analgesics (painkillers) should be taken to relieve aches and pains and to reduce fever but acetylsalicylic acid should *not* be given to children or adolescents. Adequate fluid intake should be maintained. Warm fluids soothe a sore throat and inhaling steam has a soothing effect on the lungs.

In the case of an elderly person or someone with a lung or heart disease, a physician should be called as soon as symptoms develop. In addition, a physician should be called for anyone suffering from influenza who takes a sudden turn for the worse. The drug amantadine, which can reduce the severity of an attack of type A influenza, but not of type B influenza, if given within 24 hours of onset of symptoms, may be prescribed. Antibiotics may also be used to combat secondary bacterial infection.

Once the fever has abated, the patient can get out of bed, but still needs rest. When he or she starts to regain strength, normal activities should be resumed gradually.

Informed consent

See *Consent*.

Infrared

A term denoting the part of the electromagnetic spectrum immediately beyond the red end of the visible light spectrum. Directed onto the skin, infrared radiation heats the skin and the tissues immediately below it.

The infrared wave band includes heat waves; an infrared lamp is one means of giving *heat treatment*.

Infusion, intravenous

See *Intravenous infusion*.

Ingestion

The act of taking any substance (e.g., food, drink, or medications) into the body through the mouth. The term also refers to the process by which certain cells (for example, some white blood cells) surround and then engulf small particles.

Ingrown toenail

See *Toenail, ingrown*.

Inguinal

Relating to the groin (the area between the abdomen and thigh), as in inguinal *hernia*.

Inhalation

The act of taking in breath (see *Breathing*). An inhalation is also a substance, in the form of a gas, vapor, powder, or aerosol, to be breathed in.

Inhaler

A device used for administering a drug in powder or vapor form. Inhalers are used principally in the treatment of various respiratory disorders, including *asthma* and chronic *bronchitis*. Among the medications administered in this way are *bronchodilator drugs* (used to widen the airways) and *corticosteroid drugs* (used to reduce inflammation).

Inheritance

The transmission of traits, characteristics, and disorders from parents to their children through the influence of *genes*. Genes are the units of *DNA* (deoxyribonucleic acid) in a person's cells; DNA controls all growth and functioning of the body. Half of a person's genes come from the mother, half from the father.

Children tend to resemble their parents, particularly in their physical characteristics. However, this resemblance may also apply to mental abilities, mannerisms, personality, and behavior. In addition, many disorders show a moderate to very notable tendency to "run in families."

Although there is a temptation to ascribe similarities in a family to inheritance, there are equally plausible alternative explanations for many family traits. For example, all the members of a family may be fat not through the influence of genes, but because they all eat the same fattening food and rarely exercise. Children may behave like their mother not because of inheritance, but because they imitate her. Certain abilities and behaviors (e.g., the language a person speaks) are clearly not inherited. Nevertheless, it is accepted that most physical characteristics, many disorders, and some mental abilities and aspects of personality are inherited.

MECHANISMS OF INHERITANCE

Each of a person's cells contains exactly the same genes, which come originally from the egg and sperm cells from which he or she is derived.

The genes in a cell are organized into long strands of DNA called *chromosomes*. The genes controlling most characteristics come in pairs—one gene originating from the father, the other from the mother. Everyone has 22 pairs of chromosomes (called autosomes) bearing these paired genes, in addition to two more chromosomes, the sex chromosomes. Women have two X chromosomes; men have an X chromosome and a Y chromosome.

The inheritance of normal traits and disorders can be divided into those controlled by a single pair of genes on the autosomal chromosomes (unifactorial inheritance); those controlled by genes on the sex chromosomes (sex-linked inheritance); and those controlled by the combination of many genes (multifactorial inheritance).

UNIFACTORIAL INHERITANCE

A large number of variable traits, such as eye color, blood groups, and the ability to taste certain substances, are thought to be controlled by a single pair of genes. The ways in which these traits are inherited conform to laws first elucidated in the 19th century by the Austrian monk Gregor Mendel.

HOW TO USE AN INHALER

With each type, the user puts the nozzle of the inhaler in the mouth, presses the end to release the drug, and simultaneously breathes in through the mouth. If the device is used correctly, the drug is dispersed to the bronchi. A *nebulizer* is a special type of inhaler that delivers the drug as a fine mist through a face mask.

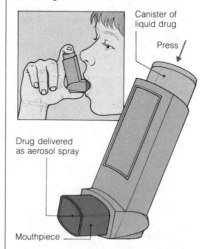

Canister of liquid drug

Press

Drug delivered as aerosol spray

Mouthpiece

Aerosol inhaler
This type of inhaler delivers the drug as an aerosol spray when the user presses the top of the canister.

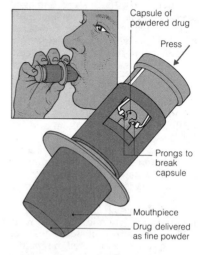

Capsule of powdered drug

Press

Prongs to break capsule

Mouthpiece

Drug delivered as fine powder

Turbo-inhaler
Here, a drug capsule is placed in the end chamber, the top of which is pressed to pierce the capsule and release the drug.

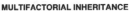

Since then, they have been referred to as the laws of Mendelian inheritance.

Either of the pair of genes controlling a trait may take any of several forms, which are known as alleles. For example, the genes controlling eye color exist as two main alleles, coding for blue and brown eye color.

Thus, an individual's gene pair for eye color may be blue/blue (giving blue eyes), brown/brown (giving brown eyes) or brown/blue (also giving brown eyes, because the brown allele is dominant over, i.e., "masks," the blue allele, which is called recessive to the brown allele).

When a couple has a child, only one of the pair of genes controlling a trait is passed to the child from each parent. For example, someone with the brown/blue combination for eye color has a 50 percent chance of passing on the blue gene, and a 50 percent chance of passing on the brown gene, to any child. This factor is combined with the gene coming from the other parent, according to dominant or recessive relationships, to determine the child's eye color. According to the combination of the parental genes, the numbers of brown- and blue-eyed offspring of a particular couple tend to conform to a certain ratio, in accordance with Mendelian laws.

Similar laws and ratios apply to the inheritance of other traits controlled by single gene pairs, and also to the inheritance of certain *genetic disorders*.

The most obvious example of sex-linked inheritance is gender itself. Male gender is caused by the existence in males of the genes on the Y chromosome, which is present only in males and is inherited by boys from their fathers. The genes on the Y chromosome almost certainly direct the development of the male primary sex organs (the testes) and all male characteristics derive from the secretion of hormones by these organs.

The X chromosome, on the other hand, is less closely associated with the female sex because it is present in both males (in a single dose) and in females (in a double dose). It seems that female gender is the natural course of development in the absence of the Y chromosome, does not require any extra genes to direct it, and that the X chromosome is concerned with general development.

Any faults in a male's genes on the X chromosome tend to be expressed outwardly, because such a fault cannot (as it can in females) be masked by the presence of a normal gene on a second X chromosome. Faults in the genes of the X chromosome include those responsible for *color vision deficiency*, *hemophilia*, and other sex-linked inherited disorders, which almost exclusively affect males.

MULTIFACTORIAL INHERITANCE

A number of traits (such as height and build) are believed to be controlled by the combined effects of many genes, along with environmental effects. Using height as an example, a simple model proposes that there are several genes determining a person's stature, some of which are "tall" genes and others "short." A person's height depends on the relative number of tall to short genes.

When two people have children, a child may, in rare cases, inherit all the tall or all the short genes from both parents, and thus be exceptionally tall or short. The laws of chance dictate, however, that, in most cases, a child will inherit a mixture of tall and short genes and thus be in the range of average stature. Nevertheless, the child of tall parents tends to inherit more tall genes than the child of short parents. Dietary and other factors also affect growth so that a person with many short genes may still attain an average stature through good diet.

Multifactorial inheritance, along with the effects of environment, may play a part in causing disorders, such as *diabetes mellitus* and *spina bifida*.

Inhibition

The process of preventing any mental or physical activity. Inhibition in the brain and spinal cord is carried out by special *neurons*, which damp down the action of other nerve cells to keep the brain's activity in balance.

In a psychological sense, certain mental activities can be described as inhibiting other thoughts or reflexes.

In *psychoanalysis*, an inhibition refers to the unconscious restraint of instinctual impulses. Such inhibition may cause symptoms, such as being temporarily unable to write because writing arouses forbidden ideas.

Injection

 Introduction of a substance into the body from a syringe through a needle. Injections may be intravenous (into a vein), intramuscular (into a muscle), subcutaneous (under the skin), or intra-articular (into a joint).

Injury

Harm to any part of the body. Injury may arise from a wide variety of causes, including physical influences (e.g., force, heat, cold, electricity, vibration, and radiation), chemical causes (e.g., poisons and caustic substances), bites, or oxygen deprivation.

INHERITANCE OF EYE COLOR

Eye color is determined by two main alleles (forms of a gene), one coding for brown eyes and the other for blue eyes. The brown allele is dominant to the blue one (which is therefore recessive).

Parents   Children   Parents   Children

Key

brown eyes   or

blue eyes

Allele for brown eyes

Allele for blue eyes

Eye color of offspring

Two brown-eyed parents (each with the brown/blue combination of alleles) have a one in four chance of producing a blue-eyed child (above left). But there is a one in two chance of having a blue-eyed child when one parent is brown-eyed (with brown/blue alleles) and the other is blue-eyed (above).

(See *Accidental death; Bites, animal; Bites, human; Bleeding; Burns; Cold injury; Dislocation, joint; Electrical injury; First aid; Fracture; Head injury; Heatstroke; Poisoning; Radiation sickness; Snake bites; Soft-tissue injury; Spinal injury; Sports injuries; Sprain; Venomous bites and stings; Wound.*)

Inkblot test

 An outdated psychological test in which the subject was asked to interpret a number of ink blots. The most widely used example was the *Rorschach test*.

Inlay, dental

A filling of porcelain or gold made outside the mouth and used to restore a badly decayed tooth. An inlay may be needed for back teeth or to provide protection for a weakened tooth.

The dentist first makes an angular cavity in the tooth to accept the inlay. A replica of the cavity is then made, generally using a wax *impression*; the inlay is constructed on the replica and cemented in place in the tooth.

Inoculation

The act of introducing a small quantity of a foreign substance into the body, usually by injection, for the purpose of stimulating the *immune system* to produce *antibodies* (protective proteins) against the substance. Inoculation is usually done to protect against future infection. (See *Immunization*.)

Inoperable

A term applied to any condition that cannot be alleviated or cured by surgery, such as a very advanced cancer that has spread to many parts of the body or a brain tumor that is not surgically accessible.

Inorganic

A term used to refer to any of the large group of substances that do not contain carbon and to a few simple carbon compounds (e.g., *carbon dioxide* and *carbon monoxide*). Examples of inorganic substances include table salt (sodium chloride) and bicarbonate of soda (sodium bicarbonate).

Inpatient treatment

Care or therapy received by a patient admitted to a hospital.

Insanity

The common term for serious mental disorder. Today the term insanity has no technical meaning for psychia-trists, but is used in law to indicate a mental state that renders a person not legally responsible for his or her own actions. The "insanity defense" was introduced to ensure that people committing murder as a result of a mental disorder would not be given the death penalty, but would instead receive proper treatment. *Psychosis* now covers serious illnesses formerly denoted by insanity.

Insect bites

Tiny puncture wounds in the skin inflicted by blood-sucking insects, such as mosquitoes, blackflies, horseflies, sandflies, midges, gnats, fleas, lice, and bedbugs. Small eight-legged creatures commonly called arachnids, which include scorpions, spiders, ticks, and mites, can cause similar injuries.

Most bites cause only temporary pain (or itching for a day or two) although some people have severe skin reactions. In the tropics and sub-tropics, insect bites are potentially more serious because certain biting species can transmit disease (see *Insects and disease*).

CAUSES

Insects that bite do so to obtain a blood meal. The mouthparts of biting insects are specially adapted for piercing skin and sucking blood. Insect bites are most common on exposed parts of the head, hands, arms, or legs.

Although mosquitoes (which attack mainly after dark) may be the most troublesome biting insects, many bites blamed on mosquitoes are in fact caused by cat or dog fleas. These fleas inhabit various domestic locations where the pet habitually rests (e.g., carpets, sleeping baskets, or sofas) and, when their normal host is absent, they may jump onto humans to feed.

Of the more easily visible insects, horseflies can produce a particularly painful bite, while gnats can be a menace if a swarm is encountered.

SYMPTOMS

All insect bites provoke a reaction in the skin that is primarily an allergic response (see *Allergy*) to substances in the insect's saliva or its feces, which are often deposited at or near the site of the bite and rubbed in by scratching. Reactions vary from innocuous red pimples to painful swellings (which may weep) or an intensely itching rash. People vary in their reactions to the same biting insect; in some people the reaction may be extremely severe.

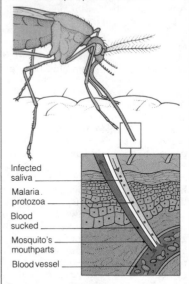

INSECT-BORNE DISEASES

Malaria is by far the most prevalent of the insect-borne diseases, affecting an estimated 200 to 300 million people worldwide.

Infected saliva

Malaria protozoa

Blood sucked

Mosquito's mouthparts

Blood vessel

Transmission of malaria
When an infected *ANOPHELES* mosquito feeds on a person's blood, it injects saliva through its mouthparts; the protozoa that cause malaria enter the blood via the insect's saliva.

AVOIDANCE

Avoiding insect bites can be particularly important for campers and hikers, anyone living in a mosquito-infested area, and travelers or residents in tropical countries.

Bites outdoors can be reduced by wearing trousers, socks, and long-sleeved shirts, and by using insect repellents.

Indoors, bites can be reduced by using insect screens over open windows and by spraying bedrooms with pressurized containers and pyre-throid insecticide before going to bed.

TREATMENT

Bites or bitten areas should be thoroughly washed with soap and water, and a soothing ointment, such as cala-mine lotion, should be applied. Scratching should be avoided. If there is a severe reaction, a physician should be called; a cream containing an *antihistamine drug* may be required.

Severe itching on the scalp or in the pubic hair suggests the possibility of a louse infestation, which is treated with insecticidal lotions (see *Lice*). In the case of flea bites, the entire residence (not just the pet) may require treatment with insecticide to kill the flea population. (See also *Mites and disease; Spider bites; Ticks and disease.*)

Insects and disease

Insects are six-legged animals with a pair of antennae, a firm exterior skeleton, and, in many cases, wings. They include such animals as ants, bees, cockroaches, fleas, flies, lice, and mosquitoes, but not mites, ticks, or spiders, which belong to another animal group, the arachnids. The insects and arachnids both belong to a larger animal group, the arthropods.

DISEASE CAUSED BY INSECTS

There are more than one million known species of insects and probably several million that have yet to be identified and named; most are either harmless or positively beneficial to humans. The majority of harmful species cause sickness by attacking crops or stored food, thus contributing to malnutrition and famine.

Other insects are a more direct cause of illness or disease. Some directly parasitize humans, living under the skin or on the body surface (see *Chigoe; Lice; Myiasis*). Others will sting if provoked, with results that range from moderate discomfort (in most cases) to a severe life-threatening reaction (see *Insect stings*).

The most troublesome insects are flies and various biting insects. Many types of flies settle first on human or animal excrement and then on food to lay eggs or to feed. They can transmit disease organisms from excrement to food via their feet and legs. This is probably important in the spread of intestinal infections such as *typhoid fever* and *shigellosis*.

Insect bites are irritating in themselves, but a much more serious risk is that an insect will spread infectious organisms as a result of its bite. Serious diseases that are spread by biting insects include *malaria* and *filariasis* (transmitted by mosquitoes), *sleeping sickness* (tsetse flies), *leishmaniasis* (sandflies), epidemic *typhus* (lice), and *plague* (rat fleas). Also, various mosquitoes, sandflies, and ticks spread a group of viral illnesses called the arthropod-borne or arboviruses. Included among such illnesses are *yellow fever*, *dengue*, and some types of viral *encephalitis*.

Organisms picked up when an insect ingests blood from an infected animal or person are able to survive or multiply in the insect. Later, the organisms are either injected into a new human host via the insect's saliva or deposited in the feces at or near the site of the bite and later rubbed in by the victim.

Most of insect-borne diseases (of which malaria is by far the most important) are confined to the tropics and subtropics.

AVOIDANCE

The avoidance of insect-borne disease is largely a matter of keeping flies off food, discouraging insect bites by the use of suitable clothing and insect repellents, and, in areas of the world where malaria is present, the use of mosquito nets and screens, *pesticides*, and antimalarial tablets.

Insect stings

A fairly small number of insects (bees, wasps, and hornets) are capable of stinging. Insect venom contains inflammatory substances that cause local pain, redness, and swelling for about 48 hours. Normally, a very large number of stings (hundreds in the case of an adult) must be received for them to be life-threatening. However, about one person in 200 is allergic to insect venom. This means that, after the person's *immune system* has been sensitized by the venom from a sting, one subsequent sting (possibly months or years later) can provoke a severe allergic reaction leading to *anaphylactic shock*. The symptoms may include a severe itchy rash (hives), dizziness, facial and throat swellings, wheezing, vomiting, breathing difficulties, and collapse.

FIRST AID: INSECT STINGS AND TICK BITES

INSECT STING

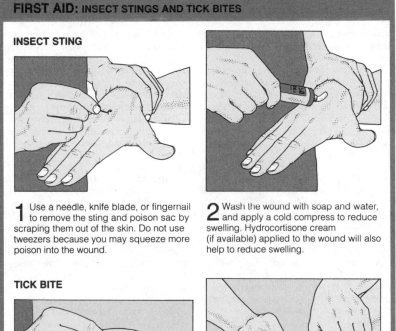

1 Use a needle, knife blade, or fingernail to remove the sting and poison sac by scraping them out of the skin. Do not use tweezers because you may squeeze more poison into the wound.

2 Wash the wound with soap and water, and apply a cold compress to reduce swelling. Hydrocortisone cream (if available) applied to the wound will also help to reduce swelling.

TICK BITE

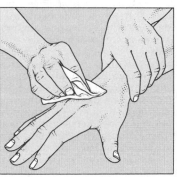

1 If the tick is still clinging to the skin, dislodge it by holding an extinguished match to its body. Do not attempt to pull it off; it might burst.

2 Use soap and warm water to wash the area thoroughly. Then rinse and dry the skin gently.

Hyposensitization—a technique for reducing sensitivity to bee or wasp venom (and some other types of allergy)—is recommended for those known to suffer hypersensitivity.

TREATMENT

A bee often leaves its sting sac in the wound. The sac should be gently scraped out with a knife blade or fingernail and not removed by grasping it with fingers or tweezers (which injects more venom). The stung area should be washed with soap and water, a cold compress should be applied, and *analgesic drugs* should be taken to ease the discomfort. If the symptoms of anaphylactic shock develop, seek emergency medical treatment, which initially consists of an injection of *epinephrine*. Any person who is known to be hypersensitive to bee or wasp venom should carry a self-injection kit. In severe cases, the victims of insect stings require *cardiopulmonary resuscitation*.

Any sting in the mouth or throat may be dangerous because swelling may obstruct breathing. Medical assistance should be sought immediately and, if possible, the victim should be given ice cubes to suck. (See also *Scorpion stings*.)

Insecurity

Lack of self-confidence and uncertainty about one's abilities, aims, and relationships with others. Repeated changes of environment (such as frequent moves of home or school) can lead to a sense of insecurity, especially in childhood. A feeling of insecurity may be a feature of *anxiety* and other neurotic mental disorders.

Insight

Being aware of one's own mental state. In a general sense, this means knowing one's own strengths, weaknesses, and abilities.

The term insight also has the specific psychiatric meaning of knowing that one's symptoms are an illness. Loss of insight may be a feature of both psychotic and neurotic disorders. In psychoanalysis, having insight is regarded as an important step toward successful treatment.

In situ

A Latin term meaning "in place." The phrase "carcinoma in situ" is used to describe tissue (particularly of the skin or cervix) that is cancerous only in its surface cells and is completely surrounded by normal cells without any signs of spread to deeper layers.

Insomnia

Trouble in sleeping. People with insomnia may have difficulty in falling asleep or in staying asleep. Most insomnia sufferers also complain of increased daytime fatigue, irritability, and find it difficult to cope. Insomnia is common: as many as one in every three adults may suffer from insomnia at some time in his or her life. *Sleeping drugs* are among the most widely used of all medicines.

CAUSES

The most common cause of insomnia is worry about a problem (such as bad news received during the day or a difficult task to cope with the following morning), but other causes are implicated in about half of all cases.

Causes include physical disorders, such as *sleep apnea*, *restless legs*, environmental factors (such as noise and light), life-style factors (such as too much coffee in the evening, lack of exercise during the day, or keeping erratic hours), or misuse of sleeping drugs (including *benzodiazepine drugs* and *barbiturate drugs*).

Insomnia also can be a symptom of a psychiatric illness. People with *anxiety* and/or *depression* may find it difficult to fall asleep; those suffering from depression typically wake early in the morning. Sleeping much less than usual is common in *mania*, in which the person is so full of drive and energy that he or she does not need much sleep. *Schizophrenia* often causes people to pace about at night, aroused by "voices" or delusions. People with *dementia* or other brain disorders may be afraid in the dark and become restless and noisy, confused by the shadows and sounds of the night.

Withdrawal symptoms from sleeping drugs, *antidepressant drugs*, *antianxiety drugs*, and some illicit drugs (see *Drug abuse*), such as heroin, may cause many weeks of insomnia.

People sometimes mistakenly believe that they are suffering from insomnia because of a misconception about the amount of sleep they need. In fact, sleep needs vary greatly, with some people requiring less than four hours and others needing more than 10. Some people who think they have insomnia are in fact "out of phase," lying awake for hours after going to bed, but sleeping normally if allowed to sleep late in the morning.

INVESTIGATION AND TREATMENT

An obvious physical or psychological cause for insomnia will be treated. For long-term insomnia with no obvious cause, *EEG* recordings of brain-wave patterns and an assessment of breathing, muscle activity, and other bodily functions during sleep may be useful in discovering the extent and pattern of the problem. Keeping a log of sleep patterns may also be helpful.

Studies have shown that many people with insomnia sleep much more than they think they do. However, they also tend to wake more frequently than normal sleepers. It is the quality, rather than the quantity, of sleep that is the problem for victims of this condition. People with insomnia should ensure that they are active during the day and should establish a regular routine and time for going to bed each night and waking in the morning. Sleeping drugs should be used only on medical advice.

Instinct

An innate primitive urge. The need for warmth, food, love, and sex, are all forms of instinct, although the instinct for survival is probably the most powerful. An instinct is distinguished from a reflex, which is an involuntary response to a stimulus (such as withdrawing one's hand from a fire).

In animals, instincts often take the form of specific inherited patterns of behavior. For example, ducks follow their mothers, and beavers build dams—activities that do not appear to have been learned.

Humans have few of these set behaviors, and instincts may be more appropriately regarded as motivators of behavior. This idea was first developed as a central part of *Freudian theory*. Freud believed that instincts arose from energy aroused in the unconscious. The aim of the instinct was to calm the aroused state by directing the energy onto some outside object (for example, sexual arousal leads to intercourse and orgasm).

Institutionalization

The loss of personal independence that stems from living for long periods in a mental hospital, prison, or other large institution. Apathy, obeying orders unquestioningly, accepting a standard routine, and loss of interests are the main features. Such features are thought to be caused by a lack of rights and personal responsibility, the attitudes of controlling staff, and the effects of drugs.

Care of the long-term sick within the community (as an alternative to hospitalization) is designed to combat the institutionalization process.

Insulin

A *hormone* produced by the *pancreas* in varying amounts depending on the level of glucose (sugar) in the blood. Carbohydrate is absorbed as glucose, increasing the blood glucose level and stimulating the pancreas to produce insulin. Insulin promotes the absorption of glucose into the *liver* and into muscle cells (where it is converted into energy). In the liver, glucose is stored as glycogen, which is reconverted to glucose in response to stress or exercise. Insulin thus prevents a buildup of blood glucose and ensures that various tissues have sufficient amounts of glucose.

Diabetes mellitus occurs when the pancreas produces little or no insulin, causing *hyperglycemia* (abnormally high blood glucose). An *insulinoma* is a rare benign tumor that causes excessive production of insulin.

INSULIN THERAPY

Insulin supplements have been used in the treatment of diabetes mellitus since the first isolation of insulin by Canadian researchers Frederick Banting and Charles Best in 1922. Insulin preparations are produced from pig or ox pancreas or by *genetic engineering* techniques from microorganisms. Various short-, intermediate-, or long-acting preparations are available.

Insulin is used in all cases of insulin-dependent diabetes mellitus (total absence of insulin production) and, occasionally, when oral hypoglycemic drugs (see *Hypoglycemics, oral*) are unable to control non-insulin-dependent diabetes mellitus (deficient production of insulin), such as during serious illness, major surgery, or pregnancy. Insulin therapy is used to prevent hyperglycemia and *ketosis* (a buildup of certain acids in the patient's blood), which, in severe cases, may cause coma.

Insulin is given to mimic the body's production of the natural hormone. Insulin injections may be self-administered before meals to act on the increase in blood glucose that occurs after eating. Alternatively, an insulin pump (see *Pump, insulin*) may be used to deliver insulin throughout the day and night; the dose is increased before each meal.

Adjustment of the dose is often needed when there are variations in diet and exercise, and during illness (especially when there has been vomiting). Regular self-monitoring of glucose levels, either by blood or by urine tests, is necessary to ensure adequate control.

POSSIBLE ADVERSE EFFECTS

Insulin injections may cause irritation or dimpling of the skin. Too high a dose will cause *hypoglycemia* (abnormally low blood glucose) with symptoms (such as dizziness, sweating, irritability, and a feeling of weakness) that are relieved by consuming food or a sugary drink. Severe hypoglycemia may cause coma, for which emergency treatment with an injection of glucose or *glucagon* (a hormone that opposes the effects of insulin) is necessary. Allergic reactions to insulin, causing rash or breathing difficulty, are rare. Pig or ox insulin may make the body produce *antibodies* which reduce the effectiveness of the insulin preparation.

Insulinoma

A rare benign tumor of the insulin-producing cells of the *pancreas*. Such a tumor can produce abnormal quantities of *insulin* so that the amount of glucose in the blood (which is reduced by insulin) can fall to dangerously low levels. This is called *hypoglycemia* and, unless sugar is given immediately, can cause *coma* and death.

Blood insulin levels are normally low during fasting; insulinoma can be diagnosed by finding high levels after a period of fasting. A drug (diazoxide) is administered to prevent hypoglycemia until surgery can be performed to remove the tumor.

Intelligence

The ability to understand concepts and to reason them out. There is much confusion about the precise definition of intelligence. Many people use the word to mean a special degree of knowledge. The widespread use of *intelligence tests* has led to the idea that intelligence is a single quality.

Many scientists prefer to divide intelligence into various factors. Some see it as having three basic parts—speed of thought, learning, and problem-solving. Others argue that a general factor of intelligence exists, made up of seven special abilities—understanding the meaning of words, fluency with words, working with numbers, visualizing things in space, memory, speed of perception, and reasoning ability. Other researchers go further, dividing intelligence into more than 100 different factors.

Intelligence can also be considered as having three entirely separate forms—abstract intelligence (understanding ideas and symbols); practical intelligence (aptitude in dealing with practical problems, such as repairing machinery); and social intelligence (coping reasonably and wisely with human relationships). Personality plays an important role in this last type of intelligence.

AGE AND INTELLIGENCE

Intelligence, however it is defined, increases up to the age of about 6 years

---

MEASURING INTELLIGENCE

Intelligence is difficult to define precisely and to measure satisfactorily. Nevertheless, various tests have been devised that provide an estimate of a person's mental abilities. Most such tests measure an individual's ability in several areas of mental functioning that are generally thought to be important components or indicators of intelligence—for example, mathematical ability, logical reasoning, vocabulary, comprehension, general knowledge, memory, perceptual ability and pattern recognition, and the ability to understand relationships between concepts or objects. The questions at right are hypothetical examples (at various levels of difficulty) of those that might be asked in a typical intelligence test.

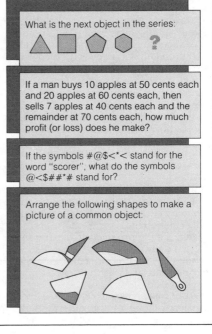

What is the next object in the series:

If a man buys 10 apples at 50 cents each and 20 apples at 60 cents each, then sells 7 apples at 40 cents each and the remainder at 70 cents each, how much profit (or loss) does he make?

If the symbols #@$<*< stand for the word "scorer", what do the symbols @<$##*# stand for?

Arrange the following shapes to make a picture of a common object:

and then stabilizes. Intelligence quotient (IQ), as measured by intelligence tests, continues to increase to about the age of 26, stays the same until about the age of 40, and then gradually declines (the drop occurring later in a person with an intellectually demanding job).

HEREDITY AND INTELLIGENCE

The role of heredity in intelligence is much argued, but there is no doubt that intelligence is inherited in a manner similar to height. Environment also plays a major part, as does physical health and personality. Intelligent parents tend to have intelligent children, but, even within one family, some children may be brighter than others. Adopted children from deprived social backgrounds, even though they may have IQs closer to their biological than their adopted parents, often score higher than would be expected had they been reared by their biological parents.

Extremes of intelligence occur in *mental retardation* (defined by a low IQ) and in the very gifted (defined by scores over 140).

People with very high IQs are often very successful, but not always. Personality and social adjustment are just as important.

Intelligence tests

Tests designed to provide an estimate of a person's mental abilities.

TYPES

WECHSLER TESTS These are the most widely used of all tests today. There are two basic versions—the Wechsler Adult Intelligence Scale (WAIS) and the Wechsler Intelligence Scale for Children (WISC). Each is divided into verbal and performance sections, which can be used separately or combined to produce an overall score. The verbal sections are concerned with language skills and include measures of vocabulary, general knowledge, verbal reasoning, and verbal memory. The performance sections include measures of constructional ability and visual-spatial and perceptual ability (interpretation of shapes).

The performance sections of the test may be used separately for people with language problems. Performance testing can measure basic intellectual ability whereas verbal testing tends to be more culture-bound because it tests skills that reflect social background.

STANFORD-BINET TEST This is a revised version of one of the oldest intelligence tests, devised by the French-

man Alfred Binet (1857-1911). It is still widely used, mainly as a measure of scholastic ability.

OTHER TESTS Numerous tests that concentrate on testing one particular aspect of intelligence have been devised. The Goodenough-Harris test assesses performance by asking a child to make a picture of a man; the child's score depends on the complexity of the drawing, such as the detail included and the body proportions.

SCORING

In most intelligence tests, scoring is based on the notion of mental age (MA) in relation to actual chronological age (CA), since intelligence normally increases with maturity. The intelligence quotient (IQ) is therefore MA divided by CA, multiplied by 100 to simplify the results. The tests are

devised to ensure that three quarters of people have an IQ between 80 and 120. They are also standardized so that the score indicates the same relative ability at different age levels. Regardless of age group, an IQ of 65 indicates that a person is in the bottom 1 percent of his or her age group; an IQ of 135 indicates the person is in the top 1 percent of his or her age group.

USES

Intelligence tests are useful in predicting whether a person has the ability to cope with certain jobs or to pass certain examinations. They may therefore be used to assess school or job aptitude. However, intelligence tests have been criticized for their alleged bias regarding gender and race. The tests are also used to define the legal

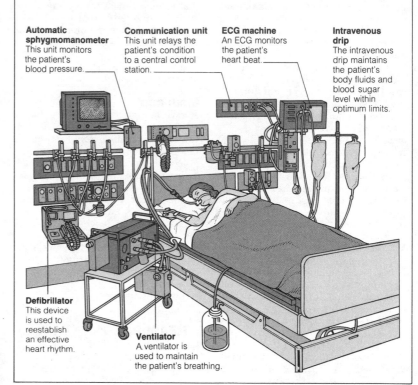

A TYPICAL INTENSIVE-CARE UNIT

Modern intensive-care units are designed so that postoperative and seriously ill patients can be monitored continuously. Such units are generally staffed by medical and nursing specialists and equipped with a wide variety of sophisticated machines fitted with automatic alarms to indicate any emergency. Each patient's blood pressure, heart rate and other vital functions are recorded electronically on a central console which is always observed by at least one staff person. This ability to check on all patients at once means any deterioration in a patient's condition can be detected instantly and treated immediately.

Automatic sphygmomanometer This unit monitors the patient's blood pressure.

Communication unit This unit relays the patient's condition to a central control station.

ECG machine An ECG monitors the patient's heart beat.

Intravenous drip The intravenous drip maintains the patient's body fluids and blood sugar level within optimum limits.

Defibrillator This device is used to reestablish an effective heart rhythm.

Ventilator A ventilator is used to maintain the patient's breathing.

notion of *mental retardation* and to assess the effects of *dementia* or other brain disease. In particular, a large difference in verbal and performance scores is helpful in assessing the degree of brain disease. Children with a particular difficulty may be tested so remedial teaching can be planned.

Intensive care

The constant, close monitoring of seriously ill patients, which enables immediate treatment to be given if the patient's condition deteriorates.

The intensive-care unit of a hospital contains electronic monitoring equipment that allows continuous assessment of vital body functions, such as blood pressure and heart and respiratory rates. The urine output, fluid balance, and blood chemistry of patients in intensive-care units are recorded regularly. Medical and nursing staff are in a high ratio to patients.

Intensive care is most often needed for patients who are on artificial *ventilation*, who may be unconscious and not breathing, or suffering from a respiratory illness. Close monitoring in an intensive care unit is also required for people recovering from a *myocardial infarction* (heart attack) or from major surgery, for patients in *shock* who are not responding to emergency treatment, and for those with acute *kidney failure* who require *dialysis*. (See also *Coronary care unit*.)

Inter-

A prefix that means between, as in *intercostal* (between the ribs).

Intercostal

The medical term for between the *ribs*, as in the intercostal muscles, thin sheets of muscle between each rib.

Intercourse, painful

Pain during *sexual intercourse*, known medically as dyspareunia. The problem can affect both men and women,

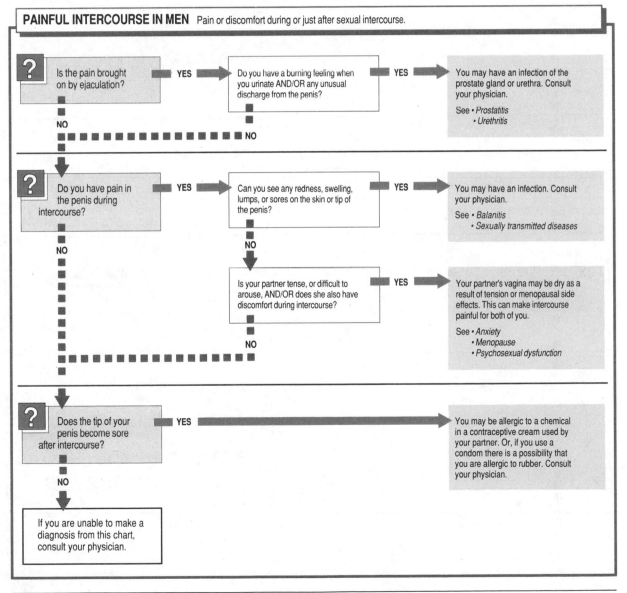

PAINFUL INTERCOURSE IN MEN Pain or discomfort during or just after sexual intercourse.

? Is the pain brought on by ejaculation? — **YES** → Do you have a burning feeling when you urinate AND/OR any unusual discharge from the penis? — **YES** → You may have an infection of the prostate gland or urethra. Consult your physician.
See • *Prostatitis*
• *Urethritis*
NO

? Do you have pain in the penis during intercourse? — **YES** → Can you see any redness, swelling, lumps, or sores on the skin or tip of the penis? — **YES** → You may have an infection. Consult your physician.
See • *Balanitis*
• *Sexually transmitted diseases*
NO

Is your partner tense, or difficult to arouse, AND/OR does she also have discomfort during intercourse? — **YES** → Your partner's vagina may be dry as a result of tension or menopausal side effects. This can make intercourse painful for both of you.
See • *Anxiety*
• *Menopause*
• *Psychosexual dysfunction*
NO

? Does the tip of your penis become sore after intercourse? — **YES** → You may be allergic to a chemical in a contraceptive cream used by your partner. Or, if you use a condom there is a possibility that you are allergic to rubber. Consult your physician.
NO

If you are unable to make a diagnosis from this chart, consult your physician.

PAINFUL INTERCOURSE IN WOMEN Pain or discomfort during or just after sexual intercourse.

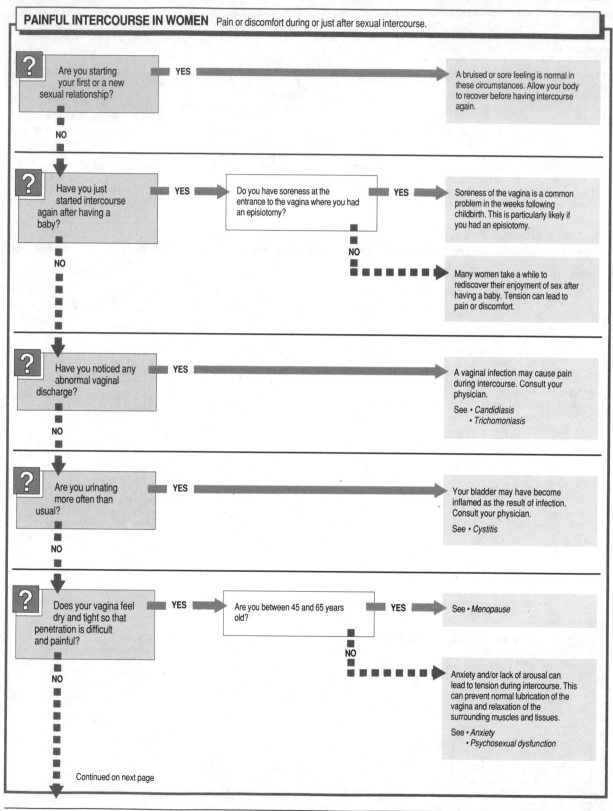

Are you starting your first or a new sexual relationship?

YES → A bruised or sore feeling is normal in these circumstances. Allow your body to recover before having intercourse again.

NO

Have you just started intercourse again after having a baby?

YES → Do you have soreness at the entrance to the vagina where you had an episiotomy?

YES → Soreness of the vagina is a common problem in the weeks following childbirth. This is particularly likely if you had an episiotomy.

NO → Many women take a while to rediscover their enjoyment of sex after having a baby. Tension can lead to pain or discomfort.

NO

Have you noticed any abnormal vaginal discharge?

YES → A vaginal infection may cause pain during intercourse. Consult your physician.

See • Candidiasis
     • Trichomoniasis

NO

Are you urinating more often than usual?

YES → Your bladder may have become inflamed as the result of infection. Consult your physician.

See • Cystitis

NO

Does your vagina feel dry and tight so that penetration is difficult and painful?

YES → Are you between 45 and 65 years old?

YES → See • Menopause

NO → Anxiety and/or lack of arousal can lead to tension during intercourse. This can prevent normal lubrication of the vagina and relaxation of the surrounding muscles and tissues.

See • Anxiety
     • Psychosexual dysfunction

NO

Continued on next page

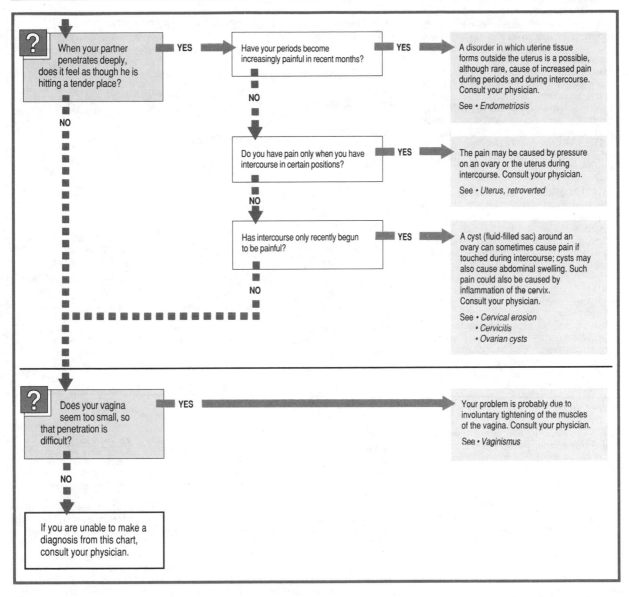

When your partner penetrates deeply, does it feel as though he is hitting a tender place?

YES → Have your periods become increasingly painful in recent months?

YES → A disorder in which uterine tissue forms outside the uterus is a possible, although rare, cause of increased pain during periods and during intercourse. Consult your physician.

See • *Endometriosis*

NO →

Do you have pain only when you have intercourse in certain positions?

YES → The pain may be caused by pressure on an ovary or the uterus during intercourse. Consult your physician.

See • *Uterus, retroverted*

NO →

Has intercourse only recently begun to be painful?

YES → A cyst (fluid-filled sac) around an ovary can sometimes cause pain if touched during intercourse; cysts may also cause abdominal swelling. Such pain could also be caused by inflammation of the cervix. Consult your physician.

See • *Cervical erosion*
      • *Cervicitis*
      • *Ovarian cysts*

NO

Does your vagina seem too small, so that penetration is difficult?

YES → Your problem is probably due to involuntary tightening of the muscles of the vagina. Consult your physician.

See • *Vaginismus*

NO →

If you are unable to make a diagnosis from this chart, consult your physician.

---

causing pain that may be superficial (around the external genitals) or deep (within the pelvis—the basin-shaped bony structure in the lower trunk).

CAUSES

Superficial pain is usually due to a problem that affects the external genitals. *Sexually transmitted diseases* (such as genital *herpes*, *gonorrhea*, or *chlamydial infections*) cause pain felt on the penis or around the vulval area. *Spermicides* may sometimes cause a burning sensation in both men and women.

In men, superficial pain during sexual intercourse may be caused by anatomical abnormalities, for example *chordee* (bowed erection) or *phimosis* (tight foreskin). *Prostatitis* (inflammation of the prostate gland) may cause a sharp, stabbing pain from the tip of the penis. Prostatitis may also cause a widespread pelvic ache or a burning sensation.

In some women, scarring (after tears from delivery or a poorly healed *episiotomy* repair, for example) may cause painful intercourse. Insufficient vaginal lubrication, especially after the *menopause*, is another cause of painful intercourse in women.

Psychosexual dysfunction may also cause pain during intercourse. For example *vaginismus*, a condition in which the muscles of the vagina go into spasm and thus prevent insertion of the penis, is usually psychological in origin.

In women, deep pain on intercourse is frequently caused by pelvic disorders (such as *fibroids*, *ectopic pregnancy*, or *pelvic inflammatory disease*) or by disorders of the *ovary* (such as *ovarian cysts*).

Endometriosis can cause thickening of tissue within the uterus, resulting in deep pain during intercourse. Varicose veins in the pelvis and disorders of the *cervix* (such as tumors or infections) can also cause deep pain during intercourse.

Cystitis commonly causes pain during sexual intercourse, especially in women. Other *urinary tract infections* may also cause pain.

TREATMENT

Treatment is directed at the underlying cause of the pain (for example *antibiotic drugs* will combat an infection, while a lubricant will help vaginal dryness). *Analgesic drugs* (painkillers) may also be helpful.

If the discomfort is psychological in origin, special counseling may be required (see *Sex therapy*).

Interferon

The name given to a group of proteins produced naturally by body cells in response to viral infections and other stimuli. Interferon inhibits viral multiplication (see illustration) and increases the activity of natural killer cells—types of *lymphocytes* that form part of the body's *immune system* (natural defenses).

USE AS DRUG

One type of interferon has been approved for use in the treatment of a type of *leukemia*. This substance is currently under investigation for use in the treatment of various types of cancer, especially *Kaposi's sarcoma* (a type of skin cancer that is common in people who have *AIDS*).

Interferon is also being assessed as a treatment for life-threatening viral infections, particularly those occurring in people who have *immunodeficiency disorders*.

Interferon is produced from a culture of human cells exposed to a specific virus or is synthesized in the laboratory from specific *nucleic acids* (genetic material). It is given by injection or taken as a nasal spray. Possible adverse reactions include fever, headache, aching muscles, fatigue, nausea and vomiting, hair loss, and abnormal bleeding.

Intern

In Canada, the term refers to a physician in the first or second year of hospital training after graduation from medical school. All provinces require an internship or its equivalent before medical licensing.

Internist

A physician with *residency* training and qualification by examination in the diagnosis and non-surgical treatment of diseases in adults, particularly those of the internal organs. In Canada, most internists further specialize in the diseases of a particular

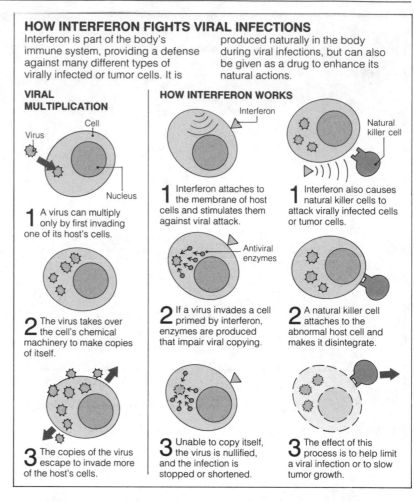

HOW INTERFERON FIGHTS VIRAL INFECTIONS

Interferon is part of the body's immune system, providing a defense against many different types of virally infected or tumor cells. It is produced naturally in the body during viral infections, but can also be given as a drug to enhance its natural actions.

VIRAL MULTIPLICATION

Cell
Virus
Nucleus

1 A virus can multiply only by first invading one of its host's cells.

2 The virus takes over the cell's chemical machinery to make copies of itself.

3 The copies of the virus escape to invade more of the host's cells.

HOW INTERFERON WORKS

Interferon

1 Interferon attaches to the membrane of host cells and stimulates them against viral attack.

Antiviral enzymes

2 If a virus invades a cell primed by interferon, enzymes are produced that impair viral copying.

3 Unable to copy itself, the virus is nullified, and the infection is stopped or shortened.

Natural killer cell

1 Interferon also causes natural killer cells to attack virally infected cells or tumor cells.

2 A natural killer cell attaches to the abnormal host cell and makes it disintegrate.

3 The effect of this process is to help limit a viral infection or to slow tumor growth.

organ system, such as the skin (*dermatology*), the joints (*rheumatology*), the cardiovascular system (*cardiology*), and the digestive system (*gastroenterology*).

Intersex

A group of abnormalities in which the affected person has ambiguous genitalia (abnormal external sex organs that could be of either sex) or external genitalia that have the opposite appearance to the chromosomal sex of the individual. (See *Sex determination*.)

Interstitial pulmonary fibrosis

Scarring and thickening of the deep lung tissues, leading to shortness of breath. The most important form of interstitial pulmonary fibrosis (IPF) is known as idiopathic IPF, diffuse IPF, or fibrosing alveolitis.

CAUSES

Although the precise cause of idiopathic IPF is unknown, this form of

the condition is probably an *autoimmune disorder* (caused by the body's *immune system* attacking its own tissues).

Less common causes of IPF include occupational exposure to mineral dusts and chemical fumes, radiation therapy, reactions to certain drugs, and allergic *alveolitis*.

SYMPTOMS AND DIAGNOSIS

The symptoms of IPF are progressive shortness of breath, cough, chest pain, and clubbing of the fingers, as well as symptoms of any underlying disease. The diagnosis, which is based on symptoms and a physical examination, is confirmed by *chest X ray* and lung *biopsy* (removal of a sample of tissue for microscopic analysis).

TREATMENT AND OUTLOOK

Treatment of idiopathic IPF often includes *azathioprine* and *corticosteroid drugs*, which suppress the immune system. In other cases, treatment is directed to the underlying cause.

The outlook for recovery is generally poor for occupational dust diseases and for idiopathic IPF, in which the lungs progressively stiffen. Progression of the disease may lead to *heart failure* and *bronchopneumonia*.

When IPF is caused by allergic alveolitis, however, the condition is more easily treated.

Interstitial radiation therapy

Treatment of a malignant tumor by inserting radioactive material into the growth or into neighboring tissue. Using this method, also known as brachytherapy, radiation can be directed to the diseased area more accurately than is possible with radiation therapy using X rays and there is less risk of radiation damage to healthy tissue.

HOW IT IS DONE

The patient is given a general anesthetic. Radioactive material (usually artificial radioisotopes) contained in wires or small tubes is then implanted into or near the diseased tissue. If the tumor is in an easily accessible area (such as the mouth), the containers may be pushed in by means of a special needle; for a tumor deep in the body, a surgical procedure is necessary. The material is left in place for variable amounts of time (and sometimes permanently), depending on the radioactive substance and the tumor being treated. (See also *Intracavitary therapy; Radiation therapy*.)

Intertrigo

Inflammation of the skin caused by two surfaces rubbing together. Intertrigo is most common in obese people and usually occurs on the inner thighs, in the armpits, on the underside of the breasts, in folds of the abdomen, and between fingers and toes. The affected skin is red and moist. There may be scales or blisters and affected skin may have an odor. The condition is made worse by sweating. Intertrigo is sometimes accompanied by seborrheic *dermatitis* or *candidiasis* (thrush).

Treatment consists of weight reduction, keeping affected areas as clean and dry as possible, and, if dermatitis or candidiasis is present, applying a cream containing a *corticosteroid drug* or an *antifungal drug*.

Intestinal imaging

See *Barium X-ray examinations*.

Intestinal lipodystrophy

See *Whipple's disease*.

Intestine

Part of the *digestive system*. The intestine is the major part of the digestive tract and extends from the exit of the stomach to the anus. The intestine forms a long tube divided into two main sections—the small intestine and the large intestine. The function of the intestine is to break down and absorb food and water into the bloodstream and to carry away the waste products of digestion.

STRUCTURE

The small intestine is about 6.5 m in length and 3.5 cm in diameter. It has three sections—the *duodenum* (a short, curved segment fixed to the back wall of the abdomen) and the *jejunum* and *ileum* (two larger, coiled, and mobile segments). The bile and pancreatic ducts enter the duodenum (see *Biliary system*). The walls of the intestine consist of circular and longitudinal muscles with an internal lining (the mucosa) and an external covering (the serosa). *Peristalsis* (the rhythmic contraction of the muscles) forces partially digested food along the intestine. The mucosa consists of many *villi* (small, fingerlike projections) covered with millions of fronds that create a large surface area for the absorption of substances into the blood.

The large intestine, which frames the loops of the small intestine, is about 1.5 m long and 4 to 7 cm in diameter. Unlike the small intestine, much of it is fixed in position, the muscles run in bands rather than forming a continuous sheet along its length, and there are no internal villi. The main section, the *colon*, is divided into an ascending, a transverse, a descending, and a pelvic portion (the sigmoid colon) that hangs down into the pelvis. The *appendix* hangs from a pouch (the *cecum*) between the small intestine and the colon. The final section before the *anus* is the *rectum*.

FUNCTION

The small intestine is concerned with the digestion of food and the absorption of food into the bloodstream. Some digestion occurs in the stomach, but more digestive enzymes and bile are added to the partly digested food in the duodenum. Glands within the walls of each section of the small intestine produce mucus and more enzymes, all of which help to break down the food into easily absorbable chemical units. The numerous blood vessels in the intestinal walls then carry the digested food to the *liver* for distribution to the rest of the body.

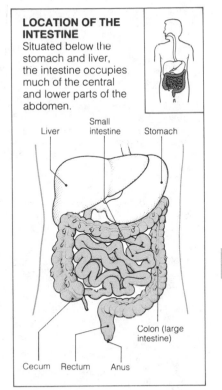

LOCATION OF THE INTESTINE

Situated below the stomach and liver, the intestine occupies much of the central and lower parts of the abdomen.

Liver — Small intestine — Stomach

Colon (large intestine)

Cecum — Rectum — Anus

Unabsorbed material leaves the small intestine in the form of liquid and fiber. As this material passes through the large intestine, water, vitamins, and mineral salts are absorbed into the bloodstream, leaving *feces* made up of undigested food residue, small amounts of fat, secretions from the stomach, liver, pancreas, and intestinal wall, and bacteria. The feces are compressed and pass into the rectum. Distention of the rectum usually produces the desire to empty the bowel.

Intestine, cancer of

A malignant tumor in the intestine. Both the small and large intestines may develop carcinoid tumors (leading to *carcinoid syndrome*) and *lymphomas*. Cancer of the small intestine is extremely rare, but cancer of the large intestine is one of the most common of all cancers. In Canada, there are some 8,700 cases of cancer of the large intestine each year. (See *Colon, cancer of; Rectum, cancer of*.)

Intestine, obstruction of

A partial or complete blockage of the small or large intestine. Without treatment, complete obstruction of the intestine is usually fatal.

DISORDERS OF THE INTESTINE

The intestine is subject to various structural abnormalities and to the effects of many infective organisms and parasites; it may also be affected by tumors, impaired blood supply, and other disorders.

CONGENITAL DEFECTS

Babies are sometimes born with an obstruction to the flow of the intestinal contents. This may be due to *atresia* (congenital closure), *stenosis* (narrowing), *volvulus* (twisting of loops of bowel), or blockage by meconium (fetal intestinal contents). Early surgery may be required.

INFECTION AND INFLAMMATION

The general term for inflammation of the stomach and intestines is *gastroenteritis*. This is caused most commonly by viral or bacterial infections, which can range from the trivial to the life-threatening. They encompass many cases of *food poisoning* and travelers' diarrhea as well as serious diseases such as *typhoid fever* and *cholera*. Protozoal infections (caused by simple, single-celled parasites) include *giardiasis* and *amebiasis*.

Intestinal worm infestations affect approximately one quarter of the world's population, principally in the tropical and subtropical regions. Endemic infestation in Canada is limited to a few species of *roundworm* (of which *pinworm* is the most prevalent) and *tapeworm*.

Two important inflammatory conditions of the intestine, not caused by infection, are *ulcerative colitis* (mainly affecting the colon) and *Crohn's disease* (which may affect any part of the digestive tract but usually the small intestine). Sometimes, inflammation is confined to a localized area, such as in *appendicitis* and *diverticular disease*.

TUMORS

Tumors of the small intestine are rare, but *lymphomas*, carcinoid tumors (producing *carcinoid syndrome*), and benign growths occur. By contrast, tumors of the large intestine are very common (see *Intestine, cancer of*). Certain forms of familial *polyposis* (in which benign polyplike tumors grow in the colon) may progress to cancer.

IMPAIRED BLOOD SUPPLY

Like other organs, the intestine is dependent on an adequate blood

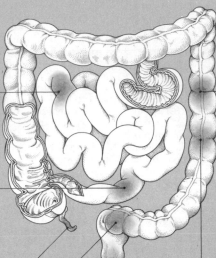

Worms
Infestations typically occur in the middle part of the small intestine.

Crohn's disease
This disease usually affects the last part of the small intestine.

Appendicitis
Inflammation of the appendix, which hangs from the cecum.

Bowel cancer
Cancers of the large bowel most often affect the lower colon and rectum.

Diverticular disease
The descending colon is the part of the intestine most commonly affected by this disease.

Ulcerative colitis
This disorder usually affects the descending colon or rectum.

supply. *Ischemia* (lack of blood) may result from several causes. Causes include partial or complete obstruction of the arteries in the abdominal wall (from diseases such as *atherosclerosis*, *thrombosis*, or *embolism*) or from the blood vessels being compressed or trapped, as in *volvulus*, *intussusception*, or *hernias* (protrusion of intestines through the abdominal wall). Loss of blood supply to a segment of intestine may cause *gangrene* (tissue death) requiring immediate surgery.

OBSTRUCTION

Intestinal obstruction may be caused by pressure from the outside, disease of the intestinal wall (such as cancer, Crohn's disease, or diverticular disease), or internal blockage (such as from *gallstones* or intussusception). One of the most common causes is paralytic *ileus*, in which intestinal contractions cease and the intestinal contents are no longer transported.

OTHER DISORDERS

Peptic ulcer of the duodenum affects about 10 percent of the population at some time in their lives. Ulceration of the small intestine occurs in typhoid

and Crohns' disease and may cause bleeding into the intestine or even perforation. Ulceration of the large intestine occurs in amebiasis and in ulcerative colitis.

Diverticula are small pouches protruding from the inside of the bowel. They are usually harmless, but, in diverticular disease, may become inflamed. *Malabsorption* and *celiac disease* result from changes to the intestinal lining. Finally, *irritable bowel syndrome* is associated with persistent abdominal pain and either constipation or diarrhea (or both) and is the most common intestinal disorder in developed countries.

INVESTIGATION

Intestinal disorders are investigated by physical examination, and by techniques such as *barium X-ray examination*, *sigmoidoscopy*, or possibly *colonoscopy*, and by laboratory examination of the feces or of a *biopsy* specimen taken from the intestinal lining.

CAUSES

The most common cause of intestinal obstruction is paralytic ileus (see *Ileus, paralytic*), in which the rhythmic muscle contractions of the intestine stop, the intestine dilates, and the intestinal contents are no longer moved along the digestive tract.

Other common causes are a strangulated *hernia*, intestinal *atresia* (a congenital malformation), stenosis (narrowing) of the intestine, *adhesions* (bands of scar tissue), *volvulus* (twisting or knotting of the intestine), and *intussusception* (telescoping of a section of intestine).

Intestinal obstruction also occurs in diseases (such as *Crohn's disease*, *diverticular disease*, and tumors) that affect the intestinal wall. Less commonly, internal blockage of the intestinal canal is caused by impacted food, *fecal impaction, gallstones,* or by some accidentally swallowed object.

SYMPTOMS

The location and degree of obstruction dictate the symptoms. A blockage in the small intestine usually causes intermittent cramplike pain in the center of the abdomen, which tends to be more severe the higher the obstruction. Pain is accompanied by increasingly frequent bouts of vomiting and by failure to pass wind or feces.

An obstruction in the large intestine, particularly in the colon, causes pain, distention (swelling) of the abdomen, and failure to pass wind or feces. In some cases, the obstruction is intermittent or partial, allowing feces to pass and giving temporary abatement of symptoms.

DIAGNOSIS AND TREATMENT

The diagnosis is usually based on the patient's symptoms and on a physical examination. Abdominal *X rays* will confirm the diagnosis.

The contents of the intestine are removed through a flexible tube passed down the throat. In some cases, surgery may be necessary to correct the obstruction. The actual type of operation depends on the nature and site of the blockage to the flow of intestinal contents.

OUTLOOK

The prospects for a full recovery after surgery are often excellent but they will depend on the cause of the obstruction and on the age and general health of the patient.

Intestine, tumors of

Tumors of the intestine may be cancerous or benign (noncancerous).

Cancerous tumors commonly affect the large intestine (see *Colon, cancer of; Rectum, cancer of*); the small intestine is only rarely affected. *Lymphomas* and carcinoid tumors (leading to *carcinoid syndrome*) are cancers that may occur in the intestine. Noncancerous tumors of the intestine include *polyps* in the colon, and *adenomas, leiomyomas, lipomas,* and *angiomas* in the small intestine. These noncancerous tumors are usually symptomless and are often discovered incidentally when a *barium X-ray examination* is being performed for some other reason.

Intoxication

A general term for a condition resulting from *poisoning*. Intoxication customarily refers to the effects of excessive drinking (see *Alcohol intoxication*), but also includes *drug poisoning*, poisoning from the accumulation of the by-products of *metabolism* in the body, or the effects of industrial poisons (such as lead intoxication and solvent intoxication).

Intra-

A prefix that means within, as in the term intramuscular (within a muscle). (See also *Inter-*.)

Intracavitary therapy

Treatment of a malignant tumor in a body cavity by placing radioactive material or *anticancer drugs* within the cavity. Intracavitary *radiation therapy* (also called brachytherapy) is mainly used to treat cancer of the uterus, cervix (neck of the uterus), vagina, or rectum. Radioactive material (usually in the form of artificial radioisotopes embedded in wires or small tubes) is introduced into the cavity and left there for a period of time.

Intracavitary chemotherapy may be used to treat a malignant effusion (a collection of fluid that contains cancerous cells). A needle, sometimes with a catheter (fine tube) attached, is passed through the wall of the abdomen or the chest into the abdominal cavity or pleural cavity (the space around the lungs). The needle is used first to draw off the effusion from the cavity, and then to inject *anticancer drugs* directly into the cavity. (See also *Interstitial radiation therapy*.)

Intracerebral hemorrhage

Bleeding into the brain from a ruptured blood vessel. An intracerebral hemorrhage is one of the three principal main mechanisms by which a *stroke* can occur.

INCIDENCE AND CAUSES

Intracerebral hemorrhage used to be a common cause of stroke, but with improvements in the treatment of *hypertension* (high blood pressure) it now accounts for only one in every 10 strokes. Most victims are middle-aged or elderly people with untreated hypertension (high blood pressure) or *atherosclerosis* (narrowing of arteries caused by deposits of fatty material) in the brain. Unlike most cases of *subdural* and *extradural hemorrhage* (bleeding between the surface of the brain and the skull), an intracerebral hemorrhage can occur without any injury or blow to the head.

The ruptured artery is usually in the cerebrum (the main mass of the brain), although sometimes it is in other structures of the brain (such as the cerebellum or the brain stem). The escaped blood seeps outward, forming a circular or oval mass up to a few centimetres in diameter. As bleeding continues and the volume of escaped blood increases, brain tissue in the blood's path is disrupted and adjacent brain tissues are displaced.

SYMPTOMS

The symptoms are sudden headache, weakness, and confusion, and often loss of consciousness. Usually the victim falls unconscious to the ground with no warning. Signs resulting from disruption of brain tissue (speech loss, facial paralysis, or one-sided weakness) may develop over periods of minutes or hours.

DIAGNOSIS, TREATMENT, AND OUTLOOK

Diagnosis is by *CT scanning*. Surgical treatment is usually impossible due to the inaccessibility of the rupture, so treatment is aimed at life-support and gradual reduction of blood pressure.

Large hemorrhages are usually fatal; overall, only about 25 percent of patients survive. Recurrent bleeding from the same site is uncommon. For the survivor of an intracerebral hemorrhage, rehabilitation and outlook are as for any type of stroke.

Intractable

A term to describe any condition that does not respond to treatment.

Intramuscular

A medical term meaning within a muscle, as in an intramuscular injection, in which a drug is injected deep within a muscle. Such injections are usually given into the upper, outer part of the buttock. The drug is absorbed from the muscle into the bloodstream.

Intraocular pressure

The balance between the rate of production and the rate of removal of aqueous humor within the *eye*. It is the intraocular pressure that maintains the shape of the eyeball. Aqueous humor enters the eye from the ciliary body, which constantly produces the fluid, and exits from the drainage angle (a network of tissue between the iris and cornea).

If drainage is impeded, intraocular pressure builds up and leads to *glaucoma*. Intraocular pressure is usually measured by *tonometry* during a routine eye examination. If the ciliary body is damaged (as after prolonged inflammation), less fluid is produced and the eye becomes soft.

Intrauterine contraceptive device

See *IUD*.

Intrauterine growth retardation

Poor fetal growth, usually due to failure of the *placenta* to provide adequate nutrients or sometimes to a fetal defect. Intrauterine growth retardation causes the fetus to be smaller than expected for the length of *gestation*.

Intrauterine growth retardation may be due to a chromosomal defect, such as *Down's syndrome*, which causes the fetus to be "small for dates." A maternal infection, such as *rubella* (German measles), in which the virus passes through the placenta, can also cause poor fetal growth. In most cases, though, the fetus is otherwise normal.

Maternal conditions such as *preeclampsia*, *hypertension* (high blood pressure), or chronic *kidney failure* can affect fetal growth, as can the mother's diet. Cigarette smoking, malnutrition and alcoholism are other major causes of intrauterine growth retardation.

DIAGNOSIS AND TREATMENT

The obstetrician can check whether the uterus is smaller than expected during a prenatal examination; *ultrasound scanning* may be performed to estimate the fetal growth. The mother may be required to rest, and tests of placental function may be needed, including blood tests and electrical *fetal heart monitoring*.

If intrauterine growth retardation is diagnosed, the pregnancy is carefully monitored and the underlying cause of the placental insufficiency treated, if possible. If the baby's growth is slowing, *induction of labor* or a *cesarean section* may be necessary.

OUTLOOK

Because babies suffering intrauterine growth retardation have been chronically undernourished in the uterus, they are usually underweight and may be premature if labor has been induced. Being prone to hypoglycemia (low blood glucose), *hypothermia*, and infection, they are usually transferred to an *incubator* immediately after birth and provided with special care.

Intravenous

A term meaning within a vein, as in *intravenous infusion* (slow introduction of a substance into a vein) and intravenous *injection* (rapid introduction of a substance into a vein).

Intravenous infusion

The slow introduction of a volume of fluid into the bloodstream. The fluid passes down from a plastic or glass container through tubing into a cannula (thin plastic tube) inserted into a vein, usually in the patient's forearm. The rate at which the fluid drips into the circulation is controlled by an adjustable valve.

An intravenous infusion, commonly known as a drip, is used to give blood (or plasma) to replace that lost in an accident or during an operation (see *Blood transfusion*). An intravenous infusion can also be used to replace or maintain body fluids in patients who are unable to drink or eat. In this case, the fluid is usually a mixture of glucose (sugar) and saline (salt solution). Other uses include the provision of more varied and concentrated nutrients to people unable to digest food normally (see *Feeding, artificial*) and the administration of certain drugs.

Intravenous pyelography

See *Urography*.

Introitus

A general term for the entrance to a body cavity or space, most commonly the vagina.

Introvert

A person more concerned with his or her inner world. Introverts prefer to work alone, are shy, quiet, and withdrawn when under stress. (See also *Extrovert*; *Personality*.)

Intubation

Most commonly, the process of passing an *endotracheal tube* (breathing tube) into the trachea (windpipe). Endotracheal intubation is performed if a patient requires mechanical *venti-

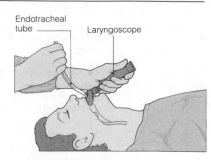

Endotracheal intubation
Guided by an anesthetist, the endotracheal tube is passed through the patient's mouth and down the throat into the trachea.

lation to deliver oxygen to the lungs— for example, because he or she is in a coma, is anesthetized, or has severe respiratory disease.

The anesthetist looks down the patient's throat with a laryngoscope (a viewing instrument) to identify the vocal cords. He or she then passes an endotracheal tube through the patient's mouth and down the throat between the vocal cords into the trachea. Alternatively, the tube may be passed through the nose. The external end of the tube is secured by tape. An inflatable cuff may be used to provide an airtight seal at the bottom of the tube within the trachea.

The term intubation is also used to refer to the placement of a gastric or intestinal tube in the stomach for purposes of suction or the giving of nutrients (see *Feeding, artificial*).

Intussusception

A condition in which part of the intestine telescopes in on itself, forming a tube within a tube (like pulling a shirt sleeve partially inside out), usually resulting in intestinal obstruction (see *Intestine, obstruction of*).

Intussusception most commonly occurs at the junction between the *ileum* (last part of the small intestine) and the *cecum* (the first part of the large intestine).

CAUSES AND INCIDENCE

It is not known exactly why this condition occurs, but in some cases there is a definite association with a recent infection. In other cases intussusception may start at the site of a *polyp* or *Meckel's diverticulum* (a small, pouch-like projection from the ileum).

Intussusception occurs most commonly in babies after the age of 1 month. Half of all cases occur in the first year, and three quarters before the age of 2. The condition affects approximately two babies per 1,000.

SYMPTOMS

An affected child usually develops severe abdominal colic and screams intermittently. Vomiting is a common feature, and blood and mucus are often found in the feces. In severe cases of intussusception, the blood supply to the intestine becomes blocked and *gangrene* (tissue death) followed by *peritonitis* (inflammation of the membrane covering the organs in the abdomen) or *perforation* (bursting) may follow.

DIAGNOSIS AND TREATMENT

A barium enema (see *Barium X-ray examinations*) will usually reveal the obstruction. Sometimes the barium enema actually treats the condition; the pressure applied when the enema is introduced can force the prolapsed segment back into position. Otherwise, an operation is carried out. In most cases, the intestine is gently squeezed to push out the inner segment, permitting surgery on the cause that led the segment of bowel to telescope.

Invasive

Having the tendency to spread throughout body tissues; the term is usually applied to malignant tumors or to harmful microorganisms. An invasive medical procedure is one in which body tissues are penetrated by an instrument. *Angiography* is an example. (See also *Noninvasive*.)

In vitro

The performance of biological processes in the laboratory rather than in the body; in vitro literally means "in glass." Tests successfully carried out in vitro do not always work the same way in the body.

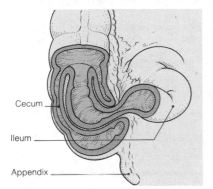

Cecum

Ileum

Appendix

Intussusception

This disorder is characterized by part of the intestine telescoping in on itself. It usually occurs at the junction between the ileum and cecum.

In vitro fertilization

A method of treating *infertility* in which an egg is surgically removed from the ovary and fertilized outside the body. In vitro (in glass) refers to the glass Petri dish that is used in the fertilization process.

The first successful birth as a result of in vitro fertilization (IVF) occurred in England in 1978.

WHY IT IS DONE

In vitro fertilization may be performed when the woman's *fallopian tubes* are permanently blocked or absent. IVF may also be carried out if the man's sperm count is very low or if it is thought that antibodies in the woman's cervical mucus are killing the sperm.

HOW IT IS DONE

Stages in the procedure are shown in the illustrated box below. After IVF, the woman is monitored for a few days to determine if the eggs have been implanted in the uterine wall. Once this occurs, the pregnancy usually continues normally, although the early miscarriage rate is high, and multiple births may occur because more than one of the eggs "takes."

It is unlikely that in vitro fertilization will become a widespread treatment of infertility, at least within the near future. Currently, this highly specialized procedure is available only at a small number of centers. It is expensive and the success rate is limited. Recent research has shown that half or more of all eggs have abnormal chromosomes and cannot develop into normal embryos; after fertilization, the eggs begin to divide, but the pregnancy miscarries.

PROCEDURE FOR IN VITRO FERTILIZATION

Fertilization of eggs outside a woman's body can be used to treat some types of infertility. The main stages involved in the procedure of in vitro fertilization are illustrated below.

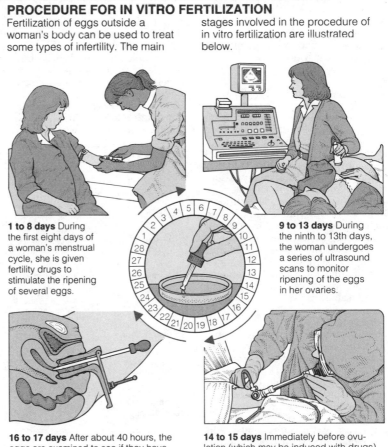

1 to 8 days During the first eight days of a woman's menstrual cycle, she is given fertility drugs to stimulate the ripening of several eggs.

9 to 13 days During the ninth to 13th days, the woman undergoes a series of ultrasound scans to monitor ripening of the eggs in her ovaries.

16 to 17 days After about 40 hours, the eggs are examined to see if they have been fertilized and have started to develop into embryos. If they have, several embryos (usually at the two- or four-cell stage) are placed in the woman's uterus through the vagina.

14 to 15 days Immediately before ovulation (which may be induced with drugs), ripe eggs are removed by laparoscopy or by ultrasound-guided needle aspiration through the vagina or abdomen. The eggs are mixed with the man's sperm in a dish, which is then put in an incubator.

Only about 10 percent of couples undergoing in vitro fertilization achieve pregnancy on the first attempt, and many attempts may be needed before a successful pregnancy is achieved. Nevertheless, success rates are continuing to improve, and modifications of the technique such as GIFT (see *Infertility*) are simpler and cheaper than the original method.

In vivo

Biological processes occurring within the body. (See also *In vitro*.)

Involuntary movements

Uncontrollable movements of the body, usually affecting the face, head, limbs, and trunk. These movements occur spontaneously and may be slow and writhing (see *Athetosis*); rapid, jerky, and random (see *Chorea*); or predictable, stereotyped, and affecting one part of the body, usually the face (see *Tic*). They may be a feature of a disease (e.g., *Huntington's chorea*) or a side effect of certain drugs used to treat psychiatric conditions.

Iodine

An element essential for the formation of the *thyroid hormones*, triiodothyronine (T_3) and thyroxine (T_4). These hormones control the rate of *metabolism* (internal chemistry) and growth and development. About 100 to 300 micrograms are needed daily. A dietary shortage of iodine may lead to *goiter* (enlargement of the thyroid gland) or to *hypothyroidism* (underactivity of the thyroid gland). Iodine deficiency in the newborn can lead to *cretinism*. The amount of iodine in food depends on the amount in animal feed and in the soil; shortages occur in limestone areas. Shortages can be overcome by consuming bread or table salt fortified with iodide or iodate.

MEDICAL USES

Iodine is sometimes given to people who have consumed food or drink contaminated with radioactive iodine. In such cases, absorption by the body of nonradioactive iodine reduces the absorption of the radioactive iodine.

Radioactive iodine is sometimes used to damage, and thus to reduce, the activity of the thyroid gland in cases of *thyrotoxicosis* (a toxic condition resulting from overactivity of the thyroid gland). Iodine compounds are used as *antiseptics*, in radiopaque contrast media used in some X-ray procedures (see *Imaging techniques*), and in some *cough remedies*.

POSSIBLE ADVERSE EFFECTS

Iodine supplements have possibly caused thyrotoxicosis in some people who have taken them after a long period on a low iodine diet. In rare cases, iodine can cause allergic reactions, e.g., rash, facial swelling, abdominal pain, vomiting, and headache.

Ion

A particle (either an atom or a group of atoms) that carries an electrical charge; positive ions are called cations and negative ions are called anions. Important cations in the body include sodium, potassium, hydrogen, and calcium. Important anions include bicarbonate, chloride, and phosphate.

ROLE IN THE BODY

Many vital body processes depend on the movement of ions across cell membranes. For example, the exchange of sodium for potassium across the membranes around nerve and muscle cells is the mechanism by which nerve impulses are transmitted and by which muscle contraction occurs. Calcium also plays an important role in muscle contraction as well as being involved in blood clotting and bone growth.

Sodium is the principal cation in extracellular fluid (which surrounds all cells in the body), where it affects the flow of water into and out of cells (see *Osmosis*) and thereby influences the concentration of body fluids.

The levels of sodium, potassium, and calcium are regulated by the kidneys, which control the amount lost from the body in the urine. The level of calcium is also affected by hormonal effects on bones.

The acidity of the blood and other body fluids depends on the level of hydrogen cations, which are produced by various metabolic processes. To prevent these fluids from becoming too acidic, hydrogen cations are neutralized by bicarbonate anions in the extracellular fluid and blood, and by phosphate anions inside cells (see *Acid-base balance*).

ION DISTURBANCES

For the body to function normally, the level of each ion must be maintained within narrow limits; any substantial deviation can cause symptoms, such as muscle weakness caused by hypokalemia (too low a level of potassium cations in the blood).

Dehydration caused by insufficient water intake or excessive water loss (from diarrhea, vomiting, or sweating) increases the concentration of all ions. This condition may cause the patient to suffer thirst, muscle cramps, dizziness, and faintness.

IMPORTANT IONS AND THEIR ROLES

Cations (positively charged ions)	Major roles in body
Ammonium	Acid-base balance; produced by protein metabolism
Calcium	Nerve conduction; muscle contraction; blood clotting; bone and tooth formation; heart action
Hydrogen	Acid-base balance; component of stomach acid
Magnesium	Nerve conduction; muscle contraction; bone and tooth formation; enzyme activation; protein metabolism
Potassium	Nerve conduction; muscle contraction; water balance; acid-base balance
Sodium	Nerve conduction; muscle contraction; water balance; acid-base balance
Anions (negatively charged ions)	
Bicarbonate	Acid-base balance; neutralizes stomach acid
Chloride	Acid-base balance; water balance; component of stomach acid
Phosphate	Acid-base balance; bone and tooth formation; protein metabolism; energy metabolism; structure of cell membranes

Ionizer

A device that produces *ions* (electrically charged particles). Ionizers that produce negative ions can be used to neutralize positive ions in the atmosphere. Some people believe that use of an ionizer reduces symptoms, such as headaches and fatigue, that may result from a buildup of positive ions generated by electrical machines.

Ipecac

A drug used to induce vomiting in the treatment of *poisoning*. Ipecac (also known as ipecacuanha) is derived from a plant native to South and Central America. Ipecac is not given if poisoning has been caused by corrosive or petroleum-based substances, if the victim is not fully conscious, or if the victim is less than 1 year old.

Ipratropium

An *anticholinergic* drug used primarily in the treatment of asthma and bronchitis. It works by relaxing the muscles surrounding the bronchioles (smaller air passages in the lungs). Ipratropium is only given by aerosol or nebulizer spray.

Common side effects are dry mouth and headache.

IQ

Abbreviation for intelligence quotient, an age-related measure of intelligence (see *Intelligence tests*).

Iridectomy

A procedure performed on the *eye* to remove part of the *iris*. The most common type of iridectomy, known as a "peripheral iridectomy," is usually performed to treat acute *glaucoma*. A small opening is made, surgically or with a laser, near the root (outer edge) of the iris to form a channel through which aqueous humor can drain.

In a complete iridectomy a sector of iris is removed. This type of iridectomy is used, for example, if the iris adheres to the underlying lens.

Iridectomy is sometimes performed to remove tumors and to improve the vision of children who have small central cataracts.

Iridencleisis

A surgical procedure that was used in the 1940s and 1950s to control chronic simple *glaucoma* by creating an artificial channel for the drainage of aqueous humor. Iridencleisis has now largely been replaced by *trabeculectomy*, which is a more reliable surgical procedure.

Iridocyclitis

Inflammation of the *iris* and ciliary body. Iridocyclitis is more usually known as "anterior *uveitis*." (See also *Eye* disorders box.)

Iris

The colored part of the *eye* that lies behind the cornea. The iris is connected at its outer edge to the ciliary body and has a central perforation called the *pupil*, through which light enters the eye and falls on the retina.

The iris, a loose framework of transparent *collagen* (a fibrous protein) and muscle fibers, constantly contracts and dilates to alter the size of the pupil and to control the amount of light that passes through the pupil and reaches the retina.

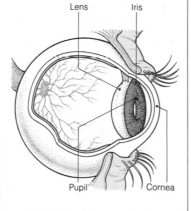

LOCATION OF THE IRIS

The iris lies behind the cornea and in front of the lens. The outer edge of the iris is connected to the ciliary body; at the center is an aperture called the pupil.

Lens   Iris

Pupil   Cornea

Iritis

An inflammation of the *iris*, now often termed an "anterior *uveitis*."

Iron

A mineral which is essential for the formation of certain *enzymes* (proteins that stimulate chemical reactions), *hemoglobin* (the oxygen-carrying pigment in red blood cells), and *myoglobin* (the oxygen-carrying pigment in muscle cells).

Iron is contained in a variety of foods, such as liver, meat, cereals (especially whole-grain), fish, green leafy vegetables, nuts, and beans. During pregnancy, iron supplements may be necessary for the healthy development of the baby.

Iron deficiency leading to anemia (see *Anemia, iron deficiency*) is usually caused by abnormal blood loss, such as from *menorrhagia* (heavy periods) or a *peptic ulcer*, but may also be due to a diet that is low in iron or from which iron is poorly absorbed.

Iron supplements may cause nausea, abdominal pain, constipation, or diarrhea. They may also color the feces black.

Excessive intake of iron over a prolonged period may cause *cirrhosis* of the liver.

Iron-deficiency anemia

See *Anemia, iron-deficiency*.

Iron lung

A large machine, properly called a Drinker respirator, formerly used to maintain breathing, especially in people paralyzed by *poliomyelitis*. The iron lung has been replaced by less cumbersome and more efficient means of maintaining breathing (see *Ventilation*).

Irradiation

See *Radiation hazards; Radiation therapy*.

Irradiation of food

The treatment of food with ionizing *radiation* to kill bacteria, molds, insects, and other parasites. Irradiation improves the keeping qualities of food and is a means of controlling some types of *food poisoning*.

Bombarding food with ionizing radiation sterilizes the food by killing microorganisms. However, the process does not destroy bacterial toxins and it may destroy or alter vitamins. It does not render food radioactive. The process is unsuitable for high-fat dairy produce and eggs, in which it causes changes in taste.

Irradiation also inhibits the ripening process and the sprouting of vegetables.

Irradiation of food in Canada is strictly controlled. Only certain foods are allowed to be irradiated and the government regulates the dose and isotope used to produce the radiation. The legislation specifies that only wheat, flour, potatoes, onions, spices, and dehydrated seasoning preparations are permitted to be irradiated and must be labeled according to government regulations.

The effects of irradiation on food additives and on pesticide residues have not been established, nor have the long-term effects of eating irradiated foods.

IRRIGATION TECHNIQUES

After removal of contaminated tissue, a wound may be cleansed either by forced syringe (or catheter) irrigation or by using an irrigation chamber.

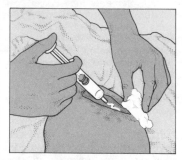

Forced syringe irrigation
A syringe (sometimes with a catheter attached) is used to flush irrigation fluid repeatedly into and out of the wound until the drained fluid is clear.

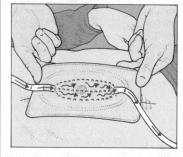

Irrigation chamber
A flexible, plastic irrigation chamber is sealed over the wound; irrigation fluid is then run through the chamber until the drained fluid is clear.

Irrigation, wound

The cleansing of a deep wound by repeatedly washing it out.

WHY IT IS DONE

A deep wound is often contaminated with infected foreign material. Unless such a wound is completely cleansed before repair, it may fail to heal, an abscess may form in it, or, in extreme cases, *gangrene* (tissue death) may result. If the wound contains agricultural soil, *tetanus* is a serious risk.

Irritable bladder

Intermittent, uncontrolled contractions of the muscles in the *bladder* wall. Irritable bladder may cause urge incontinence (see *Incontinence, urinary*).

Irritability of the bladder is commonly due to a urinary tract infection (see *Cystitis*), the presence of a cathe-ter within the bladder, a bladder stone (see *Calculus, urinary tract*), or obstruction to the outflow of urine by an enlarged *prostate gland*. In many cases of irritable bladder, however, no underlying cause for the muscular irritability and spasm is found.

Symptoms may be relieved by *antispasmodic drugs*; other treatment is directed at any underlying cause.

Irritable bowel syndrome

A combination of intermittent abdominal pain and irregular bowel habit (i.e., constipation, diarrhea, or bouts of each) that occurs in the absence of other diagnosed disease. Other names for the condition are irritable colon syndrome and spastic colon.

Although symptoms subside and even disappear for periods of time, irritable bowel syndrome is usually recurrent throughout life. Although it is not life-threatening and is unlikely to lead to complications, it can cause much distress.

CAUSES AND INCIDENCE

The cause is not fully understood, but the basic abnormality is a disturbance of involuntary muscle movement in the large intestine. However, there is no abnormality in the intestinal structure and people with irritable bowel syndrome neither lose weight nor become malnourished. Irritable bowel syndrome is the most common disorder of the intestine, accounting for more than half the patients seen by gastroenterologists.

The condition is twice as common in women as in men, usually beginning in early or middle adulthood. Sufferers are usually otherwise in good health and have had the condition for some time before seeking medical advice.

A psychological element, particularly anxiety, is believed by some physicians to be the main causative factor; emotional stress tends to exacerbate the condition. However, bowel upset is a normal reaction to stress in many people who do not suffer from the illness.

SYMPTOMS

The symptoms include intermittent cramplike pain in the abdomen, abdominal distention (swelling), often on the left side, transient relief of pain by bowel movement or passing wind, sense of incomplete evacuation of the bowels, excessive wind, and symptoms aggravated by food. Various other symptoms may also occur (which are not precisely part of the irritable bowel syndrome), such as heartburn, back pain, weakness, faintness, agitation, tendency to tire easily, reduced appetite, and palpitations.

DIAGNOSIS

The initial diagnosis is based on the patient's symptoms and a physical examination. Examination of the feces, *barium X-ray examination*, and *sigmoidoscopy* (examination of the colon through a viewing instrument passed via the anus) may be performed to exclude conditions, such as cancer (see *Colon, cancer of*; *Rectum, cancer of*) or inflammatory bowel disease (see *Crohn's disease*; *Ulcerative colitis*), that may have similar symptoms.

TREATMENT

A high-fiber diet or bulk-forming agents, such as *bran* or *methylcellulose*, may be recommended for some patients with irritable bowel syndrome. Short courses of *antidiarrheal drugs* (such as *loperamide*) may be given for persistent diarrhea. *Antispasmodic drugs* may be prescribed to relieve muscular spasm. *Hypnosis* may help some patients.

Although treatments can alleviate troublesome symptoms, irritable bowel syndrome has no cure.

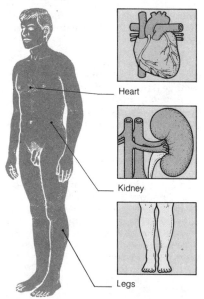

Heart

Kidney

Legs

Symptoms of ischemia
Ischemia (insufficient blood supply) of the heart causes the chest pain of angina pectoris; ischemia of blood vessels in the legs may cause a cramplike pain during exercise. Ischemia may also affect the kidneys (causing kidney failure) or the brain (resulting in a stroke).

Ischemia

Insufficient supply of blood to a specific organ or tissue. Ischemia is usually caused by disease of the blood vessels, such as *atherosclerosis* (narrowing of arteries by deposits of fatty material), but may also result from injury to a vessel, constriction of a vessel due to spasm of the muscles in the vessel wall, or inadequate blood flow due to inefficient pumping action of the heart.

The symptoms of ischemia depend on the part of the body affected.

Treatment may include *vasodilator drugs* to widen the blood vessels or, in more severe cases, an *angioplasty* or *bypass operation*.

Isocarboxazid

A monoamine oxidase inhibitor useful in treating depression especially if marked by *phobias* and other irrational fears. It produces less drowsiness than some other drugs in this group, but can be involved in *potentially serious drug interactions*. See *Antidepressant drugs* for important warning on side effects.

Isolation

Nursing procedures, also known as barrier nursing, designed to prevent a patient from infecting others or from being infected by them. In either case, the patient is usually isolated in a single room.

TYPES

COMPLETE ISOLATION This is used if a patient has a contagious disease, such as *Lassa fever*, that can be transmitted to others by direct contact and by airborne germs. All staff wear masks, gowns, caps, and gloves, which afterward are incinerated or sterilized. Bed linen, eating utensils, bedpans, and any other items that come into contact with the patient are also sterilized and, even though they wear gloves, staff members must wash their hands thoroughly after each nursing task.

PARTIAL ISOLATION This is carried out if the patient's disease is transmitted in a more limited way—for example, only by respiration (as in *tuberculosis*) or only by contact with infected skin (as in *impetigo*) or feces (as in *cholera*). In these cases, some of the precautions taken in complete isolation nursing are unnecessary.

REVERSE ISOLATION This technique, also known as reverse barrier nursing, is used to protect a patient whose resistance to infection has been severely lowered. The air supply to the room is filtered. Visiting is drastically limited.

All staff and visitors wear caps, gowns, masks, and gloves. Bed linen and all items used by the patient are sterilized. When these measures do not give enough protection (such as after a *bone marrow transplant*), the patient is placed in an isolator (plastic tent) or special room.

Occasionally, long-term reverse isolation is needed for patients with severe combined immunodeficiency (SCID) (see *Immunodeficiency disorders*); these patients are born without normal defenses against infection.

Isoniazid

An *antibacterial drug* used to prevent and treat *tuberculosis*. As a preventive measure, isoniazid may be given to close contacts of people suffering from tuberculosis. To treat the disease, isoniazid is given in combination with other antibacterial drugs, usually for at least six months.

Adverse effects, which are rare, include nausea, fatigue, numbness, twitching, and insomnia. Because isoniazid may increase the amount of pyridoxine (vitamin B_6) lost from the body, supplements of this vitamin may be given to avoid the possibility of nerve damage.

Isoproterenol

A drug that is given by injection for the emergency treatment of patients in whom a heart disorder has caused slowing of the heart rate. Isoproterenol is often given as an interim measure to increase the heart rate before a *pacemaker* can be implanted.

Isoproterenol also widens the airways in people with asthma, but this drug is now only rarely used to treat asthma because many other *bronchodilator drugs* are less likely to cause adverse effects.

Adverse effects of isoproterenol include dry mouth, dizziness, nervousness, headache, palpitations, and chest pain.

Isosorbide

A long-acting *nitrate drug* that acts as a *vasodilator drug*. Isosorbide is used to reduce the severity and frequency of *angina pectoris* (chest pain due to impaired blood supply to heart muscle). This drug is also given to treat severe *heart failure* (reduced pumping efficiency).

Adverse effects include headache, hot flashes, and dizziness.

Isotope scanning

See *Radionuclide scanning*.

Isotretinoin

A drug derived from *vitamin A* used in the treatment of severe *acne* when other treatments have proved ineffective. Isotretinoin works by reducing the formation of sebum (natural skin oils) and keratin (a tough protein that is the major component of the outer layer of skin).

POSSIBLE ADVERSE EFFECTS

Isotretinoin may cause itching, dryness and flaking of the skin, and cracking of the lips. Rarely, it may cause liver damage and an increased risk of *coronary artery disease* and *peripheral vascular disease*. Isotretinoin may damage a developing fetus; pregnancy should be avoided during treatment and for at least three months after taking the drug.

Isoxsuprine

A *vasodilator* drug intended to improve circulation through narrowed arteries, particularly in the brain and legs. There is no convincing evidence that it actually produces clinically significant improvement in circulation.

Itching

An intense, distracting irritation or tickling sensation in the skin which may be generalized (felt all over the skin's surface) or localized (confined to one area). The reason for the sensation is not fully understood.

Itching is the most prominent symptom of many skin diseases, but does not itself necessarily indicate an underlying skin disorder. People differ in their tolerance to itching, and a person's threshold can be altered by stress, emotions, or other factors. Itching is worse when the skin is warm and when there are few distractions, making it more noticeable at night.

CAUSES

GENERALIZED ITCHING Excessive bathing, which removes the skin's natural oils and may leave the skin excessively dry and scaly, is a common cause of itching. Some people experience itching after taking certain drugs, such as cocaine, codeine, and some antibiotics. Soap, detergents, and roughly textured clothing (e.g., clothing made from wool) also produce itching in some people.

Many elderly people suffer for no apparent reason from dry, itchy skin, especially on their backs. A similar condition affects some younger people in cold weather. Itching commonly occurs during pregnancy.

Many skin conditions produce an itchy rash—for example, *chickenpox*, *urticaria* (hives), *eczema*, and fungal infections (see *Tinea*). Less common causes include *psoriasis* or *dermatitis herpetiformis*. Generalized skin itchiness can be a result of *diabetes mellitus*, *kidney failure*, *jaundice*, and thyroid disorders. Disorders of the blood (such as *leukemia*) and of the lymphatic system (for example, *Hodgkin's disease*) occasionally cause itching.

LOCALIZED ITCHING Pruritus ani (itching around the anal region) occurs in adults, particularly those with such problems as *hemorrhoids*, *anal fissure*, and persistent diarrhea. Pruritus ani often results from irritation caused by overzealous cleansing after defecation. *Worm infestation* is the most likely cause of itching in children.

Another form of intense skin irritation confined to one area occurs in pruritus vulvae, which affects the external genitalia in women. The condition may be due to *candidiasis*, hormonal changes (at puberty, pregnancy, and the menopause), or to use of spermicides or vaginal suppositories, ointments, and deodorants.

Lice and *scabies* infestations and *insect bites* cause intense itching.

TREATMENT
Specific treatment depends on the underlying cause, if known. Cooling lotions, such as *calamine*, relieve irritation; *emollients* reduce dryness.

Soaps often irritate itchy skin, especially if a rash is visible. Soaps should be used only when necessary; a mild cleansing lotion or water alone is often sufficient to keep most of the skin adequately clean. Itchy skin should be handled very gently. Scratching temporarily relieves itching, but makes the itching worse in the long run. The scratching habit can be suppressed by applying a soothing lotion, ointment, or wet compress to the affected areas when the urge to scratch occurs.

-itis

A suffix meaning "inflammation of." Virtually every organ or tissue in the body can suffer inflammation (the most common form of tissue disorder), so "-itis" is by far the most common word ending in medicine. An example of its use is *bronchitis* (inflammation of the bronchi).

The term -itis is applied strictly to cases of inflammation with redness, pain, heat, and swelling. The term should not be used loosely to imply general disorder, for which the ending "-opathy" is appropriate.

IUCD

An abbreviation for intrauterine contraceptive device (see *IUD*).

IUD

An abbreviation for intrauterine contraceptive device. An IUD, alternatively called an IUCD or coil, is a mechanical device inserted into the uterus for purposes of *contraception*. IUDs are not recommended for some groups of women, but for others they are an efficient and acceptable method of contraception. The failure rate for IUDs is about 2 to 3 percent.

Several different types of IUD are available. Some are made only of molded plastic. Others have a copper wire wrapped around the stem. Most IUDs have a plastic string which, following insertion of the device, comes through the cervix into the vagina. The string makes removal easier and indicates the presence of the IUD.

HOW THEY WORK
Although it is not definitely known how IUDs work, it is thought that the main effect is to inhibit implantation of a fertilized egg in the wall of the uterus (see *Implantation, egg*).

HOW THEY ARE USED
An IUD may be inserted by a general practitioner, family planning physician, or gynecologist. The device can be inserted any time during the menstrual cycle, but the preferred time is during or just after menstruation (because it is unlikely that the woman is pregnant and because the cervix is easier to handle). After a full-term pregnancy, a woman should wait for at least six weeks before having an IUD inserted.

An IUD is inserted through the vagina and cervix into the uterine cavity. Most IUDs are loaded in a small plastic tube that is inserted through the cervical canal; the device is gently pushed out by means of a plunger. Once an IUD is in place, it provides immediate protection. The woman should check once or twice a week that the string is present. If it is not, the string has probably curled up into the uterus, but it is possible that the IUD has been expelled.

IUDs containing copper need to be replaced every three to five years.

WHO SHOULD NOT USE IUDS
Women who have never been pregnant are more likely to have complications than women who have had children. Women with no previous pregnancies usually have more pain

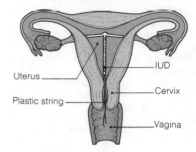

Site of an IUD
An IUD is inserted into the uterus; it has a plastic string that hangs down through the cervix and into the vagina. All types of IUDs can be inserted—by specially trained personnel—in family planning clinics, hospitals, or general practitioners' offices.

on insertion, higher expulsion rates, and a heavier menstrual flow. A woman with *fibroids* may be advised not to have an IUD. Any woman with a history of pelvic disease or infection of the fallopian tubes should not use an IUD. Women with many partners (or whose partner has other sexual partners) are at increased risk of *pelvic inflammatory disease* (PID) and should probably avoid IUDs. Young women have a higher infection rate than older women.

Women with heavy or painful periods may find the IUD makes their symptoms worse.

COMPLICATIONS
Immediately after insertion, there may be bleeding, pain, or vaginal discharge. Menstrual periods after insertion may be heavier and more painful than before.

Women who become pregnant despite having an IUD have a higher rate of *ectopic pregnancy*. PID may be severe and lead to permanent infertility. A rare complication of IUD use is a perforated uterus, in which the device works its way through the wall of the uterus into the abdominal cavity.

IVF

See *In vitro fertilization*.

IVP

The abbreviation for intravenous pyelography, also known as intravenous *urography*.

IVU

The abbreviation for intravenous *urography* (an imaging technique).

Jakob-Creutzfeldt disease
See *Creutzfeldt-Jakob disease*.

Jaundice
Yellowing of the skin and the whites of the eyes caused by an accumulation of the yellow-brown *bile* pigment *bilirubin* in the blood. Jaundice is the chief sign of many disorders of the *liver* and *biliary system*. Many babies develop jaundice soon after birth (see *Jaundice, neonatal*).

TYPES AND CAUSES
Bilirubin is formed from *hemoglobin* (the oxygen-carrying pigment in red blood cells) when old red cells are broken down, mainly by the *spleen*. The pigment is absorbed from the blood by the liver, where it is made soluble in water and is excreted in bile. The process can be upset in any of three ways, causing the main types of jaundice: hemolytic, hepatocellular, and obstructive.

HEMOLYTIC JAUNDICE In hemolytic jaundice, the amount of bilirubin produced is too great for the liver to process. This is caused by excessive *hemolysis* (breakdown of red cells), which can have many causes (see *Anemia, hemolytic*). A type of jaundice similar to hemolytic jaundice can develop as a result of a mild liver disorder called *Gilbert's disease*.

HEPATOCELLULAR JAUNDICE In hepatocellular jaundice, bilirubin builds up in the blood because its transfer from liver cells to bile is prevented, usually as the result of acute *hepatitis* (inflammation of the liver) or *liver failure*.

OBSTRUCTIVE JAUNDICE In obstructive jaundice, also known as cholestatic jaundice, bile is prevented from flowing out of the liver because of blockage of the bile ducts (see *Bile duct obstruction*) due to disorders such as *gallstones* or a tumor. Obstructive jaundice can also occur if the bile ducts are not present (as in *biliary atresia*) or have been destroyed within the liver (for example, in primary *biliary cirrhosis*). As a result, *cholestasis* (stagnation of bile in the liver) occurs and bilirubin is forced back into the blood.

SYMPTOMS AND SIGNS
In some cases, such as in acute hepatitis, jaundice is only one of several signs and symptoms. In other cases, such as in Gilbert's disease, it may be the sole sign of a disorder.

Obstructive jaundice is usually accompanied by two other characteristic features: pale feces and dark urine. The feces are pale because bilirubin, which normally colors feces brown, does not reach the intestine; the urine is dark because large amounts of water-soluble bilirubin are filtered into it from the blood. Bilirubin may also be deposited in the skin, causing itching.

In hemolytic jaundice, the color of both urine and feces is normal. In hepatocellular jaundice, the feces are normal but the urine may be dark.

DIAGNOSIS AND TREATMENT
If excessive hemolysis is suspected, *blood tests* are carried out to determine the amount of water-insoluble bilirubin. A *blood smear* indicates whether large numbers of immature red cells are present; if they are, hemolysis is the suspected cause of the jaundice.

To diagnose hepatocellular jaundice, the blood is tested and a *liver biopsy* (removal of a small sample of tissue for analysis) may be performed.

If the physician suspects obstructive jaundice, *ultrasound scanning*, *liver function tests*, and *cholangiography* may be carried out to determine if the bile ducts are diseased or blocked.

In all cases, treatment is for the underlying cause.

Jaundice, neonatal
Yellowing of the skin and whites of the eyes in the newborn period, due to the accumulation of *bilirubin* (a yellow-brown *bile* pigment) in the blood. Many babies develop *jaundice* during the first few days after birth; premature babies are especially prone to the condition.

In the newborn period, jaundice is usually due to immaturity of the *liver*, resulting in failure of the liver to excrete bilirubin efficiently. This form of jaundice is usually harmless and disappears toward the end of the first week.

Much less commonly, jaundice in babies is caused by *hemolytic disease of the newborn*, *G6PD deficiency*, infection, *hepatitis* (inflammation of the liver), *hypothyroidism* (underactivity of the thyroid gland), or *biliary atresia*.

DIAGNOSIS AND TREATMENT
Diagnosis is based on physical examination. In some cases, blood tests, urine tests, *ultrasound scanning*, and other tests may be performed.

Treatment depends on the underlying cause. Jaundiced babies usually require extra fluids and may be treated with *phototherapy*. In severe cases, exchange transfusion (a type of *blood transfusion*) may be necessary. If severe neonatal jaundice is not treated promptly, *kernicterus* (a form of brain damage) may occur.

Jaw
The lowest and only mobile bone of the face, also known as the mandible. The term jaw sometimes includes the bone that extends from the inner rims of the eyes to the mouth, more commonly known as the *maxilla*.

The mandible is U-shaped as seen from above and bears the lower teeth on its upper surface. It is connected to the base of the *skull* at the *temporomandibular joints*, which can be felt in the cheek just in front of the earlobe. Powerful muscles, arising from the temple on either side, attach to the jaw for movements needed in chewing and biting; other muscles allow side-to-side and downward movement.

Jaw, dislocated
Displacement of the lower *jaw* from one or both of the *temporomandibular joints* (the joints between the jaw and the base of the skull). A dislocated jaw is usually caused either by a blow or by yawning.

ANATOMY OF THE JAW
The U-shaped, mobile bone of the face meets the skull in front of the ears at the temporomandibular joint. The jaw bears teeth on its upper surface.

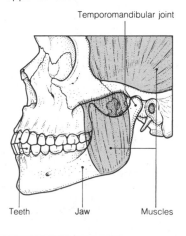

Temporomandibular joint

Teeth   Jaw   Muscles

J

The jaw is the most commonly dislocated joint because it is very unstable. Once dislocation has happened, it tends to recur.

SYMPTOMS

There is pain in front of the ear on the affected side or sides and the jaw projects forward. The mouth cannot be fully closed and, as a result, the victim drools and has difficulty eating and speaking.

TREATMENT

A second person can easily correct the dislocation. He or she should stand in front of the victim, place a thumb on the lower back teeth at each side, and press down. The lower jaw should then click back into position. To avoid causing injury when the teeth snap shut, the thumbs should be wrapped in cloth.

Recurrent dislocation requires an operation to stabilize the joint, such as strengthening the ligaments with stitches. However, surgery is rarely successful in curing the problem.

Jaw, fractured

Fractures of the *jaw* are most often caused by a direct blow to the face. Because of the shape of the jaw, fracture often occurs not only at the site of the blow, but also on the other side of the jaw.

SYMPTOMS

If the fracture is minor, the only symptoms may be some tenderness, pain on biting, and slight stiffness. In more severe injuries, teeth may be loosened or damaged, movement of the jaw may be severely limited, and there may be loss of feeling in the lower lip.

DIAGNOSIS AND TREATMENT

If a fracture is suspected, *X rays* of the area are taken. Minor fractures are normally left to heal on their own.

For severe fractures in which the bones have become displaced, surgical treatment is required. The bone fragments are first manipulated back into the correct position. Teeth too badly damaged to be saved may require extraction. The jaw is immobilized to allow healing to occur, usually by wiring the upper and lower teeth together. If the patient has no teeth, special dentures can be constructed to hold the wires.

Some fractures cannot be adequately immobilized by this method. In such cases, an incision is made in the skin to expose the jaw bone, holes are drilled in each bone fragment, and wires are inserted and twisted together. The skin incision is sewn up with the wires in position.

RECOVERY PERIOD

If the teeth have been wired together, the patient is given a liquid diet. The wires are usually removed after about six weeks.

Jealousy, morbid

Preoccupation with the sexual infidelity of one's partner. The sufferer, usually a man, becomes convinced that his partner is having an affair.

Morbid jealousy is usually due to *personality disorder, depression,* or *paranoia,* but may also occur in those suffering from *alcohol dependence* or organic *brain syndrome.*

Treatment of the underlying disorder may improve the condition, but the outlook is generally poor. Psychiatrists usually recommend separation of the partners, since morbid jealousy is a significant cause of murder.

Jejunal biopsy

A diagnostic test in which a small piece of tissue is removed from the lining of the *jejunum* (the middle, coiled section of the small intestine) for examination under a microscope.

WHY IT IS DONE

The procedure is especially useful in the diagnosis of *Crohn's disease, celiac disease, lymphoma,* and all other causes of *malabsorption* because these conditions are associated with recognizable changes in the small intestine.

HOW IT IS DONE

The patient may be sedated slightly before the procedure. A small device (Crosby capsule) is attached to a length of fine tubing; both are lubricated and the patient then swallows the capsule. The tube is guided down the esophagus through the stomach and duodenum until the capsule reaches the jejunum. An *X ray* is then performed to ensure that the capsule is in the correct position. A syringe is used to withdraw air from the tube and capsule, thereby causing a minute piece of tissue to be sucked into the capsule, where it is sheared off. The tube and capsule are withdrawn and the tissue is taken from the capsule for examination.

Jejunum

The middle, coiled section of the small *intestine,* joining the *duodenum* to the *ileum.* It is wider than the ileum and has a thicker wall, but its function is the same—the digestion of food and the absorption of nutrients from it. Among the few disorders that may affect the jejunum are *celiac disease, Crohn's disease,* and *lymphoma.*

Jellyfish stings

Jellyfish, together with corals, sea anemones, and Portuguese men-of-war, belong to a group of marine animals called coelenterates or cnidarians. These animals have tentacles armed with stinging capsules that discharge when touched. Usually, the result of a sting is no more than an itchy or mildly painful rash, but some jellyfish and Portuguese men-of-war can cause a severe sting. In rare cases, venom entering the bloodstream may cause vomiting, sweating, shock, breathing difficulties, convulsions, and collapse. Dangerous species live mainly in tropical waters.

TREATMENT

If fragments of jellyfish tentacle remain attached to the skin after a sting, vinegar should be applied to inactivate the stinging capsules; tentacle fragments may be removed with adhesive tape. The bare hands should not be used, as tentacles may remain capable of causing stings for many hours. *Analgesic drugs* (painkillers) may be taken. A severe reaction requires hospitalization and sometimes *cardiopulmonary resuscitation. Antivenin* for the more dangerous species of jellyfish may be available.

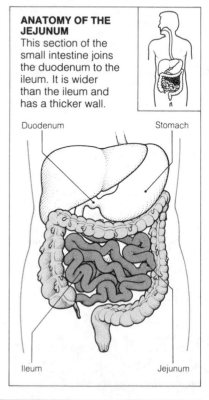

ANATOMY OF THE JEJUNUM
This section of the small intestine joins the duodenum to the ileum. It is wider than the ileum and has a thicker wall.

Duodenum

Stomach

Ileum

Jejunum

TYPES OF JOINTS

Some joints are fixed (e.g., the skull) and some allow a little movement (e.g., the vertebrae). Of the mobile joints, the hinge joint is the simplest. Pivot joints allow rotation only, while ellipsoidal joints allow all types of movement except pivotal. Ball-and-socket joints allow the widest range of movement.

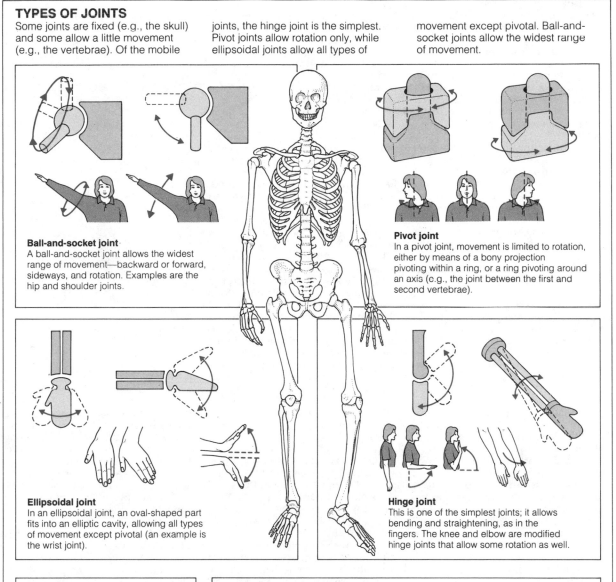

Ball-and-socket joint
A ball-and-socket joint allows the widest range of movement—backward or forward, sideways, and rotation. Examples are the hip and shoulder joints.

Pivot joint
In a pivot joint, movement is limited to rotation, either by means of a bony projection pivoting within a ring, or a ring pivoting around an axis (e.g., the joint between the first and second vertebrae).

Ellipsoidal joint
In an ellipsoidal joint, an oval-shaped part fits into an elliptic cavity, allowing all types of movement except pivotal (an example is the wrist joint).

Hinge joint
This is one of the simplest joints; it allows bending and straightening, as in the fingers. The knee and elbow are modified hinge joints that allow some rotation as well.

STRUCTURE OF A FIXED JOINT
Fixed joints are firmly secured by fibrous tissue. The joints between the bones of the skull are an example.

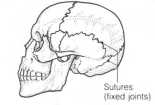

Sutures (fixed joints)

STRUCTURE OF A MOBILE JOINT
The bone surfaces are coated with very smooth cartilage to reduce friction. The joint is sealed within a tough fibrous capsule lined with synovial membrane, which produces a sticky, lubricating fluid. Each joint is surrounded by strong ligaments that support it and prevent excessive movement. Movement is controlled by muscles that are attached to bone by tendons on either side of the joint. Most mobile joints have at least one bursa (fluid-filled sac) nearby, which cushions a pressure point.

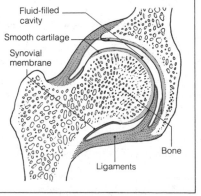

Fluid-filled cavity
Smooth cartilage
Synovial membrane
Bone
Ligaments

Jet lag

Interruption of the sleep-wake cycle, fatigue, and other symptoms caused by disturbance of normal body rhythms as a result of flying across different time zones.

Symptoms of jet lag are a desire to sleep during the local day, wakefulness at night, general fatigue, reduced physical and mental activity, and poor memory.

CAUSES

When an air traveler crosses several time zones, his or her "day" (as timed by an external clock) is longer or shorter than 24 hours, depending on the direction of the flight. Many of the traveler's *biorhythms* (natural body rhythms) do not adjust immediately to this shorter or longer day, and this results in jet lag when the flight is over.

Jet lag tends to be worse after an eastward flight (which shortens the traveler's day) than after a westward one. It is most likely to affect people over 30 who normally follow an established daily routine.

PREVENTIVE MEASURES

The symptoms of jet lag can be minimized by drinking plenty of nonalcoholic fluids during the flight and avoiding heavy meals. Also, people flying east should go to bed earlier than usual for a few days before the journey; people flying west should stay up later. It is a good idea, if possible, to arrive in the new time zone in the early evening and to go to bed early.

It may take several days to adjust to a new time zone (about half a day to one day for each time zone that has been crossed). The adjustment can be made easier by breaking up a long journey with a stopover and by resting after the flight.

The pituitary hormone *melatonin* is thought to play a part in the control of daily body rhythms, and its possible use in the prevention of jet lag is the subject of current research.

Jogger's nipple

Soreness of the nipple caused by the rubbing of clothing against it, usually during sports such as jogging or long-distance running. Jogger's nipple, which affects both men and women, can be prevented by applying petroleum jelly to the nipple before prolonged running. Wearing a clean shirt also helps because sweat can aggravate the condition. Treatment involves covering the nipple with a bandage to reduce rubbing.

Joint

The junction between two or more bones. Most joints are highly mobile, others are fixed or allow only a small amount of movement (see the illustrated box, p. 611).

DISORDERS

Common joint injuries include *sprains*, damage to the *cartilage*, torn *ligaments*, and tearing of the joint capsule.

Dislocation of a joint is usually caused by injury but is occasionally *congenital*. A less severe injury may cause *subluxation* (partial dislocation). Rarely, the bone ends are fractured, sometimes leading to *hemarthrosis* (bleeding into the joint) or *effusion* (accumulation of fluid in a joint) due to *synovitis* (inflammation of the lining of the joint).

Joints are commonly affected by forms of *arthritis* (inflammation of a joint). *Bursitis* (inflammation of a bursa) may occur as a result of local irritation or strain. Permanent joint deformities may be caused by severe injury or arthritis. Temporary deformities, usually affecting a joint in the legs, may occur during childhood but disappear as growth continues. Surgery may be required to correct certain deformities.

Joint replacement

See *Arthroplasty*.

Joule

The international unit of *energy*, work, and heat. Approximately 4,200 joules (symbol J) or 4.2 kilojoules (kJ) equal one kilocalorie (kcal); 1 kJ equals about 0.24 kcal. (See also *Calorie*.)

Jugular vein

One of three veins on each side of the neck that return deoxygenated blood from the head to the heart. Of the three (internal, external, and anterior) by far the largest is the internal jugular, which arises at the base of the skull, travels down the neck alongside the carotid arteries, and passes behind the clavicle (collarbone), where it joins the subclavian vein (the large vein that drains blood from the arms). The jugular is rarely injured because it lies deep in the structures of the neck.

Jungian theory

Ideas put forward by the Swiss psychiatrist Carl Gustav Jung (1875-1961). Originally an associate of Sigmund Freud, Jung broke away in 1913 to form his own school of analytical psychology, mainly because he did not

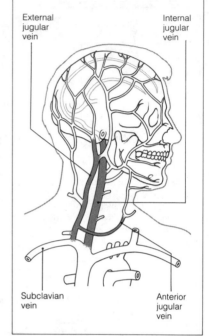

ANATOMY OF THE JUGULAR VEIN
The three veins on each side of the neck that return blood from the head to the heart.

External jugular vein

Internal jugular vein

Subclavian vein

Anterior jugular vein

believe that sexual drive was the only force behind all human activity. Instead, he theorized that certain ideas (called archetypes) inherited from experiences in our distant past were present in each person's unconscious and controlled the way in which each person viewed the world. Jung called these shared ideas the "collective unconscious."

Although Jung believed that each individual also had a "personal unconscious" containing experiences from his or her life, he regarded the collective unconscious as superior. Therapy was therefore aimed at putting people in touch with this source of profound ideas, particularly through the interpretation of dreams.

Jung's therapeutic approach was also based on his theory of personality, which postulated two basic types, the *extrovert* and the *introvert*. He believed that one of these types dominates a person's consciousness and that the other must be brought into consciousness and reconciled with its opposite for the person to become a whole individual.

Juvenile arthritis

See *Rheumatoid arthritis, juvenile*.

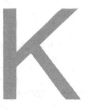

K

Kala-azar

A form of the insect-spread parasitic disease *leishmaniasis*. Kala-azar occurs in many parts of Africa, the Mediterranean area, India, and South America.

Kaolin

An *aluminum* compound used as an ingredient in some *antidiarrheal drugs*. Kaolin increases the bulk of the feces. It is also believed to adsorb *bacteria*, *viruses*, and *toxins* (poisons) from the intestine and transport them through the intestine for excretion in the feces.

Kaposi's sarcoma

A condition, characterized by malignant skin tumors, which is a prominent feature of *AIDS*. In the past, Kaposi's sarcoma developed slowly and was extremely rare. In patients with AIDS, it is highly aggressive and tumors soon become widespread.

The tumors, consisting of blue-red nodules, usually start on the feet and ankles, spread farther up the legs, and then appear on the hands and arms. In people with AIDS, tumors also commonly affect the gastrointestinal and respiratory tracts, where they may cause severe internal bleeding.

For mild cases of Kaposi's sarcoma, low-dose *radiation therapy* is usually effective. For more severe cases, *anticancer drugs* may be necessary to slow the spread of the tumors.

Kawasaki disease

An acute childhood illness that affects many systems in the body. It is also called mucocutaneous lymph node syndrome. The condition was first observed in Japan in the 1960s. It is becoming increasingly common in western countries. Kawasaki disease usually occurs in the first two years of life. The cause is unknown.

SYMPTOMS
Fever is the first symptom and usually persists for one or two weeks. Other characteristic symptoms are *conjunctivitis*, dryness and cracking of the lips, and swollen *lymph nodes* in the

neck. Toward the end of the first week of illness, the palms and soles of a Kawasaki disease victim become red, the hands and feet swell, and a rash similar to that of measles appears over the body. By the end of the second week, the skin at the tips of the victim's fingers and toes peels and the other symptoms subside.

TREATMENT AND OUTLOOK
There is no cure, but *ASA* may help prevent possible heart complications. Most children make a complete recovery. In about 1 to 2 percent of cases, however, sudden death occurs after the acute phase of the illness, usually due to *coronary artery disease*.

Keloid

A raised, hard, irregularly shaped, itchy scar on the skin. A keloid occurs because of a defective healing process in which an excess of *collagen* (a tough fibrous protein) forms at the site of a healing scar. Keloids occur more commonly in black people than in white people.

Keloids can occur anywhere on the body but are most common over the sternum (breastbone) and over the shoulder. The scars often enlarge after developing and may be unsightly. After several months most keloids flatten and cease to itch.

Injections of *corticosteroid drugs* directly into a keloid may reduce itchiness and cause some shrinkage. Surgical removal is of little use since the new scar that forms is almost always a keloid.

Keratin

A fibrous protein that is the main constituent of the outermost layer of the *skin*, *nails*, and *hair*. Keratin is a tough substance that is resistant to a wide range of chemical and environmental changes.

Keratitis

Inflammation of the *cornea* (the transparent front part of the eyeball), in contrast to *keratopathy*, noninflammatory disorders of the cornea. Keratitis usually takes the form of a *corneal ulcer*. In interstitial keratitis, which affects about 70 percent of older children with congenital *syphilis*, the inflammation affects deep corneal tissue.

Symptoms of keratitis include eye pain, excessive watering, blurring of vision, and photophobia (abnormal sensitivity to bright light). If keratitis persists for a long time, blood vessels grow into the cornea.

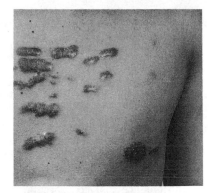

Crop of keloids over the breastbone
These overgrowths of scar tissue usually flatten out and become less noticeable over a period of months or years.

Keratoacanthoma

A harmless skin nodule, which most commonly develops on the face or arm of an elderly person.

A keratoacanthoma initially resembles a small, round wart with a soft center, and grows rapidly over a period of about eight weeks to reach a maximum size of about 2 cm across. The mature nodule has bulging sides and its center may have a whitish appearance. Without treatment, the keratoacanthoma slowly disappears after reaching its mature state, but in most cases the patient will prefer to have the nodule removed surgically.

Keratoacanthomas are fairly common. The cause is unknown, but these nodules tend to be more common in people who have had many years of exposure to strong sunlight and in people taking long-term *immunosuppressant drugs*.

Microscopic examination of a small piece of tissue may be necessary to distinguish a keratoacanthoma from a *squamous cell carcinoma* (a form of skin cancer).

Keratoconjunctivitis

Inflammation of the *cornea* associated with *conjunctivitis*. The most common form is epidemic keratoconjunctivitis, caused by a virus that usually causes painful swelling of a small *lymph node* in front of the ear. It is highly infectious and is spread mainly by sharing towels or by unsterile instruments and eye drops.

The conjunctivitis is often severe, with marked redness, swelling, or destruction of the surface layer of the conjunctiva, leaving a whitish membrane. Seven to 10 days after onset of the disorder, tiny opaque spots resembling snowflakes develop in the

K

cornea. The spots may persist for many months and sometimes interfere with vision.

There is no specific treatment for epidemic keratoconjunctivitis. The corneal opacities can sometimes be minimized by the use of eye drops containing *corticosteroid drugs*. (See also *Keratoconjunctivitis sicca*.)

Keratoconjunctivitis sicca
A condition of persistent dryness of the *cornea* and *conjunctiva* caused by deficiency in tear production. Commonly referred to as "dry eye," keratoconjunctivitis sicca occurs in *autoimmune disorders* such as *rheumatoid arthritis*, *Sjögren's syndrome*, and systemic *lupus erythematosus*; all of these conditions can damage the tear-producing glands. Prolonged dryness may cause blurred vision, burning, itching, and grittiness. In severe cases, there may be *corneal ulcers* or scarring of the cornea. The most effective treatment for keratoconjunctivitis sicca is frequent use of artificial tears (see *Tears, artificial*).

Keratoconus
An inherited condition in which abnormal corneal growth causes the central area of the *cornea* to become gradually thinned and conical. The condition affects both eyes.

Keratoconus usually starts around puberty, causing increasing *myopia* (nearsightedness) and a progressive distortion of vision that cannot be fully corrected by glasses. Hard contact lenses improve vision in the early stages but are less effective as the condition progresses.

A *corneal graft* is usually performed when vision has seriously deteriorated and contact lenses are no longer helpful. The results of corneal grafting are generally excellent.

Keratolytic drugs
Drugs that loosen and remove the tough, outer layer of the skin, which is composed mainly of *keratin* (a tough protein). Keratolytic drugs, which include preparations of *urea* and *salicylic acid*, are used in the treatment of skin and scalp disorders, such as *warts*, callosities (see *Callus, skin*), *acne*, *dandruff*, and *psoriasis*.

Keratomalacia
A disorder, caused by severe deficiency of *vitamin A*, in which the cornea becomes opaque and ulcerated. Perforation of the cornea is common, often leading to loss of the eye

through infection. Keratomalacia is a common cause of blindness in developing countries. The condition usually occurs only in severely malnourished children and is very rare in developed countries.

Prolonged lack of vitamin A first causes poor vision in dim light, severe dryness of the eyes, and a characteristic foamy patch on the corners of the conjunctiva. There may also be a gritty feeling in the eyelids and abnormal sensitivity to bright light. Treatment with large doses of vitamin A at this stage reverses the effects of the deficiency. Without treatment, the condition leads to irreparable damage and commonly to blindness.

Keratopathy
A general term used to describe a variety of disorders of the *cornea* (the transparent front part of the eyeball).

Actinic keratopathy is damage to the outer layer of the cornea by *ultraviolet light*, either from the sun or from artificial sources, such as sunlamps or arc welding torches. The outer layer of the cornea tends to strip off, exposing the nerve endings and causing severe pain. In skiers or mountaineers it is known as snow blindness.

Exposure keratopathy is damage to the cornea caused by loss of the normal protection afforded by the tear film and the blink reflex. It may occur in a variety of conditions in which the lids inadequately cover the cornea, including severe *exophthalmos*, *facial palsy*, and *ectropion*.

Keratoplasty
See *Corneal graft*.

Keratosis
A skin growth caused by an overproduction of *keratin* (the tough protein that is the major component of the outer layer of skin). Keratoses occur mainly in the elderly.

TYPES

SEBORRHEIC KERATOSES Often called seborrheic warts, these range from flat, dark brown, rough patches to small, wartlike protrusions and are covered with a greasy, removable crust. Seborrheic keratoses occur mainly on the trunk. They are completely harmless but can be unsightly.

SOLAR KERATOSES Small, wartlike, red or flesh-colored growths that appear on exposed parts of the body as a result of overexposure to the sun over a period of years. Solar keratoses may rarely develop into skin cancer, usually *squamous cell carcinoma*.

TREATMENT
Seborrheic keratoses require no treatment unless they are large and unsightly. Solar keratoses must always be removed because of the risk of skin cancer. Removal is usually by *cryosurgery* (the destruction of tissue by extreme cold) or by *curettage*.

Keratosis pilaris
A very common skin condition in which patches of rough skin appear on the upper arms, thighs, and buttocks. The openings of the hair follicles become enlarged by hard plugs of *keratin* (the tough protein that is the major component of the outer layer of skin) and the hairs that grow in them may be distorted.

The condition tends to run in families and occurs most commonly in older children, adolescents, and obese people. It is often worse in winter. Keratosis pilaris is not serious and usually clears up on its own. In severe cases, symptoms can be relieved by rubbing a mixture of salicylic acid and mineral oil into the affected areas; scrubbing these areas with a loofah may also help.

Keratotomy, radial
A procedure in which radiating incisions are made in the cornea (up to, but not through, its innermost layer) in an attempt to reduce *myopia* (nearsightedness).

The results of radial keratotomy vary and the effect is not always permanent. Serious complications may develop. The procedure is not generally recommended for people whose vision can be corrected by glasses or contact lenses.

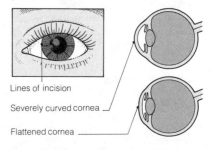

Lines of incision

Severely curved cornea

Flattened cornea

Procedure for keratotomy
Eight or more radial cuts are made in the cornea, avoiding the central zone. During healing, the scars contract, causing the cornea to become flatter and less powerful.

Kerion
A red, pustular swelling that develops as a reaction to a fungal infection, usually scalp ringworm (see *Tinea*).

The inflammation gradually subsides over six to eight weeks but, if severe, may leave a scar and permanent loss of hair from the affected area. Kerion is treated by applying a cream containing an *antifungal drug* to the swelling and by taking the antibiotic drug *griseofulvin*.

Kernicterus

A rare disorder in which newborn, especially premature, infants suffer brain damage as a result of severe jaundice (see *Jaundice, neonatal*). Kernicterus is completely preventable if neonatal jaundice is treated promptly.

In addition to showing signs of jaundice, a baby with kernicterus becomes increasingly listless and may adopt a characteristic posture with the back and neck arched backward.

Without treatment, affected babies are likely to die at the end of the first week. Less severely affected babies may survive but there will be some degree of permanent brain damage, which may possibly result in a form of *cerebral palsy*.

Ketoconazole

An *antifungal drug* taken by mouth to treat severe *fungal infections* of the lungs, brain, kidney, and lymph glands. Ketoconazole is also applied topically to treat *candidiasis* (thrush) of the skin, mouth, or vagina when other antifungal preparations have proved ineffective.

Ketoconazole tablets may cause nausea (which may be reduced if the drug is taken with food), rash, and, rarely, liver damage.

Ketoprofen

A *nonsteroidal anti-inflammatory drug* (NSAID) prescribed as an *analgesic drug* (painkiller) in the treatment of injury to soft tissues, such as muscles and ligaments. Ketoprofen is also given to reduce joint pain and stiffness in people with types of arthritis, including *rheumatoid arthritis*, *osteoarthritis*, and *ankylosing spondylitis*.

Ketoprofen may cause abdominal pain, nausea, indigestion, and an increased risk of *peptic ulcer*.

Ketosis

A potentially serious condition in which excessive amounts of ketones accumulate in the body. Ketones are substances chemically related to acetone, which is found in solvents such as nail polish remover. Ketosis results whenever glucose is not available to use as a source of energy, which forces the body to use fats instead. This, in turn, leads to fatty acids being released into the blood, where they are converted to ketones.

The underlying causes of ketosis include fasting or starvation, and untreated or inadequately controlled *diabetes mellitus* (in which lack of insulin prevents glucose from being used as fuel). Symptoms and signs include sweet, "fruity-smelling" breath, loss of appetite, nausea, vomiting, and abdominal pain. If the condition is not treated, confusion, unconsciousness, and death may follow.

Ketosis can be diagnosed by a test to detect ketones in the urine. Treatment is the same as for diabetes unless the cause is fasting or starvation, in which case gradual reintroduction of a nutritious diet is usually effective.

Kidney

The organ responsible for filtering the blood and excreting waste products and excess water in the form of *urine*. The kidneys, ureters, bladder, and urethra make up the *urinary tract*.

STRUCTURE

There are two kidneys, each about 10 to 12.5 cm long and about 170 g in weight. They lie in the abdomen below the liver on the right and the spleen on the left. The arteries that supply the kidneys arise directly from the aorta (the main artery of the body leading from the heart). Once within the kidneys, the renal arteries divide into smaller and smaller branches, ending in glomeruli (specialized capillaries that form the filtering units). Each kidney contains about one million glomeruli, which pass the filtered blood through long tubules into the medulla (the central collecting region of the kidney). The glomeruli and tubules make up the nephrons, the functioning units of the kidney. As people age, the number of functioning nephrons is reduced; this process may be speeded up by disease.

FUNCTION

The main functions of the kidney are to regulate blood and *electrolytes* and to eliminate waste products. The most important waste products are those generated by the breakdown of proteins. The kidneys also control the body's *acid-base balance*. When blood and body fluids become too acid or too alkaline, the urine acidity is altered to restore the balance. When excess water is ingested, the kidney excretes it; when water is lost (as a result of diarrhea or sweating), the kidney conserves it (see *ADH*).

K

LOCATION OF THE KIDNEYS

The kidneys are situated at the back of the abdominal cavity, just above the waist, on either side of the spinal column. The kidney on the right lies below the liver, while the kidney on the left is situated below the spleen. The arteries that supply the kidneys arise directly from the aorta.

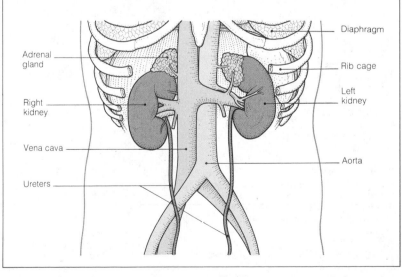

The kidney also produces several hormones, including erythropoietin, which regulates the production and release of red blood cells from the bone marrow. *Vitamin D* is converted into an active hormonal form by the kidney. *Renin*, an enzyme released by the kidney when blood pressure falls, acts on a protein in the blood to produce *angiotensin* (a powerful constrictor of small arteries that helps regulate blood pressure). Angiotensin also controls the release of *aldosterone*, an adrenal hormone that acts on the tubules to promote the reabsorption of sodium and excretion of potassium.

Kidney biopsy

A procedure in which a small portion of *kidney* tissue is removed and examined under a microscope. Kidney *biopsy*, also called renal biopsy, is usually performed as part of the investigation and diagnosis of various kidney disorders, such as *glomerulonephritis*, *proteinuria*, *nephrotic syndrome*, or acute *kidney failure*. It may also be performed to assess the kidneys' response to treatment.

HOW IT IS DONE

There are two basic techniques for performing kidney biopsy: percutaneous (through the skin) and open. The procedure for performing a percutaneous needle biopsy is shown in the illustration.

If a percutaneous needle biopsy is not advisable (e.g., if the patient has a *bleeding disorder* or only one functioning kidney), an open renal biopsy may be performed. With the patient under general anesthesia, the surgeon makes a small incision in the flank to reveal the kidney and then cuts a small wedge of tissue from the kidney. Biopsy samples of kidney tissue are sent to a pathologist for microscopic examination.

RECOVERY PERIOD

The patient may have slight pain in the back for some hours after the biopsy, and a small amount of blood may be passed in the urine. Provided there are no complications, such as severe bleeding, the patient can return home the following day.

Kidney cancer

A malignant tumor of the *kidney*. Most kidney cancers originate in the kidney itself; it is most unusual for cancer to spread to the kidney from another organ.

TYPES

There are three main types of cancer arising in the kidney.

RENAL CELL CARCINOMA Also known as hypernephroma or adenocarcinoma, this type of kidney cancer accounts for about 75 percent of all kidney tumors. It usually occurs after the age of 40 and affects twice as many men as women. The most common symptom is blood in the urine. The condition may also cause pain in the loins, a lump in the abdomen, fever, or weight loss. About 25 percent of patients survive five years or more, the rest dying because the tumor has spread to the lungs, bone, liver, and brain by the time treatment is started.

NEPHROBLASTOMA Also called Wilms' tumor, this cancer accounts for about 20 percent of all cancers in children. It is found mainly in children under the age of 4 years and is almost twice as common in males as in females. Nephroblastoma grows rapidly and is often felt as a lump in the abdomen. This cancer occasionally causes abdominal pain. Nephroblastoma frequently spreads to the lungs, liver, and brain. If treatment is started early, more than 80 percent of children survive.

TRANSITIONAL CELL CARCINOMA This type of kidney cancer arises from cells lining the renal pelvis. It sometimes develops in tobacco smokers and in people who have consumed very large quantities of *analgesic drugs* (painkillers) over the course of many years. Blood in the urine is a common symptom; *hydronephrosis* (distention of the kidney with urine) may occur due to blockage of the ureter. Survival rates vary greatly, depending in part on early detection and treatment of the tumor.

DIAGNOSIS AND TREATMENT

Diagnosis is made by intravenous *urography* or *CT scanning*. Treatment consists of *nephrectomy* (removal of the kidney) and sometimes removal of the ureter as well. In the case of a nephroblastoma, nephrectomy is followed by treatment with *anticancer drugs* and, occasionally, by *radiation therapy*.

Kidney cyst

A fluid-filled sac within the *kidney*. Most kidney cysts are noncancerous.

Single kidney cysts probably occur in about half of all people over 50. In some cases, multiple cysts develop in one or both kidneys. Most kidney cysts occur for no known reason and do not usually produce symptoms unless they become large enough to cause pain in the lower back due to pressure.

Kidney cysts also occur in polycystic kidney disease (see *Kidney, polycystic*), a hereditary condition that often leads to *kidney failure* before the victim reaches the age of 50.

DIAGNOSIS AND TREATMENT

Cysts are commonly discovered only when a person is being examined for some other reason. Treatment is not usually necessary. *Aspiration* (withdrawal of fluid by suction) of the cyst may be performed to ensure that there is no malignancy or to relieve severe pain. When the cyst is large, fluid often reaccumulates, requiring surgical removal of the cyst.

PERCUTANEOUS KIDNEY BIOPSY

This procedure is performed with a local anesthetic injected into the skin and tissues over the kidney; it is virtually painless. There is a risk of bleeding from the kidney into the abdominal cavity.

1 The kidney must be accurately located, usually by an ultrasound scan. Local anesthetic is then injected.

2 A core of tissue is taken by means of a hollow biopsy needle passed through the skin into the kidney.

A kidney glomerulus (filtering unit) as seen under a microscope.

3 The core of kidney tissue is embedded in wax and cut into thin slices, which are mounted on slides for staining and microscopic examination.

Kidney failure

The reduction in the ability of the *kidneys* to filter waste products from the blood and excrete them in the *urine*, to control the body's water and salt balance, and to regulate the *blood pressure*. Kidney failure leads to uremia (a buildup of *urea* and other chemical waste products) and other chemical disturbances in the blood and tissues, leading to symptoms of varying severity.

TYPES AND CAUSES

Kidney failure can be acute (of sudden onset) or chronic (developing more gradually). In acute kidney failure, kidney function usually returns to normal once the underlying cause has been discovered and treated; in chronic failure, function is usually irreversibly lost.

Acute kidney failure most often occurs in people suffering from physiological *shock* as a result of a severe injury or a serious underlying illness. Severe bleeding or burns can reduce blood volume and pressure to the extent that the supply of blood to the kidneys is dramatically reduced. A *myocardial infarction* (heart attack) or acute *pancreatitis* can have a similar effect. The kidneys are particularly susceptible to a reduction in the flow of blood, which can cause damage to the glomeruli (filtering units of the kidneys).

DISORDERS OF THE KIDNEY

The kidneys are susceptible to a wide range of disorders. However, only one normal kidney is needed for good health, so disease is rarely life-threatening unless it affects both kidneys and has reached an advanced stage.

Hypertension (high blood pressure) can be both a cause and effect of kidney damage. Other effects of serious disease or damage include the *nephrotic syndrome* (in which large amounts of protein are lost in the urine and fluid accumulates in body tissues) and acute or chronic *kidney failure*.

CONGENITAL AND GENETIC DISORDERS

Congenital abnormalities of the kidneys are fairly common. In *horseshoe kidney*, the two kidneys are joined at their base. Some people are born with one kidney missing, both kidneys on one side, or a kidney that is partially duplicated and gives rise to two ureters (duplex kidney). These conditions seldom cause problems. In rare cases, a baby is born with kidneys that are so underdeveloped that they are barely functional.

Polycystic disease of the kidneys is a serious inherited disorder in which multiple cysts develop on both kidneys (see *Kidney, polycystic*). In *Fanconi's syndrome* and *renal tubular acidosis* (which are rare), there are subtle abnormalities in the functioning of the kidney tubules, so that certain substances are inappropriately lost in the urine.

IMPAIRED BLOOD SUPPLY

Various diseases may damage or obstruct the small blood vessels within the kidneys, impairing blood flow. *Diabetes mellitus* and *hemolytic-uremic syndrome* are examples. In physiological *shock*, blood pressure and flow through the kidneys are seriously reduced; this can cause a type of damage known as acute tubular necrosis. The larger blood vessels in the kidney may be affected by *polyarteritis nodosa* and systemic *lupus erythematosus*. In rare cases, there is a defect of the renal artery supplying a kidney, which may lead to hypertension and tissue damage.

AUTOIMMUNE DISORDERS

Glomerulonephritis refers to an important group of autoimmune disorders in which the glomerular filtering units of the kidneys become inflamed. It sometimes develops after infection with streptococcal bacteria.

TUMORS

Benign *kidney tumors* are rare. They may cause *hematuria* (blood in the urine), although most cause no symptoms. Malignant tumors are also rare. Renal cell carcinoma, the most common type, occurs mostly in adults over 40; nephroblastoma (Wilms' tumor) affects mainly children under 4 (see *Kidney cancer*).

METABOLIC DISORDERS

Kidney stones are common in middle age. They are usually caused by excessive concentrations of various substances (such as calcium) or lack of inhibitors of crystallization in the urine. In *hyperuricemia*, there is a tendency for uric acid stones to form (see *Calculus, urinary tract*).

INFECTION

Infection of a kidney is called *pyelonephritis*. An important predisposing factor is obstruction of the flow of urine through the urinary tract, leading to stagnation and subsequent infection spreading up from the bladder. The cause of the obstruction may be a congenital defect of the kidney or ureter, a kidney or ureteral stone, a bladder tumor, or, in a man, enlargement of the prostate gland.

Tuberculosis of the kidney is caused by infection carried by the blood from elsewhere in the body, usually the lungs.

DRUGS

Allergic reactions to certain drugs can cause an acute kidney disease, with most of the damage affecting the kidney tubules. Other drugs may directly damage the kidneys if taken in large amounts for prolonged periods. For example, kidney failure can develop after many years of taking excessive amounts of analgesics. Some potent antibiotics can damage the kidney tubules, producing acute tubular necrosis.

OTHER DISORDERS

Hydronephrosis refers to a kidney swollen with urine as a result of obstruction further down the urinary tract. In the *crush syndrome*, kidney function is disrupted by proteins (released into the blood from severely damaged muscles) that block the filtering mechanisms.

INVESTIGATION

Kidney disorders are investigated by *kidney imaging* techniques such as *ultrasound scanning*, intravenous or retrograde pyelography (see *Urography*), angiography, and *CT scanning*; by *kidney biopsy* (removal of a small amount of tissue for analysis); by *blood tests*; and by *kidney function tests*, such as *urinalysis*.

Acute kidney failure may also be caused by obstruction to the urine flow as a result of a stone (see *Calculus, urinary tract*), *bladder tumor*, or enlarged prostate gland (see *Prostate, enlarged*). Certain rapidly developing types of kidney disease, such as *glomerulonephritis* and *hemolytic-uremic syndrome*, are other causes of acute kidney failure.

Chronic kidney failure can result from any disease that causes progressive damage to the kidneys, such as *hypertension* (high blood pressure), *diabetes mellitus*, polycystic kidney disease (see *Kidney, polycystic*), or *amyloidosis* (see also *Kidney* disorders box, p. 617). Long-standing obstruction to the urine flow, due to a stone, tumor, or an enlarged prostate, may also cause chronic kidney failure. Excessive use of *analgesic drugs* (painkillers) over a period of several years is another cause of the condition.

Chronic kidney failure may progress over months or years to an advanced, life-threatening condition called end-stage kidney failure.

SYMPTOMS AND SIGNS

In acute kidney failure, the most noticeable symptom may be a greatly reduced volume of urine. Production of less than 400 ml of urine per day is called *oliguria* and usually means that waste products are not being cleared effectively from the blood. Complete cessation of urine output is called *anuria* and results in a serious buildup of waste products. Some people with kidney failure pass normal amounts of urine despite loss of the filtering and cleansing function of the kidneys; this condition is called nonoliguric acute kidney failure.

Within a short time of the development of acute kidney failure, more symptoms (such as drowsiness, nausea, vomiting, and breathlessness) appear. In many cases, symptoms of the underlying cause of the kidney failure (for example, symptoms of shock such as pale skin and weak pulse) precede those of the kidney failure itself.

Symptoms of chronic failure develop more gradually and may include nausea, loss of appetite, and weakness. Unless the progress of the kidney damage is slowed or arrested, symptoms of end-stage failure may appear (including severe lethargy, weight loss, headache, vomiting, a furred tongue, unpleasant breath, intense, rashless skin itching, and, eventually, collapse, coma, and death).

COMPLICATIONS

Complications of acute kidney failure may include infections such as *pneumonia*, bleeding into the stomach, and deep vein *thrombosis*. In chronic failure, complications due to disturbances in blood chemistry may include high blood pressure (which is both a cause and a result of kidney failure), *anemia, osteomalacia, hyperparathyroidism* (overactivity of the parathyroid glands), *neuropathy* (nerve disorder), or *myopathy* (muscle disorder).

DIAGNOSIS

A person with suspected kidney failure should undergo *kidney function tests*, which include measuring the urea and creatinine (two waste products) in the blood; raised levels indi-

---

THE FUNCTION OF THE KIDNEY

The kidney is essential to the regulation of the body's fluid balance and acid-base balance. The kidney contains about 1 million nephrons, each of which consists of a glomerulus and a tubule that drain urine into the renal pelvis. Capillaries feed each glomerulus and surround each tubule.

RENAL FUNCTION AND AGE

The efficiency of the kidney diminishes with age as the number of functional nephrons is reduced.

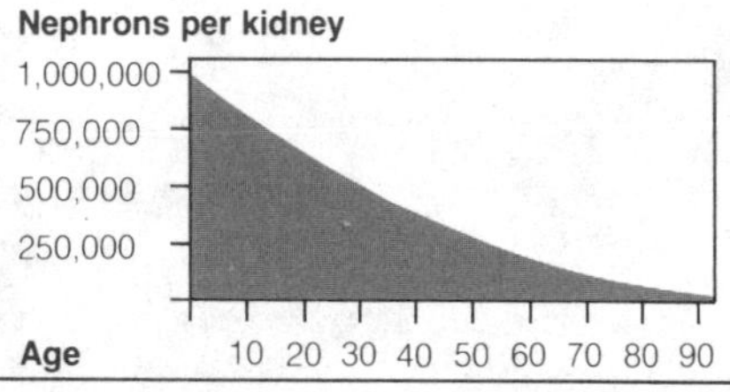

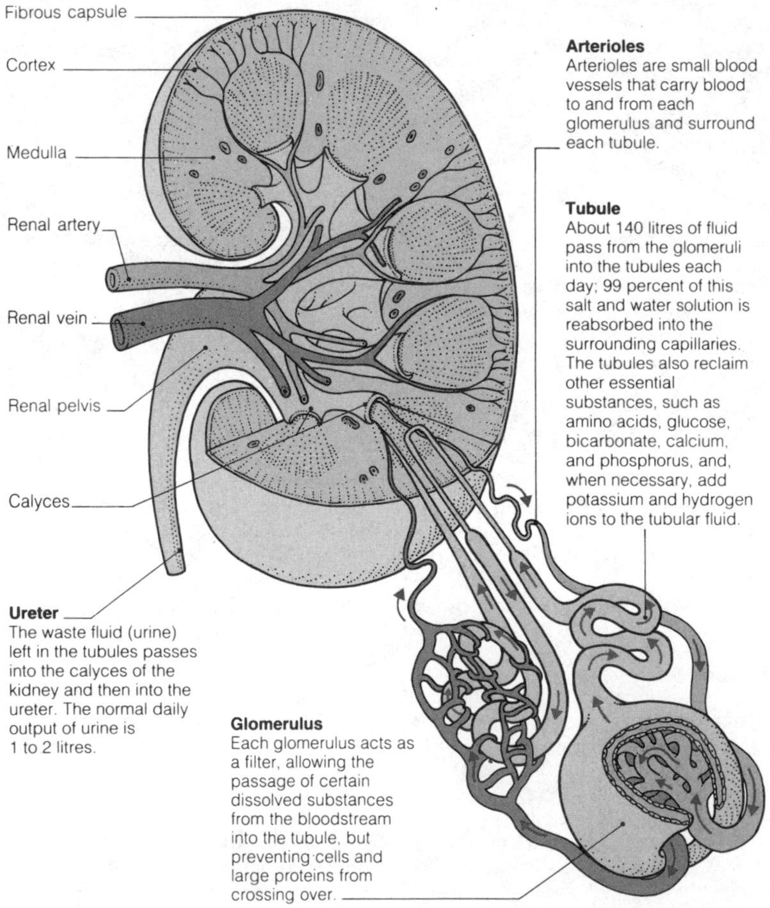

Nephrons per kidney

Arterioles
Arterioles are small blood vessels that carry blood to and from each glomerulus and surround each tubule.

Tubule
About 140 litres of fluid pass from the glomeruli into the tubules each day; 99 percent of this salt and water solution is reabsorbed into the surrounding capillaries. The tubules also reclaim other essential substances, such as amino acids, glucose, bicarbonate, calcium, and phosphorus, and, when necessary, add potassium and hydrogen ions to the tubular fluid.

Fibrous capsule

Cortex

Medulla

Renal artery

Renal vein

Renal pelvis

Calyces

Ureter
The waste fluid (urine) left in the tubules passes into the calyces of the kidney and then into the ureter. The normal daily output of urine is 1 to 2 litres.

Glomerulus
Each glomerulus acts as a filter, allowing the passage of certain dissolved substances from the bloodstream into the tubule, but preventing cells and large proteins from crossing over.

cate kidney failure. *Urinalysis* and blood pressure measurements are also performed. Unless there is an obvious cause of kidney failure (such as severe bleeding), immediate testing is carried out to determine a cause. Techniques include examination of the urine sediment and blood, intravenous *urography*, *kidney biopsy*, *ultrasound scanning*, and *radionuclide scanning*.

TREATMENT
In acute kidney failure, emergency treatment is given for any cause of shock, such as severe bleeding. Blood volume and pressure must be brought back to normal through saline *intravenous infusion* or *blood transfusions*. Surgery may be required for obstruction caused by stones, tumors, or enlargement of the prostate gland. Treatment of other causes may be complex and sometimes controversial, but may include the use of *corticosteroid drugs* and other drugs (as in the treatment of certain forms of glomerulonephritis). *Diuretic drugs* may also be given to improve urine flow and rid the body of excess fluid. In many cases of acute failure, temporary *dialysis* (artificial methods of removing waste products from the blood) may be required until the kidneys recover their function.

Dietary treatment is an important part of the treatment of all types of kidney failure. The diet must be high in carbohydrates and low in protein (the main source of waste products) to reduce the work load on the kidneys; the salt content must also be controlled. Fluid intake is carefully balanced against urine output. If the patient has been taking certain drugs (whose breakdown products are removed from the blood by the kidneys), use of these drugs may be stopped or their dosages reduced.

If hypertension develops, drugs are prescribed to keep the blood pressure under control. In end-stage kidney failure, long-term dialysis or, ideally, a *kidney transplant* is the only satisfactory form of treatment.

OUTLOOK
The outlook varies according to the cause of the failure and the patient's response to treatment. Most people eventually make a full recovery, but some require a transplant or lifelong dialysis. In chronic failure, it may be several years before such measures are required. Well over half the people with end-stage kidney failure that is treated by dialysis are able to lead comparatively normal lives for more than five years; a successful kidney transplant improves the outlook.

Kidney function tests
Tests performed to investigate urinary symptoms and kidney disorders. Kidney function tests may also be performed as part of a routine investigation before major surgery, or before prescribing drugs that are eliminated by the kidneys. The tests are also performed to determine the function of a transplanted kidney.

TYPES
Urinalysis is a simple kidney function test. Collected urine is examined under the microscope for blood cells, pus cells, and casts (cells and mucous material that accumulate within the tubules and pass into the urine). Urine may also be cultured to confirm the presence of infection, and may also be tested for substances, such as proteins, that are present only when the kidneys are diseased or damaged.

Kidney function can be assessed by measuring the concentration of substances in the blood (such as *urea* and creatinine) normally eliminated from the body via healthy kidneys. The creatinine clearance test provides an assessment of kidney function by comparing the amount of creatinine in the blood with the amount excreted in the urine over a timed interval, usually 24 hours.

Kidney function may also be assessed by *kidney imaging* techniques, which can help identify whether one or both kidneys are diseased.

Kidney imaging
Techniques for visualizing the kidneys, usually performed for diagnostic purposes.

TYPES
Ultrasound scanning provides remarkably clear pictures of the kidney. It can show an enlarged kidney, indicate the site of any blockage, and show the presence of a cyst or other tumor.

Conventional *X rays* show the outlines of the kidney and most kidney stones. Intravenous *urography* (in which a radiopaque contrast medium is injected into a vein) gives a good picture of the internal anatomy of the kidney and ureters, as well as the presence of stones.

Angiography involves injecting a radiopaque substance into the renal arteries or veins to demonstrate the kidneys' blood supply. When a radiopaque substance is injected into the arteries, the technique is known as arteriography. Digital subtraction angiography permits imaging of the renal circulation with less contrast medium and greater safety.

CT scanning provides a complete cross section of the kidney displayed as computerized X ray pictures. This is particularly useful for showing abscesses or tumors.

Radionuclide scanning is cheaper than conventional X rays and exposes the patient to less radiation. The two types usually used for the kidney are the DMSA scan and the DTPA scan. DMSA is a substance given by intravenous injection that binds to the cells of the kidney tubules and gives a single static picture of the kidneys, indicating their relative size, shape, position, and function. DTPA, also given intravenously, is filtered by the glomeruli and passes out in the urine. Pictures are taken at intervals to record its passage through the renal tract. DTPA provides similar information to that provided by the intravenous urogram, although the anatomical details are less clear.

Kidney, polycystic
An inherited disorder in which there are numerous cysts in both *kidneys*. The cysts gradually increase in size until most of the normal kidney tissue is destroyed; cysts may also occur in the liver and, rarely, in other organs. Polycystic kidney disease is distinguished from multiple simple cysts of the kidneys, which occur commonly with age (see *Kidney cyst*).

TYPES
ADULT POLYCYSTIC DISEASE This disorder shows an autosomal dominant pattern of inheritance (see *Genetic disorders*). Symptoms, which may appear at any time (but usually appear in middle age), include abdominal swelling, pain, and *hematuria* (blood in the urine). As the disease progresses, *hypertension* (high blood pressure) and *kidney failure* may result. The kidneys are replaced by very large numbers of small cysts.

JUVENILE POLYCYSTIC DISEASE This rare disorder causes *kidney failure* in infants and young children. It is usually diagnosed at birth because of massive enlargement of the kidneys. Juvenile polycystic disease shows an autosomal recessive pattern of inheritance.

TREATMENT
There is no effective treatment for preserving kidney function in polycystic kidney disease. Symptoms of kidney failure can be treated by *dialysis* (artificial purification of the blood) and *kidney transplant*.

Kidney stone
See *Calculus, urinary tract*.

K

K

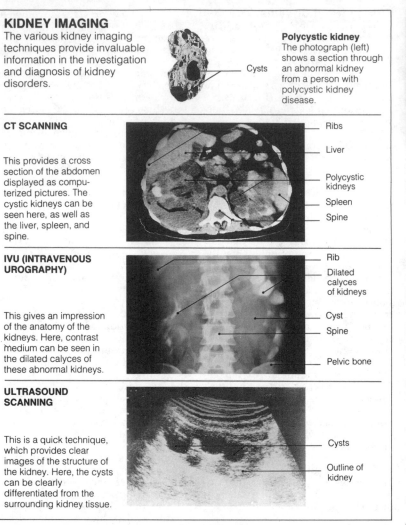

KIDNEY IMAGING
The various kidney imaging techniques provide invaluable information in the investigation and diagnosis of kidney disorders.

Cysts

Polycystic kidney
The photograph (left) shows a section through an abnormal kidney from a person with polycystic kidney disease.

CT SCANNING

This provides a cross section of the abdomen displayed as computerized pictures. The cystic kidneys can be seen here, as well as the liver, spleen, and spine.

Ribs
Liver
Polycystic kidneys
Spleen
Spine

IVU (INTRAVENOUS UROGRAPHY)

This gives an impression of the anatomy of the kidneys. Here, contrast medium can be seen in the dilated calyces of these abnormal kidneys.

Rib
Dilated calyces of kidneys
Cyst
Spine
Pelvic bone

ULTRASOUND SCANNING

This is a quick technique, which provides clear images of the structure of the kidney. Here, the cysts can be clearly differentiated from the surrounding kidney tissue.

Cysts
Outline of kidney

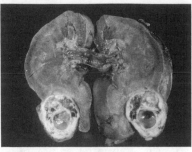

Example of a kidney tumor
A malignant tumor of one kidney (sliced in half). Surgical removal of a malignant kidney tumor is always necessary.

Kidney transplant
An operation in which the function of a diseased kidney in a person who has chronic *kidney failure* is replaced by a transplanted healthy kidney, either from a living donor (a donor's health is not adversely affected by losing one kidney) or a cadaver. About 13 percent of kidney transplants in Canada are from living donors. One healthy donor kidney is sufficient to maintain the health of the recipient.

Kidney transplantation is more straightforward than the transplantation of any other major organ and is by far the most commonly performed. Furthermore, the failure of a kidney transplant is much less serious than failure of a heart, liver, or lung transplant because kidney function can be taken over by *dialysis* (artificial purification of the blood).

HOW IT IS DONE
For a description of a kidney transplant operation, see facing page.
OUTLOOK
Kidney transplants are successful in more than 80 percent of cases. This figure rises to more than 90 percent if the donor is a close blood relative. The chief danger is rejection of the donated kidney within the first month or two after transplantation. If the kidney is rejected, the patient returns to dialysis. Further transplants may be attempted if the patient is otherwise in good health. All kidney transplant patients must take *immunosuppressant drugs* for life to prevent rejection.

Kidney tumors
Growths of the kidney. Kidney tumors may be malignant (see *Kidney cancer*) or benign.

Fibromas, lipomas, and *leiomyomas* (which are benign) often cause no symptoms and are sometimes discovered only during kidney surgery performed for another cause. A kidney may be the site of a *hemangioma* (a benign tumor composed of a collection of blood vessels), which may grow very large and may cause blood to appear in the urine; a kidney hemangioma is sometimes mistaken for cancer.

No treatment is necessary for benign tumors unless they are very large or cause pain or bleeding.

Kilocalorie
The unit of energy equal to 1,000 *calories,* sometimes abbreviated to kcal. In dietetics, a kilocalorie is sometimes called simply a Calorie (or C).

Kilojoule
The unit of energy equal to 1,000 *joules,* abbreviated to kJ. One kcal equals 4.2 kJ.

Kiss of life
A commonly used name for *artificial respiration.*

Kleptomania
A recurring inability to resist impulses to steal objects that are not necessarily wanted or needed. The condition is rare, although it is often used by shoplifters and other thieves as an excuse for stealing.

In true kleptomania, the person experiences an increasing sense of tension before committing the act of theft and then a sense of relief or pleasure while carrying it out. The act is not preplanned and little thought is given to the consequences, although later the person may suffer from anxiety and depression caused by fear of being caught.

PROCEDURE FOR A KIDNEY TRANSPLANT

The donated kidney comes from a close (living) blood relative of the patient or from any person who consented to medical use of organs after death (cadaver transplant). To prevent rejection of the kidney by the recipient's *immune system*, the tissue-type and blood group of recipient and donor must be a close match (see *Transplant surgery*).

HOW IT IS DONE

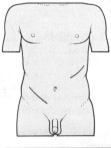

Removal
The kidney is removed via an incision under the ribs.

Insertion
The donor kidney is inserted low in the pelvis.

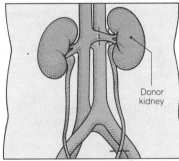

Donor kidney

1 Usually the left kidney is removed from living donors because it has a longer vein than the right and is easier to remove safely. After removal, the kidney is flushed with saline solution.

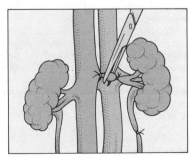

2 The surgeon may remove one or both of the patient's kidneys. Before removing a kidney, it is necessary first to clamp and cut the renal blood vessels that supply the kidney. The ureter must also be clamped and cut.

DIALYSIS AND TRANSPLANTATION IN CANADA

A significant proportion of new patients with end-stage kidney failure are suitable for a kidney transplant, but many have to remain on dialysis for some time until a suitable donor kidney becomes available. In Canada, about 13 percent of donated kidneys are from living donors. The chart shows the number of patients on dialysis and the number receiving transplants in selected years.

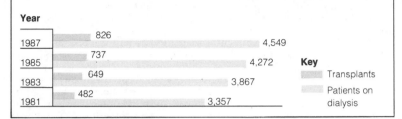

Year

Year	Transplants	Patients on dialysis
1987	826	4,549
1985	737	4,272
1983	649	3,867
1981	482	3,357

Key
▨ Transplants
▨ Patients on dialysis

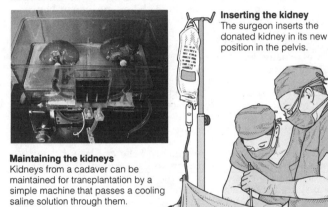

Maintaining the kidneys
Kidneys from a cadaver can be maintained for transplantation by a simple machine that passes a cooling saline solution through them.

Inserting the kidney
The surgeon inserts the donated kidney in its new position in the pelvis.

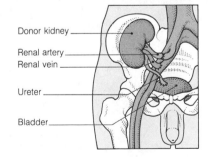

Donor kidney

Renal artery

Renal vein

Ureter

Bladder

3 The donor kidney is usually placed in the pelvis. The renal artery and vein of the donor kidney are joined to the recipient's artery and vein, and the lower end of the donor ureter is connected to the recipient's bladder. The clamps are then removed.

THE DONOR (AFTER THE OPERATION)

The health of the donor is not affected by losing one kidney; the remaining kidney enlarges to take over full function.

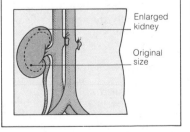

Enlarged kidney

Original size

K

Kleptomania is usually a sign of an immature personality. It may also be caused by *dementia* or result from some forms of brain damage.

Klinefelter's syndrome

A *chromosomal abnormality* in which a male has one or more extra X *chromosomes* in his cells, giving him a chromosome complement of XXY or, more rarely, XXXY, XXXXY, and so on (instead of XY). Klinefelter's syndrome affects about one in every 500 male infants born. The chances of a baby having the condition increase with the age of the mother.

SYMPTOMS AND SIGNS
The features of Klinefelter's syndrome vary in severity. Often the condition passes unnoticed until puberty, when *gynecomastia* (breast enlargement) occurs and the testes remain small. Affected males are usually infertile due to *azoospermia* (absence of sperm production).

Victims are usually tall and thin, and the body shape looks female rather than male. The incidence of *mental retardation* is higher in people with Klinefelter's syndrome than in the general population.

DIAGNOSIS AND TREATMENT
Diagnosis is confirmed by *chromosome analysis*. There is no cure for Klinefelter's syndrome. Mastectomy may be performed if gynecomastia causes psychological distress. Hormonal treatment may be used to induce secondary *sexual characteristics*, such as growth of facial hair. Parents who have had an affected child should receive *genetic counseling*.

Klumpke's paralysis
Paralysis of the lower arm, with wasting of the small muscles in the hand and numbness of the fingers (excluding the thumb) and of the inside of the forearm.

Klumpke's paralysis is caused by injury to the first thoracic nerve (one of the *spinal nerves*) in the brachial plexus (the network of nerves behind the shoulder blade); injury to this nerve is usually the result of dislocation of the shoulder.

Knee
The joint between the *femur* (thighbone) and *tibia* (shin). The *patella* (kneecap) lies across the front of the joint. The knee is a modified hinge *joint*, which is capable of bending, straightening, and slight rotation in the bent position.

STRUCTURE
Two disks of protective cartilage called menisci (see *Meniscus*) cover the surfaces of the femur and tibia. These disks reduce friction between the bones during movement and also increase the stability of the knee. The joint is partly surrounded by a fibrous capsule lined with synovial membrane, which secretes a fluid that allows the cartilage to move freely.

Strong *ligaments* on each side of the joint provide support and limit side-to-side movement. *Cruciate ligaments* within the joint, which cross over each other as they run diagonally between the femur and tibia, provide additional support, prevent overbending and overstraightening of the knee, and limit sliding movement between the bones. Bursas (fluid-filled sacs) are present above and below the patella and behind the knee. The *quadriceps muscles* (which run along the front of the thigh) straighten the knee; the *hamstring muscles* at the back of the thigh bend the knee.

DISORDERS
Sudden twisting of the knee may cause a ligament sprain or tear a meniscus. If a meniscus is torn and a fragment of the cartilage catches between the surfaces of the joint, the knee may become temporarily locked in one position.

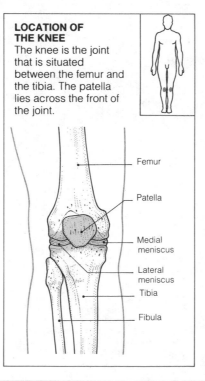

LOCATION OF THE KNEE
The knee is the joint that is situated between the femur and the tibia. The patella lies across the front of the joint.

Femur

Patella

Medial meniscus

Lateral meniscus

Tibia

Fibula

Severe damage to a joint, often as the result of a sports injury, may cause *hemarthrosis* (bleeding into the joint); minor injuries may lead to *synovitis* (inflammation of the joint lining). Repetitive activity, such as running, may cause inflammation of the tendon below the patella. Children may suffer from *Osgood-Schlatter disease*, in which the bony tibial tuberosity (the bony prominence below the knee) becomes temporarily inflamed.

Bursitis (inflammation of a bursa) usually occurs in response to local pressure on the front of the knee. Fluid escaping from a bursa behind the knee causes a *Baker's cyst*.

Arthritic conditions most likely to affect the knee are *osteoarthritis, rheumatoid arthritis,* and retropatellar arthritis (inflammation of the undersurface of the patella). A condition similar to retropatellar arthritis, known as *chondromalacia patellae* or anterior knee pain, is common in adolescents.

Fractures of the lower femur, upper tibia, or the patella disrupt normal movement of the knee. A blow to the knee may result in *dislocation* of the patella. *Knock-knee* and *bowleg*, common deformities in childhood, usually disappear with growth; in adults, these deformities may be caused by injury or disease.

Knee joint replacement
A surgical procedure to replace a diseased *knee* joint with an artificial substitute. Early replacement knees were simply large hinges. Today, most artificial knees take the form of metal and plastic implants that cover the worn cartilage. The aim of modern knee joint replacement operations is generally to preserve as much of the original joint as possible.

WHY IT IS DONE
Knee joint replacement is most often carried out in older people whose knees are severely affected by pain and impaired motion due to *osteoarthritis* or *rheumatoid arthritis*. An artificial knee is not normally recommended for younger patients because it does not restore the full range of movements and is unlikely to withstand vigorous activity.

RECOVERY PERIOD
The plaster *cast* fitted after the operation is usually removed after five days and a program of exercises is started to strengthen the *quadriceps muscles*. The patient can normally put some weight on the leg after two or three weeks.

K

PROCEDURE FOR A KNEE REPLACEMENT

The surgeon usually makes one long incision, cuts through the joint capsule and synovial membrane, and then pushes aside the patella to reach the joint. Special instruments are used to make precise measurements and to cut away areas of bone so that the artificial knee replacement components will fit and move correctly.

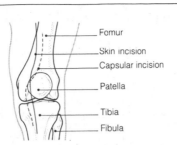

Fomur
Skin incision
Capsular incision
Patella
Tibia
Fibula

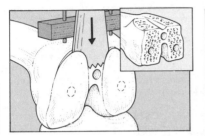

1 The lower end of the femur (thighbone) is shaped and holes are drilled into it to accept the femoral component of the prosthesis. Cutting and drilling bones are carried out using special orthopedic instruments.

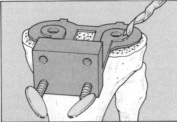

2 The upper end of the tibia (shin bone) is shaped and holes are drilled into it to accept the tibial component of the prosthesis. The cutting and drilling are again carried out using special orthopedic instruments.

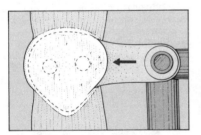

3 The back part of the patella is cut away to leave a flat surface. Small holes are then drilled into this surface to accept the patellar component of the artificial joint.

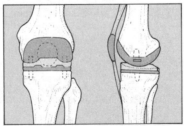

4 Having achieved a satisfactory fit using trial components, the final prosthesis is cemented in place. Excess cement is then removed and a final check is made of the joint movements.

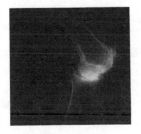

X ray of arthritic knee
Severe wear and tear of the bone and cartilage can easily be seen on this knee X ray.

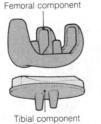

Femoral component
Tibial component

Knee prosthesis
The two main artificial knee components fit over the femur and tibia.

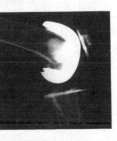

X ray of artificial knee
This X ray shows the components of the prosthesis in position after surgery.

OUTLOOK

Although knee joint replacements can relieve pain and restore some degree of movement, results of replacement are often uncertain and the durability of the artificial parts is limited. However, research continues into the development of stronger materials, better cements (glues), and better joint designs.

Knock-knee

Inward curving of the legs so that the knees touch, causing the feet to be kept farther apart than would otherwise be the case. The condition is known medically as genu valgum.

CAUSES

Knock-knee is a part of normal development in some children and is common between the ages of 3 and 5 years. It may also be the result of injury or disease. Among the common causes are diseases that soften the bones (such as *rickets* or *osteomalacia*), *rheumatoid arthritis* or *osteoarthritis* of the knee, or a fracture of the lower *femur* (thighbone) or upper *tibia* (shin) that has not healed in a straight, vertical line.

TREATMENT

In children, knock-knee usually requires no treatment unless it persists after the age of 10, when it may start to strain the joints of the lower leg. Wearing heel wedges in the shoes may help correct the line of the leg, but most people require *osteotomy*, an operation in which the tibia is cut and realigned to straighten the leg.

In adults, treatment consists of osteotomy, or, when the condition has been present for a considerable time, *knee-joint replacement*.

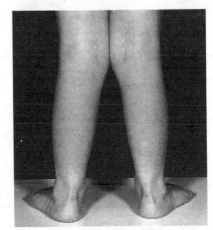

The appearance of knock-knee
This condition is common in toddlers but nearly always disappears by the age of 7.

K

K

Knuckle

The common name for a *finger* joint.

Koilonychia

A condition in which the *nails* are dry, brittle, and thin, eventually becoming concave (spoon-shaped). Koilonychia may be caused by injury to the nail; koilonychia of the toenails is very common in countries where shoes are not worn. Other causes include iron deficiency *anemia* and *lichen planus*; rarely, the condition is inherited.

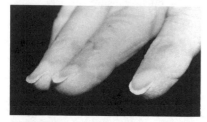

The appearance of koilonychia
In koilonychia, the nails are flattened and look fragile, bending where they protrude past the finger ends.

Koplik's spots

Tiny, gray-white spots within the mouth (on the inner lining of the cheeks) that appear during the incubation period of *measles*. If they are identified, the physician can diagnose measles before the main rash appears.

Korsakoff's psychosis

See *Wernicke-Korsakoff syndrome*.

Kraurosis vulvae

See *Vulvitis*.

Kuru

A progressive and fatal infection of the *brain* that affects some inhabitants of the highlands of New Guinea. Kuru is caused by a virus spread by cannibalism. The condition is now rare.

The disease is caused by a "slow" virus (which causes no signs of disease until many months or years after entry into the body) and the incubation period may be as long as 30 years. Symptoms include progressive difficulty in controlling movements and, eventually, *dementia*.

Kuru has aroused special interest recently because of certain similarities between the causative virus and *HIV* (the virus that causes *AIDS*). It is known that HIV can cause brain changes similar to those in kuru.

Kwashiorkor

A severe type of malnutrition in young children, occurring mainly in poor rural areas in the tropics. Kwashiorkor is chiefly confined to children between 1 and 3 years old.

The term kwashiorkor is derived from a Ghanaian word meaning "disease suffered by a child displaced from the breast."

CAUSES

The illness starts when the child is suddenly weaned onto a diet that is low in calories, protein, and certain essential micronutrients such as zinc, selenium, and vitamins A and E. The problem is often exacerbated by a poor appetite due to illness. Measles and other infections common in the tropics precipitate kwashiorkor in undernourished children.

SYMPTOMS AND SIGNS

Children with kwashiorkor have stunted growth, and a puffy appearance due to *edema* (accumulation of fluid in the tissues). Affected children are apathetic, weak, irritable, and inactive. Their skin sometimes flakes off, leaving a raw, weeping area beneath, and their hair may lose its curliness, become sparse and brittle, and turn from dark to fair.

The victim's liver often enlarges, dehydration may develop (despite the simultaneous presence of edema), and the child loses resistance against severe infection, which may be fatal. In its severe, advanced stage, the illness is often marked by jaundice, drowsiness, and a fall in the patient's body temperature.

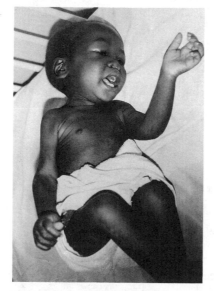

The appearance of kwashiorkor
This small child has a puffy face and legs, is listless, and has sparse hair, all of which are typical features of kwashiorkor.

TREATMENT

The priorities in severe cases are to keep the child warm, replace lost fluids, and treat any infection. Initially, the child is fed milk (in frequent small amounts) and, if possible, vitamin and mineral tablets. Zinc is given to prevent flaking of the skin. When the edema has disappeared and the child's appetite has returned, a high-calorie, protein-rich diet is given.

OUTLOOK

Most children treated for kwashiorkor recover, but those less than 2 years old are likely to suffer permanent stunting of growth. (See also *Marasmus*.)

Kyphoscoliosis

A combination of *kyphosis* (abnormal backward curvature of the spine) and *scoliosis* (curvature of the spine to one side or the other).

Kyphosis

The medical term for excessive backward curvature of the spine. Kyphosis usually affects the spine at the top of the back, resulting in either a hump or a more gradually rounded back. Less commonly, it affects normally forward-curving parts of the spine at the neck and lower back.

Kyphosis may be caused by any of a variety of spinal disorders, including *osteoporosis* (thinning of bone due to calcium loss), fracture of a vertebra, or a tumor of a vertebra (see *Spine* disorders box). In the past, the main cause of kyphosis was spinal *tuberculosis*. Treatment, which is rarely successful, is of the underlying disorder.

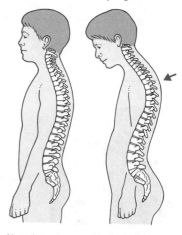

Normal curvature   Kyphosis of the thoracic spine

The appearance of kyphosis
In kyphosis, the thoracic part of the spine is excessively curved, producing a humped (rounded) appearance.

L

Labetalol

A *beta-blocker drug* used to treat *hypertension* (high blood pressure) and *angina pectoris* (chest pain caused by impaired blood supply to the heart).

Possible adverse effects include indigestion, nausea, and, in rare cases, depression and temporary impotence. Because labetalol may also mask the body's response to low blood sugar, it is prescribed with caution to diabetics. It is less likely than some other beta-blocker drugs to cause leg cramps or coldness of the hands and feet.

Labia

The lips of the *vulva* (the female external genitalia) that protect the vaginal and urethral openings. There are two pairs of labia. The outer pair, called the labia majora, are fleshy folds that bear hair and contain sweat glands. The labia majora cover the smaller, hairless inner folds, called the labia minora, which meet to form the hood of the *clitoris*.

Labile

Unstable; likely to undergo change. Vitamins are labile because they are broken down easily by such factors as heat and excess acidity. Blood pressure that has a tendency to fluctuate may be described as labile. In psychiatry, the term is sometimes used to mean emotional instability.

Labor

See *Childbirth*.

Laboratory technologist

A person trained in a school of laboratory technology, who carries out laboratory tests that produce the data necessary for physicians to diagnose, monitor, and treat disease.

Labyrinthitis

Inflammation of the labyrinth (the fluid-filled chambers in the inner *ear* concerned with balance) causing *vertigo*, a sensation that one or one's surroundings are spinning around.

CAUSES

Labyrinthitis is almost always caused by bacterial or viral infection. Viral labyrinthitis may occur during a flu-like illness or during illnesses such as measles or mumps. Bacterial labyrinthitis is commonly caused by inadequately treated *otitis media* (infection of the middle ear), particularly if a *cholesteatoma* (an infected collection of debris in the middle ear) has developed and eroded a pathway into the inner ear. Infection may also reach the inner ear (via the bloodstream) from elsewhere in the body. Less commonly, bacterial labyrinthitis results from a head injury.

SYMPTOMS

As well as vertigo, labyrinthitis may cause nausea, vomiting, *nystagmus* (abnormal jerky movements of the eye), *tinnitus* (ringing in the ears), and hearing loss.

TREATMENT

Viral labyrinthitis clears up on its own, but symptoms are relieved by *antihistamine drugs* such as meclozine. Bacterial labyrinthitis requires immediate treatment with *antibiotic drugs*; otherwise the infection may lead to permanent *deafness* or spread to cause *meningitis* (inflammation of the *meninges*, the membranes that cover the brain and spinal cord).

Surgery may be necessary to drain pus from the ear or to remove any cholesteatoma.

Laceration

A torn, irregular wound, as opposed to an *incision*, which is a straight cut. One example of a laceration is the tearing of the perineum (the area between the vagina and anus) that sometimes occurs during childbirth.

LOCATION OF THE LABIA
The labia majora extend forward from the perineum and fuse at the front at the mons pubis. The labia minora lie within.

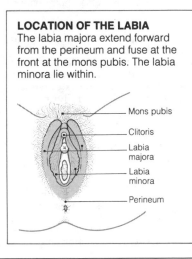

- Mons pubis
- Clitoris
- Labia majora
- Labia minora
- Perineum

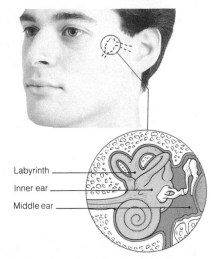

Labyrinth
Inner ear
Middle ear

Mechanism of labyrinthitis
In labyrinthitis, inflammation of the fluid-filled chambers (labyrinth) of the inner ear causes disruption of the individual's sense of balance. The inflammation is usually caused by viral or bacterial infection.

Lacrimal apparatus

The system that produces and drains *tears*, primarily needed to keep the *cornea* and conjunctiva constantly moist, and which also wash away small foreign bodies. The lacrimal apparatus includes the main and accessory lacrimal glands and the nasolacrimal drainage ducts. The main glands secrete tears during crying and when the eye is irritated; the accessory glands maintain the normal tear film.

The main lacrimal glands lie just within the upper and outer margin of the orbit and drain into the *conjunctiva* (the transparent membrane covering the white of the eye and the inside of the eyelids). The accessory glands lie within the conjunctiva, secreting directly onto its surface.

Tears sweep across the front of the eye, and drain through the lacrimal puncta, tiny openings toward the inner end of each eyelid. The puncta are connected by narrow tubes to the lacrimal sacs, which lie in shallow hollows in the lacrimal bones. These bones are situated just within the inner margin of the orbit on either side of the nose. Overlying the lacrimal sacs are flat muscles that compress the sacs during blinking. Leading from the sacs are the nasolacrimal ducts, which run down through the bone to open inside the nose.

The action of blinking sucks away excess fluid by compressing and releasing the lacrimal sacs.

L

FUNCTIONS OF THE LACRIMAL APPARATUS

Tear production must be sufficient to compensate for evaporation and maintain the tear film. Accessory lacrimal glands in the conjunctiva perform this function. The main lacrimal glands secrete when excess fluid is required. Surplus tears drain into the nose.

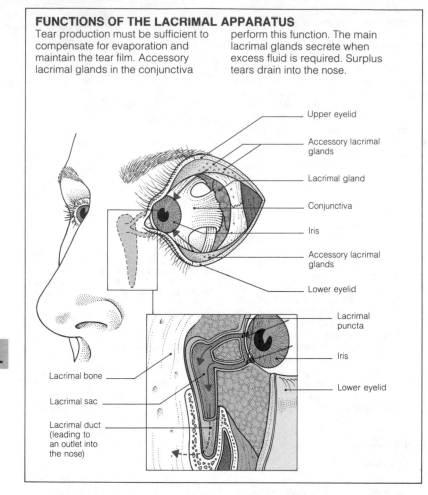

Upper eyelid

Accessory lacrimal glands

Lacrimal gland

Conjunctiva

Iris

Accessory lacrimal glands

Lower eyelid

Lacrimal puncta

Iris

Lower eyelid

Lacrimal bone

Lacrimal sac

Lacrimal duct (leading to an outlet into the nose)

Lactase deficiency

A condition in which lactase, an *enzyme* that is normally present in cells of the small intestine and which breaks down lactose (milk sugar), is missing. Lactase deficiency results in a reduced ability to digest lactose.

Lactase deficiency may be present at birth, may develop immediately after weaning, or may not become evident until puberty or later.

Congenital lactase deficiency is sometimes permanent but is more often temporary. It is caused by delayed enzyme maturation, and occurs especially in premature babies.

Permanent lactase deficiency develops in about 80 to 90 percent of blacks and Orientals and in about 5 to 15 percent of whites. Lactase deficiency may also occur as a complication of intestinal diseases (including *celiac disease* and *gastroenteritis*); in such cases, the deficiency often disappears as the disease improves.

SYMPTOMS, DIAGNOSIS, AND TREATMENT
Undigested lactose ferments in the intestine and causes severe abdominal cramps, bloating, flatulence, and diarrhea; weight loss and malnutrition may also occur.

The diagnosis can be confirmed by tests on blood and feces. Treatment is a lactose-free diet; milk must be avoided but fermented milk products, such as yogurt, can be eaten. Enzyme replacements (which break down lactose either partially or fully) may be used in some cases.

Lactation

The production and secretion of milk after childbirth. (See *Breast-feeding*.)

Lactic acid

A weak acid produced when cells break down glucose by anaerobic metabolism (chemical processes that do not require oxygen) to produce energy. Anaerobic metabolism occurs only when there is too little oxygen for the more usual aerobic metabolism (chemical processes requiring oxygen). For example, lactic acid is produced by muscles during vigorous exercise and is one of the factors that contribute to *cramp*. Lactic acid is also produced in tissues when they receive insufficient oxygen due to impairment of their blood supply in a *myocardial infarction* (heart attack) or *shock*.

Normally, lactic acid is removed from the blood by the *liver*; if lactic acid accumulates, lactic *acidosis* results.

Lactose

One of the sugars present in milk. Chemically, lactose is a disaccharide *carbohydrate*, a sugar made up of two monosaccharide (simple sugar) units.

Lactose is broken down by lactase (an *enzyme* released by the lining of the small intestine) into the monosaccharides glucose and galactose, which are then absorbed into the bloodstream. People with *lactase deficiency* have a reduced ability to digest lactose.

Lactose intolerance

The inability to digest lactose (milk sugar). Lactose intolerance may be caused by a deficiency of lactase, an enzyme found in the small intestine (see *Lactase deficiency*). Rarely, lactose intolerance occurs in a person who is not deficient in lactase.

Lactulose

A *laxative drug* used to treat *constipation* and *liver failure*. Lactulose causes water to be absorbed into the feces from the intestinal blood vessels, making the feces easier to pass. It is useful in the treatment of liver failure because it helps eliminate ammonia from the blood into the feces.

Lambliasis

Another name for *giardiasis*.

Laminectomy

Surgical removal of part or all of one or more laminae (the bony arches of the *vertebrae*) to expose the *spinal cord*. Laminectomy is performed as the first stage of spinal canal decompression, an operation carried out to relieve pressure on the spinal cord or on a nerve root leading from it (see *Decompression, spinal canal*).
HOW IT IS DONE
An incision is made in the patient's back and the laminae are exposed. Enough of one or more adjacent laminae is then chipped away to give the surgeon access to the cord. Rarely,

L

several complete laminae must be removed. In this case, *spinal fusion* (immobilization of the spine with metal rods or bone grafts) may then be necessary to prevent subsequent instability of the spine.

Lance
To incise (cut) using a *lancet* or a surgical scalpel.

Lancet
A small, pointed, double-edged knife used to open and drain lesions such as boils and abscesses.

Language disorders
Problems affecting the ability to communicate and/or comprehend the spoken and written word. See *Speech*; *Speech disorders*.

Lanolin
A mixture of a yellow, oily substance obtained from sheep's wool and purified water, used as an *emollient* in the treatment of dry skin. Lanolin is a common ingredient of bath oils and hand creams; it is also used to treat mild *dermatitis*. Occasionally, lanolin may cause an allergic reaction.

Lanugo hair
Fine, soft, downy hair that covers a *fetus*. Lanugo hair first appears in the fourth or fifth month of gestation and usually disappears by the ninth month. It can still be seen in some premature babies.

Lanugo hair sometimes reappears in adults who have cancer, particularly of the breast, bladder, lung, or large intestine. It may also occur in people with *anorexia nervosa* or be a side effect of certain drugs (especially *cyclosporine*).

Laparoscopy
A method of directly examining the interior of the abdomen by means of a laparoscope, a type of *endoscope* (viewing instrument).

WHY IT IS DONE
Laparoscopy is usually performed to determine the cause of pelvic pain or gynecological symptoms (such as suspected *ectopic pregnancy* or *pelvic inflammatory disease*) that cannot be confirmed by physical examination. It is frequently used to examine the condition of the fallopian tubes when investigating cases of *infertility*. Laparoscopy can also be used to examine the appendix, gallbladder, and liver. In cases of female *sterilization*, the procedure is usually performed using a laparoscope.

Laparotomy
An operation in which the abdomen is opened to look for the cause of an undiagnosed illness. Laparotomy strictly describes any abdominal surgery because, even when the surgeon is operating to treat a known disorder, a thorough examination of the entire abdomen is carried out.

Laparotomy is now performed less commonly than formerly because of the availability of diagnostic procedures such as *CT scanning*, *ultrasound scanning*, and *laparoscopy*.

WHY IT IS DONE
Laparotomy is usually performed when other diagnostic procedures have failed to reveal the cause of a patient's symptoms and signs. Common reasons for performing laparotomy include recurrent abdominal pain and *peritonitis* (infection within the abdominal cavity). Laparotomy may also be performed as an emergency procedure if the abdomen has been seriously injured in an accident.

HOW IT IS DONE
An incision is made in the abdomen and the abdominal cavity is opened and explored for signs of disease. Any diseased organs are repaired or removed, after which the incision is sewn up.

The recovery period depends upon the nature and extent of the disease discovered and treated.

Larva migrans
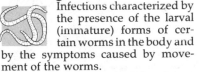
Infections characterized by the presence of the larval (immature) forms of certain worms in the body and by the symptoms caused by movement of the worms.

Visceral larva migrans, better known as *toxocariasis*, is caused by a type of worm that normally parasitizes dogs. Cutaneous larva migrans is caused by larvae of species of hookworm that normally parasitize dogs, cats, or other animals. Also known as creeping eruption, cutaneous larva migrans is contracted by walking barefoot on soil or sand contaminated with animal feces. The larvae pene-

L

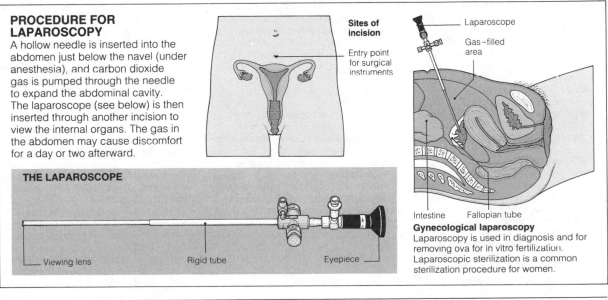

PROCEDURE FOR LAPAROSCOPY
A hollow needle is inserted into the abdomen just below the navel (under anesthesia), and carbon dioxide gas is pumped through the needle to expand the abdominal cavity. The laparoscope (see below) is then inserted through another incision to view the internal organs. The gas in the abdomen may cause discomfort for a day or two afterward.

Sites of incision

Entry point for surgical instruments

Laparoscope

Gas-filled area

Intestine　　Fallopian tube

Gynecological laparoscopy
Laparoscopy is used in diagnosis and for removing ova for in vitro fertilization. Laparoscopic sterilization is a common sterilization procedure for women.

THE LAPAROSCOPE

Viewing lens　　　Rigid tube　　　Eyepiece

LOCATION OF LARYNGEAL NERVES

Both nerves leave the brain at the base of the skull and pass down the neck. One hooks around an artery behind the right clavicle, the other hooks around the aorta; both return to the larynx.

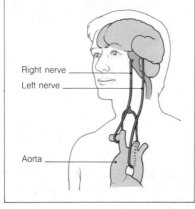

Right nerve
Left nerve
Aorta

trate the skin of the feet and move randomly, leaving intensely itchy red lines which are sometimes accompanied by blistering.

Both types of larva migrans can be treated with *anthelmintic drugs*.

Laryngeal nerve

One of a pair of nerves that carry instructions from the brain to the *larynx* (voice box) and send sensations from the larynx to the brain. Each nerve leaves the brain through a hole in the base of the skull and passes down the neck.

The right laryngeal nerve then hooks around an artery behind the right clavicle (collarbone) before returning to the larynx. The left laryngeal nerve travels farther, eventually hooking around the aorta (the major artery leaving the heart) before it too passes back to the larynx.

Damage to one or both nerves causes *vocal cord* paralysis, resulting in loss of voice and sometimes obstruction to breathing.

Laryngectomy

Surgical removal of all or part of the *larynx* (voice box) to treat advanced cancer of the larynx (see *Larynx, cancer of*). After the operation, the patient is unable to speak in the usual fashion.

WHY IT IS DONE

If cancer of the larynx is detected early, the prospects of curing it with *radiation therapy* are good. However, large tumors require surgery.

HOW IT IS DONE

With the patient under general anesthesia, an incision is made in the neck and the larynx is removed. The top of the trachea (windpipe) immediately below the larynx is then sewn to the skin around the surgical wound in the neck to form a permanent opening called a stoma, through which the patient will breathe from then on.

RECOVERY PERIOD

Immediately after the operation, a bell or buzzer and pen and paper are given to the patient so that he or she can communicate. A tube is left in the stoma for a few days so that, as the surrounding tissues heal, they do not close the opening. The air in the patient's room is humidified to reduce the production of mucus in the stoma, and any excess mucus is sucked away.

Initially, all food is passed through a thin tube running from the nose to the stomach. After about 10 days the feeding tube is removed and food (fluid or semisolid at first) can be taken normally again.

Speed of recovery depends on the patient's age and health and on whether preoperative radiation therapy has been given.

OUTLOOK

With persistence, the patient can learn from a speech therapist a new way of speaking (called esophageal speech). Air is swallowed, then expelled in a controlled way; this noise is modulated by the tongue, palate, and lips to form gruff, though distinguishable, words. The technique requires painstaking practice. Alternatively, the patient may use an electronic larynx, a device that emits a buzzing noise and is held against the top of the throat. By mouthing words, the person converts the buzz to speech.

Swimming is not possible after laryngectomy, and care must be taken when bathing.

Laryngitis

Inflammation of the *larynx* (voice box) usually caused by infection and resulting in *hoarseness*. Laryngitis may be acute, lasting only a few days, or chronic, persisting over a long period.

CAUSES

Acute laryngitis is usually caused by a viral infection, such as a cold, but it can also be due to an allergy to a drug, pollen, or some other substance.

Chronic laryngitis may be caused by overuse of the voice, by violent coughing, by irritation due to tobacco smoke, alcohol, or fumes, or by damage during surgery.

SYMPTOMS AND SIGNS

Hoarseness is the most common symptom and may progress to loss of voice. There may also be pain or a feeling of discomfort in the throat (especially during swallowing) and a dry, irritating cough. Laryngitis caused by a viral infection is often accompanied by fever and a general feeling of illness.

TREATMENT

A person with laryngitis should rest in bed, avoid tobacco and alcohol, keep the throat lining moist with humidifiers, and take drugs such as *acetaminophen*, which help to reduce fever and relieve pain.

If the symptoms do not subside within four or five days, if sputum (phlegm) is coughed up, or if hoarseness persists for several weeks, a physician should be consulted. *Antibiotic drugs* will be prescribed if there is a bacterial infection. If the physician suspects a cause other than infection, diagnostic tests may be required, possibly to check for signs of cancer (see *Larynx, cancer of*), which can be cured if treated at an early stage.

Laryngoscopy

Examination of the *larynx* (voice box) using a mirror held against the back of the palate (indirect laryngoscopy), or a viewing tube called a laryngoscope (direct laryngoscopy). A laryngoscope may be either rigid or flexible.

WHY IT IS DONE

The larynx is inspected when a person complains of persistent hoarseness or has other changes in the voice, when there is persistent stridor (a harsh noise when breathing in), or when someone has difficulty breathing in. Laryngoscopy is also used to examine people who have throat pain or difficulty in swallowing.

INDIRECT LARYNGOSCOPY This technique may be used to detect *laryngitis*, benign or malignant laryngeal tumors, and any reduction of movement in the vocal cords.

DIRECT LARYNGOSCOPY This technique allows the physician to inspect the larynx in greater detail than is possible with indirect laryngoscopy. It also allows more elaborate procedures to be performed, such as *biopsy* (removal of a sample of tissue for microscopic analysis), or removal of a foreign body or benign tumor. Direct laryngoscopy is also performed before *intubation*.

HOW IT IS DONE

Indirect and direct laryngoscopy procedures are shown in the illustrated box on facing page.

PROCEDURE FOR LARYNGOSCOPY

There are two techniques. In indirect laryngoscopy, the patient's throat is examined with the use of a mirror. In direct laryngoscopy, the patient's throat is viewed with an instrument called a laryngoscope. If a rigid laryngoscope is used, general anesthesia is required. Only mild sedation is needed if a flexible laryngoscope is used.

INDIRECT LARYNGOSCOPY

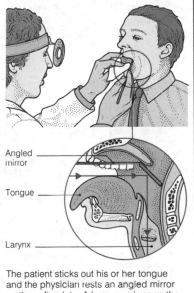

Angled mirror

Tongue

Larynx

The patient sticks out his or her tongue and the physician rests an angled mirror on the soft palate. A lamp or mirror on the physician's head illuminates the larynx, which is reflected in the mirror.

DIRECT LARYNGOSCOPY

Laryngo-scope

Larynx

A rigid laryngoscope is passed down the throat via the mouth; a flexible laryngoscope is passed via the nostril.

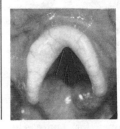

View of larynx
This view was obtained with a laryngoscope. The vocal cords (outlined in red) are at the center and the epiglottis forms the arc at the top.

LOCATION OF THE LARYNX

The larynx, commonly called the voice box, is situated deep in the throat between the pharynx and the trachea (windpipe).

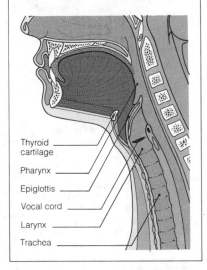

Thyroid cartilage

Pharynx

Epiglottis

Vocal cord

Larynx

Trachea

Laryngotracheobronchitis

Inflammation of the *larynx, trachea,* and *bronchi.* Laryngotracheobronchitis is caused by a virus in a quarter to a third of cases; in some other cases, a bacterial infection is involved. Laryngotracheobronchitis can be a mild disorder but can sometimes be life-threatening. It is a common cause of *croup* in young children.

Larynx

The organ in the throat responsible for voice production and for preventing food from entering the airway during swallowing. Its common name is the voice box.

STRUCTURE

The larynx, which lies between the *pharynx* (upper part of the airway) and the *trachea* (windpipe), forms part of the tube in the throat that carries air to and from the lungs. It consists of areas of cartilage (tough but flexible tissue), the largest of which is the thyroid cartilage, which projects at the front to form the Adam's apple. Below it, connecting the thyroid cartilage to the tra-

chea, is the cricoid cartilage, which is shaped like a signet ring with the seal at the back. Situated on top of the seal are the two pyramid-shaped arytenoid cartilages. Between them and the interior surface of the Adam's apple stretch two fibrous sheets of tissue, the *vocal cords.*

Attached to the top of the thyroid cartilage at the entrance to the larynx is the *epiglottis,* a leaf-shaped flap of cartilage that prevents food from entering the larynx during swallowing. The entire larynx is lined with *mucous membrane.*

FUNCTION

The most important function of the larynx is to prevent *choking.* When a person is not eating or drinking, the epiglottis stays upright, keeping the larynx open as part of the airway to the lungs; as soon as swallowing begins, the epiglottis drops like a lid over the larynx, directing food to either side. Closure of the vocal cords also helps protect the airway. The food or drink then passes down the *esophagus* to the stomach.

The secondary function of the larynx is voice production. Air from the lungs passes through the stretched vocal cords. The resultant vibrations are modified by the tongue, palate, and lips to produce *speech.*

Larynx, cancer of

A malignant tumor of the *larynx* (voice box), often causing persistent hoarseness. Laryngeal cancer represents about 2 percent of all cancers.

CAUSES AND INCIDENCE

The exact causes of laryngeal cancer are not known, but it occurs most commonly in heavy smokers. Laryngeal cancer is also associated with high alcohol consumption.

Laryngeal cancer primarily affects people over 60 and is more common in men than in women.

SYMPTOMS

Hoarseness is the main symptom, particularly when the tumor originates on the vocal cords. A tumor that develops elsewhere in the larynx often passes unnoticed until an advanced stage of the disease, when the tumor causes discomfort in the throat, difficulty in breathing and in swallowing, and the coughing up of blood.

DIAGNOSIS

Laryngoscopy (examination of the larynx with a viewing instrument) reveals any tumor on the larynx. A *biopsy* (removal of a sample of tissue

L

DISORDERS OF THE LARYNX

Disorders affecting the larynx (voice box) are common. They usually cause *hoarseness* because they interfere with the functioning of the vocal cords. Other symptoms include breathing difficulty, stridor (a harsh noise on breathing in), a painful throat, and coughing. Persistent hoarseness should be reported to a physician.

CONGENITAL DEFECTS

Rarely, a baby is born with a soft, limp larynx, a condition called laryngomalacia. The main signs are stridor and noisy breathing when feeding. The larynx usually attains a normal firmness by the age of 2.

INFLAMMATION

Laryngitis (inflammation of the larynx) is the most common laryngeal disorder in adults; symptoms are hoarseness, fever, and discomfort in the throat. In children, *croup* (inflammation and narrowing of the air passages) is very common up to the age of 4. Much rarer is *epiglottitis* (inflammation of the epiglottis, the flap of cartilage that closes the larynx during swallowing). This is a life-threatening disorder in young children.

TUMORS

Various kinds of benign growth may develop on the vocal cords. The most common is a polyp, a smooth swelling usually caused by smoking, by an infection such as influenza, or by straining the voice. Warts occasionally develop on a child's vocal cords. Both polyps and warts require removal and microscopic analysis to exclude cancer. *Singer's nodes* are small benign growths that can occur on the vocal cords of people who strain their voices. They give the voice a hoarse tone.

Malignant tumors, which cause persistent hoarseness, are usually caused by smoking and/or alcohol use (see *Larynx, cancer of*).

OTHER DISORDERS

A tumor, an infection, or, rarely, throat surgery can damage one or both of the nerves supplying the larynx, causing *vocal cord* paralysis, which results in loss of voice and may interfere with breathing.

INVESTIGATION

Disorders of the larynx are investigated by *laryngoscopy*. Sometimes a *biopsy* sample is taken for pathological analysis; X rays, especially *tomography*, may provide more information.

---

for microscopic analysis) is carried out in hospital under local or general anesthesia to determine whether the growth is benign or malignant, and also to find out whether or not the lining of the larynx shows any signs of early cancerous change.

TREATMENT

If the tumor is discovered when it is still small, the outcome is usually favorable. A small cancer of the *vocal cords* has about a 95 percent chance of cure. In these cases, *radiation therapy* or *laser treatment* may be used.

For larger tumors (and for those that do not respond to other treatment), partial or total *laryngectomy* (removal of the larynx) is considered unless the patient is frail or elderly. The cure rate of surgery varies according to the site and extent of the tumor. Any patient who has had a laryngectomy must master new techniques for producing speech.

If the tumor has spread throughout the larynx, or to other parts of the throat (or, rarely, other parts of the body), the patient is treated with radiation therapy and *anticancer drugs*. This combination relieves symptoms and often temporarily arrests the progress of the disease.

Laser

A device that produces a concentrated beam of light radiation; laser is an acronym for light amplification by stimulated emission of radiation. A laser beam is parallel, of a single specific wavelength (or sometimes of a narrow band of wavelengths), and coherent (that is, all the crests of the individual waves coincide).

Laser treatment

The use of a *laser* beam in a variety of medical procedures, for example to cut through tissue, seal small retinal tears, or destroy some tumors.

LOW-INTENSITY TREATMENT

Treatment with low-intensity beams stimulates tissue healing and reduces pain, inflammation, and swelling. It works by improving blood and lymph flow and by reducing the production of *prostaglandins* (hormonelike substances that stimulate inflammation and cause pain). Low-intensity beams are used in the treatment of muscle tears, ligament sprains, and inflamed tendons and joints.

HIGH-INTENSITY TREATMENT

High-intensity treatment destroys cells directly under the beam while leaving adjacent cells undamaged, making it useful in the treatment of some tumors. The beam cuts through tissue and, simultaneously, causes blood clotting, making it a useful surgical tool.

LASERS IN OPHTHALMOLOGY

Lasers are used in the treatment of diabetic *retinopathy* (to coagulate, and so prevent bleeding from abnormal blood vessels), to prevent and treat *retinal detachment* (by sealing small tears or areas of degeneration in the retina), to burn a hole in the iris (to reduce excess pressure in the eye in *glaucoma*), and to destroy small tumors of the retina. The laser can also be used to make a central hole (to restore vision) in the lens capsule if it becomes opaque after *cataract surgery*.

LASERS IN GYNECOLOGY

Laser beams are sometimes used to unblock fallopian tubes by removing scar tissue formed after infection or a *sterilization* procedure. Lasers are also used to destroy abnormal cells in the *cervix*.

OTHER USES

Lasers are commonly used to remove small birthmarks and tattoos; the results are variable. Early malignant tumors of the larynx can be successfully removed without damaging the vocal cords.

Many new applications are being investigated. Potential uses include the removal of atherosclerotic *plaque* from inside arteries. It may also be possible to use lasers to disintegrate bladder and kidney stones, and to remove otherwise inaccessible tumors of the brain and spinal cord.

Lassa fever

A dangerous infectious disease caused by a virus. Lassa fever, which was first reported in Lassa, Nigeria, in 1969, occurs in occasional outbreaks in West Africa; a small number of cases have been imported into Europe and North America.

USE OF A LASER

The concentrated beam of light released by a laser has a variety of medical purposes. When set to low intensity, the laser works to stimulate tissue healing and reduces pain, inflammation, and swelling. At high intensity, the beam destroys cells on which it is focused while leaving adjacent tissue unharmed. It can also cut through tissues without causing bleeding.

Argon laser

Photocoagulation of blood vessels occurs when the blue-green light from this laser is absorbed by hemoglobin.

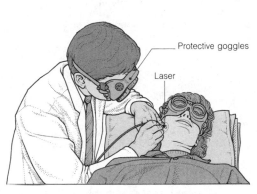

Protective goggles

Laser

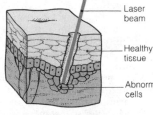

Laser beam

Healthy tissue

Abnormal cells

Focused carbon dioxide laser

This laser is ideal for precision cutting or for destroying abnormal cells because its focused beam leaves surrounding areas of tissue intact.

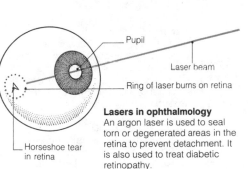

Pupil

Laser beam

Ring of laser burns on retina

Horseshoe tear in retina

Lasers in ophthalmology
An argon laser is used to seal torn or degenerated areas in the retina to prevent detachment. It is also used to treat diabetic retinopathy.

Removing skin blemishes
These photographs, taken before and after laser treatment, show removal of a port-wine stain. In some cases, treatment is less successful, leaving scars.

L

In Africa, where the virus is harbored by a type of rat, infection may be acquired by inhaling droplets of an infected rat's urine. Medical and nursing staff are at risk of acquiring the virus from the blood of an infected person or from droplets coughed into the air. However, no one in Canada has ever acquired the disease from an infected person.

SYMPTOMS AND TREATMENT

After an incubation period of three to 17 days, the illness starts with fever, headache, muscular aches, and a sore throat. Later, severe diarrhea and vomiting develop. In extreme cases, the patient's condition deteriorates rapidly in the second week.

About one quarter to one third of patients hospitalized because of Lassa fever die from the illness.

Lassa fever can be diagnosed by a blood test. Infected people must be isolated. Patients are treated by the relief of symptoms and by injections of the *antiviral drug* ribavirin and of serum containing *antibodies* active against the virus.

Lassitude

A term describing a feeling of *tiredness*, weakness, or exhaustion.

Lateral

Relating to, directed toward or coming from, or situated on, one side. Bilateral means on both sides.

Latissimus dorsi

A large, flat, triangular muscle in the back. Its fibers arise from the spines of the lower six thoracic (chest) vertebrae and from the back of the pelvis; they converge on a small tendon that is attached to the humerus (upper-arm bone) just below the shoulder. Contraction of the muscle moves the arm downward and backward.

Laughing gas

The popular name for *nitrous oxide*, a gas inhaled in combination with oxygen to produce general *anesthesia*. Laughing gas is so called because of the euphoric effects it produces.

Laurence-Moon-Biedl syndrome

A very rare inherited disorder characterized by increasing *obesity*, *retinitis pigmentosa* that may lead to blindness, *mental retardation*, *polydactyly*, and *hypogonadism*. The condition shows an autosomal recessive pattern of inheritance (see *Genetic disorders*).

Laurence-Moon-Biedl syndrome is probably caused by a disorder of the *hypothalamus* (part of the brain that controls hormone balance). There is no treatment. Parents of an affected child should seek *genetic counseling*.

Lavage, gastric

Washing out the stomach with water, usually to remove poisons.

HOW IT IS DONE

The patient is placed face down with his or her head below the level of the stomach and turned to one side. A lubricated tube is passed down the esophagus into the stomach and a funnel is attached to the top. (If the patient is not fully conscious, a tube is also passed down the throat into the trachea to prevent regurgitated water and stomach contents from entering the lungs.) Water is poured into the funnel until the stomach is filled. The top of the tube is then lowered, allowing the fluid in the stomach to drain into a bucket. This process is repeated until the water returns clear. An early sample of fluid from the stomach is kept so that the poison can be analyzed. In certain cases, an antidote is added to the water or is passed into the stomach after lavage is finished.

Lavage is not used if a corrosive poison has been swallowed because of the risk that the tube may perforate tissues. Corrosive acids or alkalis may be diluted by giving large amounts of water or milk (see *Poisoning*).

Laxative drugs

COMMON DRUGS

Bulk-forming
Methylcellulose Psyllium

Stimulant
Bisacodyl Docusate sodium
Phenolphthalein Senna

Lubricant
Mineral oil

Osmotic
Lactulose Magnesium sulfate
Sodium phosphate

> **WARNING**
> If constipation lasts for more than a week, consult your physician; you may have a serious underlying disorder.

A group of drugs used to treat *constipation*. The use of laxative drugs can often be avoided by eating a diet containing plenty of *fiber*, by drinking plenty of liquids, and by adopting proper toilet habits. Laxative drugs should generally be used only when straining should be avoided (e.g., following childbirth, abdominal surgery, or a *myocardial infarction*). Laxative drugs are sometimes used to clear feces from the intestine before surgical or investigational procedures.

TYPES

BULK-FORMING LAXATIVES These laxatives increase the volume and softness of feces by absorbing water in the intestine. Increased bulk stimulates propulsion of feces through the intestine and makes them easier to pass.

STIMULANT LAXATIVES These drugs stimulate the intestinal wall to contract and thus speed up the elimination of feces. Because the feces spend less time in the intestine, less water is reabsorbed into the blood vessels, which helps keep the feces soft.

LUBRICANT LAXATIVES These substances soften and thus facilitate the passage of feces. Liquid paraffin is the commonest substance used.

OSMOTIC LAXATIVES These laxatives cause fluid to be retained in the intestine, thus increasing the water content and volume of the feces.

POSSIBLE ADVERSE EFFECTS
If used in excess, laxative drugs may cause diarrhea. Prolonged treatment may cause dependence on the laxative drug for normal bowel action; laxative use should be stopped as soon as normal habits are reestablished.

Stimulant laxatives and lactulose may cause abdominal cramps and flatulence. Prolonged use of some osmotic laxatives is likely to cause a chemical imbalance in the blood. Lubricant laxatives may coat the intestine and impair vitamin absorption.

Lazy eye

An ambiguous name for the visual defect that commonly results from *squint*. See *Amblyopia*.

LD$_{50}$

The abbreviation for median lethal dose, the amount of a drug needed to kill 50 percent of a group of animals. This dose is determined during experiments carried out to assess the toxicity of new drugs.

Lead poisoning

Damage to the brain, nerves, red blood cells, and digestive system, caused by inhaling lead fumes or swallowing lead salts.

Acute poisoning, which is now relatively rare but sometimes fatal, occurs when a large amount of lead is taken into the body over a short period of time. Chronic poisoning results from small amounts of lead being taken in over a longer period. The body excretes lead very slowly, which therefore accumulates in the body tissues (primarily in the bones). There is some evidence that lead in amounts that are insufficient to cause detectable physical effects may cause mental impairment, particularly in children.

CAUSES AND INCIDENCE
Although interior paints sold today do not contain significant amounts of lead, poisoning has occurred in children who have licked or eaten old paint that contains high levels of lead. Adults most at risk include workers in such industries as lead smelting, soldering, demolition, battery manufacture, and pottery glazing. Inhaling the fumes from burning battery casings containing lead may also cause lead poisoning. Eating acidic food or drink that is stored or cooked in lead-glazed or lead-soldered containers has also caused lead poisoning.

Health and Welfare Canada has established limits for safe blood levels of lead in pregnant women and children, and also for allowable levels of lead in drinking water and foods; some provinces have standards for lead concentrations in air. All lead in gasoline was phased out in 1990.

SYMPTOMS AND SIGNS
Lead poisoning can cause severe, colicky, abdominal pain, diarrhea, and vomiting. There may also be *anemia*, loss of appetite, and a blue, black, or gray line along the gum margins. Lead poisoning may also produce weakness or paralysis of the limbs, but severe poisoning is now rare in Canada. Also now very uncommon is severe lead encephalopathy (disturbance of brain function due to lead poisoning), which may cause headaches, hallucinations, seizures, coma, and even occasionally death. Even if the person survives a seizure or coma, there is a high probability of brain damage.

DIAGNOSIS
Lead poisoning is suspected from the patient's condition and history, and may be confirmed by tests on the blood and urine to measure the levels of lead and other substances produced by the action of lead on the body's cells. In children, *X rays* may show characteristic areas of thickening in some bones.

TREATMENT
Treatment consists of avoiding further exposure to lead. The physician may prescribe *chelating agents* to bind to the lead and help the body excrete it at a faster rate. In mild cases, the chelating agent *penicillamine* may be used alone. In more severe cases, penicillamine may be used with other chelating agents, such as edetate calcium disodium (calcium EDTA).

Learning

The process by which knowledge or abilities are acquired, or by which behavior is modified.

Many different theories have been proposed to explain learning. Some, known as behavioral theories, emphasize the role of *conditioning* in learning. Others, known as cognitive theories, are based on the concept that learning occurs through the building of abstract "cognitive" models, using mental capacities such as *intelligence*, *memory*, insight, and understanding. Social learning theories combine aspects of both behavioral and cognitive learning theories. No one theory can account for the complexities of learning. It is probable that some things are learned by conditioning and others by complex thought processes that take account of many facts.

Learning disabilities

A range of psychological and physical problems that interfere with learning. Learning disabilities may be either general or specific.

Possible causes of a general learning disability include borderline or low *intelligence, mental retardation,* and *hyperactivity.*

Examples of specific learning disabilities include *dyslexia* (difficulty in reading), dyscalculia (inability to solve mathematical problems), and dysgraphia (writing disorders). In most cases, the cause of a specific learning disability cannot be ascertained. Some psychologists believe that specific learning disabilities in children of normal intelligence may be caused by forms of *minimal brain dysfunction,* which may be inherited.

Other problems that may cause general or specific learning disabilities include *deafness,* disorders of language or speech (see *Speech disorders*), and disorders of *vision.* Problems with schoolwork caused by emotional or environmental deprivation or by poor teaching are generally not classified as learning disabilities.

ASSESSMENT AND TREATMENT

A child with a suspected learning disability will usually be referred for psychological or medical assessment.

Treatment may be medical (such as the correction of a hearing problem), directed at improving language or speech (see *Speech therapy*), or educational (such as extra teaching or placement in a special unit or school).

Leech

A type of bloodsucking worm with a flattened body and a sucker at each end. Land leeches inhabit tropical forests and can work their way through a person's clothing to attach themselves to the ankles and lower legs. Aquatic leeches live in warm water and attach themselves to swimmers, sometimes penetrating to the bronchi and esophagus.

Leeches bite painlessly, introducing their saliva into the wound before sucking blood. When they are satiated, they drop off. Leech saliva contains an anticlotting substance, called hirudin, which may cause the wound to bleed for hours after the leech has dropped off. Leeches are thought not to transmit disease.

TREATMENT OF BITES

Attached leeches should be disturbed by applying a lighted match, alcohol, salt, or vinegar. They can then be

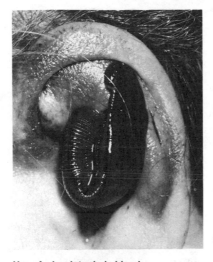

Use of a leech to drain blood
A leech is being used here to drain a hematoma (collection of blood) from a person's outer ear following an injury. Leech bites are painless, but because leech saliva contains an anticlotting agent, the wound may bleed for several hours.

pulled off gently to prevent the mouthparts from staying attached and becoming infected. A styptic pencil helps stop the bleeding after the leech has been removed. *Endoscopy* (inspection using a viewing instrument) may be necessary to remove leeches from inside the body.

MEDICAL USES

In the past, leeches were attached to the skin to "treat" many illnesses ascribed to excess blood. Today, leeches are sometimes used to drain a *hematoma* (a collection of partially clotted blood) from a wound.

Leg, broken

See *Femur, fracture of; Fibula; Tibia.*

Legionnaires' disease

A form of pneumonia (infection of the lungs) named after an outbreak that caused the death of 29 members of the American Legion who were attending a convention in a Philadelphia hotel in 1976. The bacterium responsible was isolated and named *LEGIONELLA PNEUMOPHILA.* Subsequent tests identified the organism as a common contaminant of water systems which had been responsible for earlier epidemics of pneumonia (the cause of which had not been understood at the time).

CAUSES AND INCIDENCE

The bacterium breeds most readily in warm, moist conditions; in most out-

breaks the source of infection has been the water or air-conditioning system in a large public building. Infection follows the inhalation of droplets of heavily contaminated water (from air-conditioning outlets or showers, for example). Elderly people, especially heavy smokers or drinkers, are particularly at risk.

The disease occurs both in localized outbreaks and as isolated cases. About 50 cases are reported in Canada each year, but the actual incidence may be higher. More than twice as many men as women are affected, and more than two thirds of the cases occur in people over 50 years of age.

Control of the disease relies on proper disinfection of water systems, together with keeping the water at the correct temperature.

SYMPTOMS AND SIGNS

The first symptoms develop within a week of infection; they include headache, muscular and abdominal pain, diarrhea, and a dry cough. Over the next few days pneumonia develops, resulting in a high fever, shaking chills, the coughing up of thick sputum (phlegm), drowsiness, and sometimes delirium. Like other types of pneumonia, the illness usually becomes more severe unless treated. This phase lasts about a week, after which either a gradual recovery takes place or progressively serious breathing problems develop.

DIAGNOSIS AND TREATMENT

The patient is admitted to hospital, where analysis of a sample of sputum (cultured on special media) reveals the microorganism responsible for the pneumonia. If the microorganism is *LEGIONELLA PNEUMOPHILA,* the patient is given the antibiotic *erythromycin,* often intravenously, which usually relieves symptoms quickly. Occasionally another antibiotic drug, *rifampin,* may be required.

OUTLOOK

The outcome of the disease depends on the age and general health of the patient. Younger people generally recover fully, but a substantial proportion of elderly, out-of-shape people die from the illness. Death is usually due to irreversible lung damage.

Leg, shortening of

Shortening of the leg is usually caused by faulty healing of a fractured femur (thighbone) or tibia (shin). Other causes are an abnormality present from birth, surgery on the leg, or muscle weakness associated with *poliomyelitis* or some other neurological

L

disorder. Also, a deformity of the hip, knee, or spine may make one leg effectively shorter than the other even if the two are in fact of equal length.

If the difference in leg length exceeds 4 cm, there is usually a noticeable limp; the resultant stress on the lower spine often causes *back pain*. Wearing a shoe with a raised heel can compensate for the shortened leg.

Leg ulcer

An open sore on the leg that fails to heal, usually resulting from poor arterial blood supply to, or venous drainage from, the area. Elderly people are most commonly affected.

TYPES

Venous ulcers (also known as varicose or stasis ulcers) occur mainly on the ankles and lower legs and are caused by valve failure in veins; these ulcers usually appear in conjunction with *varicose veins*.

Bedsores (also called decubitus ulcers) develop on pressure spots on the legs as a result of a combination of poor circulation, pressure, and immobility over a long period. Beginning as red painful areas, they eventually become open sores.

Leg ulcers may also be due to *peripheral vascular disease*, in which fatty deposits on the inside of arteries or thickening of the arterial walls restrict blood supply to the extremities.

Diabetes mellitus, which increases susceptibility to blood vessel disease and skin infection and impairs sensation, may lead to ulcers.

Ulcers may also develop through neglect of an infected small wound. In the tropics, infection with microorganisms can cause *tropical ulcers*.

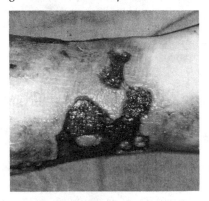

Venous ulcer on leg
This type of ulcer, also known as a stasis ulcer, is caused by impaired drainage of blood from the leg by the veins. It is usually accompanied by edema (fluid accumulation) in the lower leg.

PREVENTION AND TREATMENT

Prevention is always easier than cure. In general, anyone susceptible to leg ulcers should attempt to avoid obesity, leg injury, and immobility.

Treatment of leg ulcers depends on the cause. Whatever the source of the problem, seek medical advice at the earliest sign of trouble. If an ulcer is exuding pus, a wet dressing may be applied under the bandaging. This dressing should be changed only every three to seven days to avoid removing new skin from the area.

Leiomyoma

A benign tumor of smooth *muscle* (a type of muscle not under voluntary control). Leiomyomas usually occur in the smooth muscle of the uterus, where they gradually become replaced with fibrous tissue (hence their popular name, *fibroids*). More rarely, leiomyomas develop from smooth muscle in the wall of blood vessels in the skin.

Leiomyomas are usually multiple. Although leiomyomas are not cancerous, they may require surgical removal if they cause symptoms.

Leishmaniasis

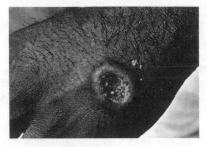

Any of a variety of diseases affecting the skin, mucous membranes, and internal organs, caused by infection with single-celled parasites called leishmania. The parasites are harbored by dogs and rodents in various parts of the world, and are transmitted from infected animals or people to new hosts by the bites of sandflies.

About 20 million people worldwide are thought to be affected. Leishmaniasis is not contracted in Canada, but travelers occasionally contract an infection abroad.

TYPES AND INCIDENCE

The most serious form of leishmaniasis, mainly affecting the internal organs, is called kala-azar or visceral leishmaniasis. It is prevalent in some parts of Asia, Africa, and South America, and also occurs in some Mediterranean countries.

In addition, there are several varieties of cutaneous leishmaniasis (mainly affecting the skin), some of which are prevalent in the Middle East, North Africa, and countries bordering the Mediterranean sea; others occur only in parts of Central and South America.

Travelers can minimize the risk of infection by taking measures to discourage sandfly bites (see *Insect bites*).

Leishmaniasis ulcer
This skin ulcer, which developed at the site of a sandfly bite, is typical of the lesions found on the skin of people who are suffering from cutaneous leishmaniasis.

SYMPTOMS

Kala-azar causes a persistent fever, enlargement of the spleen, anemia, and, later, darkening of the skin. The illness may develop any time up to two years after the initial infection, and, unless treated, the condition is sometimes fatal.

The cutaneous forms cause the appearance of a persistent ulcer at the site of the sandfly bite. The ulcer nearly always heals eventually, but can leave an ugly scar. With the South American forms, more extensive tissue damage may occur, often on the face, causing severe disfigurement.

DIAGNOSIS AND TREATMENT

Kala-azar is diagnosed by a *bone marrow biopsy* (aspirate) and/or a blood test. The cutaneous forms are diagnosed by identifying parasites in

---

LOCATION OF THE LENS
This elastic and transparent organ is situated behind the iris and is suspended on delicate fibers from the ciliary body. Its full name—the crystalline lens—differentiates it from the cornea (another lens).

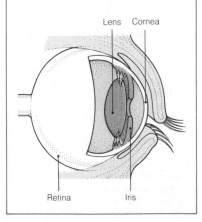

Lens   Cornea

Retina   Iris

scrapings taken from the edge of affected skin patches. All types of leishmaniasis are treated effectively with drugs, such as sodium stibogluconate, given by intramuscular or intravenous injection.

Lens

The internal optical component of the *eye*, responsible for adjusting focus. Also called the crystalline lens, it is one of two lenses in each eye; the other is the *cornea*, which provides most of the converging power needed to form an image on the *retina*.

The crystalline lens is situated behind the iris and is suspended on delicate fibers from the ciliary body. It is elastic, transparent, and slightly less convex on the front surface than on the back. Changing the curvature of the lens alters the focus so that near or distant objects can be seen sharply (see *Accommodation*).

Opacification of the crystalline lens, from any cause, is called *cataract*. (See also *Lens dislocation*.)

Lens dislocation

Displacement of the eye's crystalline *lens* from its normal position. Lens dislocation is almost always caused by an injury that ruptures some or all of the fibers that connect the lens to the ciliary body. In *Marfan's syndrome*, the fibers are particularly weak and lens dislocation is common.

A dislocated lens may slide sideways, upward, or downward, causing severe visual distortion or double vision in the affected eye, or it may slip backward into the vitreous humor. A lens dislocated forward through the pupil usually causes a form of *glaucoma* because of closure of the drainage angle of the eye. If the glaucoma is severe, the lens may need to be removed. (See also *Aphakia*.)

Lens implant

A plastic prosthesis used to replace the removed opaque lens in *cataract surgery*. There are many different designs, which may be positioned in front of the iris, clipped to the pupil, or held in place behind the pupil by delicate plastic loops.

A lens implant usually provides excellent distance vision without glasses, but glasses are usually necessary for close vision.

Lentigo

A flat, discolored area of skin similar to a freckle. Lentigines (the plural of lentigo) are usually light brown and may occur singly or in groups. Unlike freckles they are as common on covered as on exposed parts of the body, and they do not fade in winter. Lentigines are more common in middle-aged and elderly people, especially those who have been exposed to a lot of sun.

Lentigines are harmless and no treatment is necessary. If raised, darker brown areas appear within them, a physician should be consulted; there is a danger that these areas could develop into malignant melanomas (see *Melanoma, malignant*).

Leprosy

A chronic bacterial infection that causes nerve damage, mainly in the limbs and facial area, and may lead to skin damage. Contrary to popular belief, it is not highly contagious. (See *Hansen's disease*.)

Leptospirosis

 A rare disease caused by a type of spirochete (spiral-shaped) bacterium harbored by rodents and excreted in their urine. It is also known as Weil's disease.

SYMPTOMS
After an incubation period of one to three weeks, there is an acute illness with fever, chills, an intense throbbing headache, severe muscle aches, eye inflammation, and a skin rash. In most cases, the kidneys are affected, often severely. Liver damage leading to jaundice is also common.

TREATMENT
Antibiotic drugs are effective against the spirochetes. In about one third of cases improvement is prompt. However, many patients suffer a more persistent illness in which kidney and liver function recover only slowly. In these cases, the nervous system may also be affected, often producing signs of *meningitis* (inflammation of the membranes covering the brain and spinal cord).

Lesbianism

Female homosexuality. According to Alfred Kinsey's studies carried out in the 1940s, about 5 percent of women are entirely lesbian in their sexual activity, although some 15 percent have had, by the age of 45, a homosexual experience. Lesbianism is less common than male homosexuality (see *Homosexuality, male*). Masturbation, oral sex, and mutual rubbing of the clitoris are the usual means of reaching orgasm.

Lesion

An all-encompassing term for any abnormality of structure or function in any part of the body. The term may refer to a wound, infection, tumor, abscess, or chemical abnormality.

Lethargy

A feeling of *tiredness*, drowsiness, or lack of energy.

Leukemia

Any of several types of cancer in which there exists a disorganized proliferation of white *blood cells* in the bone marrow (the tissue from which all blood cells originate). The production of red blood cells, platelets, and normal white blood cells is impaired as normal cells are crowded out from the marrow by the leukemic cells (abnormal white cells).

Other organs, such as the liver, spleen, lymph nodes, testes, or brain, may cease to function properly as they become infiltrated by the leukemic cells. The number of leukemic cells circulating in the blood may be high.

Leukemias are classified into acute and chronic types (acute leukemia generally develops more rapidly than chronic leukemia). They are also classified according to the type of white cell that is proliferating abnormally. If the abnormal cells are derived from lymphocytes or from lymphoblasts (immature precursors of lymphocytes), the leukemia is called lymphocytic or lymphoblastic leukemia. If the abnormal cells are derived from other types of white blood cells or their precursors, the leukemia is known as myeloid, myeloblastic, or granulocytic leukemia.

Each year about 3,000 new cases of leukemia are diagnosed in Canada, and there are about 4,000 deaths from this cause. (See also *Leukemia, acute*; *Leukemia, chronic lymphocytic*; *Leukemia, chronic myeloid*.)

Leukemia, acute

A type of *leukemia* in which the white blood cells produced in excess within the bone marrow are immature cells called blasts. Untreated, acute leukemia can be fatal within a few weeks to months. Treatment today can often prolong life and may even provide a complete cure.

The abnormal cells may be of two types: lymphoblasts (immature *lymphocytes*) in acute lymphoblastic leukemia, and myeloblasts (immature forms of other types of white cell) in acute myeloblastic leukemia.

Various subtypes are recognized according to the nature of the abnormal cells.

INCIDENCE AND CAUSES
The incidences of the two main types (acute lymphoblastic leukemia and acute myeloblastic leukemia) at different ages are shown in the illustrated box on facing page.

Both types seem to result from a mutation in a single white cell, altering its genetic structure. The cell undergoes an uncontrolled series of divisions until billions of copies of the abnormal cell are present in the bone marrow, blood, and other tissues.

There are a number of possible causes for the original mutation. One type of acute lymphoblastic leukemia is thought to be caused by a virus similar to the one that causes *AIDS*. Exposure to certain chemicals (such as benzene and some anticancer drugs) and to atomic radiation or radioactive leaks from nuclear reactors can be a cause. Inherited factors may play a part; there is an increased incidence in people with certain genetic disorders (such as *Fanconi's anemia*) and chromosomal abnormalities (such as *Down's syndrome*). People with certain other blood disorders, such as chronic myeloid leukemia (see *Leukemia, chronic myeloid*) and primary *polycythemia*, are also at increased risk.

SYMPTOMS AND SIGNS
The symptoms and signs of both types of acute leukemia are caused by overcrowding of the bone marrow by blasts and by infiltration of organs by the abnormal cells. The overcrowding causes the marrow's failure to produce normal blood cells of all types (see illustrated box).

DIAGNOSIS
The diagnosis of acute leukemia is based on a *bone marrow biopsy* that confirms an abnormal number of blast cells. The blast cells are sometimes also seen in the blood. When acute lymphoblastic leukemia is diagnosed, a *lumbar puncture* is usually performed to examine the *cerebrospinal fluid* for the presence of blast cells.

TREATMENT
Treatment includes giving the patient transfusions of blood and platelets, and the use of *anticancer drugs* to kill the leukemic cells. These drugs tend to make the patient even more susceptible to infection, so powerful *antibiotic drugs* may also be given.

From the beginning of treatment, a catheter (tube) through which all drugs and transfusions are given is commonly inserted into a large vein near the heart. Treatment of leukemic cells in the cerebrospinal fluid is accomplished by the direct injection of drugs into the fluid and by subsequent *radiation therapy* to the head and spinal cord. Radiation therapy is more commonly given in the treatment of acute lymphoblastic leukemia than for acute myeloblastic leukemia.

The course of drug treatment may last for many weeks. When there is no evidence of leukemic cells in the blood or bone marrow, a state of remission is said to have been achieved. However, without repeated courses of treatment, the leukemia often relapses (returns). For this reason, the use of drugs is usually continued for many weeks after remission. If the leukemia relapses after the first remission, a *bone marrow transplant* may be considered. Increasingly, the practice is to offer bone marrow transplantation during the first remission to guard against relapse.

OUTLOOK
The outlook for people with acute lymphoblastic leukemia is generally better than it is for acute myeloblastic leukemia, and it is better for children than for adults. Survival rates are shown in the illustrated box.

Leukemia, chronic lymphocytic
A type of *leukemia* caused by proliferation of mature-looking *lymphocytes* (a type of white *blood cell* that plays an important role in the body's *immune system*). Although incurable, the disease is not invariably fatal.

INCIDENCE AND CAUSES
There are about 1,300 new cases of chronic lymphocytic leukemia diagnosed annually in Canada. Nearly all patients are over 50. The cause of the disorder is unknown.

SYMPTOMS AND SIGNS
Symptoms develop slowly, often over many years. Many cases are discovered by chance when a blood test is performed. In addition to features common to acute forms of leukemia (see upper section of illustrated box), symptoms and signs may include enlargement of the liver and spleen, persistent raised temperature, and night sweats.

DIAGNOSIS AND TREATMENT
Chronic lymphocytic leukemia is diagnosed by finding large numbers of lymphocytes, all of the same type, in the blood and on a *bone marrow biopsy*. The severity of the disease is assessed by the degree of liver and spleen enlargement, anemia, and lack of platelet cells in the blood. In many cases, no treatment is required if the disease is mild. In more severe cases, *anticancer drugs* are given by mouth, sometimes combined with *radiation therapy*. Other measures include transfusions of blood and platelets, *antibiotic drugs* to combat infection, and *immunoglobulin injections* to boost the patient's immune system.

OUTLOOK
The progression of chronic lymphocytic leukemia is slow. More than half the patients survive for five years from the time of diagnosis. Eventually, death may result from overwhelming infection but many patients die from causes unrelated to their leukemia.

Leukemia, chronic myeloid
A type of *leukemia*, also known as chronic granulocytic leukemia, that results from uncontrolled proliferation of the class of white *blood cell* known as granulocytes, neutrophils, or polymorphonuclear leukocytes. Large numbers of these cells, in various stages of maturity, appear in the blood.

INCIDENCE AND CAUSES
There are about 1,000 new cases of chronic myeloid leukemia diagnosed in Canada each year, mainly among middle-aged to elderly people.

The cause of chronic myeloid leukemia is not known. However, in most cases, the patient's cells contain a specific *chromosomal abnormality* known as the Philadelphia chromosome. Part of one chromosome is attached to another chromosome.

SYMPTOMS
This type of leukemia usually has two phases—a chronic phase that may last several years and a more malignant phase, called the blastic or accelerated or acute phase, in which large numbers of immature granulocytes are produced.

During the chronic phase, symptoms develop slowly; they may include tiredness, fever, night sweats, and weight loss. If the number of white cells in the blood rises very high, the blood may become excessively viscous (sticky), impairing the supply of oxygen to various organs. The effects can include visual disturbances and abdominal pain due to death of tissues within the spleen. *Priapism* (persistent, painful erection of the penis) is sometimes a feature.

The symptoms of the second phase are like those of acute forms of leukemia (see illustrated box).

LEUKEMIA

In all forms of leukemia, abnormal white cells proliferate in the bone marrow. There are four main types: acute lymphoblastic leukemia (ALL), acute myeloblastic leukemia (AML), chronic lymphocytic leukemia (CLL), and chronic myeloid leukemia (CML). Their incidence varies with age (see right). The acute types have a rapid onset. There is a risk of death from overwhelming infection or blood loss, but modern treatment has greatly improved survival rates (below) and may bring a cure.

The chronic forms of leukemia progress much more gradually but are essentially incurable.

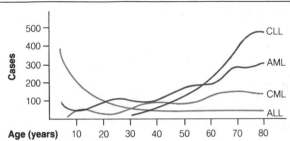

Incidence
The graphs show how the four main types of leukemia vary in incidence with age. Acute lymphoblastic leukemia (ALL) is the common type in children, chronic lymphocytic leukemia (CLL) is the most common over 40.

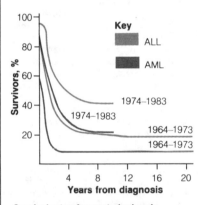

Survival rates for acute leukemia
The graphs show survival rates for acute lymphoblastic leukemia (ALL) and acute myeloblastic leukemia (AML) for cases diagnosed in the years 1964 to 1973 and 1974 to 1983. The improved survival rates are the result of better treatment.

Symptoms of acute leukemia
Symptoms are caused partly by the abnormal white cells crowding out the bone marrow (so that it fails to produce sufficient normal blood cells of all types) and partly by the invasion of other body organs by abnormal cells.

Gum bleeding
Gums may bleed as a result of insufficient production of platelet cells by the bone marrow; platelets are needed for the arrest of bleeding.

Bone tenderness
Tenderness of the bones may be felt as the bone marrow becomes packed with immature white cells.

Frequent bruising
Reduced numbers of platelets may lead to bleeding points in the skin and bruising after mild trauma.

Headache
Headache may be caused by anemia or by abnormal white cells affecting the nervous system.

Enlarged lymph nodes
The lymph nodes in the neck, armpits, and groin may be swollen with huge numbers of immature white cells. The liver, spleen, and testes may also be swollen.

Anemia
Anemia develops if there is insufficient production of red blood cells by the bone marrow. Anemia causes tiredness, breathlessness or exertion, and pallor.

Infections
White blood cells play a major part in the defense against infection. However, in acute leukemia, only immature, nonfunctioning white cells are made, so the patient may suffer from repeated chest or throat infections, herpes zoster, or skin and other infections.

HOW LEUKEMIA ATTACKS THE BODY

Leukemia is a form of cancer, but with the abnormally growing cells—mutated white blood cells—scattered throughout the body in bone marrow, rather than grouped into a single tumor. The abnormal cells may spill into the blood and may infiltrate and interfere with the function of other organs. But worse, the abnormal cells "take over" the marrow and prevent it from making enough normal blood cells—including normal white cells, red cells, and platelets. This leaves the sufferer highly susceptible to serious infections, anemia, and bleeding episodes.

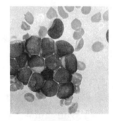

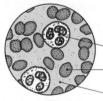

Cell photograph
Shown is blood in acute leukemia. The large cells are abnormal, immature white cells; the smaller, paler cells are red blood cells.

Normal blood smear

White cells fight infection

Red cells transport oxygen

Platelets help blood clot

Blood smear in leukemia

Abnormal white cells—susceptibility to infection

Fewer platelets—bleeding tendency

Fewer red cells—anemia

Appearance of blood in leukemia
In leukemia (above), the blood usually contains many abnormal white cells, and fewer red cells and platelets.

Normal appearance of blood
In a normal blood smear (left), there are large numbers of red cells, many platelets, and a few white cells.

L

DIAGNOSIS AND TREATMENT

The disease is sometimes not apparent until the patient has a blood test for some other reason. The diagnosis is made from the increased numbers of granulocytes in the blood and in the bone marrow (as detected by *bone marrow biopsy*). The presence of the Philadelphia chromosome, found by *chromosome analysis*, may help establish the diagnosis.

Treatment of the chronic phase includes the use of *anticancer drugs*. When the disease transforms into the acute phase, treatment is similar to that given for acute leukemia. If the number of white cells rises very high, the cells may be removed from the patient using a machine known as a cell separator.

Treatment of the acute phase is seldom successful; in many instances the patient dies of bleeding or infection. *Bone marrow transplants* are increasingly being used in an attempt to cure patients while the condition is still in the chronic phase.

OUTLOOK

The average survival time from first diagnosis is about three years. However, about one fifth of patients survive for 10 years or more. A successful bone marrow transplant may improve the outlook, but this procedure is not without its own risks.

Leukocyte

Any type of white *blood cell*.

Leukodystrophies

A rare group of inherited childhood diseases in which the *myelin* sheaths that form a protective covering around many nerves are destroyed.

Diseases within this group include metachromatic leukodystrophy (which causes impaired speech, blindness, paralysis, dementia, and death within a few years), Krabbe's disease (which results in blindness, deafness, seizures, paralysis, and death within one year), and Merzbacher-Pelizaeus disease (which causes progressive incoordination, speech difficulties, paralysis, and mental deterioration from infancy until death, which occurs in early childhood).

Leukoplakia

Raised, white patches on the mucous membranes of the mouth or vulva (the area around the vaginal opening). Leukoplakia is due to the thickening of tissue. It is most common in elderly people and is being increasingly found in people with *AIDS*.

CAUSES

Leukoplakia in the mouth, which is most common on the tongue, is usually due to tobacco-smoking (particularly pipe-smoking) or to the rubbing of a rough tooth or denture. It is not known what causes the condition to develop on the vulva.

SYMPTOMS AND TREATMENT

The patches, which develop slowly, cause no discomfort and are usually harmless. Occasionally, they result in a malignant change in the affected tissue. Because of this malignancy risk, leukoplakia should always be reported to a physician.

Leukoplakia in the mouth may clear up once the cause has been treated. If the condition persists, the patches are removed under a local anesthetic. Leukoplakia of the vulva is treated in the same way. The removed tissue is examined microscopically for any signs of malignant change. (See also *Mouth cancer*; *Vulva, cancer of*.)

Leukorrhea

See *Vaginal discharge*.

Levodopa

A drug used in the treatment of *Parkinson's disease*, a neurological disorder caused by deficiency of the neurotransmitter chemical *dopamine* in part of the brain.

HOW IT WORKS

Levodopa is absorbed into the brain and converted into dopamine. Levodopa is usually given in combination with an *enzyme*-inhibitor, such as carbidopa, that reduces the amount of levodopa broken down by the liver before it can reach the brain. This allows a lower dose of levodopa to be given and thereby reduces the risk of adverse effects.

POSSIBLE ADVERSE EFFECTS

Adverse effects include nausea, vomiting, nervousness, and agitation. Prolonged use often impairs the effectiveness of treatment or increases the severity of adverse effects.

Levonorgestrel

A *progestogen drug* used in some *oral contraceptive* preparations.

Levothyroxine

The major hormone produced by the thyroid gland, levothyroxine is sometimes called thyroxine. Its primary use is to replace the hormone when it is deficient (see *Hypothyroidism*). It may also be given to prevent the development of goiter (enlarged thyroid) in persons treated with antithyroid drugs. It is also prescribed for thyroid cancer and certain types of goiter. Dosages should be built up gradually, and it should be used with caution in people with heart problems.

LH

The abbreviation for luteinizing hormone—a *gonadotropin hormone* produced by the *pituitary gland*.

LH-RH

The abbreviation for *luteinizing hormone-releasing hormone*. This hormone is released by the *hypothalamus*.

Libido

Sexual desire. Libido is a healthy, normal feeling, especially strong in youth and gradually fading with age. Loss of libido is a common symptom of numerous physical illnesses, and of *depression*, *drug abuse*, and *alcohol abuse*.

The libido theory of the Viennese neurologist and psychoanalyst Sigmund Freud describes sexual development during childhood in terms of oral, anal, and genital stages (representing the areas of the body toward which a child's attention is directed at different ages). Freud believed that certain neurotic disorders and abnormal sexual behaviors were due to fixation of libido at one of these stages. By contrast, directing the libido (or "love energy") away from oneself and toward other people or objects was seen as a sign of maturity. (See also *Narcissism*; *Sexual desire, inhibited*.)

Lice

Small, wingless insects that feed on human blood. There are three species: PEDICULUS HUMANUS CAPITIS (the head louse), PEDICULUS HUMANUS CORPORIS (the body louse), and PHTHIRUS PUBIS (the crab, or pubic, louse). All lice have flattened bodies and measure up to 3 mm across.

HEAD LICE

These lice live on and suck blood from the scalp. Head lice leave tiny, red spots that itch intensely, leading to scratching, *dermatitis* (skin inflammation), and *impetigo* (a bacterial infection of the skin). The females lay a daily batch of tiny, pale eggs (nits) that are attached to hairs close to the scalp; the nits hatch in about seven days. The adult lice may live for up to several weeks.

Head lice affect all social classes. Children are most affected, women occasionally, and men rarely. The lice are spread by direct (although not necessarily head-to-head) contact.

Lotions containing malathion or carbaryl kill lice and nits rapidly. The lotion should be washed off 12 hours after application, and a fine-toothed comb run through the hair to remove dead lice and nits. Shampoos containing malathion or carbaryl are also effective if used repeatedly over several days. Combs and hairbrushes should be treated with very hot water to kill any attached eggs.

BODY LICE

These lice live and lay eggs on clothing next to the skin. The lice visit the body only to feed. Body lice transmit epidemic *typhus* and *relapsing fever*, diseases that are rare today but which were once common in areas affected by war or natural disaster.

These lice affect only people who rarely change their clothes. Body lice can be killed by placing infested clothes in a hot dryer for five minutes, by washing them in very hot water, or by burning them.

CRAB LICE

These lice live in pubic hair or, more rarely, in armpits, beards, or eyelashes. Crab lice are usually passed from one person to another during sexual contact. (See *Pubic lice*.)

Lichenification

Thickening and hardening of the skin that is caused by repeated scratching. Lichenification is often the result of scratching to relieve the intense itching of disorders such as atopic *eczema* or *lichen simplex*.

Lichen planus

A common skin disease of unknown cause that usually affects middle-aged people. Small, shiny, extremely itchy, pink or purple raised spots appear on the skin of the wrists, forearms, or lower legs. There is often a lacy network of white spots covering the inside lining of the cheeks.

The disease is treated with *corticosteroid drugs*. Creams, sometimes supplemented by injections in severe cases, are used to treat the skin rash. Most cases clear up within 18 months.

Lichen simplex

Patches of thickened, itchy, and sometimes discolored skin caused by repeated scratching. Typical sites are the neck, wrist, arm near the elbow, and ankles. Lichen simplex is most common in women and is psychological in origin; sufferers often rub the patches (without being aware of doing so) when agitated or under stressful circumstances. A cycle is established

in which repeated scratching to relieve itching leads to more skin thickening and itching, which then requires yet more scratching.

Treatment is with oral *antihistamine drugs* and creams containing *corticosteroid drugs* to relieve itching. Sometimes bandaging may be used to protect the skin and so break the cycle. This permits the disorder to subside and the treatment to be effective.

Lid lag

A momentary delay in the normal downward movement of the upper eyelids that occurs when the eye looks down. A characteristic feature of *thyrotoxicosis*, lid lag usually occurs in conjunction with *exophthalmos* (protrusion of the eyeball).

Lidocaine

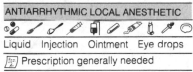

ANTIARRHYTHMIC LOCAL ANESTHETIC			
Liquid	Injection	Ointment	Eye drops
Prescription generally needed			

A local anesthetic (see *Anesthesia, local*). Lidocaine is given to numb tissues before minor surgical procedures and as a *nerve block* (to numb the area supplied by a particular nerve). It is also applied topically to relieve discomfort during the insertion of a *catheter* (tube) or an *endoscope* (viewing instrument) or to relieve irritation, for example, from *hemorrhoids*.

Lidocaine is sometimes given by intravenous injection after a *myocardial infarction* (heart attack) to reduce the risk of *ventricular fibrillation* (an irregularity of the heartbeat).

POSSIBLE ADVERSE EFFECTS

High doses given by injection occasionally cause nausea and vomiting.

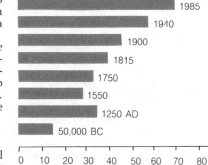

Life expectancy through history
Advances in medicine have dramatically increased life expectancy at birth. Life expectancies in England fluctuated around age 30 to 35 for many centuries, before reaching 40 in the early 19th century and climbing to over 70 in recent decades. Most developed countries follow a similar pattern.

Life expectancy

The number of years a person can expect to live. In most developed countries, life expectancy at birth is about 70 years for men and 75 years for women. Life expectancy is less in undeveloped countries, but there too it is higher for women than men. This sex difference is thought to be due to the fact that many more men than women smoked in the first half of this century. However, since then, the smoking sex ratio has evened out and there has been an increase in deaths from lung cancer in women. As a result, the sex difference in life expectancy is narrowing.

The expected age of death becomes greater the longer a person lives, so a 70-year-old may have a life expectancy of 15 years; even a 100-year-old can expect to live a year or two.

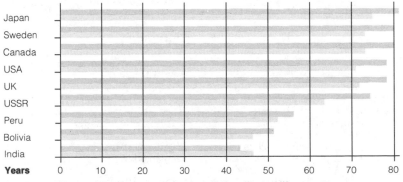

Gender and life expectancy
In rich and poor countries, life expectancy at birth is generally higher for females (gray bars) than males (pink). India is an exception.

Nationality and life expectancy
Average life expectancy at birth in most developed countries is now 70 or more; in developing countries it is 40 to 55.

LIFE EXPECTANCY AND LIFESPAN

Life expectancy should be distinguished from lifespan. Since records began, some old people have lived well beyond 70 years. Gerontologists agree that, in the absence of disease, the average normal lifespan is about 85 years (see *Aging*).

The natural lifespan is determined largely by genetic factors. People whose parents and grandparents lived to be 90 are likely to live to about this age. However, the extent to which individuals fulfil their genetic potential is affected by environmental factors, such as nutrition and accidents, as well as by disease.

The proportion of the population that attains its natural lifespan depends on the general health of that population, so life expectancy is a good means of comparing the state of health in different countries or in different parts of the same country.

Life expectancy at birth may be as low as 35 years in some developing countries. However, although statistically accurate, this figure is misleading because it reflects the high mortality in infancy. Records show that life expectancy at age 40 is not greatly different around the world.

Life support

The process of keeping a person alive by artificially inflating the lungs (see *Ventilation*) and, if necessary, maintaining the heartbeat with a *pacemaker*.

Ligament

A tough band of white, fibrous, slightly elastic tissue. Ligaments are important components of joints, binding together the bone ends and preventing excessive movement of the joint. Ligaments also support various organs, including the uterus, bladder, liver, and diaphragm, and help maintain the shape of the breasts.

INJURY

Ligaments, especially those in the *ankle joint* and *knee*, are sometimes damaged by injury. Minor sprains are treated with ice, bandaging, and sometimes *physiotherapy*. If the ligament is torn, the joint is either immobilized by a plaster *cast* to allow healing or repaired surgically. Strain of ligaments in the back may cause nonspecific *back pain*, which is usually treated with physiotherapy exercises.

Ligation

The surgical process of ligating (tying off) a blood vessel to prevent bleeding, or a duct to close it, with a length

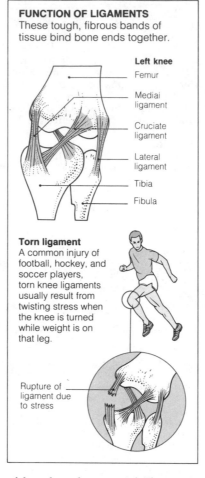

FUNCTION OF LIGAMENTS
These tough, fibrous bands of tissue bind bone ends together.

Left knee
- Femur
- Medial ligament
- Cruciate ligament
- Lateral ligament
- Tibia
- Fibula

Torn ligament
A common injury of football, hockey, and soccer players, torn knee ligaments usually result from twisting stress when the knee is turned while weight is on that leg.

Rupture of ligament due to stress

of thread or other material. The term is used in tubal ligation, a form of sterilization in which the fallopian tubes are tied off (see *Sterilization, female*).

Ligature

A length of thread or other material used for *ligation* (tying off) of a blood vessel or duct.

Lightening

A feeling experienced by many pregnant women when the baby's head descends into the pelvic cavity. Lightening usually occurs in the last three weeks of pregnancy, leaving more space in the upper abdomen and relieving pressure under the ribs.

Light treatment

See *Phototherapy*.

Limb, artificial

Artificial legs or arms, known medically as limb prostheses. Most artificial limbs are fitted to replace all or part of a limb amputated because of disease or severe injury (see *Amputation*). In some cases, however, they are required as a substitute for limbs missing from birth (see *Limb defects*).

CONSTRUCTION AND MATERIALS

Artificial limbs can be obtained ready-made. However, for the best results, they should be specially constructed to suit an individual's needs. A mold taken from the stump of the missing limb is used to make a socket for the top of the prosthesis into which the stump can fit closely and comfortably. The socket, made from wood, leather, or plastic, is attached to the stump by suction or by straps.

Each main part of an artificial limb (replacing the natural lower leg, thigh, forearm, or upper arm) is called an extension. The extension consists of an inner strut, which can be made of various materials, covered by foam rubber that is shaped to match the corresponding part of the natural limb. This unit is enclosed by an outer shell of metal, wood, or leather.

Artificial joints are usually made of plastic and metal and may incorporate sophisticated mechanisms to perform such functions as rotating the wrist, and controlling the length of stride.

Generally, artificial legs are more useful than artificial arms because the straightforward movements of the natural leg are easier to duplicate than the wide-ranging, often intricate, movements of the arm (especially the hand). Even so, the design of artificial hands is now extremely advanced. Electronic circuitry has been developed to pick up muscle and nerve impulses reaching the stump from the spinal cord. The circuitry transforms the impulses into movements of the prosthesis. People with an artificial arm or hand may have several prostheses to perform different functions. (See also illustrated box, facing page.)

Limb defects

Incomplete development of one or more limbs at birth. In some cases, an entire limb is missing. In others, only the hand or foot, or the upper or lower half of a limb, is missing. In a condition called phocomelia, hands, feet, or tiny finger or toe buds are attached to limb stumps or grow directly from the trunk. Any combination of limbs may be affected.

Limb defects are rare; the incidence is only about one in every 2,000 live births. The sedative drug *thalidomide* is known to have caused phocomelia in many of the children born to the

TYPES OF ARTIFICIAL LIMB

Different types of artificial limbs must restore as much as possible the function of the lost limb, be light enough to be worn comfortably, be easy to put on and take off, and look as normal as possible. Although ready-made prostheses are available and can be quite effective, the best artificial limbs are constructed by specialists and are specially adapted to meet an individual's particular needs.

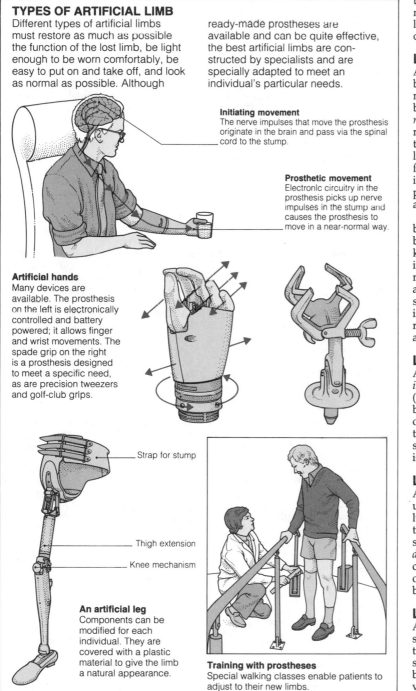

Initiating movement
The nerve impulses that move the prosthesis originate in the brain and pass via the spinal cord to the stump.

Prosthetic movement
Electronic circuitry in the prosthesis picks up nerve impulses in the stump and causes the prosthesis to move in a near-normal way.

Artificial hands
Many devices are available. The prosthesis on the left is electronically controlled and battery powered; it allows finger and wrist movements. The spade grip on the right is a prosthesis designed to meet a specific need, as are precision tweezers and golf-club grips.

Strap for stump

Thigh extension

Knee mechanism

An artificial leg
Components can be modified for each individual. They are covered with a plastic material to give the limb a natural appearance.

Training with prostheses
Special walking classes enable patients to adjust to their new limbs.

women who were given this drug during pregnancy. Limb defects may be inherited or form part of a syndrome (a group of abnormalities occurring in combination). In many cases, the cause of a limb defect is unknown.

MANAGEMENT
A child with a limb defect usually needs to attend a specialized center. Pediatricians, occupational therapists, psychologists, social workers, and other experts will treat the condition and advise on the child's development. A prosthetist will fit an artificial limb (see *Limb, artificial*) and teach the child how to use it.

Limbic system
A ring-shaped area in the center of the brain consisting of a number of connected clusters of nerve cells. The limbic system plays a role in the *autonomic nervous system* (which automatically regulates body functions), in the emotions, and in the sense of smell. The limbic system is extensive, and the different substructures within it have individual names (e.g., the hippocampus, the cingulate gyrus, and the amygdala).

Much of our knowledge of the limbic system comes from study of the behavior of animals and people known to have damage to or disease in the limbic area of the brain. The most commonly observed effects are abnormalities of emotional response, such as inappropriate crying or laughing, easily provoked rage, unwarranted fear, anxiety, and depression, and excessive sexual interest.

Limp
An abnormal, uneven pattern of *walking* in which the movements of one leg (or of the pelvis on one side of the body) are different from those of the other. A limp may involve dipping of the pelvis to one side, or failure to straighten the leg fully when the foot is placed on the ground.

Lincomycin
An *antibiotic drug* that is infrequently used to treat serious infections of the lungs, skin, bones, joints, and pelvis that are resistant to commonly prescribed antibiotics such as *penicillin drugs*. Lincomycin may, in rare cases, cause a type of *colitis* (inflammation of the intestine) called pseudomembranous colitis.

Linctus
A bland, glutinous mixture, usually sweetened, given to soothe the irritation caused by an inflamed throat. A simple linctus contains no active drug but linctuses are commonly used as vehicles for various *cough suppressants* (codeine, for example).

Lindane
A drug used in the form of a lotion or cream to treat infestation by *scabies* and some types of *lice*. Lindane, also called gamma benzene hexachloride, is used as a pesticide.

Lindane sometimes irritates the skin and causes itching. In large amounts, it can be toxic, particularly to children. Poisoning can produce vomiting, diarrhea, convulsions, liver damage, and anemia.

Linear accelerator

A device for accelerating subatomic particles, such as electrons, to a speed approaching that of light so that they have extremely high energies. A linear accelerator can also be used to generate high-energy X rays.

In medicine, high-energy electrons or X rays are used in *radiation therapy* to treat certain cancers. This method causes less damage to the healthy tissue around a tumor than does low-energy radiation therapy.

Liniment

A liquid rubbed onto the skin to relieve aching muscles and stiff joints. Some liniments contain a rubefacient (a counterirritant that increases blood flow beneath the skin). A liniment should be massaged into the skin two or three times daily; it should not be put on broken or inflamed skin.

Lip

One of two fleshy folds around the entrance to the mouth. Externally the lips are covered with skin and internally with mucous membrane, the relative transparency of which allows the red-pink of the underlying capillaries to show through.

The main substructure of the lips is a ring of muscle, whose functions include keeping food in the mouth, helping to produce speech and other sounds (whistling, for example), and kissing. Smaller muscles at the corners of the lips are responsible for facial expression.

DISORDERS

These include chapping (see *Chapped skin*), *cheilitis* (inflammation, cracking, and dryness), *cold sores* (blisters on the lips due to HERPES SIMPLEX infection), hard chancre (an early sign of *syphilis*), and *lip cancer*.

Lipancreatin

An enzyme, derived from animal tissues, used in treatment of patients with certain pancreatic disorders.

Lip cancer

A malignant tumor, usually on the lower lip. Lip cancer is largely confined to older people, especially those exposed to a lot of sunlight and those who have smoked cigarettes or a pipe

for many years. Lip cancer is the most common form of mouth cancer, but accounts for only about 1 percent of all cancers.

SYMPTOMS

A white patch develops on the lip and soon becomes scaly and cracked with a yellow crust. The affected area grows and eventually becomes ulcerated. In some cases, the cancer spreads to the lymph nodes in the jaw and neck.

DIAGNOSIS AND TREATMENT

Any lip sore that persists for longer than a month should be seen by a physician. Lip cancer (usually a *squamous cell carcinoma*) is diagnosed by *biopsy* (removal of a sample of tissue for microscopic examination).

Treatment is surgical removal, *radiation therapy*, or a combination of both. If the tumor has spread to the lymph nodes, *neck dissection* and further treatment with radiation may be necessary.

Lipectomy, suction

A type of *body contour surgery* in which excess fat is sucked out through a small incision made in the skin.

Lipid disorders

Disorders of metabolism (internal body chemistry) that cause abnormal amounts of *lipids* in the body. The most common of these disorders are the *hyperlipidemias*, which may be inherited or brought on or aggravated by diet or a disorder. There are also some very rare lipid disorders that are due solely to heredity, such as *Tay-Sachs disease*.

Lipid-lowering drugs

COMMON DRUGS
Drugs that act on the liver *Clofibrate Niacin Probucol*
Drugs that act on bile salts *Cholestyramine Colestipol*
Drug that blocks cholesterol formation *Lovastatin*

A group of drugs used to treat *hyperlipidemia* (abnormally high levels of one or more types of *lipid*, such as *cholesterol*, in the blood). Lipid-lowering drugs are given to reduce the risk of severe *atherosclerosis* (narrowing of the arteries), usually when dietary measures have not worked.

HOW THEY WORK

Some lipid-lowering drugs alter *enzyme* activity in the *liver* to prevent

the production of one or more types of lipid from fatty acids. This action reduces the level of lipids in the blood.

Other lipid-lowering drugs interfere with the absorption of *bile* salts from the intestine into the blood. Bile salts contain large amounts of cholesterol; a decrease in their concentration in the blood stimulates the liver to convert more cholesterol into bile salts, thus reducing the amount of cholesterol in the blood.

POSSIBLE ADVERSE EFFECTS

Some lipid-lowering drugs that act on the liver cause increased susceptibility to *gallstones*. Those that act on bile salts may cause nausea and diarrhea.

Lipids

A general term for *fats and oils*. Lipids, or lipins as they are sometimes called, include triglycerides (simple fats), phospholipids (important constituents of cell membranes and nerve tissue), and sterols such as *cholesterol*.

Lipoatrophy

Loss of *adipose tissue* (body fat). Patchy lipoatrophy can be caused by repeated injections of *insulin* into one area of skin. Other causes include lipodystrophies (disorders of fat metabolism) and *malabsorption* of fat.

Lipoma

A common *benign* tumor of fatty tissue. Lipomas give rise to slow-growing soft swellings. The tumors may develop anywhere in the body, but occur most commonly on the thigh, trunk, or shoulder. A person may develop one or many lipomas. The tumors are painless and harmless and do not need treatment, although they may be surgically removed for cosmetic reasons.

Liposarcoma

A rare cancer of fatty tissue that most commonly develops during late middle age. Liposarcomas usually occur in the abdomen or on the thigh, where they produce firm swellings. The tumors can generally be removed by surgery, but tend to recur.

Lipreading

A way of understanding words or conversation through the use of visual clues rather than hearing. Lipreading is invaluable in helping people who are deaf to understand more of what is said to them (see *Deafness*).

HOW IT IS DONE

The basis of lipreading is that certain speech sounds are produced by characteristic movements, positions, and relationships of the jaw, lips, and tongue. Because there are more than 40 clearly distinct sounds in the English language, facial expression and context are also important.

EFFECTIVENESS

Tests have shown that the proportion of identified words can rise from 20 to 60 percent after training. Anyone speaking to a deaf person can help improve the effectiveness of lipreading by speaking slightly more slowly than usual, by not covering the mouth when speaking, and by looking directly at the deaf person.

Lisp

The most common form of *speech disorder*. A lisp is due to protrusion of the tongue between the teeth so that the "s" sound is replaced by "th." Most children with a lisp have completely normal structures of the mouth and lips. However, sometimes the speech defect is caused by a cleft palate (see *Cleft lip and palate*). In most children, lisping disappears without treatment. If it persists after the age of about 4, *speech therapy* may be considered.

Listeriosis

A bacterial infection common in animals, including cattle, pigs, and poultry, that may also affect humans. Although the incidence of human listeriosis is low, it appears to be increasing worldwide. In 1988, 60 cases were reported in Canada. Twelve were associated with pregnancy. Many cases may be going unreported.

Listeriosis is caused by LISTERIA MONOCYTOGENES, a bacterium that is widespread in the environment, especially in soil. Possible sources of human infection include soft cheese, milk, ready-prepared coleslaw and salads, cook-chill foods, and improperly cooked meat. The bacterium is normally destroyed at pasteurizing temperatures, but if food is infected and refrigerated, the bacterium may continue to multiply. For this reason, chilled food should not be eaten after the "best before" date. Listeriosis can also be spread by direct contact with an infected live animal.

SYMPTOMS

The only symptoms in most affected adults are fever and generalized aches and pains. There may also be sore throat, conjunctivitis, diarrhea, and abdominal pain. *Pneumonia*, *septicemia*, and *meningitis* may develop in severe cases. Listeriosis can be life-threatening, particularly in the elderly, in people whose *immune system* is suppressed, in pregnant women, and in the newborn. An unborn child that is infected through its mother's blood may be stillborn. Listeriosis may be a cause of recurrent miscarriages.

DIAGNOSIS AND TREATMENT

Listeriosis is diagnosed by blood tests and by analysis of other body fluids, such as urine. Treatment is with *antibiotic drugs*, such as *ampicillin*. If listeriosis is diagnosed at an early stage and is treated promptly, the disease can be completely cured. However, severe infection, especially in the newborn, may be fatal.

Lithium

A drug used in the long-term treatment of *mania* and *manic-depressive illness*. Lithium helps prevent mood swings in mania and reduces their frequency and severity.

Lithium reduces excessive nerve activity in the brain. It is thought to work by altering the chemical balance within certain nerve cells.

POSSIBLE ADVERSE EFFECTS

High levels of lithium in the blood may cause nausea, vomiting, diarrhea, blurred vision, tremor, drowsiness, rash, and, in rare cases, kidney damage. Regular blood tests are carried out in order to monitor the level of lithium in the body.

Too much tea and coffee increases the risk of adverse effects. Too much sodium in the diet reduces the effectiveness of treatment.

Lithotomy

Surgical removal of a *calculus* (stone) from the urinary tract, especially from the bladder.

The operation of "cutting for stone" is one of the oldest known surgical procedures. Bladder stones were formerly removed by approaching the organ through incisions between the thighs rather than via the abdomen. The patient would lie back with the knees bent and legs open. Today, this *lithotomy position* is used mainly for gynecological examinations.

The operations of ureterolithotomy and *pyelolithotomy* (removal of ureteral and kidney stones respectively, by incision) are still occasionally performed. In developed countries, surgical removal of bladder stones is performed only for large stones. Instead, bladder stones are usually crushed and removed by use of a cystoscope (see *Cystoscopy*) or pulverized ultrasonically by *lithotripsy*.

Lithotomy position

Position in which a patient lies on his or her back with the knees bent and wide apart. Originally used for *lithotomy* (surgical removal of bladder stones), the position is still used for *pelvic examinations*, childbirth, and many types of pelvic surgery. Stirrups are usually used to provide support for the feet and legs.

Lithotripsy

The process of using shock waves or ultrasonic waves to break up *calculi* (stones) for excretion. There are two different procedures—extracorporeal shock wave lithotripsy (ESWL) and percutaneous lithotripsy.

WHY IT IS DONE

Lithotripsy is used to break up kidney and upper ureteral stones (see *Calculus, urinary tract*) into tiny pieces so that they can be excreted in the urine. The technique is also being used as a treatment for some types of *gallstones*.

ESWL is used to break up smaller stones; percutaneous lithotripsy is used to break up larger stones. Very large stones may be treated with a combination of the two.

HOW IT IS DONE

Both procedures may be performed under general or epidural anesthetic, although some machines do not require an anesthetic at all.

ESWL This technique uses a machine called a *lithotriptor* to produce external shock waves to break up stones. X-ray imaging systems are used to show the position of the stone and to monitor its destruction into a fine sand, which is passed out of the body in the urine or the bile over the following few weeks. ESWL has radically changed the treatment of kidney stones by eliminating the need for surgery in many cases, and is also changing the treatment of gallstones.

PERCUTANEOUS LITHOTRIPSY A nephroscope (a viewing instrument for inspecting the kidney) is inserted into the kidney via a small puncture in the flank. An ultrasonic probe is directed through the nephroscope to break up the stone, and the fragments of stone are then removed through the nephroscope. (See also illustrated box on page 644.)

RECOVERY PERIOD

There may be blood in the urine for about 12 hours after the treatment. After ESWL there may be some bruising of the skin at the entry and exit points of the shock wave. Most people can return to full activity within a week of treatment.

L

LITHOTRIPSY PROCEDURES

Calculi can sometimes be removed without major surgery. Lithotripsy uses ultrasonic or shock waves to break up the calculi. In percutaneous lithotripsy, the calculi are easily removed through a small incision. After extracorporeal shock wave lithotripsy (ESWL), stone fragments are passed in the urine.

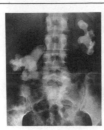

Abdominal calculi
This X ray shows two staghorn calculi in the kidneys. Before lithotripsy, stones such as these could be removed only by major surgery.

PERCUTANEOUS LITHOTRIPSY

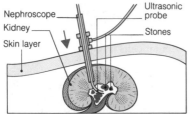
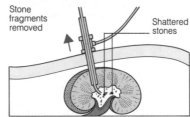

Nephroscope — Kidney — Skin layer — Ultrasonic probe — Stones

Stone fragments removed — Shattered stones

1 The surgeon first makes a small incision and inserts a nephroscope (a type of viewing tube) into the kidney.

2 A probe is passed through the nephroscope to direct ultrasound waves at the stones, causing them to shatter. Stone fragments are then removed.

EXTRACORPOREAL SHOCK WAVE LITHOTRIPSY (ESWL)

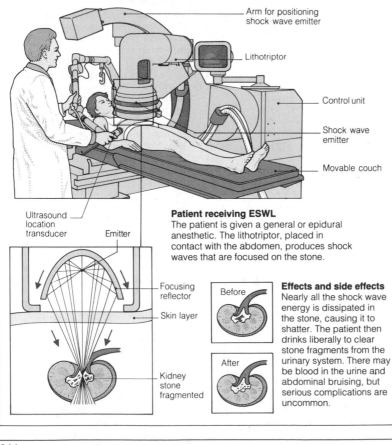

Arm for positioning shock wave emitter — Lithotriptor — Control unit — Shock wave emitter — Movable couch

Ultrasound location transducer — Emitter

Patient receiving ESWL
The patient is given a general or epidural anesthetic. The lithotriptor, placed in contact with the abdomen, produces shock waves that are focused on the stone.

Focusing reflector — Skin layer — Kidney stone fragmented

Before — After

Effects and side effects
Nearly all the shock wave energy is dissipated in the stone, causing it to shatter. The patient then drinks liberally to clear stone fragments from the urinary system. There may be blood in the urine and abdominal bruising, but serious complications are uncommon.

COMPLICATIONS
Ureteral colic (a severe spasmodic pain in the side due to obstruction of the ureter by small fragments of stone) may occur after ESWL. Patients treated for gallstones may need drug treatment to aid the final elimination of stone residues.

Lithotriptor

The machine used in extracorporeal shock wave *lithotripsy* (ESWL) to disintegrate small *calculi* (stones).

Livedo reticularis

A netlike purple or blue mottling of the skin, usually on the lower legs. It is caused by the enlargement of blood vessels beneath the skin and tends to be worse in cold weather.

Although harmless, the condition is present for life. Livedo reticularis may appear in healthy people, but is more common in those with abnormal sensitivity to cold or in people who have suffered damage to blood vessels just beneath the skin (see *Vasculitis*).

Liver

The largest and one of the most important internal organs, which functions as the body's chemical factory and regulates the levels of most of the main chemicals in blood. The liver is located in the upper right abdominal cavity, directly below the diaphragm. In adults, the liver weighs approximately 1 to 1.5 kg.

STRUCTURE
The liver is a roughly cone-shaped, red-brown organ divided into two main lobes. Each lobe consists of many lobules. Surrounding each lobule are branches of the hepatic artery and the portal vein (see illustrated box on page 646). The liver receives oxygenated blood from the hepatic artery and nutrient-rich blood via the portal vein. All the blood from the liver drains into the hepatic veins. The liver cells secrete *bile*, a fluid that leaves the liver through a network of ducts, known as bile ducts. Within the liver, the small bile ducts and branches of the hepatic artery and portal vein form a kind of conduit system called the portal tracts.

FUNCTION
The liver has many functions vital to the body. One is to produce important proteins for blood plasma. These proteins include albumin (which regulates the exchange of water between blood and tissues), complement (a group of proteins that play a part in the *immune system*), coagulation fac-

L

tors (which enable blood to clot when a blood vessel wall is damaged), and globin (a constituent of the oxygen-carrying pigment *hemoglobin*). The liver also produces *cholesterol* and special proteins that help carry fats around the body.

Another function of the liver is to take up glucose that is' not required immediately and store it as glycogen. When the body needs to generate more energy and heat, the liver (under the stimulation of hormones) converts the glycogen back to glucose and releases it into the bloodstream.

The liver also regulates the *blood level* of *amino acids*, chemicals that are the building blocks of proteins. When the blood contains too high a level of amino acids (such as after a meal), the liver converts some of them into glucose, some into proteins, some into other amino acids, and some into *urea*, which is passed to the kidney for excretion in the urine.

Along with the kidneys, the liver acts to clear the blood of drugs and poisonous substances that would otherwise accumulate in the bloodstream. The liver absorbs the substances to be removed from the blood, alters their chemical structure, makes them water soluble, and excretes them in the bile.

Bile carries waste products away from the liver and helps in the breakdown and absorption of fats in the small intestine (see *Biliary system*).

Although extremely complex in its functions, the liver is a remarkably resilient organ. Up to three quarters of its cells can be destroyed or surgically removed before it ceases to function.

Liver abscess

A localized collection of pus in the *liver*. The most common causes are a spread of bacteria from intestines inflamed by *diverticulitis* or *appendicitis*, and invasion of the liver by amebae (single-celled animal parasites) in people infected with *amebiasis*. In some cases, the source of infection cannot be identified.

An affected person is obviously ill, with a high fever, pain in the upper right abdomen, and (especially if elderly) mental confusion.

DIAGNOSIS AND TREATMENT
Ultrasound scanning usually shows the abscess. The responsible microorganisms can sometimes be identified from a blood sample or from a sample of tissue obtained by aspiration (with-drawal by suction through a needle) of the liver abscess.

A liver abscess can sometimes be treated by aspiration (sucking out the pus), using ultrasound to guide the needle through the abdominal wall. Otherwise, abdominal surgery is necessary to remove the abscess.

Liver biopsy

A diagnostic test in which a small sample of tissue is removed from the *liver*. The procedure is relatively safe, and complications are rare.

WHY IT IS DONE
The main function of the test is to diagnose liver diseases, such as *cirrhosis* and different types of *hepatitis*. A liver biopsy can also help diagnose diseases, such as *lymphomas* and various other types of tumors, which spread throughout the body and affect many organs. Liver biopsy can also provide an important check on the efficacy of treatment of diseases such as chronic active hepatitis.

HOW IT IS DONE
Most liver biopsies are performed under a local anesthetic. While the patient holds his or her breath, a slim needle is inserted into the liver via a very small incision made over the right lower ribs. The needle is removed together with a small sample of liver tissue. The structure and cells of the liver tissue are then examined by a pathologist.

A liver biopsy is sometimes performed during the course of another abdominal operation.

Liver cancer

A *malignant* tumor in the *liver*. The tumor may be primary (originating within the liver itself) or secondary (having spread from elsewhere). There are two main types of primary tumor—a hepatoma, which develops in the liver cells, and a *cholangiocarcinoma*, which arises from cells lining the *bile ducts*.

CAUSES AND INCIDENCE
Hepatomas are the most common form of cancer worldwide. They are closely linked to infection with hepatitis B (see *Hepatitis, viral*), which is common throughout Africa, the Middle East, and the Far East. When a hepatoma does occur, it is usually a complication of *cirrhosis* of the liver.

Secondary liver cancer is relatively common in Canada (about 20 times more common than primary cancer). This type of cancer often originates from cancers in the stomach, pancreas, or large intestine, which may

---

LOCATION OF THE LIVER

The liver is a roughly cone-shaped, red-brown organ that occupies the upper right-hand portion of the abdominal cavity. It lies immediately beneath the diaphragm, to which its upper side is attached. Its base is in contact with the stomach, right kidney, and intestines. Tucked within a depression on the underside of the liver is the gallbladder.

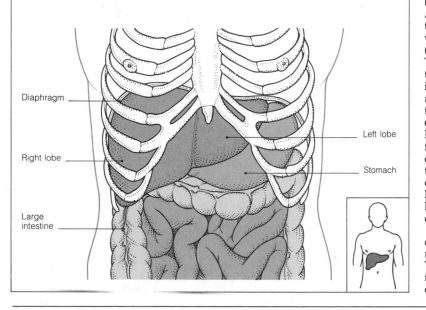

Diaphragm

Right lobe

Large intestine

Left lobe

Stomach

---

have been small and caused no symptoms (and so remained undiagnosed until they had spread to the liver).

SYMPTOMS AND SIGNS

The most common symptoms of any liver cancer are weight loss, loss of appetite, and lethargy. Many sufferers also have pain in the upper right abdomen. The later stages of the disease are marked by *jaundice* and *ascites* (fluid in the abdomen).

DIAGNOSIS

Liver tumors are usually detected as a result of *ultrasound scanning* that reveals abnormal areas in the liver. The diagnosis is confirmed by *liver biopsy* (removal of a small sample of liver tissue for microscopic analysis).

About 80 percent of hepatomas raise the production of a substance called *alpha-fetoprotein* by the liver; measurement of the blood level of this protein is used as a screening test in geographical areas where the cancer is common. *Angiography* (X rays obtained after injecting a radiopaque substance into an artery) is also used to detect hepatomas too small to be seen by other scanning techniques.

TREATMENT

A hepatoma usually remains confined to the liver for a long time. In cases where cirrhosis is not also present (which is rare in Canada), complete removal of the tumor, leading to cure, is sometimes possible. In other cases, *anticancer drugs* can help the patient survive longer. A *liver transplant* may occasionally be considered.

There is no cure for secondary liver cancer, but anticancer drugs can help slow the progress of the disease. Tying off or blocking the hepatic artery or one of its branches to deprive the tumor of its blood supply has been attempted, as has placing a catheter into the artery to administer anticancer drugs continuously.

Liver, cirrhosis of

See *Cirrhosis*.

Liver disease, alcoholic

Damage to the *liver* caused by persistent heavy *alcohol* consumption, with progression to *cirrhosis* of the liver (severe structural damage and loss of function) and death.

TYPES

Excess fat accumulation in the liver affects almost everyone with a moderate to high alcohol consumption. However, this condition is completely reversible through abstinence and, if reversed, carries a low risk of progression to cirrhosis.

LIVER STRUCTURE AND FUNCTION

The liver is a large organ with numerous functions. It absorbs oxygen and nutrients from the blood, and regulates the blood's glucose and amino-acid levels. It helps break down drugs and various toxins, and manufactures important proteins, such as albumin and blood coagulation factors. The liver also produces bile, which removes waste products and helps process fats in the small intestine.

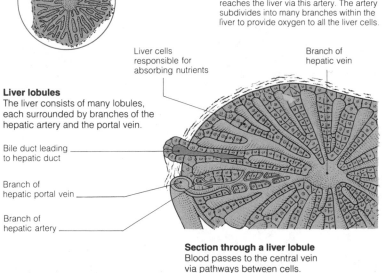

Hepatic vein
Blood leaves the liver via this vein and carries carbon dioxide and plasma proteins.

Hepatic portal vein
Blood from the intestines and spleen carries nutrients, such as fats and glucose, to the liver via this vein. The nutrients are used by the liver or stored within it.

Hepatic duct
Bile leaves the liver through a network of ducts, the bile ducts. They increase in size until they fuse to form the right and left hepatic ducts, which join and carry bile to the gallbladder.

Hepatic artery
Oxygenated blood from the heart (about one quarter of the heart's entire output) reaches the liver via this artery. The artery subdivides into many branches within the liver to provide oxygen to all the liver cells.

Liver cells responsible for absorbing nutrients

Branch of hepatic vein

Liver lobules
The liver consists of many lobules, each surrounded by branches of the hepatic artery and the portal vein.

Bile duct leading to hepatic duct

Branch of hepatic portal vein

Branch of hepatic artery

Section through a liver lobule
Blood passes to the central vein via pathways between cells.

Some persistent drinkers develop acute or chronic *hepatitis*. Individual liver cells are destroyed and there is inflammation and scarring of the liver. In people who continue to drink, there is a high risk (about 90 percent) of progression to cirrhosis; in most people who stop drinking, the liver returns to normal. Cirrhosis is irreversible, but abstinence often leads to improvement. Until the 1960s, alcoholic liver damage was thought to be caused by the malnutrition associated with alcohol dependence rather than by alcohol itself. It is now accepted that alcohol is directly toxic to the liver.

There is a clear relationship between the total amount of alcohol consumed in a population and the incidence of cirrhosis. The prevalence of alcoholic liver disease has been rising rapidly in most developed countries since about 1960, and the increase has been particularly steep in women. In Canada, around 2,000 people die each year as a result of alcoholic cirrhosis of the liver.

A person who consumes a daily average of 200 ml of alcohol (contained, for example, in about three quarters of a bottle of whisky or two and a half bottles of wine) has a 50 percent chance of developing cirrhosis within 20 years. A much lower daily average intake of 45 ml of alcohol (contained, for example, in four single whiskies or four glasses of wine) in a man, or half that amount in a woman, still carries a substantial risk.

SYMPTOMS AND DIAGNOSIS

The first symptoms or signs of liver damage are the same as those of hepatitis or cirrhosis. *Liver function tests* show a characteristic pattern of abnormalities, and *liver biopsy* (removal of a sample of tissue for microscopic analysis) may be recommended to identify the precise type of damage.

TREATMENT AND OUTLOOK

Abstinence from alcohol is the only method of returning the liver to normal or improving its function and prolonging life expectancy. Treatment methods are as for *alcohol dependence*.

Liver failure

A complication of acute *hepatitis* (inflammation of the *liver*) in which there is such a severe impairment of liver function that it affects other organs, particularly the brain. Liver failure may also refer to a critical stage in *cirrhosis* of the liver.

SYMPTOMS

The principal symptoms of acute liver failure are those of the underlying hepatitis; later, symptoms of brain dysfunction develop. Disturbance of brain function probably occurs because the liver fails to break down certain substances (such as ammonia) that build up in the blood and then poison or alter the transmission of nerve messages in the brain. Symptoms may include agitation and restlessness, followed by drowsiness, confusion, and coma—a condition known as hepatic *encephalopathy*.

When liver failure accompanies cirrhosis, other complications, such as *ascites* (fluid in the abdomen) and internal bleeding, may develop in addition to hepatic encephalopathy. The symptoms of brain dysfunction develop more slowly, and are characterized by recurrent episodes of drowsiness or confusion. These episodes are frequently precipitated by bacterial infections or by changes in drug treatment or diet.

DIAGNOSIS

A diagnosis is made from the patient's history, a physical examination, *liver function tests*, and tests for viruses that can cause acute hepatitis.

TREATMENT

Treatment of acute liver failure consists of skilled intensive care. There is no specific cure, although the use of *antibiotic drugs* and *lactulose* can reduce the number of intestinal bacteria, which are one of the main sources of toxic ammonia entering the bloodstream. A *liver transplant* is occasionally possible and suitable for certain patients. Only about a quarter of patients survive acute liver failure.

When brain dysfunction complicates cirrhosis, treatment of precipitating causes (such as infection) often leads to an improvement.

Liver fluke

Any of various species of flukes (small, flattened, worms) that infest the *bile ducts* within the *liver*.

The fluke FASCIOLA HEPATICA causes the disease fascioliasis. The adult flukes normally infest sheep and produce eggs that are passed in the sheep's feces. The eggs are eaten by snails, from which immature forms of the fluke emerge. They then become encysted (enclosed in a sac) on aquatic vegetation, particularly watercress. The disease is very rarely seen in Canada.

Fascioliasis has two stages. During the first stage, young flukes migrate through the liver, causing liver tenderness and enlargement, fever, night sweats, and sometimes a rash. In the second stage, adult worms are present in the bile ducts. This may lead to *cholangitis* (inflammation of the bile ducts) and *bile duct obstruction*, which can cause *jaundice*. In minor infections, there may be no symptoms. The disease is diagnosed from the presence of fluke eggs in the patient's

L

TABLE OF LIVER FUNCTION TESTS

Test	Significance
Serum bilirubin	Bilirubin is the yellow breakdown product of red blood cells that is passed to the liver and excreted in bile. It is the substance that gives the yellow color to the skin in jaundice. A high bilirubin level in the blood may indicate defective processing of bile by the liver or obstruction to bile flow.
Serum albumin	Albumin is one of the main proteins in blood. Made by the liver, one of its actions is to hold fluid inside the blood vessels. A low level is found in many chronic liver disorders and is often associated with ascites and ankle edema (fluid collection in the abdomen and around the ankles).
Serum alkaline phosphatase	Alkaline phosphatase is an enzyme found in bile. The blood level of this enzyme rises when there is obstruction to the flow of bile (cholestasis).
Serum aminotransferases (transaminases)	The aminotransferases are enzymes released from liver cells into the blood when the liver cells are damaged. The levels will be raised in acute and chronic hepatitis.
Prothrombin time	A normal result in this test of blood clotting depends on the presence in the blood of a protein made by the liver from a fat-soluble vitamin, vitamin K. The test result can be abnormal in two kinds of disorders—when the protein is not made because of liver cell damage, and when there is a blockage to bile flow in the liver, causing a lack of bile in the intestines (which interferes with fat and vitamin K absorption).

DISORDERS OF THE LIVER

By far the most common cause of liver disease in Canada and other developed countries is excessive consumption of alcohol (see *Liver disease, alcoholic*). Alcohol-related disorders, which include alcoholic *hepatitis* and *cirrhosis*, outnumber all other types of liver disorder by at least five to one.

Worldwide, the pattern of liver disease is different. In parts of Africa and Asia, up to 20 percent of the population are carriers of the *hepatitis B* virus; in these parts of the world, the most important liver disorders are virus-induced cirrhosis and primary *liver cancer*.

Apart from alcohol- and virus-induced liver disease, the liver may be affected by congenital defects, bacterial and parasitic infection, circulatory disturbance, metabolic disorders, poisoning, and autoimmune processes.

Liver failure (complete loss of liver function) may occur as a result of acute hepatitis, poisoning, or cirrhosis. Enlargement of the liver (hepatomegaly) and *jaundice* are two common signs of liver disease.

CONGENITAL DEFECTS

Defects of liver structure at birth principally affect the bile ducts. A choledochal cyst is a malformation of the hepatic duct (formed from the union of all the small bile ducts in the liver) which may obstruct the flow of bile in infants (causing jaundice); it requires removal. In *biliary atresia*, the bile ducts are absent, again causing jaundice.

INFECTION AND INFLAMMATION

Hepatitis is a general term for inflammation in the liver; it may be caused by viruses such as the hepatitis A, B, and non-A non-B viruses (see *Hepatitis, viral*). Bacteria may spread up the biliary system toward the liver to cause *cholangitis* or *liver abscess*. Parasitic diseases that may affect the liver include *schistosomiasis*, *liver fluke*, and *hydatid disease* (caused by various types of worm or fluke) and *amebiasis* (caused by a single-celled parasite).

POISONING AND DRUGS

Apart from alcohol, many drugs and toxins are broken down by the liver, damaging liver cells in the process. Suicidal overdose with the painkilling drug acetaminophen causes severe liver damage, which may not be obvious until up to two days after the overdose. Some medications, even in normal doses, can cause acute or chronic hepatitis by a direct toxic effect or through drug allergy.

Poisoning by certain types of mushrooms can cause acute liver failure (see *Mushroom poisoning*).

AUTOIMMUNE DISORDERS

Liver cells and bile ducts can be targets for autoimmune reactions (in which the body's immune system attacks its own tissues). A gradual destruction of liver cells is the main problem in autoimmune chronic active hepatitis (see *Hepatitis, chronic active*). The slowly progressive bile duct damage that occurs in primary *biliary cirrhosis* and sclerosing cholangitis possibly also has an autoimmune basis.

METABOLIC DISORDERS

The two main metabolic disorders affecting the liver are *hemochromatosis* (in which there is too much iron in the body) and *Wilson's disease* (in which there is too much copper).

TUMORS

The liver is a common site of malignant tumors that have spread from cancers of the stomach, pancreas, or large intestine. Enlargement of the liver and spleen is a common feature of *leukemias* and *lymphomas*. Primary tumors of the liver are much less common. (See *Liver cancer*.)

OTHER DISORDERS

In *Budd-Chiari syndrome*, the veins draining the liver become blocked by blood clots, causing painful swelling of the liver and severe *ascites* (collection of fluid in the abdomen). Obstruction of the portal vein is one cause of *portal hypertension* (high blood pressure in the portal vein), which can lead to *esophageal varices* (swollen veins in the esophagus) and ascites. Portal hypertension is also one of the usual complications of cirrhosis.

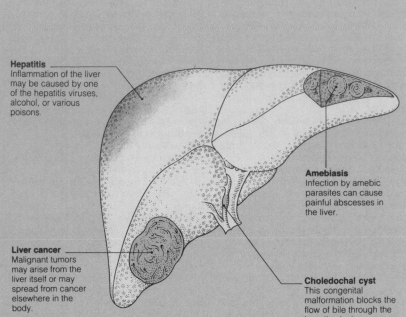

Hepatitis
Inflammation of the liver may be caused by one of the hepatitis viruses, alcohol, or various poisons.

Amebiasis
Infection by amebic parasites can cause painful abscesses in the liver.

Liver cancer
Malignant tumors may arise from the liver itself or may spread from cancer elsewhere in the body.

Choledochal cyst
This congenital malformation blocks the flow of bile through the hepatic duct.

INVESTIGATION

Disorders of the liver may be investigated by physical examination, *liver biopsy*, *liver function tests*, *ultrasound scanning*, and *CT scanning*.

feces. Treatment with the *anthelmintic drug* praziquantel may be effective.

Another species of liver fluke, *CLONORCHIS SINENSIS*, is common in the Far East. Infection is typically acquired by eating raw or under-cooked freshwater fish. The symptoms and treatment are broadly similar to those for fascioliasis.

Liver function tests

A series of tests of blood chemistry that can detect changes in the way the *liver* is making new substances, breaking down and/or excreting old ones, and whether liver cells are healthy or being damaged. The tests are widely used to help in the diagnosis of liver disease, and to assess treatment.

Liver function tests are particularly useful in distinguishing between acute and chronic liver disorders and between *hepatitis* (liver inflammation) and *cholestasis* (obstruction to the flow of bile). The most commonly performed tests are described in the table on page 647.

Liver imaging

A technique that produces images of the *liver, gallbladder, bile ducts,* and blood vessels supplying the liver to detect abnormality or disease.

TYPES

CONVENTIONAL X-RAY TECHNIQUES *Cholecystography* and *cholangiography* are techniques in which a contrast medium (an iodine-containing substance that is opaque to X rays) is introduced to show up *gallstones*, tumors, and blockages. *ERCP* (endoscopic retrograde cholangiopancreatography) is an alternative method of examining the *biliary system* by means of a contrast medium; it is especially useful in detecting blockage or narrowing of a bile duct or pancreatic duct by a stone or tumor.

Angiography shows up the blood vessels in the liver. It can be used to confirm the diagnosis of a *hemangioma* or to plan the treatment of liver tumors and other disorders.

SCANNING TECHNIQUES *Ultrasound scanning* is the most widely used of all liver imaging techniques. It is simple, safe, noninvasive, and produces excellent images, particularly of gallstones. *CT scanning* also provides good images and may be used if ultrasound has proved inconclusive.

Radionuclide scanning can indicate the presence of a cyst or a tumor. It is also useful in recording the progress of radioactive isotopes as they are excreted from the liver in bile.

Liver transplant

Replacement of a diseased *liver* with a healthy liver removed from a donor who has been declared brain dead. Liver transplantation is a technically difficult procedure, but is now accepted as a feasible and appropriate treatment for some types of advanced liver disease. The chances of surviving for many years with a transplanted liver are improving, but they are not yet as high as the chances of surviving after a *kidney transplant*.

WHY IT IS DONE

Transplantation is worth considering only for people with life-threatening or severely debilitating liver disease. However, if the disease process is too advanced, the person is unlikely to survive the operation. An assessment must be made of the likely length of survival and the quality of life with and without the operation.

In adults, the best results are obtained in the treatment of advanced liver *cirrhosis* in people with long-standing chronic active *hepatitis* or primary *biliary cirrhosis*. In acute *liver failure*, there can be difficulty in obtaining donor organs at an appropriate time, but people with a slightly less acute illness and those with *Budd-Chiari syndrome* have been successfully treated. People with primary *liver cancer* are rarely considered for transplantation because there is a high risk that the tumor will recur.

In children, congenital *biliary atresia* is the most common reason for liver transplantation.

HOW IT IS DONE

The donor organ is obtained from someone who has suffered *brain death* but whose liver is still healthy. The organ can be stored in cold salt solutions for a few hours.

A general anesthetic is given and the recipient's abdomen is opened. The diseased liver is removed, the donor organ is inserted in its place, and the major blood vessels and common bile duct are reconnected.

RECOVERY PERIOD

The first few days after the operation are spent in an *intensive-care* unit. *Immunosuppressant drugs* (particularly *cyclosporine*) are given to reduce the risk of rejection.

OUTLOOK

In some cases rejection occurs and a second transplant operation provides the only hope. There is now a 60 to 80 percent chance of surviving one year, which may mean that more than half the people now receiving a liver transplant will survive for five

years. The quality of life is generally excellent, with most people returning to near normal activity within a few weeks of the operation.

Living will

A written declaration, signed by an adult person of sound mind, that instructs his or her doctors to withhold or withdraw life-sustaining treatment if he or she suffers from an incurable and terminal condition.

Some countries have enacted legislation giving legal effect to living wills.

In Canada, no such law has been passed to date, although public opinion polls heavily support such legislation. Most legal commentators feel that a living will should be treated like any other expression of wishes by a patient.

Lobe

One of the clearly defined parts into which certain organs, such as the brain, liver, lungs, and thyroid gland, are divided. The term may also be used to describe any projecting, flat, pendulous part of the body, such as the earlobe.

Lobectomy

An operation to cut out a lobe in the brain (see *Lobotomy, prefrontal*), liver (see *Hepatectomy, partial*), lungs (see *Lobectomy, lung*), or thyroid gland (see *Thyroidectomy*).

Lobectomy, lung

An operation to remove one of the lobes of the *lung*. Lobectomy is usually performed to remove a malignant tumor, but may also be used to treat localized *bronchiectasis* that has not responded to medical treatment. In the past, lobectomy was carried out to treat *tuberculosis*.

After lobectomy, the remaining lobes expand to fill the chest cavity.

HOW IT IS DONE

With the patient under a general anesthetic, a curved incision is made, starting under the armpit and extending across the back, following the line of the lower edge of the shoulder blade. The muscles are cut through and the ribs are spread apart (or one is removed) to expose the lung. The blood vessels and bronchus (main airway) leading to the diseased lobe are then tied off and divided, and the lobe is removed. Before the incision is sewn up, a tube is inserted into the pleural space surrounding the lung to drain off fluid. The tube is usually removed after 24 hours.

L

The operation usually requires a hospital stay of several weeks; full recovery may take several months.

Lobotomy, prefrontal
The cutting of some of the fibers linking the frontal lobes to the rest of the *brain*. Prefrontal lobotomy was extensively used in the 1940s and 1950s to treat serious psychiatric disorders. However, the operation often resulted in harmful personality changes and is now used only as a last resort to treat people with severe, chronic depression. (See also *Psychosurgery*.)

Lochia
The discharge after childbirth of blood and fragments of uterine lining from the site where the placenta was attached. The discharge is bright red for the first three or four days and then becomes paler. The amount of lochia decreases as the placental site heals and usually ceases within six weeks.

Locked knee
A temporary inability to move the *knee* joint. A locked knee may be caused by a torn knee cartilage or by *loose bodies* in the joint.

Lockjaw
A painful spasm of the jaw muscles that makes it difficult or impossible to open the mouth. Lockjaw is the most common symptom of *tetanus*.

Locomotor
Relating to movement of the extremities, as in locomotor *ataxia*, the uncoordinated movements and lurching gait that occur in the later stages of untreated syphilis.

Loiasis

A form of the tropical parasitic disease *filariasis* that is caused by an infestation by the worm *LOA LOA*. Loiasis is transmitted by the bite of *CHRYSOPS* flies, which carry worm larvae or eggs. The adult worms, which are between 3 and 7 cm long, travel beneath the skin, producing itchy areas of inflammation known as Calabar swellings. The worms may also sometimes be seen moving across the front of the eye. Loiasis is treated with a course of diethylcarbamazine, which destroys the worms.

Loin
The part of the back on each side of the spine between the lowest pair of ribs and the top of the pelvis.

Loose bodies
Fragments of bone, cartilage, or capsule linings that are free to move within a *joint*. Loose bodies may occur whenever there is any damage to a joint, as in osteoarthritis (degeneration due to wear and tear), fracture, or *osteochondritis dissecans* (fragmentation of bone and cartilage due to disrupted blood supply).

SYMPTOMS AND SIGNS
Loose bodies are usually troublesome only if they lodge between joint surfaces, where they cause the joint to lock (usually only briefly), resulting in severe pain. The joint usually swells several hours later. Although the swelling subsides, further locking and swelling can recur at any time.

DIAGNOSIS AND TREATMENT
X rays or *arthroscopy* (inspection of the interior of a joint through a viewing instrument) reveal whether loose bodies are present.

Gentle manipulation may be required to unlock the joint. If locking occurs frequently, the loose bodies may be removed during arthroscopy or by surgery.

Loperamide
An *antidiarrheal drug* used in the treatment of recurrent and sudden bouts of diarrhea. Loperamide is also given to help regulate bowel action in people who have had an *ileostomy*.

Loperamide occasionally produces a rash. Other rare adverse effects, such as fever, abdominal cramps, and bloating, are often difficult to distinguish from symptoms of the disorder causing the diarrhea.

Loratidine
An antihistamine used in the treatment of allergic rhinitis (see *Rhinitis*). It may also be helpful in skin allergies. It has a long duration of action and is less likely to cause drowsiness than most antihistamines.

Lorazepam
A *benzodiazepine drug* that is used in the treatment of *insomnia* and *anxiety*. If use of lorazepam is suddenly stopped after it has been taken regularly for more than three weeks, there may be withdrawal symptoms (see *Drug dependence*).

Lordosis
Inward curvature of the *spine*, which is normally present to a minor degree in the lower back. Lordosis in the lower back can become exaggerated by poor posture (especially in someone who

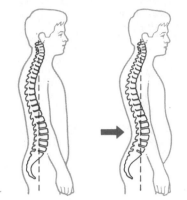

Normal and abnormal lordosis
The normal inward curvature of the spine (left) is exaggerated in abnormal lordosis (right).

is overweight and also has weak abdominal muscles) or by *kyphosis* (backward curvature of the spine) above the lower back.

Once pronounced lordosis has developed, it is usually a permanent condition and can lead to *disk prolapse* or *osteoarthritis* of the spine.

Loss of normal lordosis in the lower back or neck can occur when the back or neck muscles are in spasm. The condition corrects itself once the cause is successfully treated.

Lotion
A liquid drug preparation applied to the skin. Lotions have a cooling, soothing effect and are useful for covering large areas. Examples of drugs prepared as a lotion include *calamine* and *betamethasone*, which are used to treat skin inflammation.

Lovastatin
A *lipid-lowering* drug that works by blocking the action of an enzyme needed for the formation of cholesterol. It should be taken in conjunction with a low-cholesterol, low-fat diet. Most common side effects are gastrointestinal symptoms and headaches.

LSD
A synthetic *hallucinogenic drug* (drug that produces hallucinations) derived from ergot (a type of fungus). LSD is the abbreviation for lysergic acid diethylamide. Classified as a restricted drug under the Food and Drugs Act, LSD has no medical use, but may be used in medical research under special conditions.

LSD sometimes produces "bad trips" in which a person experiences panic, fear, and physical symptoms, such as nausea, dizziness, and weakness. In severe cases, sedation in hospital may be necessary for several days. There may be "flashbacks" to previous trips months or even years after use.

Although there is no evidence that LSD causes *psychosis* (mental illness characterized by a loss of contact with reality), it may act as a trigger in a person predisposed to mental illness, and may thus lead to lasting mental problems. There is evidence that LSD damages chromosomes.

Ludwig's angina
A rare bacterial infection of the floor of the mouth that becomes life-threatening as it spreads to the throat. The affected tissues become inflamed, swell, and harden.

The disorder is usually caused by an infected tooth or gum and is most common in people with poor *oral hygiene*. It generally results in fever, pain, swelling in the mouth and neck, and difficulty in opening the mouth and swallowing.

If the condition is not treated immediately with *antibiotic drugs*, the swollen tissues of the throat may cause difficulty in breathing. *Tracheostomy* (making a hole in the windpipe and inserting a tube through it) may be necessary to prevent asphyxiation.

Lumbago
A general term for lower *back pain*. Lumbago is a symptom that may be caused by various disorders, but in many cases no definite cause is found.

Lumbago may be caused by an intervertebral *disk prolapse*. It may also arise if a bit of *synovium* (thin membrane lining the capsule surrounding a joint) is caught between the surfaces of a small intervertebral joint, or if there is momentary *subluxation* (incomplete dislocation) of an intervertebral joint with straining of *ligaments*. Lumbago is often caused by a sudden turning or bending movement but may also begin gradually.

Lumbago is often aggravated by movement and relieved by rest. Treatment is usually bed rest, with additional measures as appropriate. (See also *Lumbosacral spasm*.)

Lumbar
Relating to the part of the back between the lowest pair of ribs and the top of the pelvis. The lumbar region of the *spine* consists of the five lumbar vertebrae between the lowest (12th) thoracic vertebra and the sacrum.

Lumbar puncture
A procedure in which a hollow needle is inserted into the lower part of the spinal canal to withdraw *cerebrospinal fluid* (the watery liquid that surrounds the brain and spinal cord) or to inject drugs or other substances. Lumbar puncture is used less often since the development of *CT scanning* and MRI (magnetic resonance imaging) as diagnostic tests.

WHY IT IS DONE
The main use of the lumbar puncture is to examine cerebrospinal fluid to diagnose and investigate disorders of the brain and spinal cord (such as *meningitis* and *subarachnoid hemorrhage*). The procedure is also used to inject drugs into the fluid (such as *anticancer drugs* to treat *leukemia* and malignant diseases of the central nervous system). Another use of lumbar puncture is to inject a contrast medium that will show up on X ray (see *Myelography*) to produce images of the spinal cord. Lumbar puncture can also be used to inject a local anesthetic to achieve extensive anesthesia without loss of consciousness.

HOW IT IS DONE
The patient lies on his or her side, chin on chest and knees drawn up to pull the vertebrae (bones of the spine) apart. The area of skin overlying the lumbar vertebrae at the base of the spine is anesthetized with a local anesthetic. A hollow needle is then inserted between two of the vertebrae and into the spinal canal and is used to withdraw cerebrospinal fluid or, depending on the purpose of the procedure, to inject drugs, an anesthetic, or a contrast medium.

After the needle is removed, the puncture site is covered with sterile tape. The procedure takes less than 20 minutes. Lumbar puncture usually causes no discomfort although some people may have a headache for a short time afterward.

L

LOCATION AND STRUCTURE OF THE LUNGS
The lungs lie in the chest within the rib cage. Air entering the body via the nose and mouth travels down the trachea to the main bronchi, which divide into smaller bronchi and then into bronchioles. These in turn lead to alveoli, where the oxygen/carbon dioxide exchange takes place. During expiration (breathing out), air leaves the body by the same routes.

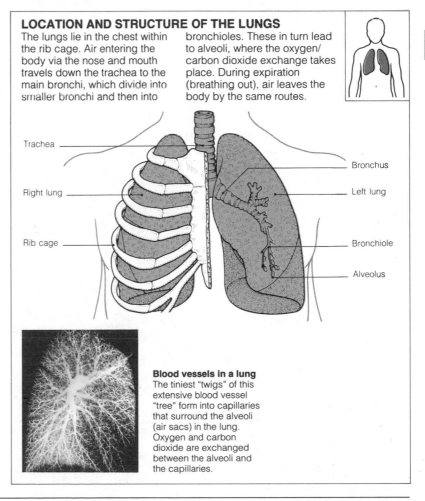

Trachea

Right lung

Rib cage

Bronchus

Left lung

Bronchiole

Alveolus

Blood vessels in a lung
The tiniest "twigs" of this extensive blood vessel "tree" form into capillaries that surround the alveoli (air sacs) in the lung. Oxygen and carbon dioxide are exchanged between the alveoli and the capillaries.

651

Lumbosacral spasm

Prolonged, excessive tightening of the muscles that surround and support the lower part of the *spine*. Lumbosacral spasm is a cause of *back pain* and may occasionally result in temporary *scoliosis* (curvature of the spine to one side). Treatment may include bed rest, *analgesic drugs* (painkillers), and *muscle-relaxant drugs*.

Lumen

The space within a tubular organ. The term is most commonly used to refer to the cavity of the intestine.

Lumpectomy

An operation to treat breast cancer (see *Mastectomy*).

Lunacy

An outdated term for serious mental disorder. It was coined because of the belief that phases of the moon ("luna" in Latin) could bring on mental illnesses, especially illnesses that seemed to come and go. Patients were called lunatics and mental hospitals were known as lunatic asylums.

Lung

The main organ of the *respiratory system*. The two lungs supply the body with the oxygen needed for *aerobic* metabolism and eliminate the waste product carbon dioxide.

STRUCTURE

The *trachea* (windpipe) branches in the chest into two main *bronchi* (air passages), which supply the left and right lungs. The main bronchi divide again into smaller bronchi and then into bronchioles, which lead to air passages that open out into grapelike air sacs called *alveoli*. It is through the thin walls of the alveoli that gases (notably oxygen and carbon dioxide) diffuse into or out of the blood.

Each lung is enclosed in a double membrane called the *pleura*, which allows the lungs to slide freely as they expand and contract during *breathing*. (See also *Respiration*.)

Lung cancer

The most common form of *cancer* in Canada, lung cancer is the leading cause of cancer deaths in men and the second most common cause (after breast cancer) in women. About 14,000 deaths from lung cancer occur annually in Canada. The peak age for this disease is 65 to 75 years. It is uncommon before the age of 40.

CAUSES

Cigarette smoking is the main cause of lung cancer. The more cigarettes smoked per day and the lower the age at which smoking started, the greater the risk. Smokers of cigars or pipes are less likely to develop the disease than people who smoke cigarettes, but they still have a significantly higher risk than nonsmokers (see *Tobacco*). Passive smoking (the inhalation of tobacco smoke by nonsmokers) has also been shown to increase the risk of developing lung cancer.

Living in an environment with a high level of air pollution or working with substances such as radioactive minerals or asbestos may cause some cases of lung cancer.

TYPES

There are several types, the most common being squamous cell carcinoma, small cell carcinoma (also called oat cell carcinoma), adenocarcinoma, and

---

DISORDERS OF THE LUNG

The lungs are continuously exposed to airborne particles, such as bacteria, viruses, and allergens, all of which can cause lung disorders. Most of these disorders do not interfere with oxygen supply; those that do are a major threat to health.

INFECTION

Infective disorders are common, especially *tracheitis* (inflammation of the lining of the windpipe) and *croup* (a virus infection of young children). *Bronchitis* (inflammation of the bronchi), *bronchiectasis* (swelling of the bronchi), and *bronchiolitis* (inflammation of the bronchioles) commonly follow colds or *influenza*. *Pneumonia* (inflammation of the lung) is usually caused by infection by viruses or bacteria. Fungal infections of the lungs, such as *aspergillosis*, *actinomycosis*, *histoplasmosis*, and *candidiasis*, are relatively uncommon.

ALLERGIES

Bronchial *asthma*, in which the muscles of the bronchi contract and obstruct the free passage of air, often occurs in sensitized people exposed to pollens, house mites, fungal spores, animal *dander*, and

many other agents. Allergic *alveolitis* (inflammation of the alveoli) may be caused by many organic dusts, such as moldy hay.

TUMORS

Lung cancer is one of the most common of all malignant tumors; in most cases it is associated with cigarette smoking. Secondary malignant tumors, which have spread from other parts of the body to the lungs, are common. However, benign tumors affecting the lung are uncommon.

INJURY

Lung injury usually results from penetration of the chest wall. *Pneumothorax* (air in the pleural cavity) and *hemothorax* (blood in the pleural cavity) are usually caused by a penetrating injury; either may cause collapse of the lung. Injury can also occur from the inhalation of poisonous dusts, gases, or toxic substances. *Silicosis* and *asbestosis* are caused by inhalation of silica and asbestos, respectively; they may lead to progressive *fibrosis* of the lung.

IMPAIRED BLOOD AND OXYGEN SUPPLY

The most serious disorder is *pulmonary embolism*, in which a

blood clot formed in one of the major veins breaks free and is carried to the lungs. The clot may block the pulmonary arteries and cause death. Heart failure may cause *pulmonary edema*, in which the lungs become filled with fluid. *Respiratory distress syndrome*, which may affect newborn babies or adults, has many causes. In this condition, leakage of fluid into the alveoli seriously interferes with the oxygen supply. *Emphysema*, in which the walls of the alveoli break down so that the area for oxygen exchange is reduced, is frequently seen in people suffering from chronic bronchitis and asthma.

INVESTIGATION

Lung disorders are investigated by *chest X ray*, *bronchoscopy*, *pulmonary function tests*, *sputum* analysis, *blood tests*, and physical examination. Sometimes a biopsy of lung tissue is taken for analysis.

large cell carcinoma; each has a different growth pattern and response to treatment. The squamous cell, small cell, and large cell types are all strongly associated with tobacco use; the relationship between adenocarcinoma and tobacco use is less clear.

SYMPTOMS AND SIGNS
The first and most common symptom is a cough, occurring in about 80 percent of people with lung cancer. About half those with lung cancer have a chronic cough due to *bronchitis*. Other symptoms include coughing up blood, shortness of breath, chest pain, and wheezing.

Lung cancer can spread locally to affect tissues immediately surrounding the lungs, or can spread to other parts of the body, especially the liver, brain, and bones. Pain may occur in these sites, and weight loss is a common symptom. Local spread may cause the collapse of a lung (see *Atelectasis*) or *pneumonia* (inflammation of the lung) or may affect the pleura (membrane covering the lung), causing *pleural effusion* (excess fluid between the lung and chest wall).

DIAGNOSIS
Lung cancer may be suspected from the patient's symptoms and from a physical examination. In most cases, however, the cancer is discovered when a *chest X ray* shows a characteristic shadow on the lung.

To confirm the diagnosis, tissue must be examined microscopically for the presence of cancerous cells (see *Cytology*). The simplest test is to examine samples of sputum (phlegm), because cancer cells may have been shed into the airways and appear in the sputum. A *bronchoscopy* (inspection of the bronchi with a viewing instrument) is usually performed to examine the condition of the lungs. A *biopsy* (removal of a sample of tissue for microscopic analysis) may be performed during bronchoscopy. Alternatively, cells for biopsy may be obtained through a needle inserted into the chest, or the chest may be opened up to allow surgical removal of part of the tumor.

TREATMENT
If lung cancer is diagnosed at an early stage, *pneumonectomy* (removal of the lung) or *lobectomy* (removal of part of the lung) may be performed. Surgery is usually possible only when the cancer is still fairly small and confined to one lung, and when the patient's general condition enables a major operation to be performed. *Anticancer drugs* and *radiation therapy* may be used to contain the spread of the tumor or to destroy cancerous cells, and are the usual treatment for small cell carcinoma.

OUTLOOK
Overall, less than 10 percent of lung cancer patients survive for five years after the disease is diagnosed. After surgery, the five-year survival rate is between 15 and 30 percent; there have been cases of long-term survival in patients treated with anticancer drugs for small cell carcinoma.

The highest chance of cure is obtained when the cancer is discovered and treated early. However, if the cancer has spread beyond the chest, a cure is highly unlikely.

Lung, collapse of
See *Atelectasis*; *Pneumothorax*.

Lung disease, chronic obstructive
A chronic condition in which there is insufficient flow of air into or out of the lungs.

CAUSES AND PREVALENCE
Bronchitis and *emphysema* are by far the commonest forms of chronic obstructive lung disease, and are usually found in the same individual. Cigarette smoking is the commonest cause of this disease, followed by asthma. In the past, occupational exposures, primarily to dusts and asbestos, were also a cause of chronic obstructive lung disease, but improved standards in the workplace have largely eliminated this risk.

In Canada, approximately 9 percent of men and 4 percent of women over the age of 65 have bronchitis or emphysema, or both. About 100,000 Canadians report they are disabled by chronic obstructive lung disease. Patients who have the disease are sometimes described as either pink puffers or blue bloaters, depending on their condition.

Pink puffers are able to maintain adequate oxygen in their bloodstream through an increase in their breathing rate, and hence remain "pink" despite serious lung damage. Pink puffers suffer from almost constant shortness of breath.

Blue bloaters are cyanotic (have a bluish discoloration of the skin and mucous membranes), because of a deficiency of oxygen in the bloodstream, and appear bloated, because of obesity and sometimes *edema* (accumulation of fluid in body tissues), mainly due to *heart failure* resulting from the lung damage.

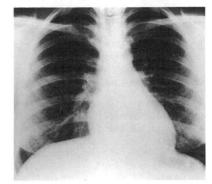

Chest X ray
This is the most important lung imaging technique. It provides information about the lungs, their blood vessels, and main airways.

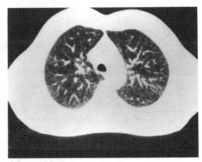

CT scanning
This shows detailed horizontal slices through the lungs. It is useful in showing the extent and spread of lung tumors.

Lung function tests
See *Pulmonary function tests*.

Lung imaging
A technique that provides images of the lungs to aid in the diagnosis of abnormalities or disease.

TYPES
CONVENTIONAL X-RAY TECHNIQUES A *chest X ray* provides an excellent image of the lungs, from which most lung disorders can be detected. *Tomography* produces a sharp image of a cross section of an organ at a particular depth and is sometimes used to visualize the interior of a lung that is obscured by an overlying diseased area, or to identify a nodule in the lung more clearly.

In pulmonary *angiography*, a contrast medium (a substance opaque to X rays) is injected into the pulmonary artery to detect *pulmonary embolism* (blockage by a blood clot). *Bronchography* (in which the contrast medium is injected into the bronchi) was formerly used to examine bronchi damaged by chronic infections; it has now been largely replaced by *bronchoscopy*.

L

SCANNING TECHNIQUES *CT scanning* provides a more detailed image of the lungs than is possible with standard X rays and plays an important role in detecting the presence and spread of *lung tumors*. *Ultrasound scanning* is sometimes used to reveal *pleural effusion* (fluid around a lung).

Other less commonly employed imaging techniques involve the use of *radionuclide scanning* to aid in detecting pulmonary embolism. Digital radiography uses a computer to process a standard X-ray film. The computer removes all unwanted elements (such as the bones of the chest) from the image, leaving a clearer view of the structures to be examined.

Lung tumors

Growths in the lung, which may be malignant (see *Lung cancer*) or benign. Benign lung tumors are less common than malignant tumors and, unlike malignant tumors, typically affect young adults and are unrelated to tobacco smoking.

The most common benign tumor is a bronchial *adenoma*, which arises in the lining of a bronchus. Adenomas often cause bronchial obstruction; coughing up of blood may also occur. Treatment involves surgical removal of the tumor.

Other rare benign tumors include *fibromas* (made up of fibrous tissue) and *lipomas* (made up of fatty tissue). No treatment is necessary unless the tumors are causing problems.

Lupus erythematosus

A chronic disease that causes inflammation of *connective tissue* (material that surrounds body structures and holds them together). The more common type, discoid lupus erythematosus (DLE), affects exposed areas of the skin. The more serious and potentially fatal form, systemic lupus erythematosus (SLE), affects many systems of the body (as well as the skin), including the joints and the kidneys.

CAUSES
Lupus erythematosus is an *autoimmune disorder* in which the body's *immune system*, for unknown reasons, attacks the connective tissue as if it were foreign, causing inflammation. It is probable that the disease can be inherited and that hormonal factors play a part. Sometimes the agent that triggers the immune response (for example, a viral infection or sunlight) can be identified. Also, certain drugs can induce some of the symptoms of SLE, particularly in elderly people;

the drugs most frequently responsible are hydralazine, procainamide, and isoniazid.

INCIDENCE
Lupus erythematosus affects nine times as many women as men, usually those of childbearing age. It occurs worldwide, although its incidence is higher in certain ethnic groups, such as blacks and Chinese. In high-risk groups the prevalence may be as high as one in 250 women.

SYMPTOMS
The symptoms of both varieties of lupus erythematosus periodically subside and recur with varying degrees of severity.

In DLE the rash starts as one or more red, circular, thickened areas of skin that later scar. They may occur on the face, behind the ears, and on the scalp, sometimes causing permanent hair loss in affected areas.

SLE causes a variety of symptoms common among which is a characteristic red, blotchy, almost butterfly-shaped rash over the cheeks and bridge of the nose. There is no scarring. Most sufferers feel ill, with fatigue, fever, loss of appetite, nausea, joint pain, and weight loss. There may also be *anemia*, neurological or psychiatric problems, *kidney failure*, *pleurisy* (inflammation of the lining of the lungs), *arthritis*, and *pericarditis* (inflammation of the membrane surrounding the heart).

DIAGNOSIS
Blood tests and sometimes a skin *biopsy* (removal of a small sample of tissue for microscopic examination) are performed to look for specific *antibodies* that are directed against the body's own tissues.

TREATMENT
Treatment aims to reduce inflammation and to alleviate symptoms; there is no cure. *Nonsteroidal anti-inflammatory drugs* may be prescribed to relieve the joint pain, antimalarial drugs for the skin rash, and *corticosteroid drugs* for fever, pleurisy, and neurological symptoms. Cytotoxic *immunosuppressant drugs* are given to patients with kidney damage or severe neurological symptoms. Sufferers whose symptoms are made worse by sunlight should avoid exposure to the sun and should use *sunscreens*.

OUTLOOK
The outlook for patients with SLE has improved dramatically over the past 20 years, although the disease may be life-threatening if the kidneys are affected. Today many people with SLE survive for longer than 10 years

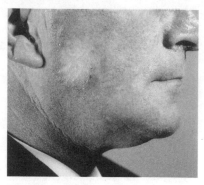
Discoid lupus erythematosus on cheek
The disease causes circular, reddened areas of skin. The patch shown here is healing at its center to form white scar tissue.

after diagnosis of the disease. This improvement may be due to earlier diagnosis, especially of mild cases, and to more effective treatment of kidney problems. Patients with drug-induced symptoms usually recover completely after discontinuation of the drug responsible.

Lupus pernio

A variant of the disease *sarcoidosis* in which purple chilblainlike swellings appear on the nose, cheeks, or ears. Lupus pernio more commonly affects women than men.

Lupus vulgaris

A form of *tuberculosis* affecting the skin, especially of the head and neck. Painless, clear, red-brown nodules appear and ulcerate. These eventually heal, leaving deep scars.

Luteinizing hormone

A *gonadotropin hormone*, also known as LH, produced by the *pituitary gland*.

Luteinizing hormone-releasing hormone

A naturally occurring hormone that is released by the *hypothalamus* in the brain; it is also prepared synthetically as a drug. Natural luteinizing hormone-releasing hormone (LH-RH) stimulates the release of *gonadotropin hormones* from the *pituitary gland*. Gonadotropin hormones, in turn, control the production of *estrogen hormones* and *androgen hormones*.

Synthetic LH-RH is given to treat abnormally early onset of puberty. It is also currently under investigation as a contraceptive and as a treatment for uterine *fibroids*, prostatic cancer (see *Prostate, cancer of*), and certain types of *breast cancer*.

HOW IT WORKS

Synthetic LH-RH reduces the amount of natural gonadotropins released from the pituitary gland and thus the amount of estrogen hormones and androgen hormones produced by the ovary and testes. This action reduces the level of cell activity in organs stimulated by these sex hormones, such as the uterus, breast, ovaries, testes, and prostate gland.

LH-RH may cause headache, nausea, hot flashes, vaginal dryness, and irregular periods.

Lyme disease

A disease characterized by skin changes, flulike symptoms, and joint inflammation. It was first described in the community of Old Lyme, Connecticut, in the US in 1975.

CAUSES AND INCIDENCE

Lyme disease is caused by the bacterium *BORRELIA BURGDORFERI*, which is transmitted by the bite of a tick that usually lives on deer but can infest dogs. Most cases have occurred in the northeastern US. A few cases have been reported in Canada.

SYMPTOMS AND COMPLICATIONS

At the site of the tick bite, a red dot may appear and gradually expand into a reddened area up to 5 mm across; in some cases, however, the bite passes unnoticed. Symptoms such as fever, headache, lethargy, and muscle pains usually develop, followed by a characteristic joint inflammation, with redness and swelling typically affecting the knees and other large joints.

The symptoms may vary in severity and occur in cycles lasting a week or so. Unless the disease is diagnosed and treated, symptoms may continue for several years, gradually declining in severity. There is usually no permanent damage to joints.

Complications affecting the heart (such as *myocarditis* and *heart block*) or nervous system (such as *meningitis*) occur in some cases.

DIAGNOSIS AND TREATMENT

Anyone in whom the above symptoms develop, particularly after a tick bite, should consult a physician. The diagnosis of Lyme disease can be confirmed by blood tests.

If diagnosed before joint inflammation occurs, the disease can be quickly cleared up with *antibiotic drugs*. If the disease is more advanced, *nonsteroidal anti-inflammatory drugs* and sometimes *corticosteroid drugs* are given and a cure may take longer.

Lymph

A milky body fluid that contains lymphocytes (a type of white blood cell), proteins, and fats. Lymph accumulates outside the blood vessels in the intercellular spaces of body tissues and is collected into the *lymphatic system* to flow back into the bloodstream. Lymph plays an important part in the *immune system* and in absorbing fats from the intestine.

Lymphadenitis

A medical term for inflammation of the lymph nodes, a common cause of lymphadenopathy (swollen glands). See *Glands, swollen.*

Lymphadenopathy

The medical term for swollen lymph nodes (see *Glands, swollen*). A condition called persistent generalized lymphadenopathy, which causes generalized swelling of the lymph nodes, develops in some people infected with HIV (the *AIDS* virus).

Lymphangiography

A diagnostic procedure that enables lymph vessels and lymph nodes (see *Lymphatic system*) to be seen on X-ray film after a contrast medium (a substance opaque to X rays) has been injected into them.

WHY IT IS DONE

Until recently, lymphangiography was frequently used to determine the extent to which a cancer had spread throughout the body (because lymph nodes trap cancer cells). However, the more straightforward techniques of *CT scanning* and *MRI* also clearly reveal abnormal lymph nodes and have largely superseded lymphangiography. Even so, in certain types of cancer (such as cancer of the testis or cervix), the additional information provided by lymphangiography is useful in planning treatment and monitoring its progress.

HOW IT IS DONE

A blue dye is injected into the web spaces between all the toes. This dye quickly finds its way into the tiny, usually invisible, lymphatic vessels, allowing the radiologist to see them. (See the illustrated box below.) Lymphangiography is sometimes performed on the arms to reveal lymph nodes in the upper body.

L

PROCEDURE FOR LYMPHANGIOGRAPHY

To plan and monitor the progress of treatment for certain types of cancer, such as of the testis or cervix, X-ray pictures of the lymph vessels and nodes can be taken to reveal the spread of the cancer throughout the body. A contrast medium is injected into the foot, from where it travels throughout the lymphatic system. The procedure takes about two and a half hours.

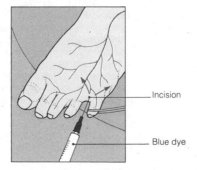

1 A blue dye is injected through a needle into the web spaces between the toes of each foot, and into the outside of the little toes. The dye spreads rapidly into the tiny lymphatic vessels along the top of the foot, and makes them visible.

Incision

Blue dye

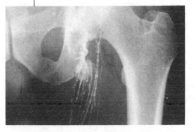

2 After the use of a local anesthetic, an incision is made over a stained lymphatic vessel in each foot. Contrast medium is injected through a needle into the vessels and passes up the legs, into the groin and abdomen. When the limit of diffusion is reached, the needles are removed and the incisions sewn.

Contrast medium spreading through lymphatic system

3 The lymph vessels and nodes containing the contrast medium show up clearly on the X-ray pictures. More lymphangiograms are taken after 24 hours.

Lymphangioma

A rare benign tumor of the skin or tongue consisting of a collection of abnormal lymph vessels. It is usually present from birth.

There are two types of lymphangioma. One consists of a group of clear blisters that may be inconspicuous at birth but are usually obvious by the age of about 2 years. If the blisters are damaged, they fill with blood, giving a red and white appearance to the lymphangioma. The growth sometimes disappears on its own, but most cases require removal.

The other type of lymphangioma, known as a cystic hygroma, is a soft swelling resembling a bunch of small white grapes that grows just beneath the skin (most commonly in the neck). A lymphangioma is usually removed when the child is about 5 years old.

Lymphangitis

Inflammation of the lymphatic vessels as a result of the spread of bacteria (commonly streptococci) from an infected wound. The inflammation is so severe that it causes tender red streaks to appear on the skin overlying the lymphatic vessels. These streaks extend progressively from the site of infection toward the nearest lymph nodes (for example, from an infected finger up the arm toward the lymph nodes in the armpits). The affected nodes become swollen and tender. Lymphangitis is usually accompanied by fever and a general feeling of illness.

Lymphangitis is a clear indication of a serious infection and requires urgent treatment with *antibiotic drugs*. (See also *Lymphadenitis*.)

Lymphatic system

A system of vessels (lymphatics) that drains *lymph* from all over the body back into the bloodstream. This system is part of the *immune system*, playing a major part in the body's defenses against infection and cancer.

STRUCTURE AND FUNCTION

All body tissues are bathed in a watery fluid derived from the bloodstream. Much of this fluid returns to the bloodstream through the walls of the capillaries, but the remainder (along with cells and small particles such as bacteria) is transported to the heart through the lymphatic system (see illustrated box, facing page).

Situated along the lymphatics are *lymph nodes*, through which the lymph flows. These nodes are, in effect, filters that trap microorganisms and other foreign bodies in the lymph. The nodes contain many lymphocytes (a type of white blood cell), which can neutralize or destroy invading bacteria and viruses. If part of the body is inflamed or otherwise diseased, the nearby lymph nodes become swollen and tender as they limit the spread of the disease (see *Glands, swollen*). If an infection is particularly virulent, the lymphatics may also be inflamed, becoming visible as thin red lines running along a limb (see *Lymphangitis*).

The lymphatic system also plays a part in the absorption of fats from the intestine. While the products of carbohydrate and protein digestion pass directly into the bloodstream, fats pass into the intestinal lymphatics (known as lacteals); the lymph in the lacteals is so rich in fat that it appears milky.

DISORDERS

In some conditions, the lymphatics to a limb become obstructed, causing lymph to accumulate and the limb to become hard and swollen, a condition known as *lymphedema*. Cancer commonly spreads via the lymphatic system. A primary tumor invades the lymphatics and fragments of tumor (metastases) break off and travel to the local group of lymph nodes, where the metastases continue to grow and produce a secondary tumor.

Lymphedema

An abnormal accumulation of *lymph* in the tissues, causing swelling of a limb. Lymphedema occurs if lymphatic vessels are blocked, damaged, or removed, resulting in disruption of the normal drainage of lymph.

CAUSES

There are various causes. In the tropical disease *filariasis*, for example, the lymphatic vessels may be blocked by parasitic worms. Blockage may also occur if cancer spreads through the lymphatic system and deposits cancer cells in the lymph vessels.

Surgical removal of lymph nodes under the arm or in the groin or radiation therapy for a tumor destroys lymph nodes and vessels, sometimes resulting in lymphedema.

Lymphedema may also occur for no known cause. It affects twice as many women as men.

SYMPTOMS AND SIGNS

In about 10 percent of women who have had a radical *mastectomy*, lymphedema develops in the arm (but not usually in the hand) on the same side as the removed breast. In some such cases, the arm becomes heavy and cumbersome. The incidence of lymphedema is much lower with newer surgical techniques.

Except after a mastectomy, lymphedema usually causes swelling of one or both legs. Starting with only a slight, intermittent puffiness around one ankle, the swelling gradually extends up the leg. In about half of all cases, the other leg also becomes affected. The swelling is usually painless, but the leg feels heavy.

TREATMENT

There is no known cure for lymphedema. Treatment consists of taking *diuretic drugs*, massaging the affected limb, wearing an elastic bandage or compression sleeve, and performing exercises with the affected leg or arm elevated. However, these measures usually produce only a slight improvement. In severe cases, when the leg or arm is so large that it causes disability, the swollen tissue and some of the overlying skin may be removed surgically.

Lymph gland

A popular name for a *lymph node*. (See also *Lymphatic system*.)

Lymph node

A small organ lying along the course of a lymphatic vessel; commonly but incorrectly known as a lymph gland.

STRUCTURE AND FUNCTION

Lymph nodes vary considerably in size, from microscopic to about 2.5 cm in diameter. Each node consists of a thin, fibrous outer capsule and an inner mass of lymphoid tissue. Penetrating the capsule are several small lymphatic vessels (which carry lymph into the gland) and a single, larger vessel (which carries it out).

Lymphoid tissue forms *antibodies* and houses *lymphocytes* (a type of white blood cell), both of which play a major role in fighting infection. Lymph nodes also contain macrophages, large cells that engulf bacteria and other foreign particles. The nodes act as a barrier to the spread of infection, destroying or filtering out bacteria before they can pass into the bloodstream. (See also *Glands, swollen*; *Lymphatic system*.)

Lymphocyte

Any of a group of white *blood cells* of crucial importance to the adaptive part of the body's *immune system*. The adaptive portion of the immune system mounts a tailor-made defense when dangerous invading organisms penetrate the body's general defenses.

L

STRUCTURE AND FUNCTION OF THE LYMPHATIC SYSTEM

The lymphatic system is a collection of organs, ducts, and tissues that has the dual role of draining tissue fluid (lymph) back into the bloodstream and of fighting infection. Lymph is drained by a system of channels (the lymphatic vessels). White cells produced by the bone marrow, thymus, and spleen are present in lymph nodes or circulate through the lymphatic system, providing defenses against infection.

The lymphatic network

The lymphatic system consists of a network of lymph nodes connected by lymphatic vessels. The nodes generally occur in clusters, mainly around the neck, armpits, and groin.

Thoracic duct

Liver

Spleen

Cisterna chyli

Lymph nodes

Lymphatic vessels

Right lymphatic duct
Thoracic duct
Right subclavian vein
Left subclavian vein
Lymph
Superior vena cava

Lymphatic drainage

Just below the neck, the thoracic duct and the right lymphatic duct drain into the two subclavian veins. These veins unite to form the inferior vena cava, which passes into the heart; in this way, the lymph fluids rejoin the circulation.

Lymphatic vessels

Collagenous capsule

Primary follicle

Artery

Vein

Lymph

White blood cells

Structure of a lymph node

Any fluid absorbed into the lymphatic system passes across at least one lymph node before it returns to the circulation. The fluid filters through a mesh of tightly packed white blood cells—some of which are grouped into primary follicles consisting of similar cells—which attack and destroy harmful organisms. Every lymph node is supplied by its own tiny artery and vein.

MOVEMENTS OF BODY FLUIDS

Lymph is constantly moving around the body, but the lymphatic system has no central pump equivalent to the heart. Lymph is circulated by the movement of the body's muscles; a system of one-way valves in the lymphatic vessels ensures that it moves in the right direction. Exertion also pushes fluid from body tissues into the bloodstream.

Heart

Arteries

Veins

Lymphatic vessels

Capillaries

Cells   Lymphatic vessel

Capillary   Tissue fluid

Fluid exchange

During a 24-hour period, approximately 24 litres of serumlike fluid pass from the bloodstream to the body's tissues. This fluid bathes the cells and provides them with oxygen and nutrients. During the same period of time, approximately 20 litres of fluid pass back from the tissues to the bloodstream, carrying carbon dioxide and other waste products. The remaining 4 litres pass from the tissues to the lymphatic system and return eventually to the circulation from there.

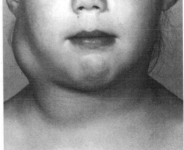

Enlarged lymph nodes

This photograph shows a girl with marked enlargement of the lymph nodes in her neck. In this case, the cause is Hodgkin's disease, a rare cancer that affects the lymph nodes. Enlargement of the nodes may also be due to infection.

L

Some lymphocytes retain a memory of invading microorganisms so that the invaders can be dealt with more rapidly when next encountered. It is this memory function that is stimulated by *vaccines*. Lymphocytes protect against the development of tumors and cause rejection of tissue in organ transplants.

TYPES

The principal types are called B-lymphocytes and T-lymphocytes.

B-LYMPHOCYTES This type accounts for about 10 percent of circulating lymphocytes. When an *antigen* (a particular foreign protein, such as a substance on the surface of a bacterium) is encountered by the immune system, certain B-lymphocytes are stimulated to enlarge and undergo cell division, transforming into cells called plasma cells. The plasma cells secrete into the blood vast numbers of tailormade *immunoglobulins* or *antibodies* that attach to the antigen on the surface of the microorganism. This starts a process that leads to the destruction of the microorganism. The protective effect of immunoglobulins is called humoral immunity.

T-LYMPHOCYTES This type accounts for more than 80 percent of circulating lymphocytes. T-lymphocytes are derived from white cells that have at some stage entered the *thymus* gland, where they were "educated" to fulfill a particular function.

There are three main groups of T-lymphocytes: killer (cytotoxic) cells, helper cells, and suppressor cells. The killer T-lymphocytes (like B-lymphocytes) are sensitized and stimulated to multiply by the presence of antigens, in this case by antigens present on abnormal body cells (e.g., cells that have been invaded by viruses, cells in transplanted tissue, and tumor cells). Unlike the B-lymphocytes, the killer cells do not produce antibodies; instead, they travel to and attach to the cells recognized as abnormal. The killer cells then release chemicals known as lymphokines, which help destroy the abnormal cells. This is called cell-mediated immunity.

Helper T-cells enhance the activities of the killer T-cells and B-cells, and also control other aspects of the immune response. In people who are infected with HIV (the *AIDS* virus) these helper T-cells are reduced in number, thus impairing the body's ability to fight certain types of infections and tumors. Suppressor T-cells have the effect of "switching off" the immune response.

MEMORY FUNCTION

Some lymphocytes do not participate directly in immune responses; instead, they serve as a memory bank for the different antigens that have been encountered in the past. These cells may survive for many years.

Lymphogranuloma venereum

A sexually transmitted disease that is caused by a *chlamydial infection*. The disease is common in tropical countries but very rare in Canada.

The first sign of infection may be a small genital blister that appears between three and 21 days after infection; this blister heals in a few days without leaving a scar. There may also be fever, headache, muscle and joint pains, and a rash.

The lymph glands, particularly in the groin, become painfully enlarged and inflamed. Abscesses may form and ulcers may develop on the skin over the affected glands; the ulcers take several months to heal.

Treatment of lymphogranuloma venereum is with *antibiotic drugs*.

Lymphoma

Any of a group of cancers in which the cells of lymphoid tissue (found mainly in the *lymph nodes* and *spleen*) multiply unchecked.

Lymphomas fall into two categories. If characteristic abnormal cells (Reed-Sternberg cells) are present, the disease is known as Hodgkin's lymphoma. All other types are called non-Hodgkin's lymphoma. (See *Burkitt's lymphoma*; *Hodgkin's disease*; *Lymphoma, non-Hodgkin's*.)

Lymphoma, non-Hodgkin's

Any cancer of lymphoid tissue (found mainly in the *lymph nodes* and *spleen*) other than *Hodgkin's disease*.

Non-Hodgkin's lymphomas vary in their malignancy according to the nature and activity of the abnormal cells. Lymphomas are most malignant when the cells are primitive or are poorly differentiated. These cells tend to take over entire lymph nodes quickly. Low-grade (less malignant) lymphomas consist of cells that are better-differentiated.

CAUSES AND INCIDENCE

In most cases of non-Hodgkin's lymphoma, the cause is unknown. Occasionally, the disease is associated with suppression of the *immune system*, particularly after organ transplantation. One type of non-Hodgkin's lymphoma, known as *Burkitt's lymphoma*, is thought to be caused by the Epstein-Barr virus; others are suspected to be caused by other viruses. Most sufferers are over 50 years old.

In most patients, there is painless swelling of one or more groups of lymph nodes in the neck or groin. The liver and spleen may enlarge and lymphoid tissue in the abdomen may be affected. Many other organs may become involved, leading to diverse symptoms ranging from headache to skin ulceration.

Unless it is controlled, spread of the disease (often marked by fever) progressively impairs the immune system, leading to death from infections. The patient may also die of an uncontrolled spread of cancer.

Diagnosis is based on a *biopsy* (removal of a sample for analysis) of lymphoid tissue, usually from a lymph node. The extent of the disease is assessed by a process called staging. A *chest X ray*, *CT scanning*, *bone marrow biopsy*, and *lymphangiography* (X rays of the lymph glands) of the abdomen may be required.

TREATMENT AND OUTLOOK

If the lymphoma is confined to a single group of lymph nodes, treatment consists of *radiation therapy*. More usually, the disease is more extensive, and *anticancer drugs* are given. In some cases both forms of treatment are used. When all else fails, a *bone marrow transplant*, along with drugs and/or radiation, may be performed.

About three quarters of patients with a low-grade localized non-Hodgkin's lymphoma survive at least five years. In more severe types of lymphoma that have spread, between 40 and 50 percent of patients survive for two years or more.

Lymphosarcoma

See *Lymphoma, non-Hodgkin's*.

Lysis

A medical term for breaking down or destruction; the term is usually applied to the destruction of cells by disintegration of their outer membrane. A common example is *hemolysis*, the breakdown of red blood cells. Lysis may be caused by chemical action, such as that of an *enzyme*, or by physical action, such as that of heat or cold. The term lysis may also describe a sudden recovery from a fever.

Lysozyme

An *enzyme* in tears, saliva, sweat, nasal secretions, breast milk, and many tissues. It destroys bacteria by disrupting their cell walls.

M

Macro-

A prefix meaning large, as in macrophage (a large cell that plays an important part in the body's defense system by engulfing bacteria and other foreign particles) or macroglossia (enlargement of the tongue).

Macrobiotics

A dietary system based on the oriental belief that foods are either yin or yang (possessed of negative or positive forces, see *Yin and yang*), and that a balance of yin and yang must be maintained for health. Foods are classified as yin or yang according to many factors, including where they are grown, their color, texture, and taste.

There are several levels of macrobiotic diet; the most extreme consists virtually entirely of whole grains. Eating such a diet may lead to severe malnutrition, *scurvy*, or *anemia* as a result of the lack of protein, vitamins, and essential minerals.

Macroglossia

Abnormal enlargement of the tongue. Macroglossia is a feature of *Down's syndrome*, of *hypothyroidism* (underactivity of the thyroid gland), and of *acromegaly*. Tumors of the tongue, such as a *hemangioma* or *lymphangioma*, also cause macroglossia, as may *amyloidosis*.

In addition to being unsightly, an abnormally large tongue can cause snoring and is sometimes responsible for *sleep apnea*. Treatment, if any, depends on the underlying cause.

Macular degeneration

A progressive disorder that affects the central part of the *retina*, causing gradual loss of central vision. Macular degeneration is a painless condition which is common in the elderly. It usually affects both eyes, either simultaneously or one after the other.

The macula is the part of the retina that distinguishes fine detail at the center of the field of vision. Degener-ation begins with partial breakdown of an insulating layer between the retina and the *choroid* (layer of blood vessels behind the retina). Fluid leakage occurs, and new blood vessels growing from the choroid destroy the retinal nerve tissue and replace it with scar tissue. The effect is a roughly circular area of blindness, increasing in size until it is large enough to obliterate two or three words at normal reading distance. Because of the loss of central vision, the patient has difficulty in seeing people's faces as well as in reading.

With early diagnosis, it is occasionally possible to seal off the leakage by *laser treatment*. In most cases, however, macular degeneration is untreatable but does not lead to complete blindness, because the patient retains vision around the edges of the visual fields.

Macule

A spot that is level with the surface of the skin and discernible only by difference in color or texture.

Magnesium

An element essential in the diet for the formation of bones and teeth, for muscle contraction, for the transmission of nerve impulses, and for the activation of many *enzymes* (substances that promote biochemical reactions in the body). There are about 35 g of magnesium in an average-sized person, much of it in the bones and teeth.

Sources of magnesium in the diet include cereals (especially wholegrain), nuts, soya beans, milk, fish, and meat.

MAGNESIUM-CONTAINING DRUGS

Magnesium compounds are used in *antacid drugs* and *laxative drugs*: magnesium carbonate and magnesium hydroxide are used in many antacids, magnesium sulfate in laxatives. Magnesium is also a constituent of some mineral supplements.

DEFICIENCY AND EXCESS

Most diets contain sufficient magnesium. Deficiency usually occurs as a result of severe kidney disease, *alcohol dependence*, an intestinal disorder that impairs the absorption of magnesium and calcium, or prolonged treatment with *diuretic drugs* or *digitalis drugs*. Symptoms of deficiency include anxiety, restlessness, tremors, palpitations, and depression. There may also be a risk of kidney stones (see *Calculus, urinary tract*) or *coronary artery disease*. Deficiency is treated with magnesium supplements.

Magnesium excess is usually the result of taking too much of a magnesium-containing antacid or laxative, and may cause nausea, vomiting, diarrhea, dizziness, and muscle weakness. Very large amounts may lead to heart damage or respiratory failure, especially in people with kidney disease. Mild magnesium excess does not usually require treatment. However, anyone who has taken a substantial overdose may require hospitalization so that breathing and heart activity can be monitored (and supported, if necessary) and drugs given to help the body excrete the excess magnesium.

Magnetic resonance imaging

See *MRI*.

Malabsorption

Impaired absorption of dietary nutrients, vitamins, or minerals by the lining of the small intestine.

CAUSES

Malabsorption can be caused by many conditions. In *lactase deficiency*, deficiency of the enzyme lactase in the intestine prevents the breakdown and absorption of lactose (a sugar in milk). In *cystic fibrosis* and chronic *pancreatitis*, damage to the pancreas prevents the production of enzymes required for the digestion and absorption of fats and other nutrients.

In *celiac disease*, many nutrients cannot be absorbed because of damage to the small intestine by sensitivity to gluten proteins. Uncommon diseases in which the intestinal lining is damaged include *Crohn's disease, amyloidosis, giardiasis, Whipple's disease*, and *lymphoma*.

Removal of portions of the small intestine can cause malabsorption, as can stomach operations that cause food to pass through the digestive tract more quickly than normal.

There are also some disorders that interfere with the passage of bile salts to the small intestine or that interfere with their uptake, thus preventing the breakdown and absorption of fats. These disorders include *bile duct obstruction*, primary *biliary cirrhosis*, and Crohn's disease.

SYMPTOMS AND DIAGNOSIS

Common effects are diarrhea and weight loss; in severe cases, there may also be malnutrition (see *Nutritional disorders*), *vitamin* deficiency, *mineral* deficiency, or *anemia*.

The diagnosis may be confirmed by examining feces for unabsorbed fat, by special tests of carbohydrate absorption (such as the xylose absorption test), and by blood tests to detect anemia and deficiencies of vitamins, minerals and other nutrients.

To determine the underlying cause of malabsorption, various other tests may be carried out, including *barium X-ray examination* of the small intestine and *jejunal biopsy* (removal of a sample of tissue from the jejunum for microscopic examination).

TREATMENT AND OUTLOOK

Treatment depends on the underlying cause. In most cases, modifications or supplements to the diet return the affected person to health. However, if there is severe, irreversible damage to the lining of the intestine, intravenous infusion of nutrients may be necessary (see *Feeding, artificial*).

Maladjustment

Failure to adapt to a change in one's environment, resulting in an inability to cope with work or social activities. Maladjustment is common and can occur at any age as a reaction to stressful situations (such as starting school, moving house, divorce, physical illness, or retirement). Maladjustment may be expressed by feelings of *depression* or *anxiety*, or by *behavioral problems in children* and adolescents.

Maladjustment is usually temporary, disappearing when the person is removed from the stressful situation or learns to adapt to it.

Malaise

A vague feeling of being unwell. Malaise is a general symptom of little value in diagnosis.

Malalignment

Positioning of *teeth* in the *jaw* so that they do not form a smooth arch shape when viewed from above or below (see *Malocclusion*).

The term malalignment is also used to refer to a *fracture* in which the bone ends are not in a straight line. The ends must then be manipulated back into position so that there is no deformity when the bone heals.

Malar flush

A high color over the cheekbones, with a bluish tinge caused by reduced oxygen concentration in the blood. Malar flush is considered to be a sign of *mitral stenosis* (narrowing of one of the heart valves), usually following *rheumatic fever*. However, malar flush is not always present in mitral stenosis, and many people with this coloring do not have heart disease.

Malaria

 A serious parasitic disease, spread by the bites of *ANOPHELES* mosquitoes. The disease produces severe fever and, in some cases, complications affecting the kidneys, liver, brain, and blood which can be fatal.

Malaria is prevalent throughout the tropics, affecting up to 300 million people worldwide each year. It is the single most important disease hazard for travelers to warm climates. The World Health Organization has undertaken a massive program of malaria control, but little progress has been made in the past 20 years. Mosquitoes have developed resistance to insecticides and, in many areas, the malaria parasites have developed resistance to antimalarial drugs.

CAUSES

The parasites responsible for malaria are *protozoa* known as plasmodia. Four species can cause disease in humans: *PLASMODIUM FALCIPARUM, PLASMODIUM VIVAX, PLASMODIUM OVALE,* and *PLASMODIUM MALARIAE*. Each species spends part of its life cycle in humans and part in *ANOPHELES* mosquitoes (see diagram facing page).

INCIDENCE

Malaria is a major health problem in much of the tropics (see map facing page). Children in affected countries suffer repeated infections, and many die. Malaria kills about 1 million infants and children every year in Africa alone. Most people living in areas where malaria is common acquire some immunity to the disease.

About 300 cases are reported annually in Canada, all attributable to exposure outside the country. Most falciparum malaria infections are contracted in Africa and most of the less dangerous vivax infections occur in visitors and immigrants from the Indian subcontinent.

SYMPTOMS

The period between being bitten by the mosquito and the appearance of symptoms is usually a week or two, but can be as long as a year if the person has been taking antimalarial drugs (which may suppress rather than prevent malaria). Symptoms, which include shaking, chills, and fever, appear only when red blood cells that are infected with parasites rupture to release more parasites into the bloodstream.

The principal symptom of infection is the classic malarial ague (fever). Except in most cases of falciparum malaria, the fever has three stages: a cold stage of uncontrollable shivering (rigors), a hot stage in which the temperature may reach 40.5°C, and finally a sweating stage that drenches the bedding and brings down the temperature. A severe headache, general malaise, and vomiting may accompany the attack. At the end of an attack, the patient is left weak and tired, and sleeps. In many cases, the parasitized red blood cells rupture at the same time in each cycle and the fever develops cyclically, occurring every other day (in vivax and ovale infections) or every third day (in malaria infections).

P. FALCIPARUM infects all ages of red blood cells, whereas the other varieties attack only young or old cells. Falciparum malaria thus affects a greater proportion of the blood cells and is therefore more severe; this form of malaria can be fatal within a few days of the first symptoms. The fever is prolonged and irregular, but symptoms are initially very like those of influenza and the severity of the illness may not be recognized. Red blood cells infected with parasites become sticky and block blood vessels in vital organs, especially the kidneys. The spleen becomes enlarged and the brain may be affected, leading to coma and convulsions. Destruction of blood cells leads to hemolytic anemia (see *Anemia, hemolytic*). Kidney failure and jaundice are common complications of falciparum malaria.

Even people who take antimalarial drugs and precautions against bites may contract malaria. Anyone in whom a fever and headache develops after returning from the tropics should see a physician as soon as possible and mention the trip abroad.

DIAGNOSIS

Malaria is diagnosed by studying blood samples taken at six- to 12-hour intervals; parasites at different stages of development can be clearly seen under a microscope.

TREATMENT

Malaria, especially falciparum malaria, is often a medical emergency that requires admission to hospital. Treatment is with antimalarial drugs. In severe cases, *blood transfusions* may be necessary.

Chloroquine, which eradicates malaria parasites from the blood, is the usual treatment for all types of malaria. However, *quinine* is commonly used to treat chloroquine-resistant falciparum malaria, which is now widespread in many tropical areas. Pyrimethamine is often used to treat

M

malaria resistant to other drugs. Patients suffering from vivax or ovale malaria must also take *primaquine* to eradicate parasites in the liver. Primaquine may cause hemolytic anemia in people who have a disorder called *G6PD deficiency.*

PREVENTION
Preventive antimalarial drugs should be taken by all visitors to the tropics, including pregnant women. Drug recommendations are continually updated, and travelers should consult a physician for up-to-date advice on the choice and dosages of drugs to be taken when visiting different parts of the world.

Chloroquine is often recommended for areas where there is no resistance to this drug; *proguanil* may be preferred for longer-term use because it has fewer side effects. Drug possibilities for chloroquine-resistant areas include a combination of chloroquine

and proguanil, or a combination of *pyrimethamine* and *dapsone.* All antimalarial drugs will need to be taken for some time before visiting a malarious region (usually for one to two weeks), and will also need to be taken for some time afterward (usually for at least four weeks).

In addition to taking preventive drugs, visitors to the tropics should make every effort to avoid *mosquito bites.* (Even persons who take antimalarial drugs may contract malaria.) Protective clothing should be worn over the arms and legs in the evening and insect repellents should be used. Other preventive measures against mosquito bites include screens over windows, insecticide sprays, and, if necessary, mosquito nets.

Malformation
A deformity, particularly one resulting from faulty development.

Malignant
A term used to describe a condition that tends to become progressively worse and to result in death. By contrast, a *benign* disorder remains relatively mild and is not usually fatal. The term malignant is primarily used to refer to a cancerous *tumor* that spreads from its original location to establish secondary tumors in other parts of the body, with potentially life-threatening results.

Malignant melanoma
See *Melanoma, malignant.*

Malingering
Deliberate simulation of physical or psychological symptoms for a particular purpose, such as obtaining time off work, or obtaining compensation. Malingering differs from *factitious disorders,* in which an individual feigns illness for no reason other than a wish

M

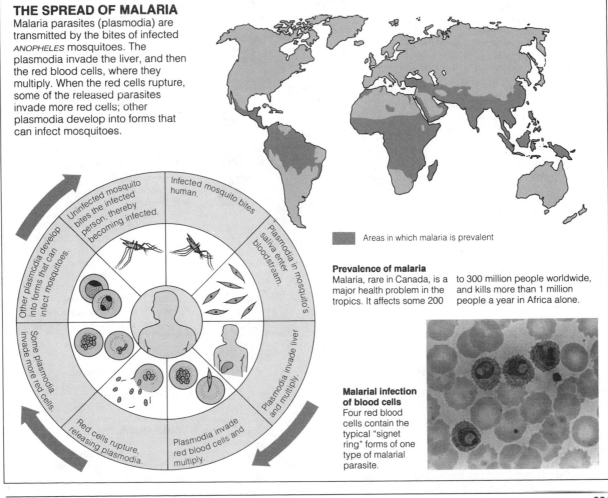

THE SPREAD OF MALARIA
Malaria parasites (plasmodia) are transmitted by the bites of infected *ANOPHELES* mosquitoes. The plasmodia invade the liver, and then the red blood cells, where they multiply. When the red cells rupture, some of the released parasites invade more red cells; other plasmodia develop into forms that can infect mosquitoes.

Uninfected mosquito bites the infected person, thereby becoming infected.

Infected mosquito bites human.

Plasmodia in mosquito's saliva enter bloodstream.

Other plasmodia develop into forms that can infect mosquitoes.

Some plasmodia invade more red cells

Red cells rupture, releasing plasmodia.

Plasmodia invade red blood cells and multiply.

Plasmodia invade liver and multiply.

Areas in which malaria is prevalent

Prevalence of malaria
Malaria, rare in Canada, is a major health problem in the tropics. It affects some 200 to 300 million people worldwide, and kills more than 1 million people a year in Africa alone.

Malarial infection of blood cells
Four red blood cells contain the typical "signet ring" forms of one type of malarial parasite.

to gain the attention associated with illness and being a patient. Malingering is also distinguished from *hypochondriasis*, in which symptoms are not under the individual's voluntary control.

Mallet finger
See *Baseball finger*.

Mallet toe
See *Claw toe*.

Mallory-Weiss syndrome
A condition in which a tear at the lower end of the *esophagus* causes vomiting of blood. Mallory-Weiss syndrome is particularly common in alcoholics after a bout of excessive drinking accompanied by retching and vomiting. Less commonly, the tear may be produced by violent coughing, a severe asthma attack, or epileptic convulsions. The damage is thought to result from violent contractions of the diaphragm during prolonged retching and vomiting.

DIAGNOSIS AND TREATMENT
Diagnosis is made by passing an *endoscope* (a viewing instrument with a light source and lens attachment) down the esophagus. The tear generally heals within 10 days and, ordinarily, no special treatment is required. In the event that the person has lost a considerable amount of blood, however, blood transfusions may be necessary.

Malnutrition
See *Nutritional disorders*.

Malocclusion
An abnormal relationship between the upper and lower sets of *teeth* when they are closed. Most people have some teeth that are slightly out of position, but a person is considered to have malocclusion only if the bite (see *Occlusion*) or appearance is adversely affected. There are three basic classes of dental malocclusion (see illustrated box).

CAUSES
Malocclusion usually develops in childhood, when the teeth and jaws are growing. Most cases of malocclusion are inherited; others result from *thumb-sucking* beyond a certain age or from a mismatch between the teeth and jaws (e.g., large teeth in a small mouth, leading to *overcrowding*).

TREATMENT
Treatment, which is usually necessary only if malocclusion is severe, may be carried out to improve appearance, to

prevent strain from an abnormal bite (which causes pain, stiffness, and sometimes *arthritis* in the jaw joints), or to make cleaning of the teeth easier and thus help prevent *periodontal disease* and decay (see *Caries, dental*).

It is sometimes possible to correct uneven contacts by smoothing down

---

CLASSES OF MALOCCLUSION
Unsatisfactory contact between the upper and lower teeth (malocclusion) is of three main classes, shown below.

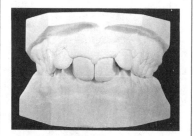

Class 1 malocclusion
In this (the most common) type, the jaw relationship is normal, but, because the teeth are poorly spaced, tilted, or rotated, the upper and lower set do not meet properly.

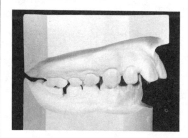

Class 2 malocclusion
In this type—called retrognathism—the lower jaw is too far back; the normal small overbite of the upper incisors is greatly increased, and the molar bite is displaced backward.

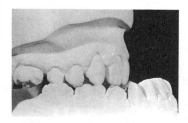

Class 3 malocclusion
In this (the least common) type—called prognathism—the lower jaw is too far forward; the lower incisors meet, or lie in front of, the upper ones, and the molar bite is displaced forward.

---

or building up opposing tooth surfaces. The usual treatment, however, is use of *orthodontic appliances* (braces) to move teeth into the proper position. In cases of dental overcrowding, some teeth may need to be extracted. *Orthognathic surgery* is used to treat severe recession or protrusion of the lower jaw. Treatment is best carried out in childhood or adolescence, when the teeth and bones of the jaw are still developing. Problems left until adulthood can be treated successfully, but may take longer to correct.

Malpractice
Malpractice is misconduct or unreasonable lack of skill on the part of a medical practitioner while rendering a professional service. Negligence is the usual basis for a finding of malpractice. A successful negligence suit must show that there was a duty of care (a professional relationship between physician and patient); that there was a breach of this standard by the physician; that there was a foreseeable or compensable injury to the patient; and that the physician's conduct was the cause of the injury. Negligence actions may be brought against hospitals and other health care providers, as well as physicians.

Malpresentation
A condition in which a baby is not in the usual headfirst position during *childbirth*. Malpresentation occurs in about 5 percent of births.

Types of malpresentation include breech presentation (in which the baby's bottom appears first), face presentation (in which the face rather than the top of the head appears first), and shoulder presentation (which occurs when the baby is lying transversely across the uterus). Breech presentations are the most common form of malpresentation.

A baby lying bottom first at the onset of labor may be born by *breech delivery* or by *cesarean section*. A baby lying transversely usually requires a cesarean section.

Malta fever
An old name for *brucellosis*.

Mammary gland
See *Breast*.

Mammography
An X-ray procedure for examining the *breast*. Mammography is used to investigate *breast lumps* and to screen women for *breast cancer*.

The main value of mammography is that it allows the detection of breast tumors that are too small to be found during a physical examination (see *Breast self-examination*). Successful treatment of breast cancer depends on early detection, and research has shown that mammography can significantly increase the early detection rate of breast cancer and can accordingly reduce death rates from this cause.

The procedure for mammography is shown in the illustrated box.

Mammoplasty

A cosmetic operation to reduce the size of extremely large or pendulous *breasts*, to enlarge small breasts, or to reconstruct a breast after part or all of it has been removed to treat *breast cancer*. Mammoplasty is performed under general anesthesia.

BREAST REDUCTION

This procedure reduces the size of the breast and raises it to correct drooping. Incisions are made in the breast and unwanted tissue is removed.

Most patients are pleased with the result. The nipple scar and the scar beneath the breast are usually hidden, but the vertical scar is usually evident and may need to be made less obvious by further surgery.

BREAST ENLARGEMENT

An implant is inserted via an incision made at the side of or below the breast. The immediate results are usually excellent, but internal scar tissue often eventually forms around the implant, altering its shape and making the breast harder. External pressure on the implant to restore its shape or sometimes another minor operation may be necessary.

BREAST RECONSTRUCTION

This operation is carried out either at the same time as a *mastectomy* (breast removal) or at a later date. Depending on the type of mastectomy, reconstruction takes one of two forms.

If the entire breast is removed, a portion of skin and underlying fat and muscle is transplanted from a site near the breast; a silicone rubber implant is incorporated at the same time.

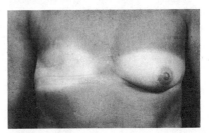

Before

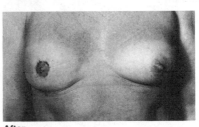

After

Reconstruction of a breast
A breast removed at an earlier mastectomy operation can be reconstructed later using a silicone rubber implant.

Increasingly often, however, surgeons remove only the tumor and surrounding tissue, leaving the overlying skin in place. An implant can then be inserted under the skin and scarring is minimal. In some cases, the size of the other breast is reduced to make the breasts look balanced.

Mandible

The lower *jaw*.

Mania

A mental disorder characterized by episodes of overactivity, elation, or irritability. Mania usually occurs as part of a *manic-depressive illness*.

SYMPTOMS

The primary symptom of mania is an abnormal increase in activity (for example, the sufferer may make elaborate plans for a constant round of social activity). Other symptoms may include: extravagant spending; repeatedly starting new tasks; less need to sleep; increased appetite for food, alcohol, sex, and energetic exercise; outbursts of inappropriate anger, laughter, or sudden socializing; and a grandiose sense of knowing better than others.

Symptoms may even extend to delusions of grandeur (for example, believing oneself to be God). When symptoms are relatively mild, the condition is called hypomania.

Manic attacks usually first appear before the age of 30, and may last for a

---

PROCEDURE FOR MAMMOGRAPHY

Mammography is simple, safe, and causes minimal discomfort. Only low-dose X-rays are used. The breast may be X-rayed from above, the side, or both; sometimes an oblique (angled) view is taken.

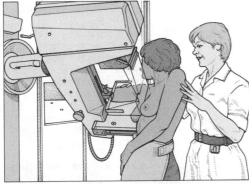

How mammography is done
In the method shown here, the breast is placed on the machine and gently compressed between the X-ray plate below and a plastic cover above. This flattens the breast so that as much tissue as possible can be imaged. Several views may be taken. In another method, the breast hangs freely and is X-rayed from the side.

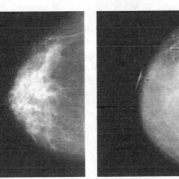

Mammograms
The normal mammogram (far left) shows a side view of a healthy breast, with the milk ducts appearing as denser areas. In the abnormal mammogram (left), an irregular, dense mass in the upper part of the breast indicates a tumor. A biopsy (removal of a tissue sample for analysis) is necessary to determine whether a tumor is cancerous.

PROCEDURE FOR MAMMOPLASTY

One of the most common cosmetic operations, mammoplasty is done to improve the appearance of the breasts by removal of excess fat and skin or by using an implant to increase their size.

BREAST REDUCTION

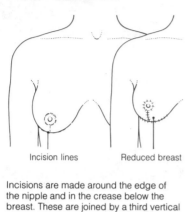

Incision lines   Reduced breast

Incisions are made around the edge of the nipple and in the crease below the breast. These are joined by a third vertical cut. Excess tissue and skin are removed, and the incisions are closed with stitches.

BREAST ENLARGEMENT

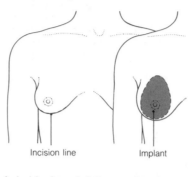

Incision line   Implant

An incision is made in the armpit or along the crease under the breast, and a pocket is created behind the breast to receive the implant. After the implant has been inserted, the incision is stitched.

few days or several months. If attacks begin after the age of 40, they are frequently more prolonged.

TREATMENT
Severe mania often leads to marked social disruption or even violence; hospital admission is usually required. Treatment is generally by means of *antipsychotic drugs*; relapses may be prevented by taking *lithium* or *carbamazepine*.

Manic-depressive illness

A mental disorder in which a disturbance of mood is the major symptom. This disturbance may be unipolar (consisting either of *depression* or *mania*) or bipolar (consisting of a swing between the two states). In a severe form of the illness, sometimes referred to as manic-depressive psychosis, mood swings may be accompanied by grandiose ideas or by extreme negative delusions.

CAUSES
Some disorders affecting the brain, certain drugs, and a clear inherited tendency are all established factors. Research has located at least one of the defective genes responsible on chromosome 11. Mood changes have been linked to changing levels of the chemical *dopamine* in parts of the brain.

PREVALENCE
Depression is very common, affecting about one in 10 men and one in five women at some time in their lives. About a third of these illnesses are severe. By contrast, mania (unipolar or bipolar) is rare, affecting only about eight per 1,000 people, men and women equally.

TREATMENT
Admission to hospital is often required for severe manic-depressive illness. *Antidepressant drugs* and/or *ECT* (electroconvulsive therapy) are effective in treating depression. *Antipsychotic drugs* (chlorpromazine and haloperidol, for example) are used to control manic symptoms. *Lithium* may be used during remission to prevent a relapse. *Group therapy, family therapy,* and individual *psychotherapy* are useful in treating neurotic disorders and in aiding recovery after a severe episode. *Cognitive-behavioral therapy* may also be helpful.

OUTLOOK
Though often crippling in the acute phase, manic-depressive illnesses have a good outlook. Abilities are not affected, and more than 80 percent of patients recover.

Repeated, severe illnesses, however, or persistent depression, can seriously disrupt life. A significant number of depressed people commit, or attempt to commit, *suicide*, whereas others suffer from social isolation, poverty, and problems caused by *alcohol dependence*. Nevertheless, the widescale use of maintenance treatment with lithium has restored many people with manic-depressive illness to near-normal health.

Manipulation

A therapeutic technique involving the skillful use of the hands to move a part of the body or a specific joint or muscle to treat certain disorders. Manipulation is an important technique in *orthopedics, physiotherapy, osteopathy*, and *chiropractic*.

Physicians and physiotherapists use manipulation to treat deformity and stiffness caused by some disorders of the bones and joints. A general anesthetic may be necessary in some cases. Manipulation may be used to realign the bones in a displaced *fracture*, to put a joint back into position following a *dislocation*, or to stretch a *contracture* (shortened muscle or tendon). The technique may also be used to increase the range of movement of a stiff joint, usually following injury. Occasionally, manipulation is helpful in the treatment of *frozen shoulder*. Manipulation does not usually relieve stiffness caused by *arthritis* (inflammation of a joint).

Mannitol

An osmotic *diuretic drug*. Mannitol is used as a short-term treatment for *glaucoma* (raised pressure in the eyeball) before corrective surgery. It is also given to reduce *edema* (accumulation of fluid) in the brain before and after surgical treatment of a *brain tumor* or an intracerebral *hematoma* (blood clot on the brain). Mannitol is occasionally used to prevent *kidney failure* following severe shock. In some cases of drug overdose, mannitol is given to increase urine production and thus hasten excretion of the overdosed drug from the body.

Possible adverse effects of mannitol include headache, nausea, vomiting, dizziness, and confusion.

Manometry

The measuring of pressure (of either a liquid or gas) by means of an instrument called a manometer.

The simplest type of manometer is a glass U-shaped tube containing mercury, oil, or water. One limb of the tube is connected to the pressure source; the other limb is either open to the atmosphere or closed. Changes in pressure cause the liquid to rise in one limb and to fall in the other. More sophisticated manometers use a coiled spring, diaphragm, or electrical transducer to measure pressure.

Manometry is used to measure *blood pressure* by means of an instrument called a *sphygmomanometer*. Other uses of manometry include measurement

M

of the pressure of *cerebrospinal fluid* in the spinal canal, measurement of pressure at the lower end of the esophagus in the diagnosis of esophageal disorders and *hiatal hernia*, and measurement of pressure in the rectum and anus in the investigation of some cases of *constipation* and fecal incontinence (see *Incontinence, fecal*).

Mantoux test
A type of skin test for tuberculosis (see *Tuberculin tests*).

Maprotiline
An *antidepressant drug*. Because maprotiline has a sedative effect, it is useful in *depression* accompanied by anxiety or difficulty sleeping. Maprotiline takes about six weeks to become fully effective. Possible adverse effects include dizziness, drowsiness, palpitations, and rash.

Marasmus
A severe form of protein and calorie malnutrition that usually occurs in famine or semistarvation conditions. In developing countries, marasmus is widespread in children under 3 years of age, usually because they have been weaned too early onto an inadequate diet, given inadequate bottle-feeding, or kept too long on unsupplemented breast milk.

Children suffering from marasmus are stunted, emaciated, and usually hungry; they have loose folds of skin on the limbs and buttocks due to loss of muscle and fat. Other signs include sparse, brittle hair, diarrhea, and dehydration.

DIAGNOSIS AND TREATMENT
Marasmus is diagnosed from a physical examination and the child's dietary history. Treatment consists of keeping the child warm and giving a high-calorie, protein-rich diet. Persistent marasmus can cause permanent mental retardation and impaired growth. (See also *Kwashiorkor*.)

Marble bone disease
See *Osteopetrosis*.

March fracture
A break in one of the *metatarsal bones* (long bones in the foot) caused by repeated jarring. Usually affecting the second or third metatarsal, march fracture is caused by running or walking long distances on a hard surface. The name is derived from the high incidence of this fracture in soldiers after long marches.

Pain, tenderness, and swelling occur around the fracture site. *X rays* may not show the fracture until healing has begun, when callus (new bone) appears as a white shadow. Treatment is rest and, occasionally, immobilization in a plaster *cast*. (See also *Stress fracture*.)

Marfan's syndrome
A rare, inherited disorder of connective tissue (material that surrounds body structures and holds them together) which results in abnormalities of the skeleton, heart, and eyes. The incidence of Marfan's syndrome is about two cases per 100,000 people. The precise cause is unknown.

SYMPTOMS AND SIGNS
The features of Marfan's syndrome usually appear after the age of 10. Affected people grow very tall and thin, the fingers are long and spidery, the chest and spine are often deformed, and the ligaments, tendons, and joint capsules are weak, leaving the sufferer "double-jointed" and susceptible to joint dislocation. In about 90 percent of cases, the heart or the aorta (major blood vessel leading from the heart) is abnormal; in more than 60 percent of sufferers, the lens of the eye is dislocated.

DIAGNOSIS
There are no specific diagnostic tests. *Echocardiography* may be used to investigate heart abnormalities, and an eye examination may be performed.

TREATMENT AND OUTLOOK
Orthopedic *corsets* or surgery may be required to correct spinal deformity. *Beta-blocker drugs* (propranolol, for example) may help to control heart problems, but heart surgery is necessary in some cases.

Affected people should receive *genetic counseling*; there is a 50 percent chance that their offspring will inherit

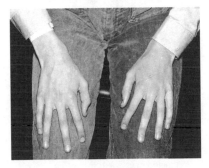

Features of Marfan's syndrome
One of the characteristic features of Marfan's syndrome is long, thin, "spider" fingers (arachnodactyly).

the disease. Women with Marfan's syndrome risk heart complications if they become pregnant.

Many sufferers do not live beyond the age of 50, and death is commonly caused by *heart failure* or rupture of an *aortic aneurysm*.

Marijuana
The flowering tops and dried leaves of the Indian hemp plant CANNABIS SATIVA. Marijuana contains the active ingredient *THC* (tetra-hydrocannabinol), which is found also in cannabis resin (hashish). The chopped leaves are usually smoked as a joint (or reefer) but can be drunk as tea or eaten in food.

EFFECTS
When marijuana is smoked, effects occur within minutes and last for an hour or more. When marijuana is eaten, the effects are not usually felt for half an hour to an hour, and may last for three to five hours.

Physical effects include a dry mouth, mild reddening of the eyes, slight clumsiness, and increased appetite. The main subjective feelings are usually of well-being and calmness, although depression occasionally occurs. Users become dreamy and relaxed, laughing readily and experiencing time as passing very slowly. Sights and sounds become more vivid, imagination increases, and random connections between things seem more relevant.

Large doses may result in panicky states, fear of death, and illusions. Rarely, true psychosis (loss of contact with reality) occurs, producing paranoid delusions, confusion, and other symptoms. These symptoms usually disappear within several days if triggered by the drug, which may merely be acting on an underlying illness. A more permanent state of apathy and loss of concern (known as amotivational syndrome) has been attributed to prolonged, regular use.

There is a possibility that regular users of marijuana may become physically dependent on it. Whether or not the drug causes brain or other physical damage is much debated. Under the Narcotics Control Act it is illegal to grow, import, possess or use marijuana in Canada.

Marital counseling
A type of professional therapy for married couples or established partners aimed at resolving problems in relationships. Usually the partners

M

attend sessions together on a regular basis. The counselor promotes communication and sorts out differences between the partners.

HOW IT IS DONE
Marital counseling today is largely based on the ideas and methods of *behavior therapy*. It is assumed that behavior in a relationship is learned. Another assumption is that both partners are responsible for problems because they have either failed to reinforce desirable behavior in their partner or have themselves failed to respond with appropriate behavior. Research evidence shows that behavioral marital therapy can be extremely effective.

Therapy starts with an analysis of the good and bad aspects of the relationship. Each of the partners then indicates how he or she would like the other to behave. In some cases, a contract may be drawn up in which each person agrees to do something that the other wants. Alternatively, a system of rewards may be set up in which each partner rewards the other for pleasing or helpful behavior.

Role play and demonstrations may be used to teach alternative ways of behaving, and training in communication skills given to promote the expression of feelings. If part of the couple's problem is sexual, the counselor may refer them for *sex therapy*.

Marrow, bone
See *Bone marrow*.

Marsupialization
A surgical procedure used to drain some types of abscess or cyst (e.g., of a *Bartholin's gland* at the entrance to the vagina) and to prevent further abscesses. Marsupialization of a Bartholin's gland abscess involves cutting out part of the abscess wall and a small piece of vaginal tissue, and then forming a pouch by stitching the opened abscess wall to the wall of the vagina.

Marsupialization is also used to treat certain types of cysts affecting the pancreas and liver.

Masculinization
See *Virilization*.

Masochism
A desire to be physically, mentally, or emotionally abused. The term is derived from the name of the 19th-century Austrian novelist Leopold von Sacher-Masoch.

The term masochism is often used specifically to refer to the achievement

of sexual excitement exclusively or preferably by means of one's own suffering. Activities include bondage, flagellation, and verbal abuse. The condition is usually chronic, and may even be life-threatening when people increase the severity of their masochistic acts. Masochists rarely seek professional treatment; when they do, it is usually at the instigation of a spouse who threatens to leave. (See also *Sadism; Sadomasochism*.)

Massage
Rubbing and kneading of areas of the body, usually using the hands. Massage is used to relieve painful muscle spasm, treat muscle injury, reduce edema (fluid retention in tissue), and, in the treatment of scars, to prevent tethering of skin and underlying tissue. Massage increases blood flow, reduces deep-seated pain by causing counter-irritation of nerve endings in the skin, relaxes muscles, and increases the suppleness of the skin.

Mast cell

A type of cell, present in most body tissues, and especially numerous in connective tissues, that plays an important part in *allergy*. In an allergic response, an allergen stimulates the release of *antibodies*, which attach themselves to mast cells. As a result, the mast cells release substances such as *histamine* (one of the chemicals responsible for allergy symptoms) into the tissue.

Mastectomy
Surgical removal of all or part of the *breast*. Mastectomy is usually performed to treat *breast cancer* and is often followed by a course of *radiation therapy* or *anticancer drugs*.

The amount of breast and surrounding tissue that is removed depends on the size and location of the tumor, on how much the cancer has spread, and on the age and general health of the patient.

SELF-MASSAGE
Although massage is most effective when carried out by another person, self-massage can still be useful; for example, it may help to alleviate pain caused by muscular tension.

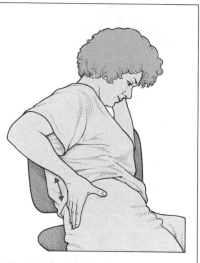

Kneading the lower back
For self-massage of the lower back, the hands should be placed with the thumbs pointing forward and the fingertips close together at the back. Firm finger pressure is required to massage this area.

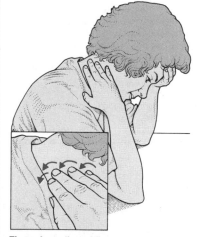

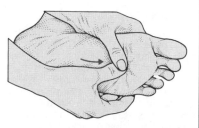

Finger kneading of the neck and foot
For neck massage, the elbows are rested on a firm surface, such as a table, and the head is supported with one hand while the fingertips of the other hand knead the back and side of the neck. After one side of the neck has been massaged, switch hands and massage the other side.

For foot massage, place one thumb over the other and knead the sole from the heel to the ball of the foot.

TYPES

Until the late 1960s, the standard operation was the radical mastectomy, which involves removal of the affected breast, the chest muscles, underarm lymph nodes, and additional fat and skin from the chest. When some of the chest muscles are left intact, the operation is known as a modified radical mastectomy.

Today, surgeons may recommend lumpectomy (in which only cancerous tissue is removed) or a quadrantectomy (in which one quadrant of the breast is removed). In many cases, however, the treatment is still a mastectomy, which consists of removing the affected breast and sometimes some of the underarm lymph nodes. Sometimes, surgeons leave the overlying skin intact, or leave plenty of surrounding skin to allow the breast to be reconstructed.

HOW IT IS DONE

Each of the operations is performed under a general anesthetic. For lumpectomy and quadrantectomy, an incision is made over the breast lump, which is cut free and removed together with some of the surrounding breast tissue.

For mastectomy, the incision extends from the armpit to encompass the entire breast. Underlying tissue is then cut free and removed, and a drainage tube is inserted. In all cases, the skin is closed with stitches or clips, which are usually removed after a week. A skin graft is sometimes needed. Some surgeons carry out a subcutaneous mastectomy, in which the skin is left intact and a silicone rubber implant is inserted to preserve the shape of the breast.

RECOVERY PERIOD

Patients may go home one to two days after lumpectomy and quadrantectomy, and can resume most activities within two weeks.

After other operations, the hospital stay is usually several days, and the drainage tube is removed on the second or third day. Analgesic drugs (painkillers) may be necessary for the first week.

OUTLOOK

Healing is usually very good after lumpectomy and quadrantectomy, with no noticeable scarring. Wound infection is uncommon. Skin scars after more radical procedures may be extensive, but usually fade within about a year.

Possible long-term complications, particularly of radical mastectomy, include *lymphedema* (accumulation of lymphatic fluid in tissues) and stiffness of the arm and shoulder.

If the entire breast has been removed, some form of prosthesis will be provided. This may be an external prosthesis, or a more permanent internal prosthesis, which may be fitted either immediately or at a later operation (see *Mammoplasty*).

Mastication

The process of chewing food. Mastication consists of two stages. In the first, the canines and incisors (front teeth) shear the food. In the second, the tongue pushes the food between the upper and lower premolars and molars (back teeth) to be ground by side-to-side and circular movements

---

TYPES OF MASTECTOMY

The type of operation depends on many factors, including the site of the tumor and the woman's health.

A small tumor may be treated by lumpectomy; other cases may require more extensive surgery.

LUMPECTOMY

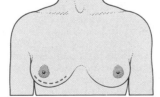

Only the area of cancerous tissue is removed. Lumpectomy is the least invasive procedure and leaves the breast looking normal.

QUADRANTECTOMY

The cancerous tissue plus a wedge of surrounding tissue is removed. The lymph nodes in the armpit may also be removed. The breast is slightly smaller after the operation.

SUBCUTANEOUS MASTECTOMY

An incision is made under the breast and internal breast tissue is removed, leaving most of the skin intact. The nipple is not involved, but the milk ducts leading to it are cut. In some cases, the appearance of the breast is restored by immediate insertion of a silicone rubber implant. More often, however, this is done later.

TOTAL MASTECTOMY

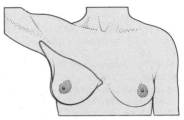

1 A large elliptical incision, encompassing the nipple and sometimes the entire breast, is made. The incision extends into the armpit.

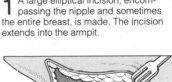

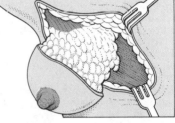

2 All the breast tissue, including the skin and some of the fat, is dissected (cut away) down to the chest muscles. The dissection is continued under the skin into the armpit, to free the upper and outer "tail" of breast tissue with its lymph nodes. All bleeding vessels are tied off before inserting a drainage tube and closing the skin with stitches or clips.

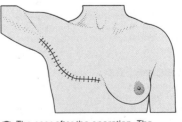

3 The scar after the operation. The woman may wear a prosthesis or may have a silicone implant inserted later.

M

of the lower jaws. During mastication, saliva is mixed with the food to help break it down for swallowing.

Any food that spills over between the gums and cheeks is scooped up by rhythmic contractions of the cheeks and lips. The muscles of mastication, which attach the lower jaw to the rest of the skull, are controlled by signals from sensory nerves in the mouth to prevent undue stress on tooth-supporting tissues.

Only gross irregularities in the positional relationship of upper to lower teeth (see *Malocclusion*) prevent normal mastication.

Mastitis

Inflammation of *breast* tissue, usually caused by bacterial infection and sometimes by hormonal changes.

CAUSES

Mastitis is usually caused by the entry of bacteria into the breast through the nipple during *breast-feeding*. This type of mastitis is most common during the first month of breast-feeding and the condition is more likely to occur if the nipples are cracked.

Mastitis can also be caused by changes in the levels of sex hormones in the body. This type of mastitis sometimes occurs in the newborn (due to high levels of hormones from the mother's circulation) and at the start of *puberty*. Fibroadenosis (chronic mastitis in which the breasts are tender and lumpy) is also thought to be due to hormonal variations.

SYMPTOMS

Pain, tenderness, and swelling occur in all types of mastitis and may be present in one or both breasts. Bacterial mastitis during breast-feeding causes redness and *engorgement* and may result in a *breast abscess*.

TREATMENT

Mastitis caused by infection is treated with *antibiotic drugs* and *analgesic drugs* (painkillers), and by *expressing milk* to relieve engorgement. Breast-feeding should be continued unless pus begins to drain from the nipple.

Symptoms of mastitis in babies and at puberty usually last for only a few weeks and clear up without specific treatment.

Mastocytosis

An unusual condition, also called urticaria pigmentosa, characterized by numerous itchy, irregular, yellow or orange-brown swellings on the skin. Mastocytosis most commonly occurs on the trunk, and is worse after bathing or scratching.

In some cases, mastocytosis affects many body organs, including the liver, spleen, and intestine. Symptoms, such as diarrhea, vomiting, and fainting may occur. Very rarely, mastocytosis leads to *anaphylactic shock*, which can be fatal.

Mastocytosis usually begins in the first year of life and disappears by adolescence. Treatment is difficult, although *antihistamine drugs* sometimes help to relieve symptoms.

Mastoid bone

The lower part of the temporal bone of the *skull*. Jutting from the lower part of the mastoid bone is a bony projection called the mastoid process. The mastoid bone is honeycombed with air cells, which are connected to a cavity called the mastoid antrum in the upper part of the mastoid. The mastoid antrum leads into the middle ear. As a result, infections of the middle ear (see *Otitis media*) occasionally spread through the mastoid bone to cause acute *mastoiditis*.

Mastoiditis

Inflammation of the *mastoid bone*, the prominent bone behind the ear.

CAUSE AND INCIDENCE

The disease is caused by the spread of infection from the middle ear (see *Otitis media*) to the mastoid antrum (a cavity in the mastoid bone), and from there to a honeycomb of air cells in the bone.

Mastoiditis has been uncommon since the advent of *antibiotic drugs*, which control middle ear infection.

SYMPTOMS AND SIGNS

Mastoiditis causes severe pain, swelling, and tenderness behind the ear, as well as pain within the ear. These symptoms are usually accompanied by fever, a creamy discharge from the ear, progressive hearing loss, and some displacement of the outer ear.

COMPLICATIONS

There is always a risk that the infection may spread, causing *meningitis*, a *brain abscess*, or clotting of blood in veins within the brain. The infection may also spread outward to damage the facial nerve and cause *facial palsy*.

DIAGNOSIS AND TREATMENT

Prompt diagnosis, based on a physical examination, is essential because of the possible complications.

Treatment is with antibiotic drugs, which usually clear up the infection. If the infection persists, an operation known as a mastoidectomy may be necessary. This procedure involves making an incision behind the ear,

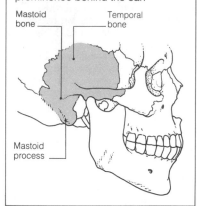

LOCATION OF MASTOID BONE
The mastoid bone is the lower part of the temporal bone. The mastoid process can be felt as a prominence behind the ear.

Mastoid bone

Temporal bone

Mastoid process

opening up the mastoid bone, and removing the infected air cells. The wound is then stitched up around a drainage tube, which is removed a day or two later.

Masturbation

Sexual self-stimulation, usually to orgasm. Masturbation is now accepted as a normal behavior. Over 90 percent of men and about 65 percent of women masturbate at some time during their lives. Massaging the penis or clitoris with the hand is the usual method.

There is no evidence that masturbation causes any physical or psychological harm, in spite of the 19th century belief that it caused insanity, blindness, or other disorders. This notion may have been based on the observation that people who are severely retarded or suffering from *schizophrenia*, *dementia*, or other forms of brain damage sometimes masturbate publicly. Such behavior is a sign not a cause of mental illness.

Maternal mortality

The death of a woman during *pregnancy* or within 42 days of *childbirth*, *miscarriage*, or induced *abortion*, from any cause related to the pregnancy. The term also describes the number of such deaths per year per 100,000 (or per 1,000 or 10,000) pregnancies.

In previous centuries, women of all social classes commonly died in childbirth; maternal mortality still remains high in developing countries. In developed countries, however, deaths and complications of childbirth have declined dramatically in this century, particularly since about the 1940s. A large proportion of this decline is due to improvements in social conditions (which have resulted in improvements in women's general health); much of the remainder is a result of medical advances in treating the complications of pregnancy and childbirth.

CAUSES

Maternal deaths may occur as a direct result of complications of pregnancy, or as an indirect result of a medical condition that has been aggravated by pregnancy. The principal direct causes include *pulmonary embolism* (blood clots in the lungs), *hypertension* (high blood pressure), *antepartum hemorrhage* or *postpartum hemorrhage*, *ectopic pregnancy* (development of the fetus outside the uterus), *eclampsia* (a condition characterized by seizures during late pregnancy), abortion, miscarriage, or *cesarean section*, and *puerperal sepsis* (infection after childbirth). Important indirect causes are heart disease, *anemia*, *hyperthyroidism* (overactivity of the thyroid gland) or *hypothyroidism* (underactivity of the thyroid gland), *diabetes mellitus*, and some cancers.

RELATED FACTORS

Maternal mortality is highest for the first pregnancy, and for the fifth and subsequent pregnancies. It is also greater in women who are younger than 20 or older than 30. Statistically, it is safest for a woman to have her first baby when she is between 20 and 25 years old; it becomes increasingly less safe after the age of 30.

Social factors also play a part; in general maternal mortality is higher among poor, less well-educated women, and among women who do not receive adequate *prenatal care*.

TRENDS

Maternal mortality has decreased considerably since about the 1940s. In Canada, the death rate has fallen from about 60 per 100,000 pregnancies in 1930, to less than 3 per 100,000 in the 1980s. This substantial decline is due largely to social improvements, better obstetric care, the development of *antibiotic drugs* and other drugs to combat infection, and the availability of *blood transfusions*. In addition, because of effective methods of *contraception*, fewer women than formerly have a large number of pregnancies.

Maxilla

One of a pair of bones that form the upper jaw. At their base the maxillae carry the upper *teeth* and form the roof of the mouth; at the top the maxillae form the floor of the orbits (the eye sockets). Each maxilla contains a large air-filled cavity (called the maxillary sinus) which is connected to the nasal cavity.

DISORDERS

The most common disorder affecting the maxilla is *sinusitis* (inflammation of the mucous membrane that lines the maxillary sinuses), usually caused by infection spreading from the nose, less commonly from a tooth. Severe sinusitis occasionally leads to *osteomyelitis* (bone infection).

The maxilla is commonly fractured in road traffic accidents, causing a variety of facial deformities, such as backward displacement of the teeth or caving in of the center of the face. Immediate surgery to reposition and secure the bones is necessary to prevent permanent disfigurement.

Various kinds of tumors may develop in the maxillary sinus, 80 percent of which are malignant. Tumors of the maxillary sinus may eventually alter the shape of the jaw, loosen the teeth, block one of the nasolacrimal ducts (causing the eye to water), push the eyeball upward or outward, or block the nose and cause a bloody, offensive-smelling discharge. Treatment is by *radiation therapy*, followed by surgical removal of the maxilla.

McArdle's disease

A rare *genetic disorder* characterized by muscular stiffness and painful cramps

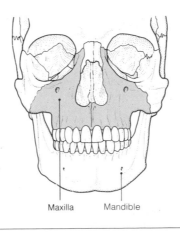

LOCATION OF THE MAXILLA
The maxilla is one of a pair of bones that together form the center of the face, the upper jaw, and the roof of the mouth.

Maxilla   Mandible

that increase during and after exertion. McArdle's disease is caused by a deficiency of an *enzyme* (a substance that promotes chemical reactions) in muscle cells that stimulates the breakdown of *glycogen* (a complex carbohydrate) to glucose (a type of sugar). This deficiency results in a buildup of glycogen in the muscles and prevents the release of glucose (an essential source of energy) during exercise.

Symptoms usually start between the ages of 20 and 30. Myoglobinuria (the presence of muscle cell pigment in the urine) occurs because of the damage to muscle cells; rarely, myoglobinuria is severe enough to cause *kidney failure*. Affected people are usually healthy apart from the need to restrict their exercise.

There is no treatment, although symptoms may be relieved by eating glucose or fructose before exercise.

Measles

A potentially dangerous viral illness that causes a characteristic rash and a fever. Measles mainly affects children but can occur at any age. One attack usually confers lifelong immunity.

CAUSES AND INCIDENCE

The measles virus is highly infective and is spread primarily by airborne droplets of nasal secretions. There is an incubation period of eight to 14 days before symptoms appear. Infected children can transmit the virus from shortly after the start of this period to up to one week after the onset of symptoms. Infants under 8 months old are rarely affected because they have acquired some immunity from their mothers.

Measles was once very common throughout the world, occurring in epidemics. It is now much less common in developed countries due to *immunization*. In Canada, where proof of immunization is required before a child can attend school, less than a thousand cases are now reported each year.

Prevention of measles is important because it can have rare but serious complications. Measles may also be serious, and sometimes fatal, in children with impaired immunity (such as those being treated for *leukemia* and those infected with the virus that causes *AIDS*).

In developing countries, measles is still common, accounting for more than 1 million deaths every year, especially in malnourished children whose defenses against infection are seriously impaired.

M

SYMPTOMS AND SIGNS

The illness starts with a fever, runny nose, sore eyes, and cough, and the sufferer is generally unwell. After three to four days a red rash appears, usually starting on the head and neck and spreading downward to cover the whole body. The spots sometimes join to produce large red blotchy areas, and the lymph glands may be enlarged. After three days the rash starts to fade and symptoms subside.

The most common complications are ear and chest infections, which usually occur with a return of fever two to three days after the appearance of the rash. Diarrhea, vomiting, and abdominal pain also occur.

Febrile convulsions are common with measles and are not usually serious (see *Convulsions, febrile*).

A serious complication, occurring in about one in 1,000 cases, is *encephalitis* (inflammation of the brain). Encephalitis causes headache, drowsiness, and vomiting, starting seven to 10 days after the appearance of the rash. Seizures and coma may follow, sometimes leading to mental retardation or even death.

Very rarely (in about one in 1 million cases) a progressive brain disorder, known as subacute sclerosing panencephalitis, develops years after the acute illness.

Measles during pregnancy results in death of the fetus in about one fifth of cases. There is no evidence that measles causes birth defects.

TREATMENT

Plenty of fluids and *acetaminophen* should be given to treat the fever. Antibiotic drugs are not required to treat the measles infection itself but may be given to treat bacterial infections that occur as complications.

IMMUNIZATION

Immunization against measles is usually offered at about 15 months of age and produces immunity in about 97 percent of cases. Side effects of the measles vaccine are generally mild. There may be slight fever, symptoms of a cold, and a rash about one week after vaccination.

The vaccine should not be given to children under the age of 1 or to those with any special risk factors (see *Immunization*).

Meatus

A canal or passageway through part of the body. The term usually refers to the external auditory meatus, the canal in the outer *ear* that leads from the outside to the eardrum.

Mebendazole

An *anthelmintic drug* used to treat *worm infestations* of the intestine. Mebendazole is under investigation as a treatment for worms that infest other areas, such as the lungs and liver, as occurs in *hydatid disease*.

Possible adverse effects include abdominal pain and diarrhea.

Meckel's diverticulum

A common congenital anomaly of the digestive tract in which a small, hollow, wide-mouthed sac protrudes from the *ileum* (the final section of the small intestine). Meckel's diverticulum occurs in 2 percent of people.

There are usually no symptoms unless the diverticulum is affected by infection, obstruction, or ulceration. The most common symptom of the condition is painless bleeding, which may be sudden and severe, making immediate *blood transfusion* necessary. In some cases, inflammation causes symptoms so similar to those of acute *appendicitis* that the disorder is diagnosed only when abdominal surgery is carried out on the victim. A Meckel's diverticulum occasionally causes *intussusception* (telescoping) or *volvulus* (twisting) of the small intestine. Diagnosis may sometimes be made by using technetium *radionuclide scanning*.

Complications are treated by removal of the diverticulum.

Meclizine

An antihistamine used primarily in treating motion sickness and the vertigo, nausea and vomiting associated with inner ear disorders (see *Labyrinthitis*). It has a longer duration of action than many other antihistamines, and may cause drowsiness and dry mouth.

Meconium

The thick, sticky, greenish-black feces passed by infants during the first day or two after birth. Meconium consists of bile, mucus, and shed intestinal cells. After the baby starts feeding, the feces gradually change in color and consistency.

Occasionally, the fetus passes meconium into the *amniotic fluid* in the uterus. This is more common in babies who experience *fetal distress* during labor or who are postmature (that is, over 40 weeks' gestation). Meconium in the amniotic fluid may be inhaled when the baby starts to breathe, sometimes blocking the airways and damaging the lungs.

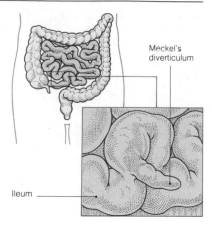

Meckel's diverticulum

Ileum

Anatomy of Meckel's diverticulum
In this birth defect, an appendixlike sac protrudes from the ileum (the last section of the small intestine).

In some babies with *cystic fibrosis*, the meconium is so thick and sticky that it blocks the intestine and causes intestinal obstruction.

Medial

A medical term meaning situated toward the midline of the body. Less commonly, the word is used to refer to the middle layer of a body structure, particularly of a blood vessel wall.

Median nerve

One of the main nerves of the arm, which runs down the arm's full length into the hand; it is a branch of the *brachial plexus*. The median nerve controls the muscles of the forearm and hand, which carry out bending movements of the wrist, fingers, and thumb, and which rotate the forearm palm-inward. This nerve also conveys sensations from the thumb, index finger, middle finger, part of the ring finger, and the region of the palm at the base of these digits.

DISORDERS

Injury to the shoulder may damage the median nerve at the point where it originates from the brachial plexus. A *Colles' fracture* may damage the median nerve just above the wrist. *Carpal tunnel syndrome* causes pressure that may damage the nerve where it passes through the wrist. The principal symptoms of any damage are numbness and muscle weakness in the areas controlled by the nerve.

Mediastinoscopy

Investigation of the *mediastinum* (the central compartment of the chest containing the heart, esophagus, and trachea) by means of an *endoscope* (a viewing tube with a light and lens) inserted into the cavity through an incision in the neck.

Mediastinoscopy is used mainly to perform a *biopsy* (removal of a small sample of tissue for microscopic analysis) of a lymph node to look for disease. Under a general anesthetic, an incision is made in the base of the neck and an endoscope is passed through it into the mediastinum. A tissue sample is removed by minute blades at the end of the endoscope and the incision is closed with stitches.

Mediastinum

The space between the lungs, including the structures in that space. The mediastinum extends from the sternum (breastbone) in front to the spine behind, and from the inlet of the thoracic duct (one of the main lymphatic vessels) at the top to the diaphragm at the bottom. The mediastinum contains the *heart*, *trachea* (windpipe), *esophagus*, *thymus* gland, the major blood vessels entering and leaving the heart, *lymph nodes* and lymphatic vessels, and nerves (including the *vagus nerve* and *phrenic nerve*).

Medical associations/ societies, provincial

In each province or territory physicians have formed an association or society that represents organized medicine in dealings with the public and the provincial government. These organizations are also recognized as divisions of the Canadian Medical Association.

Medical licensure

Each province has a college of physicians and surgeons, which acts as the governing body of all licensed physicians in the province. The colleges issue licenses to candidates who have had the required training and have passed any examinations the college deems necessary.

Medical Officer of Health

The Medical Officer of Health (the title is slightly different in some provinces) is a physician with additional training in epidemiology and public health. He or she is the executive officer of the local board of health. Responsibilities of this official include identifying, monitoring, and reducing health hazards in the region, stimulating community health and social service programs, and enforcing public health statutes and legislation.

Medical research funding

Most research in Canada is supported by agencies that consider applications from qualified researchers and fund successful proposals for a limited time. Hundreds of voluntary organizations and government agencies financially support medical research in different parts of the country. The Medical Research Council is the major federal funding agency; it funds more than 2,000 projects a year in laboratory and clinical research. Health and Welfare Canada's National Health Research and Development Program supports research in health care delivery and epidemiology. Each provincial ministry of health also funds medical research, as do many volunteer organizations seeking the cure for specific diseases.

Medical specialist

A medical specialist is a physician who has had additional training (usually four years) after internship in a specific field of medicine, such as laboratory science, cardiology, dermatology, or neurology, or in any field of surgery, such as general surgery, cardiac surgery, or ophthalmology. The medical specialist must also meet the standards of the Royal College of Physicians and Surgeons of Canada, before he or she is certified to practice as a specialist.

Medicare

This is a general term that refers to *provincial health plans*, which provide prepaid health care and are administered by each province. The Medical Care Act of 1966 requires that these programs give comprehensive coverage for all medically necessary care, that they be accessible to all Canadians even when outside the country, and that they not be administered for profit.

Medication

Any substance prescribed to treat disease. (See also *Drug*; *Medicine*.)

Medicine

The study of human diseases, including their causes, frequency, treatment, and prevention. The term is also applied to any substance prescribed to treat illness.

EARLY HISTORY

In many early cultures, medicine was closely associated with religion because disease was regarded as a punishment from the gods. As a result, the victim would turn for help to a priest, who took on the additional function of a medicine man. Medicine probably became separated from religion with the emergence of people skilled in treating injuries such as broken bones and dislocated joints. These healers attracted patients and, in time, apprentices.

By the fifth century B.C., the Greek physician Hippocrates had established medicine as a profession with a body of learning and a code of ethics to be passed on to each new generation of physicians (the Hippocratic oath is still used as an ethical guide for the medical profession). The dominant figure after Hippocrates was the second-century, Greek-born Roman physician Galen, who made valuable contributions but whose many false theories about anatomy and physiology were uncritically accepted for more than 13 centuries; these theories effectively held back advances in medical knowledge.

RENAISSANCE DISCOVERIES

With the Renaissance, medicine began to emerge from its long period of stagnation. In 1543 the Flemish anatomist and physician Andreas Vesalius (1514-1564) produced the first truly accurate anatomical text; in 1628 the English physician William Harvey (1578-1657) first demonstrated how blood circulates through the body. Also in the 17th century, the Dutch microscopist Antonj van Leeuwenhoek (1632-1723) became the first to observe and describe microorganisms and the detailed structure of blood, muscles, and sperm.

MODERN MEDICINE

Despite the medical achievements of the Renaissance and some notable later achievements, such as the discovery in the late 18th century of the principle of vaccination by the English physician Edward Jenner (1749-1823), it was not until the 19th century that the foundations of modern scientific medicine were laid. This was the result of a growing realization that medicine needed to become a true science, systematic in its approach and founded on scrupulous observation and experimentation. Significant advances in other disciplines also played an important role. For example, the first practical high-powered microscope was developed during the 19th century; the ophthalmoscope (an instrument for examining the eye) was invented in 1851; the first practical thermometer was introduced in the 1860s; and X rays were discovered in 1895, an occurrence that

M

revolutionized medical diagnosis. These developments, along with the French scientist Louis Pasteur's (1822-1895) work on the germ theory of disease, brought about an enormous advance in the understanding of a large number of diseases.

Curing and controlling disease was not a reality until the 20th century, however, when vaccines were developed against many serious diseases (including typhoid, cholera, and diphtheria); and insecticides and improved sanitation helped control diseases such as malaria, yellow fever, and sleeping sickness.

The early 20th century was also marked by the development of safe anesthesia, effective surgery, and a steady growth in the number of new drugs. In the late 1930s, the first effective antibacterial drugs (the sulfonamides) were introduced, followed in the 1940s by penicillin, streptomycin, and the tetracyclines; these drugs saved millions of lives.

Among the important recent developments are the introduction of sophisticated diagnostic techniques, such as MRI, CT scanning, and ultrasound scanning; more effective drugs and other treatments (such as radiation therapy) to treat a wider range of diseases and disorders; and developments in surgical techniques that have made it possible to perform operations such as transplanting organs and rejoining severed nerves.

Today, the boundaries between medicine and other sciences are becoming progressively less distinct; medical research is being increasingly undertaken by scientists who have little or no formal medical training. (See also *Landmarks in medicine* on this page, facing page, and page 674; entries for individual medical, surgical, and scientific specialties.)

Medicolegal

Relating to aspects of medicine and law that overlap, particularly to medical matters that come before the courts. Among the matters on which medicolegal experts advise are the laws concerning damages for injuries due to medical negligence or malpractice, medical evidence concerning the extent of injury in a civil action, the use of tests in determining paternity, the mental competence of people who have drawn up wills, and restrictions on the liberty of the mentally ill.

In recent years, new areas of medicolegal study have emerged, notably an individual's right to die (see *Brain*

LANDMARKS IN MEDICINE: DIAGNOSIS

Date	Development
c. 400 B.C.	**Disease concept** Introduced by the Greek physician Hippocrates.
1612	**Medical thermometer** Devised by the Italian physician Sanctorius.
c. 1660	**Light microscope** Single-lens microscope developed by the Dutch naturalist Antonj van Leeuwenhoek, who discovered microorganisms with it. A practicable compound microscope was not developed until the 19th century.
1810	**Stethoscope** Invented by the French physician René Laennec.
1850–1900	**Germ theory of disease** Proposed by the French scientist Louis Pasteur and developed by the German bacteriologist Robert Koch.
1851	**Ophthalmoscope** Invented by the German scientist Hermann von Helmholtz.
1895	**X rays** Discovered by the German physicist Wilhelm Roentgen. He also produced the first X-ray picture of the body.
1905	**X-ray contrast medium** First demonstrated (in retrograde pyelography) by Jean Athanese Sicard in Paris.
1906	**Electrocardiograph (ECG)** Invented by the Dutch physiologist Willem Einthoven.
c. 1932	**Transmission electron microscope (TEM)** Constructed by the German scientists Max Knoll and Ernst Ruska.
1938	**Cardiac catheterization** First performed by George Peter Robb and Israel Steinberg in New York.
1957	**Fiberoptic endoscopy** Pioneered by the South African-born physician Basil Hirschowitz at the University of Michigan.
1972	**CT scanner** Invented by the British engineer Godfrey Hounsfield of EMI Laboratories, England, and the South African-born physicist Alan Cormack of Tufts University, Massachusetts.
1975	**Monoclonal antibodies** Large-scale production method developed by the Argentinian-born scientist César Milstein at the Medical Research Council Laboratories, England.
1976	**Chorionic villus sampling** Developed by Chinese gynecologists as an aid to the early diagnosis of genetic disorders.
1981	**MRI scanner** Developed by scientists at Thorn-EMI Laboratories, England, and Nottingham University.
1985	**PET scanner** Developed by scientists at the University of California.

LANDMARKS IN MEDICINE: SURGERY

Date	Development
1545	**Basic surgical principles** Established by the French surgeon Ambroise Paré.
1842	**General anesthesia** First operation using general anesthesia performed by the American surgeon Crawford Long, who used ether. In 1845, the American dentist Horace Wells used nitrous oxide (laughing gas) as an anesthetic. In 1847, the British obstetrician James Simpson introduced chloroform anesthesia.
1870	**Antiseptic surgery** Pioneered by the British surgeon Joseph Lister, who used a carbolic acid (phenol) spray during surgery to help prevent infection.
1901	**Blood groups** ABO blood groups discovered by the Austrian pathologist Karl Landsteiner, so establishing the basis for safe transfusions.
1951	**Coronary artery bypass graft** First attempted by the Canadian surgeon Arthur Vineberg at the Royal Victoria Hospital, Montreal.
1955	**Kidney transplant** First successful kidney transplant (between identical twins) performed by a team of American surgeons—led by Joseph Murray—of the Harvard Medical School, Massachusetts.
1967	**Heart transplant** First human heart transplant performed by the South African surgeon Christiaan Barnard at the Groote Schuur Hospital, Capetown.
1976	**Coronary angioplasty** Introduced by the Swiss surgeon Andreas Grüntzig at the University Hospital, Zurich.
1987	**Fetal tissue transplant** First transplant of fetal brain tissue into brains of patients with Parkinson's disease performed by research groups in Mexico, the US, and Europe.

LANDMARKS IN MEDICINE: OTHER FORMS OF TREATMENT

Date	Development
c. 1270	**Glasses** Thought to have been invented in Italy. Contact lenses were invented in 1887 by the Swiss optician Eugen Frick.
1817	**Dental plate** Introduced by the American dentist Anthony Plantson.
1891	**Baby incubator** Introduced by the French physician Alexandre Lion.
1901	**Hearing aid (electric)** Developed by the American inventor Miller Reese Hutchinson. The first truly miniature hearing aid was introduced in 1951 by the Sonotone Corporation.
1945	**Kidney dialysis machine** Developed by the Dutch surgeon Willem Kolff to treat patients with kidney failure.
1978	**"Test-tube baby"** The first (Louise Brown) was born in England as a result of in vitro fertilization (IVF) techniques developed by the British gynecologist Patrick Steptoe and the embryologist Robert Edwards.
1979	**Shock wave lithotripsy** Pioneered by researchers at the University Hospital, Munich.

death; Euthanasia; Living will); abortion; the necessity for informed consent to any surgical procedure; the legal aspects of artificial insemination, in vitro fertilization, sterilization, and surrogacy; and the ownership of records and drug testing in the workplace. (For the medical aspects of criminal law, see Forensic medicine.)

Meditation

Concentration on an object, a word, or an idea with the intention of inducing an altered state of consciousness. Meditation of different kinds has traditionally been a feature of many religions, particularly Eastern ones.

At its deepest level, meditation can resemble a trance or be an all-engrossing spiritual experience. More commonly, by freeing the mind of excessive thought, it is a physically calming therapy for body and mind. Some clinical trials have shown that meditation can be a valuable therapy for reducing stress levels and in helping to treat stress-related disorders. The most common form of meditation practiced in the West is transcendental meditation (TM), introduced by the Maharishi Mahesh Yogi in the 1960s.

Medroxyprogesterone

A progesterone drug used in the treatment of endometriosis and certain types of breast cancer and uterine cancer (see Uterus, cancer of). Medroxyprogesterone is occasionally given to treat menstrual disorders such as mid-cycle bleeding and amenorrhea (absence of menstruation).

Injections of medroxyprogesterone are used as a contraceptive (see Contraception, hormonal methods of). Injections are given at three-monthly intervals.

Possible adverse effects include weight gain, swollen ankles, and breast tenderness.

Medulla

The innermost part of an organ or body structure; the adrenal medulla is the central region of an adrenal gland, and the medulla of bone is the bone marrow. The term medulla is also sometimes used to refer to the medulla oblongata (part of the brain stem joining the spinal cord).

Medulla oblongata

Also known as the medulla, the medulla oblongata is the lowest part of the brain stem; it is situated in the skull between the pons (above) and the spinal cord (below).

M

Medulloblastoma

A type of malignant *brain tumor* which occurs mainly in children (in whom it is the most common type of brain tumor). The tumor usually arises from the *cerebellum* (a region of the brain concerned with posture, balance and coordination). A medulloblastoma grows rapidly and may spread to other parts of the brain and to the spinal cord.

Typically, a morning headache, repeated vomiting, and a clumsy gait develop, with frequent falls caused by disturbance of the function of the cerebellum. The tumor is diagnosed by *CT scanning* or *MRI* and often responds to *radiation therapy*. This treatment, combined with surgery and the use of *anticancer drugs*, often allows survival for five years or more.

Mefenamic acid

A *nonsteroidal anti-inflammatory drug* (NSAID). Mefenamic acid is used to relieve pain after a minor operation or after injury to soft tissues (such as muscles and ligaments), and to treat joint pain and stiffness caused by types of arthritis, such as *osteoarthritis* and *rheumatoid arthritis*. This drug is also used to relieve *dysmenorrhea* (painful menstrual periods).

Possible adverse effects of mefenamic acid include abdominal pain, nausea, vomiting, and, after prolonged use, a *peptic ulcer*.

Mega-

A prefix meaning very large, as in *megacolon*, a condition in which the colon (part of the large intestine) is greatly enlarged. The prefix megalo- is synonymous with mega-.

Megacolon

A grossly distended (enlarged) colon (part of the large intestine), usually accompanied by severe, chronic constipation. Megacolon may be present at birth or may develop later in life. It is a condition that is seen in all age groups.

CAUSES
In children, the main causes of megacolon are *Hirschsprung's disease*, *anal fissures*, and psychological factors that may have developed at the time of toilet-training.

In the elderly, megacolon may be caused by long-term use of powerful *laxative drugs*, particularly those containing the substances senna, rhubarb, or cascara.

People suffering from chronic *depression* or *schizophrenia*, particularly if they live in an institution, often suffer from megacolon. Other, rarer causes include *hypothyroidism*, some neurological disorders (for example, spinal cord injury), and certain drugs (notably the narcotic drugs *morphine* and *codeine*).

SYMPTOMS
The symptoms are severe constipation and abdominal bloating; some sufferers lose their appetite, which may result in weight loss. Occasionally there is diarrhea, caused by a leakage of semiliquid feces around the obstructing hard feces.

DIAGNOSIS
Megacolon is diagnosed by *proctoscopy* (inspection of the rectum with a viewing instrument), *barium X-ray examination*, and tests of bowel muscle function. If Hirschsprung's disease is suspected, a *biopsy* (removal of a small

Date	Development
	LANDMARKS IN MEDICINE: DRUGS
1666	**Quinine** The British physician Thomas Sydenham popularized the use of Jesuits' bark (containing quinine) for treating malaria.
1785	**Digitalis** The use of digitalis to treat heart failure described by the British physician William Withering.
1796	**Smallpox vaccination** The first vaccination to be performed, by the British physician Edward Jenner. The first true vaccine (consisting of weakened microorganisms)—against chicken cholera—was developed in 1880 by the French scientist Louis Pasteur.
1805	**Morphine** Extracted from opium and used to relieve pain by the German pharmacist Friedrich Sertürner.
1899	**ASA** Developed as a drug by the German scientist Felix Hoffmann.
1911	**Salvarsan** Introduced by the German bacteriologist Paul Ehrlich to treat syphilis.
1922	**Insulin** Isolated from the dog pancreas in 1922 by Canadian researchers Banting and Best, who then showed that insulin was effective in treating human juvenile diabetes.
1928	**Penicillin** Antibacterial action first recognized by the British bacteriologist Alexander Fleming. It was produced as a drug in 1940, by the Australian-born British pathologist Howard Florey and the German-born British biochemist Ernst Chain.
1935	**Sulfonamides** Antibacterial action discovered by the German pharmacologist Gerhard Domagk.
1951	**Oral contraceptive** Developed by the American physicians Gregory Pincus and John Rock, and the Austrian-born American chemist Carl Djerassi.
1959	**Librium (chlordiazepoxide)** The first benzodiazepine minor tranquilizer, introduced by the Swiss pharmaceutical company Hoffmann-LaRoche.
1962	**Nethalide (pronethalol)** The first beta-blocking heart drug, developed by scientists at Imperial Chemical Industries, England.
1984	**Genetically engineered human insulin** Developed by scientists at Genentech, California.
1986	**Zidovudine (originally called AZT)** Introduced for treating AIDS after development by scientists at Burroughs Wellcome Research Laboratories, North Carolina.

sample of tissue for microscopic examination) of the large intestine may also be performed.

TREATMENT
In severe cases, impacted feces are removed manually. Often, however, the large intestine can be emptied by saline *enemas*.

Megalomania

An exaggerated sense of one's own importance or ability. Megalomania may take the form of a *delusion* of grandeur (such as believing oneself to be Napoleon) or of a desire to organize activities that are expensive, large in scale, and involve many people (for example, leasing an ocean liner for a party). Megalomania is not a formal category of psychiatric illness, although such bizarre ideas and behavior often occur in *mania*.

-megaly

A suffix meaning enlargement, as in *acromegaly*, a condition in which there is enlargement of the skull, jaw, hands, and feet during adulthood as a result of excessive production of growth hormone by the pituitary gland.

Megestrol

A *progestogen drug* used to treat certain types of *breast cancer* and uterine cancer (see *Uterus, cancer of*). Megestrol is usually prescribed when a tumor cannot be removed by surgery, if a tumor has recurred after surgery, or when other *anticancer drugs* or *radiation therapy* is ineffective.

Possible adverse effects include swollen ankles, loss of appetite, dizziness, headache, rash, and elevation of the blood calcium level.

Meibomian cyst

See *Chalazion*.

Meibomianitis

An inflammation of the glands on the eyelid, which causes the normal, oily secretion to thicken. Meibomianitis usually affects middle-aged people, often those with *blepharitis* (inflammation of the eyelid), and frequently leads to recurrent meibomian cysts (see *Chalazion*).

Meigs' syndrome

A rare condition in which *ascites* (fluid in the abdominal cavity) and a *pleural effusion* (fluid around one of the lungs) accompany a tumor of the *ovary*. The fluid usually disappears with removal of the tumor.

MECHANISM OF MEIOSIS

In meiosis, a cell in the testis or ovary containing 46 chromosomes divides to form four germ cells (sperm or eggs), each with 23 chromosomes. Germ cells have only half the usual chromosome content because a child can receive only half the genes of each parent.

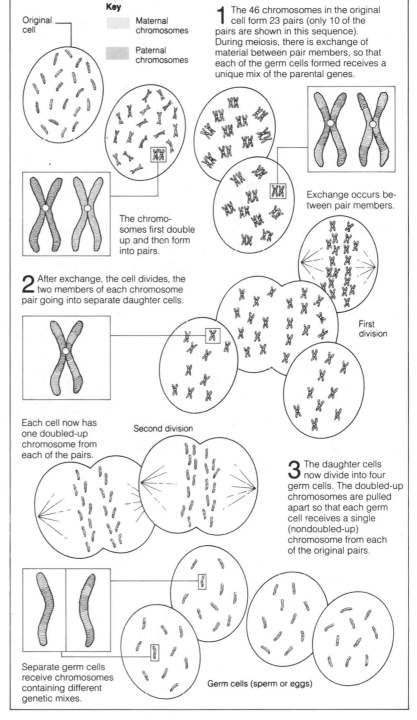

Key
Maternal chromosomes
Paternal chromosomes

Original cell

1 The 46 chromosomes in the original cell form 23 pairs (only 10 of the pairs are shown in this sequence). During meiosis, there is exchange of material between pair members, so that each of the germ cells formed receives a unique mix of the parental genes.

The chromosomes first double up and then form into pairs.

Exchange occurs between pair members.

2 After exchange, the cell divides, the two members of each chromosome pair going into separate daughter cells.

Each cell now has one doubled-up chromosome from each of the pairs.

First division

Second division

3 The daughter cells now divide into four germ cells. The doubled-up chromosomes are pulled apart so that each germ cell receives a single (nondoubled-up) chromosome from each of the original pairs.

Separate germ cells receive chromosomes containing different genetic mixes.

Germ cells (sperm or eggs)

M

Meiosis

A special type of cell division that occurs only within the ovaries and testes. The cells that undergo meiotic division are the forerunners of egg and sperm cells.

In meiosis, the *chromosomes* in the nucleus of a cell are first duplicated. In the course of two successive cell divisions, the chromosomal material is then divided into four parts, each part going into one of four daughter cells. The four daughter cells each acquire only half the original cell's chromosomal material, and each daughter cell acquires a different "selection" of this material. Consequently, every egg and sperm formed in the ovary or testis is different in its chromosomal content. As a result of meiosis, parents contribute exactly half of their chromosomal material (genes) to each child, and the selection that each child receives is unique.

Meiosis differs fundamentally from *mitosis*, the more common and simpler method of cell division, in which a cell's chromosomes are exactly duplicated into two daughter cells.

Melancholia

An old term for *depression*, derived from the Greek word for black bile, an excess of which was believed to be the cause of low spirits. The term melancholia is used today to refer to certain symptoms that occur in severe depression. These include loss of pleasure in most activities, lack of reaction to pleasurable stimuli, and inappropriate guilt feelings.

Melanin

The brown or black pigment that gives skin, hair, and the iris of the eyes their coloring. The amount of melanin present in a person depends on race and on exposure to sunlight. The pigment is produced by cells called melanocytes, whose activity is controlled by a hormone secreted by the *pituitary gland* in the brain.

Exposure to sunlight increases the production of melanin, which protects the skin against the harmful effects of ultraviolet rays and causes the skin to darken.

Localized overproduction of melanin in the skin can result in a pigmented spot, most commonly a *freckle* or mole (see *Nevus*).

Melanoma, juvenile

A raised, reddish-brown skin blemish which sometimes appears on the face or legs in early childhood. A juvenile melanoma is a form of *nevus* that grows rapidly up to about 2 cm across. Most juvenile melanomas are harmless. However, if the growth is unsightly, or if the physician suspects *skin cancer*, the melanoma can be removed surgically.

Melanoma, malignant

The most serious of the three types of skin cancer (the other two being *basal cell carcinoma* and *squamous cell carcinoma*). Malignant melanoma is a tumor of melanocytes, the cells that produce *melanin* (the pigment that colors the skin, hair, and the iris of the eyes).

CAUSES AND INCIDENCE

Malignant melanomas are most common in middle-aged and elderly people with pale skin who have been exposed to strong sunlight for many years. This type of skin cancer is more common in sunny countries such as Australia and the southern states of the US than in Canada. However, the incidence is rising here, probably because of the popularity of sunbathing. There are now about 1,700 new cases and more than 500 deaths from this cause in Canada each year.

SYMPTOMS AND SIGNS

The tumor usually develops on exposed skin, but may occur anywhere on the body, including under the nails and in the eye (see *Eye tumors*). The melanoma usually grows from an existing mole, which may enlarge, become lumpy, bleed, change color, develop a spreading black edge, turn into a scab, or begin to itch. Occasionally, a malignant melanoma may develop on normal skin.

DIAGNOSIS AND TREATMENT

Because the tumor is highly malignant and often spreads to other parts of the body, early diagnosis is essential. The diagnosis is made by a skin *biopsy* (re-

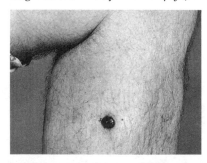

Development of malignant melanoma
Only one mole in a million becomes malignant, but change of shape, darkening, tenderness, pain, itching, and ulceration are warning signs.

moval of a small sample of tissue for microscopic analysis).

Treatment consists of surgical removal of the melanoma. To avoid an unsightly scar on exposed areas, a *skin graft* may be carried out at the same time. *Radiation therapy* or *anticancer drugs* may also be necessary.

Melanosis coli

Black or brown discoloration of the lining of the colon, associated with chronic constipation and the prolonged use of certain *laxative drugs*, such as senna, rhubarb, and cascara.

Melanosis coli is most common in the elderly and usually produces no symptoms. The discoloration disappears after the laxatives are stopped. Rarely, the condition is associated with cancer of the colon.

Melasma

See *Chloasma*.

Melatonin

A *hormone* secreted by the *pineal gland* that is thought to play a part in controlling daily body rhythms. Melatonin is currently under investigation for use in preventing *jet lag*.

Melena

Black, tarry *feces* caused by bleeding, usually in the upper gastrointestinal tract (esophagus, stomach, and duodenum). The blood is blackened by the action of secretions during digestion. Melena is a sign that should never be ignored: it is usually caused by a *peptic ulcer*, but may be an indication of cancer or another disorder of the upper gastrointestinal tract.

Iron, bismuth, or licorice may also cause blackening of the feces, which may be mistaken for melena.

Melphalan

An *anticancer drug* used mainly in the treatment of *multiple myeloma* (a cancer of the bone marrow). Melphalan is also prescribed to treat certain types of *breast cancer* and ovarian cancer (see *Ovary, cancer of*).

Possible adverse effects include nausea, vomiting, sore throat, and loss of appetite. Melphalan may also cause aplastic anemia, abnormal bleeding, and increased susceptibility to infection.

Membrane

A layer of tissue, often very thin, that covers or lines a body surface or forms a barrier. Examples include the *meninges*, which cover the surface of the brain and spinal cord; the *peritoneum*, which lines the abdominal cavity; the tympanic membrane (eardrum), which separates the *ear* canal from the middle ear; and the cell membrane, which forms the boundary of each individual *cell*.

Memory

The ability to remember. Memory is a complex process, usually thought of as having three stages—registration, storage, and recall (see box).

Many factors determine how well something is remembered, including its familiarity and how much attention has been paid to it. Techniques advertised for improving memory are generally based on teaching people methods of improving their coding systems by consciously associating new material with what is already known. For example, a person might be taught to visualize a well-known street and then think of each building as representing a new fact.

MECHANISM OF MEMORY
It is not known where in the *brain* the memory process takes place. There seems to be no set memory area; stimulating the brain with electrodes can

---

THE STAGES OF MEMORY

Stage 1
In the first stage, known as registration, information is perceived and understood. It is then retained in a short-term memory system that seems to be very limited in the amount of material it can store at one time. Unless refreshed by constant repetition, the contents of short-term memory are lost within minutes, to be replaced by other material.

Stage 2
If information is important enough, it may be transferred into the long-term memory, where the process of storage involves associations with words or meanings, with the visual imagery evoked by it, or with other experiences, such as smell or sound.

Stage 3
The final stage is recall (or retrieval), in which information stored at an unconscious level is brought, at will, into the conscious mind. The reliability of recall depends on how well the material was coded at stage 2.

---

evoke different memories from the same site. However, disturbances of the temporal lobe and limbic system typically cause memory disorders. Stimulation of a particular part of the temporal lobe in patients with *temporal lobe epilepsy* may consistently evoke the same memory.

The mechanisms for storing memory are also unknown. According to one theory, memory may be held in the chemical structure of some substance in brain cells—possibly spare *DNA* that is not being utilized to hold the genetic code. Other theories stress the role of the brain's electrical circuits in memory storage.

A good memory is usually part of a high IQ (see *Intelligence tests*), although some people have extraordinary "photographic" memories that are unrelated to their other intellectual abilities. Even some severely mentally handicapped people have phenomenal memories for specific types of information (the so-called "idiot savant"—learned idiot).

DISORDERS
Disturbances of memory can result from a problem at any of the three stages. Most disturbances are due to failure at the retention or recall stage (see *Amnesia*). In some cases, the problem occurs at the registration stage (e.g., in *mania*, because the person's attention is continually distracted, or in *depression*, because of preoccupation with personal thoughts). Some people with temporal lobe epilepsy have uncontrollable flashbacks of distant past events. The most common disorder of memory is the difficulty in recall that develops with age—so-called benign senile or senescent forgetfulness; this is entirely normal. A more severe loss of memory may be an early symptom of *dementia*.

Memory, loss of
See *Amnesia*.

Menarche
The onset of *menstruation*. Menarche usually occurs around age 13, two or three years after the first physical signs of *puberty* start to appear.

Meniere's disease
A disorder of the inner ear characterized by recurrent *vertigo*, *deafness*, and *tinnitus*. In 80 to 85 percent of cases, only one ear is affected.
CAUSES AND INCIDENCE
The disease is caused by an increase in the amount of fluid in the membranous labyrinth (the canals in the inner

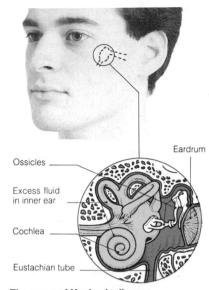

The cause of Meniere's disease
This condition is caused by excessive fluid in the labyrinth and cochlea, which may become damaged as a result.

ear that control balance). This increase damages the labyrinth and sometimes the adjacent cochlea (a spiral organ that receives sound and transmits it to the brain). The cause of the increase in fluid is not known in most cases. Meniere's disease is uncommon before the age of 50.
SYMPTOMS AND SIGNS
The main symptom is a sudden attack of vertigo, which may be so severe that the person falls to the ground. Vertigo is usually accompanied by nausea, vomiting, nystagmus (abnormal jerky eye movements), and, in the affected ear, deafness, tinnitus, and a feeling of pressure or pain. Attacks, which vary considerably in frequency, may last from a few minutes to several hours; deafness and tinnitus tend to persist between attacks.
DIAGNOSIS AND TREATMENT
Meniere's disease is usually diagnosed from the results of audiometry (see *Hearing tests*), a *caloric test*, and sometimes other tests.

During an attack, the person should rest in bed. An *antiemetic drug* (such as dimenhydrinate or cyclizine) may be given to relieve nausea and tinnitus.

Hearing tends to deteriorate progressively. If deafness becomes total, other symptoms usually disappear.

Meninges
The three membranes that cover and protect the *brain* and the *spinal cord*. The outermost layer, the dura mater,

M

is tough and fibrous; it lines the inside of the skull and forms a loose sheath around the spinal cord. The middle layer, the arachnoid mater, is elastic and weblike; it is separated from the innermost membrane, the pia mater, by the subarachnoid space, which contains *cerebrospinal fluid*. The pia mater is a thin layer that lies directly next to the brain and follows the folds and furrows of its surface.

Inflammation of the meninges, usually from infection, is called *meningitis*. Tumors of the meninges are called *meningiomas*.

Meningioma

A benign *brain tumor* that develops from the meninges (protective coverings of the brain). The tumor arises from cells in the arachnoid (middle layer of the meninges) and usually becomes attached to the dura mater (outer layer).

Meningiomas are rare, with about one new case diagnosed annually per 100,000 population. They may occur at any age. The tumor expands slowly, sometimes becoming large before it causes symptoms.

SYMPTOMS

Symptoms can include headache, vomiting, and impaired mental function from raised pressure within the skull; more specific symptoms include speech loss or visual disturbance due to pressure from the meningioma on underlying brain tissue. The tumor may invade the overlying bone, causing thickening and bulging of a region of the skull.

DIAGNOSIS AND TREATMENT

Meningiomas can be detected by skull *X ray*, *CT scanning*, and *MRI*. Because they are usually well demarcated from underlying brain tissue, meningiomas can often be completely removed by surgery. For tumors that cannot be removed surgically, treatment is by *radiation therapy*.

Meningitis

Inflammation of the *meninges* (the membranes that cover the brain and spinal cord) that usually results from infection by any of various microorganisms, usually a virus or a bacterium. Viral meningitis is relatively mild, but bacterial meningitis is life-threatening and requires prompt treatment.

CAUSES

The organisms that cause meningitis usually reach the meninges through the bloodstream from an infection elsewhere in the body. Less common

ANATOMY OF THE MENINGES
The pia mater lies on the brain, separated from the arachnoid mater by the subarachnoid space. The dura mater lines the inside of the skull.

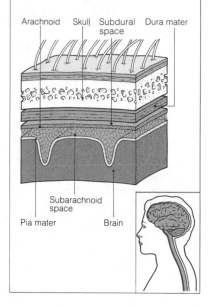

Arachnoid   Skull   Subdural   Dura mater
                     space

Subarachnoid space

Pia mater   Brain

means of transmission are through cavities in the skull from an infected ear or sinuses, or from the air following fracture of the skull.

INCIDENCE

Viral meningitis tends to occur in epidemics in the winter months. About 300 cases are reported annually in Canada, but the true incidence is probably much higher than this.

Meningococcal meningitis is the most common form of bacterial meningitis; it sometimes occurs in small epidemics, but more frequently it occurs in isolated cases. The disease affects about 300 people, mostly young children, each year in Canada. Tuberculous meningitis, which is a less common type of bacterial meningitis, is particularly prevalent among young children in parts of the world where there is a high incidence of *tuberculosis*.

SYMPTOMS

The main symptoms are fever, severe headache, nausea and vomiting, dislike of light, and a stiff neck. In viral meningitis the symptoms are mild and may resemble influenza.

In meningococcal meningitis the main symptoms develop relatively rapidly, sometimes over a few hours, and are followed by drowsiness and

sometimes loss of consciousness. In about half the cases there is also a red, blotchy skin rash.

In tuberculous meningitis, the sufferer may feel unwell for several weeks before the typical symptoms of meningitis develop.

Meningitis is diagnosed by *lumbar puncture* to remove a small sample of cerebrospinal fluid from the spinal cord for examination.

Viral meningitis requires no treatment. Bacterial meningitis is a medical emergency treated with large doses of intravenous *antibiotic drugs*.

OUTLOOK

Viral meningitis is usually not serious, clears up within a week or two, and leaves no aftereffects. Patients with bacterial meningitis who receive prompt treatment usually recover; in a few cases, however, some brain damage occurs.

PREVENTION

Vaccination may occasionally be valuable in controlling an epidemic caused by certain strains of bacteria. However, giving antibiotic drugs to people who have come into contact with sufferers is generally more effective. Vaccination against meningitis has achieved only limited success because vaccines exist against only some of the organisms responsible and the protection is of limited duration.

Meningocele

A protrusion of the meninges (protective coverings) of the spinal cord under the skin due to a congenital defect in the spine (see *Spina bifida*). Meningocele is less serious than myelocele, which is protrusion of the spinal cord and of the meninges.

Meningomyelocele

Another name for myelocele (see *Spina bifida*).

Meniscectomy

A surgical procedure in which the whole or part of a *meniscus* (cartilage disk) is removed from a joint, nearly always from the knee.

WHY IT IS DONE

Meniscectomy may be carried out when a meniscus has been damaged (usually due to injury), causing the knee to lock or give way repeatedly. Removing the damaged part of the meniscus cures these symptoms and reduces the likelihood of premature *osteoarthritis* in the joint.

HOW IT IS DONE

Arthroscopy (in which a viewing instrument is inserted into the joint

M

through a small incision) is performed to confirm that a damaged meniscus is the cause of the symptoms and to locate the area of damage. The damaged portion of the meniscus is then removed by means of instruments inserted through the arthroscope. The incision is closed with one stitch and a bandage applied.

Alternatively, the surgeon may need to open up the knee joint through an incision at the side of the patella (kneecap). After the operation, the wound is stitched and an elastic bandage and a plaster splint are applied over the knee.

RECOVERY PERIOD

After arthroscopic surgery, patients can usually go home later the same day and are able to walk normally within several days.

After an open operation, the patient stays in hospital for a few days. He or she is allowed to put weight on the affected leg after two or three days. The splint is removed after about a week, but normal activities cannot be resumed for four to six weeks.

After either type of meniscectomy, patients should do exercises that strengthen the thigh muscles, which help stabilize the knee.

OUTLOOK

The two types of meniscectomy are about equally effective in relieving symptoms and restoring the knee to normal function, although the scar after an open operation is larger. In either case, there may be an increased risk of osteoarthritis developing in later life, although the risk is less than if the damaged meniscus had been left in place.

Meniscus

A crescent-shaped disk of cartilaginous tissue found in several joints in the body. The *knee* joint has two menisci; the *wrist* joint and the *temporomandibular joints* of the jaw have one each. The main functions of the menisci, which are held in position by ligaments, are to reduce friction during joint movement and to increase joint stability.

Menopause

The cessation of *menstruation*; the term is commonly used to describe the time in a woman's life when physical and psychological changes occur as a result of reduced production of *estrogen hormones* by the ovaries.

The menopause usually occurs between the ages of 45 and 55. The follicles in the ovaries stop producing ova

(eggs) and less estrogen is produced. It is this reduced level of estrogen that causes the problems associated with the menopause. Other hormonal changes include increased amounts of *gonadotropin hormones* and *androgen hormones* in the blood.

SYMPTOMS AND SIGNS

Hot flashes and night sweats occur in about 70 percent of all menopausal women. These symptoms occur with varying frequency and severity. Women usually have flashes for between two and five years, but sometimes for longer; in about 25 percent of women flashes are so severe that medical help is sought.

Vaginal dryness is the major symptom of 20 percent of menopausal women. Dryness occurs because the vaginal skin thins and its secretions diminish with the fall in estrogen levels. The vagina itself shrinks, loses elasticity, and becomes prone to minor infections; sexual intercourse may be more difficult and painful due to dryness (see *Vaginitis*). The neck of the bladder and the urethra undergo similar changes, which can result in the "urethral syndrome," in which the woman feels the need to empty her bladder frequently.

Psychological symptoms are often attributed to the menopause, but it is not clear whether these symptoms are caused by the lack of estrogen or are a reaction to the physical symptoms and the sleep disturbance caused by

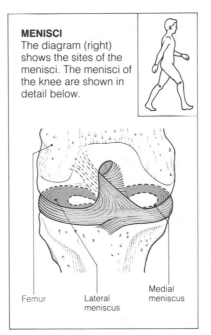

MENISCI
The diagram (right) shows the sites of the menisci. The menisci of the knee are shown in detail below.

Femur   Lateral   Medial
           meniscus   meniscus

night sweats. The most common symptoms are poor memory, poor concentration, tearfulness, anxiety, and loss of interest in sex.

Changes in *metabolism* (internal body chemistry) also occur during the menopause, but may not cause symptoms until later. The bones become thinner, especially in the first two to five years of the menopause; over a period of 10 to 15 years, *osteoporosis* (a decrease in density and increase in brittleness of the bones) may develop. Other metabolic effects of the menopause include increased levels of fats in the blood, which may result in an increase in *atherosclerosis* (narrowing of arteries by fatty deposits) and an increased incidence of *coronary artery disease* and *stroke*.

TREATMENT

If symptoms are severe, *hormone replacement therapy* is recommended to treat the physical and psychological symptoms and also to prevent menopause-related osteoporosis and heart disease. *Beta-blocker drugs* are sometimes given to women for whom hormone replacement therapy is unsuitable (for example, women who have been treated for breast cancer).

Menorrhagia

Excessive loss of blood during *menstruation*. The average amount of blood lost during a normal menstrual period is about 60 ml. A woman with menorrhagia may lose 90 ml or more. Some women regularly have menorrhagia, while others rarely or never suffer from it.

Menorrhagia may be caused by an imbalance of *estrogen hormones* and *progesterone hormone*, which control menstruation. This imbalance causes an excessive buildup of endometrium (lining of the uterus).

Any disorder that affects the uterus can cause menorrhagia, including *fibroids*, *polyps*, the presence of an *IUD*, or a pelvic infection. In some women with menorrhagia no physical cause can be found.

TREATMENT

Treatment depends on the severity of the bleeding, the age of the woman, whether or not she wants children in the future, and on any underlying disorder. A *D and C* (dilatation and curettage) may be performed to investigate the cause of menorrhagia. Hormones may be prescribed to reduce the amount of bleeding, especially if the woman is very young. If the condition is severe, a *hysterectomy* (removal of the uterus) may be considered.

M

A new technique for the treatment of menorrhagia is endometrial ablation, in which an *endoscope* is passed into the uterus and the endometrium is destroyed by *diathermy* or *laser*.

Menotropin

A *gonadotropin hormone* given as a drug to stimulate cell activity in the ovaries and testes. Menotropin is prepared from human menopausal gonadotropin, which is obtained from urine of postmenopausal women.

Menotropin is used together with human chorionic gonadotropin (see *Gonadotropin, human chorionic*) in the treatment of certain types of female and male *infertility*. Menotropin prepares the ovary for ovulation and may help stimulate sperm production.

In women, menotropin may cause multiple pregnancy, abdominal pain, bloating, and weight gain. In men, it may cause enlargement of the breasts.

Menstrual extraction

A procedure in which the endometrium (the lining of the uterus), which is ordinarily sloughed off during *menstruation*, is removed all at one time. The procedure is also known as menstrual regulation. Menstrual extraction is usually performed to terminate a possible pregnancy.

Menstrual extraction is carried out in the first two weeks after a missed period. It can be performed on an outpatient basis, with or without a local anesthetic. A plastic tube is inserted into the uterus and the contents, including any embryo if the woman is pregnant, are sucked out.

Menstruation

The periodic shedding of endometrium (lining of the uterus), accompanied by bleeding, that occurs in a woman who is not pregnant. Menstruation identifies the fertile years of a woman's life. Menstrual periods usually begin at puberty (typically between the ages of 11 and 16) and continue until the *menopause* (usually between the ages of 45 and 55).

MECHANISM

Menstruation is the end result of a complicated series of hormonal interactions. At the beginning of the menstrual cycle, *estrogen hormones* cause the endometrium to thicken to prepare the uterus for the possibility of *fertilization*; this is known as the proliferative or follicular phase.

Ovulation (egg release) usually occurs in the middle of the menstrual cycle and is accompanied by the increased production of *progesterone hormone*. The effect of this hormone is to cause the cells of the endometrium to become swollen and thick with retained fluid. These changes, which occur during the secretory (or luteal) phase of the menstrual cycle, enable a fertilized egg to implant in the endometrium. If pregnancy fails to occur, the production of estrogens and progesterone from the ovaries diminishes. The fluid-filled endometrium is not required and is shed about 14 days after the start of ovulation. Uterine contractions force the menstrual discharge to be expelled into the vagina.

Blood loss varies from cycle to cycle and from woman to woman, averaging 60 ml. The menstrual cycle, which is counted from the first day of bleeding to the last day before the next menstrual period, lasts between 24 and 35 days in 95 percent of women, the average being 28 days. The length of bleeding also varies—usually lasting from one to eight days, with the average length being five days.

Menstruation, disorders of

An abnormality in the monthly cycle of menstrual bleeding. Regular *menstruation* depends on the development of a healthy endometrium (lining of the uterus) and the regular cyclical production of *estrogen hormones* and *progesterone hormone*. This delicate balance is easily upset, making abnormal menstruation one of the most common disorders affecting women. A change in a woman's periods can indicate a problem in the pelvic area, such as *fibroids*, *endometriosis*, or *pelvic inflammatory disease*.

Dysmenorrhea (painful periods) is the most common disorder. In most women the cause is unknown.

Amenorrhea (absence of menstruation) is most frequently caused by pregnancy; it may also be caused by a hormonal imbalance, stress, starvation, and *anorexia nervosa*. Polymenorrhea (too frequent menstruation) occurs when the length of the menstrual cycle is reduced to less than 22 days. It is usually due to a hormone imbalance. Oligomenorrhea is the term used if the periods occur infrequently or if the blood loss is scanty.

Menorrhagia (excessive loss of blood) may be caused by a hormone

THE MENSTRUAL CYCLE

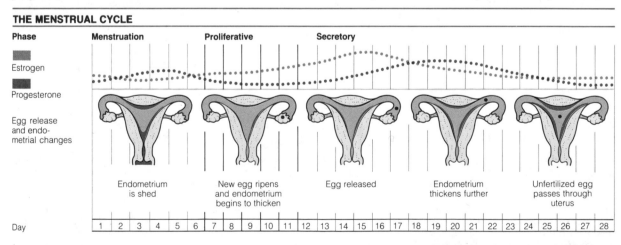

Phase	Menstruation	Proliferative	Secretory		

Estrogen

Progesterone

Egg release and endometrial changes

| Endometrium is shed | New egg ripens and endometrium begins to thicken | Egg released | Endometrium thickens further | Unfertilized egg passes through uterus |

Day | 1 | 2 | 3 | 4 | 5 | 6 | 7 | 8 | 9 | 10 | 11 | 12 | 13 | 14 | 15 | 16 | 17 | 18 | 19 | 20 | 21 | 22 | 23 | 24 | 25 | 26 | 27 | 28 |

During menstruation, estrogen and progesterone levels are low, and the unfertilized egg and endometrium are shed. Following menstruation, a pituitary hormone stimulates the ovaries to produce egg follicles. The follicles secrete estrogen, and one eventually releases an egg. The empty follicle also produces progesterone, which, with estrogen, prepares the endometrium to receive the egg. If the egg is unfertilized, follicle hormone levels fall and a new menstrual cycle begins.

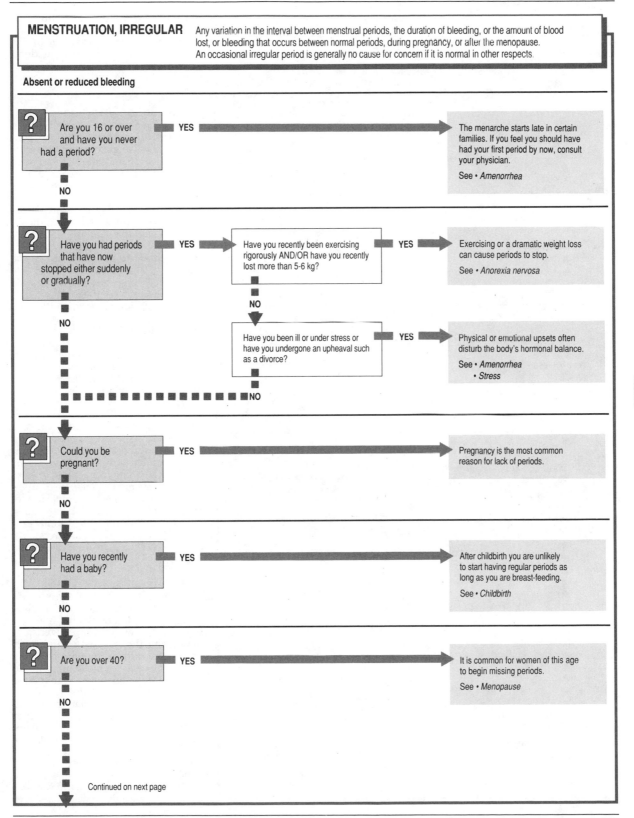

MENSTRUATION, IRREGULAR

Any variation in the interval between menstrual periods, the duration of bleeding, or the amount of blood lost, or bleeding that occurs between normal periods, during pregnancy, or after the menopause. An occasional irregular period is generally no cause for concern if it is normal in other respects.

Absent or reduced bleeding

? Are you 16 or over and have you never had a period?

YES → The menarche starts late in certain families. If you feel you should have had your first period by now, consult your physician.

See • *Amenorrhea*

NO ↓

? Have you had periods that have now stopped either suddenly or gradually?

YES → Have you recently been exercising rigorously AND/OR have you recently lost more than 5-6 kg?

YES → Exercising or a dramatic weight loss can cause periods to stop.

See • *Anorexia nervosa*

NO ↓

Have you been ill or under stress or have you undergone an upheaval such as a divorce?

YES → Physical or emotional upsets often disturb the body's hormonal balance.

See • *Amenorrhea*
• *Stress*

NO

NO ↓

? Could you be pregnant?

YES → Pregnancy is the most common reason for lack of periods.

NO ↓

? Have you recently had a baby?

YES → After childbirth you are unlikely to start having regular periods as long as you are breast-feeding.

See • *Childbirth*

NO ↓

? Are you over 40?

YES → It is common for women of this age to begin missing periods.

See • *Menopause*

NO ↓

Continued on next page

M

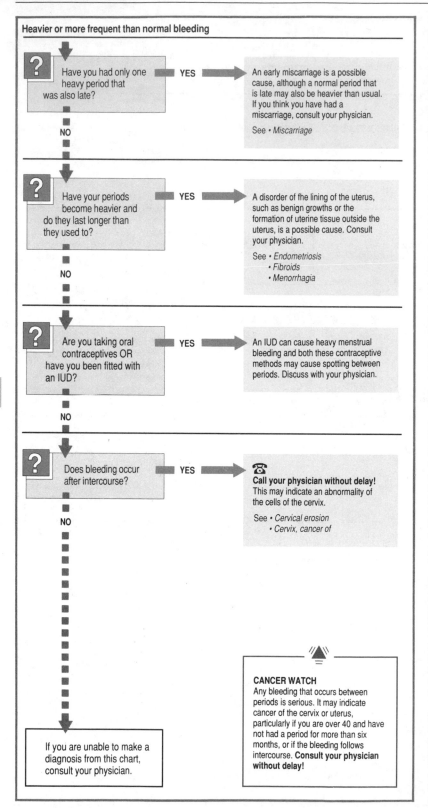

Heavier or more frequent than normal bleeding

? Have you had only one heavy period that was also late? — **YES** → An early miscarriage is a possible cause, although a normal period that is late may also be heavier than usual. If you think you have had a miscarriage, consult your physician.

See • *Miscarriage*

NO ↓

? Have your periods become heavier and do they last longer than they used to? — **YES** → A disorder of the lining of the uterus, such as benign growths or the formation of uterine tissue outside the uterus, is a possible cause. Consult your physician.

See • *Endometriosis*
• *Fibroids*
• *Menorrhagia*

NO ↓

? Are you taking oral contraceptives OR have you been fitted with an IUD? — **YES** → An IUD can cause heavy menstrual bleeding and both these contraceptive methods may cause spotting between periods. Discuss with your physician.

NO ↓

? Does bleeding occur after intercourse? — **YES** → ☎ **Call your physician without delay!** This may indicate an abnormality of the cells of the cervix.

See • *Cervical erosion*
• *Cervix, cancer of*

NO ↓

If you are unable to make a diagnosis from this chart, consult your physician.

CANCER WATCH
Any bleeding that occurs between periods is serious. It may indicate cancer of the cervix or uterus, particularly if you are over 40 and have not had a period for more than six months, or if the bleeding follows intercourse. **Consult your physician without delay!**

---

imbalance, the presence of an *IUD*, *fibroids*, or *polyps*. In some women there are extreme variations in the interval between periods, the duration of bleeding, and the amount of blood lost each month (see *Menstruation, irregular*).

Menstruation, irregular
A variation from the normal pattern of *menstruation*. Menstruation is considered to be irregular if there are wide variations in the interval between periods, in the duration of bleeding, or in the amount of blood lost.

CAUSES
Disturbance of a woman's menstrual pattern can be caused by stress, travel, or changing the method of contraception. A common cause of irregular menstruation is a disturbance of the balance of *estrogen hormones* and *progesterone hormone*, which regulate the menstrual cycle. For the first few years after menstruation starts, and for the few years before the *menopause*, cycles are often irregular and ovulation may not occur. In some cases, irregularity is due to unsuspected pregnancy or early miscarriage. Disorders of the uterus, ovaries, or pelvic cavity can also cause irregularity. (See also *Vaginal bleeding*.)

Mental Health Act
Each province or territory has a Mental Health Act that describes the conditions under which a person can be detained without consent in a psychiatric hospital. The legislation includes definitions of mental competence and procedures for determining if a person is dangerous. Some provinces have rights advisers for patients who are involuntarily detained.

Mental illness
A general term that describes any form of psychiatric disorder. Mental illness is commonly divided into two broad categories: the more severe *psychoses*, and the less disturbing *neuroses*. Whereas the former are probably caused by complex biochemical brain disease, the latter seem more related to upbringing and personality.

The concept of mental illness is also important, for legal reasons, in determining whether a person can be compulsorily admitted to hospital (see *Mental Health Act*). Mental illness is different from personality disorder, which is often characterized by antisocial behavior, or mental handicap, but can coexist with these disorders.

M

Mental retardation

Impaired intellectual function that results in an inability to cope with the normal tasks of life. The term mental handicap is sometimes preferred.

CLASSIFICATION

To be classified as mentally retarded, a person usually has an IQ below 70 (see *Intelligence tests*), will have a history of *developmental delay* in childhood, and will have been slow to acquire normal living skills. Within this group (which comprises about 2 percent of the general population) there are various degrees of severity of mental retardation, resulting in different levels of disability.

CAUSES

The more severe grades of retardation usually have a specific physical cause; their incidence is the same in all social classes. About a quarter are due to *Down's syndrome*, another quarter to other inherited or congenital conditions (such as *phenylketonuria*), and about one third result from trauma or infection around birth or early childhood. In about 15 percent of cases the cause is unknown, but the recently discovered *fragile X syndrome* may account for some of them.

By contrast, mild mental retardation usually has no specific cause, occurs more commonly in the lower social classes, and seems to run in families. Poverty and malnutrition are probably contributing factors, together with inheritance.

SYMPTOMS

The mildly retarded usually show no obvious psychological symptoms apart from slowness in carrying out mental tasks such as arithmetic or problem solving. Reading is variably impaired.

In more severely retarded people, speech is limited or absent, and *epilepsy* and other abnormalities of the nervous system are common. Fecal and urinary incontinence and self-injury may also occur.

TREATMENT

There is no specific means of eliminating the intellectual deficit, but special training and behavior modification can enhance the skills and quality of life of the mentally retarded. Many mentally retarded people are cared for in the community rather than in institutions. Family support and counseling can be crucial in preserving a stable home for a retarded person.

Anticonvulsant drugs may be needed to treat epilepsy, and *antipsychotic drugs* to treat certain types of mental illness.

The incidence of retardation should be reduced in future by prevention. Preventive measures include *genetic counseling*, the elimination of infections such as *rubella*, reducing the intake of alcohol and drugs during pregnancy, and the early identification of fetal abnormalities.

OUTLOOK

There is evidence that mentally retarded people, even those who are severely impaired, can live rewarding and emotionally stable lives. Handicap is caused not by an absolute limit on achievement, but by delay in acquiring skills; as they grow older, mentally retarded people often show improvement in personal and social function.

Menthol

An alcohol prepared from mint oils. Menthol is an ingredient of several over-the-counter inhalation preparations used in the treatment of nasal congestion caused by sinusitis and the common cold.

Meperidine

A synthetic narcotic *analgesic drug* (painkiller) similar to, but less powerful than, *morphine*. Meperidine, which is used almost exclusively in hospitals, is given as a *premedication* (a drug used to relax and sedate a person before an operation). It is also used to relieve severe pain after a major operation, during childbirth, and, occasionally, in terminal illness.

Since meperidine may cause nausea and vomiting, it is usually given with an *antiemetic drug* to control these symptoms. Used for long periods, meperidine may cause constipation.

ABUSE

Meperidine may cause euphoria and is abused for this effect. Taken regularly, it is likely to cause psychological and physical dependence (see *Drug dependence*).

Meprobamate

An *antianxiety drug* used in the treatment of *anxiety* and *stress*. Meprobamate, which also has a muscle-relaxant effect, is combined with *ASA* to relieve the pain caused by rheumatic disorders (such as *osteoarthritis*) or injury to soft tissues (such as muscles and ligaments).

Because meprobamate has a sedative effect, it may cause drowsiness and dizziness. After long-term use, its sudden discontinuation may cause a severe withdrawal reaction, symptoms of which may include seizures.

Mercaptopurine

An *anticancer drug* used to prevent the recurrence of certain types of *leukemia*, and prescribed with other anticancer drugs for leukemia victims who have not responded well to other treatment. Possible adverse effects of mercaptopurine include nausea, vomiting, mouth ulcers, and appetite loss. Rarely, it may cause liver damage, anemia, and abnormal bleeding.

Mercury

The only metallic element that is liquid at room temperature. Mercury is used in *thermometers*, *sphygmomanometers* (instruments for measuring blood pressure), and dental *amalgam*. Various compounds of mercury are used in some paints, pesticides, cosmetics, medicines, and in certain industrial processes.

Mercury poisoning

Toxic effects of mercury on the body. Some forms of mercury are absorbed into the body more readily than others and are therefore more dangerous.

If liquid mercury is swallowed, absorption via the intestines is only slight. Swallowing a small amount (e.g., from a broken thermometer) is therefore unlikely to lead to poisoning. However, liquid mercury is highly volatile and gives off a vapor that is readily absorbed into the body via the lungs. Inhalation of mercury vapor—usually as a result of industrial exposure—is the most common cause of poisoning. Mercury compounds, which are not highly volatile, may cause poisoning by absorption through the skin or intestines.

SYMPTOMS AND SIGNS

Initial symptoms of mercury poisoning depend on the part of the body affected. Mercury compounds that come into contact with the skin may cause severe inflammation. A swallowed mercury compound can cause nausea, vomiting, diarrhea, and abdominal pain.

After mercury has entered the body, it passes into the bloodstream and later accumulates in various organs, principally the brain and kidneys. Mercury deposits in the brain cause a wide range of symptoms, including tiredness, incoordination, excitability, tremors, numbness in the limbs, and, in severe cases, impairment of vision and very rarely *dementia*. Deposits of mercury in the kidneys may lead to *kidney failure*. Without treatment, severe mercury poisoning may be fatal.

M

TREATMENT

Mercury poisoning may be treated by giving *chelating agents* (such as penicillamine) to help the body excrete it at a faster rate. In some cases, purification of the blood by hemodialysis (see *Dialysis*) may also be performed, especially if the kidneys have been damaged. Inducing vomiting or pumping out the stomach is helpful only if mercury has been swallowed within the preceding few hours.

Mesalamine

A drug used to treat *ulcerative colitis* in patients who are unable to tolerate *sulfasalazine*. Possible adverse effects include nausea, diarrhea, abdominal pain, and headache.

Mescaline

A drug obtained from the Mexican peyote (or peyotl) cactus and classified as a psychedelic or *hallucinogenic drug*. The dried tops of the cactus, known as peyote buttons, have been used for centuries by Mexican and North American Indians in religious ceremonies. In modern times, mescaline has been used to study the mechanism of *psychosis*, because the drug induces temporary psychotic symptoms.

EFFECTS

The effects, which generally last for four to eight hours, are similar to those of *LSD* and psilocybin. Effects include illusions, changes in thought and mood, a sense of being in contact with the unknown, intense self-absorption, and an altered sense of time. Although the "trip" is most often pleasant and seemingly insightful, frightening ideas or experiences leading to panic and injury may occur. True psychosis, persisting after the drug has worn off, and addictive craving may occur.

Mesenteric lymphadenitis

An acute abdominal disorder in which *lymph nodes* in the *mesentery* (a membrane that anchors organs to the abdominal wall) become inflamed. Mesenteric lymphadenitis mainly affects children. Its cause is unknown but it may be related to some type of viral infection.

The main symptoms are pain and tenderness in the lower right abdomen, such as occur in appendicitis. There may be mild fever, and sometimes the condition is preceded by a sore throat, chest infection, or swollen lymph nodes in the neck.

The disorder usually clears up rapidly. *Analgesic drugs* (painkillers) may be given to reduce pain and fever. If the sufferer is no better after a few hours or if the symptoms worsen dramatically, a *laparotomy* (surgical opening of the abdominal cavity) may be carried out to rule out the possibility of appendicitis.

Mesentery

A membrane that attaches various organs to the abdominal wall. The term is used particularly to refer to the membranous fold that encloses the small intestine, attaching it to the back of the abdominal wall. The mesentery contains the arteries, veins, nerves, and lymphatic vessels that supply the large and small intestines.

Mesothelioma

A malignant tumor of the *pleura* (the membrane that lines the chest cavity and covers the lungs). There is an increased incidence of mesothelioma in people exposed to asbestos dust (see *Asbestos-induced diseases*).

Mesothelioma may cause no symptoms in some cases, whereas in others it may cause cough, chest pain, and breathing difficulty, especially if a *pleural effusion* develops.

A chest X ray may show abnormal shadowing; the diagnosis can be confirmed by examination of a sample of fluid from any effusion or by pleural *biopsy* (removal of a sample of tissue for microscopic examination).

Surgical removal of a small tumor may result in a complete cure. Usually, however, the tumor is diagnosed only after it has spread over a large area of the pleura. In such cases, there is no effective treatment, although *radiation therapy* may help to alleviate symptoms.

Mesothelium

A type of *epithelium* (surface cell layer) that covers the *peritoneum* (the membrane that lines the abdominal wall and covers the abdominal organs), the *pleura* (the membrane that lines the chest cavity and covers the lungs), and the *pericardium* (the saclike covering of the heart).

Mestranol

An *estrogen drug* used in some *oral contraceptives*.

Metabolic disorders

A group of disorders in which some aspect of the body's internal chemistry is disturbed.

Some metabolic disorders result from inherited abnormalities in which a specific *enzyme* (a substance that promotes a metabolic reaction) is absent or deficient or malfunctions in some way (see *Metabolism, inborn errors of*).

Other metabolic disorders result from disorders of the *endocrine system* in which there is underproduction or overproduction of a hormone that controls metabolic activity. Examples include *diabetes mellitus*, *Cushing's syndrome*, *insulinoma*, *hypothyroidism* (underactivity of the thyroid gland), and *hyperthyroidism* (overactivity of the thyroid gland).

Other examples of metabolic disorders are *porphyria*, *hyperlipidemia*, *hypercalcemia*, *gout*, and metabolic bone diseases (see *Osteodystrophy*), such as *osteoporosis, osteomalacia, rickets*, and *Paget's disease*.

Metabolism

A collective term for all the chemical processes that take place in the body. Metabolism is divided into catabolism and anabolism.

In a catabolic process, a complex substance is broken down into simpler ones, usually with the release of energy. An example is the "burning" of glucose in body cells to produce energy and the by-products carbon dioxide and water. In an anabolic process, a complex substance is built up from simpler ones, usually with the consumption of energy. The synthesis of complex *proteins* from *amino acids* is an anabolic process.

METABOLIC RATE

The basal metabolic rate (BMR) is the energy required to keep the body functioning at rest (that is, to maintain breathing, heartbeat, body temperature, and other basic body functions). It is measured in joules per square metre of body surface per hour.

A person's metabolic rate increases in response to factors such as exertion, stress, fear, and illness. It is controlled principally by various hormones (such as *epinephrine, norepinephrine, insulin, corticosteroid hormones*, and *thyroid hormones*), which influence the rate at which chemical processes are carried out in body cells. (See also *Metabolic disorders; Metabolism, inborn errors of*.)

Metabolism, inborn errors of

Inherited defects of body chemistry. Inborn errors of metabolism are *genetic disorders* in which the disturbance of body chemistry is caused by a single gene defect.

M

TYPES AND INCIDENCE

There are about 180 known inborn errors of metabolism, which vary in severity from harmless abnormalities to serious disorders that may cause death in a newborn baby or result in severe physical or mental handicap. Examples include *Tay-Sachs disease*, *phenylketonuria*, *galactosemia*, the *porphyrias*, *Hurler's syndrome* and various other types of *mucopolysaccharidosis*, Lesch-Nyhan syndrome, homocystinuria, hereditary fructose intolerance, glycogen storage diseases, mucolipidoses, and sphingolipidoses.

Individual disorders are rare. Most affect only one child in every 10,000 to 100,000, but the precise incidence is often unknown because sufferers may have only vague symptoms that are never investigated, or because they die before any characteristic features appear. Collectively, inborn errors of metabolism affect approximately one child in 1,000.

CAUSES

All inborn errors of metabolism are caused by abnormal functioning of a specific *enzyme* (protein that stimulates a chemical reaction) caused by a defect of a single *gene*. Most defects show an autosomal recessive pattern of inheritance (see *Genetic disorders*).

Individual disorders vary in their effects. In some cases the abnormal enzyme is nonfunctional; in others there is some residual activity.

SYMPTOMS AND SIGNS

Symptoms are usually present at or soon after birth, although in some cases they may not appear until later in childhood. Symptoms may include unexplained illness or failure to thrive in a newborn, developmental delay, floppiness, drowsiness, persistent vomiting, or seizures. Signs may include enlarged body organs, bone deformities, anemia, cataracts, persistent jaundice, unusual body odor, the recurrent development of kidney stones, or a rash brought on by sunlight. An affected child may be intolerant to specific foods.

Miscarriages, stillbirths, or deaths in early infancy suggest the possibility of an error of metabolism.

DIAGNOSIS

Investigations include tests to measure the levels of various substances in the affected child's blood, including *liver function tests* and *kidney function tests*. Chemical analysis of a *biopsy* specimen (a small piece of tissue removed from the body) may be performed to check the level and function of a specific enzyme.

Early diagnosis can be important in preventing serious complications. Routine tests are performed on the newborn for some of the more common disorders, such as phenylketonuria. Additional screening may be performed for disorders that are more common in certain countries or racial groups (e.g., Tay-Sachs disease in Ashkenazi Jews).

Certain disorders can now be diagnosed prenatally following *chorionic villus sampling* or *amniocentesis*, allowing the possibility of abortion if medically indicated.

TREATMENT

Some inborn errors of metabolism do not require treatment. Some respond to avoidance of a specific environmental factor to which an affected person is abnormally sensitive. For example, avoiding exposure to sunlight may help certain types of porphyria; avoiding food containing phenylalanine, the natural constituent in most protein-containing foods, is vital for victims of phenylketonuria.

In some cases, a vitamin supplement can help to compensate for defective enzyme function. In others, injections of the properly functioning form of the enzyme are given. Transplanting enzyme-producing cells from a donor has been effective in some cases (such as to treat Hurler's syndrome). Research is being undertaken into treating inborn errors of metabolism at the gene level, but such treatment is at present only a remote and theoretical possibility.

People with an affected close relative or child may benefit from *genetic counseling* before starting a family or planning another pregnancy.

Metabolite

Any substance that takes part in a metabolic reaction (a biochemical reaction in the body). In the breakdown of glucose to produce energy, the metabolites are glucose, oxygen, carbon dioxide, and water. The term metabolite is sometimes used to refer only to the products of a metabolic reaction. (See also *Metabolism*.)

Metacarpal bone

One of five long, cylindrical bones within the body of the hand. The bones run from the base of each digit to the wrist. On the palm of the hand, the metacarpals are covered by a thick layer of fascia (fibrous connective tissue); on the back of the hand, the metacarpals can be seen and felt through the skin. The heads of the

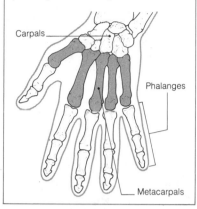

LOCATION OF METACARPAL BONES
The five metacarpals lie between the carpal (wrist) bones and the phalanges of the fingers.

Carpals

Phalanges

Metacarpals

metacarpal bones form the knuckles, standing out prominently when the hand is clenched. Fracture of the metacarpal bones is fairly common, usually as the result of a fall on the hand or a blow to the knuckles.

Metaplasia

A change in tissue resulting from the transformation of one type of cell into another. Usually harmless, but occasionally precancerous, metaplasia can affect the lining of various organs, such as the bronchi (airways) and bladder. Metaplasia of the cervix, which occurs in *cervical erosion*, can be detected by a *cervical smear test*.

Metaproterenol

See *Orciprenaline*.

Metastasis

A secondary malignant tumor (one that has spread from a primary *cancer* to affect other parts of the body); for example, a metastasis in the liver may arise as a result of the spread of a cancer originating in the colon. The term metastasis also applies to the process by which such spread occurs. The degree of malignancy of a tumor depends largely on its ability to invade surrounding normal tissue and on its ability to send metastases to other parts of the body.

Metastases can spread from one part of the body to another through the lymphatic system, in the bloodstream, or across a body cavity (such as that between the inner and outer layer of the peritoneal membrane in the abdomen).

M

Metatarsal bone

One of five long, cylindrical bones within the foot. The bones make up the central skeleton of the foot and are held in an arch by surrounding ligaments. Fracture of the metatarsal bones may be caused by a heavy object falling on the foot, by a twisting injury in which the foot turns over on its outside edge, or by prolonged walking or running on a hard surface (see *March fracture*).

Metatarsalgia

Pain in the foot. Causes include a fracture of one of the *metatarsal bones*, *flatfeet*, or a *neuroma* (benign tumor) of one of the nerves in the foot.

Metatarsophalangeal joint

The joint between each *metatarsal bone* and its adjoining toe bone (see *Phalanges*). The metatarsophalangeal joint at the base of the big toe is commonly affected by *gout* and by *hallux rigidus* (immobility due to *osteoarthritis*). *Hallux valgus* is a deformity of the big toe that may result in a *bunion*.

Metformin

An oral hypoglycemic drug used in the treatment of non-insulin-dependent *diabetes mellitus*. Metformin lowers the blood sugar level by reducing the production of glucose by cells in the liver and by increasing the sensitivity of cells to *insulin* so that they take up glucose more efficiently from the blood.

Metformin is usually prescribed in addition to another hypoglycemic drug when that preparation alone has failed to control the diabetes. Possible adverse effects include loss of appetite, a metallic taste in the mouth, nausea, vomiting, and diarrhea.

Methadone

A synthetic narcotic *analgesic drug* (painkiller) that resembles *morphine*. Methadone causes only mild symptoms when it is withdrawn and is therefore used to relieve withdrawal symptoms in people undergoing a supervised heroin or morphine detoxification program.

Possible adverse effects include nausea, vomiting, constipation, dizziness, and dryness of the mouth.

Methane

A colorless, odorless, highly flammable gas that occurs naturally in the gas from oil wells and in coal mines, where it is an explosion hazard. Methane is produced by the decompo-

LOCATION OF METATARSAL BONES

The five metatarsals lie between the tarsal bones (which form the ankle and back of the foot) and the phalanges of the toes.

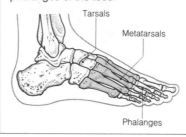

Tarsals

Metatarsals

Phalanges

sition of organic matter; it is one of the gases present in intestinal gas (see *Flatus*). By itself methane is not poisonous, in contrast to "coal gas" (which contains carbon monoxide). Cases of gas poisoning are, therefore, much less common than previously. Large quantities of methane may cause death simply by displacing oxygen in the air breathed.

Methanol

A poisonous type of *alcohol* used as a solvent or paint remover, and as an ingredient in some types of antifreeze. Also known as wood alcohol or methyl alcohol, methanol may cause blindness or death if drunk.

POISONING

Methanol poisoning usually occurs as a result of substituting it for ordinary alcohol (ethanol or ethyl alcohol), although its inebriating effect is weaker.

Symptoms, which develop 12 to 24 hours after drinking the methanol, include headache, dizziness, nausea, vomiting, and unconsciousness. The symptoms are caused by the breakdown in the liver of methanol into formaldehyde and formic acid. These substances may also damage the retina and the optic nerve, causing blurred vision. If drunk repeatedly, or after a single large dose, methanol may cause permanent blindness.

TREATMENT

If somebody has drunk methanol and is conscious, vomiting should be induced and medical help obtained. Treatment may include pumping out the stomach (see *Lavage, gastric*) and inducing vomiting, although these methods are effective only within about two hours of having drunk the methanol (before it has been absorbed into the bloodstream). In addition,

ethanol may be given by injection into the bloodstream because it slows the rate at which the liver breaks down the methanol. An *intravenous infusion* of sodium bicarbonate may be used to neutralize acid products in the blood. Occasionally, purification of the blood by *dialysis* is also necessary.

Methimazole

An antithyroid drug used in treating *hyperthyroidism*. Methimazole has a slow onset and long duration of action; rash and itching are fairly common side effects. (See *Thyroid hormones*.)

Methocarbamol

A *muscle-relaxant drug* used to relieve stiffness caused by muscle injury and back pain. Methocarbamol is sometimes given to treat the symptoms of *tetanus* (lockjaw). During prolonged treatment, methocarbamol may cause drowsiness, dizziness, and, in rare cases, liver damage.

Methotrexate

An *anticancer drug* used in the treatment of *lymphoma* (cancer of the lymph nodes) and certain forms of *leukemia*. Methotrexate is also used to treat some cancers of the uterus, breast, ovary, lung, bladder, and testis. It is sometimes used to treat severe *psoriasis* when other treatments have proved ineffective.

Methotrexate may cause nausea, vomiting, diarrhea, and mouth ulcers. It may also cause anemia, increased susceptibility to infection, and abnormal bleeding.

Methotrimeprazine

A *phenothiazine* drug used to treat the aggressive behavior, confusion, and hallucinations of patients with schizophrenia or dementia. Methotrimeprazine may also be used as an *analgesic*. It often produces drowsiness and drug-induced *Parkinsonism*.

Methoxsalen

A treatment for *psoriasis*. Used in conjunction with ultraviolet light, methoxsalen stimulates the growth of skin cells and the production of pigment. It has been used in some countries to promote sun tanning, but this use is prohibited in Canada because of the risk of burns. Anyone taking methoxsalen should take precautions to limit exposure to sunlight.

Methyclothiazide

A thiazide *diuretic drug*.

M

Methyl alcohol

Another name for *methanol*, a poisonous type of alcohol.

Methylcellulose

A bulk-forming *laxative drug* commonly used to treat *constipation, diverticular disease*, and *irritable bowel syndrome*. Methylcellulose is also used to increase the firmness of feces in chronic watery *diarrhea* and to regulate their consistency in people who have had a *colostomy* or *ileostomy*.

Methylcellulose preparations are also sometimes used together with appropriate dieting to treat *obesity*. The bulking agent swells to give a feeling of fullness, thus encouraging adherence to a slimming diet.

In eye drop form, methylcellulose is given to relieve dryness of the eyes caused by exposure to the sun, wind, and other irritants.

POSSIBLE ADVERSE EFFECTS

Methylcellulose may cause bloating, flatulence, and abdominal pain, or even bowel obstruction if sufficient amounts of fluids are not taken.

Methyldopa

An *antihypertensive drug* used in the treatment of *hypertension* (high blood pressure), usually in conjunction with other drugs from this group. Methyldopa is one of the few antihypertensive drugs that are known to be safe to take during pregnancy.

Possible adverse effects of methyldopa include drowsiness, depression, and nasal congestion.

Methylprednisolone

A *corticosteroid drug* used in the treatment of severe *asthma*, skin inflammation, *inflammatory bowel disease*, and types of arthritis, including *rheumatoid arthritis*. Possible adverse effects are typical of drugs belonging to the corticosteroid drug group.

Methysergide

A drug used to prevent *migraine* and cluster *headaches* (recurrent severe headaches). Methysergide is usually given only under hospital supervision when other treatments have been ineffective, and the headaches are seriously disrupting normal life.

Long-term treatment with methysergide may cause abnormal tissue growth in the lungs, around the ureters, or around blood vessels (resulting in chest pain, kidney failure, or leg cramps). Other possible adverse effects include dizziness, drowsiness, nausea, and diarrhea.

Metoclopramide

An *antiemetic drug* used to prevent and treat nausea and vomiting. Metoclopramide is helpful for the relief of the nausea that sometimes accompanies *migraine* headaches. It is also prescribed to relieve *acid reflux* and to treat nausea and vomiting caused by *anticancer drugs, radiation therapy*, or anesthetic drugs (see *Anesthesia, general*).

Metoclopramide is often given with a *premedication* (drug used to relax and sedate a person before an operation) to encourage normal propulsion of food through the stomach, thereby reducing the risk of inhaling vomit when under an anesthetic.

HOW IT WORKS

Metoclopramide reduces nerve activity in the part of the brain that stimulates vomiting. It also increases the speed with which fluid and food pass from the stomach.

POSSIBLE ADVERSE EFFECTS

Adverse effects of metoclopramide can include dryness of the mouth, sedation, or diarrhea. Large doses of this drug may cause uncontrollable movements of the face, mouth, and tongue.

Metolazone

A *diuretic drug* used to treat *hypertension* (high blood pressure). Metolazone is also given to reduce *edema* (fluid retention) in people with *heart failure* (reduced pumping efficiency), kidney disorders, *cirrhosis* of the liver, or *premenstrual syndrome*.

Metolazone is also a useful treatment for certain types of kidney stones (see *Calculus, urinary tract*) because it reduces the amount of calcium excreted in the urine.

ADVERSE EFFECTS

Possible adverse effects include weakness, lethargy, and dizziness caused by an increase in the amount of potassium excreted in the urine.

Metoprolol

A cardioselective *beta-blocker drug* used in the treatment of *angina pectoris* (chest pain due to impaired blood supply to heart muscle) and *hypertension* (high blood pressure). Metoprolol is also prescribed to relieve symptoms of *hyperthyroidism* (overactivity of the thyroid gland). It is occasionally given following a *myocardial infarction* (heart attack) to reduce the risk of further damage to the heart.

Possible adverse effects of metoprolol include lethargy, cold hands and feet, nightmares, and rash.

Metronidazole

ANTIBACTERIAL	ANTIPROTOZOAL

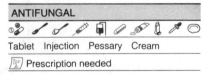

Tablet Syrup Injection Suppository

Prescription needed

An *antibiotic drug* that is particularly effective against infections caused by *anaerobic* bacteria (those that do not depend on oxygen), such as a dental *abscess* and *peritonitis* (inflammation of the membrane that lines the abdominal wall and covers abdominal organs). Metronidazole is also used to treat infections caused by *protozoa*, such as *trichomoniasis, amebiasis*, and *giardiasis*.

POSSIBLE ADVERSE EFFECTS

Adverse effects include nausea and vomiting, loss of appetite, abdominal pain, and dark-colored urine. Drinking alcohol during treatment with metronidazole often causes severe unpleasant effects, such as nausea and vomiting, abdominal pain, hot flashes, palpitations, and headache.

Mexiletine

An *antiarrhythmic drug* that is used to treat certain heart-rhythm disorders, usually after a *myocardial infarction* (heart attack). Possible adverse effects include nausea, vomiting, dizziness, and tremor.

Miconazole

ANTIFUNGAL

Tablet Injection Pessary Cream

Prescription needed

An *antifungal drug* used to treat *tinea* skin infections, such as ringworm and *athlete's foot*, vaginal *candidiasis* (thrush), and rare fungal infections.

Miconazole in the form of a cream or vaginal suppository may, in rare cases, cause a burning sensation or a rash. Injections of miconazole may cause nausea, vomiting, and fever.

Micro-

A prefix meaning small, as in microorganisms.

Microangiopathy

Any disease or disorder of the small blood vessels. Microangiopathy may be a feature of various conditions, including *diabetes mellitus*; some kidney diseases, such as *glomerulonephritis* (inflammation of the kidneys'

M

filtering units) or *hemolytic-uremic syndrome* (premature destruction of red blood cells accompanied by kidney damage); *eclampsia* (a disorder characterized by seizures in late pregnancy); *septicemia* (blood poisoning); and advanced *cancer*. When microangiopathy accompanies these conditions, the small blood vessels become distorted, resulting in red blood cells becoming damaged or destroyed. This, in turn, leads to a particular type of anemia that is called microangiopathic hemolytic anemia (see *Anemia, hemolytic*).

Another cause of microangiopathy is thrombotic thrombocytopenic *purpura*, a rare, often fatal disease that mainly affects young adults. In this condition, the small blood vessels in many organs throughout the body become blocked and the vessel walls are damaged; hemolytic anemia, fever, and a patchy, purplish rash known as purpura develop.

Microbe

A popular term for a *microorganism*, especially one that is pathogenic (causes disease).

Microbiology

The study of *microorganisms*, particularly those that are pathogenic (disease causing).

Microbiology began in the 17th century with the discovery by the Dutch microscopist Antonj van Leeuwenhoek (1632-1723) of a wide variety of organisms too small to be seen by the naked eye. However, relatively little progress was made until the 19th century when, largely due to the pioneering work of scientists such as Louis Pasteur (1822-1895) and Robert Koch (1843-1910), it was recognized that microorganisms cause many infectious diseases and are also responsible for processes such as fermentation and decay.

Microbiology continued to progress with the discovery of viruses, the development of *vaccines* and *antibiotic drugs* against many diseases, and studies of the chemical processes that are fundamental to all living cells. Recently, microbiologists have played an important role in the study of genetics by pioneering techniques of *genetic engineering*.

In hospitals, microbiologists help identify the infectious organisms responsible for a patient's illness; they also advise the attending clinicians on the sensitivity of these organisms to different drugs.

Microcephaly

An abnormally small head, usually associated with *mental retardation*. Microcephaly may occur if the brain is damaged before birth by, for example, congenital *rubella* (German measles) or if the mother is exposed to X rays in early pregnancy. Microcephaly may also result from brain damage during birth, or from injury or disease in early infancy.

Microorganism

A tiny, single-celled living organism. Most microorganisms are too small to be seen by the naked eye. In medicine, the most important microorganisms are those that are pathogenic (disease causing), even though this group constitutes a relatively small minority of the vast number of microorganisms known to exist.

The principal pathogenic microorganisms are *bacteria*, which cause a large number of disorders, including certain types of pneumonia, typhoid, diphtheria, and some types of food poisoning; *viruses* (usually classified as microorganisms although they are not true cells), which cause numerous infections, including AIDS, the common cold, influenza, and measles; *protozoa*, which are the causative agents of various diseases, including malaria, giardiasis, and amebic dysentery; *fungi*, which cause disorders such as ringworm and thrush; *rickettsiae*, which cause typhus, Rocky Mountain spotted fever, and Q fever; and chlamydiae, which cause various genital, eye, and respiratory infections (see *Chlamydial infections*).

Microscope

An instrument for producing a magnified image of a small object. There are many types of microscopes, ranging from simple, single-lens instruments (magnifying glasses) to compound microscopes and high-powered electron microscopes.

HISTORY

The single-lens microscope may date from as early as the 15th century, but the first truly powerful lenses were probably made by Antonj van Leeuwenhoek (1632-1723). His single-lens microscopes were capable of magnifying up to about 300 times. With them, he discovered microorganisms, thereby founding the science of *microbiology* and providing the basis for the development of the germ theory of disease. Probably the greatest of the early microscopists, however, was the Italian Marcello Malpighi (1628-1694), who is generally regarded as the founder of *histology*.

The compound microscope, which has two lens systems, was developed toward the end of the 16th century. However, the single-lens microscope continued to be widely used until the 19th century, when improvements in optical design and glass technology made the compound microscope a practicable instrument.

Light microscopes continued to be refined, with the development of the phase-contrast microscope, for example. However, the next major advances were instruments that used electrons instead of light—the transmission electron microscope (TEM), invented in the early 1930s, and the scanning electron microscope (SEM), invented in the mid-1960s.

LIGHT MICROSCOPES

Compound microscopes are the most widely used microscopes. They have two lens systems—the objective and the eyepiece—which are mounted at opposite ends of a tube called the body tube (see box facing page). There is also a stage to hold the specimen, a light source, and an optical condenser. The maximum practicable magnification of an ordinary light microscope is limited by the wavelength of light to about 1,500 times.

ELECTRON MICROSCOPES

TEMs are similar to light microscopes, except that they use a beam of electrons instead of light, and electromagnetic "lenses" instead of glass ones. Furthermore, because electrons are invisible, the image must be formed on a fluorescent screen or photographic film. Electron microscopes allow much higher magnifications than light microscopes. Modern TEMs can magnify up to about 5 million times, enabling tiny viruses and large molecules (such as DNA) to be seen.

The SEM works in a different way. SEMs have a lower maximum magnification (approximately 100,000 times) than do TEMs. However, unlike TEMs, SEMs produce three-dimensional images. This makes SEMs particularly valuable for studying the surface structures of cells and tissues.

OTHER MICROSCOPES

Phase-contrast and interference microscopes are types of light microscopes with modified illumination and optical systems that make it possible for unstained transparent specimens to be clearly seen. These microscopes are particularly useful for examining living cells and tissues.

Another instrument, the fluorescence microscope, is used to study the chemical composition of cells. In fluorescence microscopy, a specimen that has been selectively stained with fluorescent dyes is illuminated with ultraviolet light, which makes the stained parts glow.

Operating microscopes are low-powered compound microscopes with several modifications. They do not have a stage, and the illumination system is arranged to shine light down onto the living tissues rather than up through the specimen.

USES

The microscope is probably the single most important instrument in biological and medical science. Its applications are vast, ranging from the study of molecular structures to *microsurgery*. Microscopes have enabled scientists to examine both the structure and chemical composition of cells (a study known as *cytology*) and of tissues (histology). Microscopes are also used to investigate diseased tissues (a study known as *histopathology*), thereby playing an important role in diagnosis. And in the operating room, microscopes have enabled the development of microsurgery for a wide range of intricate procedures.

TYPES OF MICROSCOPES

Microscopes are indispensable in medicine. For many purposes, the light microscope, with a magnification of up to 1,500 times, is sufficient. Modern research increasingly requires the much higher magnifications (up to about 5 million times) of a transmission electron microscope or a scanning electron microscope.

LIGHT MICROSCOPE

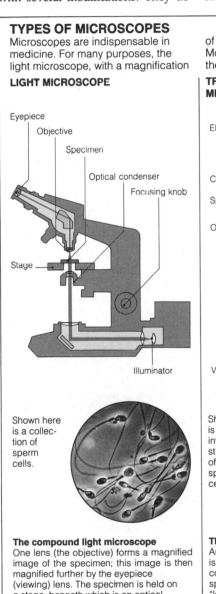

TRANSMISSION ELECTRON MICROSCOPE

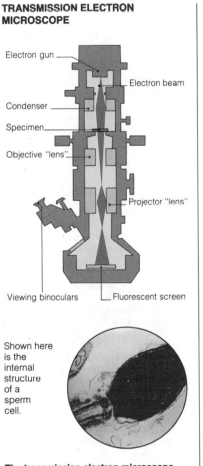

SCANNING ELECTRON MICROSCOPE

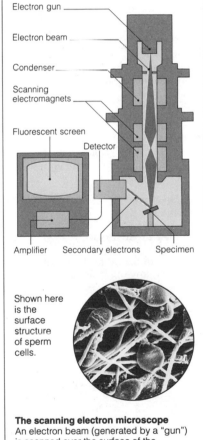

Shown here is a collection of sperm cells.

Shown here is the internal structure of a sperm cell.

Shown here is the surface structure of sperm cells.

The compound light microscope
One lens (the objective) forms a magnified image of the specimen; this image is then magnified further by the eyepiece (viewing) lens. The specimen is held on a stage, beneath which is an optical condenser that concentrates light (usually from a built-in illuminator) onto the specimen. Focusing is carried out by altering the distance between the objective and the specimen.

The transmission electron microscope
An electron beam (generated by a "gun") is concentrated by an electromagnetic condenser, then passes through the specimen. An electromagnetic objective "lens" then produces a magnified "image" of the specimen; this image is further magnified by an electromagnetic projector "lens," which also focuses the image onto a fluorescent screen, where it can be viewed through special binoculars.

The scanning electron microscope
An electron beam (generated by a "gun") is scanned over the surface of the specimen, causing the emission of a beam of secondary electrons, the intensity of which varies according to the surface features of the specimen. A detector converts the secondary electrons into an electric current, which is then amplified and used to control an electron beam that forms an image on a fluorescent screen.

M

Microsurgery

Delicate surgery in which the surgeon views the operation site through a special binocular *microscope* with pedal-operated magnification, focusing, and movements.

Microsurgery technique is used for surgery involving minute, delicate, or not easily accessible tissues. It has strikingly improved the success rate of some operations and made others possible that were previously impracticable. These operations include removing a diseased cataract from the eye and implanting a new lens (see *Cataract surgery*); transplanting a new cornea into the eye (see *Corneal graft*); replacing a diseased stapes (stirrup bone) in the middle ear to treat deafness caused by otosclerosis (see *Stapedectomy*); restoring a severed limb by rejoining disconnected blood vessels and nerves; transplanting toes to replace missing or severed fingers; and unblocking and rejoining obstructed fallopian tubes in the treatment of female *infertility*. (See also illustrated box facing page.)

Micturition

A term for passing *urine*.

Midbrain

The top part of the *brain stem,* situated above the pons. The midbrain is also called the mesencephalon.

Middle ear

See *Ear.*

Middle ear effusion, persistent

Fluid accumulation in the middle ear cavity that impairs hearing. (See *Glue ear.*)

Middle ear infection

See *Otitis media.*

Mid-life crisis

A popular phrase that describes the feelings of distress that affect some people in early middle age (35 to 45 years) after realizing that they are no longer young. The term is used most often to describe men who strive to recapture their sense of youthfulness by having extramarital affairs, suddenly changing jobs, or adopting youthful fashions. Sometimes anxiety or depression, brought on by fears of declining powers and death, can lead to psychiatric illness. Counseling and support are usually effective in helping people to come to terms with the changes of age.

Midwifery

The profession concerned with the assistance of women in *pregnancy* and *childbirth*. A midwife provides care and information throughout pregnancy, supervises labor and delivery, and cares for both mother and baby after the birth.

At present, only Quebec gives conditional recognition to midwives as a specialized branch of nursing. There is a strong movement in other provinces to follow suit.

Migraine

A severe headache, lasting anything from two hours to two days, accompanied by disturbances of vision and/or nausea and vomiting. A sufferer may experience only a single attack; more commonly, he or she has recurrent attacks at varying intervals.

CAUSES AND INCIDENCE

Migraine occurs in at least 10 percent of the population and is three times more common in women than in men. It may affect children as young as 3 years old; 60 percent of migraine sufferers have their first attack before the age of 20. It is extremely rare for migraine to appear for the first time after the age of 50.

There is no single cause of migraine. It tends to run in families, although the exact mechanism of inheritance is not understood. A number of factors, singly or in combination, may bring on an attack in a susceptible person. These factors may be stress-related (such as anger, worry, excitement, depression, shock, overexertion, changes of routine, and changes of climate), food-related (particularly chocolate, cheese and other dairy products, red wine, fried food, and citrus fruits), or sensory-related (such as bright light or loud noises). Menstruation and the contraceptive pill may also trigger migraine.

TYPES

There are two types of migraine: common and classical. In common migraine, the pain of the headache develops slowly, sometimes mounting to a throbbing pain that is made worse by the slightest movement or noise. The pain is often, but not always, on only one side of the head and usually occurs with nausea and sometimes vomiting. Many sufferers, particularly children, recover after they have vomited.

Classical migraine is comparatively rare. The headache is preceded by a slowly expanding area of blindness surrounded by a sparkling edge that increases to involve up to one half of the field of vision of each eye. The blindness clears up after about 20 minutes and is often followed by a severe one-sided headache with nausea, vomiting, and sensitivity to light. Other temporary neurological symptoms, such as weakness in one half of the body, may occur.

DIAGNOSIS

Special tests are rarely necessary. The physician can usually make a diagnosis from the patient's history and a physical examination. If there are accompanying persistent symptoms (such as tingling in a limb) or if the type of headache changes or becomes more severe, a full neurological examination may be carried out to exclude the possibility of a serious condition.

TREATMENT

If migraine attacks occur less frequently than once a month, treatment of the acute attack is all that is required. If the attacks are more frequent, preventive treatment may be necessary. The simplest form of prevention is to avoid known trigger factors; keeping a careful diary can help a sufferer pinpoint what triggers his or her own attacks.

The best treatment for an acute migraine attack is *ASA* or *acetaminophen* plus an *antiemetic drug* (often provided in suppository form). If this combination is not effective, *ergotamine* may also be prescribed. Certain ergotamine preparations may help prevent an attack if taken in the early phases before the headache begins. Most people find that they recover more quickly if they can then sleep in a darkened room.

In cases where migraine attacks occur more frequently than once a month, prophylactic drugs (for example, *beta-blocker drugs* and *calcium channel blockers*) may be prescribed.

Milia

Tiny, hard, white spots that most commonly occur in clusters on the upper cheeks and around the eyes of young adults. The cause is usually unknown although they may sometimes follow injury or blistering. They are painless and harmless.

Miliaria

Another name for *prickly heat*.

Milk

A *nutrient* fluid produced by the mammary gland of mammals. Human milk differs considerably from cow's milk in the proportions of its ingredients. It

TECHNIQUES OF MICROSURGERY

Microsurgery started with ophthalmic surgeons, whose demands for more delicate operating instruments led to the adoption of the operating microscope. The results were so favorable that surgeons working in other specialties began to use the technique for intricate operations.

The operating microscope
This surgeon is performing microsurgery with the aid of an operating microscope. The photograph (below) shows a blood vessel as seen through the microscope.

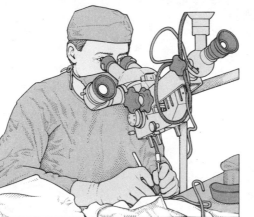

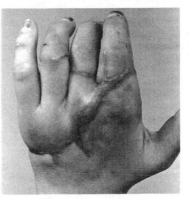

Replantation microsurgery
A major application of microsurgery is the replantation of severed fingers, toes, hands, feet, or even entire limbs. This is successful only if the severed blood vessels and nerves are accurately rejoined so that regeneration occurs.

MAIN AREAS OF OPERATION
Microsurgery is most commonly employed in ophthalmic, vascular, neurological, gynecological, urological, and otological surgical procedures, in which delicate structures are involved.

Ophthalmology
By using microsurgery, even operations on the delicate retina of the eye are now possible.

Otology
Microsurgery is routinely used for operations on the tiny bones in the middle ear.

Gynecology
With microsurgery, blockages of the fallopian tubes can often be corrected, restoring fertility.

Urology
A vasectomy (male sterilization) can sometimes be reversed by using microsurgery to rejoin the cut ends of the vas deferens.

INSTRUMENTS

Scissors   Forceps   1 cm

Clamp

Microsurgery is possible only by using extremely delicate operating instruments, such as the fine scissors, forceps, and clamp shown above (their sizes can be judged from the scale bar).

M

---

contains about the same amount of fat, but twice as much lactose (milk sugar) and half as much protein.

Virtually all babies can digest milk, but some lose the enzyme that breaks lactose down to simpler sugars (see *Lactase deficiency*). Milk allergy occurs in some infants, caused by a *food allergy* or intolerance to the proteins in the milk of cows and other animals. (See also *Breast-feeding; Feeding, infant*.)

Milk-alkali syndrome
A rare type of *hypercalcemia* (abnormally high level of calcium in the blood) accompanied by *alkalosis* (reduced acidity of the blood) and *kidney failure*. Milk-alkali syndrome is caused by excessive, long-term intake of calcium-containing *antacid drugs* and milk. It is most common in people with the symptoms of a *peptic ulcer* and associated kidney disorders.

Symptoms include weakness, muscle pains, irritability, and apathy. Treatment is to reduce the intake of milk and antacids.

Milk of magnesia
A magnesium preparation used as an *antacid drug* and *laxative drug*.

Milk teeth
See *Primary teeth*.

Minamata disease

The name given to a severe form of *mercury poisoning* that occurred in the mid-1950s in people who had eaten fish from Minamata Bay, Japan. The fish contained large amounts of mercury as a result of the water being polluted with industrial mercury waste. By the time the cause of the condition was identified and controlled, many people had suffered severe nerve damage and some had died.

Mineralization, dental

The deposition of calcium crystals and other mineral salts in developing teeth. (See *Calcification, dental*.)

Mineralocorticoid

The term used to describe a corticosteroid hormone (one produced by the cortex of the *adrenal glands*) that controls the amount of salts, including potassium and sodium, excreted in the urine. Some corticosteroid hormones (such as *aldosterone*) have only a mineralocorticoid action, whereas others (such as *hydrocortisone*) also have a glucocorticoid effect (that is, they help to regulate the body's use of carbohydrates).

The drug fludrocortisone is used if the adrenal glands produce insufficient amounts of mineralocorticoids.

Mineral oil

Mineral oil or liquid petrolatum is a lubricant derived from petroleum. It is used as a *laxative* and in some skin preparations.

Minerals

Defined in *nutrition* as chemical elements that must be present in the diet for the maintenance of health. At least 20 minerals are essential to health. Important among them are potassium, sodium, calcium, magnesium, and phosphorus. Others, such as iron, zinc, and copper, are needed in only tiny amounts (see *Trace elements*). A balanced diet usually contains all the minerals the body requires. (See also accompanying tables showing the main food sources and recommended nutrient intakes per day.)

Mineral supplements

Dietary supplements containing one or more *minerals* in tablet or liquid form. Most people obtain adequate amounts of minerals from the diet, and additional amounts do not have any beneficial effects. Taken in excess, some mineral supplements may have harmful effects.

RECOMMENDED NUTRIENT INTAKES (RNIs) EXPRESSED AS DAILY RATES

Age	Calcium (mg)	Phosphorus (mg)	Magnesium (mg)	Iron (mg)	Iodine (mcg)	Zinc (mg)
0–4 months	250[a]	150	20	0.3[b]	30	2[b]
5–12 months	400	200	32	7	40	3
1 year	500	300	40	6	55	4
2–3 years	550	350	50	6	65	4
4–6 years	600	400	65	8	85	5
7–9 years	M 700 F 700	500 500	100 100	8 8	110 95	7 7
10–12 years	M 900 F 1100	700 800	130 135	8 8	125 110	9 9
13–15 years	M 1100 F 1000	900 850	185 180	10 13	160 160	12 9
16–18 years	M 900 F 700	1000 850	230 200	10 12	160 160	12 9
19–24 years	M 800 F 700	1000 850	240 200	9 13	160 160	12 9
25–49 years	M 800 F 700	1000 850	250 200	9 13	160 160	12 9
50–74 years	M 800 F 800	1000 850	250 210	9 8	160 160	12 9
75+ years	M 800 F 800	1000 850	230 210	9 8	160 160	12 9
Pregnancy (extra) 1st Trimester	500	200	15	0	25	6
2nd Trimester	500	200	45	5	25	6
3rd Trimester	500	200	45	10	25	6
Lactation (extra)	500	200	65	0	50	6

[a] Infant formula with high phosphorus should contain 375 mg calcium.
[b] Breast milk is assumed to be the source of the mineral.

Mineral requirements
The table (above) gives the daily recommended nutrient intakes (RNIs) of minerals for which amounts have been established; when different, the RNIs for males and females are denoted by M and F.

Units
mg = milligrams (thousandths of a gram)

mcg = micrograms (millionths of a gram)

MEDICAL USES
The most commonly used mineral supplement is *iron*, which is used to treat iron-deficiency *anemia* and is sometimes needed by women who are pregnant or breast-feeding. *Iodine* is sometimes added to salt and bread in areas where there is a risk of iodine deficiency. *Calcium* supplements are sometimes provided during pregnancy and to young children.

Other types of mineral deficiency are rare among Canadians, with the possible exception of *magnesium* deficiency, which may result from alcohol dependence, kidney disease, or prolonged treatment with *diuretic drugs* or *digitalis drugs*.

Mineral supplements are sometimes needed by people suffering from an intestinal disorder that impairs the absorption of certain minerals from the diet. (See also individual mineral entries.)

MINERALS AND MAIN FOOD SOURCES

Mineral	Sources
Calcium	Soya bean products, milk, cheese, canned salmon, green vegetables, legumes
Copper	Shellfish, legumes, liver
Fluorine	Fluoridated water
Iodine	Iodized table salt, milk, dulse
Iron	Liver, lean meats, green, leafy vegetables, whole-grain cereals and breads
Magnesium	Dairy products, green, leafy vegetables, whole-grain cereals and breads, nuts
Phosphorus	Milk, meat, fish
Potassium	Widely distributed in all food
Selenium	Seafood, kidney, liver, meat
Sodium	Table salt, processed foods, widely distributed in all foods
Zinc	Oysters, liver, beef, lamb, pork

Minilaparotomy
See *Sterilization, female.*

Minimal brain dysfunction
An explanation postulated by some North American psychologists for a variety of behavioral and other problems occurring in young children for which a physical cause might be expected but for which none is found.

Minimal brain dysfunction may be a cause of difficulty in concentrating, impulsiveness, and *hyperactivity.*

Minocycline
A tetracycline *antibiotic drug* used in low doses to treat *acne*, and occasionally used to treat infections of the respiratory or urinary tracts. It may also be used to treat pneumonia and to prevent meningococcal *meningitis.*

Minoxidil
A *vasodilator drug* used to treat severe *hypertension* (high blood pressure) when other drugs have been ineffec-

tive. Prolonged treatment may cause the ankles to swell and often stimulates hair growth, especially on the face. Minoxidil in the form of a lotion has recently been introduced as a treatment for male-pattern baldness but resulting hair growth is highly variable. (See *Alopecia.*)

Miosis
Constriction (reduction in size) of the pupil of the *eye.* Miosis may be caused by certain drugs (such as pilocarpine or opium), by a disease affecting the *autonomic nervous system* (such as *Horner's syndrome*), or simply by bright light. A degree of miosis is normal in older people.

Miscarriage
Loss of the fetus before the 28th week of pregnancy or before viability (the ability to survive outside the uterus without artificial support). The medical term for miscarriage is spontaneous abortion.

INCIDENCE
The incidence of miscarriage is difficult to determine, since not all women who miscarry seek medical attention or even realize they are miscarrying. It is estimated that between 10 and 30 percent of all pregnancies end in miscarriage, with the majority occurring in the first 10 weeks.

CAUSES
A wide range of problems can cause miscarriage. Many miscarriages occur because of abnormalities of the fetus itself, such as *chromosomal abnormalities* or major developmental defects. Severe maternal illness or exposure to toxins may also cause miscarriage. Less common maternal causes include abnormalities such as inadequate progesterone secretion or an *autoimmune disorder.*

After the first three months, miscarriage is less common. Of the 3 to 5 percent of pregnancies that miscarry between 12 and 22 weeks, problems include *genetic disorders, cervical incompetence* (inability of the cervix to hold the fetus), a defect such as a septate (subdivided) uterus, and large uterine *fibroids.* Severe maternal infection can also trigger a late miscarriage.

The symptoms of miscarriage are cramping and/or bleeding. Light bleeding during the early months of pregnancy occurs in up to half of all pregnancies and is often caused by low placental implantation or *cervical erosion.* Many of these pregnancies continue uneventfully to term.

Heavy bleeding with cramping is generally more serious because it may signal impending miscarriage. Spotting and severe pain can be a symptom of either a threatened miscarriage or an *ectopic pregnancy* (a pregnancy that develops outside the uterus). A gush of clear or pinkish fluid may be caused by rupture of the amniotic sac and is a serious sign.

TYPES
Miscarriages are classified medically as different types of abortion.

THREATENED ABORTION The fetus remains alive and has not been expelled from the uterus, despite bleeding from the woman's vagina.

INEVITABLE ABORTION The fetus has died and is being expelled from the uterus. An inevitable abortion may be complete (in which case all the uterine contents are expelled) or incomplete (in which case the fetus and/or placenta are not completely expelled).

MISSED ABORTION The fetus has died but is retained with the placenta in the uterus.

M

M

DIAGNOSIS AND TREATMENT

In early pregnancy a woman in whom bleeding and cramping develop is often prescribed bed rest to minimize bleeding (although bed rest probably does not influence the outcome). *Ultrasound scanning* may be recommended to determine that the pregnancy is intrauterine (i.e., not ectopic) and that it appears to be progressing normally. A pelvic examination may be performed to find out if the size of the uterus feels appropriate and to see if the cervix is open or closed.

If a miscarriage is incomplete and bleeding is heavy, a *D and C* (scraping out of the uterus) may be required. If the miscarriage seems complete (i.e., all fetal and placental material has been expelled from the uterus), no further treatment may be needed. Missed abortion requires a D and C or *induction of labor* depending on the duration of the pregnancy. Often, women are given antibiotics and other drugs to minimize bleeding. Rh-negative women are given anti-D(Rh$_o$) immune globulin to prevent Rh complications in any future pregnancies (see *Rh incompatibility*).

After the first trimester, any cramping or spotting merits immediate medical attention; at this stage a significant number of possible miscarriages are caused by treatable problems, such as an incompetent cervix, rather than by severe fetal defects.

If there is evidence of an incompetent cervix, the cervix may be stitched shut and the suture left in position until the pregnancy is at or near full term. Prolonged bed rest may be recommended and uterine relaxants may be administered to women with uterine or cervical abnormalities.

A woman who miscarries three or more times consecutively is called a habitual aborter. Habitual abortion may be caused by genetic or hormonal abnormalities, chronic infection, an autoimmune disease, or abnormalities of the uterus. Evaluation usually includes genetic studies, tests for hormonal problems and infections, and *hysterosalpingography* (X rays of the uterus and fallopian tubes).

OUTLOOK

The majority of women who miscarry can eventually carry a pregnancy to term. Current diagnostic and treatment measures have made the outlook better than ever before. (See also *Abortion.*)

Misoprostol

See *Prostaglandin drugs.*

Mites and disease

Mites are small (less than 1.2 mm long), eight-legged animals that resemble tiny spiders. Many species have piercing and blood-sucking mouthparts and may parasitize animals and humans.

Mites can cause problems in a variety of ways. One species, the *scabies* mite, lives solely in human skin, where its burrowing causes an intense itch. Another, the house-dust mite, is common in bedding; inhaling dust containing dead mite parts and feces can cause *asthma*.

Various other types of mites inhabit grassy areas or affect crops. Chiggers (American harvest mites) can be picked up when walking through thick grass. Their bites can produce an itchy rash. Mites in grain or fruit may cause skin irritations, commonly known as grocers' itch or bakers' itch.

Certain mites transmit diseases, particularly scrub *typhus* and rickettsialpox. Both of these diseases are caused by *rickettsiae* (organisms that are intermediate between bacteria and viruses), which normally infect rodents, but which can be transmitted to humans by mites.

The use of insect repellents (such as dimethyl phthalate) is advisable when walking through mite-infested areas.

Mitosis

The way in which most cells divide, so that the *chromosomes* (inherited genetic material) within the nucleus of the original cell are exactly duplicated into two daughter cells.

Each person begins as a single cell (a fertilized egg) and, following successive mitotic divisions of this cell, is born as a multicellular being with trillions of cells, most of which contain exactly the same chromosomal material. Mitotic divisions occur in the body thousands of times every second as dead cells are replaced by new ones formed by the division and multiplication of other cells.

Mitosis can be observed in a cell culture under a microscope. The sequence of events as the original cell divides to form two daughter cells is shown on the facing page.

A minority of cells (in the ovaries and testes) undergoes a fundamentally different type of division that results in the daughter cells receiving only half of the original cell's chromosomal material. This process, called *meiosis*, occurs in the formation of egg and sperm cells.

Mitral insufficiency

Failure of the mitral valve of the *heart* to close properly, which allows blood to leak back into the left atrium (upper chamber) when pumped out of the left ventricle (lower chamber). Also known as mitral incompetence or mitral regurgitation, the disorder may occur in conjunction with *mitral stenosis* (narrowing of the valve).

In mitral insufficiency the left side of the heart must work harder to clear the regurgitated blood. Eventually, left-sided (and later, right-sided) *heart failure* may develop; generally, however, this is not a life-threatening condition. A buildup of blood from the left side of the heart can result in *pulmonary edema*.

CAUSES AND INCIDENCE

The most common cause (though much less common than it once was) is damage to the valve as a result of *rheumatic fever*. Other causes include *mitral valve prolapse* (floppy valve syndrome), damage following a *myocardial infarction* (heart attack), and stretching of the valve due to enlargement of the ventricle in left-sided heart failure. Rarely, the disorder may be present from birth or occurs as part of *Marfan's syndrome*.

SYMPTOMS AND SIGNS

The characteristic symptoms are increasing breathlessness and fatigue, sometimes accompanied by *palpitations*. Later, as right-sided heart failure develops, the ankles swell.

An occasional complication of mitral insufficiency is *endocarditis* affecting the valve. Another risk is that a thrombus (blood clot) may form in the left atrium and travel to the brain, resulting in a *stroke*.

DIAGNOSIS

The physician makes a diagnosis from the patient's history, from a characteristic heart *murmur* heard through a stethoscope, and from the results of chest *X rays*, *ECG*, and *echocardiography*. Cardiac *catheterization* is performed in some cases.

TREATMENT AND OUTLOOK

If breathlessness is troublesome, a *diuretic drug* may be prescribed to reduce fluid in the lungs and other tissues. *Digitalis drugs* may be given to increase the force of the heart's contraction and to control rhythm disturbances. *Anticoagulant drugs* may be given to prevent the formation of blood clots. Before undergoing dental or other surgery, a person with mitral valve disease should take *antibiotic drugs* to prevent a blood infection that could cause endocarditis.

Heart valve surgery is considered only if severe heart failure develops or if drug treatment fails to prevent the patient's symptoms from becoming severe and disabling.

The outlook for mitral insufficiency is good whether it is treated by drugs or by surgery. Breathlessness and fatigue cannot be relieved by treatment once there has been permanent heart damage.

Mitral stenosis

Narrowing of the orifice of the mitral valve in the *heart*. This causes the atrial portion of the left side of the heart to work harder to force blood through the narrowed valve. The consequences are similar to those of *mitral insufficiency* (failure of the valve to close properly), which may accompany stenosis.

CAUSES AND INCIDENCE

Mitral stenosis is almost always due to scarring of the valve from an earlier attack of *rheumatic fever*, although in about half the cases there is no medical record of the illness. Mitral stenosis is four times more common in women than in men.

SYMPTOMS AND SIGNS

Symptoms do not usually develop until adulthood, many years after rheumatic fever. The primary symptom is shortness of breath, which at first occurs only on exertion; as the stenosis worsens, breathing difficulty is felt with less exertion and is eventually present when the person is at rest. Other symptoms and signs include *palpitations*, *atrial fibrillation* (rapid uncoordinated, irregular heartbeat), and deeply flushed cheeks. Congestion of the lungs can lead to recurrent chest infections, coughing up of blood, and fatigue.

Possible complications are as for mitral insufficiency.

DIAGNOSIS

Mitral stenosis is diagnosed from the patient's history, by listening to heart sounds through a stethoscope, and by investigations that may include an *ECG*, chest *X rays*, *echocardiography*, and cardiac *catheterization*.

TREATMENT AND OUTLOOK

Drug treatment (with *diuretic drugs* and *digitalis drugs*) is broadly the same as for mitral insufficiency, as are the precautions to help prevent infection of the valve (see *Endocarditis*).

If symptoms persist despite drug treatment, balloon *valvuloplasty* may be considered to stretch the defective valve. Alternatively, *heart valve surgery* to repair the valve (a procedure known as mitral valvotomy) or to replace the valve may be performed. The outlook following these treatments is generally good, although they may need to be repeated after several years.

Mitral valve prolapse

A common, slight deformity of the mitral valve, situated in the left side of the *heart*, that can produce a degree of *mitral insufficiency* (leakage of the valve). Also known as "floppy valve syndrome," the condition affects up to 5 percent of the population and is most common in young to middle-aged women. Mitral valve prolapse causes a characteristic heart *murmur* which may be heard by the physician through a stethoscope during a routine examination.

The cause is often unknown, although there is some evidence that the condition is inherited. Occasionally, the valve prolapse occurs as a result of *rheumatic fever*, *coronary artery disease*, or *cardiomyopathy*.

Usually, there are no symptoms and the condition is of no consequence; treatment is not required. Occasionally, however, it may produce chest pain, *arrhythmia* (disturbance of heart rhythm), or leakage of the valve sufficient to cause *heart failure*. These conditions may require treatment with drugs, such as *beta-blocker drugs*, *diuretic drugs*, or *digitalis drugs*, or, rarely, *heart valve surgery*.

Mittelschmerz

Pain in the lower abdomen that occurs in some women at the time of *ovulation* midway through each menstrual

M

THE MECHANISM OF MITOSIS

Mitosis is the simplest type of cell division. It provides new body cells to replace those that have died. The new cells each receive an identical copy of the original cell's chromosomes.

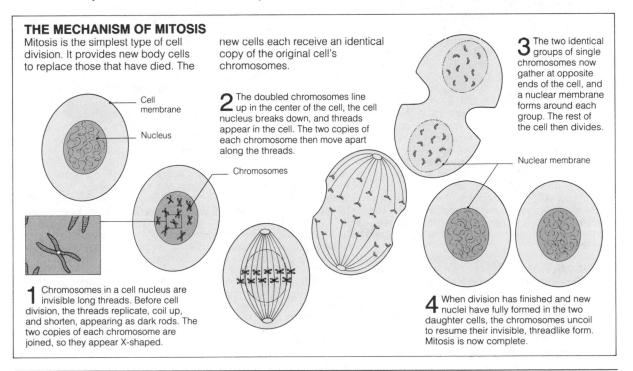

1 Chromosomes in a cell nucleus are invisible long threads. Before cell division, the threads replicate, coil up, and shorten, appearing as dark rods. The two copies of each chromosome are joined, so they appear X-shaped.

Cell membrane

Nucleus

Chromosomes

2 The doubled chromosomes line up in the center of the cell, the cell nucleus breaks down, and threads appear in the cell. The two copies of each chromosome then move apart along the threads.

3 The two identical groups of single chromosomes now gather at opposite ends of the cell, and a nuclear membrane forms around each group. The rest of the cell then divides.

Nuclear membrane

4 When division has finished and new nuclei have fully formed in the two daughter cells, the chromosomes uncoil to resume their invisible, threadlike form. Mitosis is now complete.

cycle. The pain is usually one-sided and lasts only a few hours; slight spotting (vaginal blood loss) may accompany the pain. Mittelschmerz is usually not severe. However, if it is, *oral contraceptives* may be prescribed to suppress ovulation.

MMR vaccination

Administration of a combined *vaccine* that gives protection against *measles*, *mumps*, and *rubella* (German measles). The aim of immunization is to eliminate these infections, especially congenital rubella, which can be contracted by an unborn child if the mother is infected during pregnancy. To achieve this aim, at least 90 percent of children must be vaccinated. The MMR vaccination may be given at any age after 1 year. If a child has not had the vaccination by the time of school entry, it should be offered along with the *DPT vaccination* booster. Some provinces require proof of MMR vaccination before school entry; all provinces strongly recommend it. Only a single vaccination is required; it should be given even if the child has already had one or more of three diseases.

Vaccination should be postponed if a child is suffering from an acute feverish illness. Vaccination should not be given to children who have untreated *cancer*, a history of life-threatening allergic reactions, or suppressed immunity (including those who are receiving treatment with *immunosuppressant drugs*, *radiation therapy* or high-dose *corticosteroid drugs*). Vaccination should not be given within three weeks of another live vaccine, or within three months of an *immunoglobulin injection*. Adult women given the vaccine should avoid pregnancy for at least one month.

POSSIBLE ADVERSE EFFECTS
MMR vaccination is safe and effective. Minor symptoms, such as fever, rash, and malaise, may occur—most commonly, five to 10 days after vaccination. In addition, about 1 percent of children develop mild swelling of the *parotid glands* (such as occurs in mumps) three to four weeks after vaccination; this condition is not infectious to others.

Mobilization

The process of making a part of the body capable of movement. Mobilization refers to treatment aimed at increasing mobility in a part of the body that is recovering from injury or affected by disease. Examples include exercises to treat *frozen shoulder* or joint stiffness caused by *arthritis*, and retraining in walking following a *stroke* or *fracture* of the leg.

Surgeons use the term mobilization to refer to the freeing, during an operation, of an organ or structure from surrounding *connective tissue* (material that surrounds body structures and holds them together) and fibrous adhesions (bands of tissue that join normally unconnected parts of the body). For example, in a *cholecystectomy* operation, the gallbladder has to be mobilized from the liver before it can be removed.

Molar

See *Teeth*.

Molar pregnancy

A pregnancy in which a tumor develops from placental tissue and the embryo fails to develop normally. A molar pregnancy may be benign, in which case it is called a *hydatidiform mole*, or malignant, in which case it is called an invasive mole. *Choriocarcinoma* is an invasive mole that tends to spread outside the uterus.

A different type of molar pregnancy occurs after a missed abortion (a type of *miscarriage* in which the dead embryo and placenta are not expelled from the uterus). In this case, the dead tissue is called a carneous mole.

Mold

Any of a large group of *fungi* that exist as many-celled, filamentous colonies. Some molds are the source of antibiotic drugs, such as penicillin. Others can cause disease, such as *aspergillosis*.

Mole

A type of pigmented *nevus*. (See also *Molar pregnancy*.)

Molecule

The smallest complete unit of a substance that can exist independently and still retain the characteristic properties of that substance. Almost all molecules consist of two or more atoms that are linked. A molecule of carbon dioxide comprises one carbon atom linked to two oxygen atoms. Certain unusual molecules, called monatomic molecules, consist of only one atom (e.g., molecules of inert gases such as argon and neon).

Molecules vary enormously in size and complexity. At one extreme are the small, simple ones such as oxygen, which consists of two linked oxygen atoms. At the other extreme are huge, complicated molecules such as *DNA* (deoxyribonucleic acid), which consists of thousands of atoms of carbon, hydrogen, oxygen, nitrogen, and phosphorus linked together to form a double-helix spiral structure shaped like a spiral staircase.

Molluscum contagiosum

A harmless viral infection characterized by shiny, pearly white papules (tiny lumps) on the skin surface. Each papule is circular, has a tiny central depression, and produces a cheesy fluid when it is squeezed. A crust forms before healing occurs.

The papules appear in groups, or sometimes alone, on the genitals, the inside of the thighs, the face, or elsewhere. Children or, less commonly, adults may be affected. The infection is easily transmitted by direct skin contact or during sexual intercourse.

Molluscum contagiosum usually clears up in a few months, but may require treatment by a physician.

Mongolian blue spot

A blue-black pigmented spot found singly or in groups on the lower back and buttocks at birth. The spot may be mistaken for a bruise, although it is a type of *nevus*. Mongolian blue spots are common in black or Asian children and are caused by a concentration of melanocytes (pigment-producing cells) deep within the skin. They usually disappear by the time the child is 3 or 4 years old.

Mongolism

The outdated name for the disorder now called *Down's syndrome*.

Moniliasis

See *Candidiasis*.

Monitor

To maintain a constant watch on a patient's condition so that any change can be detected early and appropriate treatment given. The term also refers to any device used to carry out monitoring, such as the cardiac monitor used in intensive-care units. A cardiac monitor displays the patient's *ECG* (a record of the heart's electrical activity) on a screen and signals the heart rate both visually and audibly.

Monoamine oxidase inhibitors

One of the two main types of *antidepressant drug*.

Monoarthritis

Inflammation of a single joint, causing pain and stiffness. Common causes are *osteoarthritis*, *gout*, and infection.

Monoclonal antibody

See *Antibody, monoclonal*.

Mononucleosis, infectious

An acute viral infection characterized by a high temperature, sore throat, and swollen *lymph nodes* (glands), particularly in the neck (hence its common name, glandular fever).

CAUSES AND INCIDENCE

Infectious mononucleosis is caused either by the Epstein-Barr virus or cytomegalovirus, both members of the herpesvirus family. The disease develops only if the virus is encountered for the first time at an age when the response of the body's *immune system* is most vigorous (that is, during adolescence and early adult life). The peak incidence of the illness occurs between ages 15 and 17. Each year, thousands of young people in Canada develop the illness. Kissing is thought to be a common method of transmitting the virus.

Once in the body, the virus multiplies in the *lymphocytes* (white blood cells that form part of the immune system). Lymphocytes are also called mononuclear cells. When infected with the virus, the lymphocytes alter their appearance and are then referred to as "atypical."

SYMPTOMS AND SIGNS

The illness usually starts with a fever and headache, followed by swelling of the lymph nodes in the neck, armpits, and groin and by a severe sore throat due to tonsillitis. The enlarged, inflamed tonsils make swallowing difficult and, in rare cases, may obstruct breathing. Occasionally, mild liver damage may occur, leading to jaundice for a few days. A physician may feel an enlarged spleen in the upper left part of the abdomen.

DIAGNOSIS

The diagnosis of infectious mononucleosis is often obvious from the symptoms and from examination of a *blood smear*, which shows many atypical lymphocytes in the blood. A test for the infection—the heterophil antibodies test—may also be carried out. This test looks for antibodies (proteins produced by the immune system to counter the virus) that possess the unique ability to cause clumping of red cells taken from sheep's blood. More specific tests are also available when the diagnosis is in doubt.

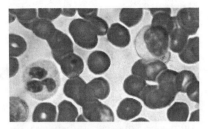

Blood smear in mononucleosis
The large cell with one nucleus, surrounded by many red blood cells, is an atypical lymphocyte (it is bigger than normal). Such cells are a feature of mononucleosis.

TREATMENT AND OUTLOOK

Almost all patients recover after four to six weeks without drug treatment. If the antibiotic *ampicillin* is given in the mistaken belief that the patient has a bacterial infection, it may produce a rash and worsening of symptoms. Rest is needed for a month or so to allow the body's immune system to destroy the virus. In rare cases, *corticosteroid drugs* are required to reduce severe inflammation, particularly if breathing is obstructed by swollen tonsils. For a period of two or three months after recovery, patients often feel depressed, lack energy, and feel sleepy during the day.

Monorchism

The presence of only one testis. Unless a testis has been removed by surgery (see *Orchiectomy*), the most probable cause of monorchism is a *congenital* absence. The term monorchism should not be used to describe a testis that has not descended into the scrotum (see *Testis, undescended*).

Monosodium glutamate

A *food additive* frequently used as a flavor enhancer and seasoning. Monosodium glutamate (MSG) is the sodium salt of an amino acid, derived from protein. Until recently, MSG was suspected to be the cause of *Chinese restaurant syndrome*, in which a sense of pressure in the face, pain in the chest, and a feeling of burning in the head and upper trunk comes on 20 minutes after a meal and lasts for about 45 minutes. Clinical trials have shown that MSG does not produce exactly this symptom pattern, although it may occasionally cause symptoms in sensitive people.

Monteggia's fracture

Fracture of the *ulna* (the bone on the inner side of the forearm) just below the elbow, with dislocation of the *radius* (the bone on the outer side of the forearm) from the *elbow* joint. Monteggia's fracture can be caused by a fall onto the arm or by a blow to the back of the upper arm.

Treatment usually requires an operation through two incisions on either side of the forearm. The fractured bone ends of the ulna are realigned and fixed with a plate and screws or a long nail to restore the length of the forearm. Then the head of the radius is replaced in the elbow joint. The incisions are sewn up and the limb is immobilized in a plaster *cast* until the fracture has healed, which usually takes about 12 weeks.

Moon face

The rounded facial appearance that is a feature of *Cushing's syndrome*.

Morbid anatomy

Also known as pathological anatomy, the study of the structural changes that occur in body tissues as a result of disease, especially the changes that are visible to the naked eye during a postmortem examination (in contrast to the tissue changes that are visible only through a microscope).

Morbidity

The state or condition of being diseased. In medical statistics, the morbidity ratio is the proportion of diseased people to healthy people in a community.

Morbilli

Another name for *measles*.

Morning-after pill

See *Contraception, postcoital*.

Morning sickness

See *Vomiting in pregnancy*.

Moron

An outdated term, derived from the Greek word for dull, for a person with mild *mental retardation*.

Morphea

A condition in which one or more hard, flat, round or oval patches develop on the skin. Morphea is a type of *scleroderma* (a disease in which there is progressive hardening of tissues), but it is confined to the skin.

The skin patches of morphea are white or reddish, measuring up to several centimetres in diameter. They usually occur on the trunk, neck, hands, or feet. Loss of hair or ulceration at the affected site may also

M

occur. The condition most often affects middle-aged women. Morphea is harmless but can be disfiguring. There is no treatment.

Morphine

The best known narcotic *analgesic drug* (painkiller), derived from the unripe seed pods of the opium poppy.

WHY IT IS USED

Morphine is given to relieve severe pain caused by *myocardial infarction* (heart attack), major surgery, serious injury, and cancer. It is occasionally used as a *premedication* (a drug used to prepare a person for surgery).

HOW IT WORKS

Morphine blocks the transmission of pain signals at specific sites (called opiate receptors) in the brain and spinal cord, thereby preventing the perception of pain. It also induces a sense of well-being or euphoria.

POSSIBLE ADVERSE EFFECTS

Morphine causes drowsiness, dizziness, constipation, nausea, vomiting, and confusion.

ABUSE

The euphoric effects of morphine are addictive and have led to its abuse. Short-term use is unlikely to cause *drug dependence*. Long-term abuse leads to a craving for the drug and *tolerance* (the need for greater amounts to have the same effect). It also causes physical dependence, with severe flu-like symptoms, such as profuse sweating, shaking, and abdominal cramps, when the drug is suddenly withdrawn (see *Withdrawal syndrome*).

Mortality

The death rate, that is, the number of deaths per 100,000 (or, occasionally, per 1,000 or per 10,000) of the population per year. The total mortality is made up of the individual mortality from different causes (such as accidents, coronary artery disease, and cancer). The study of differences in these proportions between one country and another, or between different periods in the same country, can offer valuable information about the comparative state of health of a population or about disease trends.

Mortality is often calculated for specific groups of the population. For example, *infant mortality* measures the deaths of live-born infants during the first year of life; perinatal mortality measures the deaths (including all stillbirths) during the first week (or sometimes month) of life.

Standardized mortality compares the death rate in an occupational or socioeconomic group with that for the entire population. It is a useful indicator of the relative safety of an occupation, or of whether a specific socioeconomic group is at particular risk. (See also table below, showing *Deaths and potential years of life lost by major causes; Life expectancy; Maternal mortality*.)

Mosaicism

The presence of two (or more) groups of cells containing different chromosomal material within one person.

Usually, each of a person's body cells contains 46 *chromosomes*. They include the two sex chromosomes (XX in females and XY in males). In a mosaic person, some cells may contain 46 and others 45, 47, or other numbers of chromosomes. The probable cause in most cases is a fault in cell division early in embryonic life. The diagnosis is made by *chromosome analysis* of skin or white blood cells.

Mosaicism can give rise to syndromes associated with *chromosomal abnormalities* (such as *Down's syndrome* and *Turner's syndrome*). A girl with Turner's syndrome mosaicism has some cells with a normal chromosome complement and others missing an X sex chromosome. About 3 percent of children with Down's syndrome have mosaicism. These children carry a mixture of normal cells and others containing the extra number 21 chromosome.

Depending on the proportion of abnormal cells and the type of abnormality, people with mosaicism range from looking physically normal to having features typical of a chromosomal abnormality syndrome. People with mosaicism are often less severely affected than those with the abnormality in all their cells.

Mosquito bites

Mosquitoes are flying insects found throughout the world. The females require blood from humans or animals to produce eggs; they obtain this blood through their bites. The mosquito eggs are laid and hatched in

M

The illustration shows the number of deaths and the number of potential years of life lost (PYLL) for seven causes of death, which account for almost 90 percent of all deaths. Although deaths due to cardiovascular disease far outnumber those due to accidents, they are close in PYLL because accidents occur at an earlier age, on the average.

The bars on the left show the actual number of deaths. The bars on the right show the total number of potential years of life lost (PYLL) for those dying of that cause. PYLL are calculated by subtracting the age at death from 75. (See *Accidental death*.)

DEATHS AND POTENTIAL YEARS OF LIFE LOST BY MAJOR CAUSES IN CANADA IN 1986

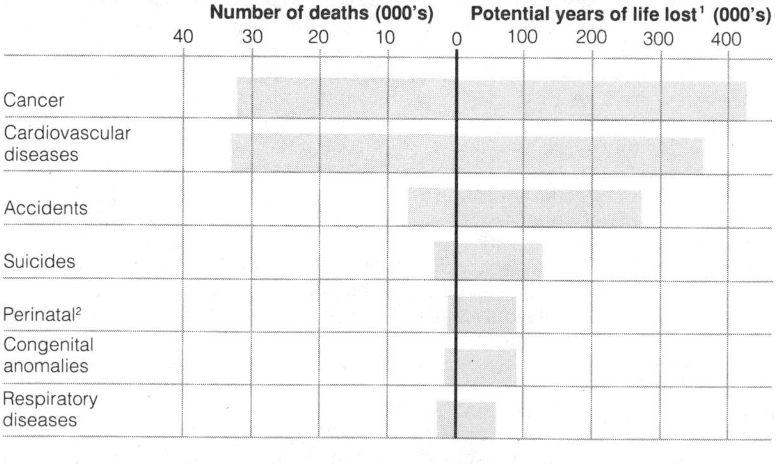

	Number of deaths (000's)	Potential years of life lost[1] (000's)
	40 30 20 10 0	0 100 200 300 400
Cancer		
Cardiovascular diseases		
Accidents		
Suicides		
Perinatal[2]		
Congenital anomalies		
Respiratory diseases		

[1] Between ages 0 and 75   [2] Excludes stillbirths

stagnating water, so mosquitoes are most prevalent close to marshes, ponds, reservoirs, and water tanks, especially after a rainy period. Male mosquitoes do not bite.

Mosquitoes are a nuisance simply because of their bites. However, the main problem with mosquitoes is disease transmission—particularly in the tropics. During a bite, a mosquito may acquire infectious organisms from the blood of an infected person; the organisms multiply within the insect and are transferred to another person during a subsequent bite.

The main disease-transmitting mosquitoes belong to three groups: *ANOPHELES*, *AEDES*, and *CULEX*. They have varying appearances and habits and transmit different diseases (see accompanying chart).

TREATMENT

Mosquito bites should be washed with soap and water, and a soothing cream applied. A physician should be consulted if mosquito bites cause a severe skin reaction.

PREVENTION

Protective measures against mosquitoes (to limit the chances of infection) should be taken in the tropics and subtropics and in any area where the insects are rampant. The most effective measures are the wearing of long sleeves and socks at dusk to reduce the amount of exposed skin, placing mosquito screens over windows, and the use of insect-repellent sprays or slow-burning coils that release a smoke containing insecticide. A mosquito net that surrounds the bed is of value in preventing mosquitoes from biting during sleep.

Attempts to control mosquitoes in the tropics have included direct attack with insecticides, efforts to limit breeding areas, and even the release of vast numbers of sterilized male mosquitoes. However, these efforts have achieved only limited success. (See also *Insects and disease; Insect bites*.)

Motion sickness

A condition produced in some people by road, sea, or air travel. In its mildest form, motion sickness may be only a feeling of slight uneasiness or discomfort, and a headache; in severe cases, there may be distress, excessive sweating and salivation, pallor, nausea, and vomiting.

Motion sickness is caused by the effect of any repetitive pronounced movement on the organ of balance in the inner ear. Other factors also play a part, however. Anxiety based on pre-

DANGEROUS MOSQUITOES

Mosquito	Appearance	Habits	Diseases transmitted
ANOPHELES species	Head and body in straight line and at an angle to surface	Mainly rural; bite at night	Malaria; filariasis
CULEX species	Body parallel to surface; head bent down; whining flight; brown color	Urban or rural; bite in evening or at night	Viral encephalitis; filariasis
AEDES species	Body shape as for *CULEX*, but tropical species are black and white	Urban or rural; bite during day	Dengue; yellow fever; viral encephalitis

vious attacks, a stuffy or fume-laden atmosphere, a full stomach, or the sight of food can make the condition worse. So, too, can focusing on nearby objects or objects flashing past; sufferers should look at a point on the horizon.

PREVENTION

Various *antiemetic drugs* are available to prevent or help control motion sickness. *Hyoscine* or cyclizine (an *antihistamine drug*) may be taken about an hour before the start of a journey. The longer-acting antihistamines (promethazine or meclozine) should be taken for a longer journey. Some drugs used for motion sickness may cause drowsiness and increase the effects of alcohol.

Motor

A term used to describe anything that brings about movement, such as a muscle or a nerve. It is usually applied to nerves (including those in the part of the brain called the cerebral cortex) that stimulate muscles to contract and thereby produce movement.

Motor neuron disease

A group of disorders in which there is degeneration of the *nerves* within the *central nervous system* that control muscular activity. This degeneration leads to weakness and wasting of the *muscles*. The cause of motor neuron disease is unknown.

TYPES

AMYOTROPHIC LATERAL SCLEROSIS Also known as ALS or Lou Gehrig's disease, this is the most common type of motor neuron disease. About one or two cases of ALS are diagnosed annually per 100,000 people in Canada. The disease usually affects

people over the age of 50 and is more common in men. About 5 to 10 percent of cases run in families.

In most cases, the first symptom is weakness in the hands and arms, accompanied by wasting of the muscles. There may also be *fasciculations* (spontaneous, irregular contractions of small areas of muscle), and muscle cramps or stiffness. In some cases, symptoms begin in the legs. Wherever the disease first appears, all four extremities soon become involved. ALS does not affect sensation or bladder function.

Other types of motor neuron disease include progressive muscular atrophy and progressive bulbar palsy, which both start with patterns of muscle weakness that differ from typical ALS but usually develop into ALS.

CHILDHOOD TYPES

Two types of motor neuron disease start in childhood or adolescence, and in most cases are inherited.

Werdnig-Hoffmann disease, also called infantile progressive spinal muscular atrophy, affects infants at birth or soon afterward; with rare exceptions, muscle weakness becomes progressively worse, leading to death.

A less severe type is chronic spinal muscular atrophy, which may begin any time during childhood and adolescence. This type causes progressive weakness but may not lead to serious disability.

DIAGNOSIS

The diagnosis of motor neuron disease may be confirmed by various tests, including *EMG* (measurement of electrical activity in muscles), muscle *biopsy* (removal of a sample of tissue for microscopic analysis), blood

M

699

tests, *myelography* (X-ray examination of the spinal cord after injection of a radiopaque substance), *CT scanning*, or *MRI*.

TREATMENT AND OUTLOOK

Motor neuron disease typically goes on to affect the muscles involved in breathing and swallowing. Involvement of these muscles usually leads to death within two to four years of onset. However, about 20 percent of sufferers survive for more than five years, and about 5 percent for more than 10 years.

Nerve degeneration cannot be slowed down, but *physiotherapy* and use of various aids may help reduce *disability*. In the late stages of the disease, the sufferer cannot speak, swallow, or move, but maintains intellect and awareness. Psychological and physical support are needed, and may be provided at home or in a *hospice*.

Mountain sickness

An illness that can affect mountain climbers, hikers, or skiers who have ascended too rapidly to heights above about 2,400 m or, more commonly, to above 3,000 m.

CAUSES

Mountain sickness is caused by the reduced atmospheric pressure—and thus reduced oxygen—at high altitude, but the exact mechanism by which reduced pressure leads to illness is not fully understood. Broadly, reduced oxygen in the blood, along with other changes in blood chemistry, affects the nervous system, muscles, heart, and lungs.

At higher altitudes the blood flow through the lungs and to the brain is greater than normal; this, combined with an apparent increase in the permeability (leakiness) of blood vessels, can lead to *edema* (accumulation of fluid) in these organs.

Mountain sickness is more likely the younger the person, the faster the ascent, and the higher the altitude.

PREVENTION

A person ascending to an altitude above 2,400 m should do so gradually, stopping for a day or two's rest after each further ascent of 600 to 900 m. Ascending higher during the rest day is permissible, provided a return to the lower level is made before night.

SYMPTOMS AND SIGNS

In most cases, mountain sickness is mild and short-lived, with symptoms such as headache, nausea, dizziness, and impaired mental processes. No further ascent should be made until the symptoms disappear.

Some cases are more severe. Sufferers develop a condition known as high-altitude pulmonary edema, in which fluid builds up in the lungs, leading to severe breathlessness, cough, and the production of frothy sputum (phlegm). In some cases, a condition known as cerebral edema develops, in which fluid builds up around the brain, causing severe headache, vomiting, unsteadiness, confusion, hallucinations, seizures, and sometimes coma.

FIRST AID AND TREATMENT

The victim must be brought down from the mountain and taken to a hospital. Any delay can result in brain damage and death. The administration of pure oxygen can help. In hospital, *diuretic drugs* are often given to help reduce edema.

The condition of patients with high-altitude pulmonary edema often improves rapidly after descending a few hundred metres. Patients with cerebral edema may take days or weeks in hospital to recover.

Mouth

The oral cavity. The mouth is the first part of the *digestive system*, where food is broken down for swallowing (see *Mastication*). It is also used in *breathing*, and converts vibrations produced by the *larynx* (voice box) into *speech*.

STRUCTURE

The roof of the mouth consists of a hard bony *palate* at the front and a soft fleshy palate behind. Most of the floor of the mouth is formed by the *tongue*, which contains specialized cells, sensitive to taste, known as taste buds. Surrounding the palate and tongue are the *teeth*, which are set in the shock-absorbent tissue of the *gums*. Enclosing them all are the cheeks and *lips*, which contain a ring of muscle that helps keep food in the mouth. The inside of the mouth is lined with mucous membrane, which is lubricated with saliva produced by three pairs of *salivary glands*.

DISORDERS

The most common deformities of the mouth, other than alignment of the teeth (see *Malocclusion*), are *cleft lip and palate* (a split in the upper lip and a gap in the roof of the mouth).

Infections of the mouth are common. Examples include an abscess around the root of a tooth (see *Abscess, dental*) and oral *candidiasis* (thrush), a fungal infection that produces sore, cream-colored patches on the lining of the mouth. Noninfective conditions that also cause discoloration include *leukoplakia* (in which there are thickened white or gray patches) and *lichen planus* (in which a white network of raised tissue develops).

Extremely common are *mouth ulcers*, painful white or yellow open sores that may develop anywhere on the mucous membrane within the mouth. *Cysts* (swellings filled with fluid or semisolid material) sometimes occur

---

ANATOMY OF THE MOUTH

The mouth has a complicated structure, reflecting its various functions. For example, the tongue, lips, teeth, and palate play an essential role in speech production. Together with the salivary glands, the same mouth parts also play a role in eating and drinking.

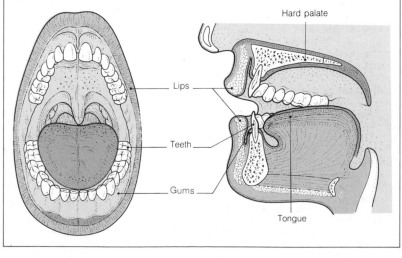

Hard palate

Lips

Teeth

Gums

Tongue

on the lining of the cheek; *ranula* are cysts on the floor of the mouth.

Any lump, sore, or ulcer in the mouth that persists for more than three or four weeks should be seen by a physician. In rare cases, the abnormality is an early sign of a malignant growth (see *Mouth cancer*).

Mouth cancer

Malignant tumors affecting the lips, tongue, and oral cavity. *Lip cancer* and *tongue cancer* are the most common types of mouth cancer. Less commonly affected by cancer are the floor of the mouth, the salivary glands, the inside of the cheeks, the gums, and the palate.

CAUSES AND INCIDENCE

The main predisposing causes of mouth cancer are poor *oral hygiene*, heavy alcohol consumption, and *tobacco smoking*. The risk to pipe and cigar smokers is as great, or greater, than the risk to cigarette smokers; chewing tobacco and inhaling snuff also predispose to mouth cancer. Irritation from ill-fitting dentures or jagged teeth are other predisposing factors.

Oral cancers represent about 5 percent of all malignancies. Men are affected twice as commonly as women, and most cases occur in men over the age of 40.

SYMPTOMS AND SIGNS

Mouth cancer usually starts with a whitish patch, called *leukoplakia*, or a small lump. These may be accompanied by a burning sensation, but are usually painless. As the tumor grows, it may develop into an ulcer or a deep, hard-edged fissure (crack), which may bleed and erode surrounding tissue. In its advanced stages, mouth cancer is usually painful.

DIAGNOSIS

Any lump, discolored patch, or other tissue change in the mouth that does not clear up within a month should be reported to a physician. In some cases, a dentist is the first person to detect a cancerous change. The diagnosis is based on a *biopsy* (removal of a small sample of tissue for microscopic analysis).

TREATMENT AND OUTLOOK

Treatment consists of surgical removal of all cancerous tissue, *radiation therapy*, or a combination of both. Extensive surgery may result in facial disfigurement and problems with eating and speaking, which may require reconstructive surgery. Radiation therapy sometimes damages the salivary glands (see *Mouth, dry*).

The rate of spread of oral cancer varies according to the site. When oral cancer in any form is detected and treated early, the outlook is good, resulting in a cure in three quarters of cases. More than half the people with oral cancer survive for more than five years after treatment.

Mouth, dry

The result of inadequate production of saliva. Dry mouth is usually a temporary condition caused by fear, infection of a *salivary gland*, or the action of *anticholinergic drugs*.

Permanent dry mouth is rare. It can occur, for unknown reasons, as part of *Sjögren's syndrome* or it may result from *radiation therapy* given to treat a tumor of the mouth. Permanent dryness of the mouth is in most cases accompanied by difficulty in swallowing and speaking, interference with taste, and tooth decay. Dry mouth may be partly relieved by spraying the inside of the mouth with artificial saliva.

Mouth-to-mouth resuscitation

See *Artificial respiration*.

Mouth ulcer

An open sore caused by a break in the *mucous membrane* that lines the mouth. Mouth ulcers take the form of round or oval, shallow, white, gray, or yellow spots with an inflamed red border. They may occur singly or in clusters anywhere in the mouth.

TYPES

The most common type of mouth ulcer is an aphthous ulcer (see *Ulcer, aphthous*), which may occur on the inside of the cheek or lip or on the tongue. Also common are ulcers caused by the *herpes simplex* virus, which also causes *cold sores*.

Rare types of mouth ulcer include those occurring in *Behçet's syndrome*, *tuberculosis*, *syphilis*, acute ulcerative *gingivitis*, *leukemia*, *anemia*, and drug allergy.

A mouth ulcer may be an early stage of *mouth cancer*. Any ulcer that fails to heal within a month, or that recurs, should be seen by a physician. *Blood tests* and/or a *biopsy* (removal of a small sample of tissue for microscopic analysis) may be required to determine the cause of the ulcer.

Mouthwash

A solution for rinsing the mouth. Various medicinal claims are made for mouthwashes, but many do no more than leave the mouth feeling fresh

and, if used vigorously, remove loose food debris from the teeth (an effect that can be achieved with water). If used for a prolonged period, mouthwashes may irritate the mouth.

Some mouthwashes are useful in certain circumstances. When the gums are too tender for proper toothbrushing, as occurs in some types of *gingivitis* (inflammation of the gums), a mouthwash containing *hydrogen peroxide* can help clean the teeth by its foaming action.

When routine dental hygiene is impossible, as is the case after oral surgery, a mouthwash containing *chlorhexidine*, used as directed by the dental surgeon, is effective against bacteria in dental *plaque* (the sticky coating on the teeth).

Fluoride mouthwashes help prevent dental caries, probably by strengthening tooth enamel, and possibly also by acting directly against plaque.

A mouthwash of warm salt water can help ease painful inflammation caused by tooth disorders, such as impacted wisdom teeth (see *Impaction, dental*) or *dry socket* (infection at the site of a tooth extraction).

Antiseptic mouthwashes intended to combat *halitosis* (bad breath) are usually ineffective because they do not treat the cause of the problem.

Movement

Bodily movements include skeletal movements and movements of soft tissues and body organs. All movement is brought about by the actions of various types of *muscles*.

SKELETAL MOVEMENTS

The simplest skeletal movement consists of a change in the relative position of two *bones*, brought about by shortening of a muscle attached to the two bones and acting across a *joint*. Simultaneously, other muscles and soft tissues, such as skin, *tendons*, and *ligaments*, are stretched.

More complex skeletal movements involve many bones, joints, and muscles, which are arranged to allow an enormous range of possible actions, from turning a screwdriver to turning a somersault. Even in a fairly simple movement, several muscles are active, some contracting to initiate and maintain a movement while others that oppose the movement contract to help prevent sudden, uncontrolled movement.

All voluntary (willed) skeletal movements are initiated in the part of the *cerebrum* (the main mass of the brain) called the motor cortex. Signals

M

MOVEMENT

During life, movement occurs constantly throughout the body. All visible movements are caused by the shortening of muscles, usually for only brief periods at a time. All movement is either voluntary (willed) or involuntary (automatic).

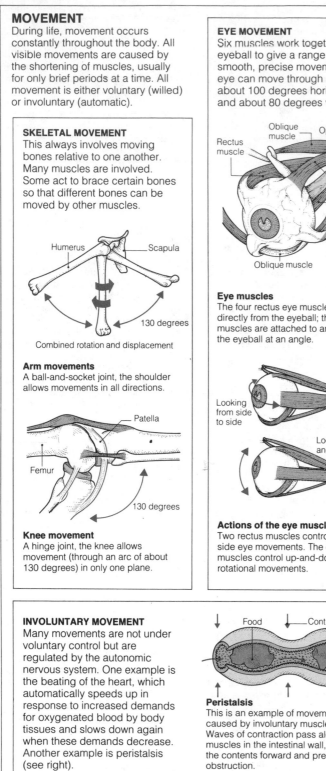

SKELETAL MOVEMENT

This always involves moving bones relative to one another. Many muscles are involved. Some act to brace certain bones so that different bones can be moved by other muscles.

Humerus — Scapula

130 degrees

Combined rotation and displacement

Arm movements
A ball-and-socket joint, the shoulder allows movements in all directions.

Patella

Femur

130 degrees

Knee movement
A hinge joint, the knee allows movement (through an arc of about 130 degrees) in only one plane.

EYE MOVEMENT

Six muscles work together on the eyeball to give a range of smooth, precise movements. The eye can move through an arc of about 100 degrees horizontally and about 80 degrees vertically.

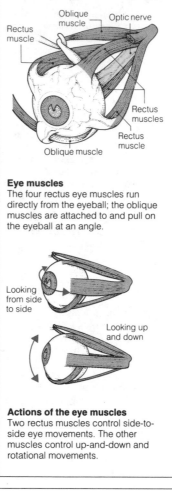

Oblique muscle — Optic nerve
Rectus muscle
Rectus muscles
Rectus muscle
Oblique muscle

Eye muscles
The four rectus eye muscles run directly from the eyeball; the oblique muscles are attached to and pull on the eyeball at an angle.

Looking from side to side

Looking up and down

Actions of the eye muscles
Two rectus muscles control side-to-side eye movements. The other muscles control up-and-down and rotational movements.

INVOLUNTARY MOVEMENT

Many movements are not under voluntary control but are regulated by the autonomic nervous system. One example is the beating of the heart, which automatically speeds up in response to increased demands for oxygenated blood by body tissues and slows down again when these demands decrease. Another example is peristalsis (see right).

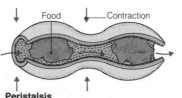

↓ Food   ↓ Contraction

Peristalsis
This is an example of movement caused by involuntary muscle action. Waves of contraction pass along muscles in the intestinal wall, forcing the contents forward and preventing obstruction.

are sent down the spinal cord along nerve fibers, and from there along separate nerve fibers to the appropriate muscles. Control relies on information supplied by sensory nerve receptors, in the muscles and elsewhere, that record the position of the different parts of the body and the amount of contraction in each muscle. This information is integrated in specific areas of the brain (including the cerebellum and basal ganglia) that control coordination, initiation, and cessation of movement. Learning complex sequences (such as piano playing) involves the establishment of unconscious patterns of nerve activity in the cerebellum.

Skeletal movements can also occur as simple *reflexes* in response to certain sensory warning signals. In these instances, the movement is automatic and less controlled, involving far fewer nerve connections.

OTHER MOVEMENTS

Not all body movements involve the skeleton. Movements of the eyes and tongue are brought about by contractions of muscles attached to soft tissues. Again, they may be voluntary movements or reflexes. Movements of the internal organs are involuntary; they include the *heartbeat* and *peristalsis* (rhythmic contractions of the walls of the digestive tract).

DISORDERS

Disorders of the nervous system, muscles, joints, or bones may impair movement. (See *Nerve injury*; *Neuropathy*; *Brain* disorders box; *Spinal cord*; *Muscles* disorders box.)

Moxibustion

A form of treatment, often used in conjunction with *acupuncture*, in which a cone of wormwood leaves (moxa) or certain other plant materials is burned just above the skin to relieve internal pain. The burning material is thought to act as a counterirritant, relieving deep-seated pain by irritating nerve endings in the skin.

MRI

Magnetic resonance imaging. MRI is a diagnostic technique that provides high-quality cross-sectional or three-dimensional images of organs and structures within the body without using X rays or other radiation.

HOW IT WORKS

During the imaging, the patient lies inside a massive, hollow, cylindrical magnet. The nuclei (protons) of the body's hydrogen atoms normally point in random directions. In a mag-

M

netic field, however, these atoms line up parallel to each other, like rows of tiny magnets. If the hydrogen nuclei are then knocked out of alignment by a strong pulse of radio waves, they produce a detectable radio signal as they fall back into alignment.

Magnetic coils in the machine detect these signals and a computer changes them into a cross-sectional or three-dimensional image based on the strength of signal produced by different types of tissue. Tissues that contain a lot of hydrogen (such as fat) produce a bright image; those that contain little or no hydrogen (such as bone) appear black.

WHY IT IS DONE

Images from MRI are similar in many ways to those produced by *CT scanning*, but MRI generally gives much greater contrast between normal and abnormal tissues.

MRI is especially useful in studying the brain and spinal cord. White and gray matter, which are relatively poorly differentiated in CT scans, are distinct and well-defined in MRI scans. MRI provides clear images of tumors of the brain and spinal cord. Also shown clearly by MRI is the internal structure of the eye and ear.

MRI also produces detailed images of the heart and major blood vessels, provides images of blood flow, and is useful for examining joints and soft tissues, particularly in the knee. The role of MRI in imaging the abdominal organs is less established.

HOW IT IS DONE

MRI is usually an outpatient procedure. During the examination the patient must lie still; children may be given a general anesthetic. A scan usually takes about half an hour.

RISKS

There are no known risks or side effects to MRI. The technique does not use radiation and can therefore be performed repeatedly with no known adverse effects. However, any person fitted with a pacemaker, hearing aid, or other electrical device should tell his or her physician before undergoing MRI, since the scanner may interfere with these devices.

OUTLOOK

MRI is a costly test that is not yet widely available; it is still the subject of continuing research. A future application of MRI, known as magnetic resonance spectroscopy, relies on the properties of other chemical elements in the body (such as phosphorus and calcium) and is able to provide information on organ function.

MAGNETIC RESONANCE IMAGING (MRI)

A valuable diagnostic technique, MRI has been in use since the early 1980s. The patient lies down surrounded by a massive electromagnet and is exposed to short bursts of powerful magnetic fields and radio waves. The bursts stimulate protons (hydrogen nuclei) in the patient's tissues to emit radio signals, which are detected and analyzed by computer to create an image of a "slice" of the patient's body.

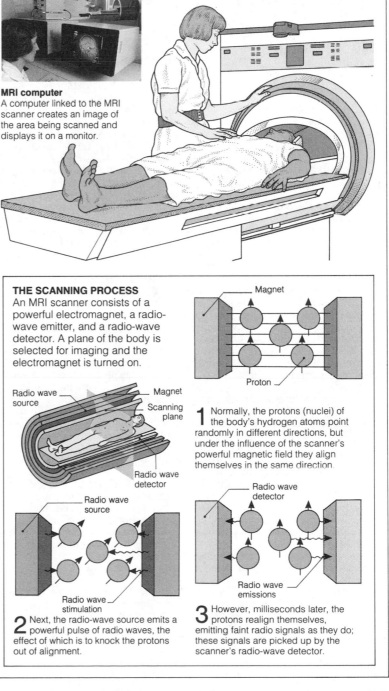

MRI computer
A computer linked to the MRI scanner creates an image of the area being scanned and displays it on a monitor.

THE SCANNING PROCESS

An MRI scanner consists of a powerful electromagnet, a radio-wave emitter, and a radio-wave detector. A plane of the body is selected for imaging and the electromagnet is turned on.

Radio wave source — Magnet
Scanning plane
Radio wave detector

Magnet
Proton

1 Normally, the protons (nuclei) of the body's hydrogen atoms point randomly in different directions, but under the influence of the scanner's powerful magnetic field they align themselves in the same direction.

Radio wave source
Radio wave stimulation

2 Next, the radio-wave source emits a powerful pulse of radio waves, the effect of which is to knock the protons out of alignment.

Radio wave detector
Radio wave emissions

3 However, milliseconds later, the protons realign themselves, emitting faint radio signals as they do; these signals are picked up by the scanner's radio-wave detector.

M

MS

The abbreviation for *multiple sclerosis*.

MSG

The abbreviation for the food additive *monosodium glutamate*.

Mucocele

A swollen sac or cavity within the body that is filled with mucus secreted by its inner lining. A mucocele of the appendix is caused by narrowing of the opening of the appendix into the intestine. A mucocele of the gallbladder, sometimes called hydrops of the gallbladder, may be caused by a gallstone obstructing its outlet.

Mucolytic drugs

Drugs that make sputum (phlegm) less sticky and easier to cough up. An example is *acetylcysteine*.

Mucopolysaccharidosis

A group of inherited metabolic disorders (see *Metabolism, inborn errors of*). The best known of these disorders is *Hurler's syndrome*; others include Hunter's, Sanfillippo's, Morquio's, Maroteaux-Lamy, and Scheie's syndromes. The mucopolysaccharidoses are rare, collectively affecting about one child in 10,000.

All mucopolysaccharidoses are *genetic disorders* in which there is an abnormality of a specific *enzyme*. This abnormality affects the way carbohydrates are handled within body cells, leading to an accumulation in the tissues of unwanted substances called mucopolysaccharides.

Depending on the disease, features include abnormalities of the skeleton and/or the central nervous system (brain and spinal cord) with mental retardation and, in some cases, a characteristic facial appearance. There may also be clouding of the cornea, liver enlargement, and joint stiffness.

No specific treatment is available. Some children with Hurler's syndrome have been successfully treated by a *bone marrow transplant*, which provides them with a continuing source of the deficient enzyme.

Some mucopolysaccharidoses cause death during childhood or adolescence. Mild varieties may allow a reasonably normal life. Parents with a seriously affected child should receive *genetic counseling* on the risk to future children and whether prenatal diagnosis of the disorder is possible.

Mucosa

Another term for *mucous membrane*.

Mucous membrane

The soft, pink, skinlike layer that lines many of the cavities and tubes in the body, including the respiratory tract, digestive tract, the urinary and genital passages, and eyelids. Mucous membranes secrete a mucus-containing fluid which keeps body structures moist and well lubricated. The fluid is produced and released onto the surface of the mucous membrane by millions of specialized cells, called goblet cells, situated within the membrane.

Mucus

The thick, slimy fluid secreted by *mucous membranes*. Mucus moistens, lubricates, and protects those parts of the body lined by mucous membrane, such as the digestive, respiratory, and genital tracts. Mucus eases swallowing, lubricates food as it passes through the digestive tract, prevents stomach acid from damaging the stomach wall, and prevents *enzymes* from digesting the intestine. In the respiratory tract, mucus moistens inhaled air and traps smoke and other foreign particles in the airways (to keep them out of the lungs). Mucus also facilitates sexual intercourse.

Mucus method of contraception

See *Contraception, natural methods of*.

Multiple myeloma

A malignant condition of middle to old age, also called myelomatosis. Multiple myeloma is characterized by the uncontrolled proliferation and disordered function of cells called plasma cells in the *bone marrow*.

Plasma cells are a type of B-*lymphocyte* (class of white blood cell) responsible for producing *immunoglobulins*, which normally help protect against infection. In multiple myeloma, the proliferating plasma cells produce an excessive amount of a single type of immunoglobulin while production of other types is impaired, making the patient prone to infection.

Multiple myeloma is rare. About 1,000 cases are diagnosed annually in Canada.

SYMPTOMS AND SIGNS

Proliferation of the abnormal plasma cells within bone causes pain and destruction of bone tissue. If the *vertebrae* are affected, they may collapse and compress nerves, causing symptoms such as numbness or paralysis. The level of calcium in the blood may increase markedly as bone is destroyed, as may the level of one or

more of the immunoglobulins secreted by the plasma cells. These changes in the blood may damage the kidneys, leading to *kidney failure*.

In addition to the increased risk of infection, patients may suffer from *anemia* and have a tendency to abnormal bleeding if healthy bone marrow is replaced by malignant plasma cells.

DIAGNOSIS, TREATMENT, AND OUTLOOK

The disease is diagnosed by a *bone marrow biopsy* (removal of a sample of tissue for microscopic analysis), which reveals an abnormal appearance; by blood or urine tests, which show an excess of specific immunoglobulins; and by X rays, which indicate areas of destroyed bone.

Treatment includes the use of *anticancer drugs* to reduce the number of abnormal plasma cells, *radiation therapy* of diseased areas of bone, and various supportive measures, including *blood transfusions* to correct anemia, *antibiotic drugs* to combat infections, and *analgesic drugs* to relieve pain.

The severity of the illness and the outlook vary, but only about one fifth of patients survive for four years or longer from the time of diagnosis.

Multiple personality

A rare disorder in which a person has two or more distinct personalities, each of which dominates at different times. The personalities are almost always very different from each other and are often total opposites, as in the story of Dr. Jekyll and Mr. Hyde.

Although multiple personality is often called split personality, a phrase also used to describe *schizophrenia*, the two disorders are unrelated. The split in schizophrenia is between thought and feeling.

Multiple pregnancy

See *Pregnancy, multiple*.

Multiple sclerosis

A progressive disease of the central *nervous system* in which scattered patches of *myelin* (the protective covering of nerve fibers) in the brain and spinal cord are destroyed. This causes symptoms ranging from numbness and tingling to *paralysis* and *incontinence*. The disease was formerly called disseminated sclerosis.

The severity of multiple sclerosis (MS) varies markedly among sufferers. It is characterized by a multiple, patchy pattern of disabilities, variable in site and time, with dramatic, unpredictable improvements. A pa-

FEATURES OF MULTIPLE SCLEROSIS

This disease can affect any area of the white matter of the brain and spinal cord. The plaques of demyelination are areas in which the fatty myelin sheaths of the nerve fibers have been destroyed. Affected fibers cannot conduct nerve impulses, so functions such as movement and sensation may be lost. The patchy distribution of plaques causes very varied effects.

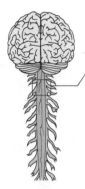

Multiple sclerosis and the spine
Multiple sclerosis often affects nerve fibers in the spinal cord, thus blocking impulses to and from the brain.

Effects of multiple sclerosis
The fiber of the nerve tract is not usually destroyed. But the loss of insulating myelin and its replacement by neuroglia alters normal ion movements, so that the fiber can no longer conduct impulses.

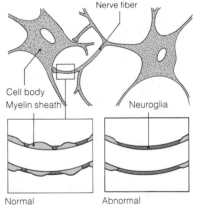

Nerve fiber

Cell body
Myelin sheath   Neuroglia

Normal   Abnormal

RANGE OF OUTLOOKS IN MULTIPLE SCLEROSIS

Dead

Bedridden

Restricted

Mild

No obvious disease

0   5   10   15   20   25   30   **Years**

Key

Rapidly progressive   Steadily progressive

Progressive with remissions   Apparent recovery

Progress of multiple sclerosis
The course and severity of multiple sclerosis vary considerably among sufferers; four of the more typical of the range of possible outcomes are illustrated (left). In the majority of cases, the disease is slowly progressive after an initial period of alternating remissions (when symptoms are mild or absent) and relapses.

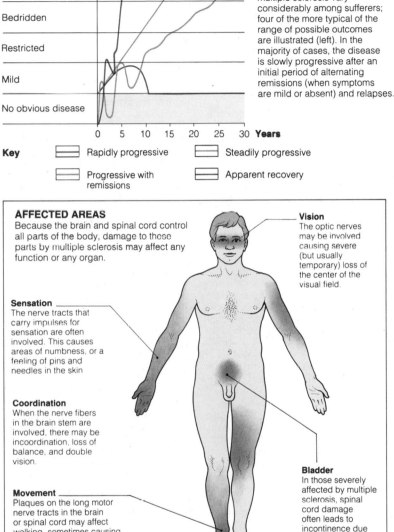

AFFECTED AREAS
Because the brain and spinal cord control all parts of the body, damage to these parts by multiple sclerosis may affect any function or any organ.

Sensation
The nerve tracts that carry impulses for sensation are often involved. This causes areas of numbness, or a feeling of pins and needles in the skin

Coordination
When the nerve fibers in the brain stem are involved, there may be incoordination, loss of balance, and double vision.

Movement
Plaques on the long motor nerve tracts in the brain or spinal cord may affect walking, sometimes causing dragging of one leg or a feeling of weakness.

Vision
The optic nerves may be involved causing severe (but usually temporary) loss of the center of the visual field.

Bladder
In those severely affected by multiple sclerosis, spinal cord damage often leads to incontinence due to loss of sphincter control in the bladder.

M

---

tient may be severely disabled one week and apparently normal the next.

CAUSES
The cause of multiple sclerosis remains unknown. It is thought to be an *autoimmune disorder* in which the body's defense system begins to treat the myelin in the central nervous system as foreign, gradually destroying it, with subsequent damage to some underlying nerve fibers.

There seems to be a genetic factor since relatives of affected people are eight times more likely than others to contract the disease. Environment may also play a part—it is five times more common in relatively temperate regions than in the tropics. Spending the first 15 years of life in a particular area seems to determine future risk. It is thought that a virus picked up by a susceptible person during this

early period of life may be responsible for the disease's later development.

INCIDENCE
Multiple sclerosis is the most common acquired (not present at birth) disease of the nervous system in young adults. In the relatively high-risk temperate areas the incidence is approximately one in every 1,000 people. The ratio of women to men sufferers is three to two.

M

SYMPTOMS AND SIGNS

Multiple sclerosis usually starts in early adult life. It may be active briefly and then resume years later. The symptoms vary according to which parts of the brain and spinal cord are affected. Spinal cord damage can cause tingling, numbness, or a feeling of constriction in any part of the body. The extremities may feel heavy and become weak. *Spasticity* (increased rigidity) and paralysis sometimes develop. The nerve fibers to the bladder may be involved, causing incontinence.

Damage to the white matter in the brain may lead to fatigue, vertigo, clumsiness, muscle weakness, slurred speech, unsteady gait, blurred or double vision, and numbness, weakness, or pain in the face.

Symptoms may occur singly or in combination and may last from several weeks to several months. In some sufferers, relapses may be precipitated by injury, infection, or physical or emotional stress.

The severity of attacks varies considerably from one person to another. In some people, the disease consists of mild relapses and long symptom-free periods throughout life, with very few permanent effects. In others, a series of flare-ups leave some disability, but there is then no further deterioration. Some sufferers become gradually more disabled from the first attack and are bedridden and incontinent in early middle life. A few people suffer gross disability within the first year.

A person paralyzed by multiple sclerosis may have additional problems, such as painful muscle spasms, urinary tract infections, constipation, skin ulceration, and changes of mood between euphoria and depression.

DIAGNOSIS

There is no single diagnostic test for multiple sclerosis; confirmation of the disease is usually by exclusion of all other possible conditions. A neurologist may perform tests to help confirm the diagnosis, including *lumbar puncture* (removal of a sample of fluid from the spinal canal for laboratory analysis), *evoked responses* (tracing electrical activity in the brain), *CT scanning*, and *MRI*.

TREATMENT

No treatment has been found to be of more than slight benefit for large numbers of patients. Individuals with MS should be encouraged to adopt as positive an outlook as possible, and to lead as active a life as their disabilities allow. *Corticosteroid drugs* may be pre-scribed to alleviate the symptoms of an acute episode; other drugs may be given to control specific symptoms, such as incontinence and depression. *Physiotherapy* often helps strengthen muscles and various aids can help patients maintain mobility and independence.

Multivitamin

A group of over-the-counter preparations containing a combination of *vitamins* that are used to supplement the intake of vitamins in the diet. (See *Vitamin supplements*.)

Mumps

An acute viral illness, mainly of childhood. The chief symptom is inflammation and swelling of one or both of the *parotid glands* situated just inside the angle of the jaw. Serious complications are uncommon. However, in teenage and adult males, mumps can be a highly uncomfortable illness in which one or both *testes* become inflamed and swollen. One attack of mumps confers lifelong immunity to future attacks.

CAUSES AND INCIDENCE

The mumps virus is spread in airborne droplets. There is an incubation period of two to three weeks between infection and the appearance of symptoms. An affected person may spread the virus to others for about a week before and up to two weeks after symptoms appear. Most infections are acquired at school or from infected family members.

Now that some provinces require proof of mumps vaccination for school entry, the incidence has dropped markedly over the last 20 years.

SYMPTOMS AND COMPLICATIONS

Many infected children have no symptoms, or are only slightly unwell with discomfort in the region of the parotid glands. In more serious cases, the child first complains of pain in this region and has difficulty in chewing; the glands on one or both sides then become swollen, painful, and tender. Fever, headache, and swallowing difficulty may develop, but the temperature falls after two to three days and the swelling subsides within a week to 10 days. When only one side is affected, the second gland often swells as the swelling of the first gland subsides.

An occasional complication of mumps is *meningitis*, which can cause headache, photophobia (abnormal sensitivity to light), drowsiness, fever, and stiff neck. Mumps menin-gitis usually clears up without any long-term effects. A less common complication is *pancreatitis*, which causes abdominal pain and vomiting.

In males after puberty, *orchitis* (inflammation of the testis) develops in about a quarter of cases. Only one testis is usually affected, becoming swollen, tender, and painful for two to four days. Subsequently, the affected testis may shrink to smaller than normal size. In rare cases, mumps orchitis affects both testes, very occasionally leading to *infertility*. There is no evidence that mumps contracted during pregnancy has any effect on the fetus.

DIAGNOSIS AND TREATMENT

Mumps is usually diagnosed from the patient's symptoms. The diagnosis may be confirmed by measuring *antibodies* to the mumps virus in the blood or by culturing the virus from samples of saliva or urine.

There is no specific treatment, but an affected child may be given *analgesic drugs* (painkillers) and plenty to drink. In moderate to severe cases, the child may need to stay in bed during the first few days of the illness and should not go to school until symptoms have subsided.

For males with severe orchitis, a physician may sometimes prescribe a stronger painkiller, and *corticosteroid drugs* to reduce inflammation.

IMMUNIZATION

A safe and effective mumps vaccine is now available in combination with measles and rubella vaccine (see *MMR vaccination*).

Males after puberty who have never had mumps or never been immunized against it should avoid contact with any infected person. If symptoms of mumps do develop, passive immunization with an *immunoglobulin* injection may provide some protection against the development of orchitis.

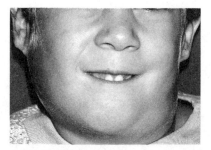

Appearance of mumps
The swelling, especially if present on both sides, may give the affected child a somewhat hamsterlike appearance.

Munchausen's syndrome

A form of chronic *factitious disorder* in which the sufferer complains of physical symptoms that are pretended or self-induced. Sufferers are not *malingering*, they simply want to play the patient role. Most afflicted people are repeatedly hospitalized for investigations and treatment.

Pain in the abdomen, bleeding, neurological symptoms (such as dizziness and blackouts), skin rashes, and fever are the usual complaints. Sufferers typically invent dramatic, but often plausible, histories and, once in the hospital, behave disruptively. Many show evidence of self-injury or of previous treatment (such as numerous scars or detailed medical knowledge). In Munchausen's syndrome by proxy, parents cause factitious disorders in their children.

It is difficult to determine the causes of Munchausen's syndrome; when challenged, sufferers may deny any allegations of deception or may immediately discharge themselves from hospital. Treatment is aimed at protecting sufferers from unnecessary operations and treatments.

Murmur

A sound caused by turbulent blood flow through the *heart*, as heard by a physician through a *stethoscope*. Murmurs are a separate phenomenon from other types of normal or abnormal *heart sounds*, which are caused mainly by sudden acceleration or deceleration of blood movement.

Heart murmurs are not necessarily a sign of disease, but an unusual sound is regarded as an indication of possible abnormality in the blood flow. Apart from "innocent" murmurs, the most common cause of extra blood turbulence is a disorder of the heart valves, such as stenosis (narrowing) or insufficiency (leakage) with regurgitation. Murmurs can also be caused by some types of congenital heart disease (see *Heart disease, congenital*), such as a *septal defect* (hole in the heart) or *patent ductus arteriosus*, by *pericarditis* (inflammation of the membrane around the heart), or by other, rarer, conditions, such as a *myxoma* in a heart chamber.

By noting the location on the chest wall at which the murmur is best heard and the timing of the murmur in relation to the basic heart sounds, and by considering these factors in conjunction with other signs and symptoms, the physician can usually arrive at a diagnosis, which may be confirmed by *echocardiography*.

Muscle

A structure composed of bundles of specialized cells capable of contraction and relaxation to create movement, both of the body itself in relation to the environment and of the organs within it. There are three types of muscle: skeletal, smooth, and cardiac.

SKELETAL MUSCLE

The largest part of the musculature consists of skeletal (voluntary) muscles; the body contains more than 600 such muscles.

Skeletal muscles are classified according to the type of action they perform. An extensor opens out a joint, a flexor closes it; an adductor draws a part of the body inward, an abductor moves it outward; a levator raises it, a depressor lowers it; and constrictor or sphincter muscles surround and close orifices.

Skeletal muscles are composed of groups of muscle fibers in an orderly

M

MUSCLE MOVEMENT

Contraction makes a muscle shorter and draws together the bones to which the muscle is attached.

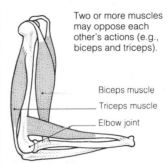

Two or more muscles may oppose each other's actions (e.g., biceps and triceps).

Biceps muscle
Triceps muscle
Elbow joint

Controlled movement at the elbow relies on coordinated relaxation and contraction of the biceps and triceps.

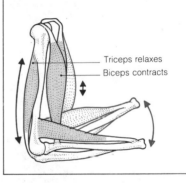

Triceps relaxes
Biceps contracts

arrangement. A small muscle may be made up of only a few bundles of fibers, while the major muscles in the body (such as the gluteus maximus that forms the bulk of the buttock) are made up of hundreds of bundles. A muscle fiber is made up of even

MUSCLE TYPES

Skeletal and cardiac muscles appear striped under the microscope, unlike smooth muscles.

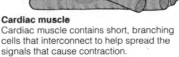

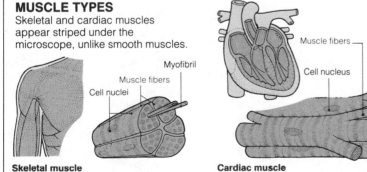

Myofibril
Muscle fibers
Cell nuclei

Skeletal muscle
Skeletal muscle consists of bundles of fibers (muscle cells), each containing contractile elements (myofibrils).

Muscle fibers — Myofibril
Cell nucleus

Cardiac muscle
Cardiac muscle contains short, branching cells that interconnect to help spread the signals that cause contraction.

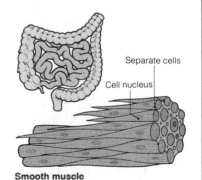

Separate cells
Cell nucleus

Smooth muscle
Smooth muscle consists of more loosely woven, tapering cells. Contraction is slower than in other muscle types.

THE BODY'S MUSCLES

The most prominent muscles in the body are the skeletal muscles, which account for 40 to 45 percent of body weight. These muscles are called voluntary because they are under conscious control; some important voluntary muscles are indicated on the illustration below.

Many internal organs, such as the heart and intestines, also consist partly or entirely of involuntary muscle, which is not under conscious control.

M

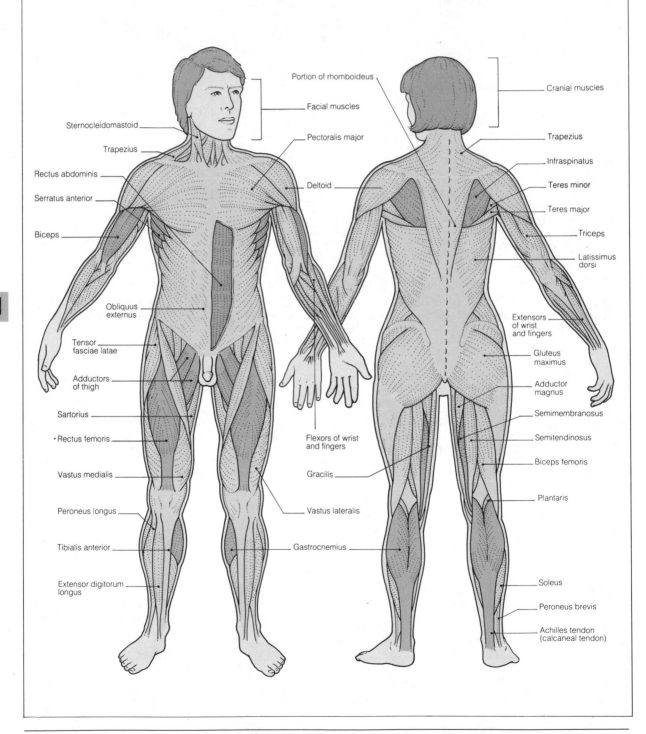

Portion of rhomboideus
Facial muscles
Sternocleidomastoid
Trapezius
Rectus abdominis
Serratus anterior
Pectoralis major
Deltoid
Biciceps
Obliquus externus
Tensor fasciae latae
Adductors of thigh
Sartorius
Rectus femoris
Vastus medialis
Peroneus longus
Tibialis anterior
Extensor digitorum longus
Flexors of wrist and fingers
Gracilis
Vastus lateralis
Gastrocnemius

Cranial muscles
Trapezius
Infraspinatus
Teres minor
Teres major
Triceps
Latissimus dorsi
Extensors of wrist and fingers
Gluteus maximus
Adductor magnus
Semimembranosus
Semitendinosus
Biceps femoris
Plantaris
Soleus
Peroneus brevis
Achilles tendon (calcaneal tendon)

smaller longitudinal units, called myofibrils, the basic working units of which are microscopic filaments of actin and myosin (two proteins that control contraction).

Movement of the skeletal muscles is under the voluntary control of the brain. Each muscle fiber is supplied with a nerve ending that receives impulses from the brain. The nerve impulses stimulate the muscle by releasing *acetylcholine*, a type of *neurotransmitter* (chemical released from nerve endings). This starts a chain of chemical and electrical events, involving sodium, potassium, and calcium ions, which results in the filaments of myosin sliding over the actin filaments in much the same way as an extendable ladder moves when it is being closed. This movement of myosin over actin filaments causes the muscle to contract (shorten).

Each muscle contains a set of specialized nerve fibers that register the force of contraction; another set in the tendon gauges the stretch. The information received by these fibers is transmitted to the brain and is vital in limiting muscle action.

Skeletal muscle is maintained in a state of partial contraction—called muscle tone. *Spasticity* is one form of abnormally increased muscle tone.

Skeletal muscle activity is affected by changes in chemical composition of the fluid surrounding the muscle cells. A fall in potassium ions causes muscle weakness; a decrease of calcium ions causes muscle spasm.

SMOOTH MUSCLE

This type of muscle is concerned with the movements of internal organs, such as *peristalsis* in the intestine and contractions of the uterus during childbirth. Many other parts of the body, such as the bronchi of the lungs, the bladder, and the walls of blood vessels, also contain smooth muscle.

Smooth muscle is composed of long, spindle-shaped cells. In most

DISORDERS OF MUSCLE

The most common muscle disorder is injury, followed by symptoms caused by a lack of blood supply to a muscle (including the heart). In addition, there are a number of other, rarer disorders of muscle.

GENETIC DISORDERS

The *muscular dystrophies* cause progressive weakness and disability. Some types appear at birth, some in infancy, and some develop as late as the fifth or sixth decade.

One type of *cardiomyopathy*, a general term for disease of the heart muscle, is inherited.

INFECTION

The most important infection of muscle is *gangrene*, which may complicate deep wounds (especially those contaminated by soil). *Tetanus* is acquired in a similar way, causing widespread muscle spasm through the release of a powerful toxin.

Viruses (especially influenza B) may also infect muscles (causing *myalgia*), as may the organism causing *toxoplasmosis*. *Trichinosis* is an infestation of muscle with the worm TRICHINELLA SPIRALIS, which is acquired by eating undercooked meat (usually pork).

INJURY

Muscle injuries, such as tears and *strains*, are very common; they cause bleeding into the muscle tissue. Healing leads to formation of a scar in the muscle, which shortens its natural length. Blunt muscle injury may result in *hematoma* formation from bleeding into the muscle. Rarely, bone may form in the blood clot, causing *myositis* ossificans.

TUMORS

Primary muscle tumors may or may not be cancerous. Noncancerous tumors are called *myomas*, those affecting smooth muscle are *leiomyomas*, and those affecting skeletal muscle are rhabdomyomas. Myomas of the uterus (see *Fibroids*) are among the most common of all tumors. Cancerous tumors are called myosarcomas and are very rare; cancers of the skeletal muscle are known as *rhabdomyosarcomas*.

Secondary tumors, which spread from a primary site of cancer elsewhere in the body, very rarely involve muscle.

HORMONAL AND METABOLIC DISORDERS

Muscle contraction depends on the maintenance of proper levels of sodium, potassium, and calcium in and around muscle cells. Any alteration in the concentration of these substances affects muscle function. For example, a severe drop in the level of potassium (hypokalemia) causes profound muscle weakness and may stop the heart. A drop in blood calcium (hypocalcemia) causes increased excitability of muscles and, occasionally, spasms.

Thyroid disease is often associated with muscle disorders, the most common being a swelling of the small muscles that move the eyes, causing a bulging eyeball (see *Exophthalmos*).

Adrenal failure causes general muscle weakness.

IMPAIRED BLOOD SUPPLY

Muscles depend on a good blood supply for normal function. *Cramp* is usually caused by a lack of blood flow, sometimes associated with severe exertion. *Peripheral vascular disease*, which restricts the blood supply,

causes *claudication* (muscle pain on exercise). *Angina pectoris* (chest pain caused by lack of blood supply to heart muscle) occurs in *coronary artery disease*.

The *compartment syndrome* is pain in muscles as a result of pressure that limits their blood supply. It may be brought on by injury or exercise, and occurs most often in athletes with well-developed muscles.

POISONS AND DRUGS

Several toxic substances can damage muscle. They include alcohol, which can cause damage following a prolonged drinking bout. Other substances that may cause muscle damage include aminocaproic acid, chloroquine, clofibrate, emetine, and vincristine.

AUTOIMMUNE DISORDERS

Myasthenia gravis is a disorder of transmission of nerve impulses to muscles; it usually begins by causing drooping of the eyelids and double vision. Other diseases with an autoimmune basis that may affect muscles are *lupus erythematosus*, *rheumatoid arthritis*, *scleroderma*, *sarcoidosis*, and *dermatomyositis*.

INVESTIGATION

Muscle disorders are investigated by *EMG* (electromyography), which measures the response of muscles to electrical impulses, and by muscle *biopsy* (removal of a sample of tissue for analysis).

M

hollow organs, these cells are arranged in bundles organized in an outer longitudinal layer and an inner circular one. However, the mechanism of contraction relies on the same sliding action of actin and myosin as in skeletal muscle.

The nerve supply to smooth muscle comes from the *autonomic nervous system*, which is not under conscious control. Hence, its alternative name—involuntary muscle. Nerves from the autonomic nervous system penetrate into the muscle, where they divide into many branches. Neurotransmitter release from these nerves initiates the process that leads to contraction.

As well as responding to neurotransmitters, smooth muscle also responds to various *hormones*, to the stretch of individual muscle fibers, and to changes in the chemical composition of the fluid surrounding the fibers (e.g., changes in acidity).

CARDIAC MUSCLE

This type of muscle, also called myocardium, is found only in the *heart*; it has unique properties that enable it to contract rhythmically about 100,000 times a day to propel blood through the circulatory system. Its structure resembles that of skeletal muscle.

Contraction of cardiac muscle is stimulated by the autonomic nervous system, by hormones, and by the stretching of muscle fibers.

To act as an efficient pump, the muscles of the heart must contract in an orderly, regular manner. Separate muscle fibers are joined end to end by areas of extensive folds that allow contractions to be transmitted rapidly from one fiber to another. The stimulus for cardiac muscle contraction is initiated in an area of the right atrium (called the sinoatrial node), which stimulates a regular rate of contraction. Specialized conducting cells in cardiac muscle form a network capable of transmitting nerve impulses throughout the cardiac muscle fibers, spreading the contraction through both atria and then both ventricles alternately (see *Heart*).

Muscle-relaxant drugs

A group of drugs used to relieve *muscle spasm* and *spasticity*. Muscle relaxant drugs are often used in combination with an *analgesic drug* (painkiller) to relieve muscle stiffness caused by types of *arthritis, back pain,* or a disorder of the *nervous system,* such as a *stroke* or *cerebral palsy*. They are occasionally used to relieve muscle rigidity caused by injury.

HOW THEY WORK

Except for *dantrolene*, muscle-relaxant drugs partly block nerve signals from the brain and spinal cord that stimulate muscles to contract.

Dantrolene acts directly on muscles by interfering with the chemical activity in muscle cells that is necessary for muscle contraction.

POSSIBLE ADVERSE EFFECTS

Because muscle-relaxant drugs reduce the strength of muscle contraction, they may cause weakness which is noticed when performing certain activities. Also, some muscle-relaxant drugs cause drowsiness. In rare cases, dantrolene causes liver damage.

Muscle spasm

Sudden involuntary contraction of a muscle. Muscle spasm is a normal reaction to pain and inflammation around a joint. Common causes of muscle spasm include muscle *strain*, other musculoskeletal injuries, pressure on a nerve from a *disk prolapse*, poor posture, and stress.

Treatment is usually directed at the cause of the spasm. In some cases, *muscle-relaxant drugs* may also be needed. (See also *Spasticity*.)

Muscular dystrophy

An inherited *muscle* disorder of unknown cause in which there is slow but progressive degeneration of muscle fibers. Different forms of muscular dystrophy are classified according to the age at which the symptoms appear, the rate at which the disease progresses, and the way in which it is inherited. (See box for main types.)

INCIDENCE

All forms of muscular dystrophy are rare. Duchenne muscular dystrophy is the most common and most severe type, affecting about one in 3,000 boys. It is inherited through a recessive, sex-linked gene (see *Genetic disorders*) so that only males are affected and only females can pass on the disease. Other types of muscular dystrophy include Becker's, limb-girdle, facioscapulohumeral, and myotonic dystrophies. These may affect children and adults and are due to autosomal or to sex-linked defects.

DIAGNOSIS

Often the physician suspects muscular dystrophy from the patient's appearance and movements, but tests are needed for confirmation. A blood test may be performed to look for high levels of certain *enzymes* released from the damaged muscle cells. An *EMG* (test of electrical activity in the muscles) and a muscle *biopsy* (removal of a sample of tissue for microscopic analysis) may be performed.

TREATMENT AND OUTLOOK

There is no effective treatment for muscular dystrophy. An affected

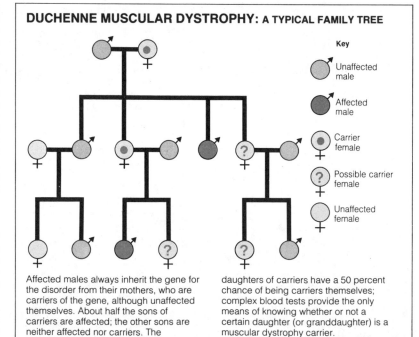

DUCHENNE MUSCULAR DYSTROPHY: A TYPICAL FAMILY TREE

Key

Unaffected male

Affected male

Carrier female

Possible carrier female

Unaffected female

Affected males always inherit the gene for the disorder from their mothers, who are carriers of the gene, although unaffected themselves. About half the sons of carriers are affected; the other sons are neither affected nor carriers. The daughters of carriers have a 50 percent chance of being carriers themselves; complex blood tests provide the only means of knowing whether or not a certain daughter (or granddaughter) is a muscular dystrophy carrier.

M

child should remain active for as long as possible to keep the healthy muscles in good condition. Sufferers should not be allowed to become overweight. Surgery to the heel tendons may assist walking in some cases. The long-term outlook depends on the type of muscular dystrophy.

PREVENTION
Parents or siblings of an affected child should receive *genetic counseling*. Carriers of sex-linked forms of muscular dystrophy can be detected because their blood contains high levels of a particular enzyme and the carrier state can be confirmed by genetic analysis.

Some types of muscular dystrophy can be diagnosed prenatally by *chorionic villus sampling* or *amniocentesis*. Women who are carriers of these types can therefore find out whether a fetus is affected and, if so, may consider terminating the pregnancy.

Musculoskeletal

Relating to muscle and/or bone. The musculoskeletal system is the bony skeleton of the body and the hundreds of muscles attached to it. (See illustrated box, p. 708.)

Mushroom poisoning

There are more than 2,000 species of mushrooms in Canada and people risk poisoning whenever they consume wild varieties. Poisonous mushrooms may look and taste like nonpoisonous ones. Cooking does not destroy the toxins of most species.

Poisonous specimens are found in northern as well as southern Canada. Before eating an unfamiliar wild mushroom, you should positively identify it as a nonpoisonous species, using a handbook.

Some types of mushroom are always poisonous, while others vary according to season; of course, individual sensitivity to the toxins also varies. It is prudent to save an uncooked piece of a mushroom: if the eaten portion makes you ill, identification of the plant and its toxins may aid in treatment.

TYPES, SYMPTOMS, AND TREATMENT
Mild gastrointestinal upset is probably the most frequent form of mushroom poisoning. In Canada, most fatal cases are caused by AMANITA VIROSA (the destroying angel) and its relatives. It looks much like the common meadow mushroom, AGARICUS CAMPESTRIS. The fungus contains highly poisonous protein substances called amatoxins, which attack cells in the lining of the small intestine, liver, and kidneys. Severe abdominal pain, vomiting, and diarrhea usually develop five to 24 hours after eating the mushroom. There is no effective antidote, and treatment consists in keeping the patient alive during the effects of the poisoning. Survivors may have permanent damage to liver, heart, or pancreas.

AMANITA MUSCARIA produces drowsiness, visual disturbances, delirium and muscle tremors usually within two hours. Treatment of this poisoning, and others that develop rapidly, is by gastric lavage (see *Lavage, gastric*). Full recovery usually occurs within 24 hours.

A third type of mushroom poisoning comes from small brown mushrooms that can be mistaken for "magic" mushrooms. Symptoms include vomiting and profuse sweating. There is an antidote for this type of mushroom poisoning; it is *atropine*.

"Magic" mushrooms are a name for any of several small species that contain the hallucinogenic substances psilocybin and psilocin. These are restricted substances in Canada, and possession of them is illegal. These mushrooms may also induce severe or even fatal poisoning.

Mutagen

Any physical or chemical agent that, when applied to a group of living cells, increases the rate of *mutation* in those cells. A mutation is a change in the genetic material within a cell,

TYPES OF MUSCULAR DYSTROPHY

Duchenne muscular dystrophy	In this type, the child is slow in learning to sit up and walk, and does so much later than normal. The condition is rarely diagnosed before the age of 3, but progresses rapidly. Affected children tend to walk with a waddle and have difficulty climbing stairs. In getting up from the floor, the child "climbs up his legs," pushing his hands against his ankles, knees, and thighs. Sometimes there	is curvature of the spine. Despite their weakness, the muscles (especially those in the calves) appear bulky; this is because wasted muscle is replaced by fat. By about the age of 12, affected children are no longer able to walk; few survive beyond their teenage years, usually dying from a chest infection or heart failure. Affected boys often have below-average intelligence.
Becker's muscular dystrophy	This type produces the same symptoms as the Duchenne type, but starts later in childhood and progresses much more	slowly. Patients often reach the age of 50. Both types of dystrophy have sex-linked inheritance.
Myotonic dystrophy	This form affects muscles of the hands and feet. Infants are floppy and slow to develop. The main feature is that the muscles contract strongly but do not relax easily. Myotonic dystrophy	is associated with cataracts in middle age, baldness, mental retardation, and endocrine problems. The condition has an autosomal dominant pattern of inheritance.
Limb-girdle muscular dystrophy	This type takes different forms. It starts in late childhood or early adult life, and progression is slow. The muscles of the hips and shoulders are mainly	affected. Other nerve and muscle conditions must be eliminated before this form of dystrophy can be diagnosed confidently.
Facioscapulohumeral muscular dystrophy	This form usually appears first between the ages of 10 and 40; it affects only the muscles of the upper arms, shoulder girdle, and face. It is inherited in an autosomal	dominant pattern. In this form of muscular dystrophy, progression of the weakness is slow, and severe disability is rare.

M

which may, under certain circumstances, give rise to a cancer or a hereditary disease.

The main mutagens are ionizing *radiation* and some chemicals. The former includes X rays, cosmic rays, and various emissions (e.g., alpha and beta particles, and gamma rays) from nuclear explosions, radioactive fallout, and reactor leaks (see *Radiation hazards*). Similar types of radiation are also emitted (at very low intensity) by certain rocks.

Many chemical *carcinogens* are thought to cause cancers by altering the genetic material within cells, thus acting as mutagens. Chief among them are chemicals in tobacco smoke.

Mutation

A change in a cell's *DNA* (the genetic material contained in *chromosomes* which provides the coded instructions for the cell's activities). Many mutations are neutral or harmless; some are harmful, giving rise to *cancers, birth defects*, and hereditary diseases. Very rarely, a mutation may be beneficial.

CAUSES

A mutation results from a fault in the replication of a cell's DNA in its daughter cells when the cell divides. A daughter cell inherits some faulty DNA, and the fault is copied each time the cell divides, creating a population of cells containing the altered DNA.

Some mutations occur by chance. A steady but low rate of random mutations is caused by natural background *radiation* from the sky and from radioactivity in rocks. Any physical or chemical agent that makes mutations more probable is known as a *mutagen*. The most important mutagens are various types of high-energy radiation (see *Radiation hazards*), and certain chemicals, including some *carcinogens* (cancer-inducing agents), such as the chemicals in tobacco smoke.

TYPES

Some mutations, known as point mutations, affect only a small part of a section of DNA (called a *gene*). Point mutations may lead to the production of defective enzymes or other proteins in the affected cells, thus disrupting their activities.

In other mutations, entire chromosomes or bits of chromosomes are deleted, added, or rearranged in affected cells. This type of mutation may produce greater disruptive effects than a point mutation.

EFFECTS

The effects of a harmful mutation depend on whether the affected cell is a "germ" cell in an ovary or testis (capable of giving rise to an egg or sperm) or whether it is a somatic cell (one of the other cells in the body).

A mutated somatic cell can, at worst, multiply to form a group of abnormal cells within a particular body region. Often these cells die out, are destroyed by the body's *immune system*, or have only a minor local effect. Sometimes, however, they may form the basis for a tumor.

A mutation in a germ cell can have a dramatically different effect. It may be passed on, via an egg or sperm, to a child, who then carries the mutation in all of his or her cells. This may lead to an obvious birth defect or to an abnormality in body chemistry. Furthermore, the child may pass on the mutation to some of his or her descendants. *Genetic disorders* (such as *hemophilia* and *achondroplasia*) stem originally from point mutations that have occurred to the germ cell of a parent, grandparent, or more distant ancestor. Some of these mutations occur frequently; about one third of all cases of hemophilia are caused by new mutations. *Chromosomal abnormalities* (such as *Down's syndrome*) generally result from mutations in the formation of a parental egg or sperm.

BENEFICIAL MUTATIONS

Very rarely, a mutation in a germ cell confers a survival advantage in the face of some environmental stress. People who inherit this mutation tend to survive longer than their peers; some of their children in turn inherit the mutation and pass it on to succeeding generations. Such mutations tend to become more common in a population over many generations as long as the original environmental stress persists.

An example is the mutation that causes sickle cell trait. Carrying this mutation protects against malaria, so it enhances a child's survival chances where malaria is prevalent. The mutation is common in Africa itself and also affects many people of African origin. A double dose of the mutation (inheriting it from both parents) can lead to *sickle cell anemia*.

Mutism

Refusal or inability to speak. Mutism may occur as a symptom of profound congenital *deafness*, severe *manic-depressive illness*, catatonic *schizophrenia*, or a rare form of *conversion disorder*. The term may also be applied to the observance of a vow of silence for religious reasons.

Elective mutism describes a rare childhood disorder usually starting before the age of 5. The child understands language and speaks properly, but refuses to speak most of the time, preferring to use nods or gestures. A shy, withdrawn personality and anxiety about social situations are important factors. In some cases, mild mental retardation or language problems may be the cause. This condition rarely lasts more than a few months.

Akinetic mutism describes a state of inert passivity that is caused by certain deep-seated tumors of the brain or by *hydrocephalus*. Though conscious and capable of following movements with their eyes, people with akinetic mutism are incontinent, require feeding, and respond at most with a whispered "yes" or "no."

Treatment of mutism depends on the underlying cause.

Myalgia

The medical term for *muscle* pain. Myalgia is common in viral illnesses (such as influenza) and also occurs in a number of rheumatic disorders, such as *rheumatoid arthritis*, systemic *lupus erythematosus*, and *polymyalgia rheumatica*. Myalgia is the main symptom of *polymyositis* and *dermatomyositis*, disorders that cause inflammation of muscle tissue.

Myalgic encephalomyelitis

A disorder of unknown cause characterized by severe muscle fatigue on exertion, also known as ME, postviral fatigue syndrome, Iceland disease, and epidemic neuromyasthenia.

CAUSES AND INCIDENCE

Much debate surrounds the cause of myalgic encephalomyelitis. Possible causes include a persistent viral infection, or damage to the *immune system* following a viral infection. Other theories are that the disease is related to a neurotic disorder, to *hysteria*, or to *hyperventilation*.

Myalgic encephalomyelitis sometimes occurs in epidemics, although isolated cases also occur. Females are affected three times more commonly than males, and the peak incidence is between the ages of 30 and 40. The diagnosis became much more frequent in the late 1980s as a result of press publicity.

SYMPTOMS

The disorder commonly follows an upper respiratory tract infection or a gastrointestinal infection, from which the sufferer does not make a full recovery. Fever and headache are fol-

M

lowed by muscle pains, tenderness, weakness, and severe muscle fatigue, particularly on exertion. There may also be general malaise, dizziness, nausea, numbness, and a sensation of pins and needles. Psychological upset, including depression, inability to concentrate, loss of memory, sleep disturbances, and panic states are common features. The condition usually clears up completely in time, but in a few cases symptoms persist over a number of years, sometimes exacerbated by stress.

DIAGNOSIS AND TREATMENT
There is as yet no diagnostic test for myalgic encephalomyelitis; the diagnosis is reached by excluding other disorders which could account for the patient's symptoms. Physical examination and laboratory tests produce normal results, although a high proportion of patients show evidence of recent or current viral infection.

There is no specific cure; treatment is of symptoms. Patients may be advised to rest early in the course of the illness, but to take exercise when they feel well enough to do so. Some sufferers may benefit from *psychotherapy*, and some from avoiding alcohol and caffeine. Many patients try self-treatment by diet, or by using antifungal treatments (believing the disease is linked to *candidiasis*).

Myasthenia gravis
A disorder in which the muscles become weak and tire easily. The eyes, face, throat, and limb muscles are most commonly affected. Typically, the sufferer has drooping eyelids, a blank facial expression, and weak, hesitant speech.

CAUSES AND INCIDENCE
Myasthenia gravis is an *autoimmune disorder* in which, for reasons that are not known, the body's *immune system* attacks and gradually destroys the receptors in muscles that are responsible for picking up nerve impulses. As a result, affected muscles fail to respond or respond only weakly to nerve impulses.

Myasthenia gravis is a rare disease; about five new cases per 100,000 people are diagnosed annually in Canada. It affects more women than men (in a ratio of three to two). Although it can occur at any age, myasthenia gravis usually appears between the ages of 20 and 30 in women, and 50 and 70 in men.

SYMPTOMS AND SIGNS
The disease may develop suddenly or gradually. It is extremely variable in

the way it affects different people and in how it affects the same person from day to day. The affected muscles become worse with use but may recover completely with rest. Symptom-free periods typically alternate with relapses of the condition.

The eye muscles are the most commonly affected, and most sufferers have drooping eyelids and double vision. Weakness is also common in the muscles of the face, throat, larynx (voice box), and neck. This causes difficulty in speaking, so that the voice becomes weak, hoarse, nasal, and slurred toward the end of a conversation. Chewing and swallowing become increasingly difficult as a meal progresses, so that the sufferer may choke or regurgitate food through the nose. Sometimes the jaw must be supported to prevent it from hanging.

In some people, the arm and leg muscles are also affected, producing difficulty in combing the hair and in climbing stairs. In severe cases of myasthenia gravis, respiratory muscles in the chest may be weakened, causing breathing difficulty.

Infection, menstruation, medications, stress, and other factors can exacerbate the condition.

Abnormalities in the *thymus* gland are present in about three quarters of affected people and, in about 10 to 15 percent of them, a *thymoma* (tumor of the thymus gland) is found.

DIAGNOSIS
The disease is diagnosed by a physical examination, the patient's history, and various tests. The most commonly used diagnostic test involves the injection of the drug edrophonium into a vein. Within a minute, power is temporarily restored to the weak muscles. *EMG*, which detects muscle weakness by measuring the muscle's electrical activity, and blood tests that reveal the presence of certain *antibodies* may also be performed.

In some patients, mainly those over 40, *CT scanning* may be performed to look for a thymoma.

TREATMENT
In mild cases of myasthenia gravis, regular medication with drugs to facilitate the transmission of nerve impulses to the muscles is often sufficient to restore the patient's condition to near normal.

In severe myasthenia gravis, thymectomy (removal of the thymus gland) often considerably improves, and sometimes cures, the condition. Otherwise, regular exchanges of the patient's antibody-containing plasma

for antibody-free plasma may be carried out. High doses of *corticosteroid drugs*, which block the immune process, are sometimes given.

OUTLOOK
In mild cases, the sufferer is able to live a comparatively normal life. In a minority of patients, progression of the disease cannot be halted and paralysis of the throat and respiratory muscles may lead to death.

Mycetoma

An uncommon tropical infection affecting skin and bone, caused by fungi or by actinomycetes (bacteria that form long chainlike colonies).

The infection is usually confined to one limb and can be highly disfiguring. It produces a hard swelling covered by the openings of multiple drainage channels, through which pus is discharged. The disease organisms form into visible "grains," which are found in the discharge.

Antibiotic drugs are the main treatment if the disease is caused by actinomycetes. Mycetoma caused by fungal infections may be difficult to treat with drugs; surgical removal of diseased tissue may be necessary.

Mycology
The study of *fungi* and *fungal infections*.

Mycoplasma
Any of a group of microorganisms which are the smallest capable of free existence. Mycoplasmas are about the same size as viruses and, like viruses, have no cell wall. However, unlike viruses, mycoplasmas can reproduce outside living cells.

Most types of mycoplasma are harmless to humans, although many cause respiratory diseases in animals such as cattle, sheep, and poultry. One species, MYCOPLASMA PNEUMONIAE, causes a form of *pneumonia* (primary atypical pneumonia) in humans. Pneumonia of this type can be treated effectively with antibiotics, such as *tetracycline drugs*.

Mycosis
Any disease caused by a fungus. (See *Fungal infections; Fungi.*)

Mycosis fungoides
A type of *lymphoma* (cancerous tumor of lymphoid tissue) that primarily affects the skin of the buttocks, back, or shoulders but can also occur in other sites. The cause of this rare disorder is unknown.

M

In its mildest form, mycosis fungoides produces a red, scaly rash that does not itch. The rash may spread slowly or remain unaltered for many years. In the more severe forms of the disease, thickened patches of skin and ulcers may develop and *lymph nodes* may enlarge.

DIAGNOSIS AND TREATMENT
A skin *biopsy* (removal of a sample of tissue for examination) is performed to confirm the diagnosis.

Mild cases of the disease are treated with *PUVA* (*psoralen drugs* plus long-wave ultraviolet light treatment) or nitrogen mustard applied to the skin. In more severe cases, *anticancer drugs* may be needed.

Mydriasis
Dilation (widening) of the pupil of the eye. Mydriasis, which occurs naturally in the dark, also occurs if a person is emotionally aroused, after the use of certain eye drops (such as those containing *atropine*), and after consumption of alcohol.

Adie's syndrome is a benign condition in which one pupil constricts slowly in response to light.

Myectomy
Surgical removal of part or all of a muscle. Myectomy may be performed to alter the power of an eye muscle to correct a *squint*, or to remove a fibroid of the uterus in an operation called a *myomectomy*. Myectomy is also part of the treatment of severely injured and infected muscles.

Myel-
A prefix that denotes a relationship to *bone marrow* (as in *multiple myeloma*, a disorder in which certain bone marrow cells proliferate) or to the *spinal cord* (as in *myelitis*, inflammation of the spinal cord). The prefix myelo- is synonymous with myel-.

Myelin
The fatty material, composed of lipid (fat) and protein, that forms a protective sheath around some types of nerve fiber. Myelin gives the characteristic appearance to the white matter of the brain, which is composed largely of myelinated nerve fibers. In addition to having a protective function, myelin acts as an electrical insulator, thereby increasing the efficiency of nerve impulse conduction.

Abnormal breakdown of myelin is called *demyelination*. It occurs in some diseases of the nervous system, notably *multiple sclerosis*.

Myelitis
Inflammation of the spinal cord. Myelitis may be the result of a viral infection—for example, *poliomyelitis* (commonly called polio), *measles*, or *herpes simplex*. The disorder starts suddenly with headache, fever, neck stiffness, and pain in the back and limbs, followed in some cases by muscle pain and weakness, and eventually by paralysis.

Transverse myelitis is a type of myelitis in which there is inflammation of the spinal cord around the middle of the back. The condition may follow a viral illness but often occurs without obvious cause. Common symptoms are back pain and gradual paralysis of the legs. Many people recover, but some are left with *spastic paralysis* of the limbs involved.

Myelocele
A protrusion of the *spinal cord* and its meninges (protective coverings) under the skin due to a congenital defect in the vertebral column (see *Spina bifida*).

Myelography
X-ray examination of the spinal cord, nerves, and other tissues within the spinal canal after injection of a contrast medium (a substance that is opaque to X rays).

WHY IT IS DONE
In the past, myelography was performed to examine the lower spinal nerves when a *disk prolapse* was suspected; it was also important in diagnosing tumors of the spinal cord, and in locating damaged nerves.

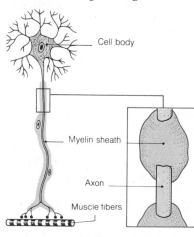

Cell body

Myelin sheath

Axon

Muscle fibers

The myelin nerve sheath
The axon is the conducting fiber of a nerve. To transmit impulses more efficiently, some nerve axons have a myelin sheath.

Myelography is being replaced today by newer imaging techniques, such as *CT scanning* and *MRI*.

HOW IT IS DONE
The patient lies on the X-ray table. After giving a local anesthetic, a *lumbar puncture* is performed, using X-ray control to guide a fine needle into the fluid-filled space that surrounds the spinal cord and spinal nerves. A small sample of spinal fluid is withdrawn for testing, and the radiopaque contrast medium is introduced. By tilting the patient head-down, the contrast medium can be moved up the spinal canal. X-ray pictures are then taken of areas where damage is suspected. The entire procedure usually takes 15 to 20 minutes. Afterward, the patient must lie down for a few hours with the head slightly raised.

Myeloma, multiple
See *Multiple myeloma*.

Myelomatosis
See *Multiple myeloma*.

Myelomeningocele
Another name for myelocele (see *Spina bifida*).

Myelopathy
A term that refers to any disease of the *spinal cord*.

Myelosclerosis
An increase of fibrous tissue within the *bone marrow*, also known as osteosclerosis or myelofibrosis. In myelosclerosis, the ability of the bone marrow to produce blood components is impaired, although this function can be partly taken over by the spleen and liver.

Myelosclerosis may be primary (i.e., occurring without any obvious cause) or secondary (resulting from some other bone marrow disease, such as *polycythemia* or chronic myeloid *leukemia*). Primary myelosclerosis most commonly occurs in middle age and has a gradual onset.

The main symptoms of myelosclerosis are those of *anemia*, caused by impaired red blood cell production by the bone marrow. Enlargement of the spleen, night sweats, itching, loss of appetite, and weight loss are other common symptoms of myelosclerosis. In secondary myelosclerosis, there may be other symptoms connected with the underlying disease.

TREATMENT
Treatment of primary myelosclerosis is aimed at the relief of symptoms,

M

mainly by means of *blood transfusions*. Only 50 percent of patients survive for more than three years after the onset of the disease. A few patients develop acute leukemia.

Treatment of secondary myelosclerosis depends on the underlying cause of the condition.

Myiasis

An infestation of the skin, deeper tissues, or intestines by fly larvae. Myiasis is primarily restricted to tropical regions of the world.

TYPES AND SYMPTOMS
In Africa, the tumbu fly lays eggs on clothing left outside to dry; the larvae that hatch from these eggs penetrate the skin to cause boillike swellings with a central small hole through which the larva breathes. Various other flies may lay eggs in open wounds, on the skin, or in the ears or nose. Sometimes the larvae penetrate deeply into the tissues, causing considerable destruction. Intestinal infestation can occur after eating contaminated food.

PREVENTION AND TREATMENT
Myiasis can largely be prevented by keeping flies away from food, by covering open wounds, and, in Africa, by thoroughly ironing clothes dried outdoors.

Cutaneous myiasis is treated by placing drops of oil over the swelling caused by the larva. The oil suffocates the larva, which is forced to come to the surface and can then be removed with a needle. Infestation in deeper tissues may require surgical treatment. Intestinal myiasis can be adequately treated with a laxative.

Myo-
A prefix that denotes a relationship to *muscle* (as in myocarditis, inflammation of the heart muscle).

Myocardial infarction
Sudden death of part of the *heart* muscle, characterized, in most cases, by severe unremitting chest pain. The disorder is popularly known as a heart attack.

Each year in Canada about 53,000 people are hospitalized for a myocardial infarction, and about 26,000 die from this cause. Myocardial infarction is the single most common cause of death in developed countries.

Men are more likely to suffer a myocardial infarction than women, and smokers are at greater risk than nonsmokers. The children of some-one who has died of a myocardial infarction are more likely than average to die from this cause. Other risk factors include increased age, unhealthy diet, obesity, and disorders such as *hypertension* (high blood pressure), *diabetes mellitus*, and *hyperlipidemias*. Most people who suffer a myocardial infarction have atherosclerosis of the coronary arteries (see illustrated box on page 716).

SYMPTOMS AND COMPLICATIONS
The characteristic symptom is sudden pain in the center of the chest (see illustrated box). The victim may also be short of breath, restless, and apprehensive, have cold clammy skin, feel nauseated or vomit (or both), or lose consciousness.

In mild cases, the pain and other symptoms are slight or do not develop at all (in which case the attack is known as a silent infarct). As a result, the episode usually passes unnoticed and may be discovered only by subsequent tests.

Damage to the heart muscle may be so severe that it leads immediately to *heart failure* (reduced pumping efficiency of the heart). *Arrhythmias* (abnormal heart rhythms) are common. Most people who die of a myocardial infarction do so within the first few hours due to a type of arrhythmia called ventricular fibrillation, which seriously interferes with the heart's pumping action. However, if the person can be brought to a hospital, arrhythmias can be controlled with drugs or electrical *defibrillation*.

Possible long-term complications include damage to the mitral valve, leading to *mitral insufficiency*, or the development of a weak area in the wall of the heart or in the muscle dividing the two sides of the heart. Complications may require surgery.

DIAGNOSIS
The diagnosis is made from the patient's history and from special tests. Those performed immediately include *ECG* and the measurement of certain *enzymes* released into the blood from damaged heart muscle. Emergency coronary artery *angiography* may be performed if surgery is being considered.

TREATMENT
If someone is thought to be having a myocardial infarction, a physician or ambulance should be called immediately. Initial treatment may include strong *analgesic drugs* (painkillers) and *oxygen therapy*. *Diuretic drugs* may be given to treat heart failure, which can lead to accumulation of fluid in the lungs. An *intravenous infusion* of fluids may need to be given for shock, and *antiarrhythmic drugs* may be given to control disturbances of heart rhythm. *Beta-blocker drugs* are given in some cases to reduce the risk of further muscle damage.

In many hospitals, patients who arrive within three to six hours of a myocardial infarction are now treated with *thrombolytic drugs* to dissolve any blood clot. Other new methods of treatment include *angioplasty* (widening of narrowed coronary arteries), which may follow the thrombolytic treatment. *Coronary artery bypass* surgery may be considered.

In the past, it was recommended that patients should rest in bed for two weeks or more following a myocardial infarction. Today, however, patients are encouraged to be out of bed within four or five days.

It is increasingly common for patients suffering from a myocardial infarction to be supervised in special hospital coronary care units. The nursing and medical staff are trained to recognize and institute early treatment for arrhythmias, and many patients find the environment reassuring. However, some specialists believe coronary care units are actually more stressful than the regular hospital rooms and recommend that some patients are cared for elsewhere in hospital or at home.

OUTLOOK
Anyone who has suffered a myocardial infarction has an increased risk of suffering another one in the following few years. Such people should have their medical condition assessed by their physicians at regular intervals for life. The chances of surviving for many years can be improved by taking appropriate action to reduce risk factors (see table on the following page).

Myocarditis
Inflammation of the *heart* muscle, usually caused by an infection. Myocarditis is often accompanied by *pericarditis* (inflammation of the outer lining of the heart).

CAUSES
The most common cause of myocarditis is a viral infection, usually due to a coxsackievirus. Mild myocarditis often accompanies viral infections of the lungs. In rare cases, myocarditis is caused by a bacterial infection.

Myocarditis is a characteristic feature of *rheumatic fever*. In rare cases, myocarditis is caused by drugs or *radiation therapy*.

FEATURES OF MYOCARDIAL INFARCTION

Myocardial infarction, in which an area of heart muscle is deprived of blood supply and suffers tissue death as a result, is a major cause of death in developed countries. Atherosclerosis of the coronary arteries is the cause in most cases of myocardial infarction.

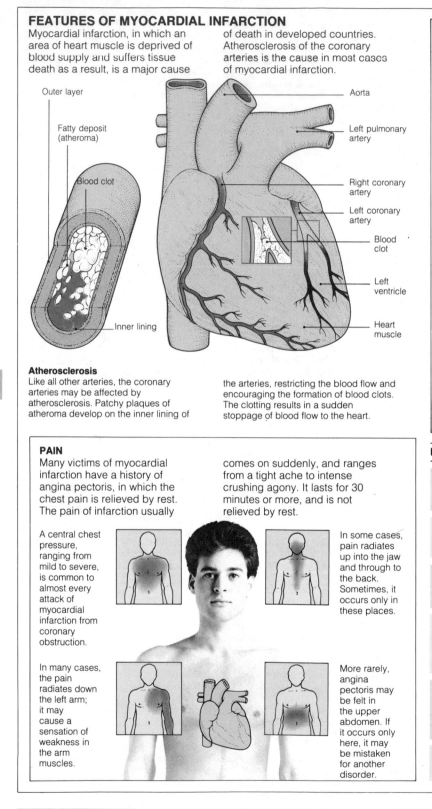

Outer layer

Fatty deposit (atheroma)

Blood clot

Inner lining

Aorta

Left pulmonary artery

Right coronary artery

Left coronary artery

Blood clot

Left ventricle

Heart muscle

Atherosclerosis

Like all other arteries, the coronary arteries may be affected by atherosclerosis. Patchy plaques of atheroma develop on the inner lining of the arteries, restricting the blood flow and encouraging the formation of blood clots. The clotting results in a sudden stoppage of blood flow to the heart.

M

PAIN

Many victims of myocardial infarction have a history of angina pectoris, in which the chest pain is relieved by rest. The pain of infarction usually comes on suddenly, and ranges from a tight ache to intense crushing agony. It lasts for 30 minutes or more, and is not relieved by rest.

A central chest pressure, ranging from mild to severe, is common to almost every attack of myocardial infarction from coronary obstruction.

In many cases, the pain radiates down the left arm; it may cause a sensation of weakness in the arm muscles.

In some cases, pain radiates up into the jaw and through to the back. Sometimes, it occurs only in these places.

More rarely, angina pectoris may be felt in the upper abdomen. If it occurs only here, it may be mistaken for another disorder.

OUTLOOK AFTER AN ATTACK

After a myocardial infarction serious enough to require medical care (some are painless and are not detected at the time they happen) the period of greatest risk is the first 20 days after the attack. Many have a long survival, especially if they can modify the risk factors that caused the heart attack.

SURVIVAL RATES

67%

55-64%

20-39%

Percentage alive after 20 days

Percentage alive after one year

Percentage alive after 10 years

RISK FACTORS

Uncontrollable factors include a family history of heart disease, old age, and being male.

Habitual cigarette smokers have a substantially increased risk of dying from myocardial infarction.

High blood pressure is a major risk factor, and the risk increases the higher the pressure.

The risk of atherosclerosis and coronary artery disease increases dramatically in those who are more than 30 percent overweight.

A raised blood cholesterol level (for which there may be a genetic tendency) increases the risk. A high-fat diet is also a factor.

Physical inactivity is also a major risk factor.

In Central and South America, the most common cause of myocarditis is the parasitic infection *Chagas' disease.* Many years after the initial infection, extensive myocarditis leads to progressive heart failure, which is fatal in many cases.

SYMPTOMS AND SIGNS
Myocarditis often causes no symptoms. Rarely, there may be a serious disturbance of the heartbeat, breathlessness, chest pain, and *heart failure* (reduced pumping efficiency of the heart). In severe cases, death may result from *cardiac arrest.*

DIAGNOSIS
Myocarditis may be suspected from the patient's history, which often includes a recent infection of the upper respiratory tract, and from a physical examination. An *ECG* will show characteristic abnormalities of the heartbeat.

In some cases, a diagnosis of myocarditis is made at a postmortem examination performed after a young person has died unexpectedly during vigorous exercise.

TREATMENT
There is no specific treatment for myocarditis. Bed rest is usually recommended. Exercise should be avoided until an ECG shows a normal pattern. *Corticosteroid drugs* are occasionally prescribed to reduce inflammation.

Myoclonus
Rapid and uncontrollable jerking or spasm of a muscle or muscles, which may occur either at rest or during movement.

Myoclonus may be associated with a disorder affecting the muscles or nervous system. It may occur during an epileptic seizure (see *Epilepsy*) or as a feature of *encephalitis* (inflammation of the brain).

Myoclonus also occurs in healthy people. An example is the twitching of the limbs that often occurs shortly before falling asleep.

Myofascial pain disorder
An ill-defined but common syndrome of localized pain or discomfort in the muscles and connective tissues of an area of the body, usually around a joint. The syndrome may be due to postural strain or injury. If no underlying disease is found, symptomatic treatment may be effective.

Myoglobin
The oxygen-carrying pigment in muscles. Myoglobin consists of a combination of iron and protein, and gives muscles their red color. Like *hemoglobin* (the oxygen-carrying pigment in red blood cells), myoglobin takes up and then stores oxygen, which it releases when the muscle tissues need oxygen to sustain contraction.

The presence of myoglobin in the urine is known as myoglobinuria. Slight myoglobinuria may occur during prolonged, vigorous exercise. Severe myoglobinuria is usually caused by the release of myoglobin from a large area of damaged muscle, such as occurs in *crush syndrome,* and may cause *kidney failure.*

Myoma
A noncancerous tumor of muscle. The most common type is a *leiomyoma,* which affects the smooth muscle of the intestine, uterus, or stomach.

Myomectomy
Surgical removal of a *myoma* (a noncancerous tumor of muscle). The term is commonly applied to the removal of *fibroids* of the uterus.

Myopathy
A disease of *muscle* that is not caused by disease of the nervous system. Most myopathies are *degenerative disorders; muscular dystrophy* is an example. Others are caused by chemical poisoning, or by a chronic disorder of the *immune system,* or occur as a side effect of a drug. (See also *Muscle* disorders box.)

Myopia
An error of *refraction* in which near objects can be seen clearly while those in the distance appear blurred. Commonly called nearsightedness, myopia is caused by the *eye* being too long from front to back. As a result, images of distant objects are focused in front of the retina.

Myopia, which tends to be inherited, usually appears around puberty and increases progressively until the early 20s, when it stabilizes. Myopia that starts in early childhood often progresses into adult life, and may become very severe.

If myopia is detected during a *vision test,* concave *glasses* (or *contact lenses*) may be prescribed to sharpen distant vision.

Myositis
Inflammation of muscle tissue that causes pain, tenderness, and weakness. Types of myositis include *pleurodynia* (a viral infection that affects muscles around the rib cage), myositis

ossificans (in which damaged muscle is replaced by bone), *polymyositis* (inflammation of muscles throughout the body), and *dermatomyositis* (inflammation of muscles plus a rash). Polymyositis and dermatomyositis are *autoimmune disorders.*

Myotomy
A procedure that involves cutting into a muscle. An example is pyloromyotomy—cutting into the muscle surrounding the lower end of the stomach to treat *pyloric stenosis* (narrowing of the stomach's exit).

Myotonia
Inability of a *muscle* to relax after the need for contraction has passed. Myotonia occurs primarily in two forms of myotonic dystrophy: myotonia congenita and dystrophia myotonica. Myotonia congenita starts during infancy and usually improves with age. Dystrophia myotonica is a progressive disorder that starts in early adult life. Drugs, such as procainamide and quinine, may help reduce myotonia.

Myringitis
Inflammation of the eardrum. Myringitis occurs, to some degree, in every case of *otitis media.*

M

THE CAUSE OF MYOPIA
Myopia is caused by the combined power of the cornea and lens being too great in relation to the length of the eyeball.

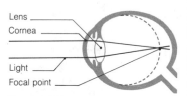

Lens
Cornea
Light
Focal point

Uncorrected myopia
With uncorrected myopia, the images of distant objects are focused in front of the retina and appear blurred.

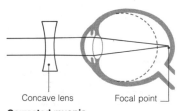

Concave lens   Focal point

Corrected myopia
To see distant objects clearly, the power of the eye must be reduced by a concave (negative) lens.

Myringoplasty

Surgical closure of a perforation (hole) in the eardrum (see *Eardrum, perforated*) by means of a tissue graft. Myringoplasty is performed to improve hearing and, sometimes, to stop a recurrent discharge from the ear. The graft is usually taken from the fibrous covering of a muscle in the temple or thigh.

Myringotomy

A surgical opening made through the eardrum to allow drainage of an accumulation of sticky fluid from the middle ear cavity.

WHY IT IS DONE

Myringotomy is usually performed on children to treat persistent *glue ear*, in which a sticky secretion fills the middle ear cavity. The fluid causes hearing loss, which may become permanent if the condition is not treated before damage occurs.

Before the advent of antibiotics, myringotomy was performed to treat acute *otitis media* (middle ear infection) by releasing the pus and thereby relieving pressure on the eardrum.

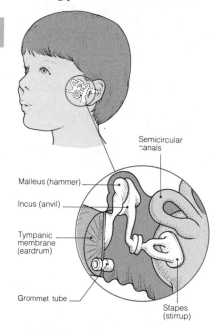

Semicircular canals

Malleus (hammer)

Incus (anvil)

Tympanic membrane (eardrum)

Grommet tube

Stapes (stirrup)

Myringotomy
This operation is performed to treat glue ear. An incision is made in the eardrum, then the thick fluid is sucked out from the middle ear cavity. A grommet (small tube) may be inserted through the eardrum and into the middle ear to equalize pressure on both sides of the eardrum. Sometimes the adenoids are removed while the patient is having the myringotomy operation.

HOW IT IS DONE

With the patient under a general anesthetic, a small incision is made in the eardrum and most of the fluid is removed by suction. At the same time, a *grommet* (small tube) may be inserted into the eardrum to equalize pressure in the outer and middle ears. In most cases, the patient can leave hospital the following day.

Mythomania

An excessive or morbid propensity for exaggerating or lying.

Mytilotoxism

Poisoning due to eating mussels contaminated with mytilotoxin.

Myxedema

A condition in which there is thickening and coarsening of the skin and other body tissues (most noticeable in the face, where the lips become swollen and the nose thickened).

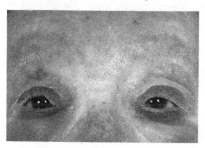

Appearance of myxedema
The person shown in this photograph has characteristics typical of myxedema, notably coarse, dry skin, sparse hair, and puffiness around the eyes.

Myxedema often results from *hypothyroidism* (underactivity of the thyroid gland) and in such cases is commonly accompanied by weight gain, hair loss, sensitivity to cold, and mental dullness. The term myxedema is sometimes used interchangeably with adult hypothyroidism.

Myxoma

A benign, jellylike tumor composed of soft mucous material and loose fibrous strands. Myxomas usually occur singly, and may sometimes grow very large.

The most common site for a myxoma is under the skin (typically in the limbs or neck). Myxomas may also develop in the abdomen, bladder, or bone. Very rarely, a myxoma may grow inside the heart, where it may lead to the formation of thrombi (blood clots) and to the obstruction of

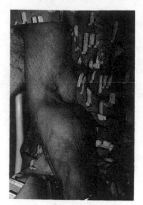

Myxoma on arm
The ball-like swelling on this woman's arm is a myxoma, a form of benign tumor, which grows under the skin.

blood flow through the heart. Myxomas can usually be successfully removed by surgery.

Myxomatosis is a highly infectious viral disease of rabbits in which numerous myxomas develop throughout the body; this disease does not affect humans.

Myxomycetes

A group of microorganisms making up a class of fungi. On the borderline of the plant and animal kingdoms, myxomycetes are sometimes classified as protozoa.

Myxorrhea

A flow of mucus from the bowel. The condition occurs in nervous individuals under stress.

Myxovirus

Any of a large group of RNA-containing viruses. The group includes the influenza and mumps viruses.

M

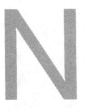

Nadolol

A *beta-blocker drug* used in the treatment of *hypertension* (high blood pressure), *angina pectoris* (chest pain due to impaired blood supply to heart muscle), certain types of *arrhythmia* (irregularity of the heartbeat), and to control symptoms of *hyperthyroidism* (overactivity of the thyroid gland).

Possible adverse effects are typical of other beta-blocker drugs.

Nail

A hard, curved plate on the fingers and toes composed of *keratin* (a tough protein that is also the main constituent of skin and hair). A fingernail takes about six months to grow from base to tip, although there are seasonal growth variations. Toenails take twice as long to grow.

DISORDERS

The nails are susceptible to damage through injury, usually as a result of crushing or pressure on the nail. Sometimes the nails become abnormally thick and curved—a condition called *onychogryphosis* which mainly affects the big toes of elderly people.

Nails may be damaged by bacterial or fungal infections, especially *tinea* and *candidiasis*. In *paronychia* the nail folds are infected. The nails may also be affected by skin disease or by more generalized illnesses.

Examples of the effects of skin disease on the nails include pitting of the nails in *alopecia* areata, pitting and *onycholysis* (separation of the nail from its bed) in *psoriasis*, and scarring and onycholysis in *lichen planus*.

Nail abnormalities may be signs of more generalized disease. Brittle, ridged, concave nails are a sign of iron-deficiency *anemia*, onycholysis is seen in *thyrotoxicosis*, and fibrous growths on the nails are a sign of *tuberous sclerosis*. Splinterlike black marks develop beneath the nails (denoting bleeding into the nail bed) in *endocarditis* and *bleeding disorders*.

Abnormalities of nail color may also signify disease. A greenish discoloration may be caused by bacterial infection under the nail; blue nails may be a sign of heart or respiratory disease; and yellow nails that are hard and curved develop in *bronchiectasis* and *lymphedema*. Nails may also be discolored by nail polish or nicotine.

DIAGNOSIS

Nail disorders are usually diagnosed by inspecting the nails and skin, along with a more extensive physical examination if necessary. Laboratory examination of nail clippings may be performed.

TREATMENT

Treatment of nail disorders is difficult. Creams and lotions seldom penetrate sufficiently; oral medication may take months to be effective.

Nail-biting

A common activity that does not indicate any underlying medical condition. Many children bite their nails during their first years at school, but most grow out of it. Nail-biting sometimes continues as a nervous habit in adolescents and adults. Persistent nail-biting may make the nails unsightly and cause pain and sometimes bleeding.

Various preparations with an unpleasant taste can be painted on the nails, but many people become accustomed to the taste.

ANATOMY OF A NAIL

The nail bed is the area from which the nail grows. At the base of each nail, a half-moon shape, the lunula, is crossed by a flap of skin, the cuticle. The skin that surrounds the nail is the nail fold. The nail is composed of keratin, a tough protein also found in skin and hair.

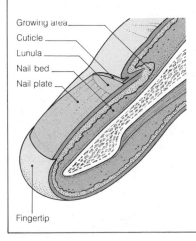

Growing area
Cuticle
Lunula
Nail bed
Nail plate

Fingertip

Nalidixic acid

An *antibiotic drug* used to treat and, occasionally, to prevent *urinary tract infection*. Nalidixic acid is effective against some types of bacteria that are resistant to other antibiotics.

Possible adverse effects include nausea, vomiting, increased sensitivity to sunlight, blurred vision, drowsiness, and dizziness.

Naloxone

A drug that blocks the action of *narcotic drugs*. Naloxone reverses breathing difficulty caused by an overdose of a narcotic drug. It is given to people who have been given high doses of a narcotic drug during surgery. Naloxone is also given to newborns affected by narcotic drugs given to relieve maternal pain during childbirth.

Possible adverse effects include abdominal cramps, diarrhea, nausea, vomiting, and tremors.

Nandrolone

An anabolic steroid (see *Steroids, anabolic*). Nandrolone is sometimes used with *growth hormone* in the treatment of *short stature*. It is also used to treat certain types of *anemia*.

Possible adverse effects include swollen ankles, nausea and vomiting, jaundice, and aggressive behavior. In men, nandrolone may cause difficulty in passing urine. In women, it may cause irregular menstruation and abnormal hair growth.

Naphazoline

A sympathomimetic decongestant that reduces nasal congestion by causing blood vessels to constrict (narrow). Naphazoline comes in liquid or spray form. Overuse can lead to irritation, and rebound congestion may occur after the drug is stopped.

Naproxen

A *nonsteroidal anti-inflammatory drug* (NSAID). Naproxen is used to relieve joint pain and stiffness in different types of *arthritis*. It is also prescribed to hasten recovery following injury to soft tissues, such as muscles or ligaments. Possible adverse effects of naproxen include nausea, abdominal pain, and *peptic ulcer*.

Narcissism

Intense self-love. The term is derived from the Greek myth of Narcissus, who so loved to stare at his own reflection in the water that he fell in and drowned. According to *psychoanalytic theory* there is an early stage in child

N

development when the *ego* (self) feels omnipotent. Failure to deal with the frustrations of discovering that this is not so may later result in *neurosis*.

A narcissistic personality disorder is characterized by an exaggerated sense of self-importance, constant need for attention or praise, inability to cope with criticism or defeat, and poor relationships with other people.

Narcolepsy

A *sleep* disorder characterized by chronic, excessive daytime sleepiness with recurrent episodes of sleep occurring several times per day. Attacks may last from a few seconds to more than an hour and may be mildly inconvenient or severely disabling, often interfering with work and daily life. *Cataplexy* (sudden loss of muscle tone without loss of consciousness) occurs in about three quarters of cases. Other symptoms may include *sleep paralysis* and vivid hallucinations.

Diagnosis is made by the examination of an *EEG* (electrical recording of brain activity). In narcolepsy, the REM (rapid eye movement) state, which normally occurs only during *sleep*, intrudes into wakefulness. Narcolepsy is often inherited. Treatment usually involves regular naps, along with *stimulant drugs* to control drowsiness and sleep attacks, and *antidepressant drugs* to suppress cataplexy.

Narcosis

A state of stupor, which is usually caused by a drug (see *Narcotic drugs*) or other chemical. Narcosis resembles sleep, being marked by reduced awareness and by diminished ability to respond to external stimulation. However, a person in narcosis cannot be roused completely.

Narcotic drugs

COMMON DRUGS

Codeine Diamorphine Dihydrocodeine Meperidine Morphine Oxycodone

A type of *analgesic drug* (painkiller) used to treat moderate and severe pain. Abuse of narcotic drugs for their euphoric effects often causes *tolerance* (the need for greater amounts to have the same effects), and physical and psychological *drug dependence*.

Nasal congestion

Partial blockage of the nasal passage caused by swelling of the *mucous membrane* that lines the *nose*. Swelling of the mucous membrane may be accompanied by the accumulation of thick nasal mucus, which further impedes breathing.

Nasal congestion produces the familiar feelings of a stuffy, "full" nose. There is a frequent desire to blow the nose, but blowing usually has little effect on the congestion.

CAUSES

Nasal congestion is a symptom of the common cold (see *Cold, common*) and of hay fever (see *Rhinitis, allergic*). In these conditions, the swelling is due to inflammation of the membrane that lines the inside of the nose. Inflammation may become persistent in certain disorders, such as chronic *sinusitis* or nasal *polyps*. Nasal congestion may also be caused by certain drugs, such as *reserpine*.

TREATMENT

A very simple, effective, and time-honored method of alleviating nasal congestion is to inhale the steam from a basin of hot water. This loosens the mucus, which enables the sufferer to blow it out through the nose. *Decongestant drugs* in the form of nasal drops and sprays should be used sparingly since prolonged use can make congestion worse. Decongestant tablets and syrups may be recommended for long-term use.

Persistent nasal congestion should be investigated by a physician.

Nasal discharge

The spontaneous emission of fluid from the *nose*. Nasal discharge is commonly caused by inflammation of the mucous lining and is often accompanied by *nasal congestion*.

In allergic *rhinitis*, the discharge consists of runny, clear mucus. Infection of the nasal passage itself, such as occurs in a cold (see *Cold, common*), or an infection that has spread from the sinuses (see *Sinusitis*) usually causes a thicker discharge of mucus, often mixed with pus. A persistent runny discharge of recent onset may be an early indication of a tumor (see *Nasopharynx, cancer of*).

Bleeding from the nose (see *Nosebleed*) is usually caused by injury or a foreign body in the nose. In rare cases, bleeding from the nose may be a sign of an underlying bleeding disorder or a tumor. A discharge of cerebrospinal fluid from the nose may follow a fracture at the base of the skull (see *Skull, fracture of*).

NASAL FEEDING

Feeding through a *nasogastric tube*. (See also *Feeding, artificial*.)

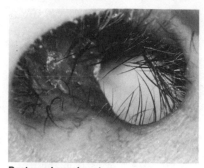

Destroyed nasal septum
This photograph of the left nostril was taken with a light shone into the right nostril. There is a hole in the septum.

Nasal obstruction

Blockage of the nasal passage, which interferes with breathing.

The most common cause of nasal obstruction is inflammation of the *mucous membrane* that lines the passage (see *Nasal congestion*). Other causes include severe deviation of the *nasal septum*, nasal *polyps*, a *hematoma* (a collection of clotted blood) usually caused by injury, and, rarely, a malignant tumor. In children, enlargement of the *adenoids* is the most common cause of nasal obstruction.

Nasal septum

The central partition inside the *nose* that divides it into two. The nasal septum consists of cartilage at the front and bone at the rear, both of which are covered by *mucous membrane*.

DISORDERS

A deviated septum (twisting of the septum to one side) may be present from birth or may be caused by a blow or blows to the nose. The condition is rarely troublesome, but surgery to straighten the septum may be recommended if breathing is obstructed.

Injury may cause a *hematoma* (a collection of clotted blood) to form between the cartilage of the septum and the wall of one nasal cavity. The hematoma may obstruct breathing to varying degrees. Sometimes, a hematoma becomes infected, causing an *abscess*, which may require surgical drainage. Occasionally, an abscess develops on a child's septum without prior injury.

Rarely, a hole may be eroded in the septum by *tuberculosis*, *syphilis*, *Wegener's granulomatosis*, or as a result of sniffing *cocaine*.

Nasogastric tube

A narrow plastic tube that is passed through the nose, down the esophagus, and into the stomach.

WHY IT IS USED
One of its most common uses is to suck or drain digestive juices from the stomach when the intestine is blocked (as in *pyloric stenosis*) or is not working properly (as may occur after an abdominal operation). A nasogastric tube is also used to give liquid nourishment to very ill patients who cannot eat (see *Feeding, artificial*), to obtain specimens of stomach secretions for examination, and to wash out the stomach after a drug overdose or after swallowing a poison (see *Lavage, gastric*).

HOW IT IS USED
Inserting the tube is a quick, simple procedure that causes little discomfort and does not require an anesthetic. After it has been lubricated, the tube is passed into one nostril and then, while the patient is swallowing, slid down the throat and into the stomach. To ensure that the tube is in the stomach, a sample of fluid is withdrawn through a syringe and tested on litmus paper for acidity. The stomach contents are then either sucked out through the syringe or a suction device or are allowed to drain freely into a container; fluids for lavage or feeding are introduced through a funnel. If the tube is to be left in place for some time, the protruding end is taped to the face.

Nasopharynx
The passage connecting the nasal cavity behind the *nose* to the top of the throat behind the soft *palate*. Part of the respiratory tract, the nasopharynx forms the upper section of the *pharynx*. During swallowing, the nasopharynx is sealed off (to prevent food from entering it) by the action of the soft palate pressing against the back of the throat.

The nasopharynx contains the lower openings of the *eustachian tubes*

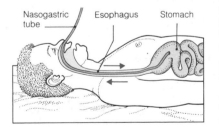

Using a nasogastric tube
The tube is passed via a nostril and the esophagus into the stomach. Substances may be delivered into the stomach via the tube, or the stomach contents may be removed through it.

(passages connecting the back of the nose to the middle ear) and, in children, the *adenoids*. The adenoids can enlarge to such an extent that the nasopharynx becomes completely blocked, forcing the child to breathe through his or her mouth.

Nasopharynx, cancer of
A malignant tumor that originates in the *nasopharynx* (uppermost part of the throat, behind the nose) and usually spreads to the nasal cavity, nasal sinuses, base of the skull, and lymph nodes in the neck.

Cancer of the nasopharynx is rare in the West but common in the Far East; it is most common between the ages of 40 and 50 and affects twice as many men as women. One cause is believed to be the *Epstein-Barr virus*.

SYMPTOMS AND SIGNS
Common first signs are recurrent nosebleeds, a persistently runny nose, and voice change. There may also be a bloody nasal discharge, loss of smell, double vision, deafness, paralysis of one side of the face, and severe facial pain.

DIAGNOSIS AND TREATMENT
The diagnosis is made from a *biopsy* (removal of a small sample of tissue for microscopic analysis). *X rays* may also be taken to determine the extent of the cancer. Treatment of cancer of the nasopharynx is with *radiation therapy*. The outlook depends on when treatment begins; one third of sufferers survive for more than five years.

Natural childbirth
See *Childbirth, natural*.

Naturopathy
A form of *alternative medicine* based on the principle that disease is due to the accumulation of waste products and toxins (poisons) in the body, and that symptoms reflect the body's attempt to rid itself of these substances. Practitioners of naturopathy believe that health is maintained by avoiding anything artificial or unnatural in the diet or in the environment.

Nausea
The sensation of needing to vomit. Although nausea may occur independently of vomiting, the causes are the same (see *Vomiting*).

Navel
A popular term for the *umbilicus*, the depression in the abdomen that marks the point at which the umbilical cord was attached to the fetus.

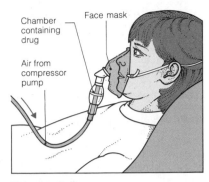

Using a nebulizer
An electric or hand-operated pump sends a stream of air or oxygen across a chamber containing the required drug. This stream of air disperses the drug into a fine mist, which is then conveyed to the face mask and inhaled by the user.

Nearsightedness
See *Myopia*.

Nebulizer
A device used to administer a drug in aerosol form through a face mask or mouthpiece. Nebulizers are used to administer *bronchodilator drugs*, especially in the emergency treatment of an attack of *asthma*. Most patients can use a nebulizer more easily than a conventional *inhaler* (a pressurized aerosol canister).

Neck
The part of the body that supports the head and serves as a passageway between the head and brain and the body.

The neck contains several vital structures: the *spinal cord* (which carries nerve impulses to and from the brain), the *trachea* (windpipe), the *esophagus*, and major blood vessels leading to and from the head. Decapitation kills because it cuts through these vital structures. Strangulation kills by compressing major blood vessels and by cutting off the air supply to the lungs.

DISORDERS
INJURY *Torticollis* (wry neck), in which the head is twisted to one side, may result from birth injury to a neck muscle or from skin *contracture* (shrinkage) after burns or other injuries.

Fractures and *dislocations* of any of the vertebrae in the neck can injure the spinal cord, causing paralysis or even death; *whiplash injuries* can also severely damage the spinal cord (see *Spinal injury*).

DEGENERATION The joints between vertebrae may be affected by *cervical*

N

osteoarthritis, causing neck pain, stiffness, and sometimes tingling and weakness in the arm and hand. Similar symptoms may be caused by a *disk prolapse*. In *ankylosing spondylitis*, fusion of the vertebrae may result in permanent neck rigidity.

CONGENITAL DEFECT *Cervical rib* (a small extra rib in the neck) often causes no symptoms until middle age, when it may result in pain, numbness, and a pins and needles sensation in the forearm and hand.

OTHER DISORDERS Because structures in the neck are so closely packed together (see the illustrated box below), any condition that causes swelling (such as inflammation, allergy, bleeding, or tumors) may, if the swelling is large enough, interfere with breathing or with swallowing.

Enlargement of the lymph nodes usually results from infection, but may be due to other conditions.

Neck pain of unknown origin is very common. As long as neurological symptoms (such as loss of sensation or muscle power) are absent, it is unlikely to be serious. Most sufferers recover within a few weeks.

Neck dissection, radical

A surgical procedure for removing cancerous *lymph nodes* in the neck. The operation is commonly required as part of the treatment of cancer of the tongue, tonsils, or other structures in the mouth and throat.

A flap of skin on the affected side of the neck is raised (under general anesthetic) to expose the underlying sternomastoid muscle. The muscle is cut through just above the clavicle (collarbone) and lifted up. The entire lymphatic system in the neck (the lymph vessels as well as the lymph nodes) is then removed, together with the internal jugular vein, the lower salivary gland, and other surrounding tissue.

Neck rigidity

Marked stiffness of the neck caused by spasm of the muscles in the neck and spine. Neck rigidity is an important clinical sign of *meningitis* (inflammation of the membranes covering the brain and spinal cord). Severe neck rigidity may cause the head to arch backward; this is especially the case in babies.

Necrolysis, toxic epidermal

A severe, blistering rash in which the surface layers of the skin peel off, exposing large areas of red raw skin over the body.

The effects of toxic epidermal necrolysis are similar to those of a severe third-degree burn, with the same potentially serious risks of widespread infection and loss of body fluid and salts from the exposed body surface.

In newborns, the condition is usually caused by staphylococci (a type of bacteria) and is called the scalded skin syndrome. Treatment is with *antibiotic drugs* and sometimes with intravenous fluid replacement.

In adults, the most common cause of toxic epidermal necrolysis is an adverse reaction to a *drug*, particularly a barbiturate, sulfonamide, or penicillin. The condition usually clears up when use of the drug is discontinued. Intravenous fluid replacement is sometimes necessary.

Necrophilia

A rare sexual perversion in which orgasm is achieved by means of sexual acts with dead bodies.

Necropsy

A little-used alternative medical term for an *autopsy* (postmortem examination of a body).

Necrosis

The death of tissue cells. Necrosis can occur as a result of *ischemia* (inadequate blood supply), which may lead to *gangrene*; infection (such as *tuberculosis*); or damage by extreme heat or cold, noxious chemicals (such as acids), or excessive exposure to X rays or other forms of *radiation*.

The appearance of dead tissue depends on the cause of the necrosis and, usually, on the type of tissue affected. For example, in necrosis due to tuberculosis, the dead tissue is soft, dry, and cheeselike; fatty tissue beneath the skin that has died as a result of damage or infection develops into tough scar tissue that may form a firm nodule.

Nelson's syndrome

A rare disorder of the *endocrine system* that causes increased skin pigmentation. Nelson's syndrome results from enlargement of the *pituitary gland*, which sometimes follows removal of both *adrenal glands*—an old treatment for *Cushing's disease*.

Nelson's syndrome is treated by *hypophysectomy* (removal or destruction of the pituitary gland).

Nematodes

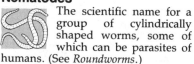 The scientific name for a group of cylindrically shaped worms, some of which can be parasites of humans. (See *Roundworms*.)

Neologism

The act of making up new words that have a special meaning for the inventor. The term also refers to the invented words themselves. Persis-

---

ANATOMY OF THE NECK

The neck contains many important structures, including the larynx, the thyroid and parathyroid glands, many lymph nodes, and the carotid arteries. The upper seven vertebrae of the spine are in the neck; a complex system of muscles is connected to these vertebrae, the clavicles, the upper ribs, and the lower jaw. Contraction of these muscles allows the head to turn and the jaw to open and close.

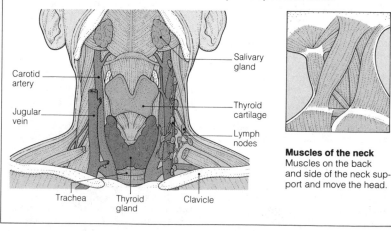

Carotid artery
Jugular vein
Trachea
Thyroid gland
Clavicle
Salivary gland
Thyroid cartilage
Lymph nodes

Muscles of the neck
Muscles on the back and side of the neck support and move the head.

tent neologism can be a feature of speech in people with *schizophrenia*, in which it occurs with other disordered thoughts.

Neomycin
An *antibiotic drug* used in the treatment of ear, eye, and skin infections, often in combination with other drugs. Neomycin is sometimes given to prevent infection of the intestine prior to surgery. Possible adverse effects include rash and itching.

Neonate
An infant under the age of one month (see *Newborn*).

Neonatology
Neonatology is a specialty in pediatrics, usually requiring two additional years of training. A premature baby, one with a serious defect such as *spina bifida*, or one in neonatal intensive care, is usually under the care of a neonatologist until he or she is discharged from the hospital.

Neoplasia
A medical term for *tumor* formation, characterized by a progressive, abnormal multiplication of cells. The term neoplasia does not necessarily imply that the new growth is *malignant*; *benign* tumors also develop as a result of neoplasia.

Neoplasm
A medical term for a *tumor* (any new, abnormal growth). Neoplasms may be *malignant* or *benign*.

Neostigmine
A drug used in the treatment of *myasthenia gravis* (a rare autoimmune disorder that causes muscle weakness). Neostigmine works by increasing the activity of *acetylcholine*, a *neurotransmitter* (chemical released from nerve endings) that stimulates the contraction of muscles.

Possible adverse effects include nausea and vomiting, increased salivation, diarrhea, abdominal cramps, blurred vision, sweating, muscle cramps, twitching, and rash.

Nephrectomy
Surgical removal of one or both of the *kidneys*.
WHY IT IS DONE
One of the most common reasons for nephrectomy is to remove a malignant tumor (see *Kidney cancer*). A kidney may also be removed if it is not functioning normally due to infection or the presence of stones (see *Calculus, urinary tract*), or is causing severe *hypertension* (high blood pressure). Nephrectomy may also be necessary if a kidney is so badly injured that bleeding cannot be stopped.
HOW IT IS DONE
Nephrectomy is carried out under general anesthesia. The patient lies on his or her side, bent sharply at the waist over an angled operating table. An incision is made along the lower edge of the ribs, from the spine to the front of the abdomen, in order to expose the kidney. The *ureter* and renal blood vessels are tied off, and the kidney is removed. The incision is stitched up after insertion of a drainage tube, which is left in position for 24 to 48 hours.
OUTLOOK
A person's kidney function becomes virtually normal about six months after removal of a single kidney because the remaining kidney (providing it is healthy) takes over the entire work load. If both kidneys are removed, the patient requires *dialysis* or a *kidney transplant*.

Nephritis
Inflammation of one or both *kidneys*. Nephritis may be caused by infection (see *Pyelonephritis*), by abnormal responses of the *immune system* (see *Glomerulonephritis*), or by metabolic disorders, such as *gout*. (See also *Kidney* disorders box.)

Nephroblastoma
A cancer, also known as *Wilms' tumor*, which is found mainly in children under 4 years of age. (See *Kidney cancer*.)

Nephrocalcinosis
The deposition of calcium within the substance of one or both *kidneys*. Nephrocalcinosis is not the same as kidney stones (see *Calculus, urinary tract*), in which calcium particles develop within the drainage channels of the kidney.

Nephrocalcinosis may occur in any condition in which the blood level of calcium is raised—for example, *hyperparathyroidism* (overactivity of the parathyroid gland) and *renal tubular acidosis* (in which the kidney produces urine of lower than normal acidity). Nephrocalcinosis may also develop as a result of taking excessive amounts of certain *antacid drugs* or *vitamin D*.

Treatment in nephrocalcinosis is of the underlying cause so that further calcification may be prevented.

Nephrolithotomy
The surgical removal of a *calculus* (stone) from the *kidney* by cutting into the main part of the kidney. Nephrolithotomy may be performed through an abdominal incision, or through a puncture incision made through the skin of the back directly into the kidney (a technique known as percutaneous nephrolithotomy). Instruments are used to grasp and remove the calculus; large calculi may need to be broken up before removal.

Other methods used for removing calculi from the kidneys are *pyelolithotomy* (a surgical procedure in which a calculus is removed through a cut at the renal pelvis) and *lithotripsy* (a nonsurgical procedure in which ultrasonic waves are used to break up calculi for excretion).

Nephrology
The medical specialty concerned with the normal functioning of the *kidneys*, and with the causes, diagnosis, and treatment of kidney disease.

Methods of investigating the kidneys include kidney *biopsy*, *kidney function tests*, and *kidney imaging* techniques (such as intravenous *urography*). Treatment of kidney disorders includes drugs (to control high blood pressure, inflammation, or infection), surgical intervention (for the treatment of stones and tumors), and *dialysis* or, in some cases, a *kidney transplant* (for the treatment of advanced kidney disease).

Nephron
The microscopic unit of the *kidney* consisting of a glomerulus (filtering funnel) and a tubule. There are about 1 million nephrons in each kidney. The nephrons filter waste products from the blood and modify the amount of salts and water excreted in the urine according to the body's needs.

Nephropathy
A term for any disease or damage to the kidneys (see *Kidney* disorders box).

Obstructive nephropathy refers to kidney damage caused by a urinary tract *calculus* (stone), tumor, scar tissue, or pressure from an organ blocking urine flow and creating back pressure within the kidney.

Reflux nephropathy refers to kidney damage caused by backflow of urine from the bladder toward the kidney. It is caused by failure of the valve mechanism at the lower end of the ureter.

N

Toxic nephropathy refers to damage caused by various poisons or minerals (such as carbon tetrachloride or lead).

Nephrosclerosis

A process in which normal *kidney* structures are replaced with scar tissue. Nephrosclerosis usually represents the final healing stage of any of the various conditions that cause inflammation within the kidney. Examples of such conditions include *diabetes mellitus*, *glomerulonephritis*, and chronic *pyelonephritis*.

Nephrosis

See *Nephrotic syndrome*.

Nephrostomy

The introduction of a small tube into the *kidney* to drain urine to the abdominal surface, thus bypassing the ureter and bladder. Nephrostomy is sometimes performed after an operation (typically removal of a *calculus*) on the ureter or kidney-ureter junction.

Nephrotic syndrome

A collection of symptoms and signs that results from damage to the glomeruli (filtering units of the *kidney*), causing severe *proteinuria* (loss of protein from the bloodstream into the urine). Loss of large amounts of protein in the urine lowers the protein content of the blood, resulting in *edema*.

CAUSES

Nephrotic syndrome may be caused by *diabetes mellitus*, *glomerulonephritis* (inflammation of the glomeruli), *amyloidosis* (a condition in which amyloid, an abnormal protein, collects in tissues), severe *hypertension* (high blood pressure), reactions to poisons (e.g., lead and carbon tetrachloride), and adverse *drug* reactions.

SYMPTOMS

Edema causes marked swelling of the legs and face. Fluid may also collect in the chest cavity (producing *pleural effusion*) or within the abdomen (causing *ascites*). Anorexia, lethargy, and diarrhea may also occur.

TREATMENT

Treatment is of the underlying condition. A low-sodium diet may be recommended, and *diuretic drugs* may be given to reduce edema. If the concentration of protein in the blood is particularly low, protein may need to be given intravenously.

Nerve

A bundle of nerve fibers which travel to a common location. Nerve fibers, also called axons, are the filamentous projections of many individual *neurons* (nerve cells).

The most obvious nerves in the body are the peripheral nerves, which extend from the *central nervous system* (consisting of the *brain* and *spinal cord*) to other parts of the body.

STRUCTURE

There are 12 pairs of *cranial nerves* (which link directly to the brain) and 31 pairs of *spinal nerves* (which join the spinal cord). All these nerves are peripheral nerves.

In the shoulder and hip regions, the spinal nerves join to form plexuses, from which branch the main nerves to the limbs, such as the median nerve in the arm and the sciatic nerve in the leg. Most nerves divide at numerous points along their length to send branches to all parts of the body, particularly to the sense organs, the skin, skeletal muscles, internal organs, and glands.

FUNCTION

Nerve fibers may have a sensory function, carrying information from a receptor or sense organ at the far end of the nerve toward the central nervous system (CNS), or they may have a motor function, carrying instructions from the CNS to a muscle or to a gland.

Messages are carried by electrical impulses propagated along the fibers. Some nerves carry only sensory or motor fibers, but most carry both.

Nerve functioning is sensitive to cold, pressure, and to a wide variety of injuries (see *Nerve injury*). The peripheral nerves can be damaged by infection, inflammation, poisoning, nutritional deficiencies, and metabolic disorders (see *Neuropathy*).

Nerve block

The injection of a local anesthetic into or around a nerve to produce anesthesia (loss of sensation) in a part of the body supplied by that nerve.

WHY IT IS DONE

A nerve block is performed when it is not possible to inject anesthetic directly into the tissues that are being treated because the area is painfully inflamed or because there is a risk of spreading infection.

Nerve block may also be used to anesthetize a large area, or an area which is not suitable for injection because it is deep within the body or is covered with bone.

HOW IT IS DONE

The local anesthetic is injected at an accessible area into or around the nerve at a point remote from the area to be treated (for example, the palm of the hand may be anesthetized by giving injections at sites up the arm, thus blocking the ulnar and the median nerves).

A nerve may be blocked as it leaves the spinal cord. This is done in *epidural anesthesia*, which is used mainly in childbirth, and in *spinal anesthesia*, which is used mainly for surgery of the lower abdomen and limbs. A caudal block is a type of nerve block in which an anesthetic is injected around nerves leaving the lowest part of the spinal cord. It produces anesthesia in the buttock and genital areas, and is occasionally used in childbirth, especially in a *forceps delivery*.

In a pudendal nerve block, an anesthetic is injected into nerves passing under the pelvis into the floor of the vagina. This type of nerve block is sometimes used in a forceps delivery. (See also *Anesthesia, local*.)

Nerve injury

Damage or severance of some or all of the conducting fibers within a *nerve* as a result of trauma. (See *Neuropathy* for nerve damage from causes other than injury.)

Nerves may be damaged in many different injuries, including knife wounds, bullet wounds, penetrating injuries (such as from flying glass, for example), or from accidental contact with powered devices (such as rotary saws and propellers).

PERIPHERAL NERVE INJURY

If injury to a peripheral nerve (i.e., a nerve outside the brain or spinal cord) results in severence of some, but not all, of the individual fibers within the nerve, the cut fibers degenerate on both sides of the injury, leading to loss of power in the muscles and loss of sensation in the skin area supplied by the fibers.

In cases of partial severence in which the ends of the severed fibers are still aligned, new fibers can regenerate along the channels left by the degenerated fibers. These fibers begin to grow within a few days of an injury and continue at a rate of about 2.5 cm per month.

If injury results in total severence of a nerve, the individual fibers try to regenerate but, in the absence of directing channels, simply bunch up to form a lump of tissue; there is no recovery of function.

Regenerating nerve fibers sometimes pass down the wrong channels; as a result, when function is restored, actions may differ from what was intended (for example, an attempt to move the index finger may move the middle finger as well). Movement skills and the interpretation of sensations may need to be relearned.

BRAIN AND SPINAL CORD INJURY

Nerve tracts within the brain and spinal cord are structurally different from the peripheral nerves, and severed fibers in these tracts do not regenerate. For example, it is impossible for vision to be restored if the *optic nerves* are cut.

TREATMENT

Surgery can sometimes repair a severed nerve, but such treatment is possible only for peripheral nerves. Using *microsurgery*, the neurosurgeon ensures that the severed fibers are meticulously brought together and stitched into place with delicate needles and sutures. Careful realignment of the nerve ends gives the fibers the best chance of regenerating along the correct channels. Even with the best surgical repair, recovery is rarely complete.

A program of *physiotherapy* is needed to keep paralyzed muscles healthy and free from *contractures* (abnormal shortening) during the recovery period.

Nerve, trapped

Compression or stretching of a *nerve*, causing numbness, tingling, weakness, and sometimes pain in the area supplied by the nerve.

Common examples of a trapped nerve include *carpal tunnel syndrome*, in which symptoms appear in the thumb, index, and middle fingers as a result of pressure on the median nerve as it passes through the wrist; a *disk prolapse*, in which pressure on the nerve root leading from the spinal cord produces symptoms in the back and legs; and *crutch palsy* (sometimes called Saturday night palsy), in which the radial nerve is pressed against the humerus (upper arm bone), producing symptoms in the wrist and hand.

A damaged nerve may take some time to heal, causing symptoms to persist. Surgical decompression to relieve pressure on the nerve may be necessary in severe cases.

Nervous breakdown

A popular term used to describe unusual behavior that is thought to be part of a crisis of severe *anxiety* or tension or part of a psychiatric illness. The term has no technical meaning, but is often applied to people subject to sudden tearfulness, episodes of shouting and screaming, marked social withdrawal, and concern about the possibility of illness.

Nervous energy

A popular term for the increased drive and activity of individuals who are always restless, anxious, and on the go. The term has no technical meaning.

Nervous habit

A nontechnical term for a minor repetitive movement or activity. Sometimes a nervous habit consists of involuntary twitches and facial tics, such as in *Gilles de la Tourette's syndrome* and some forms of *dyskinesia*.

Voluntary nervous habits, such as *thumb-sucking* and nose picking, are common in young children, but usually disappear naturally with time. Also common is *nail biting*, which often persists into adult life (20 percent of adults bite their nails). Such habits are thought to be a means of releasing inner tension.

All nervous habits increase during tension or anxiety, and may be severe in some forms of *depression, anxiety disorder*, or drug withdrawal.

Nervous system

The body's information-gathering, storage, and control system.

STRUCTURE

The nervous system is organized like a computer system that controls a highly complex machine. The central processing unit for the system is the *central nervous system* (CNS), comprising the *brain* and *spinal cord*, which consists of billions of interconnecting *neurons* (nerve cells).

Input of information to the CNS comes from the sense organs. Output (motor) instructions go to the skeletal muscles, muscles controlling speech, internal organs and glands, and the sweat glands in the skin. The cables along which this information is carried are the *nerves* that fan out from the CNS to the entire body. Each nerve is a bundle of the axons (filamentous projections) of many neurons.

In addition to these anatomical divisions of the nervous system, there are various functional divisions. Two of the most important are the *autonomic nervous system*, which is specifically concerned with the automatic (unconscious) regulation of internal body functioning, and the somatic nervous system, which controls the skeletal muscles responsible for voluntary (willed) movement.

FUNCTION

The overall function of the nervous system is to gather information about the external environment and the body's internal state, to analyze this information, and to initiate appropriate responses aimed at satisfying certain drives. The most powerful drive is for survival. Many survival responses, which range from avoiding physical pain and danger to shivering in response to cold, are initiated unconsciously and automatically by the nervous system.

Other drives are more complex, revolving around a need to experience positive emotions (such as pleasure and excitement) and to avoid negative emotions (such as pain, anxiety, and frustration).

In carrying out its functions, the nervous system has access to many built-in programs, but it can also improve its performance through *learning*, which relies on *memory*.

The nervous system functions largely through automatic responses to various stimuli (see *Reflex*), although voluntary actions can also be initiated through the activity of higher, conscious areas of the brain. Certain higher functions (such as visual perception, memory, thought, and speech) are extremely complex and not understood in detail. In general, all nervous activity is based on the transmission of impulses through complex networks of neurons.

DISORDERS

Disorders of the nervous system may result from damage to or dysfunction of its component parts (see *Brain* disorders box; *Nerve injury*; *Neuropathy*; *Spinal cord*). Disorders of the nervous system may also be due to impairment of sensory, analytical, or memory functions (see *Agnosia*; *Amnesia*; *Anosmia*; *Deafness*; *Numbness*; *Vision, disorders of*) or of motor functions (see *Aphasia*; *Ataxia*; *Dysarthria*).

Netilmicin

An *antibiotic drug* usually prescribed only in hospital to treat serious infection, when other antibiotic drugs have been ineffective. In rare cases, netilmicin can damage the inner ear or the kidneys.

Nettle rash

A common name for *urticaria*.

Neuralgia

Pain caused by irritation of, or damage to, a *nerve*. The pain usually occurs in brief bouts, may be very severe, and

NERVOUS SYSTEM

The nervous system detects and interprets changes in conditions inside and outside the body and responds to them. The central nervous system analyzes information and initiates responses; the peripheral nervous system gathers information and carries the response signals. Some responses are involuntary; others are dictated by conscious thought. All nervous system activity consists of signals passed through pathways of interconnected neurons (nerve cells).

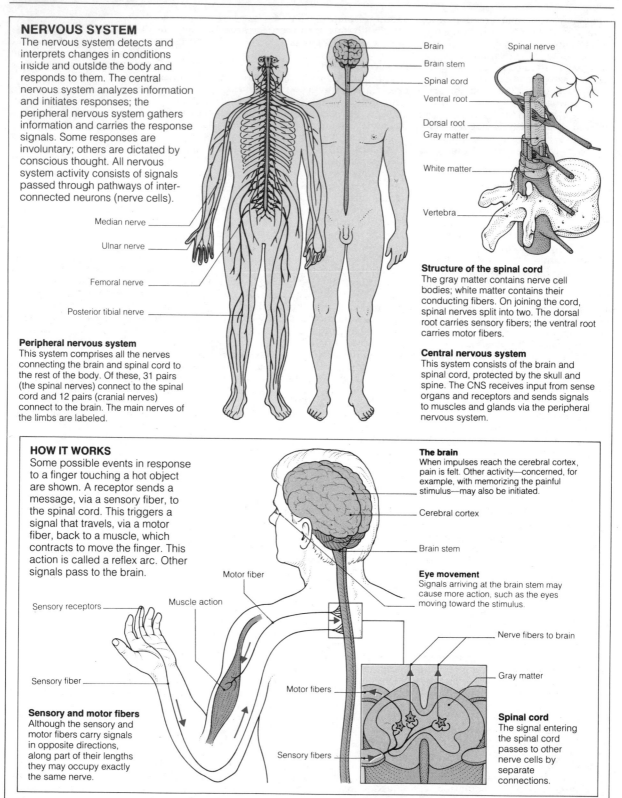

Median nerve

Ulnar nerve

Femoral nerve

Posterior tibial nerve

Brain

Brain stem

Spinal cord

Ventral root

Dorsal root

Gray matter

White matter

Vertebra

Spinal nerve

Peripheral nervous system

This system comprises all the nerves connecting the brain and spinal cord to the rest of the body. Of these, 31 pairs (the spinal nerves) connect to the spinal cord and 12 pairs (cranial nerves) connect to the brain. The main nerves of the limbs are labeled.

Structure of the spinal cord

The gray matter contains nerve cell bodies; white matter contains their conducting fibers. On joining the cord, spinal nerves split into two. The dorsal root carries sensory fibers; the ventral root carries motor fibers.

Central nervous system

This system consists of the brain and spinal cord, protected by the skull and spine. The CNS receives input from sense organs and receptors and sends signals to muscles and glands via the peripheral nervous system.

HOW IT WORKS

Some possible events in response to a finger touching a hot object are shown. A receptor sends a message, via a sensory fiber, to the spinal cord. This triggers a signal that travels, via a motor fiber, back to a muscle, which contracts to move the finger. This action is called a reflex arc. Other signals pass to the brain.

Motor fiber

Muscle action

Sensory receptors

Sensory fiber

Cerebral cortex

Brain stem

Motor fibers

Sensory fibers

Nerve fibers to brain

Gray matter

The brain

When impulses reach the cerebral cortex, pain is felt. Other activity—concerned, for example, with memorizing the painful stimulus—may also be initiated.

Eye movement

Signals arriving at the brain stem may cause more action, such as the eyes moving toward the stimulus.

Sensory and motor fibers

Although the sensory and motor fibers carry signals in opposite directions, along part of their lengths they may occupy exactly the same nerve.

Spinal cord

The signal entering the spinal cord passes to other nerve cells by separate connections.

N

can often be felt shooting along the affected nerve.

Some types of neuralgia are features of a specific disorder. Sufferers from *migraine* commonly suffer from a form of neuralgia consisting of attacks of intense, radiating pain around the eye. Postherpetic neuralgia is a burning pain that may recur at the site of an attack of *herpes zoster* (shingles) for months or even years after the illness.

Other types of neuralgia result from disturbance of a particular nerve. In glossopharyngeal neuralgia, intense pain is felt at the back of the tongue and in the throat and ear. The structures in this area are served by the glossopharyngeal nerve. The pain may occur spontaneously or may be brought on by talking, eating, or swallowing; its cause is generally unknown. The same is true of *trigeminal neuralgia*, a severe paroxysm of pain affecting one side of the face supplied by the trigeminal nerve.

TREATMENT
The pain of neuralgia is sometimes relieved by *analgesic drugs* (painkillers), such as acetaminophen. Glossopharyngeal, trigeminal, and postherpetic neuralgia sometimes respond to *carbamazepine*.

Neural tube defect
A developmental failure affecting the spinal cord or brain in the *embryo*.
INCIDENCE
From 9 to 16 per 10,000 live-born babies in Canada have a neural tube defect. The condition is slightly more common in girls than in boys. Many more fetuses are affected but do not survive to birth.

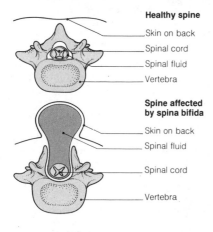

Neural tube defect
This defect leads to failure of the bony arch to fuse over the back of the spinal cord, thus causing spina bifida.

CAUSES AND OUTLOOK
Early in embryonic development, a ridge of nervous tissue forms along the back of the embryo. As development continues, this material differentiates into the spinal cord and body nerves at the lower end and into the brain at the upper end. At the same time, the bones that make up the spine gradually surround the spinal cord. If any part of this sequence goes awry, many defects can result. The worst is *anencephaly* (total lack of a brain). Much more common is *spina bifida*, in which the vertebrae (spinal bones) do not form a complete ring to protect the spinal cord.

Genetic factors play a part in neural tube defects, which show multifactorial *inheritance*. Couples who have had an affected child or who have a family history of neural tube defect should seek *genetic counseling*.

Many physicians believe that the risk of recurrence can be reduced by giving vitamin and folic acid supplements to the woman before conception and during the early part of pregnancy.

Ultrasound scanning and *amniocentesis* allow accurate prenatal testing for neural tube defects in high-risk pregnancies. Many hospital clinics screen all pregnant women by means of a blood test which will identify a considerable proportion of fetuses with neural tube defects that would otherwise remain unsuspected.

Neurapraxia
A type of *nerve injury* in which the outward structure of a nerve appears intact, but in which some of the conducting fibers have been damaged or have degenerated and thus do not transmit signals to muscles.

Neurasthenia
An outdated term that literally means "nervous exhaustion." It was once used to describe a number of physical and mental symptoms, including loss of energy, insomnia, aches and pains (especially in the chest and abdomen), *depression*, irritability, and reduced concentration.

Neuritis
A term that literally means inflammation of a nerve. True nerve inflammation may be caused by infection (for example by a virus in *herpes zoster* or by a bacterium in *Hansen's disease*). The term neuritis is also often applied to nerve damage or disease from causes other than inflammation.

Thus, it has become virtually synonymous with *neuropathy*, a term for all disorders of the peripheral nerves.

Neuroblastoma
A tumor of the *adrenal glands* or the sympathetic nervous system (part of the *autonomic nervous system*). Most neuroblastomas develop in the adrenal glands or in the sympathetic nerves along the back wall of the abdomen. Less commonly, neuroblastomas develop in the sympathetic nerves of the chest or neck, or, very rarely, in the brain.

Neuroblastomas are the most common extracranial (outside the skull) solid tumor of childhood. About 80 percent of cases develop during the first 10 years of life, most commonly in the first four years. The incidence is 8.3 cases per 1 million children.
SYMPTOMS AND SIGNS
The symptoms vary according to the site of the tumor and the extent to which it has spread. Common symptoms include weight loss, general aches and pains, paleness, and irritability. There may also be tumors of the abdomen, neck, eyes, or skin. In some cases, the tumor secretes the hormones *epinephrine* and *norepinephrine*, which may cause diarrhea, high blood pressure, and flushing of the skin.
DIAGNOSIS
The condition is diagnosed from the symptoms and signs, and from X rays, blood tests, and urine tests. In some cases, it may be necessary to perform a *biopsy* (removal of tissue for microscopic examination) of the bone marrow and any accessible tumors.
TREATMENT AND OUTLOOK
Treatment consists of the surgical removal of the tumor, followed by *radiation therapy* and possibly also by *anticancer drugs*.

The outlook varies greatly because neuroblastomas range from being relatively harmless to highly malignant. Overall, however, about one third of those affected survive for at least five years after treatment.

Neurocutaneous disorders
A group of conditions characterized by abnormalities of the skin as well as abnormalities of the nerves and/or the central nervous system.

The best known of these disorders is *neurofibromatosis*, in which there are brown patches on the skin and numerous fibrous nodules on the skin and nerves. Another example is *tuberous sclerosis*, which is characterized by

N

STRUCTURE OF A NEURON

A neuron (nerve cell) consists of a cell body and several branching projections called dendrites. Every neuron has a filamentous projection called an axon (nerve fiber). Axons vary in length from a fraction of a centimetre to about a metre. An axon branches at its end to form terminals, via which signals are transmitted to target cells, such as the dendrites of other neurons, muscle cells, or glands. Bundles of the axons of many neurons are known as nerves or, within the brain or spinal cord, as nerve tracts or pathways.

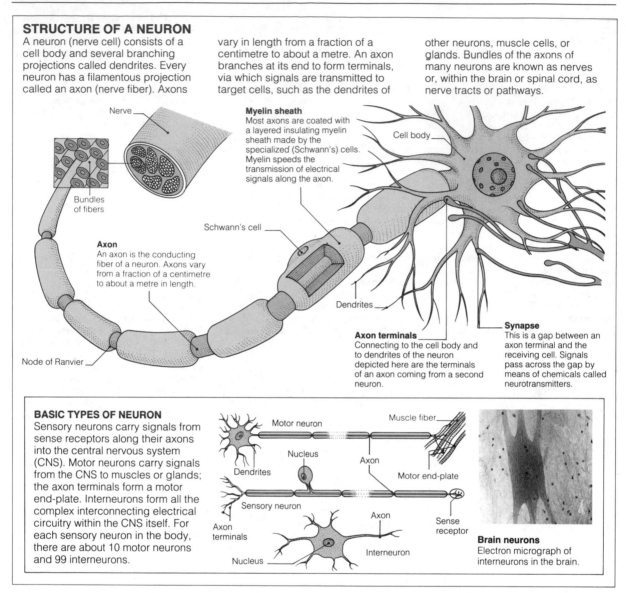

Nerve

Bundles of fibers

Myelin sheath
Most axons are coated with a layered insulating myelin sheath made by the specialized (Schwann's) cells. Myelin speeds the transmission of electrical signals along the axon.

Cell body

Schwann's cell

Axon
An axon is the conducting fiber of a neuron. Axons vary from a fraction of a centimetre to about a metre in length.

Dendrites

Node of Ranvier

Axon terminals
Connecting to the cell body and to dendrites of the neuron depicted here are the terminals of an axon coming from a second neuron.

Synapse
This is a gap between an axon terminal and the receiving cell. Signals pass across the gap by means of chemicals called neurotransmitters.

BASIC TYPES OF NEURON
Sensory neurons carry signals from sense receptors along their axons into the central nervous system (CNS). Motor neurons carry signals from the CNS to muscles or glands; the axon terminals form a motor end-plate. Interneurons form all the complex interconnecting electrical circuitry within the CNS itself. For each sensory neuron in the body, there are about 10 motor neurons and 99 interneurons.

Motor neuron
Muscle fiber
Nucleus
Axon
Dendrites
Motor end-plate
Sensory neuron
Axon
Axon terminals
Sense receptor
Interneuron
Nucleus

Brain neurons
Electron micrograph of interneurons in the brain.

small skin-colored swellings over the cheeks and nose, mental deficiency, and epilepsy.

Neurodermatitis
An itchy, eczemalike skin condition caused by repeated scratching. (See also *Lichen simplex*.)

Neuroendocrinology
The study of the interactions between the *nervous system* and the *endocrine system*, which control internal body functions and the way in which the body responds to the external environment. Investigations range from recording the electrical activity of neurosecretory cells to experiments showing the relationship between hormones and behavior.

Neurofibromatosis
An uncommon inherited disorder, also called von Recklinghausen's disease, characterized by numerous neurofibromas (soft, fibrous swellings that grow from nerves) and by *café au lait spots* on the skin.

SYMPTOMS AND SIGNS
Neurofibromas may develop anywhere on the skin and sometimes elsewhere in the body. These swellings may be tiny or be as large as several centimetres in diameter. They are sometimes unsightly. Café au lait spots are most common on the skin of the trunk and pelvis.

If neurofibromas occur in the central nervous system, they may cause *epilepsy* and other complications, sometimes affecting vision and hearing. In some cases, neurofibromatosis leads to bone deformities. Rarely, neurofibromas become cancerous.

TREATMENT
Surgical removal of neurofibromas is necessary only if there are complications. Anyone who has this disorder, and parents of an affected child, should seek *genetic counseling* if they are planning a pregnancy.

Neurology

The medical discipline concerned with the study of the *nervous system* and its disorders, particularly with their diagnosis and treatment.

Neurologists are trained to examine the nerves, reflexes, motor and sensory functions, and muscles to determine a disorder's cause and extent. To aid diagnosis, extensive use is made of modern imaging techniques (such as *CT scanning* and *MRI*).

In the past, relatively few disorders of the nervous system could be treated effectively. Today, with a better understanding of the biochemical and structural bases of neurological disorders, treatments have been developed for *migraine, Parkinson's disease*, and the control of *pain*. Neurologists have become specialists in the care and support of patients with progressive disorders, such as *multiple sclerosis* and *muscular dystrophy*. (See also *Neuropathology; Neurosurgery*.)

Neuroma

A benign tumor of *nerve* tissue. In most cases, the cause is unknown; rarely, a neuroma develops as a result of damage to a nerve.

A neuroma may affect any nerve in the body. Symptoms vary according to the nerve involved. In most cases, there is intermittent pain in the areas of the body supplied by the affected nerve. The same areas may also become numb and weak if the neuroma develops in a confined space and presses on the nerve.

If symptoms are troublesome, the tumor may be surgically removed. (See also *Acoustic neuroma*.)

Neuron

The term for a nerve cell. The *nervous system* contains billions of neurons, which act in various combinations to do everything from writing a symphony to scratching a fleabite. The neurons are analogous to the wires in a complex electrical machine.

There are three main types of neuron—interneurons, motor neurons, and sensory neurons (see illustrated box on facing page).

The function of a neuron is to "fire" (transmit an electrical impulse along its axon) under certain specific conditions. The electrical impulse causes the release of a chemical called a *neurotransmitter* from the axon terminals. This neurotransmitter may make a muscle cell contract, cause an endocrine gland to release a hormone, or affect an adjacent neuron.

EFFECTS OF NEUROTRANSMITTERS

Different stimuli excite different types of neurons to fire. Sensory neurons may be excited by physical stimuli, such as cold, pressure, or light of a certain wavelength. The activity of most neurons is controlled by the effects of neurotransmitters released from adjacent neurons. The ability of a neuron to fire depends on a small difference in electrical potential between the inside and outside of the cell. Under the direct influence of an excitatory neurotransmitter, a sudden change occurs in this potential at one point on the cell's membrane. The change, called an "action potential," then flows along the membrane (and thus along the axon of the cell) at up to 430 km per hour. A neuron may be able to fire in this way several times every second.

Other neurotransmitters stabilize neuronal membranes, preventing an action potential. Thus, the firing pattern of a neuron depends on the balance of excitatory and inhibitory influences acting on it.

LIFE SPAN

If the cell body of a neuron is damaged or degenerates, the cell dies and is never replaced. A baby starts life with the maximum number of neurons. The number of neurons decreases continuously thereafter. People seem to be born with an excess number of neurons, so problems arise only when disease, injury, or persistent alcohol abuse affects the *central nervous system*, dramatically increasing the rate of neuron loss.

If a peripheral nerve is damaged, its individual fibers have the ability to regenerate themselves (see *Nerve injury; Neuropathy*).

Neuropathic joint

A joint that has been damaged by a series of injuries, which pass unnoticed because of loss of sensation in the joint due to *neuropathy* (nerve damage caused by disease).

Neuropathic joints develop in a number of conditions, including *diabetes mellitus* and untreated *syphilis*.

When sensation to pain is lost, abnormal stress and strain on a joint do not stimulate the protective reflex spasm of the surrounding muscles; this failure of the protective reflex spasm allows exaggerated movement that can damage the joint. Severe recurrent damage to a joint may lead to *osteoarthritis*, swelling, and deformity. Pain is minimal, however, because of the lack of sensation.

DIAGNOSIS AND TREATMENT

Severe joint degeneration and deformity are visible on *X rays*. An orthopedic *brace* or *caliper splint* may be necessary to restrict abnormal joint movement. Occasionally, an *arthrodesis* (a surgical operation to fuse a joint) is performed. The nerve damage is irreversible.

Neuropathology

The branch of *pathology* that is concerned with the causes and effects of disorders of the *nervous system*. (See also *Neurology*).

Neuropathy

Disease, inflammation, or damage to the peripheral *nerves*, which connect the central nervous system (brain and spinal cord) to the sense organs, muscles, glands, and internal organs.

Symptoms caused by neuropathies include numbness, tingling, pain, or muscle weakness, depending on the nerves affected.

TYPES

Most nerve cell axons (the conducting fibers that make up nerves) are insulated by a sheath of a fatty substance called *myelin*, but some are unmyelinated. Most neuropathies arise from damage or irritation either to the axons or to their myelin sheaths. An axon may suffer thinning of, complete loss of, or patchy loss of its myelin sheath. This may cause a slowing of or a complete block to the passage of electrical signals.

Various types of neuropathy are described according to the site and distribution of damage. For example, a distal neuropathy starts with damage at the far end of a nerve (farthest from the brain or spinal cord). A symmetrical neuropathy affects nerves at the same places on each side of the body. Some neuropathies are described according to their underlying cause (for example, diabetic neuropathy and alcoholic neuropathy).

The term neuritis is now used virtually interchangeably with neuropathy. Polyneuropathy (or polyneuritis) literally means damage to several nerves; mononeuropathy (or mononeuritis) indicates damage to a single nerve. *Neuralgia* describes pain caused by irritation or inflammation of a particular nerve.

CAUSES

In some cases of neuropathy there is no obvious or detectable cause. Among the many specific causes are *diabetes mellitus*, dietary deficiencies (particularly of B vitamins), persistent

N

729

excessive alcohol consumption, and metabolic upsets such as *uremia*. Other causes include *Hansen's disease* (leprosy), *lead poisoning*, or poisoning by drugs.

Nerves may become acutely inflamed. This often occurs after a viral infection (e.g., in *Guillain-Barré syndrome*). Neuropathies may result from *autoimmune disorders* such as *rheumatoid arthritis*, systemic *lupus erythematosus*, or *polyarteritis nodosa*. In these disorders, there is often damage to the blood vessels supplying the nerves. Neuropathies may occur secondarily to malignant tumors, such as *lung cancer*, or with *lymphomas* and *leukemias*. There is also a group of inherited neuropathies, the most common being *peroneal muscular atrophy*.

SYMPTOMS
The symptoms of neuropathy depend on whether it affects mainly sensory nerve fibers or motor nerve fibers.

Damage to sensory nerve fibers may cause numbness and tingling, sensations of cold, or pain, often starting in the hands and feet and spreading toward the center of the body. Damage to motor fibers may cause muscle weakness and muscle wasting.

Damage to nerves of the *autonomic nervous system* may lead to blurred vision, impaired or absent sweating, episodes of faintness associated with falls in blood pressure, and disturbance of gastric, intestinal, bladder, and sexual functioning, including incontinence and impotence.

Some neuropathies are linked with particular symptoms (e.g., diabetic neuropathy and alcoholic neuropathy may both cause severe pain).

DIAGNOSIS
To determine the extent of damage, studies of nerve conduction are performed, together with *EMG* tests, which record the electrical activity in muscles. To determine the cause of neuropathy, *blood tests, X rays*, nerve or muscle *biopsy* (removal of a small sample of tissue for microscopic analysis), and various other diagnostic tests may be required.

TREATMENT
When possible, treatment is aimed at the underlying cause of the neuropathy. For example, in diabetes mellitus, scrupulous attention to the control of the blood sugar level affords the best chances for recovery. Other people may need to stop drinking alcohol, or, if a nutritional deficiency has been diagnosed, may be given injections of vitamins such as thiamine (see *Vitamin B complex*).

If treatment is successful and the cell bodies of the damaged nerve cells have not been destroyed, a full recovery from the neuropathy is possible.

Neuropsychiatry
The branch of medicine that deals with the relationship between psychiatric symptoms and neurological disorder. This may include the effects of head injury and alcohol on the brain, or specific disorders such as brain tumors, infections, inherited illnesses, and disorders affecting the brain in childhood and causing mental handicap.

Increasingly, new techniques of *brain imaging* are demonstrating abnormalities of brain structure and function in disorders which produce psychiatric symptoms.

Neurosis
A term commonly used to describe a range of psychiatric disorders in which the sufferer remains in touch with reality.

Neurotic symptoms are distressing to the afflicted person, who is aware of a change from his or her usual psychological state. By contrast, people suffering from psychotic illnesses usually do not recognize that they are ill (see *Psychosis*). Neurotic symptoms generally do not lead to distinctly abnormal behavior, although they can severely limit work or social activities. They tend to fluctuate in intensity, often in response to social or personal stresses. No physical abnormality has been shown to underlie them.

The major neurotic disorders are mild forms of *depression; anxiety disorders*, including *phobias* and *obsessive-compulsive behavior; hypochondriasis;* and *dissociative disorders*.

Neurosurgery
The specialty concerned with the surgical treatment of disorders of the *brain, spinal cord*, or other parts of the *nervous system*. Many generalized nervous system disorders do not respond to surgical treatment, but neurosurgery can deal with most conditions in which a localized structural change interferes with nerve function.

Conditions treated by neurosurgery include tumors of the brain, spinal cord, or meninges (membranes that surround the brain and spinal cord), certain abnormalities of the blood vessels that supply the brain, such as an *aneurysm* (balloonlike swelling at a weak point in an artery), bleeding

inside the skull (see *Extradural hemorrhage; Intracerebral hemorrhage;* and *Subdural hemorrhage*), *brain abscess*, some birth defects (such as *hydrocephalus* and *spina bifida*), certain types of *epilepsy*, and nerve damage caused by illness or accidents. Neurosurgeons are also concerned with the surgical relief of otherwise untreatable *pain*.

Neurosyphilis
Infection of the brain or spinal cord that occurs in untreated *syphilis* many years after the initial infection.

Damage to the spinal cord due to neurosyphilis may cause tabes dorsalis, characterized by poor coordination of leg movements when walking, urinary incontinence, and intermittent pains in the abdomen and limbs. Damage to the brain may cause *dementia* and muscle weakness, which in rare cases progresses to total paralysis of the limbs (in which case it is called general paralysis of the insane).

Neurotoxin
A chemical that damages nervous tissue. The principal effects of neurotoxic nerve damage are numbness, weakness, or paralysis of the part of the body supplied by the affected nerve.

Neurotoxins are present in the venom of certain snakes (see *Snake bites*), and are released by some types of bacteria (such as those that cause *tetanus* and *diphtheria*). Some chemical poisons, such as arsenic and lead, are also neurotoxic.

Neurotransmitter
A chemical released from nerve endings that transmits impulses from one *neuron* (nerve cell) to another neuron or to a muscle cell. Neurotransmitters are released from nerve endings in response to electrical impulses traveling down neurons. Scores of different chemicals fulfil this function in different parts of the *nervous system* (see illustrated box on facing page).

Many neurotransmitters, such as *norepinephrine*, act as both neurotransmitters and *hormones*, being released into the bloodstream to act on their target cells at a distance.

One of the most important neurotransmitters is *acetylcholine*. This chemical is released by neurons connected to skeletal muscles, causing them to contract, and also by neurons that control the sweat glands and the heartbeat. Acetylcholine also transmits messages between neurons in the brain and spinal cord. Interference

HOW NEUROTRANSMITTERS WORK

When an electrical impulse travels down a nerve cell axon, it causes the release of a chemical neurotransmitter at the axon terminals. The chemical is not the same in every case; acetylcholine, norepinephrine, dopamine, and serotonin are all important examples.

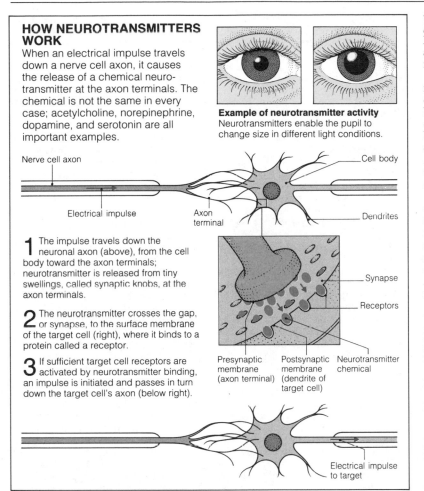

Example of neurotransmitter activity
Neurotransmitters enable the pupil to change size in different light conditions.

Nerve cell axon

Cell body

Electrical impulse

Axon terminal

Dendrites

1 The impulse travels down the neuronal axon (above), from the cell body toward the axon terminals; neurotransmitter is released from tiny swellings, called synaptic knobs, at the axon terminals.

2 The neurotransmitter crosses the gap, or synapse, to the surface membrane of the target cell (right), where it binds to a protein called a receptor.

3 If sufficient target cell receptors are activated by neurotransmitter binding, an impulse is initiated and passes in turn down the target cell's axon (below right).

Synapse

Receptors

Presynaptic membrane (axon terminal)

Postsynaptic membrane (dendrite of target cell)

Neurotransmitter chemical

Electrical impulse to target

with the action of acetylcholine on skeletal muscles is the cause of the disease *myasthenia gravis*. It is thought that depletion of the nerve cells that release acetylcholine in the brain may be a cause of *Alzheimer's disease*.

Norepinephrine has an important role in the nervous control of heartbeat, blood flow, and the body's response to stress. This substance is made by the *adrenal glands* as well as being produced by neurons. *Dopamine*, another neurotransmitter, plays an important role in parts of the brain that control movement. Malfunction of the neurons that respond to dopamine is thought to be important in causing *Parkinson's disease*. *Serotonin* is one of the main neurotransmitters in parts of the brain concerned with conscious processes.

In the last 20 years, a new group of neurotransmitters (called neuropeptides) has been discovered. These are small proteins that consist of larger molecules than the previously known neurotransmitters, which consist of very small molecules. The best studied of the neuropeptides are the *endorphins*, used by the brain to control sensitivity to pain.

Nevus

A skin blemish of various types. Nevi can be flat, slightly raised, or on a stalk, colored or not colored, and with or without hair growth. Some nevi are present at birth, others can develop at any age.

TYPES

There are two main groups of nevi: pigmented nevi and vascular nevi.

PIGMENTED NEVI These are caused by abnormality or overactivity of melanocytes (skin cells that produce the brown pigment *melanin*).

The most common type of pigmented nevus is a *freckle*, which is a small, flat, light brown to dark brown area which may occur on any part of the body that is exposed to the sun. A *lentigo* is a light brown spot very similar to a freckle. *Café au lait spots* are another type of light brown pigmented nevus.

Another common type of pigmented nevus is a mole, sometimes called a melanocytic nevus. Moles are brown to dark brown in color and of different sizes. They are unusual at birth, but commonly develop during childhood and young adulthood. Adults have an average of 15 to 20 moles. In rare cases, moles become cancerous (see *Melanoma, malignant*).

Hairy, pigmented nevi sometimes develop on the shoulders of young men. Another type of pigmented nevus is a halo nevus, in which the skin surrounding the blemish lightens in color to give a characteristic halo appearance. Juvenile melanomas (see *Melanoma, juvenile*) are red-brown nevi that occur in childhood.

Some nevi have a bluish coloration; these so-called blue nevi are often found on the backs of the hands of young girls. Most black and Asian infants are born with one or more blue-black spots on their lower backs (see *Mongolian blue spot*).

VASCULAR NEVI These are caused by an abnormal collection of blood vessels. They include port-wine stains and strawberry marks (see *Hemangioma* and *Spider nevus*).

TREATMENT

Most nevi are harmless and do not require treatment. However, if a nevus suddenly appears, grows, bleeds, or changes color, medical advice should be sought without delay to exclude the possibility of *skin cancer*.

Newborn

An infant at birth and during the first few weeks of life.

INITIAL EXAMINATION

Immediately after birth, the newborn baby is briefly checked by the nurse, midwife, or physician in attendance. This examination includes checking the heart rate with a *stethoscope* and establishing that breathing is normal. The *Apgar score* and other tests are performed to check that the baby is in good health. At this time too the baby's sex is noted and a check made for any obvious *birth defect*.

NURSING PROCEDURE

The baby is labeled with his or her name and date of birth. A record is also made of the birthweight, length, and head circumference, and a handprint or footprint is usually made.

N

At birth, the baby is usually covered with vernix, a white substance that lubricates its passage from the uterus. The vernix is wiped off and the baby is wrapped in a blanket and given to the mother to hold and feed, or is placed in a warm cot. If very small or sick, the baby will be kept in an *incubator* and treated in a neonatal special-care or intensive-care unit.

The frequency of the baby's urine and *meconium* (feces passed by the newborn) is recorded. During the second week of life, two special blood tests are performed: a blood sample is removed from all babies to check for *phenylketonuria* (see *Guthrie test*) and *hypothyroidism*.

MEDICAL EXAMINATION
Within 24 hours of birth (or sooner if there is any cause for concern), the baby is usually given a complete medical examination by the pediatrician. This examination assesses the baby's general health and identifies any birth defects (such as cleft palate). The skull, eyes, face, abdomen, heart, spine, hips, genitals, and limbs are checked, and the baby's posture, movements, behavior, cry, reflexes (see *Reflex, primitive*), and responsiveness are noted.

ABNORMALITIES IN THE NEWBORN
The baby may have a swollen or misshapen head due to pressure during labor. Less commonly, there may be more notable evidence of *birth injury*, such as *cephalhematoma* (swelling of the scalp caused by bruising around the skull). Most problems caused by the pressure of delivery resolve themselves within a few days.

Jaundice (see *Jaundice, neonatal*) is extremely common in the newborn, especially if the baby is breast-fed. Usually appearing on the second or third day, the jaundice generally disappears over the next few days. In most cases, jaundice in the newborn is harmless. However, the condition may be serious if it appears during the first 24 hours or occurs in a very premature infant.

Some newborn girls have slight vaginal bleeding or discharge, and babies of either sex may have enlargement of the breasts. These harmless conditions are caused by maternal sex hormones that reached the fetus through the placenta. Any extra hormones soon leave the baby's body.

The umbilical cord, which may be painted with antiseptic to prevent infection, usually dries and drops off within a week or so of birth. Infections of the cord stump sometimes occur.

Minor, harmless abnormalities of the newborn include *milia* (tiny, white spots on the face), *hemangioma*, *mongolian blue spot*, and a blotchy, red rash (see *Urticaria, neonatal*) that may occur around the second day. (See also *Postmaturity*; *Prematurity*.)

Niacin
See *Vitamin B complex*.

Niacinamide
See *Vitamin B complex*.

Nickel
A metallic element which is present in the body in minute amounts. Its exact role is poorly understood. Nickel is thought to activate certain *enzymes* (substances that promote biochemical reactions). It may also play a part in stabilizing chromosomal material in the nuclei of cells.

Disease due to a deficiency of nickel is unknown. However, exposure to nickel may cause *dermatitis* (inflammation of the skin). *Lung cancer* has been reported in workers in nickel refineries.

Nicotine
A drug in tobacco which acts as a stimulant and is responsible for dependence on tobacco. Nicotine has no medical use, but certain of its derivatives are used as pesticides.

After inhalation, the nicotine in tobacco smoke passes rapidly into the bloodstream. Nicotine in chewing tobacco is absorbed more slowly through the lining of the mouth. After entering the bloodstream, nicotine acts on the nervous system until the drug is eventually broken down by the liver and excreted in the urine.

EFFECTS
Nicotine acts primarily on the *autonomic nervous system*, which controls involuntary body activities such as the heart rate. The effects of the drug vary from one person to another, and also depend on dosage and past usage. In someone unused to smoking, even a small amount of nicotine may slow the heart rate and cause nausea and vomiting. However, in habitual smokers, the drug increases the heart rate and narrows the blood vessels (the combined effect of which is to raise blood pressure). Nicotine also stimulates the *central nervous system*, thereby reducing fatigue, increasing alertness, and improving concentration.

Regular use of tobacco results in tolerance to nicotine, so that a higher intake is needed to bring about the same effects. This process is, however, less noticeable with tobacco than with other addictive drugs.

NICOTINE AND DISEASE
Although it is the tar in tobacco smoke that damages lung tissue and causes lung cancer, smoking is also clearly associated with *coronary artery disease*, *peripheral vascular disease*, and other cardiovascular disorders. It is uncertain whether these disorders are caused by the nicotine or by the carbon monoxide content of the smoke.

Excessively large amounts of nicotine can cause poisoning, which may result in vomiting, seizures, and, very occasionally, death.

WITHDRAWAL
Because most smokers are physically dependent on nicotine, stopping smoking commonly causes withdrawal symptoms; the victim usually experiences drowsiness, headaches, fatigue, and difficulty concentrating. To reduce these symptoms in a person who is trying to stop smoking, a physician may prescribe nicotine chewing gum, which is less harmful to the circulatory system. (See also *Tobacco smoking*.)

Nicotinic acid
A form of niacin (see *Vitamin B complex*). Apart from its use as a vitamin supplement, nicotinic acid is also prescribed as a *lipid-lowering drug* and as a *vasodilator drug*. High doses are used to treat certain types of *hyperlipidemia*. Low doses are used to improve circulation in disorders such as *peripheral vascular disease*.

Adverse effects, which are more common with high doses, include flushing, dizziness, nausea, palpitations, and itching.

Nifedipine
A *calcium channel blocker* used mainly to prevent and treat *angina pectoris*. Nifedipine is also often used to treat *hypertension* (high blood pressure) and disorders affecting the circulation, such as *Raynaud's disease*. Possible adverse effects include *edema* (accumulation of fluid in tissues), flushing, headache, and dizziness.

Night blindness
The inability to see well in dim light. Many people with night blindness have no discernible eye disease. The condition may be an inherited functional defect of the retina, an early sign of *retinitis pigmentosa*, or a result of vitamin A deficiency.

Nightmare

An unpleasant vivid dream, often accompanied by a sense of suffocation. Nightmares occur during REM (rapid eye movement) *sleep* in the middle and later parts of the night, and are often clearly remembered if the dreamer awakens completely.

Nightmares are very common, especially in children aged between 8 and 10, and are particularly likely to occur when the child's breathing is slightly difficult because of a cold or illness, or when there is anxiety over separation from parents or home. In adults, nightmares may be a side effect of certain drugs, including *beta-blocker drugs* and *benzodiazepine drugs*. Traumatic experiences (such as accidents, torture, or prolonged imprisonment) seem to be particularly associated with disturbing and repeated nightmares. However, there is no specific relationship to psychiatric illness.

Nightmares should not be confused with hypnagogic *hallucinations*, which occur while falling asleep, nor with *night terror*, which occurs in NREM (nonrapid eye movement) sleep and is not remembered the next day.

Night terror

A disorder, occurring mainly in children, consisting of abrupt arousals from sleep in a terrified state. Night terror (also called sleep terror) usually starts between the ages of 4 and 7, and gradually disappears in early adolescence.

Episodes occur during NREM (nonrapid eye movement) *sleep*, usually half an hour to three and a half hours after falling asleep.

Sufferers wake up screaming in a semiconscious state and remain frightened for some minutes. They do not recognize familiar faces or surroundings, and usually cannot be comforted. Physical signs of agitation, such as sweating or an increased heart rate, are also common. The sufferer gradually falls back to sleep and has no memory of the event the following day.

Though distressing to parents, night terror in children has no serious significance. In adults, it is likely to be associated with an *anxiety disorder*.

Nipple

The small prominence at the tip of each *breast*. Each of a woman's nipples contains tiny openings through which milk can pass. The nipple and the surrounding areola are darker than the surrounding skin, darkening more and increasing in size during *pregnancy*. Muscle in the nipple allows it to become erect.

DISORDERS

Structural defects of the nipple are rare. One or both nipples may be absent, or there may be additional nipples along a line extending from the armpit to the groin.

An inverted nipple is usually an abnormality of development. It can be corrected by drawing out the nipple between finger and thumb daily for several weeks. Inversion of a previously normal nipple in an adult is much more significant and may be due to *breast cancer*.

Cracked nipples are common during the last months of pregnancy and during the period when a woman is *breast-feeding*. Daily washing, drying, and moisturizing of the nipple can help to prevent cracking. In addition to causing discomfort, cracks may lead to infective *mastitis*.

Papilloma of the nipple is a benign swelling attached to the skin by a stalk. *Paget's disease of the nipple* appears initially as persistent eczema of the nipple. It is caused by a slowly growing cancer arising in a milk duct, and surgical treatment is required.

Discharge from the nipple occurs for a variety of reasons. A clear, straw-colored discharge may develop in early pregnancy. A milky discharge may occur after the period of breast-feeding is over. *Galactorrhea* (discharge of milk in someone who is not pregnant or breast-feeding) may be caused by a hormone imbalance; rarely, it may be due to a galactocele (a cyst under the areola). A discharge containing pus indicates a breast *abscess*. A bloodstained discharge may be due to *fibroadenosis* or cancer.

Nitrate drugs

COMMON DRUGS
Isosorbide dinitrate Nitroglycerin

A group of *vasodilator drugs* used in the treatment of *angina pectoris* (chest pain due to impaired blood supply to heart muscle) and severe *heart failure* (reduced pumping efficiency).

Possible adverse effects of nitrate drugs include headache, flushing, and dizziness. *Tolerance* (the need for greater amounts of a drug to have the same effect) may develop when the drug is taken regularly.

Nitrazepam

A *benzodiazepine drug* used in the short-term treatment of *insomnia*. Nitrazepam is long-acting and may cause a hangover effect, with drowsiness and lightheadedness, the following day. Regular use over several weeks can lead to a reduction in its effectiveness as the body adapts.

Nitrazepam can lead to *drug dependence* and to withdrawal symptoms, such as nervousness and restlessness.

Nitrites

Salts of nitrous acid (a nitrogen-containing acid). To preserve meat, sodium nitrite is added in small amounts together with potassium nitrate (saltpeter) and salt to inhibit the growth of potentially harmful bacteria. During the curing process, the nitrate is converted into nitrite which combines with muscle pigment to form the characteristic red color of cured meats (bacon, salt beef, etc.).

If consumed in large amounts, nitrites can cause dizziness, nausea, and vomiting.

Within the intestine, nitrites are converted to substances called nitrosamines. In laboratory investigations, nitrosamines have been shown to cause cancer in animals. However, there is no conclusive proof that they have the same effect in humans or that eating food containing nitrites is harmful to health. Vegetarian diets may contain significantly more nitrites than a typical "mixed" diet.

N

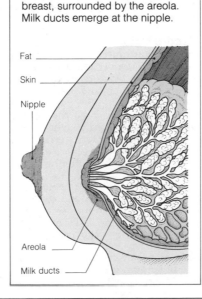

LOCATION OF THE NIPPLE
The protrusion at the tip of the breast, surrounded by the areola. Milk ducts emerge at the nipple.

Fat

Skin

Nipple

Areola

Milk ducts

Nitrofurantoin

An *antibacterial drug* used in the treatment of *urinary tract infection*.

Nitrofurantoin should be taken with food to reduce the risk of irritating the stomach, which can cause abdominal pain and nausea. More serious adverse effects, such as breathing difficulty, numbness, and jaundice, occur rarely.

Nitrogen

A colorless, odorless gas that makes up 78 percent of the Earth's atmosphere. Atmospheric nitrogen has no biological action, although in scuba diving, bubbles of nitrogen gas may form in body fluids if a diver ascends to the surface too rapidly, causing the "bends" (see *Decompression sickness*).

Although nitrogen gas cannot be utilized by the body, compounds of nitrogen are essential to life. Probably the most important of such compounds are *amino acids*, the building blocks of *proteins*, which represent the fundamental structural substances of all cells and tissues. Because humans cannot make some (so-called essential) amino acids, they must be obtained from the diet in the form of animal and plant proteins. The proteins are then broken down into their constituent amino acids so that they can be absorbed and reconstituted into the specific proteins needed by the body. These processes of protein breakdown and reconstitution produce a variety of nitrogen-containing waste products, primarily *urea*, which is excreted from the body in the urine. (See also *Nitrate drugs*; *Nitrites*.)

Nitroglycerin

Nitroglycerin is one of the oldest potent drugs in continuous use. A tablet placed under the tongue gives rapid although temporary relief of the pain of *angina pectoris*. Common side effects are flushing and headache; because of its *vasodilatation* effect it may also cause fainting. To lengthen the duration of its action, nitroglycerin is available as an ointment that allows it to be absorbed through the skin and also in the form of slow-release tablets.

Nitrous oxide

A colorless gas (sometimes called laughing gas) with a sweet smell. Nitrous oxide is used with oxygen to provide *analgesia* (pain relief) and light anesthesia (see *Anesthesia, general*) at the site of a serious accident or during dental procedures, childbirth, and minor surgery. For major surgery requiring deeper anesthesia, a nitrous oxide and oxygen mixture needs to be combined with other drugs.

The advantages of the combination of nitrous oxide and oxygen over other agents are its rapid action and nonflammability. Possible adverse effects include nausea and vomiting during the recovery period.

Nits

The eggs of lice. Both head lice and pubic lice produce eggs, which they glue to the base of hairs growing from their host's head or pubic area. The nits are tiny, measuring about 0.5 mm in diameter. They are yellow when newly laid, and white when hatched. Hatching takes place within eight days; the empty eggshells are carried outward as the hair grows.

Louse infestations are often diagnosed from the presence of nits. The distance from the base of hairs to the furthest nits provides a rough approximation of the duration of the infestation. (See *Lice*; *Pubic lice*.)

Nizatadine

Nizatadine is used in the prevention and treatment of ulcers of the stomach and duodenum. Unlike most other antiulcer drugs, it can be taken along with anticoagulants and anticonvulsants. The most prominent side effect is drowsiness.

NMR

Abbreviation for nuclear magnetic resonance. The preferred term for this technique is magnetic resonance imaging, abbreviated to *MRI*.

Nocardiosis

An infection caused by a funguslike bacterium. The infection usually starts in the lung and spreads via the bloodstream to the brain and tissues under the skin. The causative organism is present in the soil in all parts of the world and is acquired by inhalation.

Nocardiosis is rare except in people with *immunodeficiency disorders* or those already suffering from another serious disease.

The infection causes a pneumonia-like illness, with fever and cough. It fails to respond to normal, short-term, antibiotic treatment, and signs of progressive lung damage occur. Brain abscesses may follow. The condition is diagnosed by microscopic examination of sputum (phlegm). Treatment, which may have to be continued for 12 to 18 months, is with *sulfonamide drugs*, sometimes in conjunction with other antibacterial drugs, for example *trimethoprim*.

Nocturia

The disturbance of a person's sleep at night by the need to pass *urine*. In most people, a moderately full *bladder* does not usually disturb sleep, although light sleepers are more likely than others to wake to empty their bladders. Drinking alcohol in the evening stimulates urine production and may result in nocturia.

A common cause of nocturia is enlargement of the prostate gland (see *Prostate, enlarged*), which obstructs the normal outflow of urine and causes the bladder to empty incompletely.

Another common cause is *heart failure* (reduced pumping efficiency) leading to the retention of excess fluid in the legs during the day, which is absorbed into the bloodstream when the patient lies down at night and carried to the kidneys to make more urine.

Also common is *cystitis* (inflammation of the bladder), in which irritation of the bladder wall increases its sensitivity so that smaller volumes of urine trigger a desire to pass urine.

Rarer causes of nocturia include *diabetes mellitus*, in which greater volumes of urine are produced both day and night; chronic *kidney failure*, in which the normal ability of the kidney to produce a reduced quantity of more concentrated urine at night is lost; and *diabetes insipidus*, in which the kidneys fail to concentrate the urine owing to lack of a particular pituitary hormone.

Nocturnal emission

Ejaculation that occurs during sleep, commonly called a "wet dream." Nocturnal emission is normal in male adolescents and is a common cause of unnecessary anxiety. Nocturnal emissions may also occur in adult males whose sexual activity is limited.

Node

A small, rounded mass of tissue that may be normal or abnormal. The term most commonly refers to a *lymph node*, a normal structure in the lymphatic system. Abnormal nodes are often called *nodules*.

Nodule

A small lump of tissue, usually more than 5 mm in diameter. A nodule may protrude from the skin's surface or it may form deep under the skin. Nodules may be either hard or soft.

COMPARATIVE NOISE LEVELS

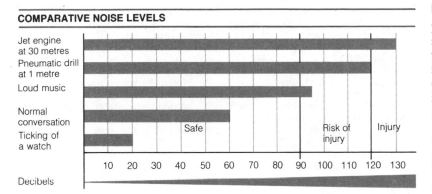

Noise

Sound that is disordered and irregular (producing an unpleasant sensation), that is unwanted, or that interferes with the ability to hear.

Hearing may be damaged by exposure to intensely loud noise for a short period (such as an explosion at close range) or by prolonged exposure to lower levels of noise (such as might occur in a machine room or foundry). Any noise above 90 decibels may cause damage; the louder the noise, the shorter the time required for damage to occur (see chart).

HOW NOISE DAMAGES HEARING

Exposure to a sudden very loud noise, usually above 130 decibels, can cause immediate and permanent damage. Normally, muscles in the *middle ear* respond to loud noise by altering the stiffness of the ossicles (the chain of bones that pass vibrations to the inner ear), thus reducing their efficiency and damping down the intensity of the noise. But when the noise occurs without warning, these protective reflexes have no time to respond. The full force of the vibrations is carried to the inner ear, causing severe damage to delicate hair cells in the cochlea. Occasionally, loud noises can rupture the *eardrum*. More commonly, damage from loud noise occurs over a period of time, with gradual destruction of the hair cells of the cochlea and permanent hearing loss.

SYMPTOMS OF NOISE DAMAGE

Sound at 90 decibels or above may cause pain and temporary deafness lasting for minutes or hours. This is a warning that hearing may be damaged unless the source of the noise is removed or unless suitable precautions are taken. Prolonged *tinnitus* (ringing or buzzing in the ears) occurring after a noise has ceased is an indication that some damage has probably occurred.

Prolonged exposure to loud noise leads initially to a loss of ability to hear certain high tones. Later, deafness extends to all high frequencies, and the perception of speech becomes impaired. Eventually, lower tones are also affected.

PREVENTION OF NOISE DAMAGE

Regulations governing maximum noise levels apply to places of work. People who cannot avoid exposure to loud noise (for example, workers using pneumatic drills) should wear ear protection. People who are persistently exposed to loud noise may have their hearing monitored regularly. Noise from low-flying aircraft may disturb sleep and interfere with social activities such as conversation. Regulations exist to control noise levels around airports; some have nighttime "noise" curfews.

Noma

Also known as cancrum oris, death of tissue in the lips and cheeks caused by bacterial infection. Noma is most often seen in (and largely confined to) young, severely malnourished children in developing countries. It may complicate other diseases, especially *measles*, and sometimes occurs during the last stages of *leukemia*.

SYMPTOMS

The first symptom is inflammation of the gums and the inner surface of the cheeks. Without treatment, this leads to severe ulceration (with a foul-smelling discharge) and eventual destruction of the bones around the mouth, and loss of teeth. Healing occurs naturally after a time, but scarring may be severe.

TREATMENT

Penicillin drugs and improved nutrition halt the progress of the disease. Plastic surgery may be necessary to reconstruct damaged bones or to improve facial appearance.

Noninvasive

A term used to describe any medical procedure that does not involve penetration of the skin or entry into the body through any of the natural openings; examples include *CT scanning* and *echocardiography*. The term noninvasive is sometimes also applied to benign tumors that do not spread throughout body tissues.

Nonspecific urethritis

Also called nongonococcal urethritis, inflammation of the urethra due to a cause or causes other than *gonorrhea*. Worldwide, nonspecific urethritis is the most common type of *sexually transmitted disease*.

CAUSES

The name nonspecific urethritis was given to the disorder at a time when few laboratory tests were available for the detection of microorganisms. Today, almost 50 percent of cases are known to be caused by CHLAMYDIA TRACHOMATIS (see *Chlamydial infections*); a few are caused by HERPESVIRUS HOMINIS (the virus that causes *herpes simplex*) or TRICHOMONAS VAGINALIS infections (see *Trichomoniasis*). In the remainder of cases, the cause remains unknown.

SYMPTOMS

Nonspecific urethritis has an incubation period of about two to three weeks. In men, the infection usually causes a clear or a purulent urethral discharge often accompanied by pain or discomfort on passing urine. Sometimes these symptoms are very mild or even absent. The equivalent condition in women is called nonspecific genital infection. This does not usually cause symptoms unless there are complications.

DIAGNOSIS AND TREATMENT

Laboratory tests are performed to identify the organism responsible for the infection. Because a woman may have no symptoms, a diagnosis often rests on the fact that she has a male partner with nonspecific urethritis.

Treatment is difficult because in many cases the cause of the infection cannot be determined. The cure rate is approximately 85 percent. *Antibiotic drugs*, including oxytetracycline and erythromycin, are given. Because relapses are common, however, follow-up visits may be advised for three months after treatment.

COMPLICATIONS

In men, *epididymitis*, *prostatitis*, and *urethral stricture* (narrowing of the urethra) can occur as complications of nonspecific urethritis.

N

In women, *salpingitis* (inflammation of the fallopian tubes) and cysts of the *Bartholin's glands* may occur. *Ophthalmia* neonatorum, a type of conjunctivitis, sometimes develops in babies born to women with chlamydial cervicitis.

Reiter's syndrome (in which there is arthritis and conjunctivitis as well as urethritis) occurs as a complication in about 5 percent of men who develop nonspecific urethritis.

Nonsteroidal anti-inflammatory drugs

COMMON DRUGS

Diclofenac Diflunisal Fenoprofen Flurbiprofen Ibuprofen Indomethacin Ketoprofen Mefenamic acid Naproxen Piroxicam

> **WARNING**
> Report abdominal pain, heartburn, or indigestion to your physician.

A group of drugs that produce *analgesia* (pain relief) and reduce inflammation in joints and soft tissues, such as muscles and ligaments. The name is commonly abbreviated to NSAIDs.

WHY THEY ARE USED
NSAIDs are widely used to relieve symptoms caused by types of arthritis, such as *rheumatoid arthritis, osteoarthritis*, and *gout*. They do not cure or halt the progress of disease but improve mobility of the affected joint by relieving pain and stiffness.

NSAIDs are also used in the treatment of back pain, menstrual pain, headaches, pain after minor surgery, and soft tissue injuries.

HOW THEY WORK
NSAIDs reduce pain and inflammation by blocking the production of *prostaglandins* (chemicals that cause inflammation and trigger transmission of pain signals to the brain).

POSSIBLE ADVERSE EFFECTS
NSAIDs sometimes cause adverse effects such as nausea, indigestion, diarrhea, and *peptic ulcer*.

Norepinephrine

A *hormone* secreted by certain nerve endings (principally those of the *sympathetic nervous system*) and by the medulla (center) of the *adrenal glands*. Norepinephrine's primary function is to help maintain a constant blood pressure by stimulating certain blood vessels to constrict (narrow) when the blood pressure falls. For this reason, an injection of norepinephrine may sometimes be given in the emergency treatment of *shock* or severe bleeding. (See also *Epinephrine*.)

Norethindrone

A *progestogen drug* used primarily as an ingredient of some *oral contraceptives*. Norethindrone is sometimes prescribed to postpone menstruation.

It is also used to treat *premenstrual syndrome*, menstrual disorders, such as *menorrhagia* (heavy periods), *endometriosis*, and certain types of *breast cancer*. Norethindrone is occasionally given by injection as a long-acting contraceptive.

Possible adverse effects include swollen ankles, weight gain, depression and, rarely, jaundice.

Norgestrel

A *progestogen drug*.

Nortriptyline

An *antidepressant drug* that also has a sedative effect. Nortriptyline is also used in the treatment of nocturnal *enuresis* (bed-wetting) in children over the age of 7 years.

Nose

The uppermost part of the respiratory tract and the organ of *smell*.

STRUCTURE
The nose is an air passage connecting the nostrils at its front to the *nasopharynx* (the upper part of the throat) at the rear. The *nasal septum*, which is made of cartilage at the front and bone at the rear, divides the passage into two chambers.

Two small bones, the nasal bones, project from the front of the cranium and form the top of the bridge of the nose; the remainder of the bridge is cartilage. The roof of the nasal passage is formed by bones at the base of the skull, the walls by the maxilla (upper *jaw*), and the floor by the hard *palate*. Projecting from each wall are three conchae (thin, downward-curling plates of bone); the conchae are covered with *mucous membrane*, which considerably increases the surface area of the nasal passage.

The bones surrounding the nose contain air-filled, mucous membrane-lined cavities known as paranasal *sinuses*, which open into the nasal passage. In each wall of the nose is the opening to a nasolacrimal duct, which drains away the tears that bathe the front of the eyeball.

Projecting into the roof of the nasal passage through tiny openings are the hairlike nerve endings of the *olfactory nerves*, which are responsible for the sense of smell.

FUNCTION
One of the main functions of the nose is to filter, warm, and moisten inhaled air before it passes into the rest of the respiratory tract. Just inside the nostrils, small hairs trap large dust parti-

ANATOMY OF THE NOSE

The nose is involved in breathing and also in the sense of smell; it is a hollow passage connecting the nostrils and the top of the throat. The upper part of the nose transmits sensations of smell.

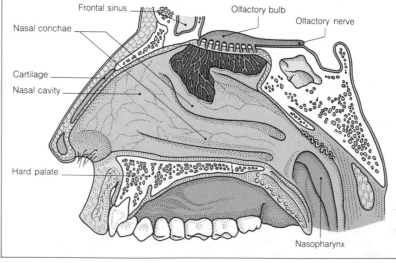

DISORDERS OF THE NOSE

The nose is susceptible to a wide range of disorders. Infections and allergic conditions, leading to stuffiness or sneezing and sometimes some loss of smell, are common. Because of its prominent position, the nose is also particularly prone to injury.

CONGENITAL DEFECTS

In choanal atresia, one or both nasal cavities fail to develop fully. If both sides are affected, the baby cannot breathe properly. An abnormality affecting one side may not cause any problems until later in life.

Syphilis that is transmitted to a fetus during pregnancy may lead to a failure of full development of the nasal bones.

INFECTION

The common *cold*, a virus infection, causes inflammation of the lining of the nasal passages and excessive production of mucus, leading to nasal congestion. Small *boils* (infected hair follicles) are common just within the nostril, where they may cause severe pain. Backward spread of infection from the nose occasionally causes *cavernous sinus thrombosis*, a serious condition that, without antibiotics, may be fatal.

TUMORS

Hemangiomas (benign tumors of blood vessels) commonly affect the nasal cavity in babies. Many disappear spontaneously before puberty.

Basal cell carcinoma and *squamous cell carcinoma* (types of skin cancer) may occur in and around the nostril. The nose may also be invaded by cancers originating in the sinuses.

INJURY

Fracture of the nasal bones (see *Nose, broken*) is a common sports injury that may require surgery. *Nosebleeds* are also common, particularly in children; they may be caused by fragile blood vessels, infection of the lining of the nose, or a blow to the nose.

DRUGS

Repeated sniffing of cocaine interferes with the blood supply to the mucous membrane lining the nose and can cause perforation of the nasal septum. Persistent taking of snuff can irritate or damage the nasal lining.

ALLERGIES

Allergic rhinitis (hay fever) is one of the most common allergies—the most common causative allergens being pollens, animal dander, house mites, and fungal spores. (See *Rhinitis, allergic.*)

OBSTRUCTION

A nasal *polyp* (a projection of swollen mucous membrane) may block a nostril, causing a sensation of congestion.

Young children frequently insert foreign bodies, such as beads, peas, or pebbles, into their nostrils. Objects often become stuck, causing obstruction and a discharge.

INVESTIGATION

To inspect the inside of the nose, the physician uses a speculum to open up the nostrils. If a fracture is suspected, *X rays* are taken. For suspected cancer, nasal endoscopy and a *biopsy* are performed.

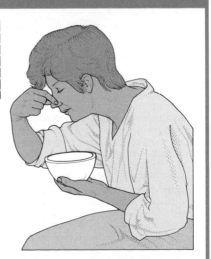

N

cles and even larger foreign bodies and induce sneezing to remove them. Smaller dust particles are filtered from the air by the microscopic hairs of the conchae. All air entering the nose passes over the blood vessels and mucus-secreting cells on the surface of the conchae. The mucus on the conchae flows inward, carrying harmful microorganisms and other foreign bodies back toward the nasopharynx so that they can be swallowed and destroyed by the gastric acid in the stomach.

The nose detects smells by means of the olfactory nerve endings, which, when stimulated by inhaled vapors, transmit this information to the olfactory bulb in the brain.

The nose also acts as a resonator, helping to give each voice its individual characteristic tone. (See also *Nose* disorders box.)

Nosebleed

Loss of blood from the mucous membrane that lines the nose, most often from inside one nostril only.

Nosebleeds are most common during childhood, when they are usually insignificant and easily stopped. They occur infrequently in healthy young adults, but become more common and more serious during old age.

CAUSES

The most common causes of a nosebleed are a blow to the nose, fragile blood vessels, or the dislodging of crusts that have formed in the mucous membrane as a result of a common cold or other infection. Rarely, recurrent nosebleeds are a sign of an underlying disorder, such as *hypertension*

FIRST AID: NOSEBLEED

WARNING
If a nosebleed starts after a heavy blow to the head, it could indicate a fractured skull. Take the victim to hospital immediately.

1 Sit the victim up, ensuring that he or she leans forward slightly with the mouth held open so that blood or clots do not obstruct the airway.

2 Pinch the lower part of the nostrils for about 15 minutes. The victim should breathe through the mouth.

3 The nostrils should be released slowly and the victim should avoid touching or blowing the nose. If the bleeding has not stopped after 20 minutes, seek medical attention.

(high blood pressure), a *bleeding disorder*, or a tumor of the nose or of the paranasal sinuses.

TREATMENT
Most nosebleeds can be controlled by simple first aid measures (see the illustrated box on page 737).

If first aid treatment fails to stop bleeding within 20 minutes, a physician should be consulted. He or she may pack the affected nostril firmly with gauze (to apply constant pressure to the wound) or may cauterize the wound. In rare cases, surgery may be needed to stop the bleeding.

Nose, broken

Fracture of the nasal bones or dislocation of the cartilage that forms the bridge of the *nose*. A blow from the side may knock the bones or cartilage out of position or cause displacement of the *nasal septum*. A frontal blow tends to splay the nasal bones outward, depressing the bridge. Usually, the fracture is accompanied by severe swelling of overlying soft tissue. Such swelling can mask a minor fracture, which may be detected only when *X rays* are taken.

A fractured nose is painful and remains tender for about three weeks after the injury.

TREATMENT
Resetting is usually carried out either before the swelling has started, or after it has subsided, usually about 10 days after the injury. Occasionally, the displaced bone can be manipulated into position under a local anesthetic, but usually a general anesthetic is needed. A plaster splint is sometimes required during healing.

Nose reshaping
See *Rhinoplasty*.

Notifiable diseases

Medical conditions that must be reported by the physician responsible for the affected person to the local health authorities.

Notification of certain potentially harmful infectious diseases is important because it enables health officers to take the necessary steps to control the spread of infection (e.g., by isolation or by offering *immunization* to contacts). Notification also allows monitoring of the occurrence of infectious diseases and provides valuable statistics on the *incidence* and *prevalence* of diseases. Such information may be used in formulating health policies such as immunization programs or improvements in sanitation.

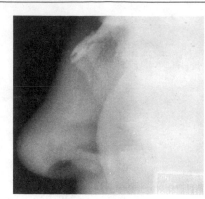

X ray showing broken nose
The nasal bones under the bridge of the nose and part of the ethmoid bone, which forms the top part of the nasal septum (partition between the two sides of the nose), have been broken.

Examples of notifiable infectious diseases are *food poisoning, hepatitis, measles, malaria, rabies, tuberculosis,* and *pertussis* (whooping cough).

Some categories of diseases other than infections must also be notified. These include some *birth defects* and certain forms of *handicap*. *Cancers* are registered nationally, and cancer data is now pooled in an international registry. Certain types of *occupational disease* are also notifiable; examples include *lead poisoning, mercury poisoning, cadmium poisoning,* and *anthrax*.

NSAID
The commonly used abbreviation for *nonsteroidal anti-inflammatory drugs*.

NSU
The commonly used abbreviation for *nonspecific urethritis*.

Nuclear energy

The energy released as a result of changes in the nuclei of atoms. It is also known as atomic energy and is principally released in the form of heat, light, and ionizing *radiation*, such as gamma rays.

Nuclear energy is released in certain natural processes, examples of which include the spontaneous decay of naturally occurring radioactive substances (such as uranium ores) and the nuclear reactions that power the sun and other stars. Nuclear energy is also released in man-made devices, for example nuclear reactors and nuclear weapons.

Nuclear magnetic resonance
See *MRI*.

Nuclear medicine

Techniques that use radioactive substances to detect or treat disease. The most important application of nuclear medicine is in diagnosis. Radioactive materials, which may be injected or swallowed, are taken up by body tissues or organs in different concentrations, and a radioactivity detector, such as a gamma camera, is used to discover and map the distribution of radiation within the body.

This diagnostic technique requires only a small amount of radiation. Yet, within a few hours, it is able to produce images that reflect bodily functions—not simply anatomy. (See *Radionuclide scanning*.)

CASES OF NOTIFIABLE INFECTIOUS DISEASES IN CANADA (1988)	
Disease	**Number of cases**
Gonococcal infections	20,376
Salmonellosis (See *Food poisoning*)	11,626
Campylobacteriosis (See *Food poisoning*)	11,098
Giardiasis	9,075
Hepatitis B	3,132
Shigellosis	2,096
Tuberculosis	2,031
Amebiasis	1,989
Syphilis	1,583
Hepatitis A	1,533
Pertussis (whooping cough)	1,106
AIDS	801
Hemophilus influenzae*	646
Mumps	639
Measles	609
Rubella (German measles)	559
Bacterial meningitis (all forms)	521
Malaria	300
Viral meningitis	290
Typhoid	58
Legionnaires' disease	52
Leprosy	24
Brucellosis	11
Diphtheria	11
Botulism	5
Rabies	0

*The organism, *Hemophilus influenzae*, is a cause of meningitis and upper respiratory tract infections in children

In techniques for treatment, higher doses of radiation are used. Diseased tissues are destroyed by exposing them to an external radioactive source or by inserting a radioactive substance into a body tissue or cavity. (See *Interstitial radiation therapy; Intracavitary therapy; Radiation therapy*.)

Nucleic acids

Substances found in all living matter that have a fundamental role in the propagation of life. Nucleic acids provide the inherited coded instructions (or "blueprint") for an organism's development; they also provide some of the apparatus by which these instructions are carried out.

There are two types of nucleic acid, called deoxyribonucleic acid (DNA) and ribonucleic acid (RNA). In all plant and animal cells (including humans'), it is the DNA that permanently holds the coded instructions; RNA helps transport, translate, and implement the instructions. The DNA is the main constituent of *chromosomes*, which are carried in the nucleus (central unit) of the cell.

STRUCTURE

DNA and RNA are similar in structure. Both have long, chainlike molecules. The main difference is that DNA usually consists of two intertwined chains, whereas RNA is generally single stranded.

The basic structure of DNA (see illustrated box) has been likened to a very long rope ladder, the chains of the DNA forming the two sides of the ladder, with interlinking structures between the chains forming the rungs. The ladder is not straight, however, but twisted into a helical (spiral) shape, which gives it great stability. This shape is called a double helix.

If the two DNA chains are separated, it is found that each has a "backbone" (the side of the ladder) consisting of a string of sugar and phosphate chemical groups. Attached to each sugar in this string is a chemical called a base. The base can be any of four types, called adenine, thymine, guanine, and cytosine (or A, T, G, and C), and each forms half of one rung of the DNA ladder. The four bases can occur in any sequence along the chain (a sequence might be, for example, GTCGTATTTAGTCC). The sequence itself, which may be many millions of individual bases long, provides the code for the activities of the cell, just as the sequence of letters on this page provides a message for its readers (see *Genetic code*). Because the

A DNA molecule consists of two intertwined strands, the margins of which are chains of sugar and phosphate groups. The chains are linked by pairs of substances called bases, of which there are four types—adenine, guanine, thymine, and cytosine. An adenine on one chain is always paired with thymine on the second; similarly, cytosine is always paired with guanine. The sequence of bases in one chain thus exactly determines the sequence in the other chain.

Nucleotides
Each base, along with the sugar and phosphate groups to which it is attached, forms a unit called a nucleotide.

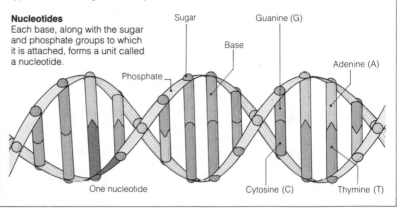

Sugar
Guanine (G)
Base
Adenine (A)
Phosphate
One nucleotide
Cytosine (C)
Thymine (T)

two bases that form each rung of the ladder conform to certain pairings (A always pairs with T, and G with C), the sequence of bases on one chain determines the sequence on the second chain. This is of fundamental importance for the copying of DNA molecules when a cell divides.

RNA is like a single strand of DNA, except that the nucleotide base thymine in DNA is replaced by another base, uracil, in RNA, and the sugar and phosphate chain in RNA is chemically slightly different.

FUNCTION

DNA controls a cell's activities by specifying and regulating the synthesis of *enzymes* and other proteins in the cell, with different *genes* (sections of DNA) regulating the production of different proteins. For a particular protein to be made, an appropriate section of DNA acts as a template for an RNA chain. This "messenger" RNA then passes out of the nucleus into the cell cytoplasm, where it is decoded to form proteins (see *Genetic code; Protein synthesis*).

In mitotic division, identical copies of a cell's DNA must go to each of the two daughter cells. The structure of DNA makes this possible.

Starting at one end of the molecule, the two chains separate, or "unzip." As they do so, two more chains are formed (side by side with the original chains) by the linking of free, unlinked, nucleotides that are present in cells. Because only certain base pairings are possible, the new double chains are identical to the original DNA molecule. Thus a dividing cell provides an exact copy of its DNA to its daughter cells. Each of a person's cells carries the same DNA replica that was present in the fertilized ovum, so the DNA message passes from one generation of cells to the next.

Nucleus

The central core, structure, or focal point of an object.

The nucleus of a living *cell* is a roughly spherical unit at the center of the cell. It contains the *chromosomes* (composed mainly of *nucleic acid*) responsible for directing the cell's activities, and is surrounded by a mem-

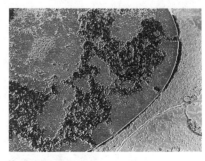

Nucleus
This photomicrograph shows a typical nucleus (at left). The nuclear envelope, which separates nucleus from cytoplasm, consists of two layers of membrane broken by pores.

N

739

NUMBNESS AND TINGLING   Loss of feeling and/or a pins and needles sensation in any part of the body

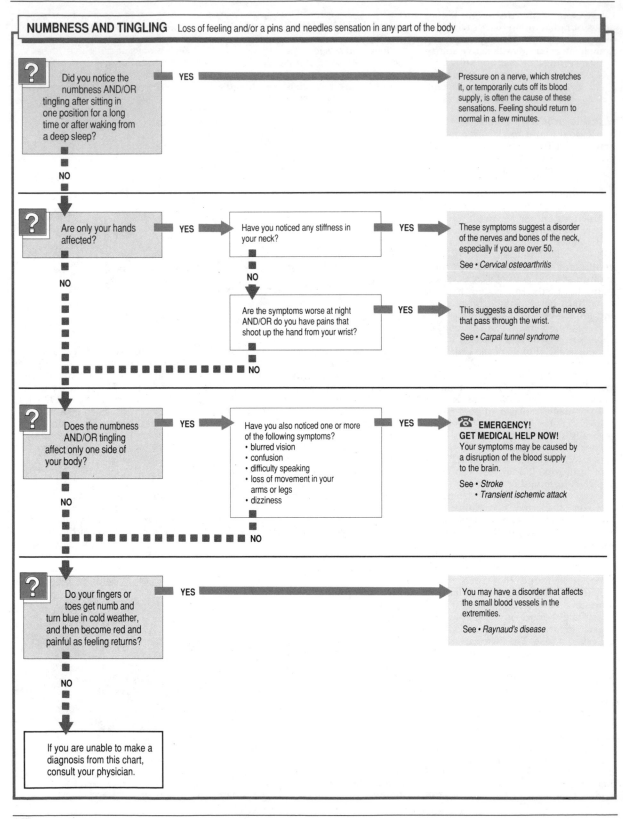

Did you notice the numbness AND/OR tingling after sitting in one position for a long time or after waking from a deep sleep?

YES → Pressure on a nerve, which stretches it, or temporarily cuts off its blood supply, is often the cause of these sensations. Feeling should return to normal in a few minutes.

NO

Are only your hands affected?

YES → Have you noticed any stiffness in your neck?

YES → These symptoms suggest a disorder of the nerves and bones of the neck, especially if you are over 50.

See • *Cervical osteoarthritis*

NO

Are the symptoms worse at night AND/OR do you have pains that shoot up the hand from your wrist?

YES → This suggests a disorder of the nerves that pass through the wrist.

See • *Carpal tunnel syndrome*

NO

NO

Does the numbness AND/OR tingling affect only one side of your body?

YES → Have you also noticed one or more of the following symptoms?
• blurred vision
• confusion
• difficulty speaking
• loss of movement in your arms or legs
• dizziness

YES → ☎ **EMERGENCY!**
GET MEDICAL HELP NOW!
Your symptoms may be caused by a disruption of the blood supply to the brain.

See • *Stroke*
    • *Transient ischemic attack*

NO

NO

Do your fingers or toes get numb and turn blue in cold weather, and then become red and painful as feeling returns?

YES → You may have a disorder that affects the small blood vessels in the extremities.

See • *Raynaud's disease*

NO

If you are unable to make a diagnosis from this chart, consult your physician.

N

ESSENTIAL NUTRIENTS

Proteins	The main structural component of tissues and organs. We need proteins for growth and repair of cells. Each protein contains hundreds and sometimes thousands of units called amino acids in specific combinations. In the body there are 20 amino acids; 12 of these are manufactured by the body itself and	the remaining eight are obtained from a balanced diet. A vegetarian diet containing eggs, milk, and cheese provides sufficient amounts of all essential amino acids. A vegan diet, which also excludes dairy products, needs careful planning to prevent protein deficiency (see *Vegetarianism*).
Carbohydrates	The two carbohydrate food groups, sugars and starches, are the main energy sources required for metabolism (chemical processes that take place in cells). Carbohydrates should make up at	least half of the diet. Unrefined (unprocessed) carbohydrates found in cereals and fruit are usually richer in fiber and nutrients than are refined carbohydrates, such as sugar and white flour.
Fats	Fats provide energy for metabolism and are a structural component of cells. Most people in developed countries eat too much fat; fats should constitute no more than 30 percent of total calorie intake. There are three types of dietary fats: saturated fats (found mostly in meat and dairy products), monosaturated fats (found in olive oil and avocados), and polyunsaturated fats (found in fish and vegetable oils). Saturated fats	tend to increase the amounts of unwanted types of cholesterol in the blood whereas polyunsaturated fats and monosaturated fats have the opposite effect. Studies have indicated that a high level of low-density lipoprotein cholesterol in the blood is associated with coronary artery disease. Our bodies produce enough cholesterol for our needs; any excess is primarily due to eating too much saturated fat.
Fiber	This is the indigestible structural material in plants. Although fiber passes through the intestine unchanged, it is an essential part of a healthy diet. A low-fiber diet may lead to constipation, diverticular disease, and other disorders. High-fiber diets (including plenty	of fruit, raw vegetables, grains, and cereals) provide bulk without excess calories. Low-fiber diets tend to be high in refined carbohydrates and fats, and thus are more likely to encourage obesity, heart disease, and other undesirable conditions.
Water	Our bodies are composed of about 60 percent water. Water constitutes a high proportion of many foods and is essential to maintain metabolism	(chemical processes in cells) and normal bowel function. It also determines the volume of blood in the circulation.
Vitamins	Regulators of metabolism. Vitamins ensure the healthy functioning of the brain, nerves, muscles, skin, and bones. Although vitamins do not supply energy, some enable energy to be released from food. A healthy, balanced diet contains enough vitamins for most people's needs and supplements are not	usually necessary. Indeed, some vitamins (especially A, D, E, and K) are dangerous if taken in excess. The body can store only relatively small amounts of water-soluble vitamins (B and C), but even on a very restricted diet, vitamin deficiency is rare until several months have elapsed.
Minerals	A balanced diet provides enough minerals for most people. Calcium is necessary for the maintenance of healthy teeth and bones. Other minerals, such as zinc and magnesium, are needed in minute amounts to control cell metabolism.	The only mineral commonly required as a supplement is iron, which is used to prevent anemia in women who have heavy periods. Sodium chloride (table salt) is needed to maintain fluid balance; excess may cause *hypertension*.

brane. This membrane has small pores through which various substances can pass between the nucleus and the cytoplasm (the rest of the cell).

The nucleus of an atom, composed of protons and neutrons, accounts for nearly all the mass of an atom but only a tiny proportion of its volume. *Nuclear energy* is produced through changes in the mass and structure of atomic nuclei.

A nerve nucleus is a group of *neurons* (nerve cells) within the brain and spinal cord that work together to perform a particular function.

Nudophobia

An abnormal fear of being in an unclothed state.

Numbness

Loss of sensation in part of the body caused by interference to the passage of impulses along sensory *nerves*.

CAUSES

Numbness can occur naturally and harmlessly (such as when blood supply to a nerve in the leg is cut off temporarily by sitting cross-legged), it can be induced artificially (e.g., by a dentist anesthetizing a nerve before filling a tooth), or it may be the result of a disorder or damage to the *nervous system* or its blood supply.

Multiple sclerosis can cause loss of sensation in any part of the body through damage to nerve pathways in the central nervous system (CNS). In a *neuropathy*, it is the peripheral nerves (nerves outside the CNS) that are damaged. In a *stroke*, pressure on, or reduced blood supply to, nerve pathways in the brain often causes loss of feeling on one side of the body.

Severe cold, as in *frostbite*, causes numbness by a direct action on the nerves. Numbness may also be a feature of various psychological disorders, such as *anxiety*, *panic attack*, or a hysterical *conversion disorder*.

DIAGNOSIS AND TREATMENT

Examination by a physician usually reveals an area of sensory loss or impairment that corresponds to the skin distribution of a single peripheral nerve, several nerves, or a sensory area in the CNS. The distribution of the affected area may suggest the site and mechanism of nerve damage.

Nurse

A person trained in *nursing care*. There are more than 220,000 registered nurses in Canada; about 87 percent are women. Most nurses are now being trained in community colleges

N

FOOD SOURCES OF ESSENTIAL NUTRIENTS

PROTEIN

Food	Protein content (g of protein per 100 g of food)
Yeast extract (Baker's yeast)	50
Beef, lean, roast	31
Tuna, canned	28
Wheat germ	27
Cheese, cheddar	26
Chicken, lean, roast	26
Peanuts, shelled, roasted	24
Cod, grilled	17
Cottage cheese, low-fat	13
Brazil nuts, shelled	12
Eggs, boiled	12

FAT

Food	Fat content (g of fat per 100 g of food)
Oils, cooking and salad	100
Butter and margarine	81
Brazil nuts, shelled	67
Peanuts, shelled, roasted	49
Sausage, pork, cooked	42
Beef, lean with fat, roast	40
Low-fat spread	39
Cream, whipping	38
Cheese, cheddar	32
Chocolate, milk	30
Egg yolk	30

CARBOHYDRATE

Food	Carbohydrate content (g of carbohydrate per 100 g of food)
Sugar, white	100
Rice, white, uncooked	87
Cornflakes	84
Pasta, uncooked	84
Honey	81
Flour, white	80
Apricots, dried, stoned	67
Chocolate, milk	57
Beans, green, uncooked	45
Bread, whole wheat	37
Prunes	34

FIBER

Food	Fiber content (g of fiber per 100 g of food)
Bran	44
Apricots, dried, stoned	24
Prunes	14
Peas, boiled	12
Blackcurrants	9
Brazil nuts, shelled	9
Bread, whole wheat	9
Peanuts, shelled, roasted	8
Beans, green, uncooked	7
Sweet corn	6
Celery	5

The tables (above) list a selection of foods that are good sources of protein, carbohydrate, fat or fiber together with the amount of the nutrient concerned in 100 g of each food. The figures given here are averages, because the exact nutrient content of many foods depends on variable factors such as the method of preparation. (See also *Vitamins* and *Minerals*.)

and vocational schools rather than hospital nursing schools. Many nurses practice in specialized areas such as emergency care, surgical nursing, and psychiatric nursing. (See *Canadian Nurses Association*.)

Nursing
Care of the sick or injured (see *Nursing care*), or an alternative name for *breast-feeding*.

Nursing care
The process of looking after the physical or emotional needs of patients with the aim of restoring, improving, maintaining, or promoting well-being. Nurses assist patients to recover from illness and injury, encourage them to regain their independence, and, in cases of terminal illness, help patients to meet death with as little distress and as much dignity as possible.

Nursing home
A type of long-term care facility for the elderly or those with special needs for chronic medical care. Nursing homes may be private or public facilities.

There are more than 3,000 facilities for long-term care in Canada. Strictly speaking not all are nursing homes; some emphasize residential arrangements and independent living. Standards in provincial long-term care facilities are monitored by provincial accreditation and inspection.

Nutrient
Essential dietary factors, such as carbohydrates, proteins, certain fats, vitamins, and minerals.

Nutrition
The scientific study of food and the processes by which it is digested and assimilated. Until about 30 years ago, nutritionists were mainly concerned with dietary deficiencies and with the minimum amounts of nutrients required for health. Of course this is still the main concern for developing countries, but in Western societies the focus is now on the dangers of too much fat or sugar in the diet, and the possible ill effects of food additives.

A good diet supplies adequate but not excessive quantities of *proteins, carbohydrates, fats, vitamins, minerals,* dietary *fiber*, and water. The basis of a good diet is variety because no one food contains all the nutrients we need. Often, too, nutrients are interdependent: they cannot function alone. For example, calcium and phosphorus are both needed for forming and maintaining bones and teeth. The daily diet should include foods from each of the four basic food groups: milk and milk products; vegetables and fruits; breads and cereals; meat, fish, poultry, and legumes.

Personal requirements of nutrients and *energy* vary, depending on individual body size, age, sex, and lifestyle. For example, an average woman requires about 2,000 cal (8,400 kJ) daily compared with about 2,750 cal (11,550 kJ) for an average man. (See also *Energy requirements*.)

Nutritional disorders

Nutritional disorders may be caused by a deficiency or excess of one or more of the elements of *nutrition*, or by the presence of a *toxin* (poisonous element) in the diet.

NUTRITIONAL DEFICIENCY

A diet that is deficient in *carbohydrate* is almost invariably also deficient in *protein*. Inevitably, such a diet leads to the development of protein-calorie malnutrition. This particular deficiency is most often seen in developing countries in Africa and Asia as a result of poverty and famine (see *Kwashiorkor*; *Marasmus*).

Inadequate intake of protein and calories may also occur in people who restrict their diet in an attempt to lose weight (see *Anorexia nervosa*); it can also occur because of mistaken beliefs about diet and health (see *Food fad*) or because of loss of interest in food associated with *alcohol dependence* or *drug dependence*.

Deficiency of specific nutrients is commonly associated with a disorder of the digestive system, such as *celiac disease*, *Crohn's disease*, or pernicious anemia (see *Anemia, megaloblastic*).

NUTRITIONAL EXCESS

Obesity results from taking in more *energy* from the diet than is used up by the body. Limiting foods high in fat, salt, and sugar reduces the risk of obesity, as well as *cardiovascular disorders*, dental *caries*, *diabetes mellitus*, and *hypertension*. Nutritional disorders may also result from an excessive intake of *minerals* and *vitamins*. An excessive intake of *fat* is thought to be a contributory factor in *coronary artery disease* and it has been linked to some forms of *cancer*.

TOXIC EFFECTS

Naturally occurring toxins can interfere with the digestion, absorption, and/or utilization of nutrients, or can cause specific disorders due to their toxic effects (e.g., the *ergot* fungus found on rye can cause ergotism).

Industrial pollutants, pesticides, fertilizers, and other chemicals may also contaminate food.

Nymphomania

A *psychosexual disorder* in which a woman is dominated by an insatiable appetite for sexual activity with numerous different male partners. Nymphomaniacs are often distressed by their own behavior and their inability to see men as anything other than objects for sexual conquest. Nymphomania is thought to be an expression of some deep psychological disorder.

The equivalent behavior in men is called satyriasis or Don Juanism. It is said to be caused by intense *narcissism* and by feelings of inferiority.

Nystagmus

A condition in which there is involuntary movement of the eyes; the movement is usually horizontal, but can be vertical or rotatory. In almost all cases, both eyes move together.

CAUSES AND TYPES

In the most common type, called jerky nystagmus, the eyes repeatedly move slowly in one direction and then rapidly in the other, giving a jerking effect. Less commonly, nystagmus is "pendular," with the eyes moving evenly from side to side.

Nystagmus is usually congenital and is not associated with any abnormality of the eyes; the cause is unknown. Because a steady gaze is impossible, there is almost always a moderate to severe defect of visual acuity. Nystagmus also occurs in *albinism* and as a result of any very severe defect of vision present at birth, such as congenital *cataract*.

Persistent nystagmus appearing later in life usually indicates the presence of a disorder of the nervous system (such as *multiple sclerosis*, a *brain tumor*, or an *alcohol-related disorder*) or a disorder of the balancing mechanism in the inner ear. Adult-onset nystagmus is occasionally seen as an occupational disorder in people who work in poor light (coal miners, for example). Nystagmus may also occur as a normal effect of attempts to follow a sequence of objects rapidly passing the eyes. This phenomenon is generally known as "optokinetic nystagmus."

Electronystagmography, a method of recording eye movements, may be performed to identify the different types of nystagmus.

N

Nystatin

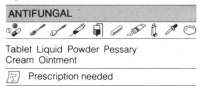

ANTIFUNGAL

Tablet Liquid Powder Pessary
Cream Ointment

Prescription needed

An *antifungal drug* used in the treatment of *candidiasis* (thrush). Nystatin may be safely used during pregnancy. High doses of nystatin taken by mouth may cause diarrhea, nausea, vomiting, and abdominal pain.

NUTRITIONAL DISORDERS

Nutritional disorders can result from too much or too little food. Obesity resulting from excessive energy intake is one of the most common. Malnutrition resulting from inadequate protein and energy intake is common among young children in developing countries.

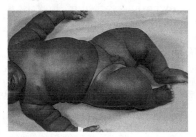

Obesity
This photograph shows an obese 8-month-old baby boy. He weighs 14.8 kg, the average for a 3-year-old child.

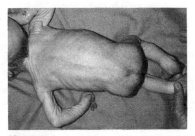

Marasmus
This baby has marasmus, a form of malnutrition resulting from insufficient intake of protein and energy.

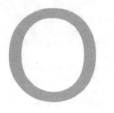

Oat cell carcinoma

See *Small cell carcinoma*.

Obesity

A condition in which there is too much body fat. A person is usually not considered obese unless he or she weighs 20 percent or more over the maximum desirable weight for his or her height, or has a body mass index (calculated by dividing one's weight in kilograms by one's height in metres squared) of 27 or more (see *Weight* tables). In Canada, it is estimated that 29 percent of the men and 19 percent of the women over the age of 18 are at increased risk of developing health problems because of excess weight.

The reasons why some people become obese are unclear. Although obesity occurs when the net energy intake exceeds the net energy expenditure (that is, when more calories are taken in than are being used by the body), overweight people do not always eat more than thin people.

A person's energy requirements are determined partly by his or her basal metabolic rate (the amount of energy needed to maintain vital body functions at rest—see *Metabolism*) and partly by his or her level of physical activity. Obesity may develop in people who have a low basal metabolic rate, or who are less physically active and so need fewer calories.

It is thought that genetic factors play a part in the development of obesity; children of obese parents are 10 times more likely to be obese than children with parents of normal weight. Some hormonal disorders are accompanied by obesity, but the overwhelming majority of obese people do not suffer from such disorders.

COMPLICATIONS

Obesity increases a person's chance of becoming seriously ill. *Hypertension* (high blood pressure) and *stroke* are twice as likely to occur in obese people than in lean people. *Coronary artery disease* is more common, particularly in obese men under the age of 40. Adult-onset *diabetes mellitus* is five times more common among obese people, the risk increasing with the degree and duration of obesity. Increasing degrees of extra weight in men are associated with an increased risk of cancer of the colon, rectum, and prostate. With increasing weight, women show a progressive increase in risk of cancer of the breast, uterus, and cervix. *Osteoarthritis* may be aggravated by obesity. Extra weight on the hips, knees, and back places undue strain on these joints. Weight loss does not reverse the disease but does help relieve stress and pain.

TREATMENT

The first line of treatment for obesity is a slimming diet (see *Weight reduction*). An obese person should follow a diet that provides 500 to 1,000 calories less than his or her energy requirements. The body meets this deficit by using up some of the excess stored fat. About 0.5 kg of body fat supplies about 3,500 cal, so a daily deficit of 1,000 cal would result, on average, in a loss of about 1 kg in a week. Water loss during the first one to two weeks further increases the loss of weight.

Regular exercise (especially *aerobics*) helps increase weight loss by causing the body to burn extra calories and by increasing the metabolic rate.

Fad diets may cause a dramatic weight loss within a short period of time, but, in almost all cases, the weight is quickly regained when normal eating habits are resumed. The use of drugs as *appetite suppressants* was once popular, but is now rarely recommended by physicians.

Radical procedures are sometimes performed on severely obese people who have failed to lose weight. *Wiring of the jaws* may be carried out to restrict food intake. An operation in which part of the stomach is stapled together may be performed to reduce the size of the stomach and make the person feel full after eating a small amount of food. Intestinal bypass operations, in which a large part of the small intestine is bypassed by cutting the jejunum and joining it to the ileum, are occasionally performed to reduce the length of the digestive tract and allow less food to be absorbed. However, because of the risk of adverse effects, such procedures are attempted only if the person's health is in danger.

OUTLOOK

Some people who have been seriously obese for much of their lives can lose weight without regaining it. As when trying to give up smoking or alcohol, the essential element is motivation.

Obsessive-compulsive disorder

A *neurosis* in which sufferers are constantly troubled by persistent ideas (obsessions) that make them carry out repetitive, ritualized acts (compulsions). Obsessive-compulsive disorder usually starts in adolescence and runs a fluctuating course.

CAUSES AND INCIDENCE

The condition is partly inherited, but environmental factors also play a part. Personality traits of orderliness and cleanliness are said to be related, as is a tendency for other neurotic symptoms. Certain forms of brain damage, especially when due to *encephalitis*, can result in obsessional symptoms.

Obsessive-compulsive disorder is rare, although minor obsessional symptoms probably occur in about one sixth of the population.

SYMPTOMS

People with this disorder usually suffer from both obsessions and compulsions, often accompanied by *depression* and *anxiety*.

Obsessions are recurrent thoughts or feelings that come into the mind seemingly involuntarily. Sufferers regard these thoughts as senseless and sometimes unpleasant, but are unable to ignore or resist them. Thoughts of violence, fears of being infected by germs or dirt, and constant doubts (e.g., whether the front door is shut) are the most common obsessions. One form is obsessional rumination, in which a person broods constantly over a word, phrase, or an unanswerable problem.

Compulsions are repetitive, apparently purposeful acts that are carried out in a ritualized fashion. They are performed for the purpose of warding off fears or relieving anxiety and are thus the physical form of an obsessional state. Sufferers do not usually derive any pleasure from performing the activities, but feel increasingly anxious if they try to resist the compulsion. Handwashing, counting, and checking are the most common compulsions.

Compulsive acts may have to be performed so many times in a particular way that they seriously disrupt work and social life. It may take some sufferers two or three hours just to get up and wash in the morning. In addition, the constant use of soap may irritate the skin.

TREATMENT

In the past, obsessive-compulsive symptoms were treated by *psychoanalysis*. Today, treatment is usually by *behavior therapy*, sometimes in combination with *antidepressant drugs* (especially *clomipramine*).

OUTLOOK
At least two thirds of all people who have obsessive-compulsive disorder respond well to therapy. Symptoms may recur under stress but can usually be controlled. In severe cases, the affected person may become housebound and severely handicapped by indecision.

Obstetrics
The branch of medicine concerned with *pregnancy* and *prenatal care, childbirth,* and *postnatal care*. Obstetrics also involves the study of the structure and function of the female *reproductive system*. There is thus an overlap with *gynecology*, and most obstetricians are also gynecologists.

Obstructive airways disease
See *Lung disease, chronic obstructive.*

Occiput
The lower back part of the head, where it merges with the neck.

Occlusion
Blockage of any passage, canal, opening, or vessel in the body. Occlusion may be the result of disease (in *pulmonary embolism*, for example) or it may be induced for medical reasons (see *Embolism*). The term is also used to refer to the covering of the better-seeing eye during treatment of *amblyopia*.

In dentistry, occlusion is the relationship between the upper and lower teeth when the jaw is shut. In an ideal occlusion: the upper incisors and canines (front teeth) slightly overlap the lower ones; the front two upper incisors are aligned centrally with the front two lower incisors, and the remaining upper teeth are positioned in an alternating pattern relative to the equivalent lower teeth; the outer ridges of the lower premolars and molars (back teeth) fit into the hollows in the corresponding upper teeth.

In practice, very few people have an ideal occlusion, but unless the variation from the ideal is very marked, the arrangement of the teeth usually enables food to be bitten and chewed efficiently. (See also *Malocclusion*.)

Occult
A term meaning hidden or obscure. Occult blood in a sample of feces is invisible to the naked eye but can be detected by chemical tests.

Occult blood, fecal
The presence in the feces of blood that cannot be seen by the naked eye but can be detected by chemical tests. It may be a sign of various disorders of the gastrointestinal tract, including *esophagitis*; *gastritis* (inflammation of the stomach lining); *stomach cancer*; intestinal cancer (see *Intestine, cancer of*); rectal cancer (see *Rectum, cancer of*); *diverticular disease*; *polyps* in the colon; *ulcerative colitis*; or the taking of drugs that irritate the stomach or intestine, such as *ASA*. Bleeding gums or *hemorrhoids* may also cause occult blood in the feces, although in most cases of hemorrhoids the blood is visible.

DETECTION
Screening for cancer of the colon or rectum can be performed by testing the feces for occult blood. A thin film of feces is smeared on a chemically coated paper and a drop or two of oxidizing agent is placed on it. If blood is present, the feces-covered paper turns blue. (See also *Feces, abnormal; Rectal bleeding*.)

Occupational disease and injury
Illnesses, disorders, or injuries that occur as a result of work practices or of exposure to chemical, physical, or biological factors (such as dusts, poisons, or radiation) in the workplace. The efforts of specialists in this field have made serious occupational diseases much less common than formerly, but new hazards are continually appearing. Overall, occupational diseases still make up an important and fairly common group of conditions.

TYPES
Some of the main types of occupational diseases are described below.

DUST DISEASES The name *pneumoconiosis* is used to refer to *fibrosis* of the lung that is caused by inhaled inorganic and organic dusts. Pneumoconiosis includes various diseases associated with mining (including coal and quartz mining), china clay processing, metal grinding, and foundry work.

Asbestosis (see *Asbestos-induced diseases*) is a similar hazard in the asbestos, mining, milling, and manufacturing industries, and in the demolition and maintenance of plants and buildings where asbestos has been used. This has been seen particularly in shipbuilding. Formerly a problem in Quebec, safety precautions and air monitoring have virtually eliminated industrial asbestosis.

Allergic *alveolitis* is a lung condition caused by inhalation of organic dusts (often containing fungal spores). It is often occupationally related (such as *farmers' lung* in agricultural workers.

CHEMICAL POISONING Many industrial chemicals can cause damage to the lungs if inhaled, or to the liver, kidneys, bone marrow, or other organs if they reach the bloodstream via the lungs or skin.

Exposure to the fumes of cadmium (used, for example, in the welding and electroplating industries) may damage the kidneys. Beryllium (used in high-technology industries) can damage the lungs. Lead and its compounds (used in metal processing and other industries) and benzene (used in various industries where solvents are used) can damage the bone marrow, leading to *anemia* and other blood abnormalities. Carbon tetrachloride and vinyl chloride (used in the manufacture of chemicals and plastics) are causes of liver disease. Many of these compounds can also cause kidney damage.

OCCUPATIONAL SKIN DISEASE Contact *dermatitis* (skin inflammation) can occur as a result of an allergy or of direct irritation by chemicals contacting the skin at work. Many substances may be responsible, from wet cement to chemicals used in the rubber goods industry. Other skin problems may also be occupationally related (for example, severe itching caused by fiberglass, or *squamous cell carcinoma* due to exposure to tar).

RADIATION HAZARDS People with outdoor occupations in sunny climates are at increased risk of skin disease, such as *basal cell carcinoma*.

Workers in the *nuclear energy* industry and in some health care professions should use precautions to reduce the risk of developing a disease caused by ionizing radiation (see *Radiation hazards*).

INFECTIOUS DISEASES Some rare infectious diseases are more common than average in people with certain occupations. Examples include *brucellosis* and *Q fever* (acquired from livestock) in farmworkers, and *psittacosis* (acquired from birds) in pet shop owners. *Leptospirosis* is more common than average in sewer workers, miners, ditchdiggers, and fishermen, who acquire the disease from rats, and, increasingly, in farmworkers, who acquire it from cattle. Viral *hepatitis* and *AIDS* are hazards for people who work with blood and blood products.

MISCELLANEOUS Disorders caused by repetitive actions or by overuse of parts of the body range from *writer's* cramp to *carpal tunnel syndrome* and *singer's nodes. Raynaud's phenomenon* is associated with the handling of vibrating tools. The so-called White finger disease due to continued use of a chain saw is a permanent and crippling form of Raynaud's phenomenon. However, improved vibration damping in the saws and greater consciousness of the problem in chain saw operators have reduced the frequency and severity of the disability. *Deafness* may be caused by exposure to noise, and *cataracts* by exposure to the radiation associated with intense heat. Farming still ranks as one of the most dangerous common occupations. Injuries and fatalities can be caused by machinery, especially tractors and their power takeoffs. (See also *Farmer's lung*.)

DIAGNOSIS AND PREVENTION

Sometimes the link between a disease and occupation may be obvious; sometimes it may become apparent only when a patient with mysterious symptoms mentions his or her occupation to the physician. Part of every medical history is a question regarding the patient's occupation. Even when an occupational disease is suspected, extensive investigation at the workplace may be required to determine the exact cause. In more serious cases, the patient may have to leave his or her occupation. In all cases, measures to prevent a recurrence should be taken. Sufferers may be able to claim benefit under Workers' Compensation legislation or may be able to sue an employer for negligence.

Occupational medicine

A branch of medicine concerned with the effects of a person's job on his or her health, and with the effects of health on the capacity to work. Occupational medicine includes the prevention of *occupational disease and injury*, and the promotion of general health in the working population.

Occupational medicine has a long history. As early as the Middle Ages, it was recognized that miners were at risk of lung diseases caused by dust, and attempts were made to improve their working conditions by increasing ventilation. The scope of occupational medicine widened during the industrial revolution as research revealed the hazards of working with metals, such as lead and mercury, and with various other materials, such as phosphorus.

The occupational physician uses epidemiological techniques (see *Epide-*

miology) to analyze patterns of absenteeism, injury, illness, and causes of death in working populations, and clinical techniques to investigate and monitor the health of a particular work force. Health risks can be reduced in two ways: by primary prevention—the reduction of exposure to harmful substances by correct work practices, attention to dust control, use of safe work stations, and the disposal of wastes—and by secondary prevention, which involves regular screening of workers for early evidence of occupational disorders, such as dust diseases or damage to the liver from chemicals.

Today, the occupational physician is also increasingly concerned with psychological stress at work, with the investigation of the hazards (known and unknown) of new technologies, and with promoting healthy personal habits in workers.

Occupational therapy

Treatment aimed at enabling people disabled by physical illness or a serious accident to relearn muscular control and coordination, to cope with everyday tasks (such as dressing), and, when possible, to resume some form of employment. Treatment, carried out by specially trained therapists, usually starts in hospital and may be continued at an outpatient clinic or in the person's home.

Ocular

Relating to or affecting the *eye* and its structures. The term is also used to refer to the eyepiece of an optical device, such as a microscope.

Oculogyric crisis

A state of fixed gaze, lasting for minutes or hours, in which the eyes are turned in a particular direction (usually upward). The fixed-eye position is sometimes associated with spasm of the muscles of the tongue, mouth, and neck.

The crisis may occur in people with *parkinsonism* or those who have had *encephalitis*. It may also be induced by drugs (such as *reserpine* or the *phenothiazine* derivatives). An oculogyric crisis is often precipitated by emotional stress.

Oculomotor nerve

The third *cranial nerve*. The oculomotor nerve stimulates only motor functions. This nerve controls all the muscles that move the eye, except for two—the superior oblique muscle

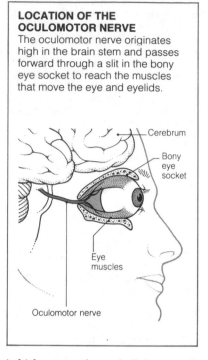

LOCATION OF THE OCULOMOTOR NERVE
The oculomotor nerve originates high in the brain stem and passes forward through a slit in the bony eye socket to reach the muscles that move the eye and eyelids.

Cerebrum

Bony eye socket

Eye muscles

Oculomotor nerve

(which rotates the eyeball downward and outward and is controlled by the *trochlear nerve*) and the lateral rectus muscle (which moves the eye outward and is controlled by the *abducent nerve*). The oculomotor nerve also supplies the muscle that constricts the pupil, the ciliary muscle (which focuses the eye), and the muscle that raises the upper eyelid.

The oculomotor nerve may be damaged as a result of a fracture of the base of the skull or of a disorder that distorts the brain, such as a tumor. Depending on the severity of damage, the following symptoms may occur: *ptosis* (drooping of the upper eyelid), *squint*, dilation of the pupil, inability to focus the eye, double vision, and slight protrusion of the eyeball.

Oedipus complex

A term used in *psychoanalytic theory* to describe the unconscious sexual attachment of a child for the parent of the opposite sex and the consequent jealousy of, and desire to eliminate, the parent of the same sex. The name is derived from the Greek myth in which, unknowingly, Oedipus kills his father Laius and marries his mother Jocasta.

Sigmund Freud believed that the Oedipus complex (sometimes called the Electra complex in females) was present in all young children and that normal psychological development depended on a child identifying with the parent of the same sex and, later, making sexual attachments with the opposite sex outside the family.

Oils

See *Fats and oils*.

Ointment

A greasy, semisolid skin preparation. Ointments are used to apply drugs to an area of skin or to act as a protective agent. Most ointments contain petrolatum or wax and have an *emollient* (soothing, moisturizing) effect.

Olecranon

The bony projection at the upper end of the *ulna* (the inner bone of the forearm) that forms the point of the *elbow*. The olecranon is commonly known as the "funny bone"; a blow to the nerve that passes across it produces a tingling sensation that passes down the forearm to the fourth and fifth fingertips.

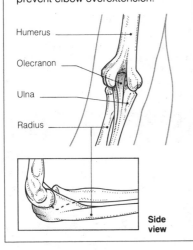

LOCATION OF THE OLECRANON
This is the curved projection at the upper end of the ulna. It acts to prevent elbow overextension.

Humerus
Olecranon
Ulna
Radius

Side view

Olfactory nerve

The first *cranial nerve*, which conveys *smell* sensations (as nerve impulses) from the *nose* to the *brain*. Each of the two olfactory nerves detects smells by means of hairlike receptors (nerve endings specialized in detecting stimuli) in the mucous membrane lining the roof of the nasal cavity. Nerve fibers pass from the receptors through tiny holes in the roof of the nasal cavity and come together to form two

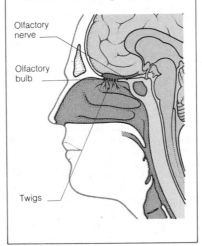

LOCATION OF THE OLFACTORY NERVE
Each olfactory bulb lies on top of a thin bony plate in the roof of the nose and connects to the brain via an olfactory nerve. Nerve twigs pass through the bony plate to enter the nasal lining.

Olfactory nerve
Olfactory bulb
Twigs

structures called the olfactory bulbs. From the bulbs, nerve fibers travel to the olfactory center in the brain.

Damage to the olfactory nerves, which is usually caused by a head injury, may result in loss or impairment of the sense of smell.

Oligo-

A prefix meaning few, little, or scanty, as in oligospermia (too few sperm in the semen). The prefix olig- is synonymous with oligo-.

Oligodendroglioma

A rare, slow-growing type of primary *brain tumor* that mainly affects young or middle-aged adults. Symptoms, diagnosis, and treatment are as for other types of brain tumor. Surgical removal of the tumor can, in some cases, lead to a complete cure. About one third of patients survive for five years or more.

Oligohydramnios

A rare condition in which there is an abnormally small amount of *amniotic fluid* surrounding the fetus in the uterus during pregnancy.
CAUSES
Amniotic fluid is produced by the *placenta*, swallowed by the fetus, and excreted as fetal urine. Oligohydramnios may occur if the placenta is not functioning properly, as occurs in se-

vere *preeclampsia*. Oligohydramnios may also occur if there is an abnormality of the fetal urinary tract.
TREATMENT AND OUTLOOK
In some cases, the underlying disorder can be treated, but sometimes it cannot (particularly if the fetus is abnormal). If oligohydramnios occurs early in pregnancy, it usually results in *miscarriage*. If the condition occurs later in pregnancy, the pressure of the uterus on the fetus may cause a deformity, such as *talipes* (clubfoot). If oligohydramnios occurs in an overdue pregnancy, induction of labor or a cesarean section may be performed.

Oligospermia

A deficiency in the number of *sperm* per unit volume of seminal fluid; there are normally more than 20 million sperm per millilitre of semen. Oligospermia may be temporary or permanent. It is a major cause of *infertility*, especially when present with certain other disorders of the sperm.
CAUSES
Oligospermia may be caused by a number of different disorders, including *orchitis* (inflammation of a testis), failure of a testis to descend into the scrotum (see *Testis, undescended*), and, infrequently, a *varicocele* (varicose vein of the testis). Stress, cigarette smoking, alcohol abuse, and treatment with some types of drugs may cause temporary oligospermia.
DIAGNOSIS AND TREATMENT
A sperm count is performed as part of *semen analysis*. Treatment is of the underlying cause. *Gonadotropin hormones* may be prescribed for a short period if the cause of the oligospermia is unknown. (See also *Azoospermia*.)

Oliguria

The production of a smaller-than-normal quantity of *urine* in relation to the volume of fluid taken in. Oliguria may be due simply to excessive sweating without adequate fluid replacement in a hot climate. In other cases, oliguria may be a sign of abnormal kidney function. (See *Kidney failure*.)

Olive oil

An oil obtained from the fruit of the olive tree OLEA EUROPAEA. Warm olive oil may sometimes be used to soften *earwax* before the ears are syringed. Olive oil is also used for its *emollient* (soothing, moisturizing) effect in the treatment of *cradle cap* in babies.

O

-oma

A suffix that denotes a tumor, as in lipoma, which is a benign tumor of fatty tissue.

Omentum

An apronlike double fold of fatty membrane that hangs down in front of the intestines. In addition to acting as a fat store, the omentum may limit the spread of infection within the abdominal cavity by adhering to the affected area.

Omphalocele

An alternative name for *exomphalos*.

Onchocerciasis

 A tropical disease that is caused by infestation with the worm ONCHOCERCA VOLVULUS. The disease, which is a type of *filariasis*, affects more than 20 million people in parts of Africa and Central and South America. Many sufferers are blinded by the disease.

CAUSES AND SYMPTOMS

Onchocerciasis is transmitted from person to person by small, fiercely biting, black simulium flies. These flies breed in, and always remain near, fast-running streams (thus giving the disease its alternative name of "river blindness").

The transmission of the disease and the life cycle of the worm are shown in the box (below). Blindness can occur as a result of an allergic reaction to dead microfilariae in or near the eyes.

TREATMENT AND PREVENTION

The microfilariae are quickly killed by the drug diethylcarbamazine. This drug must be used with great care, however, because of the severe reactions caused by the dead larvae.

Travelers to areas where the disease is prevalent should take measures to discourage *insect bites*.

Oncogenes

Genes, found in all cells, that are involved in the control of normal cell proliferation. Abnormalities of these genes have been shown to be one of the steps responsible for cells becoming cancerous. Of the full human complement of 50,000 genes, fewer than 100 are probably oncogenes.

Cancerous cells differ from healthy ones in various ways. Their growth is unrestrained, and they infiltrate and destroy normal tissues (see *Cancer*). These differences are induced by *mutations* (alterations) in certain key genes—the oncogenes—which cause them to be "switched on." Switching on of a cell's oncogenes may increase its rate of multiplication, alter its responsiveness to hormonal growth factors, or increase its invasiveness.

Oncogenes may be switched on by the various environmental factors that are known to cause cancer, such as ultraviolet light, radioactivity, tobacco smoke, alcohol, asbestos particles, carcinogenic chemicals, and certain viruses. To transform a cell from normal to malignant seems to require the switching on of between two and four oncogenes. Thus, cancer of the cervix may develop in a woman who smokes and whose cervix has been infected with papillomavirus (a potentially cancer-causing virus), whereas either of these factors by itself might not be sufficient to cause cancer.

Oncology

The study of the causes, development, characteristics, and treatment of *tumors*, particularly *cancers* (malignant tumors). Because there are many different types of tumors, deriving from virtually any tissue in the body, oncology encompasses a range of experimental techniques and investigative approaches. These include surveying the frequency and distribution of tumors, testing new treatments, investigating biochemical processes involved in tumor formation, and studying abnormal genes.

Physicians specializing in the study and treatment of cancer are known as oncologists. They are concerned with diagnosing the type of cancer and determining its exact location and rate of spread. They will then be responsible for the prescription and monitoring of *radiation therapy* and *anticancer* drug treatment as well as for follow-up care and referral for surgery.

Onychogryphosis

Abnormal thickening, hardening, and curving of the *nails*, which occurs mainly in elderly people. Its cause is unknown, but onychogryphosis is associated with *fungal infection* or with poor circulation.

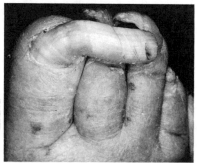

Onychogryphosis
This extraordinary thickening and overgrowth, resembling the claws of the mythological griffin, may affect toenails or fingernails.

Onycholysis

Separation of the *nail* from its bed, beginning at the tip. Onycholysis is a feature of many skin conditions, including *psoriasis*, *dermatitis*, and some *fungal infections*.

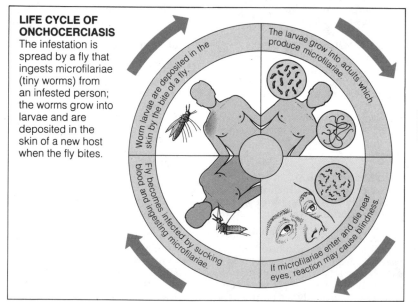

LIFE CYCLE OF ONCHOCERCIASIS
The infestation is spread by a fly that ingests microfilariae (tiny worms) from an infested person; the worms grow into larvae and are deposited in the skin of a new host when the fly bites.

Worm larvae are deposited in the skin by the bite of a fly.

The larvae grow into adults which produce microfilariae.

Fly becomes infected by sucking blood and ingesting microfilariae.

If microfilariae enter and die near eyes, reaction may cause blindness.

Oophorectomy

Removal of one or both *ovaries*.

WHY IT IS DONE

Oophorectomy is performed to treat *ovarian cysts* or ovarian cancer (see *Ovary, cancer of*). In women under 40, the surgeon attempts to preserve ovarian function by performing only a partial oophorectomy.

Both ovaries may be removed during a *hysterectomy* if disease has spread from the uterus to the ovaries. Removing both ovaries can also reduce the risk of ovarian cancer in women past the menopause. Occasionally, both ovaries may be removed in a patient with *breast cancer*, as the growth of the cancer may be dependent on hormones produced by the ovary.

HOW IT IS DONE

Oophorectomy is performed under general anesthesia and usually takes less than one hour. The ovaries are removed through an incision in the lower abdominal wall.

RECOVERY PERIOD

There is some pain and tenderness around the operation site. Most activities can be resumed within about a month of surgery, and sexual intercourse after about six weeks.

OUTLOOK

There are usually no adverse effects when one ovary or part of an ovary is removed because *ovulation* and hormone production continue. If both ovaries are removed before the menopause, *hormone replacement therapy* may be necessary.

-opathy

A suffix that denotes a disease or disorder. An example of its use is in the word neuropathy (a disorder of the peripheral nerves). The suffix *-pathy* is synonymous with -opathy.

Open heart surgery

Any operation on the *heart* in which the heartbeat is temporarily stopped and the heart's function is taken over by a mechanical pump.

The early heart surgeons carried out limited operations while the heart continued to beat. In such "closed" operations it was possible, for example, for a surgeon to insert a finger or a specially designed knife into the heart to open the channel of a narrowed valve.

With the development of reliable *heart-lung machines* in the 1950s, much more elaborate heart surgery became possible. Once the pump was connected, the surgeon could open the heart, repair defects, and even reconstruct the main chambers. During the operation, the heart is kept cool through techniques of surgical *hypothermia*, which help to prevent any damage occurring to the heart muscle from lack of oxygen.

The main applications of open heart surgery have been the correction of congenital heart defects (see *Heart disease, congenital*), surgery for heart valve insufficiency or narrowed heart valves (see *Heart valve surgery*), and *coronary artery bypass* surgery.

Operable

A term applied to any condition that is suitable for surgical treatment, such as an accessible benign tumor that requires removal because it is causing symptoms. (See also *Inoperable*.)

Operating room

A hospital room in which surgical procedures are performed. The room is designed to reduce the risk of infection in open surgical wounds. A ventilation system provides a constant supply of clean, filtered air, the walls and floors are easily washable and are cleaned at least once daily, and there are adjoining rooms with foot- or elbow-operated faucets where surgeons, assistants, and nurses use sterile brushes and bactericidal soaps to scrub their hands and forearms before putting on sterile gowns, masks, and gloves. Often built into the walls are lightboxes for viewing images obtained by such techniques as *X-ray*, *CT scanning*, or *MRI*.

EQUIPMENT

During an operation using general anesthesia, the anesthetic machine stands at the head of the operating table (see *Anesthesia, general*), connected by tubes to oxygen and various anesthetic gases.

The surgeon's sterile instruments, covered with sterile towels before use, are arranged on stainless steel wheeled tables. There is also a surgical *diathermy* machine, which controls bleeding. If required, other equipment, such as a *heart-lung machine* (which can take over the function of the patient's heart and lungs), is brought into the operating room.

Operation

Any surgical procedure, usually carried out with instruments but sometimes using only the hands (as in the manipulation of a simple fracture). Operations range from procedures performed quickly under local anesthesia (e.g., draining a skin abscess) to surgery lasting several hours performed under general anesthesia (e.g., a heart or liver transplant).

Ophthalmia

An old term for *Ophthalmitis*.

Ophthalmitis

A term for any inflammatory *eye* disorder. It is also used to describe the following two specific disorders.

Neonatal ophthalmitis (also called ophthalmia neonatorum) is a discharge of pus from the eyes of an infant that starts within 21 days of birth. In many cases the cause is an infection (such as *gonorrhea* or a *chlamydial infection*) acquired during birth. The condition is treated with *antibiotic drugs*.

Sympathetic ophthalmitis is a rare condition in which a penetrating injury to one eye is followed at least 10 days later by severe *uveitis* (inflammation of the iris and choroid) that threatens blindness in the uninjured eye. The condition can be treated with *corticosteroid drugs*, but in some cases, removal of the injured eye is necessary to save the sight of the other eye.

Ophthalmology

The study of the *eye*, and the diagnosis and treatment of the disorders that affect it. Ophthalmology includes not only the assessment of *vision* and the prescription of *glasses* or *contact lenses* to correct defects, but also the surgery required to treat eye disorders, such as *cataracts*, *glaucoma*, *retinal detachment*, and obstruction of the tear ducts.

Physicians who specialize in care of the eyes are called ophthalmologists. Ophthalmologists frequently work closely with other physicians because many disorders of the retina at the back of the eye are signs of nonoptical disorders, such as *hypertension* (high blood pressure), *atherosclerosis* (narrowing of arteries by fatty deposits), or *diabetes mellitus*. Careful analysis of a person's field of vision (see *Eye, examination of*) can reveal defects that indicate neurological damage, such as that caused by a brain tumor. (See also *Optician*; *Optometry*; *Orthoptics*.)

Ophthalmoplegia

Partial or total paralysis of the muscles that move the *eyes*. Ophthalmoplegia may be caused by disease of the muscles themselves (as in *Graves' disease*) or by one of the conditions affecting the brain or the nerves supplying the eye muscles.

O

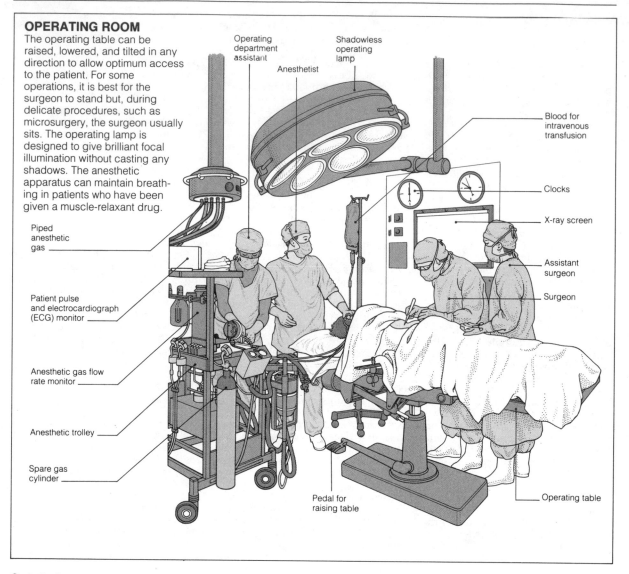

OPERATING ROOM
The operating table can be raised, lowered, and tilted in any direction to allow optimum access to the patient. For some operations, it is best for the surgeon to stand but, during delicate procedures, such as microsurgery, the surgeon usually sits. The operating lamp is designed to give brilliant focal illumination without casting any shadows. The anesthetic apparatus can maintain breathing in patients who have been given a muscle-relaxant drug.

Operating department assistant

Anesthetist

Shadowless operating lamp

Blood for intravenous transfusion

Clocks

X-ray screen

Assistant surgeon

Surgeon

Operating table

Pedal for raising table

Piped anesthetic gas

Patient pulse and electrocardiograph (ECG) monitor

Anesthetic gas flow rate monitor

Anesthetic trolley

Spare gas cylinder

O

Ophthalmoscope
An instrument used to examine the inside of the *eye*. The ophthalmoscope contains a deflecting prism or a perforated angled mirror, which allows illumination and viewing of the entire area of the retina, the head of the optic nerve, the retinal arteries and veins, and the vitreous humor. (See illustration on facing page.)

Opiate
Any drug derived from, or chemically similar to, *opium* is described as an opiate. The term opiate is also used in the term opiate *receptor* to refer to a specific site on a cell's surface with which opiate drugs combine to initiate their effects.

Opium
A substance obtained from the unripe seed pods of the poppy plant *PAPAVER SOMNIFERUM*. Opium has an analgesic (painkilling) effect and may also cause sleepiness and euphoria.

Opium and its derivatives, which include *codeine* and *morphine*, are among the drugs collectively known as *narcotic drugs*.

Opportunistic infection
Infection caused by organisms that do not usually produce disease in healthy people; or widespread infection by organisms that normally produce only a mild, local infection.

Many of the causative organisms are normally present on or in the human body and cause disease only when the host's *immune system* (natural defenses) is impaired. This impairment may be due to treatment with anticancer and immunosuppressant drugs, to radiation therapy, or to diseases such as leukemia. Opportunistic infections also affect premature or malnourished infants and people with *immunodeficiency disorders*.

Opportunistic infections, especially *pneumocystis pneumonia*, are the cause of death in most *AIDS* patients. Many fungal infections (e.g., *cryptococcosis* and *candidiasis*) and some viral infections (e.g., *cytomegalovirus* and *herpes simplex*) are opportunistic infections.

Opportunistic infections are often unavoidable because the underlying

OPHTHALMOSCOPE

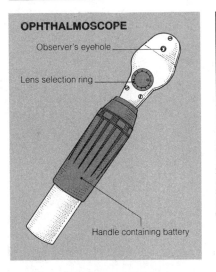

Observer's eyehole

Lens selection ring

Handle containing battery

Each optic nerve is a bundle of long fibers originating from nerve cells in the retina and passing to the back of the brain. Because of the arrangement of the nerve fibers, disease or injury at any point causes a unique pattern of visual loss. Charting the pattern of visual loss allows accurate location of damage to the nerve.

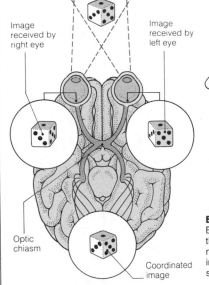

Image received by right eye

Image received by left eye

Optic nerve

Lens

Retina

Optic chiasm

Coordinated image

Binocular vision
Because the eyes are a distance apart, they form slightly different images of a nearby object. The fusion of these two images into one provides the illusion of solidity. This is called stereopsis.

defects in the host's defenses cannot easily be rectified. However, treatment with appropriate antimicrobial drugs may be lifesaving.

Optic atrophy

A shrinkage or wasting of the *optic nerve* fibers, which results in partial or complete loss of vision. Optic atrophy is caused by disease or injury to the optic nerve and may occur without prior signs of nerve disease, such as inflammation or swelling.

Optic disk edema

See *Papilledema*.

Optician

A person who fits and sells *glasses* or *contact lenses* according to the prescription of an optometrist or ophthalmologist.

Optic nerve

The second *cranial nerve*; the nerve of *vision*. The optic nerve consists of a collection of about 1 million nerve fibers that transmit impulses from the *retina* (the layer of light receptors at the back of the eye) to the *brain*.

The two optic nerves converge to a junction behind the eyes, where fibers from the inner halves of the retinas cross over. Nerve fibers from the right halves of both retinas pass to the right side of the occipital lobes at the back of the brain, while those from the left halves go to the left side.

Disorders of the optic nerve include *optic neuritis* (inflammation of the optic nerve), and *papilledema*, which is caused by pressure on the nerve from disease within the orbit (eye socket) or a brain tumor.

Optic neuritis

Inflammation of the *optic nerve*, often causing sudden loss of part of the *visual field*. Optic neuritis is usually accompanied by pain on moving the eyes and tenderness when the eyes are touched. In some cases, however, there may be little or no pain.

The cause of optic neuritis often remains uncertain, but most cases are thought to be due to *demyelination* (destruction of the myelin sheaths) of the optic nerve fibers, which occurs in *multiple sclerosis*. The condition may also result from inflammation or infection of tissues around the optic nerve.

Optic neuritis causes loss of vision, usually in the central part of the visual field. Vision usually improves substantially within six weeks, but each attack causes damage to a proportion of the optic nerve fibers; recurrent attacks usually lead to permanent loss of *visual acuity*.

Treatment with *corticosteroid drugs* may aid the return of vision but seems to have little effect on the long-term outcome of the inflammatory process.

Optometry

Optometry is practiced by optometrists, health care professionals who diagnose disorders and diseases of the eyes and visual system and prescribe or provide treatment including glasses, contact lenses, orthoptics, and low vision therapy. Optometrists are trained in a four-year course of basic and clinical science. If an optometrist detects a medical condition, he or she will refer the patient to a physician for further treatment.

Oral

Concerning the mouth; taken through or applied in the mouth.

Oral contraceptives

COMMON DRUGS

Estrogens
Ethinyl estradiol Mestranol

Progestogens
Ethynodiol diacetate Norethindrone

> **WARNING**
> If you vomit or have diarrhea while taking an oral contraceptive, follow the advice for missing a pill. If you have missed two consecutive periods, you should have a pregnancy test.

A group of oral drug preparations containing a *progestogen drug*, often combined with an *estrogen drug*, taken by women to prevent pregnancy. All types of oral contraceptives—combined pills, phased pills, and mini-pills—are commonly known as "the pill." Combined pills (including phased pills) contain an estrogen and a progestogen. The minipill contains only progestogen.

HOW THEY ARE TAKEN

Combined oral contraceptives need to be taken in a monthly cycle for as long as a woman wishes to avoid pregnancy. The first course of pills is started on the first day of a period or on the fifth day after bleeding starts. Additional contraceptive precautions for the first 14 days are needed if the combined or phased pill is begun on day five, and are usually recommended when starting the minipill.

The way each course of pills is usually taken is described in the illustrated box at right. Some brands of phased pills contain seven additional inactive pills, which may contain an iron supplement, so that the habit of taking a pill each day is not broken. It is possible to take a combined or a phased pill continuously and thus avoid bleeding, but most physicians do not recommend this. In some women, oral contraceptives may cause menstruation to cease.

MISSING A PILL

For maximum contraceptive effect, each type of pill should be taken at approximately the same time each day. This is particularly important with the minipill, which should be taken within three hours of the chosen time each day.

A forgotten combined or phased pill should be taken as soon as it is remembered even if this means taking two pills the next day. Pills for the rest of the course should be taken at the correct time. An additional form of contraception should be used for 14 days after missing a pill.

If the minipill is taken more than three hours late, extra precautions should be taken for 14 days.

EFFECTIVENESS

Used correctly, oral contraceptives have a failure rate of less than one pregnancy per 100 woman-years (i.e., the number of pregnancies among 100 women using the method for one year is less than one). Allowing for incorrect use or other factors, the actual failure rates may be as high as between two and three pregnancies per 100 woman-years for the combined or phased pill, and between two and a half and four pregnancies for the minipill.

Certain other drugs (such as *barbiturate drugs, anticonvulsant drugs*, and some *antibiotic drugs*) may impair the effectiveness of oral contraceptives. A woman should always inform her physician if she is taking other medication.

In addition to providing excellent protection against pregnancy, the main advantage of oral contraceptives is that they do not interfere with the spontaneity of sex.

Estrogen-containing pills protect against cancer of the uterus and ova-

---

HOW ORAL CONTRACEPTIVES WORK

The combined and phased pills increase the levels of estrogen and progesterone in the body, which interferes with the production by the pituitary gland of two *gonadotropin hormones* called follicle-stimulating hormone (FSH) and luteinizing hormone (LH). This action in turn prevents ovulation.

The minipill works mainly by making the mucus that lines the inside of the cervix (neck of the uterus) so thick that it is impenetrable to sperm.

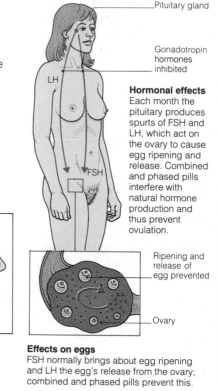

Hormonal effects
Each month the pituitary produces spurts of FSH and LH, which act on the ovary to cause egg ripening and release. Combined and phased pills interfere with natural hormone production and thus prevent ovulation.

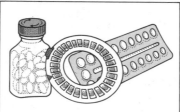

Pill packaging
Most oral contraceptives come in packs that clearly indicate the day on which each pill should be taken.

Effects on eggs
FSH normally brings about egg ripening and LH the egg's release from the ovary; combined and phased pills prevent this.

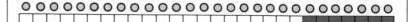

Combined pill
This pill contains an estrogen and a progestogen drug in fixed doses. A course usually consists of one pill per day

for 21 days, followed by seven pill-free days, during which bleeding may occur. A new course is then started, whether or not bleeding has occurred.

Phased pill—a typical program
These pills contain both an estrogen and a progestogen drug, but are divided into two or three groups or phases. The dose

of the progestogen drug, and sometimes of estrogen as well, changes from phase to phase. A course lasts for 21 days followed by seven pill-free days.

Minipill—progestogen only
These pills contain only a progestogen drug in a fixed dose. The pills are taken continuously, one every day with no

pill-free days. Bleeding usually occurs during the last few days of each cycle. The minipill has a slightly higher failure rate than the combined and phased pills.

O

ries, *ovarian cysts*, *endometriosis*, and iron-deficiency *anemia*. They also tend to make periods regular, lighter, and relatively free of menstrual pain.

The main disadvantages of oral contraceptives are that they are medically unsuitable for some women and that they may produce adverse effects.

CONTRAINDICATIONS

Estrogen-containing pills increase the risk of certain disorders and are not usually prescribed if a woman suffers from *hypertension* (high blood pressure), *hyperlipidemia* (high levels of fat in the blood), *liver* disease, *migraine*, *otosclerosis* (an ear disorder), or if she has previously had a *thrombosis* (abnormal blood clot).

The chances of a thrombosis occurring are increased in women who smoke and who are over the age of 35. An estrogen-containing pill is not usually given during the first few weeks after childbirth or in the four weeks before major surgery because of the increased risk of thrombosis. *Obesity* also makes a woman on the pill more susceptible to thrombosis.

Oral contraceptives are not usually prescribed to a woman who has a personal or family history of heart or circulatory disorders, or who suffers from unexplained vaginal bleeding.

Combined or phased pills may interfere with milk production and should not be taken during breast-feeding. The minipill is usually considered unsuitable for a woman who has had an *ectopic pregnancy*.

POSSIBLE ADVERSE EFFECTS

Estrogen-containing pills may sometimes cause nausea and vomiting, weight gain, depression, swelling of the breasts, reduced sex drive, increased appetite, cramps in the legs and abdomen, headaches, and dizziness. A more serious adverse effect of these pills is the risk of a thrombosis causing a *stroke* or a *pulmonary embolism*. Estrogen-containing pills may also aggravate heart disease or cause hypertension, *gallstones*, *jaundice*, and, very rarely, *liver cancer*.

Medical evidence suggests that cancer of the cervix is more common in women taking estrogen-containing pills, and several studies in the late 1980s pointed to a link between prolonged use of oral contraceptives and the development of breast cancer in women under 35. This may be outweighed by reduced risk of other cancers of the reproductive system.

All forms of oral contraception can cause bleeding between periods, but this is especially true of the minipill.

Other possible adverse effects of the minipill are irregular periods, ectopic pregnancy, and ovarian cysts.

There is no evidence that use of an oral contraceptive reduces a woman's fertility permanently (although menstruation may be irregular or absent for some months after stopping the pill). Likewise, there is no evidence that a fetus can be harmed if conceived while the woman is taking the pill or has recently stopped doing so.

Adverse effects usually disappear after a few months of taking the pill. If they persist, it may be necessary to change to a different type of pill or to an alternative method of contraception. Because adverse effects are more likely to occur with high doses of estrogen, low-estrogen preparations are prescribed whenever possible. The minipill may be used by women who suffer adverse effects even with low estrogen doses or who should not take estrogen drugs for other medical reasons. Women taking oral contraceptives should receive regular checkups, including blood pressure and weight checks and *cervical smear tests*. (See also *Contraception*.)

Oral hygiene

Measures that keep the *mouth* and *teeth* clean and healthy. Good oral hygiene reduces the incidence of tooth decay (see *Caries, dental*), prevents *gingivitis* and other *gum* disorders, and helps to prevent *halitosis* (bad breath). Oral hygiene can be broadly divided into personal and professional care.

PERSONAL CARE

The most important aspect of personal oral hygiene is daily removal of dental *plaque* (a sticky, bacteria-containing substance) by thorough *toothbrushing* and use of dental floss (see *Floss, dental*). Use of a *fluoride* mouthwash or of an oral irrigator (a device that produces a forceful jet of water) may also be helpful, but these aids cannot remove plaque or replace brushing and flossing. *Disclosing agents* can help make tooth cleaning more efficient by showing the location of plaque. Dentures must always be kept scrupulously clean by brushing every surface and soaking in a cleansing solution.

PROFESSIONAL CARE

A dentist or a dental hygienist removes stubborn plaque and *calculus* (a hard mineral deposit that forms on the teeth above and below the gums) by *scaling* and polishing. These procedures are usually carried out during a routine checkup.

Oral surgery

The branch of surgery concerned with the treatment of deformity, injury, or disease of the teeth, jaws, and other parts of the mouth and face.

All oral surgeons have a degree in general dentistry and further training in oral and maxillofacial (jaw and face) surgery. Many oral surgeons also have medical degrees, although this is not required.

Among the dental procedures carried out by oral surgeons are the extraction of severely impacted wisdom teeth (see *Impaction, dental*) and *alveolectomy* (removal of tooth-bearing bone from the jaw) to improve the fitting of dentures.

More complicated oral surgery includes *orthognathic surgery* to correct deformities of the jaw that result in an abnormal relationship between the upper and lower teeth; repairing a broken jaw; plastic surgery to correct *cleft lip and palate*; and the removal of certain types of benign tumors from tissues within the mouth.

Orbit

The socket in the *skull* that contains the eyeball, protective pads of fat, and various blood vessels, muscles, and nerves involved with eye function. An opening in the back of the orbit allows the *optic nerve* to pass from the eyeball into the *brain*.

DISORDERS

INJURY A fracture of the orbit may be caused by a blow of great force, as in a car crash or sports injury. In a fracture

O

LOCATION OF THE ORBITS
The orbits are the deep cavities in the skull in which the eyeballs and muscles that move the eyes are protectively enclosed.

Orbit   Skull   Hole for optic nerve

of the orbit, the eyeball itself often escapes damage because it is squeezed backward by protective muscles during reflex blinking. Many such fractures heal without treatment, but some result in facial deformity requiring corrective surgery. Surgery may also be needed to reinforce the floor of the orbit if a fracture causes downward displacement of the eye.

INFECTION Rarely, bacteria infect the fatty tissue lining the orbit, causing orbital *cellulitis*. Usually the infection originates in a nearby sinus, but sometimes it spreads in the blood from a facial infection. The affected eye protrudes and is extremely painful and red. There is also severe swelling of the lids and conjunctiva (the membrane lining the inside of the lids and the white of the eye). Orbital cellulitis is a serious disorder. The pressure on the eye may damage it and there is a slight risk that the infection may spread inward to cause *meningitis* (inflammation of the membranes covering the brain). Prompt treatment with high doses of *antibiotic drugs* usually clears up the condition.

Orchiectomy

The surgical removal of one or both of the *testes*.

WHY IT IS DONE
Orchiectomy may be performed to treat testicular cancer (see *Testis, cancer of*), to treat gangrene due to torsion (see *Testis, torsion of*), or to reduce production of the hormone testosterone as part of the treatment of cancer of the prostate gland (see *Prostate, cancer of*). Because the prostate gland depends on male sex hormones for its normal growth, orchiectomy is often effective in reducing the growth of a prostatic cancer. It is especially effective in controlling the symptoms of secondary tumors in the bones.

HOW IT IS DONE
Under general or spinal anesthesia, the scrotum is cut open, the blood vessels and nerves leading to the scrotum are cut free, the testis is cut away from surrounding tissue and removed, and the skin is stitched.

After the operation, *analgesic drugs* (painkillers) may be needed and an *ice pack* may be applied to the scrotum for the first 24 hours to prevent excessive swelling.

OUTLOOK
Complete healing can be expected without complications. Removal of one testis does not affect sex drive, potency, or the ability to have children. The patient is advised to wear

an athletic support and to avoid vigorous exercise for a month or so after the operation.

Orchiopexy

An operation in which an undescended testis (see *Testis, undescended*) is brought down into the scrotum. Orchiopexy is usually performed when the boy is between 2 and 5 years old to avoid the risk of subsequent infertility or even cancer of the testis (see *Testis, cancer of*).

Under general anesthesia, an incision is made in the groin and the testis is gently freed and maneuvered down into the scrotum. The base of the testis is then usually attached to the scrotum with a few stitches to prevent it from retracting. Pain and swelling are relieved with *analgesic drugs*.

Orchitis

Inflammation of a *testis*. Orchitis may be caused by infection with the virus that causes *mumps*.

Orchitis develops in about one quarter of males who contract mumps after puberty. It is characterized by swelling and severe pain in the affected testis and a high fever. In *epididymo-orchitis* (which has different causes), the tube that carries sperm from the testis is also inflamed.

Treatment is with *analgesic drugs* (painkillers) and *ice packs* to reduce swelling and pain; *antibiotic drugs* may be given, but not for mumps orchitis. The condition usually begins to subside after three to seven days. Occasionally, orchitis is followed by shrinking of the testis.

Orciprenaline

A *bronchodilator drug* used in asthma and chronic lung disease that dilates the airways in the lungs while having little effect on the heart. The drug is usually taken through an inhaler, although it can also be taken orally.

Orf

A skin infection, caused by a pox virus, which is occasionally transmitted to humans from sheep and goats. Orf usually produces a single fluid-filled blister on the arm or the hand. Without treatment, the condition will persist for several weeks. Application of the antiviral drug *idoxuridine* hastens recovery.

Organ

A collection of various *tissues* integrated into a distinct structural unit that performs specific functions. For

example, the brain consists of nerve tissue and supporting tissue (called neuroglia) organized to receive, process, and send out information.

Organ donation

The agreement of a person (or his or her relatives) to the surgical removal of one or more organs for use in *transplant surgery*. Most organs used for transplantation are removed immediately after a *donor* has died, but kidneys may also be taken from living donors. Kidney donation by living donors is usually confined to the relatives of transplant patients. Relatives are more likely to have a tissue-type (see *Tissue-typing*) that is compatible with that of the patient. Donation of kidneys by unrelated living donors raises ethical problems, especially when organs are sold as is the case in some undeveloped countries.

Before taking a kidney from a living donor, the surgeon will explain carefully the risks of donation, removing the kidney only after the donor has given clear voluntary consent.

The range of organs removed after death is much greater, including the cornea, heart, lungs, liver, pancreas, and kidneys. Most organs can be transplanted successfully only if they are removed immediately after death; the best results often require surgical removal of organs before the donor's heart has stopped beating. In practice, this means that most donations of major organs are made from patients who die in an intensive-care unit and are certified as "brain dead" while their heart and lung function is maintained by a machine (see *Death*).

People who want to donate some or all of their organs after death should make their intentions clear to their relatives and sign a donor card. In most Western countries the demand for donated organs is far greater than the supply. Some countries have introduced laws that allow physicians to remove organs after death unless the patient has specifically forbidden it. In Canada the supply of donor organs continues to depend on voluntary donations. (See also *Corneal graft; Heart-lung transplant; Heart transplant; Heart valve surgery; Kidney transplant; Liver transplant*.)

Organic

Related to a body *organ*; having organs or an organized structure; or related to *organisms* or to substances from them. In chemistry, the term refers to any of the group of compounds that contain carbon, with the exception of carbon oxides (such as carbon dioxide), carbon sulfides, and metal carbonates (such as calcium carbonate).

The term organic also signifies the presence of disease, in contrast to a *functional disorder* or a *psychosomatic* complaint. (See also *Inorganic*.)

Organic brain syndrome
See *Brain syndrome, organic*.

Organism
A general term for any individual animal or plant. Medically, the most important organisms are humans and disease-causing *microorganisms*, such as *bacteria, fungi, protozoa,* and *viruses*.

Orgasm
Intense sensations resulting from the series of muscular contractions that occur at the peak of sexual excitement. Orgasm is usually followed by physical relaxation and often by drowsiness.

In men, contractions of the muscles of the inner pelvis massage seminal fluid from the prostatic area into the urethra, from which it is forcefully propelled from the urethral orifice (see *Ejaculation*). Following orgasm, the penis becomes soft again and there is a refractory period during which there is no physical response to further sexual stimulation.

Orgasm in women is associated with irregular contractions of the voluntary muscles of the walls of the vagina and, in some women, of the uterus, followed by relief of congestion in the pelvic area. Orgasm usually lasts about three to 10 seconds, but can last up to a minute in some women. It is generally believed that there is no refractory phase in women. Some women experience multiple orgasms if stimulation is continued.

Both men and women may have problems with orgasm (see *Ejaculation, disorders of; Orgasm, lack of*).

Orgasm, lack of
The inability to achieve *orgasm* during sexual activity. Lack of orgasm, also sometimes called anorgasmia, is reported more commonly in women than in men. In either sex, failure to achieve orgasm may result from inhibition of sexual desire (see *Sexual desire, inhibited*), or from an inability to become aroused or to maintain arousal (see *Frigidity; Impotence*). In men, there may be a problem in achieving orgasm despite normal arousal (see *Ejaculation, disorders of*).

In women, lack of orgasm is the most common sexual problem. Between 30 and 50 percent of women experience difficulty with orgasm at some time in their lives. Some 10 to 15 percent are unable to achieve orgasm under any circumstances; others experience orgasm only occasionally or under special circumstances.

CAUSES
Lack of orgasm in women during *sexual intercourse* may result from problems with sexual technique, psychological factors, or pain during intercourse (see *Intercourse, painful*).

Problems with sexual technique may be due to inexperience on the part of either the man or the woman, poor sex education, or lack of familiarity with the body's sexual responses. Some women fail to reach orgasm because they do not receive, or do not allow, sufficient foreplay to become properly aroused.

In general, women take longer than men to reach orgasm (about 13 minutes for a woman compared to less than three minutes for the average man). In some cases, a woman may experience difficulty in reaching orgasm because of premature ejaculation by her partner. Problems may also arise if a woman has a new partner who is unfamiliar with her particular sexual responses.

Some women are able to achieve orgasm through *masturbation* but not during sexual intercourse.

Psychological factors that may contribute to lack of orgasm in women include anxiety or early sexual trauma. Some women are unable to relax during sex because they are ashamed of their bodies, have inhibitions about the sex act, have deep-seated guilt feelings about sexual pleasure, fear pregnancy, feel uncertain about intimacy, or fear "losing control" during orgasm. Anxiety about sexual performance and psychological pressures to achieve orgasm may have an inhibitory effect, which in time sets up a cycle of failure.

Problems in a long-term relationship may be due to underlying feelings of hostility, boredom, or distrust in one or both of the partners.

TREATMENT
Women may be helped to achieve orgasm or to increase the frequency of orgasm through *sex therapy* or *marital counseling. Psychotherapy* may be helpful for women in whom the problem is related to deep-seated feelings of guilt or insecurity.

Ornithosis
A disease of birds caused by the microorganism CHLAMYDIA PSITTACI. Ornithosis can be transmitted to humans, causing *psittacosis*, a feverish illness accompanied by pneumonia.

Orphan drugs
Drugs that have been developed to treat rare conditions but are not manufactured because the potential sales are small while the cost of performing the necessary safety tests is high.

Certain orphan drugs can be obtained for therapeutic use if the physician makes application to Health and Welfare Canada. In some countries, changes in the law have made it profitable to provide certain orphan drugs.

An example of an orphan drug is tetrahydroaminoacridine (THA). Although clinical trials suggest THA may improve orientation and memory in people who have *Alzheimer's disease*, it has not been manufactured because the patent has expired.

Orphenadrine
A *muscle-relaxant drug* used to relieve painful muscle spasm caused by injury to soft tissues (such as muscles and ligaments). Orphenadrine is also given to reduce muscle rigidity in *Parkinson's disease*.

Possible adverse effects of orphenadrine include dryness of the mouth and blurred vision.

Ortho-
A prefix meaning normal, correct, or straight. It occurs, for example, in the term orthopedics, which is derived from the Greek for "straight child" because this branch of surgery was originally concerned with correction of skeletal deformities in children.

Orthodontic appliances
Devices, commonly known as braces, worn to correct *malocclusion* (an abnormal relationship between the upper and lower *teeth*). Braces are most commonly fitted during childhood and adolescence when the teeth and jaws are still developing.

WHY THEY ARE USED
Braces are commonly used to correct the position of overcrowded teeth (see *Overcrowding, dental*), which may splay outward, tilt inward, or be twisted sideways. Another common use is to correct the position of *buck teeth* (projecting upper front teeth). Braces can also be used to reposition upper and lower premolars and

O

molars (back teeth) when a faulty relationship between the upper and lower jaws prevents the teeth from meeting properly and interferes with chewing.

TYPES

FIXED APPLIANCES These braces, which cannot be removed by the wearer, exert a continuous pressure and can move teeth in any direction. They are usually fitted to all the upper and/or lower teeth and are used when many teeth need repositioning. The tooth-moving part of a fixed appliance is the arch wire, an adjustable, high-tensile steel wire, threaded through a bracket on each tooth.

To allow extra force to be applied to specific teeth, some brackets may be fitted with small hooks to which headgear (straps that fit around the back and over the top of the head) can be attached when the wearer is in bed.

Fixed appliances are kept in the mouth until the teeth have moved into the correct position, which may take a year or more. Thereafter, a fixed or removable retainer plate may need to be worn for anywhere from six months to five years to hold the teeth in their correct place until tooth and jaw growth stop in late adolescence.

Fixed appliances give more precise control over tooth movement than removable braces, but are more expensive and take longer to fit and adjust. Such appliances also trap dental *plaque* and make cleaning of the teeth more difficult.

Some people can be treated with lingual (also called "invisible") braces, which are fitted to the inner arch (tongue side) of the teeth, and pull rather than push the teeth into place.

REMOVABLE APPLIANCES These braces are used when only one or a few teeth need correcting. They consist of a plastic plate that covers the roof of the mouth (or, much less commonly, the floor of the mouth) with attachments that anchor over the back teeth. Force is applied by means of springs, wire bows, screws, or rubber bands fitted to the plate, sometimes combined with the use of headgear.

Occasionally, a special type of removable appliance is used in younger children before facial growth has stopped. Such braces consist of interconnected upper and lower plates that force the jaw into a position of slight tension against the pull of the surrounding muscles, translating this force to move the teeth.

Potential disadvantages of removable appliances are that their bulk may interfere with speech and that wearers may remove them so often that they become ineffective.

Orthodontics

A branch of *dentistry* concerned with the prevention and treatment of *malocclusion* (an abnormal relationship between the upper and lower *teeth*). In most cases, the orthodontist performs orthodontic procedures on children and adolescents while the teeth are still developing and are relatively maneuverable. However, adults may also be able to benefit from orthodontic treatment.

Diagnosis of the exact type of malocclusion involved may require making models of the teeth (see *Impression, dental*) to see clearly how they come together when clenched,

---

HOW ORTHODONTIC APPLIANCES WORK

The tooth sockets are remarkably responsive to sustained pressure against the teeth. Orthodontic appliances, which may be fixed or removable, provide such pressure. Even gentle pressure applied in a particular direction will move teeth. As they move, bone is remodeled so that the new position is stable.

FIXED APPLIANCES

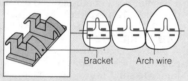

Bracket   Arch wire

Appearance of brackets and wires
Brackets are fixed appliances cemented to the outer surface of the teeth; they have slots into which arch wires can be fitted.

By careful design of the arrangement of wires and springs, force can be exerted in any direction to move a tooth into the desired position.

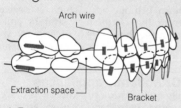

Arch wire

Extraction space

Bracket

1 Teeth are removed to create space and an appliance is made to correct the alignment of the remaining teeth and to close gaps between them.

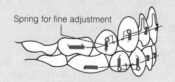

Spring for fine adjustment

2 Once the teeth in the upper and lower jaws are aligned, the appliance is adjusted to tip or rotate the teeth to give a good appearance and bite.

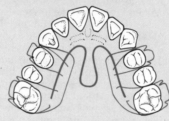

Overcrowding
This is frequently associated with malocclusion (poor alignment between upper and lower teeth). Some teeth have to be extracted to make room for others to be straightened.

REMOVABLE APPLIANCES

These are easier to keep clean than fixed appliances and are less obtrusive, but they may interfere with speech; their efficiency relies on patients using them as directed. This type exerts pressure to push the teeth at the sides outward.

Bow device
This simple wire spring acts by exerting force to straighten the tooth. Many bow devices are more complicated.

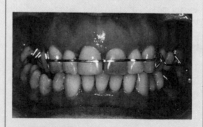

A removable bow
One of the many forms of orthodontic wire appliance, this bow device exerts pressure on the teeth at the sides, which straightens and moves them outward.

taking X rays of the head to relate the position of the teeth to that of the facial bones, and taking X rays of the jaws to study their structure and relationship.

Orthodontic treatment consists of moving poorly positioned teeth by means of gentle pressure exerted by *orthodontic appliances* (dental braces). In some cases, the orthodontist may first need to extract certain teeth, often the premolars, to provide growing room for the teeth being moved.

Orthognathic surgery
An operation to correct deformity of the jaw and the severe *malocclusion* (an abnormal relationship between the upper and lower teeth) that is invariably associated with it.

Orthognathic surgery, which usually requires a stay in hospital, is performed while the patient is under a general anesthetic.

A jaw that projects too far can be shortened by removing a block of bone from each side and maneuvering the front of the jaw backward. A jaw that is too short can be remedied by dividing the bone on each side, sliding the front of the jaw forward, and inserting bone grafts (taken from elsewhere in the body) into the gaps.

After repositioning, the jaw bones often require splinting (see *Splinting, dental*) until healing occurs.

Orthopedics
The branch of surgery concerned with disorders of the *bones* and *joints* and their associated *muscles*, *tendons*, and *ligaments*. Orthopedic surgeons perform many tasks, including setting broken bones and putting on casts; treating joint conditions such as dislocations, slipped disks, arthritis, and back problems; treating bone tumors and birth defects of the skeleton; and surgically repairing or replacing hip, knee, or finger joints.

Orthopnea
Breathing difficulty brought on by lying flat. Orthopnea is a symptom of *heart failure* (reduced pumping efficiency) and is caused by *pulmonary edema* (accumulation of fluid in the lungs). Orthopnea also occurs with *asthma* and chronic obstructive lung disease (chronic *bronchitis* with or without *emphysema*).

Orthoptics
A technique used to measure and evaluate *squint*, mainly in children. Orthoptics includes assessment of monocular and binocular vision, eye exercises, and measures to combat *amblyopia* (lazy eye).

Os
An anatomical term for a bone, as in os coxae, the hip bone. The term os is also used to refer to an opening in the body, usually the cervical os (entrance to the *uterus*).

Osgood-Schlatter disease
Painful enlargement of the tibial tuberosity, the bony prominence of the *tibia* (shin) just below the knee. Osgood-Schlatter disease occurs most commonly in children (usually boys) aged between 10 and 14. It can be caused by repeated exercise and is a consequence of excessive, repetitive pulling of the *quadriceps muscle* (at the front of the thigh) on the patellar tendon attached to the tibial tuberosity. There is usually pain above and below the knee, which is worse during strenuous activity, and the tibial tuberosity is tender when touched.

Osgood-Schlatter disease usually clears up completely without treatment; if pain is severe, the knee may be immobilized in a plaster *cast*.

Osmosis
The passage of a solvent (e.g., water) through a semipermeable membrane (one that acts like a sieve) from a less concentrated (weaker) solution to a more concentrated (stronger) one. Osmosis occurs whenever solutions of different strengths are separated by a semipermeable membrane and con-

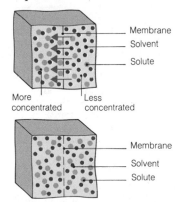

More concentrated / Less concentrated

Same concentration

Osmosis
If two solutions, consisting of different concentrations of a solute (e.g., salt) in a solvent (e.g., water), are separated by a semipermeable membrane, solvent moves from the weaker to the stronger solution until the two solutions attain equal concentration.

tinues until the solutions are of equal strength unless the movement of solvent is opposed by applying pressure to the stronger solution. The pressure needed to stop all such movement is called osmotic pressure.

Semipermeable membranes are widespread in the body—they surround all cells. These membranes allow water, salts, simple sugars (such as glucose), and amino acids (but not proteins) to pass through. Consequently, osmosis plays an important part in regulating the distribution of water and other substances.

Ossicle
A small bone, particularly the malleus (hammer), incus (anvil), and stapes (stirrup)—the three tiny bones in the middle *ear* that conduct sound from the eardrum to the inner ear.

Ossification
The process by which *bone* is formed, renewed, and repaired. Ossification begins in the embryo and continues throughout life. There are three main types of ossification: bone growth, during which new bone is formed mainly from *cartilage* at the *epiphyses* (bone ends); bone renewal, which occurs as part of the normal regeneration process; and bone repair, which fuses broken bones after a *fracture*.

Osteitis
Inflammation of bone. The most common cause is infection (see *Osteomyelitis*). Other causes are *Paget's disease* and *hyperparathyroidism* (overactivity of the parathyroid glands).

Osteo-
A prefix that denotes a relationship to bone, as in *osteoporosis*, a condition in which the bones thin and weaken.

Osteoarthritis
A common *joint* disease aggravated by mechanical stress. Osteoarthritis is characterized by degeneration of the cartilage that lines joints or by formation of *osteophytes* (bony outgrowths), which lead to pain, stiffness, and occasionally loss of function of the affected joint.

INCIDENCE
Osteoarthritis occurs in almost all people aged over 60, although not all have symptoms. Various factors lead to the development of osteoarthritis earlier in life, including an injury to a joint or a *congenital* joint deformity. Severe osteoarthritis affects three times as many women as men.

SYMPTOMS

Osteoarthritis causes pain, swelling, creaking, and stiffness of one or more joints. The hips, knees, and spine are most commonly affected. Pain and stiffness may interfere with activities such as walking and dressing, and may disrupt sleep.

Weakness and shrinkage of surrounding muscles may occur if pain prevents the joint from being used regularly. Affected joints become enlarged and distorted by osteophytes, which are responsible for the characteristic gnarled appearance of hands affected by osteoarthritis.

DIAGNOSIS

A diagnosis is generally made from the patient's symptoms, and from a physical examination that reveals joint tenderness, swelling, and pain on movement. An *X ray* can confirm loss of cartilage and formation of osteophytes and can also allow assessment of the extent of the degenerative process.

TREATMENT

There is no cure for osteoarthritis. Symptoms can be relieved by *analgesic drugs* (painkillers) and by *nonsteroidal anti-inflammatory drugs*. An injection of a *corticosteroid drug* can sometimes ease a painful joint. Many sufferers are overweight, and weight loss often gives substantial relief of symptoms. *Physiotherapy*, including exercises and heat treatment, can often relieve symptoms. If the condition is severe, various aids can make coping at home easier (see *Disability*).

Surgical treatment for severe osteoarthritis includes *arthroplasty* (joint-replacement surgery) and *arthrodesis* (immobilization of a joint).

Osteochondritis dissecans

Degeneration of a *bone* just under a joint surface, causing fragments of bone and cartilage to become separated from surrounding bone.

Osteochondritis dissecans commonly affects the knee and usually starts in adolescence. The exact cause is unknown but the disorder is thought to be caused by damage to a small blood vessel beneath the joint surface, which may be initiated by injury. The separated fragment sometimes reattaches but usually forms a *loose body* within the joint. Symptoms include aching discomfort and intermittent swelling of the affected joint. The presence of a loose body may cause locking of a joint.

X rays show damage to the joint and reveal the presence of any loose

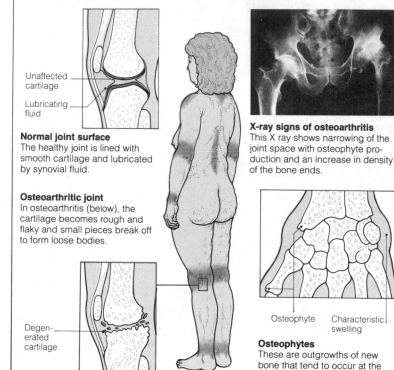

OSTEOARTHRITIS

This differs from rheumatoid arthritis and has a better outlook. It results from excessive wear on joints, sometimes due to obesity or to slight deformity or misalignment of bones in a joint. Inflammation from a disease, such as gout, may also proceed to osteoarthritis. Weight-bearing joints, such as those in the neck, the lower back, and the knees and hips, are the areas most commonly affected by this type of arthritis.

Normal joint surface
The healthy joint is lined with smooth cartilage and lubricated by synovial fluid.

Unaffected cartilage

Lubricating fluid

Osteoarthritic joint
In osteoarthritis (below), the cartilage becomes rough and flaky and small pieces break off to form loose bodies.

Degenerated cartilage

X-ray signs of osteoarthritis
This X ray shows narrowing of the joint space with osteophyte production and an increase in density of the bone ends.

Osteophyte   Characteristic swelling

Osteophytes
These are outgrowths of new bone that tend to occur at the margins of the joint surfaces in osteoarthritis.

bodies. If a fragment has not completely separated, the joint may be immobilized in a plaster *cast* to allow reattachment. Loose bodies of the knee are removed during *arthroscopy*.

The cavity left in the bone by a detached fragment disrupts the smoothness of the joint surface, increasing the likelihood of developing *osteoarthritis* in later life.

Osteochondritis juvenilis

Inflammation of an *epiphysis* (growing area of *bone*) in children and adolescents. The exact cause is unknown, but the condition is thought to be due to disruption of the blood supply to the bone.

There are several distinct types of osteochondritis juvenilis, each involving different bones in the body. *Perthes' disease* affects the epiphysis of the head of the femur (thigh bone).

Scheuermann's disease affects epiphyses of several adjoining vertebrae. Other types affect certain bones in the foot and wrist.

SYMPTOMS AND SIGNS

Osteochondritis juvenilis causes localized pain and tenderness and, if the epiphysis forms part of a joint, restricted movement. Inflammation leads to softening of the bone, which may result in deformity because of surrounding pressure. X rays of the affected area show a patchy appearance and flattening of the bone.

TREATMENT AND OUTLOOK

Immobilization by use of an orthopedic *brace* or plaster *cast* may be used to relieve the patient's pain and reduce the risk of suffering deformity. In some cases of Perthes' disease, an operation is required to relieve the pressure on the diseased bone to prevent more deformity.

O

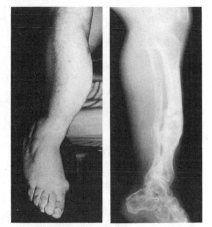
Osteogenesis imperfecta
Affected children may suffer recurrent fractures of the limbs that lead to deformity and shortening, and to abnormal growth. At right is an X ray of the leg of a sufferer.

The bone usually regenerates within three years and rehardens. In many cases, however, deformity is permanent and increases the likelihood of the development of *osteoarthritis* in later life.

Osteochondroma

A benign *bone* tumor made up of a stalk of bone capped with cartilage. It grows from the side of a bone, usually at the end of a long bone in the region of the knee or shoulder. The osteochondroma develops in late childhood and early adolescence, and stops growing when the skeleton is fully developed.

The tumor, which appears as a hard round swelling near a joint, causes problems only if it interferes with the movement of tendons or the surrounding joint. In such cases, surgical removal of the tumor may be necessary. Large osteochondromas can interfere with skeletal growth, causing deformity.

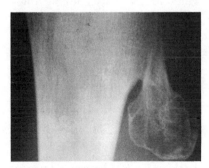
X ray of osteochondroma
The X ray shows a typical osteochondroma protruding from the bone. The tumor has a bony stalk and a cap made of cartilage.

Osteochondrosis

See *Osteochondritis juvenilis*.

Osteodystrophy

Any generalized *bone* defect caused by a *metabolic disorder* (an abnormality of the body chemistry). Examples include *rickets*, a childhood condition in which the bones fail to harden properly due to a deficiency of *vitamin D*; *osteomalacia*, the equivalent condition in adults; *osteoporosis* (a decrease in bone density) when it is caused not by aging but by the hormonal disorder *Cushing's syndrome* or by an excessive intake of *corticosteroid drugs*; and bone cysts and reduction of bone mass, which occasionally occur in chronic *kidney failure* or *hyperparathyroidism* (overactivity of the parathyroid glands) due to a disturbance in calcium metabolism in the body.

An osteodystrophy is usually reversible in adults if the underlying cause can be treated effectively before bone deformity occurs.

Osteogenesis imperfecta

A *congenital* condition characterized by abnormal brittleness of *bones* caused by an inherited defect in the development of the *connective tissue* that forms the basic material of bone. The fragile bones are unusually susceptible to *fractures*.

SYMPTOMS AND SIGNS
Severely affected infants, born with multiple fractures and a soft skull, do not usually survive. Those who are less severely affected suffer from many fractures during infancy and childhood, often caused by only minimal force. A physician examining such children may sometimes find it

difficult to determine whether the cause is osteogenesis imperfecta or *child abuse*. Very mild cases may not be detected until adolescence or later.

A common accompanying sign of the disorder is abnormal thinness of the sclera (whites of the eyes), making them appear blue. In addition, sufferers of osteogenesis imperfecta may be deaf due to *otosclerosis*.

TREATMENT AND OUTLOOK
Fractures are generally treated in the usual way, by immobilization; otherwise, there is no specific treatment for the condition. The fractures usually heal quickly but may cause severe shortening and deformity of the limbs, resulting in stunted, abnormal growth. Skull fractures may cause brain damage or death.

Parents who have a child with osteogenesis imperfecta should seek *genetic counseling* in order to estimate the risk of recurrence in any future pregnancies.

Osteogenic sarcoma

See *Osteosarcoma*.

Osteoid osteoma

A *bone* disorder in which an abnormal area of bone causes deep pain. An osteoid osteoma measures only about 0.5 cm in diameter, and most commonly affects a long bone of the arm or leg. The diagnosis can be made from an *X ray*.

Pain, which is typically worse at night, can usually be relieved by *ASA*. The condition is cured by removing the affected area of bone. (See also *Osteoma*.)

O

Osteoma

A benign tumor of *bone*. An osteoma is hard, usually small, and may occur on any bone. The tumor is usually harmless, but surgical removal may be necessary if an osteoma causes symptoms by pressing on surrounding structures.

Osteomalacia

Softening, weakening, and demineralization of the *bones* in adults due to *vitamin D* deficiency (in children, the condition is called *rickets*).

The development of healthy bone requires an adequate intake of calcium and phosphorus from the diet, but these minerals cannot be absorbed by the body without a sufficient amount of vitamin D. This vitamin is obtained from certain foods and from the action of sunlight on the skin; a deficiency results in softening and weakening of the bones, which then become vulnerable to distortion and *fractures*.

CAUSES

Osteomalacia is usually caused by any of the following, alone or in combination: an insufficient amount of vitamin D in the diet (due to a lack of butter, fortified margarine, fish, eggs, or fish liver oils), insufficient exposure to sunlight, or inadequate absorption of vitamin D from the intestine (see *Malabsorption*), which may be caused by a disorder such as *celiac disease* or by intestinal surgery. Rare causes include *kidney failure*, *acidosis* (increased acidity of body fluids), and certain inherited *metabolic disorders*.

Osteomalacia is rare in developed countries. Most commonly affected are people with an inadequate diet, the housebound elderly, and dark-skinned immigrants living in countries that have much less sunlight than their countries of origin.

SYMPTOMS AND SIGNS

Osteomalacia causes pain in the bones (particularly those in the neck, legs, hips, and ribs), muscle weakness, and, if the blood level of calcium is very low, *tetany* (muscle spasms) in the hands, feet, and throat. If the bones become greatly weakened, they may break after a minor injury.

DIAGNOSIS AND TREATMENT

Osteomalacia is diagnosed from the symptoms and signs, along with blood tests, urine tests, and bone *X rays*. In some cases, a bone *biopsy* (removal of a small sample of bone for microscopic analysis) is performed.

Treatment consists of a diet that is rich in vitamin D and regular supplements of the vitamin. Supplements are usually taken as tablets; if tablets cannot be absorbed by the intestine, injections may be necessary. In some cases of osteomalacia due to malabsorption, calcium supplements may also be taken.

Osteomyelitis

Infection of *bone* and *bone marrow*, usually by bacteria. Osteomyelitis can affect any bone in the body, is more common in children, and most often affects the long bones of the arms and legs and the vertebrae. In adults, the disorder usually affects the pelvis and the vertebrae. In developed countries, adequate nutrition and a generally high resistance to infection have made osteomyelitis, which may be acute or chronic, much rarer than it once was.

ACUTE OSTEOMYELITIS

The infecting microorganism (usually the bacterium *STAPHYLOCOCCUS AUREUS*) is carried to the bone in the bloodstream, having entered the bloodstream via a skin wound or as a result of infection elsewhere in the body (usually in the nose or throat). The infected bone and bone marrow become inflamed and pus forms, causing fever, severe pain and tenderness in the infected bone, and inflammation and swelling of the skin over the affected area.

The diagnosis may be confirmed by blood *cultures*, bone scanning (see *Bone imaging*, and bone *X rays*). Treatment is with high doses of *antibiotic drugs* over several weeks or months. With prompt antibiotic treatment, acute osteomyelitis usually clears up completely. If the condition fails to respond to antibiotic treatment, an operation is performed to expose the bone, to clean out the areas of infected and dead bone, and to drain the pus.

CHRONIC OSTEOMYELITIS

This form may develop when an attack of acute osteomyelitis is neglected or fails to respond to treatment. It may also occur after a compound *fracture* or, occasionally, as a result of the spread of *tuberculosis* from another part of the body.

Chronic osteomyelitis causes constant pain. Complications include persistent deformity and, in children, arrest of growth in the affected bone. In the later stages of the disease (which may have been recurring for many years), *amyloidosis* (harmful deposits of a starchy substance in vital organs) may develop.

Chronic osteomyelitis requires surgical removal of all affected bone, sometimes followed by a *bone graft* to replace the removed bone; antibiotic drugs are also prescribed. If the cause is *tuberculosis*, antituberculous drugs are prescribed for at least one year.

Osteopathy

A system of diagnosis and treatment that emphasizes the role of the musculoskeletal system (bones, muscles, tendons, tissues, nerves, and spinal column) in the healthy functioning of the human body.

The osteopath uses various manual techniques, as well as traditional diagnostic and therapeutic procedures, to diagnose and treat dysfunction. Manual techniques include manipulation and the application of rhythmic stretching and pressure to restore movement to the joints.

There is no school of osteopathy in Canada, and provincial regulations governing licensing and practice vary widely. Very few osteopaths practice in Canada.

Osteopetrosis

A very rare inherited disorder in which *bones* harden and become more dense. The growth of healthy bone is a balance between the activity of two types of bone cells: bone-forming osteoblasts and bone-reabsorbing osteoclasts. In osteopetrosis, there is a deficiency of osteoclasts, which results in the disruption of normal bone structure.

The mildest form of osteopetrosis may not cause any symptoms. More severe forms can result in greater susceptibility to fractures, stunted growth, deformity, and *anemia*. Pressure on nerves may cause blindness, deafness, and facial paralysis.

Bone marrow transplants have been attempted on an investigational basis. The transplant supplies the recipient with cells from which healthy osteoclasts might develop.

Osteophyte

A localized outgrowth of *bone* that forms at the boundary of a joint. Osteophytes are a characteristic feature of *osteoarthritis* and are, in part, responsible for the deformity and the restricted movement of affected joints.

Osteoporosis

Loss of protein matrix tissue from *bone*, causing it to become brittle and easily fractured.

Osteoporosis needs to be distinguished from *osteomalacia*, which is

OSTEOPOROSIS

In osteoporosis, the density of bones decreases, and their brittleness increases, although there is no change in size or composition. Women past the menopause are the most commonly affected because their ovaries no longer produce estrogen, which helps to maintain bone mass. The risk of the condition is greater in a woman who undergoes the menopause early, or whose mother had osteoporosis.

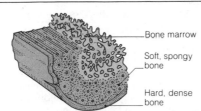

Normal bone cross section
Bone consists of fibers of collagen (a protein), which give elasticity, and calcium, which gives hardness.

Osteoporotic bone
Thinning is mainly due to loss of collagen, which takes calcium with it. Both hard and spongy bone tissue are affected.

Bone loss with age
The graph on the right shows how the percentage of bone lost increases in both sexes from age 30 onward, with the losses particularly marked in women after the menopause. By age 75, about half of all women have sustained at least one fracture due to osteoporosis, a much higher proportion than in men.

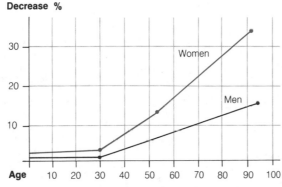

Spine affected by osteoporosis
The X ray shows generalized thinning of the vertebrae, giving a characteristic "codfish" appearance to the spine.

demineralization of bone due to vitamin D deficiency. The two conditions may be present at the same time, causing severe bone weakness.

Osteoporosis is a natural part of aging. By the age of 70, the density of the skeleton has diminished by about one third, even though the bones may remain the same size and retain the same composition (see Osteoporotic bone in box above). For hormonal reasons, significant osteoporosis is more common in women than in men. Also, for reasons that are unknown, the disorder is more common in white people than it is in black people.

CAUSES

Bone naturally becomes thinner as a person ages, but women are especially vulnerable to osteoporosis after the *menopause* because their ovaries no longer produce *estrogen hormones*, which help maintain bone mass.

Other causes of osteoporosis include removal of the ovaries; a diet deficient in calcium, which is essential for bone health; certain hormonal disorders (such as *Cushing's syndrome*) or prolonged treatment with *corticosteroid drugs*; and prolonged immobility. Osteoporosis is more common in heavy smokers and drinkers and, for unknown reasons, is associated with chronic *bronchitis* and *emphysema*.

SYMPTOMS AND SIGNS

In many cases, osteoporosis produces no obvious symptoms; the first sign is often a fracture after a fall that would not cause a fracture in a young adult. Typical sites for such fractures are just above the wrist and the top of the femur (thigh bone). Another type of fracture that occurs in osteoporosis is a spontaneous fracture of one or several vertebrae, which causes the bones to crumble, leading to a progressive loss of height or to pain due to compression of a spinal nerve.

DIAGNOSIS

The condition is diagnosed from the symptoms and from bone *X rays*. In some cases, blood tests and a bone *biopsy* may also be necessary.

PREVENTION AND TREATMENT

Bone tissue that has already been lost cannot be easily replaced, but more bone loss can be minimized by preventive measures.

Hormone replacement therapy to compensate for reduced estrogen production after the menopause has been shown to prevent osteoporosis in women.

Exercise helps to build bones, but anything less than three brisk 5-km walks a week (or the equivalent) is unlikely to be of much benefit in preventing osteoporosis.

Both men and women should ensure that their *calcium* intake is adequate. The richest dietary sources of calcium are milk and milk products, green leafy vegetables, citrus fruits, sardines, and shellfish. Calcium tablets may be needed. It is best not to smoke, and to drink alcohol in moderation only.

Osteosarcoma

A malignant tumor of *bone* that spreads rapidly to the lungs and, less commonly, to other areas. Osteosarcoma occurs mainly in adolescents and the elderly. In young people, osteosarcoma develops for no known reason; in elderly people, it is a late, rare complication of *Paget's disease*.

SYMPTOMS

The most common site of the tumor in young people is in a long bone of the leg or arm, or around the knee, hip, or shoulder. The first symptom is usually a painful visible swelling of the affected bone (if it is near the surface) or a deep-seated pain (if the affected bone cannot be felt through the skin).

As a complication of Paget's disease, an osteosarcoma may develop in several bones; its pain may be indistinguishable from that caused by the original disease.

DIAGNOSIS AND TREATMENT

Diagnosis of this malignancy is usually based on X rays of the bone. Other *bone imaging* techniques (e.g., *MRI*) may also be used.

Osteosarcoma is sometimes treated by *radiation therapy*, but it is usually necessary to remove the affected bone surgically. In most cases, this means *amputation* of one of the patient's limbs; in some cases, a prosthesis (see *Limb, artificial*) can be fitted immediately after the amputation has taken place. Instead of amputation, it is sometimes possible to remove affected bone and replace it by a *bone graft* or by an artificial bone.

Treatment with *anticancer drugs* is usually given for several months after surgery to destroy any cancer cells that may have spread to other parts of the body. With this additional treatment, the outlook is good; about half of all patients whose disease is discovered early are cured.

Osteosclerosis

Increased *bone* density, usually detected on an X ray as an area of extreme whiteness.

Localized osteosclerosis may be caused by a severe injury that compresses the bone; by *osteoarthritis*, in which bone around affected joints thickens; by chronic *osteomyelitis*, in which healthy bone next to the infected area thickens and becomes more dense; or by an *osteoma* (benign bone tumor), which consists of a hard, dense, usually harmless outgrowth of normal bone tissue.

Osteosclerosis occurs throughout the body in *osteopetrosis*, an inherited bone disorder.

Osteotomy

An operation in which a *bone* is cut to change its alignment or to shorten or lengthen it.

WHY IT IS DONE

Osteotomy is sometimes performed on a *hallux valgus* (a deformity of the big toe) that has caused a *bunion*. Another use is to straighten a long bone that has healed crookedly after a *fracture* or to shorten the uninjured leg after a fractured leg has shortened during healing (see *Leg, shortening of*). Osteotomy can also be used to correct the deformity caused by congenital dislocation of the hip (see *Hip, congenital dislocation of*) when this condition has not been detected and treated early enough to avoid surgery. Osteotomy is also sometimes used to correct *coxa vara* (a hip deformity).

HOW IT IS DONE

Under general anesthesia, bones are straightened by cutting through them and repositioning the ends; sometimes a wedge of bone is inserted or removed to achieve the correct alignment. Bones can be lengthened by making an oblique cut and displacing the two parts slightly before rejoining them. Bones can be shortened by cutting out a section of bone and rejoining the two parts.

After the operation, bones that were corrected during surgery are held in position by a metal plate or nail or by a plaster *cast* or *splint*.

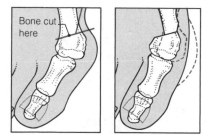

Example of an osteotomy
This procedure is performed to correct a hallux valgus (outward protrusion of the joint at the base of the toe), usually because it has caused a bunion. Part of the top of the first metatarsal bone is removed.

Ostomy

The term used to describe a surgical opening or junction of two hollow organs (e.g., *colostomy* and *ileostomy*).

Otalgia

The medical term for *earache*.

OTC

OTC is an abbreviation for "over-the-counter." It refers to drugs that can be purchased from the pharmacy without a physician's prescription.

Otitis externa

An *ear* infection causing inflammation of the outer ear canal, also known as swimmer's ear.

CAUSES

Generalized infection, affecting the whole canal and sometimes also the pinna (external ear), may be caused by fungi, which produce a persistent inflammation known as otomycosis, or by bacteria. Bacterial infection may also cause a localized infection in the form of a *boil*. Sometimes the ear becomes inflamed as part of a generalized skin disorder, such as atopic *eczema* or seborrheic *dermatitis*.

Malignant otitis externa is an uncommon and occasionally fatal form of the disorder caused by the bacterium *PSEUDOMONAS AERUGINOSA*. This form usually affects elderly diabetics, whose resistance to infection is reduced, and spreads rapidly into surrounding bones and soft tissue.

SYMPTOMS AND SIGNS

Otitis externa usually causes redness and swelling of the skin of the ear canal, a discharge from the ear, and sometimes an area of eczema around the opening of the ear. The ear may itch only in the early stages, but can become painful. Occasionally, pus blocks the ear, causing deafness.

DIAGNOSIS AND TREATMENT

The physician examines the ear with an *otoscope* (a viewing instrument) and may take a sample of any pus for laboratory analysis.

Often the only treatment required is a thorough cleaning and drying of the ear by the physician, sometimes using suction apparatus. In some cases, local application of preparations containing *antibiotic drugs*, *antifungal drugs*, or *corticosteroid drugs* is needed. Oral antibiotic drugs may be prescribed for the treatment of severe bacterial infections. A person with otitis externa should avoid getting the ear canal wet until the infection has cleared up.

Otitis media

Inflammation of the middle *ear* (the cavity between the eardrum and the inner ear).

CAUSES

The inflammation occurs as the result of a viral or bacterial upper respiratory tract infection extending up the eustachian tube, the passage that connects the back of the nose to the middle ear. The tube may become blocked by the inflammation or sometimes by enlarged *adenoids*, which are often associated with infections of the nose and throat. As a result, fluid produced by the inflammation—along with pus in bacterial infections—is not drained off through the tube but accumulates in the middle ear.

The chronic phase of otitis media (otitis media with effusion) follows an upper respiratory infection that has produced acute otitis media.

INCIDENCE

Children are particularly susceptible to otitis media, partly because of the shortness of their eustachian tubes. About one in six children suffers from the acute form in the first year of life and about one in 10 in each of the next six years. Some children have recurrent attacks. Chronic otitis media is much less common because, in most cases, attacks of acute middle ear infection clear up with treatment.

SYMPTOMS AND SIGNS

Acute otitis media is marked by sudden, severe earache, a feeling of fullness in the ear, deafness, tinnitus (ringing or buzzing in the ear), and fever. Sometimes the eardrum bursts, relieving the pain and resulting in a discharge of pus. In this case, healing usually occurs in a few days.

In chronic otitis media, pus constantly exudes from a perforation in the eardrum and there is some degree of deafness. Complications of the condition include *otitis externa* (inflammation of the outer ear); damage to the bones in the middle ear, causing more deafness (sometimes total) in the affected ear; or a *cholesteatoma* (a matted ball of sometimes infected skin debris). In rare cases, infection spreads inward from an infected ear, causing *mastoiditis* or a *brain abscess*.

Inadequately treated otitis media may sometimes lead to a continual production of sticky fluid in the middle ear, a condition that is known as *glue ear*.

DIAGNOSIS

The diagnosis is usually made from examining the ears with an *otoscope* (a viewing instrument). A swab may be taken of any discharge so that the organism responsible for the infection can be cultured and identified.

Acute otitis media usually responds to treatment with *antibiotic drugs* and *analgesic drugs* (painkillers).

Chronic otitis media may be treated by *myringotomy* (surgical creation of an opening in the eardrum) and by sucking out pus and infected debris from the ear as necessary. Antibiotic eardrops may also be needed. A cholesteatoma should always be removed surgically.

Oto-

A prefix that denotes a relationship to the ear, as for example, in *otorrhea* (a discharge from the ear) and *otosclerosis* (hardening of the ear).

Otoplasty

Cosmetic or reconstructive surgery on the outer *ear*. Otoplasty is usually performed to flatten protruding ears. It may also be done to construct or repair a missing or badly damaged ear.

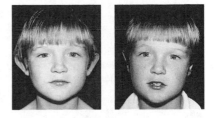

Otoplasty for protruding ears
A strip of skin is removed from behind each ear. The underlying cartilage is remodeled and the edges of the wound are stitched together.

PROTRUDING EARS

Otoplasty may be performed under general or local anesthesia. A strip of skin is removed from behind the ear. The underlying cartilage is then remodeled and the two edges of the wound are stitched together, pulling the ear closer to the head. After the operation, a dressing is kept on the ear until the wound has healed, usually 10 to 14 days later. The scar is hidden in the crease between the ear and scalp.

LACK OF AN OUTER EAR

Some children are born with part or all of the outer ear missing, and may also lack an external ear passage; in some cases there is also underdevelopment of the same side of the face.

Treatment involves transferring a piece of rib cartilage, which is sculpted to resemble the normal ear, to a pocket of skin where the ear is to be placed. The procedure usually involves three operations. Hearing in the reconstructed ear may be abnormal but if the child has a normal range of hearing in the other ear, no attempt need be made to improve hearing in the reconstructed ear.

Otorhinolaryngology

The surgical specialty concerned with diseases of the *ear*, *nose*, and *throat*. It is commonly known as ENT surgery.

ENT specialists commonly treat *sinus* problems, *otitis media* (middle ear infection), *glue ear*, *tonsillitis*, and minor hearing loss. Other disorders treated include *otosclerosis*, *Meniere s disease*, airway problems in children, uncontrollable nosebleeds, and cancer of the larynx and sinuses.

Otorrhea

The medical name for a discharge from the ear (see *Ear, discharge from*).

Otosclerosis

A disorder of the middle *ear* that causes progressive *deafness*. Otosclerosis often runs in families.

O

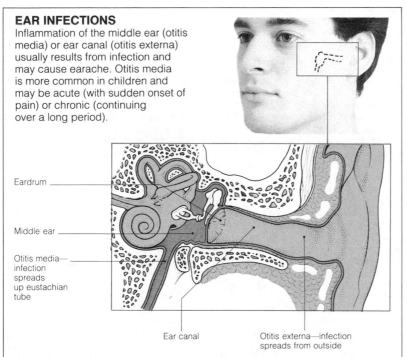

EAR INFECTIONS

Inflammation of the middle ear (otitis media) or ear canal (otitis externa) usually results from infection and may cause earache. Otitis media is more common in children and may be acute (with sudden onset of pain) or chronic (continuing over a long period).

Eardrum

Middle ear

Otitis media—infection spreads up eustachian tube

Ear canal

Otitis externa—infection spreads from outside

Otitis media
This usually occurs through spread of infection from the back of the nose to the middle ear via the eustachian tube.

Otitis externa
The ear canal is susceptible to infection if it is moist (after swimming) or damaged by attempts to remove earwax.

CAUSES AND INCIDENCE

Otosclerosis occurs when, for unknown reasons, an overgrowth of bone immobilizes the stapes (the innermost bone of the middle ear). This prevents sound vibrations from being passed to the inner ear, resulting in conductive deafness. In most cases of otosclerosis, both ears are ultimately affected.

About one person in 200 is affected by the disease, which usually starts in early adulthood. It is more common in women than in men and often develops during pregnancy.

SYMPTOMS AND SIGNS

Sound is heard as muffled but is more distinguishable when there is background noise. Affected people tend to talk quietly. Hearing loss progresses slowly over a period of 10 to 15 years and is often accompanied by *tinnitus* (noises in the ear) and rarely by *vertigo* (a spinning sensation). Some sensorineural deafness (caused by damage spreading to the inner ear) may eventually occur, making high tones difficult to hear and causing the sufferer to speak loudly.

DIAGNOSIS AND TREATMENT

The diagnosis is based on abnormal results of *hearing tests*. A *hearing aid* can markedly improve hearing, but the condition can be cured only by *stapedectomy* (an operation in which the stapes is replaced by an artificial substitute).

Otoscope

An instrument for examining the *ear*. An otoscope includes magnifying lenses, a light, and a speculum (a funnel-shaped tip that is inserted into the

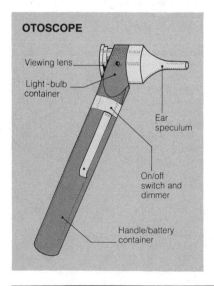

OTOSCOPE

Viewing lens

Light-bulb container

Ear speculum

On/off switch and dimmer

Handle/battery container

ear canal). The instrument allows easy inspection of the outer ear canal and the eardrum. With an otoscope it is also possible to detect certain diseases of the middle ear through the semi-transparent eardrum.

Ototoxicity

Toxic damage to the inner *ear*. High doses of certain drugs (especially aminoglycoside *antibiotic drugs*) can damage the cochlea and the semicircular canals in the inner ear, impairing hearing and balance.

Outpatient treatment

Medical care given to a person on a day basis in a hospital or clinic.

Ovarian cyst

An abnormal, fluid-filled swelling in an *ovary*. Ovarian cysts are common and, in about 95 percent of cases, benign (noncancerous). Many ovarian cysts disappear without treatment.

TYPES

The most common type of ovarian cyst is a follicular cyst, in which the egg-producing follicle of the ovary enlarges and fills with fluid. Cysts may also occur in the corpus luteum, a yellow mass of tissue that forms from the follicle after *ovulation*.

Other types of ovarian cysts include *dermoid cysts* and malignant cysts (see *Ovary, cancer of*).

SYMPTOMS AND SIGNS

Ovarian cysts often cause no symptoms, but some cause abdominal discomfort, pain during intercourse, or menstrual irregularities including *amenorrhea* (lack of menstruation), *menorrhagia* (heavy periods), or *dysmenorrhea* (painful periods). Severe abdominal pain, nausea, and fever, which necessitate surgery, may develop if twisting or rupture of an ovarian cyst occurs.

DIAGNOSIS AND TREATMENT

A cyst may be discovered during a routine *pelvic examination*. *Ultrasound scanning* or a *laparoscopy* (an examination of the abdominal cavity through a viewing instrument) may be necessary to confirm the diagnosis as well as to determine the size and position of the cyst.

Simple cysts (which are thin-walled and filled with fluid) often go away on their own. Complex cysts (such as dermoid cysts) do not, and commonly require surgical removal. In many cases, it is only the cyst that needs to be removed, but if a cyst is large it is sometimes necessary to remove the entire ovary.

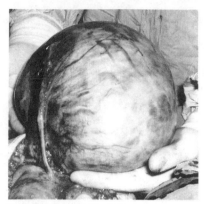

Removal of an ovarian cyst
This photograph shows a surgeon removing a very large ovarian cyst. Most ovarian cysts are much smaller than this.

Ovary

One of a pair of almond-shaped glands situated on either side of the *uterus* immediately below the opening of the *fallopian tube*. Each ovary is about 3 cm long and 2 cm wide and contains numerous cavities called follicles in which egg cells (see *Ovum*) develop. In addition to producing ova, the ovaries also produce the female· sex hormones *estrogen* and *progesterone*.

DISORDERS

Absence or failure of normal development of the ovaries is a rare disorder, and one that is usually caused by a chromosomal abnormality (see *Turner's syndrome*).

Oophoritis (inflammation of the ovary) may be caused by the *mumps* virus or by other infections; for example *gonorrhea* or *pelvic inflammatory disease*.

Ovarian cysts may develop at any age; about 95 percent of them are benign. Polycystic ovary syndrome (see *Ovary, polycystic*), in which multiple ovarian cysts form, is a disorder thought to be due to the body's inappropriate hormonal stimulation of the ovaries. The cysts may produce small amounts of male sex hormones, leading to *amenorrhea* (absence of menstruation), *infertility*, and *hirsutism*.

Cancer of the ovary (see *Ovary, cancer of*) occurs mainly in women over 50 and usually causes few symptoms (if any) in the early stages. However, it can cause abdominal discomfort, pain during intercourse and other symptoms similar to those of an ovarian cyst, an abnormal fluid-filled swelling. Physicians find that ovarian failure, in which the ovaries cease

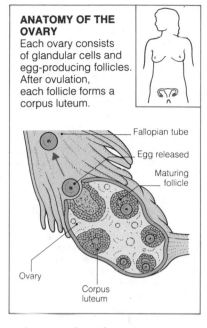

ANATOMY OF THE OVARY

Each ovary consists of glandular cells and egg-producing follicles. After ovulation, each follicle forms a corpus luteum.

Fallopian tube

Egg released

Maturing follicle

Ovary

Corpus luteum

to function altogether, causes premature *menopause* in about 5 percent of all women.

Ovary, cancer of

A malignant growth of the *ovary*. Cancer of the ovary can occur at any age but is most common after the age of 50, the postmenopausal years. There are about 2,000 cases of this cancer diagnosed in Canada each year. It is three times more common in women who have never had children and less common in women who have taken *oral contraceptives*. In Canada, ovarian cancer is the fifth leading cause of cancer death in women, after cancer of the breast, lung, colon and stomach.

The growth may be primary (arising in the ovary) or may be a secondary growth that has spread to the ovary from some other part of the body, often the breast.

SYMPTOMS AND SIGNS

In most cases, ovarian cancer causes no symptoms until the condition is fairly widespread. The first symptom is usually vague abdominal discomfort and swelling. There may be digestive disturbances, such as nausea and vomiting, abnormal vaginal bleeding, and ascites (excess fluid in the abdominal cavity). A physical examination may reveal a swelling in the pelvis.

DIAGNOSIS

A *laparoscopy* (examination of the abdominal cavity through a viewing instrument) or *laparotomy* (opening of the abdomen wall for an exploratory operation) may be necessary to confirm the diagnosis.

TREATMENT

Ovarian cancer is treated by the surgical removal of the growth or of as much of the malignant tissue as possible. This usually involves *salpingo-oophorectomy* (removal of the ovaries and fallopian tubes) and *hysterectomy* (removal of the uterus). Surgery is usually followed by *radiation therapy* and *anticancer drugs*.

OUTLOOK

If the growth is confined to one or both ovaries, 60 to 70 percent of patients survive for at least five years. If the growth is more widespread, only about 10 to 20 percent of patients survive for five years. New drug combinations may improve this survival rate, however.

Ovary, polycystic

A condition, also called Stein-Leventhal syndrome, which is characterized by oligomenorrhea (scanty menstruation) or *amenorrhea* (absence of menstruation), *infertility*, *hirsutism* (excessive hairiness), and *obesity*. Often, but not always, there are multiple *ovarian cysts*. The condition may sometimes occur in the absence of hirsutism or obesity.

In most women with polycystic ovaries, menarche (the onset of menstruation) occurs at the normal age. After a year or two of regular menstruation, the periods become highly irregular, and then cease. Hirsutism, which often becomes evident around menarche, occurs in about 50 percent of cases, as does obesity.

CAUSE

The condition is due to an imbalance between luteinizing hormone (LH) and follicle-stimulating hormone (FSH), which are two *gonadotropin hormones* produced by the *pituitary gland*; there is excessive stimulation of the ovaries by LH and a relative deficiency of FSH. This results in lack of *ovulation* and in increased production of *testosterone* by the ovaries.

DIAGNOSIS

Tests to determine the level of hormones in the blood are needed to confirm the diagnosis. *Ultrasound scanning* of the ovaries and/or *laparoscopy* (examination of the abdominal cavity with a viewing instrument) may be helpful.

TREATMENT

The condition may be treated with *clomiphene* (an anti-estrogen drug), *progestogen drugs*, *LH-RH* (luteinizing hormone–releasing hormone), or *oral contraceptives*. In rare cases, surgical removal of a wedge of ovarian tissue is performed. The method of treatment used depends on the severity of the symptoms and on whether the woman wishes to become pregnant. Spontaneous ovulation is not unusual in women with polycystic ovary.

OUTLOOK

Women with polycystic ovaries often have a high level of estrogen in the body, which increases the risk of endometrial cancer (see *Uterus, cancer of*). Treatment with progesterone may be recommended to restore hormonal balance and decrease the risk of this cancer.

Overbite

Overlapping of the lower front *teeth* by the upper front teeth. A slight degree of overbite is normal because the upper jaw is larger than the lower one. In *malocclusion*, overbite may be greater than normal or may be reversed (with the lower teeth projecting in front of the upper ones).

Overbreathing

A common name for *hyperventilation*, abnormally deep or rapid breathing, usually caused by anxiety.

Overcrowding, dental

Excessive crowding of the *teeth* so that they are unable to assume their normal positions in the jaw.

CAUSES

Dental overcrowding is commonly inherited, and may occur either because the teeth are relatively too large for the jaw or because the jaw is too small to accommodate the teeth.

Overcrowding may also be caused, or be aggravated by, premature loss of primary molar (back) teeth. Prema-

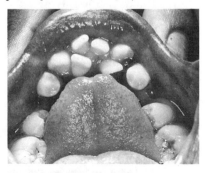

Severe case of overcrowding
The front teeth are crowded together because the two molars, just behind them, have grown too far forward.

ture loss of these teeth can cause the permanent teeth growing beneath them to move out of position and leave insufficient space for the developing permanent teeth further forward in the mouth.

PROBLEMS
Overcrowding of the teeth may lead to *malocclusion* (an incorrect relationship between the upper and lower teeth). Overcrowding may also prevent certain teeth from erupting through the gum (see *Impaction, dental*). The risk of dental decay (see *Caries, dental*) is increased when the teeth are overcrowded because cleaning of the teeth is more difficult than normal. Difficulty in cleaning the teeth, together with greater stress on tissues supporting the teeth, also increases the risk of *periodontal disease*.

TREATMENT
A dentist or orthodontist decides whether one or more teeth should be extracted to allow room for others to grow. In many cases, the remaining teeth must be fitted with an *orthodontic appliance* to move them into their correct positions.

Overuse injury
A term for any injury that has been caused by repetitive movement of part of the body. An alternative term is repetitive strain injury.

A common example of an overuse injury is *epicondylitis*, painful inflammation of one of the epicondyles (bony prominences) at the elbow, caused by the pull of the attached forearm muscles during gardening, painting, or playing certain sports (see *Golfers' elbow; Tennis elbow*).

Overuse injuries of the finger and wrist joints may affect assembly-line workers and typists. Musicians are also prone to a variety of problems; the thumb may be affected in players of woodwind instruments and the neck may be affected in violinists.

Symptoms, which usually disappear with rest, include pain and stiffness in the affected joints and muscles. A recurrence of the injury can sometimes be avoided by a change in the technique used during the causative activity.

Overweight
A condition in which there is excess body fat, which creates an increased risk of health problems. Serious overweight is a factor in diseases such as *diabetes mellitus* and *hypertension*. (See *Obesity, Weight* and Weight charts.)

Ovulation
The development and release of an *ovum* (egg) from a follicle within the *ovary*. Ovulation occurs midway through the menstrual cycle and is regulated by hormones. During the first half of the cycle, follicle-stimulating hormone (FSH) causes several ova to mature in the ovary. At mid-cycle, luteinizing hormone (LH) causes one ripe ovum to be released. The follicle then forms a small mass of tissue called the corpus luteum, which secretes *progesterone* late in the cycle.

After its release, the ovum travels along the *fallopian tube* and, if *fertilization* does not occur, is shed during *menstruation*. Regular menstruation usually means that ovulation is occurring, except around *puberty* and when nearing the *menopause*.

Some forms of contraception (see *Contraception, natural methods of*) are based on predicting when ovulation occurs each month and avoiding sexual intercourse at this time. Signs of ovulation include a rise in body temperature and changes in the amount and consistency of cervical mucus; there may also be mild abdominal pain (see *Mittelschmerz*).

If a woman does not ovulate, she cannot conceive. Investigation of female *infertility* includes tests to determine whether ovulation occurs.

Ovum
 The egg cell (female cell of reproduction). Each ovum measures about 0.1 mm in diameter. There are about one million immature ova present in each *ovary* at birth; only about 200 per ovary ever mature to be released at *ovulation* during a woman's fertile years. If *fertilization* occurs, the ovum develops into an *embryo*.

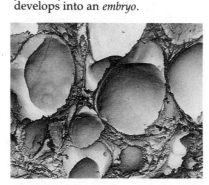

Developing ova
This section of a human ovary shows several eggs at various developmental stages. Only about 1 in 20 eggs matures enough to be released at ovulation each month.

Oxazepam
A *benzodiazepine drug* used as a short-term treatment for *anxiety* and tension, and to encourage sleep. It may also be of value in relieving the symptoms of acute alcohol withdrawal. Like other benzodiazepines, oxazepam may cause dependence if taken regularly for more than two weeks (see *Drug dependence*).

Oxprenolol
A *beta-blocker drug* used in the treatment of *angina pectoris* (chest pain due to inadequate blood supply to the heart muscle), *hypertension* (high blood pressure) and cardiac *arrhythmias* (irregularity of the heartbeat). Oxprenolol may also be prescribed to relieve palpitations and tremor caused by *anxiety* and to control symptoms of *hyperthyroidism* (overactivity of the thyroid gland).

Possible adverse effects are typical of drugs in the beta-blocker group.

Oxtriphylline
A *bronchodilator drug* used in the treatment of asthma and chronic lung disease. It is often used in conjunction with other bronchodilator drugs. The drug may cause nausea, vomiting and dizziness, and monitoring its levels in the blood is often advisable.

Oxybutynin
An *anticholinergic drug* used to reduce spasm of the bladder muscle for the relief of symptoms associated with an overactive bladder. It is used in conjunction with bladder-training procedures such as timed voiding. By enlarging bladder capacity, oxybutynin reduces urinary frequency, urgency and incontinence. Dry mouth is the most common side effect, but the drug may also cause drowsiness and blurred vision. Oxybutynin has been taken for up to two years without problems.

Oxycodone
A narcotic useful in control of pain after ASA and acetaminophen have failed to give relief. Oxycodone may cause nausea, drowsiness, and dizziness. Psychologic and physiologic dependence may occur with long-term use.

Oxygen
A colorless, odorless gas that makes up 21 percent of the Earth's atmosphere. Oxygen is essential for almost all forms of life, including humans, because it is necessary for the meta-

bolic "burning" of foods to produce energy—a process known as *aerobic* metabolism.

To reach the body cells, where aerobic metabolism takes place, oxygen in the air is absorbed through the lungs and into the blood, where it binds to the *hemoglobin* in red blood cells. In this form, the oxygen is distributed throughout the body, being released from the hemoglobin and taken up by cells in areas where the oxygen level is low.

Oxygen is used therapeutically to treat conditions such as severe *bronchitis* or *hypoxia* (inadequate oxygen in the body tissues). In some cases, high pressure oxygen (see *Hyperbaric oxygen treatment*) is used to treat the bends (*decompression sickness*) or poisoning from *carbon monoxide*. (See also *Ozone*.)

Oxygen tent

A plastic sheet that is placed over a hospital bed to enable a patient to receive *oxygen therapy*. Small oxygen tents, sometimes called croupettes, are occasionally used for infants and toddlers who require humidified (moistened) oxygen but who will not tolerate wearing a face mask. Oxygen is passed into the tent after being humidified by bubbling it through water. Children may find oxygen tents uncomfortably cold or may be frightened by being in an enclosed space.

Oxygen is sometimes administered to infants via a perspex box placed over the head.

Oxygen therapy

Supplying a person with oxygen-enriched air to relieve severe *hypoxia* (inadequate oxygen in body tissues).

In hospitals, oxygen is usually piped to a terminal at the patient's bedside and is administered as necessary through a face mask or through nasal cannulas (tubes inserted into the nostrils). The concentration of oxygen is varied according to the patient's needs.

People at home can be supplied with oxygen in cylinders for use during acute attacks of hypoxia, as occur in severe *asthma* for example. People with persistent hypoxia due to severe chronic *bronchitis* or *emphysema* may benefit from long-term oxygen therapy. These patients may be supplied with a machine called an oxygen concentrator, which separates oxygen from the air and remixes it in a higher-than-normal concentration. Oxygen-rich air is

then piped to different rooms for prolonged inhalation.

People receiving oxygen therapy should not smoke, since smoking not only presents a fire risk but also reduces the oxygen-carrying capacity of the blood and aggravates the underlying condition for which the oxygen is being given. (See also *Hyperbaric oxygen treatment*.)

Oxymetazoline

A *decongestant drug* which is used in the treatment of allergic *rhinitis* (hay fever), *sinusitis*, and the common *cold*. By restricting the small blood vessels in the nose, it reduces swelling and congestion in the nasal passages. Oxymetazoline eye drops act in a similar way. Oxymetazoline has a longer lasting effect than many other decongestant drugs, but it may irritate the nose. Prolonged use causes rebound congestion (increased congestion after the drug is withdrawn).

Oxytetracycline

A tetracycline *antibiotic drug*. Oxytetracycline is used to treat *chlamydial infections*, such as *nonspecific urethritis*, *psittacosis*, and *trachoma*. It is prescribed for a variety of other infections, including *bronchitis*, pneumonia caused by *mycoplasma*, *syphilis*, and *cholera*. Oxytetracycline may also be used to treat severe *acne*.

POSSIBLE ADVERSE EFFECTS
Nausea, vomiting, diarrhea, skin rash, or increased sensitivity of the skin to sunlight are possible adverse effects. Oxytetracycline may discolor developing teeth and is therefore not prescribed for children under 12 or for pregnant women.

Oxytocin

A *hormone* produced by the *pituitary gland*. Oxytocin causes uterine *contractions* during labor and stimulates the flow of milk in women who are *breast-feeding*.

USE AS A DRUG
Synthetic oxytocin can be used to induce childbirth (see *Induction of labor*). It is sometimes used to help expel the placenta (afterbirth) after delivery or to empty the uterus after an incomplete *miscarriage* or a fetal death. Oxytocin is sometimes given as a nasal spray to stimulate milk flow, and it is sometimes used to test the well-being of the fetus if the mother is at high risk because of diabetes or high blood pressure. In such cases the response of the baby's heart rate to the drug-induced contractions is moni-

tored. If there are fetal difficulties, labor may be induced or a cesarean section performed.

POSSIBLE ADVERSE EFFECTS
Contractions may be stronger and more painful than usual, increasing the need for stronger *analgesic drugs* (painkillers). Rare adverse effects, particularly with excessive or prolonged use, include nausea, vomiting, palpitations, seizures, and coma.

Oxyuriasis

An alternative name for enterobiasis or *pinworm infestation*.

Ozena

A severe and rare form of *rhinitis* (inflammation of the mucous membrane in the nose) in which the membrane atrophies (wastes away) and a thick nasal discharge dries to form crusts. Ozena often causes severe *halitosis* (bad breath).

Ozone

A rare form of oxygen, ozone is a poisonous, faintly blue gas that is produced by the action of electrical discharges (such as lightning) on oxygen molecules.

Ozone occurs naturally in the upper atmosphere (about 15 to 30 km above the Earth's surface), where it screens the Earth from most of the sun's harmful ultraviolet radiation. Evidence suggests that the ozone layer is being depleted by various environmental chemicals, notably the chlorofluorocarbons (CFCs) in aerosols. The result of this depletion is that stronger and more potent forms of ultraviolet radiation are now reaching the Earth's surface. Increased ultraviolet levels could lead to an increase in the incidence of skin cancer and cataracts.

O

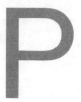

Pacemaker

A device that supplies electrical impulses to the *heart* to maintain the *heartbeat* at a regular rate. A pacemaker consists of a small electronic device and power source connected to the heart via an electrical wire.

In a healthy heart, the heartbeat is maintained by a nucleus of specialized heart tissue called the sinoatrial node, which sends out regular electrical impulses that pass through the heart muscle and trigger heart contractions. An artificial pacemaker is implanted when a person's sinoatrial node is not functioning properly, or when there is some impairment to the passage of the normal electrical impulses (see *Heart block; Sick sinus syndrome*).

The two basic types of pacemaker—fixed rate and demand—are described in the illustrated box. More advanced types can increase the heart rate during exercise. Related devices are being developed that can convert an abnormal rhythm back to normal.

IMPLANTATION

Implantation is carried out under a local anesthetic. Patients can expect complete healing without complications and should return to normal work and activity as soon as possible. Vigorous exercise should be avoided for two weeks after the operation.

Modern microelectronic circuits require little power, and the lithium batteries used in pacemakers have a long life. Unless the demand on the battery is excessive, a pacemaker will usually operate quite satisfactorily for several years. Battery replacement requires only a minor operation.

PRECAUTIONS

Modern pacemakers are relatively insensitive to interference but may be affected by powerful electromagnetic pulses. Anyone fitted with a pacemaker should avoid powerful radio or radar transmitters and should not pass through security screens at air-

ports. Precautions may also be required if *diathermy* machines are to be used during physiotherapy or surgery. *TENS* is an unsuitable method of pain relief for people with a pacemaker.

Paget's disease

A common disorder of middle-aged and elderly people in which the normal process of *bone* formation is disrupted, causing the affected bones to weaken, thicken, and become deformed. Also known as osteitis deformans, Paget's disease usually involves only limited areas of the skeleton. The bones usually affected are the pelvis, skull, clavicle (collarbone), vertebrae, and long bones of the leg.

CAUSE AND INCIDENCE

The normal maintenance of healthy bones by the body involves a balance between the actions of cells that break down bone tissue and those that rebuild it. In Paget's disease, this balance is disturbed. The disease varies in frequency from one part of the country to another, suggesting an infective cause, which is thought to be viral. Overall, Paget's disease affects about 3 percent of the population over

---

PACEMAKERS

A pacemaker may be external (worn on a belt) or internal (implanted in the chest), like those shown below.

Transvenous implantation
An insulated wire is inserted into a major vein in the neck and guided down into the heart until the electrode at its far end is positioned within the part of the heart muscle to be stimulated. The free end is connected to the pacemaker, which is fitted into a pocket created under the skin of the abdomen or below the collarbone.

External pacing is used only as a temporary measure. There are two main methods of implantation.

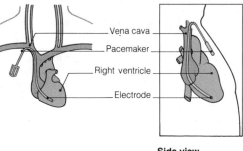

Vena cava
Pacemaker
Right ventricle
Electrode

Side view
The pacemaker is usually well hidden by overlying tissue.

Epicardial implantation
The electrode is attached to the outer surface of the part of the heart muscle to be stimulated and the pacemaker is fitted into a pocket constructed underneath the skin of the abdomen.

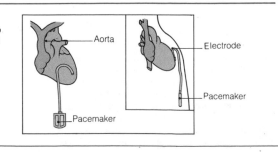

Aorta
Electrode
Pacemaker
Pacemaker

TYPES OF PACEMAKERS
Two main types are shown. In some cases, an external programmer can adjust the rate.

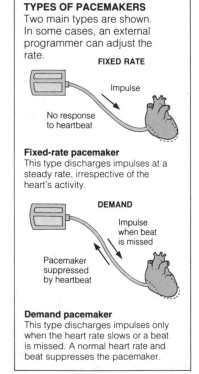

FIXED RATE
Impulse
No response to heartbeat

Fixed-rate pacemaker
This type discharges impulses at a steady rate, irrespective of the heart's activity.

DEMAND
Impulse when beat is missed
Pacemaker suppressed by heartbeat

Demand pacemaker
This type discharges impulses only when the heart rate slows or a beat is missed. A normal heart rate and beat suppresses the pacemaker.

the age of 40, the incidence increasing with age. The disorder has a tendency to run in families and affects more men than women.

SYMPTOMS AND SIGNS

Paget's disease often causes no symptoms and is usually discovered from an X ray taken for some other reason. The most common symptoms are bone pain and deformity, especially bowing of the legs. Affected bones are prone to fracture.

Changes in the skull may lead to leontiasis (distortion of the facial bones that produces a rather lionlike appearance) and to inner-ear damage, sometimes resulting in deafness, tinnitus, vertigo, or headaches. Enlarged vertebrae may press on the spinal cord, causing pain and sometimes paralysis of the legs. If the pelvis is affected, severe arthritis of the hips can result. Occasionally, *bone cancer* may develop, and, in rare cases, when many bones are involved, increased blood flow through the affected bones may cause *heart failure*.

DIAGNOSIS

X rays reveal areas of porous, thickened bone. *Blood tests* that show an elevated level of the *enzyme* alkaline phosphatase (which is associated with bone cell formation) give an indication of the extent and activity of the disease.

TREATMENT AND OUTLOOK

Most people with the disorder do not require treatment, and many others simply need to take *analgesic drugs* (painkillers). In severe cases, the hormone *calcitonin* may be prescribed. It relieves pain, reduces alkaline phosphatase levels, and promotes normal bone formation. Other drugs that have the same effect (including disodium etidronate and plicamycin) may also be used. Surgery may be required to correct deformities or to treat arthritis.

Paget's disease of the nipple

A rare type of *breast cancer* in which the tumor starts in the milk ducts of the nipple. Paget's disease of the nipple looks similar to *eczema* and causes itching and a burning sensation. A sore that will not heal may develop on the nipple. In most cases, only one nipple is affected. Without treatment, the tumor may gradually spread further into the breast.

Anyone who develops eczema of the nipple should consult a physician, who may arrange for a *biopsy* (removal of a sample of tissue for microscopic examination) to be taken.

Pain

A localized sensation that can range from mild discomfort to an unbearable and excruciating experience. Pain is the result of stimulation of special sensory nerve endings usually following injury or caused by disease.

THE MECHANISM OF PAIN

The basic mechanism of pain is shown in the illustrated box on page 770. The skin contains many specialized nerve endings (nociceptors). Stimulation of these receptors leads to transmission of pain messages to the brain. Nociceptors have different sensitivities, some responding only to severe stimulation, such as cutting or heating the skin to a high temperature; others respond to warning stimuli, such as firm pressure, stretching, or temperatures not high enough to burn. Pain receptors are present in structures other than the skin, including blood vessels and tendons. Most internal organs have few, if any, nociceptors. The large intestine, for example, can be cut without causing any pain. It does, however, have nociceptors that respond to stretching, which, in severe cases, may cause pain.

PSYCHOLOGICAL ASPECTS OF PAIN

Pain is usually associated with distress and anxiety, and sometimes with fear. People vary tremendously in their pain thresholds (the level at which the pain is felt and the person feels compelled to act). The cause and circumstances of the pain may also affect the way it is perceived by the sufferer. The pain of cancer, because of fear of the disease, may seem much greater and cause more suffering than similar pain resulting from persistent indigestion. Unexplained pain is often worse because of the anxiety it can cause; once a diagnosis is made and reassurance given, the pain may be perceived as less severe.

The experience of pain may be reduced by arousal (e.g., an injury sustained during competitive sport or on the battlefield may go unnoticed in the heat of the moment); strong emotion can also block pain. Some people believe that mental preparation for pain (e.g., in childbirth or in experiments to test pain) can greatly reduce the response.

A person's response to pain is greatly modified by past experience; the outcome of previous episodes of pain may affect the way the individual copes with subsequent pain. Factors such as insomnia, anxiety, and depression, which often accompany incapacitating illness, lower tolerance

to pain. Treatment for these symptoms may be given together with treatment for the pain.

Cultural differences exist in the expression of pain. In some parts of the world, self-inflicted torture and the ability to withstand great pain are a mark of a person's strength and character. However, the pain of even mild torture inflicted by captors may be perceived as much worse than a similar degree of pain that occurs under different circumstances.

TYPES OF PAIN

Many adjectives are used to describe different types of pain, such as throbbing, penetrating, gnawing, aching, burning, and gripping. The extent to which a patient is accurately able to describe his or her pain to the physician is highly variable, even though an accurate description can be a vital clue to the diagnosis.

Attempts have been made to categorize pain according to intensity, ranging from a minor cut or sore throat at the lower end of the scale to childbirth or renal colic at the upper.

If the pain comes from an internal organ it is often difficult for the sufferer to pinpoint its origin with any precision. For example, in the early stages of appendicitis, pain may be felt in the region above the navel. In the later stages, when infection has caused inflammation of the peritoneum (lining of the abdominal cavity), the pain becomes localized above the right groin.

Pain may be felt at a point some distance from the disorder; this phenomenon is known as *referred pain* (see illustrated box, p. 770). Following amputation of a limb, pain may seem to come from the amputated limb (see *Phantom limb*); in some cases, the person can localize the pain site, such as in a toe despite having had the leg amputated. (See also *Endorphins*; *Enkephalins*.)

Painful arc syndrome

A condition in which pain occurs when the arm is raised from the side of the body between 45 degrees and 160 degrees.

Painful arc syndrome is usually caused by inflammation of a tendon or a *bursa* around the shoulder joint. The pain is caused by the inflamed tendon or bursa being squeezed between the upper parts of the *scapula* (shoulder blade) and the *humerus* (upper-arm bone). Treatment includes *physiotherapy* and the injection of *corticosteroid drugs* into the tender area.

P

Painkillers
See *Analgesic drugs*.

Pain relief
The treatment of *pain*, usually with *analgesic drugs*. Methods of treatment depend on the severity, duration, location, and cause of the pain.

DRUG TREATMENT
Mild analgesic drugs, available over-the-counter, are usually effective in the treatment of mild or moderate pain, such as may be caused by *headache, toothache*, or *dysmenorrhea* (menstrual pain). *Acetaminophen, ASA*, and *codeine* are the most widely used

drugs in this group. Pain accompanied by inflammation, as may be caused by *arthritis* or *sports injuries*, is often alleviated by a *nonsteroidal anti-inflammatory drug* (NSAID).

Severe pain, such as may be caused by serious injury or kidney stones (see *Calculus, urinary tract*), may require

---

PAIN
Pain mechanisms exist to provide a useful warning of possible injury or to caution against repeating an action that has led to injury. Certain

diseases, such as arthritis and extensive cancer, may set off these same mechanisms, causing chronic pain that has no apparent function.

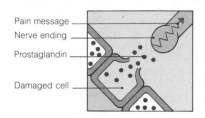

Initiation of pain signals
The signals are set off by stimulation of special nerve endings—by pressure, heat, or release of chemicals, including prostaglandins, by damaged cells.

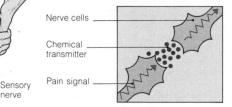

Signal transmission to brain
Within the brain and spinal cord, pain signals pass between nerve cells by means of chemicals that cross the gaps between the cells.

Reflex action
The nerve pathways that warn of noxious stimuli (through the sensation of pain) may also initiate automatic, reflex actions that help prevent harm.

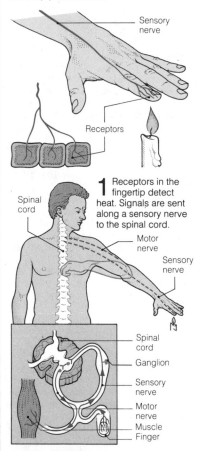

1 Receptors in the fingertip detect heat. Signals are sent along a sensory nerve to the spinal cord.

2 The signals arriving in the spinal cord pass instantaneously to a motor nerve that connects to a muscle in the arm. The signals received via the motor nerve cause the muscle in the arm to contract, moving the arm away from the source of danger (the flame).

Perception of pain
When an injury occurs, signals pass along nerve pathways concerned with pain, first to the spinal cord and then to the thalamus in the brain; there the pain is perceived.

REFERRED PAIN
A referred pain is one felt in a site other than an injured or diseased part. Sensory nerves from certain body areas converge before they enter the brain, causing confusion about the source of pain signals.

Tooth to ear region
A toothache may be felt in the ear, because the same sensory nerve supplies both parts.

Diaphragm to right shoulder
Inflammation of the diaphragm, often due to pneumonia, may be felt as a pain in the right shoulder.

Heart to left arm
Angina, a pain caused by reduced blood supply to the heart muscle, is often felt in the left shoulder or arm.

Knee to hip
Disorders affecting the knee, such as arthritis, may be felt as pain in the hip.

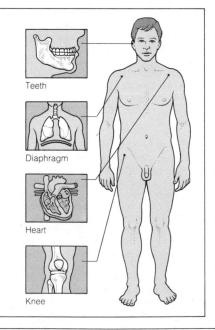

---

treatment with *narcotic drugs*, such as *morphine* or *pethidine*. Narcotic analgesics are also used to prevent pain after surgery. Long-term use of narcotic analgesics may be necessary to prevent or relieve pain in *cancer*. Narcotic analgesics or local anesthetic agents may be used to relieve pain during *childbirth*.

NONDRUG TREATMENT

Massage, ice packs, or *poultices* may be used for the relief of localized pain caused by muscle spasm, inflammation, or injury.

Chronic or recurrent pain that has not responded to drug treatment may be relieved by *TENS, acupuncture* or *hypnosis*. TENS is also sometimes used to relieve pain during childbirth.

Surgical procedures are sometimes performed to relieve pain when other treatments have failed. Surgery may involve destruction of nerves that transmit pain (as is done in a *cordotomy*). Alternatively, nerve fibers in the thalamus (the part of the brain that responds to pain) may be cut to prevent perception of pain.

Palate

The roof of the mouth, which separates the mouth from the nasal cavity above. Covered with *mucous membrane*, it consists, in the front, of the hard palate, whose substructure is a plate of bone forming part of the *maxilla* (upper jaw). At the rear is the soft palate, a flap of muscle and fibrous tissue that projects into the *pharynx*

LOCATION OF THE PALATE
The palate forms the floor of the nasal cavity and roof of the mouth, providing a surface against which the tongue can push during chewing and swallowing.

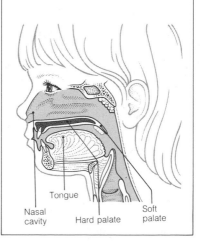

Nasal cavity — Hard palate — Tongue — Soft palate

(throat). During swallowing, the soft palate presses against the rear wall of the pharynx, preventing food from ascending into the nose.

About one in 500 babies is born with a gap along the midline of the palate (see *Cleft lip and palate*).

Palliative treatment

Therapy that relieves the symptoms of a disorder but does not cure it. For example, treatment for the symptoms of advanced cancer may be palliative rather than curative.

Pallor

Abnormal paleness of the skin and mucous membranes, particularly discernible in the face. Pallor has many possible causes and is only sometimes a symptom of disease.

In some people, pallor is due to a deficiency of the skin pigment *melanin*. Melanin deficiency may occur in people, such as nightworkers or miners, who spend very little time in daylight. It is also a feature of the inherited condition *albinism*.

Pallor may also be caused by constriction (narrowing) of small blood vessels in the skin, which may occur in response to shock, severe pain, injury, heavy blood loss, fainting, or extreme cold. Cutting off the blood flow to the skin ensures that the brain and other vital organs are adequately supplied and that body heat is at least temporarily conserved.

In *anemia*, pallor results from lack of the blood pigment *hemoglobin* in blood vessels in the skin.

Certain kidney disorders, such as *pyelonephritis* and *kidney failure*, produce a sallow pallor, as does *hypothyroidism*. Rare conditions that give rise to pallor include *lead poisoning*.

Palpation

A technique, used in *physical examination*, in which certain parts of the body are felt with the hands. By palpation, the physician is able to assess the condition of the skin and of the underlying organs.

Palpitation

Awareness of the *heartbeat* or a sensation of having a rapid and unusually forceful heartbeat.

CAUSES

Palpitations are usually felt after strenuous exercise, in tense situations, or after a severe scare, when the heart is beating harder and/or faster than normal. When palpitations are experienced at rest or in a calm mood,

they are usually due to *ectopic heart beats* (premature beats followed by an unusually prolonged pause) and are felt as a fluttering or thumping in the chest, sometimes with a brief but alarming sense that the heart has stopped beating.

Ectopic heart beats do not usually indicate heart disease, however; they are often caused by such things as drinking alcohol, a high intake of caffeine, or heavy smoking.

Palpitations may be caused by cardiac *arrhythmias* (irregularities of the heartbeat). An example of an arrhythmia is atrial *tachycardia*, a condition in which the heart suddenly starts to beat very rapidly; the affected person may feel faint and breathless. The pulse may be as high as 200 beats per minute but remains regular. In *atrial fibrillation*, the atria (upper chambers of the heart) beat in a disorganized manner and the impulses passed to the ventricles (lower, pumping chambers) are very irregular. *Hyperthyroidism* (overactivity of the thyroid gland) may cause palpitations by speeding up the heartbeat.

DIAGNOSIS AND TREATMENT

If palpitations last for several hours or recur over several days, or if they cause chest pain, breathlessness, or dizziness, a physician should be consulted as soon as possible, as there may be a serious underlying disorder. Recurrent palpitations may be investigated by means of a 24-hour *ECG* and by *thyroid function tests*. Treatment depends on the underlying cause.

Palsy

A term applied to certain forms of *paralysis*. Examples are *cerebral palsy*, *facial palsy*, and Erb's palsy (paralysis of the upper arm and shoulder on one side of the body).

Panacea

A remedy for all diseases; a cure-all. No such remedy is known, despite claims to the contrary made by numerous quacks through the ages.

Pancreas

An elongated, tapered *gland* that lies across the back of the abdomen, behind the stomach. The broadest part of the pancreas (called the head) is situated on the right-hand side, in the loop of the duodenum. The main part of the gland (called the body) tapers from the head, extending toward the left and slightly upward; the narrower end (called the tail) terminates near the spleen.

P

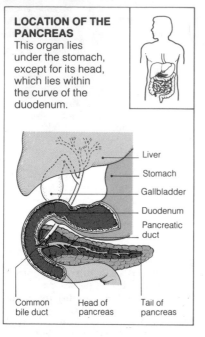

LOCATION OF THE PANCREAS
This organ lies under the stomach, except for its head, which lies within the curve of the duodenum.

Liver
Stomach
Gallbladder
Duodenum
Pancreatic duct
Common bile duct
Head of pancreas
Tail of pancreas

STRUCTURE
Most of the pancreas consists of exocrine tissue, embedded in which are "nests" of endocrine cells (the islets of Langerhans). The exocrine cells secrete digestive *enzymes* into a network of ducts that meet to form the main pancreatic duct. This duct joins the common bile duct (which carries bile from the gallbladder) to form a small chamber, called the ampulla of Vater, which opens into the duodenum. The islets of Langerhans are surrounded by many blood vessels into which they secrete *hormones*.

FUNCTION
The pancreas has two functions: digestive and hormonal. The exocrine tissue secretes various digestive enzymes that break down carbohydrates, fats, proteins, and nucleic acids (see *Digestive system*). Most of these enzymes are inactive until activated in the duodenum by other enzymes. Also secreted is sodium bicarbonate, which neutralizes stomach acid entering the duodenum. The endocrine cells in the islets of Langerhans secrete the hormones *insulin* and *glucagon*, which regulate the level of glucose in the blood. (See also *Pancreas* disorders box.)

Pancreas, cancer of
A malignant tumor of the exocrine tissue of the *pancreas* (the main tissue in the gland). The cause of the condition is unknown, although it has been linked to heavy smoking and to certain dietary factors, such as a high intake of fats or alcohol.

The incidence of pancreatic cancer has increased threefold during the past 50 years, and there are now about 2,700 cases diagnosed in Canada per year, mostly in people over 50.

SYMPTOMS
The most common symptom is pain in the upper abdomen, often spreading to the back. Other common symptoms are loss of appetite, weight loss, and jaundice. There may also be indigestion, nausea, vomiting, diarrhea, and tiredness. In most cases, the symptoms do not appear until the cancer is well advanced, often not until it has spread to other parts of the body (typically to the liver or lungs).

DIAGNOSIS
Diagnosis of pancreatic cancer usually requires *ultrasound scanning* or *CT scanning* of the upper abdomen, or endoscopic examination of the ducts of the pancreas (see *ERCP*). In some cases, the condition is detected during exploratory surgery on the abdomen (see *Laparotomy*).

TREATMENT AND OUTLOOK
If the condition is detected in its early stages, surgical removal of the malignant tissue (see *Pancreatectomy*) along with *radiation therapy* and *anticancer drugs* may result in a cure. However, in most cases the cancer is not diagnosed until it is well advanced, and little can be done apart from relieving the pain with *analgesic drugs* (painkillers), alleviating any other symptoms, and bypassing the growth if it is causing obstruction of the bile duct or bowel. In such cases, the outlook is poor; death occurs in about 90 percent of the cases within a year of diagnosis.

Pancreatectomy
Removal of all or part of the *pancreas*. Pancreatectomy may be performed to treat *pancreatitis* (inflammation of the pancreas), localized cancer of the pancreas (see *Pancreas, cancer of*), or cancer of the ampulla of Vater (the small chamber formed by the union of the common bile duct and pancreatic duct which opens into the duodenum). Rarely, it is done to treat some endocrine tumors, such as *insulinomas* (insulin-producing tumors).

The amount of the gland that is removed depends on the disorder involved and/or on how much of the pancreas is affected. Obstruction of the pancreatic duct may require removal of only the tail of the gland (the narrower end, nearest the spleen) and the linking of the duct with a small piece of small intestine. Disease of the head of the pancreas (the broader end, situated in the loop of the duodenum) may necessitate removal of both the pancreatic head and the duodenal loop (an operation known as Whipple's operation).

COMPLICATIONS
Pancreatectomy may lead to *diabetes mellitus*, which requires insulin therapy, and *malabsorption*, which requires oral supplements of *pancreatin* (a preparation of digestive enzymes produced by the pancreas).

Pancreatin
An oral preparation of digestive *enzymes* obtained from the pancreas of pigs. Pancreatin is used to supplement deficiency of these enzymes and thus prevent *malabsorption* of fats, carbohydrates, and proteins. Pancreatin may be required following *pancreatectomy* or by people suffering from pancreatic disorders, such as chronic *pancreatitis*, cancer of the pancreas (see *Pancreas, cancer of*), and *cystic fibrosis*.

Pancreatitis
Inflammation of the *pancreas*, which may be acute or chronic. Acute pancreatitis is less damaging, although attacks may recur. Chronic pancreatitis causes permanent damage to the pancreas due to the formation of fibrous scar tissue.

CAUSES
The main causes of acute pancreatitis are alcohol abuse and *gallstones*. Less commonly, pancreatitis results from a viral infection (such as *mumps* or *hepatitis*), injury (such as may be caused by a strong blow to the abdomen), surgery on the biliary tract, or certain drugs (such as *diuretic drugs* and *sulfonamide drugs*).

Chronic pancreatitis is most commonly caused by alcohol abuse. In rare cases, chronic pancreatitis occurs in people with *hyperlipidemias* (a group of disorders characterized by high levels of fat in the blood) or *hemochromatosis* (a disorder in which there is an excess of iron in the body). Chronic pancreatitis may also rarely be inherited or result from a severe attack of acute pancreatitis.

SYMPTOMS AND DIAGNOSIS
Acute pancreatitis produces a sudden attack of severe upper abdominal pain, often accompanied by nausea and vomiting. In many cases, the pain spreads to the back. The pain of acute pancreatitis is usually made worse by movement, and may be relieved by

P

DISORDERS OF THE PANCREAS

Serious disruption of pancreatic function occurs only when the secretory tissue of the gland has been damaged or destroyed in advanced disease. The most common pancreatic disorder is *diabetes mellitus*, in which the insulin-producing cells in the gland are destroyed.

CONGENITAL AND GENETIC DISORDERS

About 85 percent of people with the genetic disorder *cystic fibrosis* produce totally inadequate quantities of pancreatic digestive enzymes. This failure results in *malabsorption* of fats and proteins and may cause steatorrhea (excess fat in the feces) and muscle wasting.

Genetic factors are thought to play some part in diabetes mellitus, although they are not the primary cause of the disease.

Chronic *pancreatitis* (inflammation of the pancreas) may, in rare cases, be hereditary; chronic pancreatitis often causes diabetes.

INFECTION

Acute pancreatitis may result from certain viral infections, especially with the *mumps* or *hepatitis* viruses. Other viruses, such as coxsackieviruses and echoviruses, may also cause pancreatitis. In some cases, coxsackievirus infection may contribute to the development of diabetes.

TUMOR

Pancreatic cancer is one of the more common cancers (see *Pancreas, cancer of*). It is difficult to diagnose and, in most cases, has spread extensively by the time it is detected.

TRAUMA

Injury to the pancreas—as a result of a blow to the abdomen, for example—may cause acute pancreatitis. The mechanism by which this happens is not fully established, but it is believed that pancreatic enzymes (most of which are inactive until they reach the intestine) are released within the gland and then activated, with the result that they digest the pancreas.

POISONS AND DRUGS

Excessive alcohol intake is a common cause of pancreatitis. It can also be caused by various drugs, such as sulfonamides, estrogens (including estrogen-containing contraceptive pills), and thiazide *diuretic drugs*; *corticosteroid drugs* may also cause pancreatitis.

AUTOIMMUNE DISORDERS

The cause of the damage to the pancreas in diabetes mellitus remains controversial. However, there is increasing evidence that, possibly in response to a viral infection, the body's immune system produces *antibodies* (proteins with a role in the defense against infection) that inappropriately attack and destroy the pancreatic cells.

OTHER DISORDERS

Other than alcohol overuse, the condition most commonly associated with pancreatitis is *gallstones*. These occasionally block the exit of the pancreatic duct into the duodenum, which leads to inflammation of the pancreas.

INVESTIGATION

Diagnosis of pancreatic disorders may involve *ultrasound scanning* of the abdomen, tests to measure levels of pancreatic enzymes in the blood or duodenum, and endoscopic examination of the gland (see *ERCP*).

---

adopting a sitting position. An attack, which usually lasts for about 48 hours, is accompanied by the release of digestive enzymes from the pancreas directly into the blood; measurement of these enzymes is an important diagnostic test. *Ultrasound scanning* or *CT scanning* may also be performed.

Chronic pancreatitis usually produces the same symptoms as acute pancreatitis, although the pain may last from hours to several days, and attacks become more frequent as the condition progresses. However, in some cases there may be no pain and the principal signs may be *malabsorption* (due to a deficiency of pancreatic enzymes) or *diabetes mellitus* (due to insufficient *insulin* production by the pancreas). Measuring pancreatic enzyme levels in the blood is of little value in diagnosing chronic pancreatitis, although measurement of the output of such enzymes into the duodenum (by means of a fine tube passed through the stomach) may be useful. Abdominal *X rays* or scans are the usual diagnostic methods, along with endoscopic examination of the pancreatic ducts (see *ERCP*) to determine the extent of tissue damage.

COMPLICATIONS

If acute pancreatitis causes severe damage to the gland, *hypotension* (low blood pressure), *heart failure*, *kidney failure*, *respiratory failure*, and *ascites* (accumulation of fluid in the abdomen) may occur. In some cases, cysts or abscesses may develop in the damaged gland.

Chronic pancreatitis may also lead to the development of ascites and cysts. Other possible complications include obstruction of the common bile duct (see *Bile duct obstruction*), permanent diabetes mellitus, and blood clots in the splenic vein, which drains the spleen and pancreatic veins.

TREATMENT

There is no specific remedy for acute pancreatitis. Treatment consists of narcotic *analgesic drugs* to relieve pain, and the administration of fluids and salts by *intravenous infusion*. Patients are not allowed to eat or drink because this would stimulate pancreatic activity and make the symptoms worse. A recurrence of the condition can sometimes be prevented by treating an underlying cause. Occasionally, surgery is necessary to remove the pancreas (see *Pancreatectomy*) or to remove any gallstones.

Chronic pancreatitis is treated by providing pain relief, by controlling diabetes mellitus with insulin, and by giving *pancreatin* (a preparation of pancreatic enzymes). In some cases, pancreatectomy may be necessary to relieve pain.

Pancreatography

Imaging of the pancreas or its ducts. Methods include *CT scanning*, *ultrasound scanning*, or *X rays* taken after the injection of a radiopaque contrast medium into the pancreatic ducts either during exploratory surgery or through the use of an endoscope during endoscopic retrograde cholangiopancreatography (see *ERCP*).

P

P

Pandemic

A term applied to a disease that occurs over a large geographical area (sometimes worldwide) and affects a high proportion of the population; a widespread *epidemic*.

Panic attack

A brief period of acute *anxiety*, often dominated by an intense fear of dying or losing one's reason. Panic attacks occur unpredictably at first, but tend to become associated with certain places, such as a crowded supermarket or a cramped elevator.

The symptoms begin suddenly and usually include a sense of breathing difficulty, chest pains, palpitations, feeling light-headed and dizzy, sweating, trembling, and faintness. *Hyperventilation* (fast, shallow breathing) often accompanies and worsens the symptoms, leading to *pins and needles*, and to feelings of *depersonalization* and *derealization*.

Although unpleasant and frightening, panic attacks last for only a few minutes, cause no physical harm, and are rarely associated with serious physical illness. The symptoms of hyperventilation may be relieved by covering the mouth and nose with a small paper bag and breathing into the bag for a few minutes.

In general, panic attacks are a symptom of an *anxiety disorder*, *agoraphobia*, or other *phobias* (if they lead to avoidance of certain situations). Less often they are part of a *somatization disorder* or *schizophrenia*. The cause of panic attacks is unknown but increasingly they are treated by *behavior therapy*, particularly if they are associated with specific phobias. Relaxation exercises may be of some help.

Papain

A naturally occurring mixture of *enzymes*, including one, chymopapain, found in pawpaws. Papain breaks down proteins and has been used to remove clotted blood and dead tissue from wounds and ulcers, and as a meat tenderizer. Chymopapain is used in *chemonucleolysis* (injection of the enzyme into a prolapsed intervertebral disk).

Papilla

Any small, nipple-shaped projection from the surface of a tissue, such as the mammary papilla (the nipple of the breast) and the lingual papillae (the numerous projections on the surface of the tongue, some of which contain taste buds).

Papilledema

Swelling of the head of the *optic nerve*, also known as optic disk edema, which is visible when the eye is examined with an *ophthalmoscope*. Papilledema usually indicates a dangerous rise in the pressure of *cerebrospinal fluid* in the skull, sometimes caused by a *brain tumor*. Swelling of the head of the optic nerve may also arise from conditions affecting the nerve itself, including damage due to the restriction of blood supply. It may be followed by *optic atrophy*.

Papilloma

A usually nonmalignant tumor, often resembling a wart, that arises from the *epithelium* (the cell layer that forms the skin and mucous membranes, and that lines most of the hollow organs of the body). Although papillomas may develop from epithelial tissue anywhere in the body, they most commonly affect the skin, tongue, larynx (voice box), urinary tract, and digestive tract.

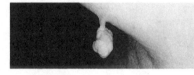

Skin papilloma
This harmless type of growth is common in elderly people. It can easily be snipped off at skin level and the base cauterized by your physician.

Pap smear

See *Cervical smear test*.

Papule

A small, solid, slightly raised area of skin. Papules are usually less than 0.5 cm in diameter and may be raised or flat, have a smooth or warty texture, and be either pigmented or the color of the surrounding skin. Many skin conditions, including *acne* and *lichen planus*, start with papules.

Par-/para-

Prefixes with several meanings: beside or beyond, as in the parathyroid glands (which are situated behind the thyroid at its sides); closely related to or closely resembling, as in paratyphoid fever (a disease that is similar to typhoid); faulty or abnormal, as in paresthesia (abnormal sensation); or associated with an accessory capacity, as in paramedical workers (personnel who supplement the work of physicians).

Para-aminobenzoic acid

Also known as PABA, it is a common ingredient of *sunscreens*.

Para-aminosalicylic acid

A drug that was formerly commonly used in the treatment of *tuberculosis*. Para-aminosalicylic acid (PAS) has now been largely superseded by other antituberculous drugs.

Paracentesis

A procedure in which a body cavity is punctured with a needle from the outside. Paracentesis is performed to remove fluid for analysis, to relieve pressure due to excess fluid, or to instill drugs. The procedure is quick and relatively painless, and is usually carried out under local anesthesia.

Paracentesis is most often performed on the abdomen, to aid the diagnosis of conditions causing *ascites*, in which fluid collects in the abdominal cavity. It is commonly performed on the thorax, and sometimes on other sites, including the pericardium and the scrotum.

Paraffinoma

A tumorlike swelling under the skin caused by prolonged exposure to paraffin. Paraffinomas may occur in the lungs due to inhalation of paraffin, usually in someone who uses liquid paraffin as a laxative. Paraffinomas were an uncommon side effect of augmentation *mammoplasty* (enlargement of the breast) before silicone replaced paraffin wax in this operation.

Paraldehyde

An unpleasant-smelling sedative drug used to stop prolonged epileptic seizures and occasionally to treat alcohol withdrawal. Paraldehyde can be administered as an enema or by injection. A glass syringe must be used to inject it, because paraldehyde dissolves plastic.

Paralysis

Complete or partial loss of controlled movement caused by the inability to contract one or more *muscles*. Weakness, rather than complete loss of movement, is often referred to as *paresis*. Paralysis may be temporary or permanent, and can affect anything from a small facial muscle to many of the major muscles in the body. Loss of feeling in the affected parts may accompany inability to move them.

TYPES
Paralysis of one half of the body is called *hemiplegia*; paralysis of all four

limbs and the trunk is called *quadriplegia*. *Paraplegia* is paralysis of both legs and sometimes part of the trunk. *Palsy* is an outdated term for paralysis; it is still used in the names of certain disorders (such as *cerebral palsy*).

Paralysis may be flaccid, which gives the limbs a floppy disposition, or spastic, in which case the affected parts of the body are rigid.

CAUSES

Muscles that control movement of the body are stimulated to contract by impulses originating in the motor cortex of the *brain*. These impulses travel via the spinal cord and peripheral nerves to reach the muscles. Paralysis may be caused by any form of injury or disorder anywhere along this nerve pathway, or by a muscle disorder.

BRAIN DISORDERS A very common cause of paralysis is a *stroke*, in which damage to part of the brain is caused by bleeding from or blood clotting in a blood vessel that supplies that area of the brain. Because motor nerve fibers cross in the brain stem, paralysis occurs on the side opposite to the site of the brain damage.

Hemiplegia can be caused by any brain disorder in which the portion of the brain that controls movement is damaged—for example, by a *brain tumor*, *brain abscess*, *brain hemorrhage*, *cerebral palsy*, or *encephalitis* (brain infection).

Some forms of paralysis are caused by damage to those parts of the nervous system concerned with the fine control of movement (such as the *cerebellum* and *basal ganglia*). *Parkinson's disease* is caused by lack of dopamine in the basal ganglia.

SPINAL CORD DISORDERS Paralysis can be caused by damage to the spinal cord within a spine fractured in a road traffic accident. Pressure on the spinal cord may cause paralysis in *disk prolapse* or *cervical osteoarthritis*. Muscles supplied by nerves below the damaged area are affected.

Diseases affecting the spinal cord (such as *multiple sclerosis*, *poliomyelitis*, *myelitis*, *Friedreich's ataxia*, *meningitis*, and deficiency of *vitamin B$_{12}$*) may also cause paralysis.

PERIPHERAL NERVE DISORDERS A group of disorders, known as *neuropathies*, affect the peripheral nerves and cause varying degrees of paralysis. Neuropathies may be caused by a variety of conditions, including *diabetes mellitus*, vitamin deficiency, liver disease, cancer, and the toxic effects of some drugs or metals (such as lead). A neuropathy may also sometimes occur as an in-herited disorder. Another type of neuropathy that often causes paralysis of the shoulder, arm, or hand can result from an injury to the *brachial plexus* (a nerve network that serves the arm and hand).

MUSCLE DISORDERS *Muscular dystrophy* causes progressive muscular weakness and may lead to paralysis. Temporary paralysis sometimes occurs in *myasthenia gravis*.

TREATMENT

The underlying cause is treated if possible. *Physiotherapy* is used to prevent joints from becoming locked into useless positions, which is important in both temporary and permanent paralysis. When the paralysis is temporary (such as in a mild stroke), physiotherapy is used to retrain and strengthen the muscles and joints so that some degree of mobility is possible after recovery.

For paralyzed people confined to bed or a wheelchair, nursing care is essential to avoid complications of prolonged *immobility*—such as bedsores, deep vein thrombosis, urinary tract infections, constipation, and limb deformities. (See also *Disability*.)

Paralysis, periodic

A rare, inherited condition that affects young people. Periodic paralysis is characterized by episodes of weakness and paralysis of limb muscles, which occur every six weeks or so and may last from a few minutes to two days. Episodes often begin during the night and wake the sufferer.

The exact cause of periodic paralysis is unknown, although in many cases there is a drop in the level of potassium (which is essential for normal muscle function) in the blood. A meal that is rich in carbohydrates often triggers an attack.

The frequency of attacks can be lessened by reducing the intake of carbohydrates and by taking *acetazolamide* or potassium-sparing *diuretic drugs*. An episode can sometimes be curtailed by taking potassium or by exercising gently at the first sign of muscle weakness. The condition often disappears without treatment by the age of 30.

Paramedic

A person trained to provide emergency resuscitation after an accident or when someone has collapsed from a myocardial infarction (heart attack) or other medical condition. Paramedics work from ambulances and in the emergency room. The term is also used as an abbreviation for paramedical, to describe any health care worker other than a physician, nurse, dentist, or podiatrist. Examples of paramedical staff include physiotherapists, X-ray and radiation oncology technologists and laboratory technicians.

Paranoia

A condition whose central feature is the *delusion* (a false idea not amenable to reasoned argument) that people or events are in some way specially connected to oneself. The term is also used popularly to describe feelings of persecution.

A person suffering from paranoia gradually builds up an elaborate set of beliefs based on the interpretation of chance remarks or events. Typical themes include persecution, jealousy (see *Jealousy, morbid*), love, and grandeur (belief in one's own superior position and powers).

TYPES AND CAUSES

Chronic paranoia may result from brain damage, alcohol abuse, amphetamine abuse, *schizophrenia*, or *manic-depressive illness*. The condition is especially likely to develop in people with paranoid *personality disorder*—suspicious, oversensitive people who seem emotionally cold.

Acute paranoia, lasting for less than six months, may occur in people who have experienced radical changes in their environment, such as immigrants, refugees, or people leaving home for the first time.

In shared paranoia (see *Folie à deux*), delusion develops as a result of a close relationship with someone who already has a delusion.

SYMPTOMS

The feelings and activities of a person with paranoia often seem relatively normal in that they are appropriate to his or her beliefs. There are usually no other symptoms of mental illness apart from occasional *hallucinations*. In time, however, anger, suspicion, and social isolation may mark an increasing change toward difficult and eccentric behavior. Paranoid individuals rarely see themselves as ill or needing help. As a result, they usually receive treatment only at the instigation of relatives or friends.

TREATMENT AND OUTCOME

When acute illness is treated early with *antipsychotic drugs*, the outlook is good. In long-standing paranoia, delusions are usually firmly entrenched, although antipsychotic drugs may make them less prominent.

P

Paraparesis

Partial *paralysis* or weakness of both legs and sometimes part of the trunk. The cause is disease in or injury to the nervous system.

Paraphilia

See *Deviation, sexual*.

Paraphimosis

Constriction of the *penis* behind the glans (head) by an extremely tight foreskin that has been retracted (pulled back), causing swelling and pain. Paraphimosis often occurs as a complication of *phimosis* (an abnormally tight foreskin).

In many cases, the foreskin can be returned manually to its normal position. The swelling in the glans may be reduced by first applying an ice pack and then squeezing the glans. If manual return proves impossible, an injection or an operation to cut the foreskin may be necessary. *Circumcision* (surgical removal of the foreskin) is usual to prevent recurrence.

Paraplegia

Weakness or *paralysis* of both legs and sometimes of part of the trunk, often accompanied by loss of sensation and by loss of urinary control.

Paraplegia is a result of nerve damage in the *brain* or *spinal cord*. It is usually caused by a motor vehicle accident, sports accident, fall, or gunshot wounds. Twice as many men as women are victims, and the incidence is highest between the ages of 19 and 35 years.

Parapsychology

The branch of *psychology* dealing with experiences and events that cannot be accounted for by scientific understanding. Such paranormal phenomena include telepathy (the communication of thoughts from one person's mind to another), telekinesis (the movement of objects simply by thinking), clairvoyance (the ability to "see" events at a distance without using one's eyes), and precognition (being able to see into the future). These are all forms of extrasensory perception (ESP).

The basis of many paranormal experiences can probably be explained by mental disturbances. Thought broadcasting (in which individuals have the impression that their thoughts can be heard by others) is a common symptom of *schizophrenia*. Other apparently paranormal experiences are a result of coincidence or self-deception, while some, such as psychic surgery (removal of objects from the body apparently without an incision) are no more than sleight-of-hand trickery.

Paraquat

A poisonous defoliant weedkiller. The forms of paraquat that are generally available to the public are almost harmless. However, much more concentrated solutions are available for agricultural purposes and these can cause potentially fatal poisoning if swallowed, inhaled, or absorbed through the skin.

The main symptom of paraquat poisoning is difficulty in breathing. In severe cases, there may be respiratory failure, acute or progressive lung damage, and kidney failure, which may be fatal.

Marijuana is sometimes contaminated with paraquat. Smoking contaminated supplies can cause any or all of the following disorders: stinging eyes, a burning sensation in the mouth and throat, vomiting, and ulcers in the mouth.

TREATMENT

If paraquat poisoning is known or suspected, medical help should be obtained immediately. First aid treatment consists of getting the victim to eat charcoal or fuller's earth (a clay-containing earthy substance), which inactivates paraquat. Medical treatment may include hemodialysis (removal of toxic substances from the blood, see *Dialysis*) and other emergency measures to remove the chemical from the body.

If paraquat has been splashed into the eyes or onto the skin, it should be washed away with plenty of water.

Parasite

Any organism living in or on any other living creature and deriving advantage from doing so, while causing disadvantage to the host. The parasite satisfies its nutritional re-

---

PARASITES

| Head louse | Bedbug | Cat flea | Tapeworm | Hookworm |

ECTOPARASITES (present in skin or on body surface)

Common examples	Activities	How acquired
Head lice Ticks Bedbugs Cat fleas Dog fleas Aquatic leeches	Suck host's blood.	Through contact with other people (lice, scabies mites, warts), animals (ringworm fungi, ticks), vegetation (ticks, mites), or water (aquatic leeches). Bedbugs live in bedroom walls or mattresses and visit humans at night. Cat and dog fleas may visit humans when the pet is absent.
Scabies mites	Burrow in skin.	
Ringworm fungi	Multiply in skin.	
Wart viruses		

ENDOPARASITES (live within body)

Tapeworms Flukes Roundworms Hookworms	Adults live in human gut, blood vessels, bile ducts, or elsewhere and produce eggs that are passed out of the body.	By eating infected meat, swallowing eggs on food, contaminated fingers with fecal material, or contact with infected water.
Various disease-causing protozoa, fungi, bacteria, and viruses	Organisms multiply locally or spread throughout the body, causing disease.	By inhalation, water- or food-borne transmission, sexual transmission, or blood-borne infection, among other mechanisms.

quirements from the host's blood or tissues or from the host's diet, which allows the parasite to reproduce.

Parasites may remain permanently with their host or may spend only part of their life cycles in association. Some parasites cause few symptoms, others cause disease and even the eventual death of the host.

Animal parasites of humans include various *protozoa* (single-celled animals), *worms, flukes, leeches, lice, ticks,* and *mites. Viruses* and disease-causing *fungi* and *bacteria* are also essentially parasites. Some types of bacteria actually benefit their hosts (e.g., by helping to control the populations of more harmful organisms) and so are not strictly parasites.

Parasitology

The scientific study of organisms that treat others as their living environment (see *Parasite*), especially the study of their life cycles and reproductive behavior, the ways in which they cause disease, and their susceptibility to drug treatment and other methods of control. Although viruses and many types of bacteria and fungi are parasites, their study is conducted under the general title of *microbiology*.

Medical parasitology is concerned primarily with parasites of humans, especially the protozoa, worms, and arthropod parasites (insects and related animals) such as lice and the scabies mite.

Parasuicide

See *Suicide, attempted.*

Parasympathetic nervous system

One of the two divisions of the *autonomic nervous system.* In conjunction with the other division (the sympathetic nervous system), the parasympathetic system controls the involuntary activities of the organs, glands, blood vessels, and other tissues in the body.

Parathion

An agricultural organophosphate insecticide which is highly poisonous to both humans and animals. Poisoning may occur by absorption through the skin (as in agricultural work), by inhalation, or by swallowing.

Symptoms of poisoning include nausea, vomiting, abdominal cramps, involuntary defecation and urination, excessive salivation and sweating, blurred vision, headache, confusion, and muscle twitching. If poisoning is severe, there may also be difficulty breathing, palpitations, seizures, and unconsciousness. Without treatment, parathion poisoning may be fatal.

TREATMENT
If parathion has been swallowed, treatment consists of inducing vomiting or of washing out the stomach (see *Lavage, gastric*). If poisoning occurred by skin absorption, the victim's clothing is removed and contaminated areas of skin are thoroughly washed.

To counteract the effects of the poison, injections of *atropine* and pralidoxime may be given. It may also be necessary to support the victim's breathing with *oxygen therapy* and/or artificial *ventilation.* With rapid treatment, people may survive doses of parathion much greater than the usual fatal dose, but correct initial diagnosis is essential.

Parathyroidectomy

The surgical removal of abnormal tissue from the *parathyroid glands.* Parathyroidectomy may be performed to treat *hyperparathyroidism* (excess secretion of parathyroid hormone) when it is caused by an *adenoma* (a small, benign tumor) of a parathyroid gland or, less commonly, by a general overgrowth of the glands or by parathyroid cancer.

In the case of an adenoma, usually only one of the glands is involved and needs to be removed. If all the glands are enlarged and overactive, all but one or part of one gland may need to be removed. Removal of all parathyroid tissue leads to *hypoparathyroidism*, causing a dangerously low level of calcium in the blood which may result in *tetany* (painful, cramplike spasms).

The operation is performed under general anesthesia. An incision is made in the neck, just beneath the Adam's apple. A section of tissue that is suspected of being abnormal is taken and examined to decide how much parathyroid tissue should be removed. This is then cut out, and the incision sewn up.

The average hospital stay for parathyroidectomy is less than a week. Patients can expect complete healing without complications, although some people need treatment for hypoparathyroidism.

Parathyroid glands

Two pairs of oval, pea-sized glands, that lie behind the lobes of the *thyroid gland* in the neck. Some people have only a single parathyroid gland or have extra glands in the neck or chest.

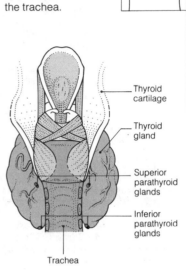

LOCATION OF THE PARATHYROID GLANDS
These glands are situated in the neck, behind the thyroid and to each side of the trachea.

Thyroid cartilage
Thyroid gland
Superior parathyroid glands
Inferior parathyroid glands
Trachea

FUNCTION
The glands produce parathyroid hormone, which helps control the level of calcium in the blood. This requires constant regulation, since even small variations from normal can impair muscle and nerve function.

If the level of calcium in the blood drops, the parathyroid glands respond by increasing their output of parathyroid hormone. This causes the bones to release more calcium into the blood, the intestines to absorb more from food, and the kidneys to conserve calcium. These actions quickly restore the blood calcium level. If the blood level of calcium rises, the glands reduce their output of hormone, reversing the above processes.

In rare cases, the parathyroid glands may become overactive (see *Hyperparathyroidism*), causing erosion of the bones and *calculi* (stones) in the urinary tract; or they may become underactive (see *Hypoparathyroidism*), resulting in tetany (painful spasms) or seizures.

Parathyroid tumor

A growth within a *parathyroid gland.* Parathyroid tumors may cause excess secretion of parathyroid hormone into the bloodstream, thereby leading to increased levels of calcium in the blood and to symptoms of *hyperparathyroidism*. Most parathyroid tumors are benign *adenomas*. Cancers of the parathyroid are very rare and are not highly malignant, although occasionally they may spread to other organs in the body.

TREATMENT AND OUTLOOK

An adenoma that is causing hyperparathyroidism will be surgically removed (see *Parathyroidectomy*). In most cases, surgery gives a complete cure. Occasionally, however, a tumor may recur or the patient may need treatment for *hypoparathyroidism*.

In people who have parathyroid cancer, surgery allows long-term survival without recurrence, provided the entire tumor can be completely removed before it has spread.

Paratyphoid fever

An illness identical in most respects to *typhoid fever*, except that it is caused by a slightly different bacterium, SALMO- NELLA PARATYPHI, and is usually less severe. The causative organism is spread in a way similar to the typhoid bacterium, but long-term carriers of infection are less common.

Parenchyma

The functional tissue of an organ, as distinct from accessory structures such as the *stroma* (framework) and the capsule (fibrous outer layer) that hold the organ together.

Parenteral

A term applied to the administration of drugs or other substances by any route other than via the gastrointestinal tract. Examples of parenteral routes of administration include injection into a blood vessel or muscle or insertion of a suppository into the vagina.

Parenteral nutrition

An alternative name for intravenous feeding. (See *Feeding, artificial*.)

Paresis

Partial *paralysis* or weakness of one or several muscles.

Paresthesia

Altered sensation in the skin without a stimulus (see *Pins and needles*).

Parietal

A medical term that refers to the wall of a part of the body. Examples are the parietal peritoneum (the membrane that lines the walls of the abdomen and pelvis and the underside of the

---

CAUSE OF PARKINSON'S DISEASE

This disorder results from damage, of unknown origin, to the basal ganglia (nerve cell clusters in the brain). The difference between the healthy state and Parkinson's disease is shown below.

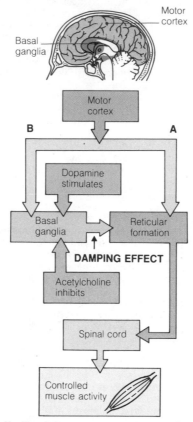

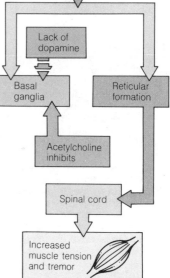

Healthy state
During movement, signals pass from the brain's cortex, via the reticular formation and spinal cord (pathway A), to muscles, which contract. Other signals pass, by pathway B, to the basal ganglia; these damp the signals in pathway A, reducing muscle tone so that movement is not jerky. Dopamine, a nerve transmitter made in the basal ganglia, is needed for this damping effect. Another transmitter, acetylcholine, inhibits the damping effect.

Parkinson's disease
In Parkinson's disease, degeneration of parts of the basal ganglia causes a lack of dopamine within this part of the brain. The basal ganglia are thus prevented from modifying the nerve pathways that control muscle contraction. As a result, the muscles are overly tense, causing tremor, joint rigidity, and slow movement. Most drug treatments increase the level of dopamine in the brain or oppose the action of acetylcholine.

---

diaphragm); the parietal bones (the two joined bones that form a large part of the skull); and the parietal lobes of the brain (the parts of the cerebral hemispheres that are covered by the parietal bones).

Parkinsonism

Any neurological disorder characterized by a masklike face, rigidity, and slowness of movements. The most common type, which is of unknown cause, is *Parkinson's disease*.

Causes of parkinsonism include *antipsychotic drugs*, the rare *encephalitis lethargica* infection, *carbon monoxide* poisoning, *cerebrovascular disease*, and certain *drugs* of abuse.

Parkinson's disease

A neurological disorder that causes muscle tremor, stiffness, and weakness. The characteristic signs of Parkinson's disease are trembling, a rigid posture, slow movements, and a shuffling, unbalanced walk.

CAUSES AND INCIDENCE

Parkinson's disease is caused by degeneration of or damage to nerve cells within the *basal ganglia* in the brain. The way this affects muscle tension and movement is shown in the illustrated box on facing page.

About 70,000 Canadians suffer from Parkinson's disease. It is present in one person in 200 over the age of 40, and in one in 100 over the age of 60. It is somewhat commoner in men. Because the disease usually has a gradual onset, parkinsonism in its early stages is often overlooked, and the actual prevalence may be higher than the figures given here.

SYMPTOMS AND SIGNS

The disease usually begins as a slight tremor of one hand, arm, or leg. In the early stages, the tremor is worse when the hand or limb is at rest; when it is used, the shaking virtually stops.

Later, the disease affects both sides of the body, and causes stiffness and weakness as well as trembling of the muscles. Symptoms include a stiff, shuffling, unbalanced walk that may break into uncontrollable, tiny, running steps; a constant trembling of the hands, more marked at rest and sometimes accompanied by shaking of the head; a permanent rigid stoop; and an unblinking, fixed expression. Eating, washing, dressing, and other everyday activities become very difficult.

The intellect is unaffected until late in the disease, although speech may become slow and hesitant; handwriting usually becomes very small. Depression is common.

TREATMENT

Although there is no cure for Parkinson's disease, much can be done for sufferers to improve their morale and mobility through exercise, special aids in the home, and encouragement. Organizations exist to provide help and advice for sufferers and their families. No other treatment is usually needed during the early stages.

Later, treatment is with drugs, which minimize symptoms but cannot halt the degeneration of brain cells. Such treatment is often complex because several different types of drugs may need to be administered in various combinations.

Levodopa, which the body converts into *dopamine*, is usually the most effective drug and is often the first drug to be tried. The beneficial effects of levodopa often suddenly wear off and an alternative drug may then be given; levodopa can usually be reintroduced some weeks later.

Drugs used in conjunction with, or as substitutes for, levodopa include *benztropine*, *bromocriptine* and *amantadine*. Other drugs, such as *anticholinergic drugs*, provide effective relief for specific symptoms, such as tremor. (See also *Selegiline*.)

Occasionally, an operation on the brain may be performed to reduce tremor and rigidity. This operation is reserved for relatively young, active sufferers who are otherwise in good health and who are in the early stages of the illness.

OUTLOOK

Untreated, the disease progresses over 10 to 15 years to severe weakness and incapacity. However, with modern drug treatment, a person suffering from Parkinson's disease can obtain considerable relief from the illness and a much improved quality of life. About one third of patients eventually show signs of *dementia*.

Experiments involving transplantation of dopamine-secreting tissues are now taking place, using either the patient's own adrenal glands or brain tissue taken from fetuses after abortion. As yet, the results have been very variable, with only a few surgeons claiming substantial improvement in their patients.

Paronychia

An infection of the skin fold at the base or side of the *nail*. Paronychia may be acute or chronic. The acute form is usually caused by bacteria. Chronic paronychia is usually caused by *CANDIDA ALBICANS* (a yeast).

The condition is most common in women—particularly those who have poor circulation and whose work involves frequent contact with water. Paronychia is also likely to develop in people with skin disease that affects the nail fold.

Treatment is with *antifungal drugs* or *antibiotic drugs*. It is important to keep the hands as dry as possible (by wearing rubber gloves for wet work and by drying the hands thoroughly each time they are washed). If an abscess forms, surgical drainage may be necessary.

Parotid glands

The largest of the three pairs of *salivary glands* (the other two are the sublingual glands and the submandibular glands). The parotid glands lie, one on each side, above the angle of the jaw, below and in front of the ear. The parotid glands continuously secrete saliva, which passes along the duct of

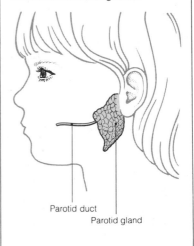

the gland and into the mouth through an opening in the inner cheek, level with the second upper molar tooth. The output of saliva is increased by the thought, sight, or smell of food.

DISORDERS

Certain conditions, including *dehydration* and *Sjögren's syndrome*, may cause reduced secretion of saliva by the gland, resulting in a dry mouth.

Parotitis, inflammation of one or both glands, is usually due to infection with the *mumps* virus but may also be caused by a bacterial infection due to poor oral hygiene, by dehydration, or by severe illness. In some cases, an *abscess* forms in the gland.

Calculi (stones) may block the duct of the parotid gland, causing a painful swelling of the gland. Painless enlargement may be caused by *sarcoidosis*, *tuberculosis*, a *lymphoma*, or a benign tumor. Rarely, carcinoma (a type of malignant tumor) of the gland causes a hard, painful growth.

Paroxysm

A sudden attack, worsening, or recurrence of symptoms or of a disease; a *spasm* or *seizure*.

Parrot fever

A common name for *psittacosis*.

Parturition

The process of giving birth (see *Childbirth*).

P

Pasteurization

The process of heating foods, usually milk and milk products, to destroy pathogenic (disease-causing) microorganisms and to reduce the number of nonpathogenic organisms, thus protecting against putrefaction and fermentation. The process is named after its inventor, the French scientist Louis Pasteur (1822-1895).

For milk, the conditions are specified by law. Batch pasteurization involves keeping the milk for *not less than* 30 minutes at a minimum temperature of 61.6°C. In continuous pasteurization, known as the high-temperature short-time process (HTST), the milk is held for at least 15 seconds at a temperature of at least 71.7°C. Other foods, such as ham, may also be pasteurized to preserve them. In general, pasteurization is preferred to sterilization, which changes the taste and texture of foods.

Patella

The medical name for the kneecap, the triangular bone at the front of the *knee*. The patella is held in position by the lower end of the *quadriceps muscle* (the main muscle at the front of the thigh), and by the patellar tendon, which attaches it to the tibia (shin).

Dislocation of the patella is usually due to a congenital abnormality, such as underdevelopment of the lower end of the femur (thigh bone) or excessive laxity of ligaments that support the knee. Fracture is usually caused by a direct blow.

Inflammation and roughening of the undersurface of the patella, resulting in knee pain that worsens when bending the knee or climbing stairs, is caused by *chondromalacia patellae* in adolescents and by *arthritis* in adults.

Patent

A term meaning open or unobstructed, as in *patent ductus arteriosus*, a condition in which the ductus arteriosus (a blood vessel that enables blood to bypass the lungs in the fetus) remains open after birth.

The term patent medicine is sometimes used to refer to proprietary drugs protected by a patent.

Patent ductus arteriosus

A *heart* defect in which the ductus arteriosus fails to close at birth. Patent ductus arteriosus accounts for about 8 percent of all heart defects present from birth (see *Heart disease, congenital*), affecting about 60 babies per 100,000.

PATERNITY TESTING USING GENETIC FINGERPRINTING

Genetic fingerprinting is replacing older techniques of paternity testing because it gives a decisive result in more cases.

Blood samples are taken from the mother, child, and suspected father, and some DNA (hereditary material) from each is specially processed.

PATERNITY ESTABLISHED

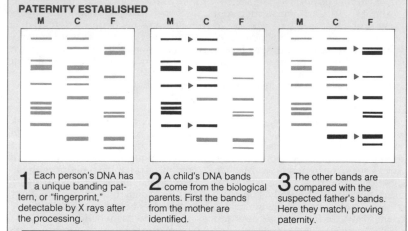

1 Each person's DNA has a unique banding pattern, or "fingerprint," detectable by X rays after the processing.

2 A child's DNA bands come from the biological parents. First the bands from the mother are identified.

3 The other bands are compared with the suspected father's bands. Here they match, proving paternity.

PATERNITY DISPROVED

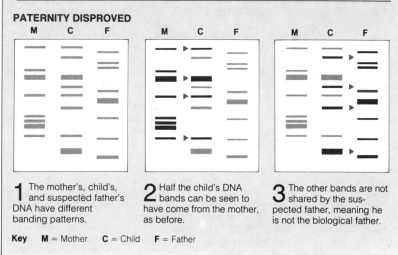

1 The mother's, child's, and suspected father's DNA have different banding patterns.

2 Half the child's DNA bands can be seen to have come from the mother, as before.

3 The other bands are not shared by the suspected father, meaning he is not the biological father.

Key   **M** = Mother   **C** = Child   **F** = Father

CAUSES

The ductus arteriosus is a channel between the pulmonary artery and the aorta (two large vessels emerging from the heart). In the fetus, blood pumped by the right side of the heart flows through the ductus arteriosus and bypasses the lungs (see *Fetal circulation*). At or shortly after birth, the ductus usually closes and blood passes to the lungs. In some babies born prematurely or with breathing difficulties, or in babies whose ductus has an abnormal structure, this closure may fail to happen, producing a patent ductus arteriosus. Some of the blood pumped by the left side of the heart and intended for the body is directed via the ductus to the lungs. As a result, the heart must work harder to pump sufficient blood to the body.

SYMPTOMS AND SIGNS

When a large amount of blood is misdirected, strain is placed on the heart; as a result, the baby fails to gain weight, becomes short of breath on exertion, and may have frequent chest infections. Eventually, *heart failure* (reduced pumping efficiency) may develop.

DIAGNOSIS AND TREATMENT

The diagnosis is made from hearing a characteristic *murmur* through a stethoscope, from *chest X rays*, and from an *ECG* and *echocardiography*.

The drug indomethacin often causes the duct to close in premature babies. If this treatment fails, the channel is closed surgically. The operation is straightforward, carries little risk, and enables the child to thrive normally.

Paternity testing
The use of blood tests to help decide whether a particular man is or is not the father of a particular child. Tests are carried out on blood samples taken from the child, from the man who is suspected to be the father, and, sometimes from the child's mother.

The investigation may be requested, or ordered by a court, in any of various legal situations in which the paternity of a child is disputed.

The blood samples are examined for the presence of various genetically determined substances. These substances may include the proteins found on the surface of red blood cells that determine *blood groups*, other proteins in the blood plasma, *histocompatibility antigens*, and short lengths of *DNA*, the genetic material itself. Comparison of these genetic markers in the different blood samples can provide useful information. For example, if a particular marker is present in the child but not in the mother, it must be determined by a gene present in the real father. If the man who is claimed to be the father does not display this marker in his blood, he can be excluded from paternity.

Techniques have advanced to the stage where it is now possible, through extensive tests, to exclude a wrongly named father in nearly 100 percent of cases. Until recently it was never possible to prove beyond reasonable doubt that a man was the father of a particular child; the new technique of *genetic fingerprinting* (see illustrated box on facing page) has dramatically changed this situation. An investigator may now be able to state that the similarities between a man and a child's DNA could have occurred by chance with a probability of just one in 30 billion, which would amount to positive proof of paternity.

Patho-
A prefix denoting a relationship to disease, as in pathogen, a disease-causing agent.

Pathogen
Any agent, particularly a *microorganism* (and particularly a parasite bacterium), that causes disease.

Pathogenesis
The processes by which a disease (or disorder) originates and develops. Pathogenesis applies particularly to the cellular and physiological events involved in these processes.

Pathognomonic
A medical term applied to a symptom or sign that is itself characteristic of a specific disease or disorder, and is therefore sufficient to establish a diagnosis. For example, Koplik's spots (small red spots with white centers) on the lining of the mouth are pathognomonic of measles.

Pathological
Relating to disease or to *pathology* (the study of disease).

Pathology
The study of disease, its causes, mechanisms, and effects on the body. Various factors can cause pathological changes in tissues and cells. These factors include pathogens (disease-causing microorganisms), poisonous chemicals, *radiation*, *inflammation*, degeneration (see *Degenerative disorders*), the accumulation of abnormal substances (see *Infiltrate*), metabolic defects (see *Metabolic disorders*; *Metabolism, inborn errors of*), nutritional disorders, and *carcinogens*.

The study of the pathological changes that occur in cells is known as cytopathology (a branch of *cytology*); histopathology (a branch of *histology*) is concerned with changes in tissues. Both rely on examining cell or tissue samples under the *microscope*.

A physician who specializes in this subject is called a pathologist. Pathologists conduct the laboratory studies of tissues and cells that help other physicians reach accurate diagnoses, and supervise other laboratory personnel in the testing and microscopic examination of blood and other body fluids.

Pathologists are resposible for conducting autopsies to determine causes of death and to determine what effects a disease or a particular type of treatment has had on the body. It was the growth of postmortem pathology in the 18th and 19th centuries that formed the basis of modern scientific medicine. Study of the body after death enabled a patient's symptoms to be linked with observable changes in the internal organs. It also made it possible for physicians to assess the accuracy of their diagnoses and the effects of their treatment.

Pathology, cellular
Also called cytopathology, the branch of *cytology* concerned with the effects of disease on cells.

Pathology, chemical
Also called clinical biochemistry, the branch of pathology concerned with examining abnormalities in the chemistry of body tissues in disease.

Pathophysiology
The study of the effects of disease on body functions (e.g., how bronchitis impairs lung function).

-pathy
A suffix that denotes a disease or disorder, as in myopathy, any disorder of the muscles.

Peak-flow meter
A piece of equipment that measures the maximum speed at which air can flow out of the lungs. Because narrowed airways slow the rate at which air can be forced from the lungs, a peak-flow meter is useful in assessing the severity of *bronchospasm* (narrowing of the airways in the lungs).

The most common use of a peak-flow meter is to monitor patients with *asthma* and to assess their response to treatment with *bronchodilator drugs*. A peak-flow meter is also useful in confirming whether people who suffer from intermittent coughing or breathing difficulty without wheezing have asthma.

People with asthma are encouraged to measure their peak flow every day as a means of monitoring their health, just as diabetics measure their blood sugar level. A diary of readings is kept to record the difference in airflow when symptoms are present and during other times in the day.

The peak flow is measured by taking a deep breath in and then breathing out with maximum effort through the mouthpiece of the meter.

Peau d'orange
A condition in which the skin resembles orange peel. The skin remains a normal color but develops a dimpled appearance due to retention of fluid in the nearby lymph vessels. Causes of blockage of the lymph vessels include *breast cancer* in the region of the nipple and *elephantiasis*.

Pectoral
A medical term that means relating to the chest, as in the major and minor pectoral muscles.

P

781

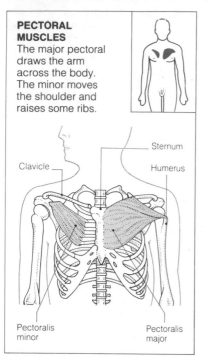

PECTORAL MUSCLES
The major pectoral draws the arm across the body. The minor moves the shoulder and raises some ribs.

Clavicle

Sternum

Humerus

Pectoralis minor

Pectoralis major

The pectoralis major is a large, fan-shaped muscle that covers much of the upper part of the front of the chest; it arises from the sternum (breastbone) and cartilages of the second to sixth ribs, and converges on the humerus (upper-arm bone) just below the shoulder. The main function of the pectoralis major is to move the arm across the body.

The pectoralis minor is a smaller, triangular muscle that underlies the pectoralis major; it arises from the third to fifth ribs, and converges on the scapula (shoulder blade), which it moves down and forward.

Pediatrics

The branch of medicine concerned with the growth and development of children, and with the diagnosis, treatment, and prevention of childhood diseases.

Pediatrics as a specialty is subdivided into neonatology (the care of newborn infants), community pediatrics (preventive medicine and developmental pediatrics), the care of disabled and handicapped children, and other subspecialties, such as pediatric cardiology, neurology, or gastroenterology. The specialty of pediatric surgery is concerned with the diagnosis and treatment of small children with congenital and acquired disorders that may require surgery.

Pediculosis

Any type of louse infestation. (See *Lice*; *Pubic lice*.)

Pedophilia

A sexual perversion in which illegal sexual activity with a prepubertal child is the preferred recurrent means of reaching orgasm. Pedophiles are almost exclusively male and may be heterosexual, bisexual, or homosexual. They are rarely diagnosed as suffering from psychosis, but often show personality problems and little concern for the effect of their behavior on the child.

Pedophiles commonly fantasize about sex with a child. Fondling of children is more common than intercourse. Actual research is rudimentary. However, the incidence of child prostitution and of child sexual abuse within families seems much higher than was previously thought. Nearly 10 percent of women in some studies have reported some form of sexual interference in childhood or early adolescence. (See also *Child Abuse*; *Incest*.)

Pellagra

A potentially fatal nutritional disorder caused by a deficiency of niacin (see *Vitamin B complex*), resulting in dermatitis, diarrhea, and dementia. Pellagra occurs primarily in poor rural communities in parts of India and southern Africa where people subsist on corn.

CAUSES
Although the niacin content of corn is no lower than that of some other cereals, much of the vitamin occurs in an unabsorbable form unless it is first treated with an alkali such as lime water. (People living in communities in Mexico who prepare the cereal in this way before making tortillas do not suffer from the disease.)

Corn is also low in tryptophan, an amino acid that is converted into niacin in the body. Certain disorders, such as *carcinoid syndrome* (which increases the breakdown of tryptophan) and *inflammatory bowel disease* (which reduces its absorption from the intestine) may also cause pellagra.

SYMPTOMS
The first symptoms are weakness, weight loss, lethargy, depression, irritability, and inflammation and itching where the skin is exposed to sunlight. In acute attacks, weeping (leaking) blisters may develop on the affected skin; the tongue becomes bright red, swollen, and painful. In chronic cases, the exposed skin darkens, thickens, and becomes rough and dry. Diarrhea is a common symptom, and severe mental disturbance, including confusion and memory loss, may develop.

DIAGNOSIS AND TREATMENT
Pellagra is diagnosed from the patient's physical condition and dietary history. Daily intake of a regulated amount of niacin and a varied diet rich in protein and carbohydrates are usually enough to bring about a complete cure.

Pelvic examination

Examination of a woman's external and internal genitalia. A pelvic examination may be performed as part of a general *physical examination*, during contraceptive counseling, or to investigate the cause of symptoms, such as abdominal pain, vaginal bleeding or discharge, urinary incontinence, or infertility. During labor, pelvic examinations are performed to help assess the position and descent, and the well-being, of the baby.

The main aspects of a pelvic examination are shown in the illustrated box on the next page.

Pelvic floor exercises

A program of exercises to strengthen the muscles and tighten the ligaments at the base of the abdomen. These muscles and ligaments, which form the pelvic floor, support the uterus, vagina, bladder, urethra, and rectum. Slackening of the pelvic floor is common during childbirth and is also a part of the aging process.

Performing pelvic floor exercises, especially during pregnancy and following childbirth, tones these structures and may prevent prolapse of the uterus (see *Uterus, prolapse of*) and urinary stress incontinence (see *Incontinence, urinary*). Pelvic floor exercises can also help women who are having difficulty achieving orgasm.

One exercise, carried out during urination, involves stopping and starting the flow of urine several times by contracting and then relaxing the muscles around the vagina, each time for a count of six. Another exercise involves placing two fingers inside the vagina and contracting the muscles around the fingers. The exercises should be done two or three times a day for at least a month.

Pelvic infection

An infection in the female reproductive system. Severe or recurrent pelvic infection is referred to as *pelvic inflam-*

PROCEDURE FOR PELVIC EXAMINATION

The examination is usually performed with the woman lying on her back with knees bent. If it is carried out because of uterine prolapse or incontinence, she may be asked to lie on her side. The physician usually begins by inspecting the external genitals for ulceration or swelling and then does an internal examination.

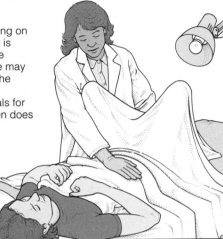

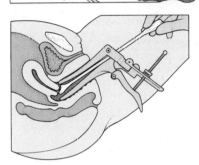

Use of speculum
A speculum is inserted into the vagina to hold apart the vaginal walls; this gives the physician a clear view of both the vagina and cervix. A *cervical smear* test may also be performed at this time.

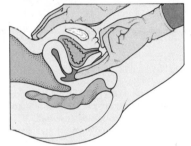

Manual examination
The physician inserts two fingers into the vagina and palpates (feels) the abdomen to evaluate the size and position of the uterus and ovaries, and to detect any abnormal pelvic swelling or tenderness.

matory disease (PID). Pelvic infection can result in damage to the fallopian tubes and can cause female *infertility*.

Occasionally, conditions affecting surrounding organs, such as *inflammatory bowel disease*, can damage the female genital tract.

Pelvic inflammatory disease

Infection of the internal female reproductive organs.

Pelvic inflammatory disease (PID) is a common cause of pelvic pain in women. The infection may not have any obvious cause, but often occurs in patients who have just had a sexually transmitted disease, such as a *chlamydial infection* or *gonorrhea*. PID may also occur after miscarriage, abortion, or childbirth. *IUD* users have a higher incidence of PID, as do young, sexually active women.

SYMPTOMS AND SIGNS
Abdominal pain and tenderness, fever, and irregular menstrual periods are common symptoms of PID. The pain often occurs immediately after menstruation and may be worse during intercourse. There may also be malaise, vomiting, or backache.

DIAGNOSIS AND TREATMENT
The physician may detect tenderness on internal pelvic examination and will take swabs to identify microorganisms that may be causing the condition. A *laparoscopy* (examination of the abdominal cavity using a viewing instrument) may be performed to confirm the diagnosis or to detect any abscess. *Antibiotic drugs* are prescribed to clear the infection, and *analgesic drugs* (painkillers) may also be required. If the woman has an IUD, it may need to be removed.

OUTLOOK
Some women have repeated attacks of PID with or without reinfection. PID may cause *infertility* or increase the risk of *ectopic pregnancy*, primarily due to scarring in the fallopian tubes that prevents the egg from traveling down the tube into the uterus.

Pelvic pain

See *Abdominal pain*.

Pelvimetry

Assessment of the shape and dimensions of a woman's pelvis. Pelvimetry is most commonly carried out in about the 37th week of pregnancy to determine whether a woman is likely to have difficulty delivering her baby. Pelvimetry may also be performed after childbirth in women who have required a cesarean section. Such assessment determines whether future deliveries should be vaginal or by cesarean section.

A rough indication of the size of the pelvic outlet can be obtained by manually checking the distance between the ischial tuberosities (the prominent bones in the lower pelvis) during a pelvic examination. More precise measurement is possible using radiological pelvimetry (use of X rays to assess pelvic dimensions). However, excessive exposure to X rays in pregnancy may increase the risk of subsequent development of leukemia or other cancers in unborn children. The procedure is therefore carried out only in certain circumstances, such as a breech presentation, even though the X-ray exposure involved in pelvimetry is minimal.

Pelvis

The ring of bones in the lower trunk, bounded by the coccyx and the hip bones. The pelvis protects abdominal organs, such as the bladder, rectum, and, in women, the uterus.

STRUCTURE
The pelvis consists of two innominate bones (hip bones), which are joined by rigid sacroiliac joints to the sacrum (the triangular spinal bone below the lumbar vertebrae) at the back; the hip bones curve forward to join at the pubic symphysis at the front. Attached to the pelvis are the muscles of the abdominal wall, the buttocks, the lower back, and the insides and backs of the thighs.

Each innominate bone consists of three fused bones: the ilium, ischium, and pubis. The ilium, the largest and uppermost of these bones, consists of

P

P

STRUCTURE OF THE PELVIS

The pelvis is a basin-shaped bony structure at the base of the trunk. It consists of the sacrum and coccyx at the back and, at the sides, the two hip bones, which curve around to meet at the front. The pelvis supports the upper half of the body and protects the lower abdominal organs. The female pelvis is shallower and wider.

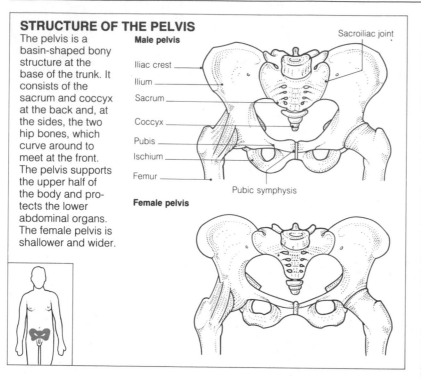

Male pelvis

Sacroiliac joint

Iliac crest

Ilium

Sacrum

Coccyx

Pubis

Ischium

Femur

Pubic symphysis

Female pelvis

a wide, flattened plate with a long curved ridge (called the iliac crest) along its upper border. The ischium is the bone that bears much of the body weight when sitting. The pubis is the smallest pelvic bone; from the ischium it extends forward and round to the pubic symphysis, where it is joined to the other pubis bone by tough fibrous tissue. All three bones meet in the acetabulum, the cup-shaped cavity that forms the socket of the hip joint.

The pelvis differs considerably between men and women. In women, the pelvis is generally shallow and broad, and the pubic symphysis joint is less rigid than a man's. These differences facilitate childbirth. In men, the pelvis is usually larger and built more heavily to bear a greater body weight.

DISORDERS

Fractures of the pelvis may be caused by a direct blow, or by a force transmitted through the femur (thigh bone). Considerable force is required to cause such a fracture, and it is usually the result of a motor vehicle accident; motorcycle riders are particularly at risk. The fracture itself often heals without problems, but it is frequently accompanied by damage to internal organs within the pelvis, especially the bladder.

Osteitis pubis (inflammation of the pubic symphysis) is usually caused by repeated stress on the pelvis. It is most common in soccer players as a result of continually kicking a ball. The symptoms include pain in the groin and tenderness over the front of the pelvis. In most cases, the condition clears up with rest.

Pemoline

A central nervous system *stimulant drug* used in the treatment of *narcolepsy* (a rare condition characterized by paroxysms of sleep) and *hyperactivity* in children. Pemoline may cause insomnia, loss of appetite, and, in rare cases, drowsiness, depression, and hallucinations.

Pemphigoid

An uncommon, chronic skin disease in which large blisters form on the skin. The blisters in pemphigoid are sometimes intensely itchy, unlike those in *pemphigus*, a similar but more serious disorder. Pemphigoid, which is considered to be an *autoimmune disorder* (one in which the body reacts against its own tissues), primarily affects elderly people.

The diagnosis is confirmed by a skin *biopsy* (removal of a small sample of tissue for microscopic analysis). Treatment is usually a long-term course of *corticosteroid drugs* or, in some cases, *immunosuppressant drugs*.

Pemphigus

An uncommon, serious skin disease in which blisters appear on the skin and on mucous membranes in the mouth and sometimes elsewhere. Pemphigus primarily affects people between the ages of 40 and 60.

SYMPTOMS AND SIGNS

The blisters usually begin in the mouth, and sometimes in the nose, and then appear on the skin. They rupture easily, forming raw, often painful areas that may become infected and that later crust over. Apparently unaffected skin may also blister after gentle pressure. When the blisters occur over a great area of the body, the resultant severe skin loss can lead to secondary bacterial infection and, sometimes, death.

DIAGNOSIS AND TREATMENT

A diagnosis of pemphigus is confirmed by a skin *biopsy* (removal of a small sample of tissue for microscopic analysis).

The usual treatment is with *corticosteroid drugs* given over long periods to keep the disease under control. Other *immunosuppressant drugs* may also help. *Antibiotic drugs* may need to be taken for secondary infections.

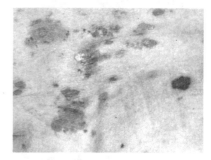

Pemphigus on the back
The typical appearance is of numerous large, raw areas of skin where the fragile blisters have broken down.

Penicillamine

An *antirheumatic drug* used to treat *rheumatoid arthritis* when symptoms are not relieved by *nonsteroidal antiinflammatory drugs* (NSAIDs).

Penicillamine is not one of the *penicillin drugs*, but rather a *chelating agent* used in the treatment of copper, mercury, lead, or arsenic poisoning. It is used to treat *Wilson's disease* (a rare brain and liver disorder caused by copper deposits in these tissues), primary *biliary cirrhosis* (a liver disorder), and has also been given to people with cystinuria (excessive excretion of cystine in the urine) to prevent stones from forming in the urinary tract.

POSSIBLE ADVERSE EFFECTS
Penicillamine frequently causes allergic rashes, itching, nausea, vomiting, abdominal pain, and loss of taste. . Infrequently, it causes blood disorders or impaired kidney function. Regular blood and urine tests are carried out during treatment.

Penicillin drugs
The first group of *antibiotic drugs* to be discovered. Natural penicillins are derived from the mold PENICILLIUM; other pencillin drugs are synthetic preparations.

Penicillin drugs are used in the treatment of many infections, including *tonsillitis, pharyngitis, bronchitis,* and *pneumonia.* Penicillins are also given to prevent the recurrence of *rheumatic fever* and to treat bacterial *endocarditis, syphilis, gonorrhea,* and acute ulcerative *gingivitis.*

POSSIBLE ADVERSE EFFECTS
The most common adverse effect is an allergic reaction that causes a rash. Any person who has had an allergic reaction to one type of penicillin is not usually prescribed any other type. Another common adverse effect of penicillin drugs is diarrhea. Prolonged use may cause yeast infections.

Penile implant
A prosthesis inserted into the *penis* to help a man suffering from *impotence* to achieve intercourse. Penile implants are usually used only for men who are permanently impotent.

One treatment involves inserting a silicone splint in the tissues of the upper surface of the penis. The penis can be inserted into the vagina, but does not increase in size.

Alternatively, an inflatable prosthesis may be implanted in the penis. This type makes the penis larger and firmer for intercourse and is operated by squeezing a small bulb placed in the scrotum.

Penile warts
See *Warts, genital.*

Penis
The male sex organ through which urine and semen pass. The penis consists mainly of three cylindrical bodies of erectile tissue (spongy tissue full of tiny blood vessels) that run the length of the organ. Two of these bodies, the corpora cavernosa, lie side by side in the upper part of the penis. The third, the corpus spongiosum, lies centrally beneath them, expanding at its end to form the tip of the penis, the glans.

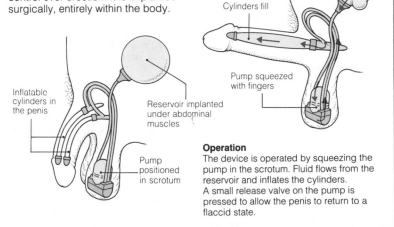

INFLATABLE PENILE IMPLANT
There are various types of penile implant for the treatment of impotence. The type below gives full control over erection. It is implanted surgically, entirely within the body.

Liquid is pumped from the reservoir

Cylinders fill

Pump squeezed with fingers

Inflatable cylinders in the penis

Reservoir implanted under abdominal muscles

Pump positioned in scrotum

Operation
The device is operated by squeezing the pump in the scrotum. Fluid flows from the reservoir and inflates the cylinders. A small release valve on the pump is pressed to allow the penis to return to a flaccid state.

Through the center of the corpus spongiosum runs the *urethra,* a narrow tube that carries urine and semen out of the body through an opening at the tip of the glans. Surrounding the erectile tissue is a sheath of fibrous connective tissue enclosed by skin. Over the glans, the skin forms a loose fold called the *foreskin,* which is sometimes removed (see *Circumcision*).

DISORDERS
The most common congenital abnormality of the penis is *hypospadias,* in which the urethra opens on the undersurface of the penis anywhere from the base of the glans to the root. In male *pseudohermaphroditism,* which is also a congenital problem, the penis is very small and there is usually also hypospadias.

Balanitis (inflammation of the glans and foreskin) is usually caused by *candidiasis,* although other organisms, including those that cause *gonorrhea* and *syphilis,* may cause inflammation. Balanitis may lead to *phimosis,* in which the foreskin is abnormally tight, or *paraphimosis,* in which the foreskin retracts at erection but is too tight to move back over the glans.

Penile warts (see *Warts, genital*) are caused by a sexually transmitted virus. Cancer of the penis (see *Penis, cancer of*) is a rare disorder; the incidence is higher in uncircumcised than in circumcised men.

Impotence (failure to attain or maintain an erection) is usually psychological in origin. However, it may be caused by nerve damage associated with *diabetes mellitus, alcohol dependence, atherosclerosis,* or spinal cord injury. The causes of *priapism* (prolonged, painful erection) and of *Peyronie's disease,* in which the erect penis bends to one side, are unknown.

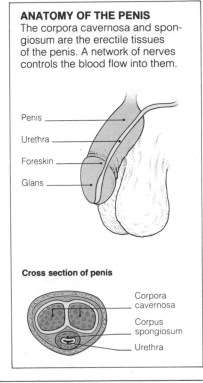

ANATOMY OF THE PENIS
The corpora cavernosa and spongiosum are the erectile tissues of the penis. A network of nerves controls the blood flow into them.

Penis
Urethra
Foreskin
Glans

Cross section of penis

Corpora cavernosa
Corpus spongiosum
Urethra

P

Penis, cancer of

A rare form of malignant tumor that is more common in uncircumcised men whose personal hygiene is poor. Viral infection and smoking have both been shown to be additional factors.

The tumor usually starts on the glans (head) of the penis or on the foreskin as a dry, painless, wartlike lump or a painful ulcer, and develops into a cauliflowerlike mass. The growth usually spreads slowly, but a highly malignant tumor can spread to the lymphatic glands in the groin within a few months; the glands swell and the skin over them may ulcerate. Any growth or sore area on the penis that persists for more than two or three weeks should be reported to a physician. A *biopsy* (removal of a sample of tissue for microscopic analysis) will show whether the condition is due to cancer or to some other cause, such as warts (see *Warts, genital*) or *syphilis*.

Cancer of the penis can generally be treated successfully by *radiation therapy* if it is reported early. Otherwise, surgical removal of part or all of the penis may be necessary.

Pentazocine

A narcotic *analgesic drug* (painkiller) used to relieve moderate or severe pain caused by injury, surgery, cancer, or childbirth.

Possible adverse affects are typical of other narcotic analgesics. Such effects include dizziness, drowsiness, nausea, vomiting, and occasionally hallucinations. Dependence may develop in people who take high doses for prolonged periods.

Pentobarbital

A *barbiturate drug* formerly used to treat *insomnia*. Pentobarbital was also used as a *premedication* (drug used to prepare a person for an operation). Possible adverse effects, including a tendency to prolonged sedation or "hangover," are typical of other barbiturate drugs.

Peppermint oil

An oil obtained from the peppermint plant MENTHA PIPERITA. Peppermint oil is prescribed to relieve abdominal colic, particularly in *irritable bowel syndrome*. It may occasionally cause *heartburn*. Peppermint oil is also used as a flavoring in some drug preparations.

Pep pills

A popular name for *stimulant drugs*, particularly *amphetamine drugs*.

Peptic ulcer

A raw area that occurs in the gastrointestinal tract as a result of erosion by acidic gastric juice. Peptic ulcers may occur in the esophagus, stomach, or duodenum. Rarely, they develop in the jejunum (as occurs in *Zollinger-Ellison syndrome*) or in the ileum (as may occur in *Meckel's diverticulum*). Peptic ulcers, which may be single or multiple, usually measure about 10 to 25 mm across and about 0.25 mm deep. The typical symptom is a gnawing pain in the abdomen when the stomach is empty.

CAUSES AND INCIDENCE

The lining of the duodenum is constantly at risk of erosion from acid produced by the stomach wall. The lower esophagus is at risk only when reflux of acid juice from the stomach occurs (see *Acid reflux*). Peptic ulcers in the jejunum occur only when there is a massive outpouring of gastric acid. In a Meckel's diverticulum, a peptic ulcer may develop if misplaced gastric lining grows in the diverticulum.

Some of the main factors that may be involved in causing peptic ulcer are shown in the illustrated box, page 787. In some people, there is a strong family history of peptic ulceration. Psychological stress may play a part in making an existing ulcer worse.

The incidence of gastric ulcers is about equal in men and women, but more males than females suffer from duodenal ulcers. Middle age is the most likely time for either type of ulcer to develop, although the peak age for the development of duodenal ulcers is somewhat earlier than the peak age for gastric ulcers.

SYMPTOMS

Many people found to have a peptic ulcer suffer no symptoms, but a greater number complain of a burning or gnawing pain in the abdomen, which sometimes wakes them at night. The pain of a duodenal ulcer is often relieved by eating, but usually recurs a few hours later.

Other symptoms accompanying both types of ulcer include loss of appetite (although in some cases a duodenal ulcer increases the appetite), belching, feeling bloated, weight loss, nausea, and vomiting (which usually relieves the pain).

The most common complication of a peptic ulcer is bleeding from the ulcer. Severe bleeding results in hematemesis (vomiting of blood) and melena (black feces), and is a medical emergency. Chronic bleeding may cause iron-deficiency *anemia*.

Rarely, an ulcer may perforate (make a hole in) the wall of the digestive tract and extend to the pancreas, usually causing pain that spreads through to the back. If digestive juices leak through the perforation or if the perforation is on the front wall of the duodenum, the juices may cause *peritonitis* (inflammation of the abdominal lining), producing sudden, severe pain and requiring emergency hospital admission.

Chronic ulcers can cause extensive scarring of the stomach or duodenum, which may narrow the outlet of the stomach into the duodenum (a condition called *pyloric stenosis*) and thus obstruct the passage of food. This may cause vomiting and rapid weight loss.

A small number of gastric ulcers are malignant and should be removed as soon as they are diagnosed.

DIAGNOSIS

The condition can be diagnosed with certainty only after a *barium X-ray examination* or *endoscopy* (inspection through a viewing instrument) of the stomach and duodenum.

TREATMENT

Antacid drugs neutralize excess acidity and assist in the healing of ulcers. Such drugs ultimately relieve pain if taken regularly, and, along with the other self-help measures listed in the illustrated box, may be enough to heal the ulcer. If not, and if symptoms persist, professional treatment is necessary. This usually consists of *ulcer-healing drugs* (such as cimetidine, ranitidine, or famotidine), which reduce acid production, or sucralfate, which may form a protective covering on the ulcer.

In more than two thirds of cases, the drugs promote healing within six to eight weeks of the start of treatment. In the remaining one third, long-term drug treatment is usually required; very rarely, if the ulcer fails to respond to medication, surgery is necessary. Usually surgery takes the form of a *vagotomy* (cutting of the fibers of the vagus nerve that controls digestive acid production) and pyloroplasty (widening of the outlet of the stomach into the duodenum).

Occasionally, a partial *gastrectomy* (surgical removal of a portion of the stomach) is performed to treat the ulcer and reduce acid production.

Substantial bleeding from an ulcer sometimes requires a *blood transfusion*. Perforation, peritonitis, or obstruction usually necessitates surgery to correct the problem. In some cases of perforation, however, passing a suc-

P

SITES AND CAUSES OF PEPTIC ULCER

A peptic ulcer develops in about one in 10 people in Canada at some time in their lives. Some of the mechanisms involved in causing ulcers are shown below. Most ulcers respond to self-help measures or to drug treatment, but occasionally surgery is necessary.

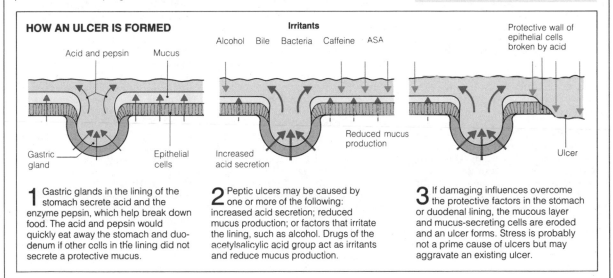

Gastric ulcer
This photograph of an ulcer in the wall of the stomach was taken via a viewing tube passed down the esophagus.

Gallbladder   Stomach

Duodenum   Pancreas

Site of ulcers
Peptic ulcers are most common in the first part of the duodenum or lower half of the stomach; esophageal ulcers also occur.

ULCER CARE

Self-help methods

Avoid smoking, the most important step in self-help.

Avoid drinking alcohol, coffee, and tea.

Avoid using ASA and nonsteroidal anti-inflammatory drugs.

Eat several small meals a day, at regular intervals, rather than two or three large ones.

Drug treatment

Antacids neutralize acid in the stomach.

H_2-blockers, such as ranitidine, cimetidine, and famotidine, reduce acid secretion by blocking receptors on acid-producing cells.

Drugs such as sucralfate work by forming a protective coat over the ulcer crater.

HOW AN ULCER IS FORMED

Acid and pepsin   Mucus

Gastric gland   Epithelial cells

1 Gastric glands in the lining of the stomach secrete acid and the enzyme pepsin, which help break down food. The acid and pepsin would quickly eat away the stomach and duodenum if other cells in the lining did not secrete a protective mucus.

Irritants
Alcohol   Bile   Bacteria   Caffeine   ASA

Increased acid secretion

Reduced mucus production

2 Peptic ulcers may be caused by one or more of the following: increased acid secretion; reduced mucus production; or factors that irritate the lining, such as alcohol. Drugs of the acetylsalicylic acid group act as irritants and reduce mucus production.

Protective wall of epithelial cells broken by acid

Ulcer

3 If damaging influences overcome the protective factors in the stomach or duodenal lining, the mucous layer and mucus-secreting cells are eroded and an ulcer forms. Stress is probably not a prime cause of ulcers but may aggravate an existing ulcer.

---

tion tube into the stomach via the nose to drain off digestive juices may be sufficient treatment. Peritonitis, however, inevitably requires emergency hospital treatment.

Peptide

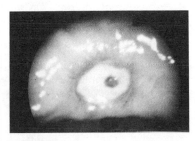

A fragment of protein consisting of two or more *amino acids*. Peptides are formed by the linking of amino acids by chemical bonds (peptide bonds) between the amino and carboxyl groups of adjacent acids.

Larger peptides, consisting of many linked amino acids, are known as polypeptides; still longer chains of amino acids, made up of linked polypeptides, are called *proteins*.

Peptides are widely distributed in the body's endocrine and nervous systems. Many *hormones* are peptides, including some *gastrointestinal hormones* and several pituitary hormones, such as *oxytocin*, *ADH* (antidiuretic hormone), and *ACTH* (adrenocorticotropic hormone). In the nervous system, peptides are found in nerve

cells throughout the brain and the spinal cord; examples include *endorphins* and substances involved in the control of the pituitary gland.

Perception

The interpretation of a sensation. People receive information about the environment through the five senses—*taste, smell, hearing, vision,* and *touch*—but interpreting the information depends on other factors.

First, the information must be organized into a pattern. In vision, for example, objects must be distinguished from their background and recognized as moving or stationary. Each object then requires identification (e.g., as a chair or a friend), a process that relies on memory. The final interpretation depends on an individual's attitudes, expectations, and mood. Valued objects often appear larger, and hungry people are more likely to notice food sooner than those who have just eaten.

Hallucinations, which are a symptom of *psychosis*, are false perceptions that occur in the absence of sensory stimuli.

Percussion

A diagnostic technique for examining the chest or abdomen by tapping it with the fingers and listening to the resonance of the sound produced. In this way, the condition of internal organs can be deduced. For example, a fluid-filled lung produces a dull note when tapped, and *pneumothorax* (air in the pleural cavity) produces a hollow sound quite distinctive to a physician. (See also *Examination, physical*.)

Percutaneous

A medical term meaning through the skin. Percutaneous procedures include the injection of drugs into veins, muscles, or other body tissues, and biopsies in which tissue or fluid is removed with a needle.

Perforation

A hole made in an organ or tissue by disease or injury. Among the more common types of perforation due to a disorder are a hole in the wall of the stomach or duodenum (the first part of the small intestine) caused by a *peptic ulcer*, and a rupture of the eardrum, usually caused by middle-ear infection (see *Eardrum, perforated*).

Perforating *wounds* that penetrate through outer layers of tissue to damage an internal organ or cavity usually require exploratory surgery to check for and remove any foreign material.

Peri-

A prefix meaning around, as in pericardium, the membranous sac that surrounds the heart.

Pericarditis

Inflammation of the *pericardium* (the membrane that surrounds the *heart*), leading, in many cases, to chest pain and fever. In addition to inflammation, there may be an effusion (increased amount of fluid) in the

pericardial space, which separates the two smooth layers of the pericardium. This excess fluid may compress the heart, restricting its action.

Long-standing inflammation can cause constrictive pericarditis, in which the pericardium becomes scarred, thickens, and contracts, interfering with the heart's action.

CAUSES

Pericarditis has many possible causes. These include certain bacterial, viral, and fungal infections; *myocardial infarction* (heart attack); cancer spreading from a nearby tumor in the lung or breast or by way of the blood from a remote site; and injury to the pericardium from a penetrating wound or after *open heart surgery*. Pericarditis sometimes accompanies *rheumatoid arthritis*, systemic *lupus erythematosus*, and *kidney failure*. It can also occur for no known reason.

SYMPTOMS AND SIGNS

The characteristic symptom of pericarditis is pain behind the sternum (breastbone), sometimes spreading to the neck and shoulders. The pain often becomes more severe if the person takes a deep breath, changes posture, or even swallows; sitting up and leaning forward sometimes relieves it. Fever is another fairly common symptom.

When pericarditis is due to infection, pus may accumulate in the pericardial space. When, rarely, the cause is a tumor, blood may collect there. If heart action is impeded, heart output and blood pressure fall—a condition known as cardiac tamponade. This results in breathing difficulty and in swollen neck veins. The main symptom of constrictive pericarditis is *edema* (accumulation of fluid in the tissues) of the legs and abdomen, causing them to swell.

DIAGNOSIS

The condition is diagnosed from information obtained during a physical examination (which includes listening to the heart with a stethoscope), and from the result of an *ECG* and chest *X rays*. *Echocardiography* may be used to confirm that enlargement of the heart shown on X rays is due to effusion.

TREATMENT

Treatment is aimed at the underlying cause whenever possible. *Analgesic drugs* (painkillers) or *anti-inflammatory drugs* may be given to relieve pain. If effusion is seriously affecting heart action, the excess fluid is drawn off through a needle inserted through the chest wall into the pericardial space.

Severe constrictive pericarditis may require surgical removal of the thickened pericardium.

Pericardium

The membranous bag that completely envelops the *heart* and the roots of the major blood vessels that emerge from the heart. The pericardium has two layers. The outer layer is tough, inelastic, and fibrous. It is attached to the diaphragm below and to the sternum (breastbone) in front. The inner layer is separated into two sheets. Of these, the inner is firmly attached to the heart and the outer is attached to the fibrous layer. The space between the smooth, inner surfaces of these sheets is called the pericardial space. This contains a small quantity of fluid that lubricates the heart.

Perimetry

A visual field test to determine the extent of peripheral vision. Perimetry, which is not usually done as a routine procedure, may be performed to provide vital information in certain neurological disorders, such as a brain tumor (See *Eye, examination of*.)

Perinatal

Relating to the period just before or just after birth. Perinatal is often defined more precisely as the period from the 28th week of pregnancy to the end of the first week after birth. Perinatal mortality is a statistical expression of the number of stillbirths and infant deaths occurring during the first week after birth.

Perinatology

A branch of *obstetrics* and *pediatrics* concerned with the study and care of mother and baby during pregnancy and the early days after birth.

The perinatologist specializes in the management of high-risk pregnancies and births, and in the investigation and treatment of prenatal conditions that might endanger the life or well-being of the fetus, such as *Rh incompatibility*, *spina bifida*, or some biochemical disorder. The perinatologist is also skilled in the assessment of placental function and in looking after the health of the expectant mother.

Perineum

The area bounded internally by the pelvic floor (the muscles that form the supportive base of the pelvis) and the surrounding bony structures. The perineum is pierced by the genito-

P

urinary and digestive organs. Externally, the perineum is represented by the area between the thighs that lies behind the genital organs and in front of the anus.

Periodic fever

An inherited condition causing recurrent bouts of fever. (See *Familial Mediterranean fever*.)

Period, menstrual

See *Menstruation*.

Periodontal disease

Any disorder of the periodontium (the tissues surrounding and supporting the *teeth*). The most common type of periodontal disease is chronic *gingivitis* (inflammation of the *gums*), which, if untreated, leads to *periodontitis* (inflammation of the periodontal membranes around the base of the teeth and erosion of the bone holding the teeth).

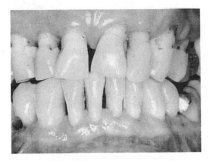

Periodontal disease
The gums are inflamed and have receded. Many of the teeth are eroded at their bases; the tooth sockets may also be decayed.

Periodontics

The branch of *dentistry* that is concerned with the study and treatment of diseases that affect the periodontium (the structures that surround and support the teeth), particularly *gingivitis* (inflammation of the *gums*) and *periodontitis* (inflammation of the periodontium).

A periodontist makes considerable use of *dental X rays* in diagnosis (to detect loss of bony support in which the teeth are embedded) and is concerned with *preventive dentistry*. Treatment includes dental *scaling*, dental *curettage*, *gingivectomy*, and root planing (removal of *calculus* from the root surface).

Periodontitis

Inflammation of the periodontium (the tissues that support the teeth). There are two types. Periapical periodontitis is a complication of neglected dental *caries* and affects the area around a root tip. Chronic periodontitis is a complication of untreated *gingivitis* (inflammation of the gums). This type affects the whole of the periodontium and is the major cause of tooth loss in adults.

CAUSES
If dental caries is untreated, enamel and the dentin beneath it are eventually destroyed, allowing bacteria to enter the tooth pulp. From there, bacteria spread to the root tip and into the surrounding tissues, sometimes leading to the formation of a dental *abscess*, *granuloma*, or dental *cyst*.

If gingivitis, which is usually the result of poor *oral hygiene*, is neglected, inflamed gum tissue at the base of the teeth becomes damaged and pockets form between the gums and the teeth. Dental *plaque* (a sticky deposit of mucus, food particles, and bacteria) and dental *calculus* (a hard, mineralized coating that forms from plaque and saliva) then collect in these pockets. The bacteria in the plaque and calculus attack the periodontal tissues, causing them to become inflamed and detached from the teeth. The bacteria also eventually erode the bones surrounding the teeth. In time, the teeth become loose and fall out.

SYMPTOMS AND SIGNS
In periapical periodontitis, there may be localized toothache, especially when biting. An abscess may cause some bone and ligament destruction, thus causing the tooth to become loose; a large dental cyst may cause visible swelling of the jaw.

In chronic periodontitis, the signs of gingivitis are present (red, soft, shiny, tender gums that bleed easily) along with an unpleasant taste and bad breath. The deepening pockets in the gums gradually expose the sensitive dentin of the roots of the teeth, causing aching when hot, cold, or sweet foods or liquids are consumed.

Occasionally, there is a discharge of pus from the gums or a gumboil (see *Abscess, dental*); in late stages of chronic periodontitis, there may be bone loss and loosening of teeth.

DIAGNOSIS
In periapical periodontitis, the dentist usually finds a deep cavity beneath a filling, and *dental X rays* may show bone destruction around the root tip.

The extent of chronic periodontal disease is assessed by measuring the depth of the gum pockets and by taking X rays to determine the extent of bone loss.

TREATMENT
Periapical periodontitis is treated either by draining pus through the root canal and then cleaning and filling the tooth or, if the tooth cannot be saved, by dental *extraction*. A minor operation may be required to remove dental cysts or large granulomas. Root canal treatment may also be necessary.

If chronic periodontal disease has not reached an advanced stage, regular, scrupulous cleaning of the teeth can prevent further plaque and calculus formation, and thus halt destruction of the tissues surrounding the teeth. The dentist removes existing plaque and calculus by *scaling* and, in some cases, root planing. In some cases, *gingivectomy* (surgical trimming of the gums) may be required to reduce the size of the gum pockets. Curettage (see *Curettage, dental*) may be carried out to remove the diseased lining from the pocket so that healthy underlying tissue will reattach itself to the tooth. Loose teeth can sometimes be anchored to firmer ones by splinting (see *Splinting, dental*).

Period pain

See *Dysmenorrhea*.

Periosteum

The tissue that coats all the bones in the body except the surfaces inside joints. Periosteum contains small blood vessels that supply nutrients to the underlying bone, and nerves that respond to pain caused by injury or disease. New bone is produced by the periosteum in the initial stages of healing after a *fracture*.

Periostitis

Inflammation of the *periosteum* (connective tissue covering bone). The usual cause is a blow that presses directly onto bone. Rarely, periostitis is caused by infection, such as syphilis. Symptoms include pain, tenderness, and swelling over the affected area of bone.

Peripheral nervous system

All the nerves that fan out from the central nervous system (brain and spinal cord) to the muscles, skin, internal organs, and glands (see *Cranial nerves*; *Nerve*; *Spinal nerves*).

Peripheral vascular disease

Narrowing of blood vessels in the legs, and sometimes in the arms, restricting blood flow and causing pain in the affected area. In severe cases,

P

HOW PERIPHERAL VASCULAR DISEASE DEVELOPS

The disease usually starts with the formation of atheromas (fatty plaques) on artery walls. Smokers are among those at highest risk.

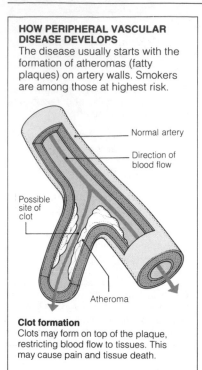

Normal artery

Direction of blood flow

Possible site of clot

Atheroma

Clot formation
Clots may form on top of the plaque, restricting blood flow to tissues. This may cause pain and tissue death.

gangrene (death of tissue supplied by the vessels) may develop, requiring amputation of the limb.

TYPES AND CAUSES

In most cases, peripheral vascular disease is caused by atherosclerosis, in which fatty plaques form on the inner walls of arteries. Factors that contribute to the risk of atherosclerosis, such as hypertension and inadequately controlled diabetes mellitus, are associated with peripheral vascular disease. However, the greatest risk factor is tobacco smoking; more than 90 percent of patients are, or were, moderate to heavy cigarette smokers.

Diseases affecting the peripheral arteries that are not caused by atherosclerosis include Buerger's disease, which mainly affects smokers, and Raynaud's disease. Deep vein thrombosis and varicose veins are diseases of peripheral veins.

SYMPTOMS AND COMPLICATIONS

When narrowing of the arteries develops gradually because of atherosclerosis, the first symptom is usually an aching, tired feeling in the leg muscles when walking. This occurs most often in the calf, but may be felt anywhere in the leg. Typically, the pain is relieved by resting the leg for a few minutes, but recurs after roughly the same amount of walking as before. This symptom is called intermittent claudication. Prolonged use of the arms may produce a similar symptom.

As the disease worsens, the amount of activity possible before symptoms develop decreases, until eventually pain is present at rest. This pain may be severe and continuous, disturbing sleep. By this stage, the affected leg is dangerously short of blood supply; the foot and lower leg are cold and often numb, the skin is dry and scaly, and leg ulcers tend to develop after minor injury. In the final stage there is gangrene, which usually starts in the toes and then spreads up the leg.

Sometimes, sudden arterial blockage occurs. This may be caused by the rapid development of a clot on top of a plaque of atherosclerosis, by a dissecting aneurysm (splitting of an arterial wall), or by an embolism arising from a clot formed in the heart and carried to obstruct a peripheral artery. Blockage causes sudden severe pain in the affected limb, which becomes cold and either pale or blue. There is no pulse in the limb, and movement and sensation in it are lost.

DIAGNOSIS

The diagnosis is based on blood pressure readings taken at the ankle, calf, upper thigh, and arm, and on blood flow measurements using Doppler ultrasound or plethysmography.

TREATMENT

Giving up smoking is by far the most important aspect of treatment. Exercise is also extremely important; sufferers should walk for up to an hour each day, stopping whenever claudication occurs and resuming when it stops.

Regular inspection of the feet and scrupulous care of them (ideally by a podiatrist) are essential to prevent infection, which can lead to gangrene. Feet should be washed and stockings changed daily. Shoes should fit well to avoid pressure on the feet, and toenails should be cut straight across.

Surgery on the diseased blood vessels is sometimes required. Arterial reconstructive surgery may be performed to bypass affected vessels. Endarterectomy may be carried out to remove fatty deposits from blood vessel linings. The newer technique of balloon angioplasty is increasingly successfully being used to widen diseased blood vessels in peripheral vascular disease.

In severe cases in which gangrene has developed, amputation is necessary, usually just below the knee in order to leave a stump suitable for a prosthesis. (See Limb, artificial).

Peristalsis

Wavelike movement as a result of rhythmic (but involuntary) contraction and relaxation of the muscles in the walls of the digestive tract and of the ureters. Peristalsis is responsible for the movement of food and waste products through the digestive system and for transporting urine from the kidneys to the bladder.

Peristalsis in the esophagus moves food toward the stomach, and is effective even when the body is upside down. In the stomach, peristalsis helps to mix food with gastric juices and moves the partly digested food into the duodenum. In the small intestine, peristalsis changes to a slow back-and-forth churning motion that allows more time for absorption of nutrients.

In the large intestine, peristaltic contractions occur only about once every 30 minutes. Two or three times a day, usually following a meal, a strong, sustained wave of peristalsis passes over the colon. This forces the contents into the rectum and may prompt the urge to defecate.

Peritoneal dialysis

See Dialysis.

Peritoneum

The two-layered membrane that lines the wall of the abdominal cavity and covers the abdominal organs. The peritoneum contains blood vessels, lymph vessels, and nerves.

The most important functions of the peritoneum are to support the abdominal organs, to produce a lubricating fluid that allows the organs to glide smoothly over each other and the abdominal wall, and to protect against infection. The peritoneum also absorbs fluid and acts as a natural filtering system—a function made use of in peritoneal dialysis.

The peritoneum may become inflamed as a complication of an abdominal disorder (see Peritonitis).

Peritonitis

Inflammation of the peritoneum (the membrane that lines the wall of the abdomen and covers the abdominal organs). Peritonitis is a serious, usually acute, and painful condition, almost always due to irritation and bacterial infection caused by another abdominal disorder.

CAUSES

The most common cause of peritonitis is perforation of the stomach or intestine, which allows bacteria and di-

HOW PERISTALSIS HAPPENS

The walls of many body passages contain a special type of muscle called smooth muscle. The muscle fibers contract in sequence, sending waves of contraction along the walls of the passage.

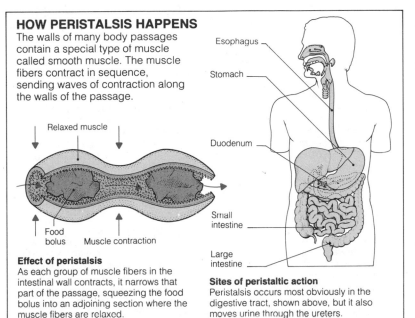

Effect of peristalsis
As each group of muscle fibers in the intestinal wall contracts, it narrows that part of the passage, squeezing the food bolus into an adjoining section where the muscle fibers are relaxed.

Sites of peristaltic action
Peristalsis occurs most obviously in the digestive tract, shown above, but it also moves urine through the ureters.

gestive juices to escape from the digestive tract into the abdominal cavity. Perforation is usually the result of a *peptic ulcer, appendicitis,* or *diverticulitis.* Less commonly, intestinal contents may leak into the abdominal cavity after surgery on the intestine. Peritonitis may also be associated with acute *salpingitis,* with *cholecystitis,* or with *septicemia.*

SYMPTOMS AND SIGNS

Peritonitis is usually marked by severe abdominal pain, which may be either localized (in one place) or generalized (affecting the entire abdomen). In some cases, however, pain may be mild or absent. After a few hours, the muscles in the abdominal wall go into spasm, making the abdomen feel hard, and *peristalsis* (wavelike contractions of the intestinal muscles) stops (see *Ileus, paralytic*). Other symptoms include fever, bloating, nausea, and vomiting. Dehydration and shock may occur.

DIAGNOSIS AND TREATMENT

The condition is diagnosed from a *physical examination* and requires immediate admission to hospital. Prompt surgery may be needed to deal with any underlying cause—for example, removal of a perforated appendix (see *Appendectomy*) or repair of a perforated peptic ulcer. When the cause of the peritonitis is unknown, an exploratory operation called a *laparotomy* may be performed. *Antibiotic drugs* are often given, some-

times delaying surgery. Dehydration is treated by an *intravenous infusion* of fluid.

OUTLOOK

In most cases, the patient makes a full recovery following treatment. Occasionally, however, an abscess develops within the abdomen, requiring more surgery. Intestinal obstruction, resulting from the formation of *adhesions* (fibrous bands of scar tissue between loops of the intestine), may occur later.

Peritonsillar abscess

See *Quinsy.*

Permanent teeth

The second *teeth,* which usually start to replace the primary teeth at about the age of 6. There are 32 permanent teeth, 16 in each jaw. Each set of 16 consists of four incisors (biting teeth) at the front, flanked by two canines (eye teeth), and four premolars and six molars (grinding teeth) at the back of the mouth. (See also *Eruption of teeth.*)

Pernicious anemia

A type of *anemia* caused by a failure to absorb *vitamin B_{12},* which is essential for normal red blood cell production in the bone marrow. A deficiency leads to the production of abnormal, large, red cells. The vitamin is also essential for normal nerve cell metabolism. (See *Anemia, megaloblastic.*)

Pernio

An alternative term for *chilblain.*

Peroneal muscular atrophy

A rare, inherited disorder characterized by wasting of the muscles, first in the feet and calves and then in the hands and forearms. The condition, also known as Charcot-Marie-Tooth disease, is a result of degeneration of some of the peripheral nerves. It can affect either sex, but is more common in boys, and usually appears in late childhood or adolescence.

SYMPTOMS AND SIGNS

Wasting of the muscles stops abruptly halfway up the arms and legs, giving them the appearance of inverted bottles; sensation may be lost in the affected areas. Muscle weakness in the legs causes a characteristic high-stepping walk and clawing of the toes.

TREATMENT AND OUTLOOK

No treatment is available but the condition tends to progress so slowly that the sufferer rarely becomes completely incapacitated; sometimes the deterioration stops for no apparent reason. Life expectancy for an affected person is normal.

Perphenazine

A *phenothiazine*-type *antipsychotic drug* used to relieve symptoms in certain psychiatric disorders, such as *schizophrenia* and to sedate agitated or extremely anxious patients. Perphenazine is occasionally used as an *antiemetic drug* to relieve severe nausea and vomiting caused by anesthesia, *radiation therapy,* chemotherapy, or certain drugs. It has also been prescribed to relieve persistent hiccups.

Possible adverse effects include abnormal movements of the face and limbs, drowsiness, blurred vision, stuffy nose, and headache. Long-term use may cause *parkinsonism.*

Personality

The sum of a person's traits, habits, and experiences. There is much disagreement about precisely what personality is, what defines it, and how it can be assessed. However, the following aspects are usually considered to be important in any definition: temperament, intelligence, and emotion and motivation.

The notion of temperament originates from that of the four ancient humors, which divided people into choleric, melancholic, sanguine, and phlegmatic types. This classification reflects differences in the nature and speed of an individual's responses.

For example, some people are easily angered, while others are placid and react slowly. Intelligence defines a person's capabilities in comparison with a theoretical norm, while emotion and motivation describe feelings, attachments to others, moral standards, and aspirations.

The development of personality seems to depend on the interaction of two basic factors: heredity (the qualities a person is born with) and environment (a person's life experiences that affect his or her ways of thinking and behaving).

Personality disorders

A group of conditions characterized by a general failure to learn from experience or to adapt appropriately to changes, resulting in personal distress and impairment of social functioning.

Personality disorders are not forms of illness, but ways of behaving that may become especially obvious during periods of stress. They are usually first recognizable in adolescence and continue throughout life, often leading to *depression* or *anxiety*. Some people realize that they have personality problems; others fail to see their personalities as in any way unusual or difficult, blaming circumstances, bad luck, or other people for their constant failures in life.

TYPES

Specific types of personality disorders are divided into three groups; there is often overlap among types, particularly within each group.

The first group is characterized primarily by eccentric behavior. Paranoid people show unwarranted suspiciousness and mistrust of others, schizoid people are cold emotionally and have difficulty forming social relationships, and schizotypal personalities show oddities of behavior similar to those of *schizophrenia* victims, although somewhat less severe.

In the second group, behavior tends to be dramatic and emotions intensely expressed. Histrionic individuals are very excitable and constantly crave stimulation, narcissists have an exaggerated sense of their own importance (see *Narcissism*), and those with *antisocial personality disorder* consistently fail to conform to the accepted social standards of behavior. There may be a history of recurrent conflicts with the law.

People in the third group characteristically show anxiety and fear. Included in this group are dependent personalities, who lack self-confidence and cannot function independently (see *Dependence*); compulsive people, who are perfectionists, rigid in their habits, and emotionally cold (see *Obsessive-compulsive disorder*); and passive-aggressive types, who resist demands from others to improve their performances at work and at home.

TREATMENT AND OUTLOOK

The usual forms of treatment are counseling, individual *psychotherapy*, and *behavior therapy*. Treatment is, however, difficult and patients may not comply. It may prove difficult for people with personality disorders to attain goals, such as avoiding the complications of drug abuse or hospitalization, or maintaining personal relationships and jobs. Drug therapy is used only for treating additional illnesses.

Personality tests

Questionnaires designed to define various *personality* traits or types. Personality tests are used to assist in research, and have been used to assess the suitability of candidates or employees for positions in colleges or industry. The validity and reliability of the tests are uncertain.

The Minnesota Multiphasic Personality Inventory (MMPI) has more than 500 questions, some relating to psychiatric symptoms (such as *depression* or *paranoia*) and others relating to underlying personality traits (such as *intelligence*). Another personality test is said to measure "extraversion-introversion" (how outgoing or reserved a person is) and "neuroticism" (predisposition to developing neurotic illness). Closely related to this test is a third questionnaire, in which a person is rated on pairs of factors, such as tense versus relaxed, or timid versus adventurous.

Perspiration

The production and excretion of sweat from the *sweat glands*. Perspiration is another name for sweat.

Perthes' disease

Inflammation of an epiphysis (growing area) of the head of the *femur*. A type of *osteochondritis juvenilis*, Perthes' disease is thought to be due to disrupted blood supply to the bone.

The condition is most common in children aged from 5 to 10, especially in boys, and usually affects one hip. Symptoms include pain in the thigh and groin, and a limp on the affected side. Movement of the hip is restricted and painful. X rays may show flattening, then fragmentation, and, at a later stage, shrinking of the head of the femur.

TREATMENT AND OUTLOOK

Treatment may consist of rest for a few weeks until the pain subsides, followed by splinting of the hip to reduce pressure on the femur, or an operation to change the angle of the head of the femur so that it fits more securely into the pelvis.

Perthes' disease usually clears up by itself within three years, but may leave the hip permanently deformed. Severe deformity may increase the likelihood of *osteoarthritis* later in life.

Pertussis

A distressing infectious disease, also known as whooping cough, which mainly affects infants and young children. The main features of the illness are paroxysms of coughing (during which air is expelled from the chest), often ending in a characteristic "whoop" (during which breath is rapidly drawn in again).

CAUSES AND INCIDENCE

Pertussis is mainly caused by a bacterium, BORDETELLA PERTUSSIS, that is spread from an infected person to others in coughed-out airborne droplets. The disease leads to inflammation of the entire respiratory tract. The illness occurs worldwide. Infants are susceptible from birth, and the illness is most dangerous in the newborn, especially in premature babies. Adults are occasionally affected. Half of all cases occur before the age of 2.

In developed countries, most infants are vaccinated in the first year of life. However, the vaccine is not completely effective in preventing the illness, and not all children are suitable for vaccination.

About 1,000 cases of pertussis are reported in Canada each year.

PREVENTION

The belief that pertussis vaccine is ineffective and unacceptably dangerous is now seen to have been mistaken. Because the illness is potentially serious, it is important that as many infants as possible who are suitable for vaccination be vaccinated. The risks of vaccination are far less than the dangers of having pertussis.

The vaccine is usually given in combination with diphtheria and tetanus vaccines (see *DPT vaccination*). In Canada, DPT vaccination is usually given to infants at around 3, 5, and 9 months of age.

Vaccination against pertussis may cause an infant to become mildly

P

feverish or fretful for a day or two, but this is no cause for concern. Very rarely, in about one in 100,000 cases, an infant may have a severe reaction, with high-pitched screaming or *seizures*. About one in 300,000 babies may suffer permanent brain damage. To lessen these already very small risks, the vaccine is not given to an infant who has a history of seizures, who has a feverish illness, or who has suffered a previous reaction to the vaccine.

Infants should be kept away from anyone with pertussis.

SYMPTOMS AND COMPLICATIONS
After an incubation period of one to three weeks, the illness starts with a mild cough, sneezing, nasal discharge, fever, and sore eyes; this is the period when the child is most infectious. After a few days, the cough becomes more persistent and severe, especially at night. Whooping occurs in most but not all cases. Sometimes the cough induces vomiting. In infants, there is a risk of temporary *apnea* (cessation of breathing) after a coughing spasm.

The illness continues for up to 10 weeks and can be exhausting for the whole family, especially if the child's coughing continues at night.

COMPLICATIONS
Coughing may cause nosebleeds and bleeding from blood vessels on the surface of the eyes. Recurrent vomiting may cause *dehydration* and malnourishment. Chest complications include the development of *pneumonia*, *pneumothorax* (a form of collapsed lung), and *bronchiectasis* (permanent widening of the airways).

DIAGNOSIS
Pertussis is usually diagnosed from the symptoms but the causative bacterium can be grown from a swab taken from the back of the nose (pernasal swab) early in the illness.

TREATMENT
Antibiotic drugs are not particularly helpful once the severe coughing stage of the illness has begun. However, if the illness is recognized early, *erythromycin* is often given. This drug reduces the child's infectivity to others and may shorten the length of the illness.

A child with pertussis should be kept warm, given small, frequent meals and plenty to drink, and protected from stimuli that can cause coughing (such as drafts or smoke). An infant or child who becomes blue or persistently vomits after coughing needs to be admitted to hospital.

Perversion
See *Deviation, sexual*.

Pes cavus
See *Clawfoot*.

Pessary
Any of a variety of devices placed in the vagina. Some types of pessaries are used to correct the position of the uterus (see *Uterus, prolapse of*).

Pesticides
Poisonous chemicals used to eradicate pests of any kind. The most frequently used types are herbicides (weedkillers), insecticides, and fungicides.

Pesticide poisoning, especially in children, may result from swallowing an insecticide or a garden herbicide, such as a chlorate preparation (see *Chlorate poisoning*). Pesticide poisoning also occurs in agricultural workers, often as a result of inhalation or absorption of the chemical through the skin—as in *paraquat* or *parathion* poisoning, for example. Spraying and dusting of farmland increased dramatically in the 1980s.

Exposure to pesticides can also occur indirectly, through eating food in which chemicals have accumulated as a result of repeated spraying of crops. Some authorities blame such foods for insidious long-term damage to health. (See also *DDT*; *Defoliant poisoning*; *Lindane*.)

Petechiae
Red or purple, flat, pinhead spots that occur in the skin or mucous membranes. Petechiae are caused by a localized hemorrhage from small blood vessels. They occur in *purpura* (a group of bleeding disorders) and sometimes in bacterial *endocarditis*.

Pethidine
A synthetic narcotic *analgesic drug* (painkiller) similar to, but less powerful than, *morphine*. Pethidine is given as a *premedication* (a drug used to relax and sedate a person before an operation). It is also used to relieve severe pain after major operations, during childbirth, or, occasionally, in terminal illness.

Since pethidine may cause nausea and vomiting, it is usually given with an *antiemetic drug*.

ABUSE
Pethidine may cause euphoria and is sometimes abused for this effect. Taken regularly, it is likely to cause psychological and physical dependence (see *Drug dependence*).

Petit mal
A type of seizure that occurs in *epilepsy*. Petit mal attacks occur in children and adolescents but rarely persist into adult life. They are characterized by a momentary loss of awareness, occasionally with drooping of the eyelids. Petit mal attacks may occur many times a day, sometimes lasting as long as half a minute each. Treatment is successful with an appropriate *anticonvulsant drug*.

Petroleum jelly
A greasy substance obtained from petroleum, also known as petrolatum or soft paraffin. Petroleum jelly is commonly used as an *ointment* base, as a protective dressing, and as an *emollient* to soothe the skin.

PET scanning
Positron emission tomography, a diagnostic technique based on the detection of positrons (positively charged electrons) emitted by labeled substances introduced into the body. PET scanning produces three-dimensional images that reflect the metabolic and chemical activity of tissues being studied. The images therefore give information about function as well as about structure.

HOW IT WORKS
Substances that take part in biochemical processes in the body are labeled with radioisotopes (radioactive forms of elements, such as carbon 11, nitrogen 13, or oxygen 15). These substances are injected into the bloodstream and are taken up in greater concentrations by areas of tissue that are more metabolically active. In the tissue, the substances emit positrons, which, in turn, release photons. It is the detection of these photons that actually forms the basis of PET scanning.

By surrounding the patient with an array of detectors linked to a com-

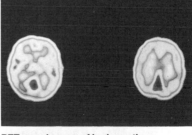

PET scan images of brain sections
Features within the brain appear as light or dark areas according to their uptake of radioactively labeled glucose.

P

puter, the origin of the photons can be computed and a picture built of the distribution of the radioisotope.

WHY IT IS DONE

PET scanning is particularly valuable for investigating the brain. It is used for detecting tumors (which are more or less metabolically active than surrounding brain tissue), for locating the origin of epileptic activity within the brain, and for examining brain function in various mental illnesses.

OUTLOOK

PET scanning equipment is expensive to buy and operate, and is available in only a few centers. However, because PET scanning can provide valuable information not obtainable by other techniques, its use is likely to become more widespread.

Peutz-Jeghers syndrome

An extremely rare, inherited condition in which numerous polyps occur in the gastrointestinal tract and small, flat, brown spots appear on the lips and in the mouth. The syndrome usually produces no symptoms but occasionally the polyps cause abdominal pain, bleed, or lead to *intussusception* (in which the intestine telescopes in on itself and causes obstruction).

Tests may include *barium X-ray examination* and *endoscopy* (inspection through a viewing instrument) of the gastrointestinal tract. Bleeding polyps may be removed.

Peyote

A cactus plant, found in northern Mexico and the southwestern US, of which the dried blossoms are prepared as a *hallucinogenic drug*. The active ingredient is *mescaline*, which produces visual hallucinations and altered consciousness lasting for several hours.

Peyronie's disease

A disorder of the *penis* in which there is thickening of part of the sheath of fibrous connective tissue. Peyronie's disease causes the penis to bend at an angle during erection, usually to one side, commonly making intercourse difficult and painful. The disorder most often affects men over 40 and the cause is unknown.

The thickened area can usually be felt as a firm nodule when the penis is flaccid. Eventually, some of the erectile tissue (spongy tissue within the penis responsible for erection) may also thicken.

In some cases, Peyronie's disease improves without treatment. Local injections of *corticosteroid drugs* sometimes improve the condition. If it persists, the thickened area may be removed surgically and replaced with a graft of normal tissue. In some cases, however, this operation creates more scarring and thereby makes the problem worse.

pH

A measure of the acidity or alkalinity of a solution. The pH scale ranges from 0 to 14, 7 denoting neutrality; the smaller the pH value below 7, the more strongly acidic a solution is; the larger the value above 7, the more strongly alkaline it is.

The pH of body fluids must be maintained very near 7.4 (close to neutrality) for the body's metabolic reactions to proceed properly (see *Acid-base balance*). If the pH falls below about 7.3, the condition is called *acidosis*; if it rises above about 7.5, it is called *alkalosis*.

Phagocyte

 A cell capable of surrounding, engulfing, and digesting microorganisms (such as bacteria and viruses), foreign particles that have entered the body (such as dust inhaled into the lungs), and cellular debris.

Phagocytes form part of the body's *immune system* (natural defenses against infection) and are found in the blood, spleen, and lymph nodes, in the alveoli (small air sacs) within the lungs, and elsewhere. Some types of white *blood cells*, especially granulocytes and some monocytes, are "free" phagocytes, able to wander through the tissues and engulf organisms and debris.

Phalanges

The small bones that make up the skeleton of the fingers, thumb, and toes. Each finger has three phalanges, the thumb and big toe have two, and the other toes have three. The phalanges join at hinge joints moved by muscle tendons.

Phallus

Any object that may symbolize the male penis.

Phantom limb

The perception that a limb is still present after *amputation*. Impulses from the nerves in the victim's remaining stump are interpreted by the brain as if they were coming from the original limb.

Pharmaceutical

Any medicinal *drug*. The term is also used in relation to the manufacture and sale of drugs.

Pharmacist

A licensed, trained health professional who prepares drugs and dispenses them according to physicians' prescriptions and provincial regulations. Pharmacists also ensure that patients have accurate information about prescription drugs and advise on the use of "over-the-counter" drugs.

Pharmacokinetics

The term used to describe how the body deals with a *drug*, including how the drug is absorbed into the bloodstream, distributed to different tissues, broken down, and excreted from the body.

Pharmacology

The branch of science concerned with the discovery and development of drugs; their chemical structure and composition; the ways in which they act in the body; their uses in the prevention or treatment of disease; and with their side effects and toxicity in long-term treatment.

Pharmacologists continually undertake research to help develop new drugs and find new uses for existing drugs. They are concerned with devising methods of synthesizing naturally occurring drugs, producing and sufficiently testing completely new synthetic drugs, finding new combinations of drugs, and modifying existing drugs to extend or improve their effectiveness.

Most drugs today come in prepackaged forms and dosages, but clinical pharmacologists working in hospitals often develop special preparations to meet special needs, and give advice on dosages, methods of administration, contra-indications and side effects.

Pharmacopeia

Any book that lists and describes almost all drugs used in medicine, especially an official national publication. In Canada, the Canadian Pharmaceutical Association publishes an updated pharmacopeia yearly.

Used as a standard book of reference by physicians and pharmacists, a pharmacopeia describes sources, preparations, doses, and tests that can be used to identify individual drugs and to determine their purity.

P

Pharmacopeias may also contain additional information, such as how a drug works, and its possible adverse effects on the patient.

Pharmacy

The practice of preparing drugs, making up prescriptions, and dispensing them; the term is additionally used to describe a place where this activity is carried out.

Pharyngeal diverticulum

An alternative term for a pharyngeal pouch. (See *Esophageal diverticulum*.)

Pharyngeal pouch

An abnormal blind-ending sac that bulges back and down from the top of the esophagus. (See *Esophageal diverticulum*.)

Pharyngitis

Inflammation of the *pharynx* (the part of the throat between the tonsils and the larynx), the chief symptom of which is a *sore throat*. Pharyngitis may be acute or chronic.

CAUSES

Pharyngitis is most often caused by a viral infection. Sometimes it is due to a bacterial infection (e.g., a *streptococcal infection*), rarely to *chlamydial infection* or to infection with *mycoplasma*.

Pharyngitis often occurs as part of a cold (see *Cold, common*) or *influenza*, and may also be an early feature of mononucleosis (see *Mononucleosis, infectious*) or *scarlet fever*. *Diphtheria* is a rare, but serious, cause of pharyngitis.

Pharyngitis may also be caused by swallowing substances that scald, corrode, or scratch the lining of the throat. Inflammation of the pharynx can be aggravated by smoking or by excessive consumption of alcohol.

SYMPTOMS AND SIGNS

In addition to a sore throat, there may be discomfort when swallowing, slight fever, earache, and tender, swollen lymph nodes in the neck. In severe acute cases, the fever may be high and the soft palate and throat may swell so much that breathing and swallowing become difficult. One potential complication is edema (an accumulation of fluid in the tissues) of the larynx (voice box), which is a life-threatening condition.

TREATMENT

Other than gargling with warm salt water, avoiding lying flat, and taking *analgesic drugs* (painkillers), no treatment is usually required; pharyngitis most often clears up on its own. Antiseptic lozenges and sprays may ag-gravate the condition and should therefore be avoided.

Particularly severe and/or prolonged sore throats should be reported to a physician, who may send a throat *swab* sample for analysis and prescribe *antibiotic drugs*. Severe edema of the larynx may require *intubation* (establishment of an air passage by placing a tube through the larynx into the trachea) or *tracheostomy* (creating an opening in the trachea to insert a breathing tube).

Pharynx

The passage that connects the back of the mouth and the nose to the esophagus. This muscular tube, lined with *mucous membrane*, forms part of the respiratory and digestive tracts. The uppermost part, the *nasopharynx* (an air passage), connects the nasal cavity to the region behind the soft *palate* of the mouth. The middle section, the oropharynx (a passage for both air and food), runs from the nasopharynx to below the tongue. The remaining portion, the laryngopharynx (a passage for food only), lies immediately behind and to each side of the larynx and merges with the esophagus.

DISORDERS

Acute *pharyngitis* (inflammation of the pharynx), which causes sore throat, is the most common disorder affecting

---

LOCATION OF THE PHARYNX
The pharynx, or throat, plays an essential part in breathing and eating and can change shape to help form vowel sounds in speech. It has a mucous membrane lining.

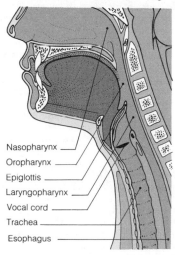

Nasopharynx
Oropharynx
Epiglottis
Laryngopharynx
Vocal cord
Trachea
Esophagus

---

the pharynx. A foreign body, such as a fish bone, may become lodged in the pharynx, causing pain and *choking*.

A pharyngeal pouch (also called Zenker's diverticulum) is a rare disorder in which a small sac develops in the rear wall of the laryngopharynx, the lowest section of the passage (see *Esophageal diverticulum*).

Malignant tumors of the nasopharynx (see *Nasopharynx, cancer of*), though common in the Far East, are rare in the West, as are cancers of the oropharynx and laryngopharynx (see *Pharynx, cancer of*). The latter two have been linked with smoking and heavy drinking.

Pharynx, cancer of

A malignant tumor of the *pharynx* (the passage that connects the back of the mouth and the nose with the esophagus). Pharyngeal cancer usually develops in the squamous (flattened, scalelike) cells of the *mucous membrane* which lines the passage. Tumors of the nasopharynx, the uppermost part of the passage, have different causes and symptoms from those occurring elsewhere in the pharynx (see *Nasopharynx, cancer of*).

CAUSES AND INCIDENCE

In the West, almost all pharyngeal cancer is related to smoking (of pipes and cigars as well as cigarettes) and to drinking alcohol. The highest incidence of pharyngeal cancer is in those who both smoke and drink.

The incidence of this disease rises with age, and the disorder is more common in men.

SYMPTOMS AND SIGNS

Malignant tumors of the oropharynx (the middle section of the pharynx, running from behind the soft palate to below the tongue) usually cause swallowing difficulty, often with a sore throat and earache. In addition, blood-stained sputum (phlegm) may be coughed up. Sometimes the disease causes no more than the feeling of a lump in the throat or a visible enlarged lymph node in the neck.

Cancer of the laryngopharynx (the lowest part of the pharynx, which lies behind the larynx and merges with the esophagus) initially causes an uncomfortable sensation of incomplete swallowing. As the tumor spreads, symptoms include a muffled voice, hoarseness, and increased difficulty in swallowing. A sensation of incomplete swallowing may have a different, harmless cause, but this symptom should in all cases be reported to a physician.

P

DIAGNOSIS
Diagnosis is made from abnormalities found by *biopsy* (removal of a small sample of tissue for analysis). The biopsy is often performed in conjunction with *laryngoscopy*, *bronchoscopy*, and *esophagoscopy* (inspection by means of a viewing tube of the larynx, lungs, and esophagus).

TREATMENT AND OUTLOOK
The growth may be removed surgically or treated with *radiation therapy*. *Anticancer drugs* may also be given. The outlook varies according to the site and type of tumor, its degree of malignancy, the stage of the disease, and the age of the patient.

Phenazopyridine
An analgesic drug that relieves pain in the urinary tract due to inflammation or injury. Phenazopyridine may cause abdominal pain, and may color the urine orange or red.

Phencyclidine
A drug of abuse, commonly known as *angel dust*.

Phenelzine
A monoamine oxidase inhibitor *antidepressant drug*. Like other drugs of this type, phenelzine may cause a dangerous increase in blood pressure if taken with certain drugs, foods, or drinks. For this reason, it is usually given only when other antidepressant drugs have proved ineffective.

Phenelzine may cause dizziness and, rarely, jaundice and rash. Headache, unexplained sweating, nausea, and vomiting may indicate a dangerous rise in blood pressure.

Phenobarbital
A *barbiturate drug* used mainly as an *anticonvulsant drug*. Although phenobarbital has to some extent been replaced by newer anticonvulsant drugs, it is still often used in combination with *phenytoin* to treat *epilepsy*.

Possible adverse effects from taking phenobarbital include drowsiness, clumsiness, dizziness, excitement, and confusion.

Phenothiazine drugs

COMMON DRUGS
Chlorpromazine Fluphenazine Perphenazine Thioridazine Trifluoperazine

A group of drugs widely used to treat psychotic illnesses (see *Antipsychotic drugs*) and to relieve severe nausea and vomiting (see *Antiemetic drugs*).

Phenoxymethylpenicillin
A synthetic *penicillin drug*. Phenoxymethylpenicillin is an *antibiotic drug* which is commonly prescribed to treat a variety of bacterial infections, including pharyngitis, tonsillitis, gum infection, and tooth abscess.

Possible adverse effects include rash and nausea. A few people develop a serious allergic reaction in which there is wheezing, breathing difficulty, and swelling around the mouth and eyes.

Phentermine
An appetite suppressant similar to the *amphetamines*.

Phenylbutazone
A *nonsteroidal anti-inflammatory drug* (NSAID) used to relieve the symptoms of *ankylosing spondylitis*. Because of the risk of adverse effects, phenylbutazone is prescribed only under hospital supervision when other similar drugs have proved ineffective. (Phenylbutazone is sometimes given illegally to improve the performance of lame horses.)

POSSIBLE ADVERSE EFFECTS
Phenylbutazone may cause nausea, fluid retention, rash, and *peptic ulcer*. It may also increase the risk of *blood disorders*, such as agranulocytosis (lack of granulocytes, a type of white blood cell). Regular blood tests are therefore carried out if treatment lasts for longer than one week.

Phenylephrine
A *decongestant drug* commonly used in the treatment of seasonal allergic *rhinitis* (hay fever) and the common *cold*. Phenylephrine has a bronchodilator effect and is included in several preparations used to treat *asthma* and chronic *bronchitis*. In the form of eye drops, phenylephrine is used to dilate the pupils during examination of or surgery on the eyes.

POSSIBLE ADVERSE EFFECTS
Eye drops may irritate the eyes. High doses or prolonged use of nasal preparations may cause headache and blurred vision; suddenly to stop taking the drug may lead to worsening of nasal congestion.

Phenylketonuria
An inherited disorder in which the *enzyme* that converts phenylalanine (an amino acid) into tyrosine (another amino acid) is defective. Unless phenylalanine is excluded from the diet, it builds up in the body and causes severe mental retardation.

INCIDENCE AND DIAGNOSIS
About one baby in 16,000 has phenylketonuria (PKU). All newborn babies are routinely given the *Guthrie test* (sometimes called a PKU test), in which a sample of blood is taken from the baby's heel so that the level of phenylalanine can be checked. If the level of phenylalanine is high, more sensitive tests are carried out during the first few weeks of life.

SYMPTOMS AND SIGNS
Affected newborn babies show few signs of abnormality, but unless phenylalanine is avoided they develop neurological disturbances, including *epilepsy*, early in infancy. Affected children have an unpleasant, musty, mousy smell due to the excretion in the sweat and urine of a breakdown product of phenylalanine. Skin, hair, and eye coloring is often lighter than in other members of the family; 90 percent of affected children have blond hair and blue eyes. Some skeletal changes are associated with phenylketonuria, such as a small head, short stature, and flat feet. About one third to half the patients have eczema.

TREATMENT
The condition is effectively treated by restricting the intake of phenylalanine, which is a natural constituent of most protein-containing foods. Babies must be given special milk substitutes. After weaning, they are given a very low-protein, mainly vegetarian, diet. Some physicians believe that a strict low-protein diet should be followed throughout life. Others maintain that a normal diet can be introduced when a child is 10 to 12 years old; the special diet must be reintroduced during pregnancy, to prevent brain damage in the fetus.

Phenylpropanolamine
A *decongestant drug* commonly used in the treatment of seasonal allergic *rhinitis* (hay fever), *sinusitis*, and the common *cold*.

High doses or prolonged use may cause anxiety and nausea; suddenly to stop taking the drug may lead to worsening of the congestion.

Phenytoin
An *anticonvulsant drug* commonly used as a long-term treatment for *epilepsy*. Phenytoin is also given to treat *trigeminal neuralgia* and infrequently to control certain types of *arrhythmia* (irregularity of the heartbeat).

Prolonged use of phenytoin may cause slurred speech, dizziness, confusion, and overgrowth of the gums.

P

Pheochromocytoma

A rare tumor of cells secreting the hormones *epinephrine* and *norepinephrine*, which regulate heart rate and blood pressure. The tumor increases production of these hormones, causing intermittent or sustained *hypertension* (high blood pressure). Pheochromocytomas may be single or multiple, and usually develop in the medulla (core) of one or both *adrenal glands*. Sometimes they occur in similar tissue in the brain and elsewhere. The tumors may develop at any age but are most common in young to middle-aged adults.

SYMPTOMS AND SIGNS

Most patients have hypertension. At most times, there are usually no other signs or symptoms, but pressure on the area of the tumor, emotional upset, a change in posture, or taking *beta-blocker drugs* can cause a surge of hormones from the tumor. This surge in hormones brings on a sudden rise in blood pressure, rapid pulse, palpitations, headache, nausea, vomiting, clammy skin, and sometimes a feeling of impending death.

DIAGNOSIS AND TREATMENT

Diagnosis of pheochromocytoma involves blood and urine tests to check for excessive epinephrine and norepinephrine and related substances. *CT scanning* and *radioisotope scanning* may be used to locate tumors.

Treatment consists of surgical removal of the tumors. Before surgery, drugs are usually given to control the patient's blood pressure. The outlook after treatment is very good in almost all cases. In some patients, hypertension recurs and requires treatment with drugs.

Pheromone

An odorous substance, released in minute quantities by an animal, that affects the behavior or development of other individuals of the same species. Although humans also give off distinctive body odors, it is questionable whether or not these are true pheromones, able to alter the behavior of other humans.

Phimosis

Tightness of the foreskin, preventing it from being drawn back over the underlying glans (head) of the *penis*.

In uncircumcised males, some degree of phimosis is normal until the age of 6 months. In some boys it persists for several years, sometimes making it difficult to pass urine and causing the foreskin to balloon out on urination. Phimosis prevents proper cleaning of the glans, leading to *balanitis* (infection of the glans). There may also be an increased risk of cancer (see *Penis, cancer of*). Phimosis makes erection painful and may lead to *paraphimosis* (constriction of the penis behind the glans). Phimosis is treated by *circumcision*.

Phlebitis

Inflammation of a vein, often accompanied by clot formation. The preferred medical name for this condition is *thrombophlebitis*.

Phlebography

The obtaining and interpretation of X-ray images of veins after they have been injected with a radiopaque substance. Phlebography is an alternative name for *venography*.

Phlebotomy

Puncture of a vein for the purpose of removing blood (see *Venipuncture; Venesection.*)

Phlegm

See *Sputum*.

Phobia

A persistent, irrational fear of, and desire to avoid, a particular object or situation. Many people have minor phobias—an illogical fear of spiders for example—that may cause them some distress but that do not impair their ability to cope with everyday life. It is only when a fear causes significant disturbance and interferes with normal social functioning that it is considered a psychiatric disorder.

TYPES

Simple phobias, also known as specific phobias, are the most common. These may involve fear of particular animals (most often dogs, snakes, spiders, or mice) or of particular situations, such as enclosed spaces (*claustrophobia*), heights, or air travel. Animal phobias usually start in childhood, but other forms may develop at any time. Treatment is not usually required, unless the feared object is so common that it is not easily avoided (e.g., fear of escalators in a person who lives in a large city).

Agoraphobia (fear of open spaces or of entering public places) is a more serious type of phobia, often causing severe impairment and disruption of family life. It is the most common phobia for which treatment is sought. The disorder usually starts in the late teens or early 20s.

Social phobia, which is relatively rare, is fear of being exposed to the scrutiny of others. Examples include fear of eating, speaking, or performing in public, using public toilets, or writing in the presence of others. The disorder usually begins in late childhood or early adolescence.

CAUSES

According to some theories, simple phobias are a form of learned response (see *Conditioning*). People with such phobias have often been brought up by someone with a similar fear or have had an early frightening experience that has become associated with the feared object or situation. According to other theories, the phobia has a symbolic meaning (e.g., a fear of snakes may result from repressed sexual feelings).

SYMPTOMS

Exposure to the feared object or situation causes intense *anxiety* and sometimes a *panic attack*. Phobic individuals may also suffer from *depression* and generalized anxiety and may indulge in minor obsessional rituals (see *Obsessive-compulsive disorder*). People with agoraphobia or social phobia may attempt to relieve their anxiety with alcohol, barbiturate drugs, or antianxiety drugs, and may become psychologically dependent on them, thus compounding the problems.

TREATMENT

The most effective treatment is *behavior therapy*, sometimes combined with *antidepressant drugs*. People with social phobia may benefit from training in social skills.

Phocomelia

A type of *limb defect* in which the feet and/or the hands are joined to the trunk by short, stubby stumps resembling seal fins. The condition is rare and has occurred mostly in children whose mothers took the drug *thalidomide* early in pregnancy.

Phosphates

Salts containing phosphorus and oxygen. Phosphates are an essential part of the diet and are present in many foods, including cereals, dairy products, eggs, and meat.

FUNCTION

About 85 percent of the body's phosphorus is combined with calcium to form the structure of bone and teeth. The remainder is deposited in small amounts in most of the body's tissues and plays a part in maintaining the acid-alkaline balance of the blood, urine, saliva, and other body fluids.

P

ATP (adenosine triphosphate) is a phosphate compound which stores energy for chemical reactions in cells.

DISORDERS

In most people, the kidneys maintain a constant level of phosphates in the body by regulating the amount excreted in the urine. A slight deficiency of phosphates in the diet is compensated for by a reduction in the amount lost in the urine.

Hypophosphatemia (an abnormally low level of phosphates in the blood) may occur in some forms of kidney disease, *hyperparathyroidism*, long-term treatment with *diuretic drugs*, *malabsorption*, or prolonged starvation. It causes bone pain, weakness, seizures, and, in severe cases, coma and death.

DRUG THERAPY

Phosphates may be taken by mouth in the form of drug preparations or milk to treat hypophosphatemia. Phosphates are also used to treat *hypercalcemia*. Diarrhea is a possible side effect of phosphate drugs.

Phosphorus poisoning

There are two forms of phosphorus—yellow and red. Yellow phosphorus is readily absorbed by the body and is highly poisonous. Red phosphorus cannot be absorbed and is nontoxic.

Yellow phosphorus is used in matches, fireworks, some insecticides, and certain rodent poisons. It may cause serious burns if it comes into contact with the skin. Most cases of poisoning occur in industrial workers who accidentally ingest the chemical or inhale its vapor. Acute poisoning, due to absorption of comparatively large amounts of phosphorus over a short period, causes damage to the liver, kidneys, central nervous system, and other organs.

Symptoms of acute phosphorus poisoning include burning abdominal pain, an odor of garlic on the breath, nausea, vomiting, bloody diarrhea, jaundice, and symptoms of *kidney failure* and *liver failure*. In severe cases, or untreated milder ones, delirium, seizures, unconsciousness, and death may occur within about 48 hours.

Chronic poisoning, due to taking in small amounts of phosphorus over a relatively long period, may cause gradual destruction of the jaw bones (a condition known as phosphonecrosis or phossy jaw), *cirrhosis* of the liver, and kidney damage. This is now very uncommon.

Treatment of acute poisoning consists of washing out the stomach (see *Lavage, gastric*) with copper sulfate, along with injections of calcium and treatment for liver and kidney failure.

Photocoagulation

The destructive heating of tissue by intense light focused to a fine point, as in *laser treatment*. Photocoagulation is used to treat disorders of the retina, especially diabetic retinopathy.

Photophobia

An uncomfortable sensitivity or intolerance to light. Photophobia occurs with some eye disorders, such as *corneal abrasion*, *corneal ulcer*, acute *iritis* (inflammation of the iris), and congenital *glaucoma* (raised pressure in the eyeball). Photophobia is also a feature of *meningitis* (inflammation of the membranes that surround the brain and spinal cord).

Photosensitivity

Abnormal reaction to sunlight. Photosensitivity usually takes the form of a skin rash that occurs as a reaction to the effects of light on the skin. This reaction often occurs because a substance has been ingested, or applied to the skin. Examples of such substances, called photosensitizers, are certain drugs, dyes, chemicals used in perfumes and soaps, and plants such as buttercups, parsnips, and mustard.

Photosensitivity is also a feature of certain disorders that affect internal organs as well as the skin, such as systemic *lupus erythematosus* and *porphyria*. In such disorders, exposure to light may worsen the condition.

TREATMENT

Known photosensitizers should be avoided when possible. If the reaction occurs independently of photosensitizers, a susceptible person should avoid exposure to sunlight, especially between 10 a.m. and 4 p.m. (when the light is at its most intense) and should use *sunscreen* preparations.

Phototherapy

Treatment with light, involving the use of sunlight, nonvisible ultraviolet light, visible blue light, or *lasers*.

Moderate exposure to sunlight is the most basic form of phototherapy. This is helpful in treating about 75 percent of people with *psoriasis*.

A newer form of phototherapy, *PUVA*, combines the use of long-wave ultraviolet light with a *psoralen drug* (e.g., methoxsalen), which sensitizes the skin to light. PUVA is particularly effective in treating psoriasis and is also used in treating some other skin diseases (e.g., *vitiligo* and *mycosis fungoides*). Short-wave ultraviolet light, sometimes combined with application of coal tar, may also be used to treat psoriasis. Several treatments are given; the exposure time is gradually increased according to the reaction of the patient's skin to the therapy.

Visible blue light is used in the treatment of jaundice in the newborn (see *Jaundice, neonatal*), which is caused by accumulation of the bile pigment bilirubin as a result of an insufficiently developed liver. The light is thought to cause the chemical breakdown of bilirubin, allowing it to be excreted in the urine. With his or her eyes shielded, the infant is completely exposed to the light for 12 hours or more; he or she may need additional fluids to compensate for water loss.

Phototherapy is also used to treat *seasonal affective disorder syndrome*.

Phrenic nerve

Either of the two principal nerves supplying the *diaphragm*. Each nerve carries motor impulses to, and some of the sensory impulses from, the diaphragm, and plays an important part in controlling breathing. The phrenic nerves arise from the third, fourth, and fifth cervical nerves in the neck, and pass down through the chest each to one side of the diaphragm. Injury

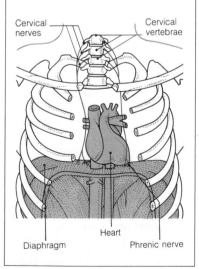

LOCATION OF PHRENIC NERVES
There are two phrenic nerves, one on each side of the body. Each follows a tortuous course from its origin in the neck, through the chest, to the diaphragm.

Cervical nerves

Cervical vertebrae

Heart

Diaphragm

Phrenic nerve

P

to, or surgical cutting of, one of the nerves results in paralysis of one half of the diaphragm. The phrenic nerve may be deliberately crushed to produce temporary paralysis of the diaphragm after an operation to repair a *hiatal hernia*, or as a rare treatment for intractable *hiccups*. In the past, crushing was performed to treat lung disorders such as *tuberculosis*.

Physical examination
See *Examination, physical*.

Physical medicine and rehabilitation
A branch of medicine concerned with the care of patients who have been disabled as a result either of injuries, or of illness, especially strokes or other neurological disorders. The physician responsible for the patient makes a careful assessment before drawing up a rehabilitation program and enlisting the help of other professionals (for example, physiotherapists, nurses, occupational therapists, and speech therapists).

Physician
A person licensed to practice medicine. (See *Intern; Medical licensure; Medical specialist; Resident physician*.)

Physiology
The study of the functioning of the body, including the physical and chemical processes of its cells, tissues, organs, and systems, and their various interactions. Along with *anatomy* (the study of body structure), physiology constitutes the foundation of all medical science.

Strictly, physiology is concerned with normal functioning, but the boundary between normality and abnormality is not always distinct. Thus a specialty has developed called pathophysiology, which is concerned with the functional changes associated with diseases and disorders. There are also other physiological specialties, such as renal physiology (the study of kidney function), and endocrine physiology (the study of the functions of endocrine glands).

Physiotherapy
Treatment of disorders or injuries with physical methods or agents.

Physiotherapy is used to prevent or reduce joint stiffness and to restore muscle strength in the treatment of arthritis or after a fracture has healed. It is also used to reduce pain, inflammation, and muscle spasm and to retrain joints and muscles after stroke or nerve injury.

Methods of treatment used by physiotherapists include exercises, which may be active or passive (see illustrated box), *massage, heat treatment* (including *ultrasound treatment* and short-wave *diathermy*), cold (see *Ice packs*), water (see *Hydrotherapy*), and electrical currents (as in *TENS*).

Physiotherapy is also concerned with the maintenance of breathing capacity in people with impaired lung function or the prevention and treatment of pulmonary complications following surgery. Physiotherapists help treat severe respiratory diseases (such as chronic *bronchitis*) and care for the respiratory needs of patients who are on *ventilators* or recovering from major operations. Techniques used include *breathing exercises, percussion, postural drainage*, and the administration of oxygen, drugs, or moisture to the lungs through a *nebulizer*.

Physostigmine
A drug used in the form of eye drops to treat *glaucoma* (raised pressure in the eyeball).

Phytomenadione
Also called phytonadione, this compound is a synthetic form of vitamin K, which is essential for blood clotting. It is used in treating bleeding disorders, and is the only drug that can reverse the bleeding induced by oral *anticoagulant drugs*. The most common side effect is flushing.

Phytonadione
See *Phytomenadione*.

Pica
A craving to eat substances (such as earth, coal, chalk, or wood) that are not food. Pica sometimes occurs dur-

P

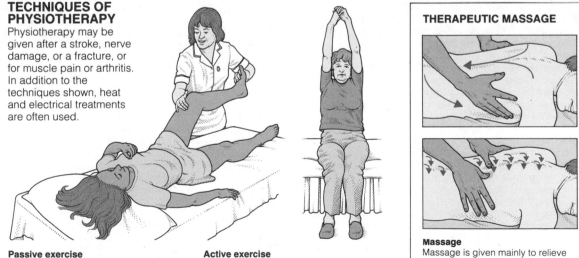

TECHNIQUES OF PHYSIOTHERAPY
Physiotherapy may be given after a stroke, nerve damage, or a fracture, or for muscle pain or arthritis. In addition to the techniques shown, heat and electrical treatments are often used.

Passive exercise
The therapist moves the affected part. This preserves joint mobility and is valuable after nerve injuries and in the treatment of diseases such as polio.

Active exercise
The patient is taught to contract and relax certain muscle groups or to perform specific movements (e.g., exercising the arm muscles after a stroke).

THERAPEUTIC MASSAGE

Massage
Massage is given mainly to relieve muscle pain and spasm. Long, sweeping strokes can be alternated with "circling" techniques.

ing pregnancy and may be a feature of various nutritional or iron-deficiency disorders. It may also occur in severe psychiatric disorders.

Pickwickian syndrome

An unusual disorder characterized by extreme *obesity*, abnormally shallow breathing, excessive sleepiness, and *sleep apnea*. It is named after the fat boy Joe in Charles Dickens' "Pickwick Papers." The cause of the disorder is unclear. Symptoms usually improve with weight loss.

PID

See *Pelvic inflammatory disease.*

Pigeon toes

A minor abnormality in which the leg or foot is rotated, forcing the foot and toes to point inward.

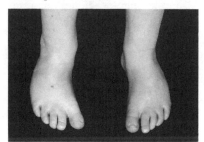

Appearance of pigeon toes
This is a common condition in toddlers. In almost all cases it requires no treatment and corrects itself by about the age of 7.

Pigmentation

Coloration of the skin, hair, and iris of the eyes by *melanin* (a brown or black pigment produced by special cells called melanocytes). The greater the amount of melanin present, the darker the coloration. The amount of melanin produced is determined by heredity and by exposure to sunlight. Blood pigments can also color skin (such as in a bruise).

ABNORMALITIES OF PIGMENTATION
LIGHTENED SKIN Patches of pale skin occur in various skin disorders. In *psoriasis*, *pityriasis alba*, and *pityriasis versicolor*, skin scales flake off, resulting in loss of melanin. In *vitiligo*, areas of skin stop producing melanin.

The rare, inherited condition *albinism* is caused by generalized melanin deficiency, resulting in pale skin and white hair. In *phenylketonuria*, another genetic condition, sufferers have a reduced melanin level, making them paler-skinned and fairer-haired than other members of the family.

DARKENED SKIN Patches of dark skin mingled with lighter areas may follow an episode of *eczema* or psoriasis, or may occur in pityriasis versicolor. In *chloasma*, hormonal changes cause dark areas to develop on the face; this condition may occur in women who are taking oral contraceptives, or during pregnancy or the menopause. Dark facial patches may also be caused by some perfumes and cosmetics, particularly when they contain chemicals that cause *photosensitivity*. Such discolorations usually fade with time.

Permanent areas of pronounced deep pigmentation are usually due to an abnormality of the melanocytes, as is the case with freckles and moles (see *Nevus*). *Acanthosis nigricans*, which may be inherited or acquired, is characterized by dark patches of velvetlike, thickened skin, primarily in body creases.

Darkening of the skin, unrelated to sun exposure, may occur in certain hormonal disorders, such as *Addison's disease* and *Cushing's syndrome*.

OTHER SKIN DISCOLORATION Some abnormal skin pigmentation is caused by an excessive blood level of other pigments. An excess of the bile pigment bilirubin in *jaundice* turns the skin yellow, and too much iron in *hemochromatosis* turns the skin bronze. Discoloration may also be caused by an abnormal collection of blood vessels, such as the one that produces a portwine stain (see *Hemangioma*).

Piles

The common name for *hemorrhoids*.

Pill, contraceptive

See *Oral contraceptives*.

Pilocarpine

A drug obtained from PILOCARPUS plants, used to treat *glaucoma* (raised pressure in the eyeball). Because pilocarpine causes the pupils to constrict, it is also used to reverse dilation (widening) of the pupils (which may be caused by drugs given during surgery or examination of the eyes).

Pilocarpine may initially cause blurred vision, headache, and irritation of the eyes.

Pilonidal sinus

A pit in the skin, often containing hairs, in the upper part of the cleft between the buttocks. Pilonidal sinus is probably caused by hair fragments burrowing inward. The condition is usually harmless, but the pit can become infected, resulting in recurrent painful abscesses.

Treatment of an infected sinus is by surgical removal of a wide area around the infection; the wound is usually left open to allow slow healing. Recurrence is common; plastic surgery is occasionally required.

Pimozide

An *antipsychotic drug*, which is also used in the treatment of *Gilles de la Tourette's syndrome*. Pimozide may cause sedation, dry mouth, constipation, and blurred vision.

Pimple

A common name for a small *pustule* or *papule*. Pimples are usually found on the face, neck, or back, particularly in adolescents suffering from *acne*.

Pindolol

A *beta-blocker drug* used in the treatment of *angina pectoris* (chest pain due to inadequate blood supply to the heart muscle), *arrhythmias* (irregularities of the heartbeat), and *hypertension* (high blood pressure). In addition, pindolol is currently under investigation for the control of *glaucoma* (raised pressure in the eyeball).

Pindolol is less likely than some beta-blocker drugs to cause *bradycardia* (abnormally slow heartbeat). Otherwise, possible adverse effects are typical of other beta-blocker drugs.

Pineal gland

A tiny, cone-shaped structure within the brain, whose sole function appears to be the secretion of the hormone *melatonin*. The amount of hormone secreted varies over a 24-hour cycle, being greatest at night. Control over this secretion is possibly exerted through nerve pathways from the retina in the eye; a high light level seems to inhibit secretion. The exact function of melatonin is not understood, but it may help to synchronize circadian (24-hour) and other *biorhythms*.

The pineal gland is situated deep within the brain, just below the back part of the corpus callosum (the band of nerve fibers that connects the two halves of the cerebrum). In rare cases, it is the site of a tumor.

Pinguecula

A small, benign, yellowish spot on the *conjunctiva* over the exposed areas of the white of the eye. Pingueculas are sometimes attributed to ultraviolet radiation in sunlight, and are common in elderly people. Some pingueculas are removed for cosmetic reasons.

P

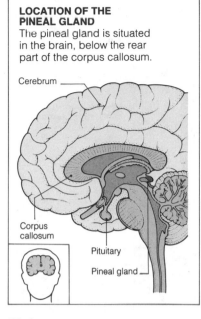

LOCATION OF THE PINEAL GLAND
The pineal gland is situated in the brain, below the rear part of the corpus callosum.

Cerebrum

Corpus callosum

Pituitary

Pineal gland

Pinkeye
A common name for *conjunctivitis*.

Pink puffer
A term sometimes used by physicians to describe some patients with chronic lung disease (see *Lung disease, chronic obstructive*).

Pinna
The fleshy part of the outer *ear*, consisting of a flap of cartilage and skin. It is also known as the auricle. The pinna appears to have little practical value; its loss barely affects hearing. Cosmetic problems of the pinna (e.g., *cauliflower ear*) can usually be corrected by plastic surgery (see *Otoplasty*).

Pins and needles
Medically called paresthesia, a tingling or prickly feeling in an area of skin. It is usually associated with *numbness* (loss of sensation) and occasionally with a burning sensation.

Temporary pins and needles are caused by a disturbance in the conduction of impulses through nerves that carry sensation from the skin to the brain (e.g., after sleeping with an arm bent awkwardly under the body). Persistent pins and needles may be caused by *neuropathy* (any of a group of nerve disorders).

Pinta
A skin infection occurring in some remote villages in tropical America. The organism responsible, *TREPO-*

NEMA CARATEUM, is closely related to the bacterium that causes *syphilis*. It is uncertain how the disease is transmitted. A large spot, surrounded by smaller ones, appears on the face, neck, buttocks, hands, or feet, and, one to 12 months later, is followed by red skin patches that turn blue, then brown, and finally white. A *penicillin drug* or *tetracycline* clears up the infection, but the skin may be left permanently disfigured.

Pinworm infestation
A common infestation with a small parasitic worm, *ENTEROBIUS VERMICULARIS*, that lives in the intestines. Pinworms primarily affect children and are the most common worm parasite of children in temperate areas. Possibly one fifth of all children in Canada are affected by this parasite at any time.

The female adult pinworms are white and about 10 mm long. They lay eggs in the skin around the anus, and their movements cause tickling or itching in the anal region, often at night, which may cause the child to scratch. Eggs are transferred directly via the fingers to the mouth to cause reinfestation, or are carried on toys or blankets to other children. Swallowed eggs hatch in the intestine and the worms reach maturity after a period of two to six weeks.

DIAGNOSIS AND TREATMENT
Adult worms can sometimes be seen in the feces or on the buttocks. Pin-

worm eggs for microscopic examination can be obtained by applying a piece of sticky paper to the anal area.

Ointments may be used to relieve anal itching. An *anthelmintic drug*, in combination with good hygiene, usually clears up the problem. Treatment of all members of the family is advisable.

Preventative and self-help measures include the wearing of pyjamas to discourage scratching, keeping the fingernails short, and washing the hands scrupulously before all meals. Sheets and nightwear should be changed frequently, washed at high temperature, and ironed.

Piperazine
An *anthelmintic drug* used to treat roundworm and *pinworm infestation*. Piperazine paralyzes the worms, which are then expelled with the feces. The drug is usually taken once a day for seven days to clear pinworms and as a single dose for roundworms. A laxative drug may also be given to speed up the expulsion.

Possible adverse effects of piperazine include abdominal pain, nausea, vomiting, and diarrhea.

Piroxicam
A *nonsteroidal anti-inflammatory drug* (NSAID) used to relieve the symptoms of types of arthritis, such as *osteoarthritis*, *rheumatoid arthritis*, and *gout*. Piroxicam is also used to relieve pain in *bursitis*, *tendinitis*, and after minor surgery.

 P

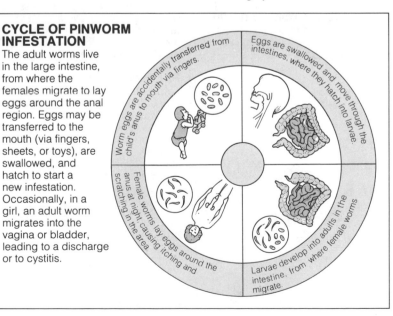

CYCLE OF PINWORM INFESTATION
The adult worms live in the large intestine, from where the females migrate to lay eggs around the anal region. Eggs may be transferred to the mouth (via fingers, sheets, or toys), are swallowed, and hatch to start a new infestation. Occasionally, in a girl, an adult worm migrates into the vagina or bladder, leading to a discharge or to cystitis.

Possible adverse effects of piroxicam include nausea, indigestion, abdominal pain, swollen ankles, *peptic ulcer*, and liver problems.

Pituitary gland

Sometimes referred to as the master gland, the pituitary is the most important of the *endocrine glands* (glands that release hormones directly into the bloodstream). The pituitary regulates and controls the activities of other endocrine glands and many body processes (see *Endocrine system*).

STRUCTURE

The pituitary is a pea-sized structure that hangs from the base of the brain, just below the optic nerves. It is attached by a short stalk of nerve fibers to the *hypothalamus*, a region of the brain that controls the function of the pituitary by nervous stimulation and by hormone-releasing factors. The pituitary consists of three lobes known from their relative positions as the anterior, intermediate, and posterior.

FUNCTION

The different lobes of the pituitary produce a range of hormones.

The anterior pituitary produces six hormones: *growth hormone*, which stimulates growth; *prolactin*, which stimulates production of milk after giving birth (see *Breast-feeding*); *ACTH* (adrenocorticotropic hormone), which stimulates hormone production by the adrenal glands; TSH (thyroid-stimulating hormone), which stimulates hormone pro-

HORMONES SECRETED BY THE PITUITARY GLAND

Growth hormone stimulates cell division and protein synthesis in tissues such as bone and cartilage, leading to growth.

Thyroid-stimulating hormone (TSH) stimulates the thyroid gland to secrete various hormones vital to body metabolism.

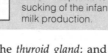
Adrenocorticotropic hormone (ACTH) stimulates the adrenal glands to secrete hormones, with multiple effects on metabolism.

Prolactin stimulates female breast development, and, in response to sucking of the infant, milk production.

Luteinizing and follicle-stimulating hormones (LH and FSH) help control the function of male and female sex organs.

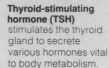
Melanocyte-stimulating hormone (MSH) controls skin darkening by stimulating pigment cells.

Antidiuretic hormone (ADH) acts on the kidneys to decrease water loss in the urine and thus reduces urine volume.

Oxytocin stimulates contraction of the uterus during childbirth and milk release from the breasts.

duction by the *thyroid gland*; and the *gonadotropins* FSH (follicle-stimulating hormone) and LH (luteinizing hormone), which stimulate the *gonads*.

The intermediate part of the pituitary secretes one hormone, melanocyte-stimulating hormone (MSH), which controls darkening of the skin.

The posterior pituitary produces two hormones—*ADH* (antidiuretic hormone), which increases reabsorption of water into the blood by the kidneys and therefore decreases urine production; and *oxytocin*, which stimulates contractions of the uterus during labor and the secretion of milk during breast-feeding.

Pituitary tumors

Growths that arise in the *pituitary gland*. Pituitary tumors are rare, comprising about 10 percent of primary *brain tumors*. Most are benign (noncancerous). However, because the pituitary is situated in a bony hollow at the base of the skull, enlargement of the tumor is upward, where it tends to press on the *optic nerves*, causing visual field defects.

CAUSES AND TYPES

The causes of pituitary tumors are unknown. The most common type is called an endocrine inactive tumor. As it grows, it leads to destruction of some of the hormone-secreting cells in the gland, which causes hypopituitarism (reduced hormone production). This often leads to a failure of

sexual function, with cessation of menstrual periods in women and reduced sperm production in men.

Other types of tumors cause the gland to produce too much of a particular hormone. For example, a tumor of the anterior pituitary can cause excess growth hormone production, leading to *gigantism* or *acromegaly*. Too much thyroid-stimulating hormone (TSH) can lead to *hyperthyroidism*. Excess adrenocorticotropic hormone (ACTH) can cause *Cushing's syndrome*. Finally, an increased production of prolactin can cause *galactorrhea* (abnormal milk production), absence of menstrual periods, and infertility in women. In men, it can cause impotence, infertility, feminization, and galactorrhea. Tumors that affect the posterior pituitary may disrupt production of antidiuretic hormone (ADH) and lead to *diabetes insipidus*.

The diagnosis is made from measurements of the levels of different hormones in the blood and urine, from *CT scanning* or *MRI* of the brain, and usually also from visual field testing (see *Vision tests*).

Treatment may be by surgical excision, by *radiation therapy*, by replacement of missing hormones, or by a combination of these techniques. The drug *bromocriptine* is sometimes used to treat pituitary tumors that secrete prolactin or growth hormone because this medication suppresses production of these hormones.

P

LOCATION OF PITUITARY GLAND

This master gland is itself controlled by the hypothalamus, located immediately above it.

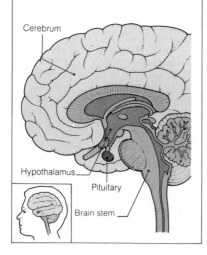

Cerebrum

Hypothalamus

Pituitary

Brain stem

DISORDERS OF THE PITUITARY GLAND

Any abnormality of the pituitary gland usually means that it produces either too much or too little of one or more hormones, and this causes changes elsewhere in the body. Locally, serious effects may be caused by enlargement of the gland; for example, it may press on the nearby optic nerves and cause visual defects.

CONGENITAL AND GENETIC DISORDERS

Deficiency of *growth hormone* may be a genetic disorder, or it may be due to congenital absence or undergrowth of the pituitary, or to damage to the gland sustained during birth. Whatever the cause, deficiency of growth hormone leads to *short stature*.

Congenital growth hormone deficiency may also be associated with deficiency of other pituitary hormones, notably *ACTH* (adrenocorticotropic hormone), *gonadotropin hormone*, and thyroid-stimulating hormone (TSH).

TUMORS

Pituitary tumors are usually benign but may cause either overproduction of pituitary hormones (hyperpituitarism) or underproduction (hypopituitarism).

INJURY

Birth injury may cause loss of pituitary function, as may head injuries at any age.

IMPAIRED BLOOD SUPPLY

Rarely, the pituitary may suffer deprivation of its blood supply as a result of pressure on its blood vessels from a growing tumor. This may cause a sudden loss of pituitary function, which may be fatal, or a more gradual loss, which produces signs of general underactivity of the gland. A similar deprivation of blood supply may occur as a complication of massive blood loss associated with childbirth (Sheehan's syndrome). This may lead to failure of milk production, and a wide range of secondary effects due to the resultant underactivity of other endocrine glands.

Impaired blood supply may also occur from *vasculitis*, or from pressure on the gland from an *aneurysm* of a nearby artery.

RADIATION

Radiation therapy for a pituitary tumor may cause general underactivity of the gland.

INVESTIGATION

Techniques used to investigate pituitary disorders include analysis of the levels of pituitary hormones in the blood or urine, and of hormones from other endocrine glands under pituitary control; *X rays*, *CT scanning*, or *MRI* of the pituitary; and *angiography*, to show displacement of blood vessels by a pituitary tumor. A visual field test (see *Vision tests*) may be done.

Pityriasis alba

A common skin condition of children and adolescents in which irregular, fine, scaly, pale patches appear on the face, usually the cheeks.

Pityriasis alba is caused by mild *eczema* and is often more pronounced after exposure to sun because the patches tan poorly. The condition usually clears up with emollients.

Pityriasis rosea

A common mild skin disorder in which flat, scaly-edged, round or oval, dark pink or copper-colored spots appear over the trunk and upper arms. The rash may be associated with a viral infection, and is preceded about a week beforehand by a single, larger, round spot (called a herald patch) on the trunk.

Pityriasis rosea is not contagious. The condition mainly affects children and young adults. Its cause is unknown.

The rash, which lasts for about six to eight weeks, can occasionally cause itching but is otherwise symptomless. Although the rash usually clears up without treatment, a physician should be consulted to rule out other conditions that cause similar rashes.

Calamine lotion alleviates mild itching; more severe itching can be relieved by *antihistamine drugs*.

Pityriasis versicolor

See *Tinea versicolor*.

Pivampicillin

A penicillin-type antibiotic drug. (See *Penicillin drugs*.)

Pivmecillinam

A penicillin-type antibiotic drug used mainly in the treatment of cystitis. (See *Penicillin drugs*.)

Pizotyline

An *antihistamine drug* used to prevent migraine headaches in people who suffer frequent, disabling attacks. The exact mechanism of action is not known but pizotifen is thought to block the effects of the chemicals histamine and serotonin on blood vessels in the brain.

Possible adverse effects include nausea, dizziness, drowsiness, dry mouth, and muscle pains. Pizotifen increases appetite, and prolonged use often causes weight gain.

PKU test

See *Guthrie test*; *Phenylketonuria*.

Placebo

A chemically inert substance given in place of a *drug*. Some physicians may prescribe a placebo if symptoms, such as fatigue, are not caused by an illness that requires drug treatment. The benefit gained from taking a placebo occurs because the person taking it believes it will have a positive effect.

Since the effectiveness of any drug may be due in part to this "placebo effect," which is based on a person's expectations of the drug, many new drugs are tested against a placebo preparation. The placebo is made to look and taste identical to the active preparation; volunteers are not told which preparation they are taking. A comparison of the results enables a more accurate assessment of the drug's efficacy.

Placenta

The organ that develops in the uterus during *pregnancy* and links the blood supplies of the mother and baby for the exchange of nutrients and oxygen.

STRUCTURE

The placenta develops from the chorion (the outermost layer of cells that develops from the fertilized egg). It is firmly attached to the lining of the woman's uterus and is connected to the baby by the umbilical cord. By the end of pregnancy it is about 20 cm wide and 2.5 cm thick. Shortly after the baby is born, the placenta is expelled with other redundant tissues (all together being given the common name, "afterbirth").

P

FUNCTION OF THE PLACENTA

The mother's and baby's blood do not completely mix in the placenta, but are brought sufficiently close so that exchange of nutrients and oxygen (from mother to baby) and waste products (from baby to mother) can occur between the two blood circulations.

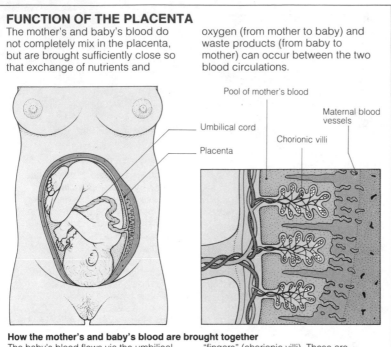

How the mother's and baby's blood are brought together
The baby's blood flows via the umbilical cord to the placenta, where it enters numerous tiny blood vessels arranged in "fingers" (chorionic villi). These are surrounded by a pool of maternal blood brought to the placenta by a major artery.

FUNCTION

The placenta acts as an organ of respiration and excretion for the fetus. It transfers oxygen from the mother's circulation into the fetus's circulation, and removes waste products from the fetus's blood into the mother's blood for excretion by her lungs and kidneys. The placenta also conveys nutrients from mother to baby.

The placenta produces hormones such as *estrogen*, *progesterone*, and human chorionic gonadotropin (HCG; see *Gonadotropin, human chorionic*). High levels of HCG appear in the woman's urine during early pregnancy and detection of them in the urine forms the basis of *pregnancy tests*. The hormones enter the mother's blood to help her body adapt to the conditions of pregnancy; they also prepare the breasts for lactation (see *Breast-feeding*).

Placenta previa

Implantation of the *placenta* in the lower part of the *uterus*, near or over the cervix. Placenta previa occurs in about one in 200 pregnancies; it is less common in first pregnancies.

The condition varies in severity, depending on how much of the placenta is situated close to the cervix. In some cases, mild placenta previa is detected during routine *ultrasound scanning* but has no adverse effect on the pregnancy. More severe placenta previa often causes sudden painless vaginal bleeding in late pregnancy, when placental tissue separates from the uterus.

If the bleeding is slight and the pregnancy still has several weeks to run, bed rest may be all that is necessary. If the bleeding stops, the woman may be allowed to get up but she will probably be advised to remain in hospital until the baby is born because of the risk of sudden severe hemorrhage. The baby is usually delivered by *cesarean section* at the 38th week.

If the bleeding is heavy or if the pregnancy is near term, an immediate delivery is carried out.

Placenta, tumors of

See *Choriocarcinoma; Hydatidiform mole*.

Plague

 A serious infectious disease that mainly affects rodents but is transmissible to humans by the bites of rodent fleas. Plague has been a scourge to people since early history. One of the largest pandemics (world-wide epidemics) was the "black death" of the 14th century, which killed 25 million people in Europe alone. Today, human plague occurs sporadically in various parts of the world. Now, however, outbreaks can be treated with antibiotic drugs.

CAUSES, TYPES, AND INCIDENCE

The bacterium responsible for the disease, YERSINIA PESTIS, circulates among rodents and their fleas. The great pandemics of the past were caused by spread of plague from wild rodents to rats in cities and then to humans (via rat fleas) when the rats died. Today, human disease is usually the result of being bitten by fleas from wild rodents. A bite from an infected flea leads to bubonic plague, a form of the disease which is characterized by swollen lymph glands (called "buboes"). Pneumonic plague, which affects the lungs, can occur as a complication of bubonic plague; it is also spread from person to person in infected droplets expelled during coughing.

In recent years, outbreaks of plague have been confined mainly to parts of Africa, South America, and Southeast Asia, but some 10 to 50 cases of human plague occur in the US each year. Plague is very rare in Canada.

PREVENTION

There is a constant risk of plague spreading to urban rat populations, and the main measures to prevent this are rat control and surveillance of the disease in wild rodents. Hikers in parts of the world where plague is present should not touch rodents or any carcass.

A vaccine against plague is available for people in high-risk occupations.

SYMPTOMS AND SIGNS

Bubonic plague usually starts, two to five days after infection, with fever, shivering, and severe headache. Soon the buboes appear. These are smooth, oval, reddened, intensely painful swellings usually in the groin, less commonly in the armpits, neck, or elsewhere. There may be bleeding into the skin around the buboes, resulting in dark patches. The victim may have seizures and, in about half the cases, will die if not treated. Occasionally, *septicemia* (blood poisoning) is an early complication and may cause death before buboes appear.

In pneumonic plague, there is severe coughing that produces a bloody, frothy sputum (phlegm) and labored breathing. Death is almost inevitable unless the disease is diagnosed and treated early.

SPREAD OF PLAGUE

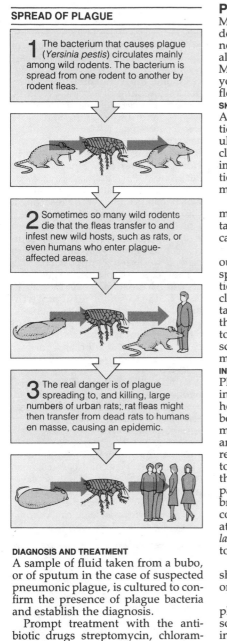

1 The bacterium that causes plague (*Yersinia pestis*) circulates mainly among wild rodents. The bacterium is spread from one rodent to another by rodent fleas.

2 Sometimes so many wild rodents die that the fleas transfer to and infest new wild hosts, such as rats, or even humans who enter plague-affected areas.

3 The real danger is of plague spreading to, and killing, large numbers of urban rats; rat fleas might then transfer from dead rats to humans en masse, causing an epidemic.

DIAGNOSIS AND TREATMENT

A sample of fluid taken from a bubo, or of sputum in the case of suspected pneumonic plague, is cultured to confirm the presence of plague bacteria and establish the diagnosis.

Prompt treatment with the antibiotic drugs streptomycin, chloramphenicol, or tetracycline reduces the risk of death to less than 5 percent.

All contacts of anyone who has pneumonic plague are watched closely and their temperatures checked regularly for a week. Antibiotic drugs are given as a preventive measure, and at the first suspicion of illness.

Plantar wart

A growth on the sole of the foot. (See *Wart, plantar*.)

Plants, poisonous

Many plants, including common garden and house plants, are poisonous. Others can cause a severe allergic reaction after skin contact. Most cases of poisoning occur in young children who eat berries or flowers.

SKIN CONTACT

Among the plants that can cause reactions are nettles, hogweed, primula, and poison ivy. Some people claim to be immune to poison ivy, but immunity may be lost after sensitization due to casual contact. Poison ivy may sometimes grow as a large vine.

Itching, burning, and blistering may develop at the site of skin contact. In some people, skin reactions can be extremely severe.

First aid treatment includes thorough washing of the affected area, sponging with alcohol, and application of calamine lotion. Washing any clothing that may have come in contact with the plant is also advised. In the case of a severe reaction, it is wise to consult a physician, who may prescribe *corticosteroid drugs* to be taken by mouth or injection.

INTERNAL POISONING

Plants that are poisonous to eat include aconite, castor beans, water hemlock seeds, and many types of berry, including the berries of ornamental yew and holly. Young children are the most commonly affected as a result of eating colorful berries. Symptoms of poisoning vary according to the plant but may include abdominal pain, vomiting, excitement, flushing, breathing difficulties, delirium, and coma. Medical help should be sought at once. The usual treatment is gastric *lavage* and measures to relieve symptoms as they arise.

Fatal poisoning is rare. Children should be taught not to sample berries or any type of non-food plant.

Paradoxically, many poisonous plants throughout the world are also a source of useful drugs. Examples include *atropine* from deadly nightshade and *digitalis drugs* from foxglove. (See also *Mushroom poisoning*.)

Plaque

The term given to an area of *atherosclerosis* (fatty deposits within arteries). The atheromatous plaques give no indication of their presence until they become so large that they reduce blood flow in a vessel or until some disturbance of the surface of the plaque develops, causing *thrombosis* (clotting of blood) at the site. When

POISON IVY

Leaves grow in threes on this plant found upright and as a climbing vine in semi-open areas. Its glossy green leaves turn bright red in fall, when its greenish yellow berries become creamy white.

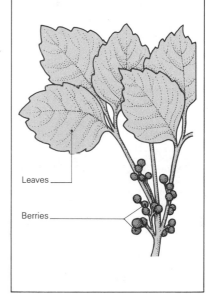

Leaves

Berries

this occurs in a small- or medium-sized vessel, blockage is likely (see *Peripheral vascular disease*). Plaques in the coronary arteries (which supply blood to the heart muscle) are the cause of *coronary artery disease*.

Plaque, dental

A rough sticky coating on the teeth that consists of saliva, bacteria, and food debris. It is the chief cause of tooth decay (see *Caries, dental*) and *gingivitis*; if allowed to accumulate, plaque forms the basis of a hard deposit (see *Calculus, dental*).

Plaque begins to form on teeth within a few hours of cleaning and is responsible for the furry feeling of unbrushed teeth. Salivary mucus, consisting mainly of proteins, forms on the teeth. Bacteria that live in the mouth then multiply within this mucus, gradually building up a layer of plaque. Some of these microorganisms, particularly STREPTOCOCCUS MUTANS, break down the sugar in the remains of carbohydrate food that stick to the mucus, adding to the plaque and also creating an acid that can rapidly erode tooth enamel.

P

DEVELOPMENT OF PLAQUE

Plaque starts with a deposit of salivary mucus on the teeth. The mucus is colonized by various types of bacteria. Initially, the predominant bacteria are spherical cocci. After a day or two, long filamentous colonies of bacteria spread over the surface of the teeth.

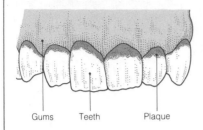

Gums   Teeth   Plaque

Areas of plaque buildup
Plaque develops predominantly at the margin of teeth and gums. If the gums are inflamed or otherwise unhealthy, the plaque tends to develop more rapidly.

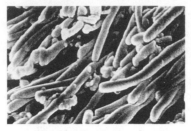

Mature plaque
This picture, taken with a scanning electron microscope, shows a mass of filamentous bacterial colonies in plaque, magnified about 2,000 times.

Plaque should be thoroughly removed at least once a day by *toothbrushing* and use of dental floss (see *Floss, dental*). It can be made more visible by the use of harmless dyes known as *disclosing agents*.

Plasma

The fluid part of *blood* which remains if the blood cells are removed. Plasma is a solution that contains many important nutrients, salts and proteins.

Plasmapheresis

A procedure, also called plasma exchange, for removing or reducing the concentration of unwanted substances in the *blood*. Blood is withdrawn from the patient in the same way as for *blood donation*, and the plasma portion of the blood is removed by special machines called cell separators. The blood cells are then mixed with a plasma substitute and returned to the circulation in the same way as for *blood transfusion*. It usually takes about two hours.

The main use of plasmapheresis is the removal of damaging *antibodies* or antibody-antigen particles (known as immune complexes) from the circulation in some *autoimmune disorders*, such as *myasthenia gravis*, *Goodpasture's syndrome*, and rapidly progressive kidney disease which is sometimes associated with systemic *lupus erythematosus*.

Plasma proteins

All the proteins present in *blood* plasma. Plasma proteins include *albumin*, fibrinogen and other substances important to *blood clotting*, and *immunoglobulins* (proteins with a role in the *immune system*).

Apart from their specific roles, the plasma proteins help maintain blood volume by preventing loss of water from the blood into the tissues. The proteins keep the water in the blood by a phenomenon called osmotic pressure (see *Osmosis*).

Plasminogen activator

See *Tissue plasminogen activator*.

Plaster cast

See *Cast*.

Plaster of Paris

A white powder composed of a calcium compound that reacts chemically with water, giving off heat and producing a paste that can be molded and shaped before it sets. Plaster of Paris is used for constructing *casts* to immobilize parts of the body and for making dental models (see *Impression, dental*).

Plastic surgery

Any operation carried out to repair or reconstruct skin and underlying tissue that has been damaged or lost by injury or disease, has been malformed since birth, or has changed with aging. Every attempt is made to maintain function of the affected part of the body and to create as natural an appearance as possible.

Operations performed mainly to improve appearance in an otherwise generally healthy person are known as *cosmetic surgery*.

WHY IT IS DONE
Plastic surgery is usually performed to repair damage caused by severe burns or injuries, cancer, certain types of operation, such as *mastectomy* (breast removal), or the effects of aging.

Among the congenital conditions that may require correction by plastic surgery are *cleft lip and palate*, *hypospadias*, and imperforate anus (see *Anus, imperforate*).

HOW IT IS DONE
A variety of techniques is used to provide skin cover for damaged areas, including *skin grafts*, *skin flaps*, *Z-plasty*, and tissue expansion (in which skin is stretched by inserting a silicone balloon beneath the surface which is then gradually increased in size). These techniques may be combined with a *bone graft* or *implants* to provide underlying support.

The scope of plastic surgery has been much broadened over the past 10 years by the use of microsurgical techniques (see *Microsurgery*) to join blood vessels, thus allowing the transfer of blocks of skin and muscle from one part of the body to another.

-plasty

A suffix meaning shaping by surgery; performing *plastic surgery* on. *Rhinoplasty* is plastic surgery on the nose; *mammoplasty* is reshaping or reconstruction of the breast.

Platelet

The smallest type of *blood cell*, also called a thrombocyte. Platelets play a major role in *blood clotting*. A deficiency of platelets (a condition known as *thrombocytopenia*) can cause some types of *bleeding disorders*.

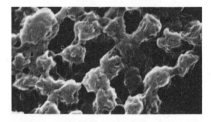

Electron micrograph of platelets
Normal and activated (spiky) platelets can be seen. Activated platelets clump to seal defects in blood vessel walls after injury.

Platyhelminth

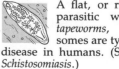 A flat, or ribbon-shaped, parasitic worm. Flukes, *tapeworms*, and schistosomes are types that cause disease in humans. (See *Liver fluke*; *Schistosomiasis*.)

P

Play therapy

A method used in the *psychoanalysis* of young children. Play therapy is based on the principle that all children's play has some symbolic significance.

The child is allowed to choose from the toys, drawing materials, and games in the therapist's room. Watching the child at play helps the therapist diagnose the source of the child's problems; the child can then be helped to "act out" thoughts and feelings that are causing anxiety. An improvement in the child's state may be indicated by changes in play, such as drawing smiling faces.

Plethora

A florid, bright-red, flushed complexion. It may be caused by dilation of blood vessels near the skin surface, or, more rarely, by *polycythemia* (excessive numbers of red blood cells).

Plethysmography

A method of estimating the blood flow in vessels by measuring changes in the size of a body part. Plethysmography may be used on the penis to establish whether a patient with *impotence* gets an erection during sleep. It is occasionally used in the investigation of deep vein *thrombosis* to detect an obstruction of the blood flow back toward the heart.

Pleura

A thin membrane with two layers, one lining the outside of the *lungs* and the other the inside of the chest cavity. Fluid between the two layers provides lubrication and thus allows smooth, uniform expansion and contraction of the lungs during breathing.

DISORDERS
Pleurisy (inflammation of the pleura) is usually caused by a lung infection, such as *pneumonia* or *tuberculosis*, and may lead to *pleural effusion* (excessive fluid between the layers of the pleura). *Pneumothorax* (air in the pleural cavity) may occur spontaneously or be caused by a penetrating injury.

Pleural effusion

An accumulation of fluid between the layers of the *pleura* (the membrane lining the lungs and chest cavity). Pleural effusion may be caused by *pneumonia, tuberculosis, heart failure, cancer, pulmonary embolism,* or *mesothelioma* (a tumor of the pleura). The effusion may affect one or both sides of the chest.

Pleural effusion causes compression of the underlying lung, leading to breathing difficulty. Diagnosis is confirmed by *chest X ray*. To determine the cause of the effusion, some of the fluid may be aspirated (removed with a needle and syringe) and examined. A *biopsy* (removal of a tissue sample for microscopic analysis) of the pleura may also be necessary.

Treatment is of the underlying cause. The fluid may need to be drained with a needle or tube to help breathing. In some cases caused by malignancy, *anticancer drugs* are injected into the pleural space to prevent a recurrence.

Pleurisy

Inflammation of the *pleura* (the membrane lining the lungs and chest cavity). Pleurisy is usually caused by a lung infection, such as *pneumonia* or a viral infection of the pleura. Rarer causes include *pulmonary embolism, lung cancer,* and *rheumatoid arthritis*.

Pleurisy causes a sharp chest pain that sometimes travels to the tip of the shoulder on the involved side. The pain, which is worse when breathing in, arises because the two inflamed membranes rub across each other. Treatment is of the underlying cause, along with *analgesic drugs* (painkillers).

Pleurodynia

Pain in the chest usually due to a viral infection. Sometimes called Bornholm disease, pleurodynia is caused by coxsackievirus B and often occurs in epidemics; it usually affects children but can occur at any age.

Symptoms include sudden severe pain in the lower chest or upper abdomen, with fever, sore throat, headache, and malaise. The disease usually settles in three or four days without treatment.

Plexus

A network of interwoven nerves or blood vessels, such as the *brachial plexus* (a network of nerves in the neck and upper arm).

Plication

A surgical procedure in which tucks are taken in the walls of a hollow organ and then stitched to decrease the organ's size. One type of plication is fundoplication, used to treat *hiatal hernia*. In this operation, the fundus (upper part) of the stomach is folded up around the lower end of the esophagus to create an inkwell-like valve to prevent reflux of gastric acid from the stomach into the esophagus.

Plummer-Vinson syndrome

Difficulty swallowing caused by the formation of webs of tissue across the upper *esophagus*, and usually occurring along with severe iron-deficiency *anemia*. The condition primarily affects middle-aged women.

The diagnosis is made by a barium swallow (see *Barium X-ray examinations*) and by inspection of the esophagus with an *endoscope* (flexible viewing instrument). Treatment of the anemia usually relieves symptoms; swallowing is relieved when the web is broken, which often occurs at the time of endoscopy.

Plutonium

A radioactive metallic element which occurs naturally only in infinitesimal amounts in uranium ores; it is produced artificially in breeder reactors by the bombardment of uranium with neutrons. Plutonium is used as a fuel in nuclear reactors and in nuclear weapons, such as the atomic bomb that was dropped on Nagasaki in 1945. The element is highly toxic if it enters the body because of its high rate of *radiation* emission (in the form of alpha particles) and its absorption in bone marrow where it may be retained for many years.

PMS

The abbreviation for *premenstrual syndrome*.

PMT

The abbreviation for premenstrual tension. (See *Premenstrual syndrome*.)

Pneumaturia

The presence of gas in the *urine*. Pneumaturia usually indicates that a *fistula* (an abnormal connection) has developed between the bladder and the intestine. Such a fistula is an unusual complication of a number of disorders, including *Crohn's disease, cancer,* or *diverticular disease*.

Pneumo-

A prefix meaning related to the lungs, to air, or to the breath. For example, pneumonia is inflammation of the lungs, and pneumothorax is air in the pleural space in the chest.

Pneumoconiosis

Any of a group of lung diseases caused by the inhalation of certain mineral dusts, primarily asbestos and silica.

Only dust particles smaller than about 0.005 mm in diameter—small

P

enough to reach the smallest air passages and alveoli (air sacs) in the lungs—are likely to cause harm. The dust particles cannot be destroyed within or completely removed from the lungs, so they accumulate and may eventually cause thickening and scarring. The lungs therefore become less efficient in supplying oxygen to the blood.

The incidence is falling due to better preventive measures (e.g., by enforcing maximum permitted dust levels in industry, by medical surveillance of exposed workers, and by use of protective clothing).

SYMPTOMS AND COMPLICATIONS

Pneumoconiosis is often detected by a *chest X ray* before it causes any symptoms. If exposure to the dust is stopped at this point, further progression of the disease may be prevented. In other cases, the main symptom initially is shortness of breath, which may gradually get worse.

In severe cases, pneumoconiosis may lead to *cor pulmonale* (right-sided heart failure resulting from lung damage).

Complications of pneumoconiosis include the development of *emphysema*, and, in people with silicosis, an increased risk of *tuberculosis*. Pneumoconiosis caused by asbestos is associated with an increased risk of *lung cancer*; smoking increases this risk of cancer.

DIAGNOSIS, TREATMENT, AND OUTLOOK

The diagnosis depends on a history of exposure to dusts, a chest X ray, medical examination, and *pulmonary function tests*.

There is no treatment for pneumoconiosis apart from treating complications, such as lung infections or cor pulmonale. Further exposure to dust must be avoided.

Anyone in whom pneumoconiosis develops at an early age or in whom progressive massive fibrosis develops at any age is at increased risk of a premature death. Industrial injury benefit can be claimed by anyone in whom pneumoconiosis develops and causes disability provided there is proof that the disability is work related.

Pneumocystis pneumonia

An infection of the lungs that is caused by the microorganism *PNEUMO-CYSTIS CARINII*, a type of protozoan (single-celled) parasite. Pneumocystis pneumonia is an *opportunistic infection* that is dangerous only to people with impaired immunity (resistance) to infection—such as people who are suffering from *AIDS* or *leukemia*. Pneumocystis pneumonia is a major cause of death in people who have AIDS.

Symptoms include fever, dry cough, and shortness of breath. They may last from a few weeks to a few months. Diagnosis is by examination of the sputum (phlegm) or a lung *biopsy* (removal of a sample of tissue for microscopic analysis). High doses of *antibiotic drugs* may help eradicate the infection, although it may recur.

Pneumonectomy

An operation to remove an entire lung. Pneumonectomy is sometimes performed to treat *lung cancer*. It once was used to treat *tuberculosis*, *bronchiectasis*, and lung infection, but these conditions are usually treated today by drugs or removal of only part of the lung (see *Lobectomy, lung*).

Before a pneumonectomy is performed, *pulmonary function tests* are carried out to make sure that the remaining lung is healthy enough to cope with the increased demands that will be placed on it.

HOW IT IS DONE

Under general anesthesia, a curved incision is made (starting under the armpit and extending across the back) following the line of the lower edge of the shoulder blade. The muscles are cut through and the ribs spread apart to expose the lung. Sometimes a rib is removed for better exposure. The arteries, veins, and bronchi leading to the lung are tied off and divided, and the lung is removed. A drainage tube is usually inserted into the space between the two layers of *pleura*, and the incision is then stitched.

The drain is usually removed the day after the operation, and the stitches are taken out after about 10 days. Many patients require artificial *ventilation* for hours to days after the operation. At home, normal activities should be resumed slowly; many people are able to return to work after about two months.

Pneumonia

Inflammation of the *lungs* due to infection. Pneumonia is a common late complication of any serious illness and is the certified cause of about 6,000 deaths in Canada each year. It is more common in males, during infancy and old age, and in those who have reduced immunity to infection (such as alcoholics).

There are two main types: lobar pneumonia and bronchopneumonia. In lobar pneumonia one lobe of one lung is initially affected. In bronchopneumonia, inflammation starts in the bronchi and bronchioles (airways) and then spreads to affect patches of tissue in one or both lungs.

CAUSES

Most cases of pneumonia are caused by viruses or bacteria. Causes of viral pneumonia include adenovirus, respiratory syncytial virus, or a coxsackievirus. The most common bacterial pneumonia is pneumococcal pneumonia caused by *STREPTOCOCCUS PNEUMONIAE*. Other causes of bacterial pneumonia include *HAEMOPHILUS INFLUENZAE*, *LEGIONELLA PNEUMOPHILIA* (see *Legionnaires' disease*), and *STAPHYLOCOCCUS AUREUS*. Pneumonia may also be caused by a *mycoplasma* (an organism that is intermediate between a bacterium and a virus) or by a *chlamydial infection*; *Q fever* is a type of pneumonia caused by a *rickettsia*.

Rarely, pneumonia may be due to a different type of organism, such as fungi, yeasts, or protozoa. These types usually occur only in people with *immunodeficiency disorders*. For example, *pneumocystis pneumonia*, caused by a protozoon, commonly occurs in people with *AIDS*.

SYMPTOMS AND SIGNS

Symptoms and signs typically include fever, chills, shortness of breath, and a cough that produces yellow-green sputum and occasionally blood. Chest pain that is worse when breathing in may occur because of *pleurisy* (inflammation of the membrane lining the lungs and chest cavity).

Potential complications include *pleural effusion* (fluid around the lung), *empyema* (pus around the lung), and, in rare cases, an *abscess* in the lung.

DIAGNOSIS

The physician gives the patient a physical examination, listening to chest sounds through a stethoscope. The diagnosis may be confirmed by a *chest X ray* and by examination of sputum and of blood for microorganisms.

TREATMENT

Patients with mild pneumonia can usually be treated at home, but hospitalization is necessary in severe cases. The drugs prescribed depend on the causative microorganism; they may include *antibiotic drugs* or *antifungal drugs*. *ASA* or *acetaminophen* may be given to reduce fever. In severe cases, *oxygen therapy* and artificial *ventilation* may be required.

P

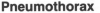

OUTLOOK
Most sufferers recover completely within two weeks. However, some elderly or debilitated people fail to respond to treatment.

Pneumonitis
A form of inflammation of the *lungs* that may cause coughing, breathing difficulty, and wheezing. Pneumonitis may be due to a wide range of causes, including an allergic reaction caused by inhalation of dust containing animal or plant material (see *Alveolitis*), and exposure to radiation (see *Radiation hazards*). Pneumonitis may also occur as a rare side effect of some drugs, such as *amiodarone*, an antiarrhythmic drug, and *azathioprine*, an antirheumatic medication.

Pneumothorax
A condition in which air enters the pleural cavity (the space between the two layers of the *pleura* which cover the *lungs* and the chest wall). The air may enter the pleural cavity from the lungs or from outside the body.

CAUSES
Spontaneous pneumothorax, which usually occurs for no apparent reason,

---

PNEUMONIA
Pneumonia is not a single disease, but the name for several types of lung inflammation caused by infectious organisms. In some cases, accidental inhalation of vomit or a liquid starts the infection. The symptoms, treatment, and outcome vary greatly, depending on the cause and on the general health of the patient.

Lobar pneumonia
In this type, which is rare in most developed countries today, the inflammation is usually confined to just one lobe of one lung—often a lower lobe.

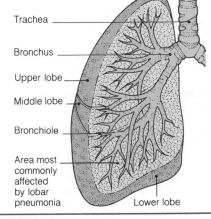

Trachea
Bronchus
Upper lobe
Middle lobe
Bronchiole
Area most commonly affected by lobar pneumonia
Lower lobe

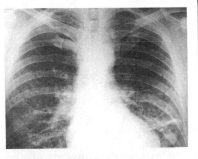

Chest X ray in bronchopneumonia
The X ray clearly shows broncho-pneumonia. The blotchy, white areas within the darker areas correspond to patches of inflamed lung.

TYPES, CAUSES, AND TREATMENT OF PNEUMONIA

Types	Causes	Symptoms	Drug treatments	Other treatments
Pneumonias always or usually caused by bacteria				
Lobar pneumonia	*Streptococcus pneumoniae*	Cough, painful breathing, high temperature, rust-colored sputum	Penicillin	Machine ventilation of the lungs to help breathing may be required in some cases. Physio-therapy to clear sputum out of the lungs may also be needed
Bronchopneumonia	*Hemophilus influenzae* or other organisms	Cough, often a fever, green or yellow sputum	Various antibiotics	
Aspiration pneumonia	Various organisms. Occurs following inhalation of sputum, vomit, liquids, and so on	Fever, cough	Various antibiotics	
Legionnaires' disease	*Legionella pneumophila*	Fever, cough, chest pain, headache, aches and pains	Erythromycin	
Pneumonias not caused by bacteria				
Viral pneumonia	Chickenpox virus, influenza virus, adenovirus and others	Cough, fever, not much sputum	Antibiotics (if lungs become infected by bacteria)	Machine ventilation of the lungs to help breathing may be required in severe cases
Psittacosis	*Chlamydia psittaci*, a bacterialike organism caught from birds	Cough, raised temperature, not much sputum	Tetracycline or erythromycin	
Q fever	*Coxiella burnetti*, a rickettsia	Cough, raised temperature, not much sputum	Tetracycline or erythromycin	
Mycoplasmal pneumonia	*Mycoplasma pneumoniae*, a bacterialike organism	Cough, raised temperature, not much sputum	Tetracycline or erythromycin	

P

is six times more common in men than in women. Most often, it occurs in thin young adults who have no underlying lung disease; in many cases, it is thought to be due to rupture of a congenital blister at the top of the lung. There is a 30 percent chance of a recurrence of spontaneous pneumothorax, usually on the same side. Pneumothorax may also be a complication of lung disease (particularly *asthma* or *emphysema*) or it may follow an injury, such as a fractured rib.

A pneumothorax may be caused accidentally when a catheter is inserted into a vein in the neck for intravenous feeding (see *Feeding, artificial*) or to monitor pressure in the heart and circulation.

SYMPTOMS

A pneumothorax may cause chest pain or shortness of breath. The degree of breathlessness is proportional to the size of the pneumothorax. Any underlying lung disease will increase breathing difficulty. If there is continual leakage of air into the pleural space, the pneumothorax may become progressively bigger and produce a tension pneumothorax, which may become life-threatening because of compression of the heart.

DIAGNOSIS AND TREATMENT

A *chest X ray* confirms the diagnosis. A small pneumothorax in a healthy adult usually disappears within a few days without treatment. A larger pneumothorax, or a small one in the presence of underlying lung disease, requires treatment. Treatment usually involves removing the air from the pleural cavity through a suction tube inserted through the chest wall for several days. A small pneumothorax can be treated by drawing out the air through a needle and syringe. If the lung fails to expand, or if the pneumothorax recurs, surgery may be required to seal the pleural cavity.

Pocket, gingival

See *Periodontitis*.

Podiatry

A health profession that specializes in care of the feet. Podiatrists are trained in a four-year course and are licensed by the provinces, in most of which they may prescribe certain medications and perform soft tissue and bone surgery. There is no school of podiatry in Canada.

Podophyllin

A drug used in the treatment of anal, genital, and skin *warts*.

Poison

A substance that, in relatively small amounts, disrupts the structure and/or function of cells. Although *toxin* is often used interchangeably with poison, toxin refers strictly and specifically to poisonous proteins produced by pathogenic (disease causing) bacteria, some animals, and certain plants. (See also *Drug poisoning; Poisoning*.)

Poisoning

Poisons enter the body by various routes. They may be swallowed, inhaled, absorbed through the skin, or injected under the skin (as with an *insect sting* or *snake bite*). Poisons may also originate within the body itself.

For example, bacteria can produce poisonous *endotoxins*, *enterotoxins*, or *exotoxins*. Various disorders, such as *kidney failure*, *liver failure*, and certain *metabolic disorders*, may cause poisonous substances to be produced or to accumulate within the body.

Poisoning may be acute or chronic. In acute poisoning, a large amount of poison enters, or is produced in, the body over a short time (as may occur in *food poisoning*). Chronic poisoning results from the gradual accumulation of a poison that is not eliminated quickly.

Inadvertent poisoning is one of the most common types of accident in the home. It occurs principally in young children, although adults sometimes unwittingly poison themselves, often by mistaking the dosage of a prescribed drug (see *Drug poisoning*) or, less commonly, by unthinkingly taking very high doses of certain vitamin or mineral supplements. Exposure to poisonous substances in industry is another important cause of unintentional poisoning in adults. *Drug abuse* is another.

Poisoning may be a deliberate attempt to commit *suicide*. However, many such attempts are unsuccessful or are actually intended to gain sympathy or attention. Taking a drug overdose (often in combination with alcohol, which increases the toxicity of many drugs) is a common method of suicidal poisoning. (See also *Poisoning* first aid box below; and articles on individual poisons.)

Polio

An abbreviation for *poliomyelitis*.

Poliomyelitis

An infectious disease once known as infantile paralysis but now usually called polio. Poliomyelitis is caused by a virus, which usually provokes no

---

FIRST AID: POISONING

DO NOT
■ make the victim vomit if he or she has swallowed corrosives.

1 If the victim is conscious, quickly ask what he or she has swallowed.

2 Call an ambulance and say what the victim has taken.

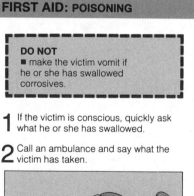

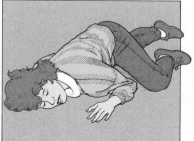

3 If the victim is unconscious but breathing, place him or her in the *recovery position*.

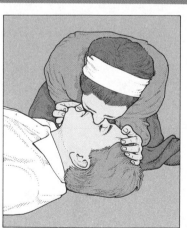

4 If the victim is not breathing, *artificial respiration* is necessary. Use the mouth-to-nose method to avoid contact with the poison.

5 If you are certain the victim has swallowed only tablets or berries, it may help to induce vomiting by placing your fingers at the back of the throat.

more than a mild illness. However, in more serious cases it attacks the *brain* and *spinal cord*. This may lead to extensive paralysis (including paralysis of the muscles involved in breathing) or may be fatal.

Since the development of effective vaccines in the 1950s, polio has virtually been eliminated from most developed countries, although cases still occur in people who have not been fully vaccinated. Polio also remains a serious risk for unvaccinated people traveling in southern Europe, Africa, or Asia. The World Health Organization is campaigning for polio to be eliminated worldwide by the year 2000.

CAUSES AND INCIDENCE
There are three closely related polioviruses. Infected people pass large numbers of virus particles in their feces, from where they may be spread indirectly, or directly via fingers, to food and thus infect others. Airborne transmission also occurs.

In countries where standards of hygiene and sanitation are low, most children become infected early in life, when the infection rarely causes serious illness, and develop immunity to polio. In countries with better standards of hygiene, children do not become immune in this manner; if they are not vaccinated, disastrous epidemics may occur.

PREVENTION
Vaccination is given during infancy, usually at about 3, 5, and 9 months, with a booster dose at about 5 years (see *Immunization*). The vaccine contains all three types of poliovirus, and immunity develops against each of them. There are two alternative types of vaccine: IPV (inactivated polio vaccine), which contains dead viruses and is given by injection, and OPV (oral poliovirus vaccine), which contains live but harmless strains of virus and is given by mouth.

There is an extremely small risk (about one in 5 million doses) that the live vaccine will cause polio in the vaccinated person or in someone who is a close contact.

SYMPTOMS AND SIGNS
Minor forms of polio are by far the most common. About 85 percent of children infected with the virus have no symptoms at all. In the rest, after an incubation period of three to five days, there is a short illness with slight fever, sore throat, headache, and vomiting. This lasts for a few days, after which most children recover completely.

In some children, however, after a short period of apparent health there is a major illness with symptoms caused by inflammation of the *meninges* (membranes covering the brain and spinal cord). These symptoms are fever, severe headache, stiffness of the neck and back, and aching in the muscles, sometimes with widespread twitching. In some cases the condition progresses, often in the course of a few hours, to extensive paralysis of muscles. The legs and lower trunk are the most frequently paralyzed. If infection spreads to the brain stem (the lowest part of the brain), the result may be swallowing and breathing problems, or even total loss of these faculties.

DIAGNOSIS
To make a firm diagnosis, the causative virus must be isolated from a sample of cerebrospinal fluid, taken by *lumbar puncture*, or from a throat swab or a sample of feces. Muscle paralysis combined with an acute feverish illness is so characteristic of severe polio that it usually enables an immediate diagnosis to be made.

TREATMENT
There is no effective drug treatment for polio. Nonparalytic patients do not usually need treatment except for bed rest and *analgesic drugs*. When muscles are paralyzed, *physiotherapy* is essential to prevent muscle damage while the virus is active. Later, during convalescence, physiotherapy is needed to help retain muscle function.

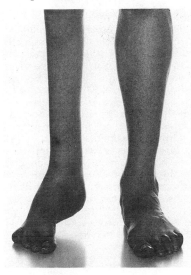

Wasted limb of polio patient
Muscle bulk is severely reduced in the paralyzed (right) leg. Muscle function can sometimes be helped by physiotherapy.

When the lower part of the body is paralyzed, the bladder does not function properly and may make catheterization (see *Catheterization, urinary*) necessary. Respiratory paralysis requires *tracheostomy* (emergency surgical creation of an opening in the windpipe to insert a breathing tube) and artificial *ventilation*.

OUTLOOK
Recovery from nonparalytic polio is complete. Of those who become paralyzed, more than half eventually make a full recovery, more than a quarter suffer only minor permanent muscle weakness, less than a quarter are left with severe disability, and less than one in 10 dies (mainly adults and those in whom the brain stem has been severely affected). Years after extensive paralysis with some recovery, there may be a "postpolio" deterioration with new weakness and pain in some of the recovered muscles.

Pollution
Contamination of the environment by poisons, microorganisms, or radioactive substances.

Serious public concern about pollution developed in the 1950s with the growing realization that *pesticides* were destroying wildlife and disturbing or poisoning the food chain, and that atmospheric nuclear tests were disseminating radioactive fallout over wide areas (see *Radiation*). This concern was strengthened by incidents of industrial pollution, such as the release of mercury waste into Minamata Bay, Japan (see *Minamata disease*); the release into the atmosphere of the poisonous chemical dioxin by a factory explosion in Italy (see *Defoliant poisoning*); damage to seabirds and beaches from oil tanker spillages; and, more recently, from acid rain caused by the burning of coal and oil, and from radioactive fallout from the nuclear reactor explosion at Chernobyl in the USSR.

A potentially serious pollutant in its long-term effects is *carbon dioxide*, large amounts of which are discharged into the atmosphere by the burning of fossil fuels. The continual increase in the atmospheric carbon dioxide level is producing what is called the "greenhouse effect," which is increasing the average global temperature, and may go on to cause future catastrophic climatic changes.

Another serious pollution effect is the gradual destruction of the *ozone* layer (which blocks harmful ultraviolet radiation from the sun) by various

P

chemicals, notably some CFCs (chlorofluorocarbons). Concern about this effect has led to a reduction in the emission of ozone-depleting chemicals in many developed countries. Other important pollutants include lead (see *Lead poisoning*), cadmium (see *Cadmium poisoning*), and some pesticides, such as *parathion*.

In Canada, primary concern about pollution that could affect human health has been the accumulation of mercury and dioxin in the Great Lakes.

Poly-
A prefix that means many or much, as in polymyositis (inflammation of many muscles) and polyuria (passing of large volumes of urine).

Polyarteritis nodosa
An uncommon disease of medium-sized arteries, also called periarteritis nodosa. Areas of arterial wall become inflamed, weakened, and liable to the formation of *aneurysms* (ballooned-out segments). Many different groups of blood vessels may be involved, including the coronary arteries that supply blood to the heart muscle, or the arteries of the kidneys, intestine, skeletal muscles, and nervous system. The seriousness of the condition depends on which organs are affected and how severely they are affected.

CAUSES AND INCIDENCE
The disease seems to be the result of a disturbance of the *immune system* (body's defenses against infection), triggered in some cases by exposure to the *hepatitis B* virus. It may develop at any age but is most common in adults. More men than women are affected.

SYMPTOMS AND COMPLICATIONS
In the early stages the patient has a fever and aching muscles and joints. There is general malaise, loss of appetite and weight, and, if blood vessels supplying nerves are affected, nerve pain. Damage to blood vessels leads to obstruction of the blood supply, causing *hypertension* (raised blood pressure), muscle weakness, ulceration of the skin, and *gangrene* (tissue death). If the coronary arteries are affected, *myocardial infarction* (heart attack) may occur. Because blood vessels supplying the intestines are frequently affected, a high proportion of patients suffer abdominal pain, nausea and vomiting, and diarrhea, and pass blood in the feces.

DIAGNOSIS
Polyarteritis nodosa is diagnosed by finding inflammation in blood vessels in a *biopsy* specimen taken from an affected organ. *Angiography* (X rays of blood vessels that have been injected with a radiopaque substance) may show areas of narrowing and scarring and/or aneurysms.

TREATMENT AND OUTLOOK
Large doses of *corticosteroid drugs*, sometimes supplemented by *immunosuppressant drugs*, are effective in improving an otherwise unfavorable outlook. Without treatment, few victims of the condition survive for five years; death often occurs from a myocardial infarction, *kidney failure*, severe bleeding into the intestine, or from complications of hypertension. With modern drug treatment, about 50 percent of patients survive for five years or more.

Polycystic kidney
See *Kidney, polycystic*.

Polycystic ovary
See *Ovary, polycystic*.

Polycythemia
A condition characterized by an unusually large number of red cells in the *blood* due to increased production of red cells by the *bone marrow*. This condition usually results from some other disorder or is a natural response to *hypoxia* (reduced oxygen in the blood and tissues). In such cases, it is called secondary polycythemia. Rarely, it occurs for no apparent reason and is called polycythemia vera or primary polycythemia.

SECONDARY POLYCYTHEMIA
Polycythemia occurs naturally in people living at (or visiting) high altitudes due to the reduced air pressure and level of oxygen. It can also result from any disorder that impairs the supply of oxygen to the blood (e.g., chronic *bronchitis*). In these cases, the low level of oxygen in the blood stimulates production of the hormone erythropoietin by the kidneys, which in turn stimulates the bone marrow to produce more red cells. The result is an increase in the oxygen-carrying efficiency of the blood, which compensates for the reduced oxygen supply. Descending to sea level, or effective treatment of an underlying disorder, soon returns the person's blood to normal.

Polycythemia can also be secondary to *liver cancer* or certain kidney disorders that cause excess production of erythropoietin. Treatment of the underlying disorder quickly returns the blood to normal.

POLYCYTHEMIA VERA
This rare disorder of the bone marrow develops primarily in people over 40.

The large number of red cells results in an increased volume and thickening of the blood, which may cause headaches, blurred vision, and *hypertension* (high blood pressure). There may also be a flushed skin, dizziness, night sweats, and widespread itching, particularly after a hot bath. Often, the sufferer's spleen is enlarged. There may also be abnormalities in the platelets in the blood, causing a tendency to bleed or to form blood clots. Other complications include *stroke* and, at a late stage, other types of bone marrow disease, such as *myelosclerosis* or acute leukemia (see *Leukemia, acute*).

The diagnosis is made from a physical examination and *blood tests* and by ruling out any other causes of polycythemia. Treatment of polycythemia vera consists of regular removal of blood through a vein (*venesection*), sometimes in combination with *anticancer drugs* or radioactive phosphorus taken by mouth to control the overproduction of red cells in the marrow.

Treatment enables most patients to survive for 10 to 15 years. Death usually occurs from a stroke or other complication of the disease.

Polydactyly
A *birth defect* in which there is an excessive number of fingers or toes. The extra digits may be fully formed and look like the other fingers or toes or they may be fleshy stumps.

Polydactyly affects about 50 babies in every 100,000. If both parents have polydactyly, there is a one in two chance that each of their children will be affected. Polydactyly often runs in otherwise normal families, but may also occur as part of the *Laurence-Biedl-Moon syndrome* or of other congenital syndromes. If there are no other

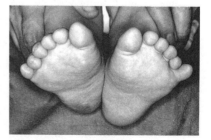

Polydactyly affecting the feet
The extra toes can cause problems with footwear and are usually removed surgically during childhood.

abnormalities, the condition presents no risk to the child's physical or mental development.

Polydipsia

A medical term for persistent excessive thirst, which occurs, for example, in untreated *diabetes mellitus* and *diabetes insipidus* (see *Thirst, excessive*).

Polyhydramnios

Excess *amniotic fluid* surrounding the fetus during pregnancy. Polyhydramnios occurs in about one in 250 pregnancies.

CAUSES

In many cases, there is no known cause for polyhydramnios. The condition sometimes occurs if the fetus has a malformation (particularly *anencephaly* or *esophageal atresia*) that makes normal swallowing impossible. Polyhydramnios may also occur if the pregnant woman has *diabetes mellitus*. Polyhydramnios occurs in about 10 percent of multiple pregnancies.

SYMPTOMS AND SIGNS

In polyhydramnios, an excess of amniotic fluid usually accumulates slowly during the second half of the pregnancy, producing symptoms from about week 32. The main symptom is abdominal discomfort. Other possible symptoms are breathlessness and swelling of the legs. The uterus is larger than usual for the duration of the pregnancy.

Less commonly, the fluid accumulates rapidly, causing abdominal pain, breathlessness, nausea, and vomiting. The abdomen becomes tense, the overlying skin is stretched and shiny, and the legs swell. Polyhydramnios may cause premature labor and the baby may not be in the usual delivery position (see *Malpresentation*).

DIAGNOSIS

Polyhydramnios is usually evident from the mother's history and a physical examination. *Ultrasound scanning* is needed to detect fetal abnormality or multiple pregnancy.

TREATMENT

Mild cases without fetal abnormality require no treatment other than extra rest. Withdrawal of amniotic fluid via a needle inserted through the abdominal wall can provide temporary relief in severe cases although the procedure may cause premature labor. If the pregnant woman has diabetes mellitus, careful attention must be paid to her diabetic control. If symptoms occur in late pregnancy, *induction of labor* may be performed to deliver the baby early.

Polymyalgia rheumatica

An uncommon disease of elderly people that is marked by pain and stiffness in the muscles of the hips, thighs, shoulders, and neck.

CAUSE AND INCIDENCE

The cause of polymyalgia rheumatica is unknown, but it may be associated with *temporal arteritis*, *rheumatoid arthritis*, systemic *lupus erythematosus*, and, sometimes, cancer. The disease affects twice as many women as men and is unusual before the age of 50.

SYMPTOMS

The pain and stiffness, which may develop gradually or suddenly, make movement difficult. Morning stiffness is notable and often makes getting out of bed a problem. Weight loss and depression may also occur.

DIAGNOSIS AND TREATMENT

The diagnosis, which is often difficult to confirm, is based on the patient's history, a physical examination, and blood tests (including an *ESR*). If temporal arteritis is suspected, a *biopsy* (removal of a small sample of tissue for analysis) may be performed on an artery at the side of the scalp.

Small doses of *corticosteroid drugs* (higher doses when temporal arteritis is present) usually bring about an improvement in the disorder within a few days. The dosage is gradually reduced and use of the drug may be discontinued within two years.

Polymyositis

A rare disease in which the muscles become inflamed and weak. Polymyositis shares the features of *dermatomyositis* except that there is no rash.

Polymyxins

A group of *antibiotic drugs* derived from the bacterium BACILLUS POLYMYXA. Polymyxins, which include *colistin* and polymyxin B, are commonly given in drop or ointment form to treat eye, ear, and skin infections. They are very infrequently given by injection to treat severe infections because in this form they may cause nerve or kidney damage.

Polyp

A growth that projects, usually on a stalk, from the lining of the nose, the cervix, the intestine, the larynx, or any other *mucous membrane*.

Polyps may need to be removed surgically if they are responsible for symptoms. Some types of polyps are liable to develop into cancer, and are removed whether or not they are causing symptoms.

Polypeptide

A compound that consists of many *amino acids* linked by *peptide* bonds.

Polypharmacy

The practice of prescribing several different drugs to one person at the same time. Drug combinations may be more effective and may reduce the risk of drug resistance. Polypharmacy increases the risk of drug interactions and, thus, the risk of adverse effects.

Polyposis, familial

A rare, inherited disorder, also known as polyposis coli, in which numerous (often a thousand or more) *polyps* are present in the colon and rectum. Without preventive treatment, the development of cancer of the colon (see *Colon, cancer of*) by the age of 40 is almost a certainty.

SYMPTOMS AND DIAGNOSIS

The polyps are not present at birth but usually appear by the age of 10 and may cause bleeding and diarrhea. However, there are often no symptoms until cancer has developed; it is therefore extremely important that a diagnosis be made as early as possible. The polyps are detected by air contrast *barium X-ray examination* and *colonoscopy* (investigation of the colon with a viewing instrument).

PREVENTION AND TREATMENT

Since there is a 50 percent chance that the children of an affected parent will inherit the disease, close medical surveillance is necessary from the age of about 10. This screening, by barium examinations and colonoscopy, is performed every two years until the age of about 40, after which time it is unlikely that polyps will appear.

Individual polyps may be cauterized during endoscopic examination. Because there is such a high risk of cancer, more radical treatment may be needed. This often takes the form of total *colectomy* (removal of the entire colon) and the creation of an artificial opening of the ileum (the lower part of the small intestine) through the abdominal wall (see *Ileostomy*). Alternatively, the end of the ileum is joined to the rectum so that a normal passage for bowel movements exists. However, the rectum must be examined regularly to detect polyps, which must be treated immediately before there is a chance for cancerous changes to occur.

Polyuria

The medical term for excessive urination. (See *Urination, excessive*.)

P

Pompholyx

An acute form of *eczema* in which itchy blisters form over the palms and/or soles. The condition, also called dyshydrotic eczema, often develops for no apparent reason but is sometimes due to an allergic response to a substance in contact with the skin. It is associated rarely with *ringworm*.

Treatment is with an astringent, which causes the skin to tighten and dry, or with topical application of a *corticosteroid drug*.

Pons

The middle part of the *brain stem*, situated between the midbrain (above) and the medulla oblongata (below).

Pore

A tiny opening. The term usually describes an opening in the *skin* that releases sweat or sebum (an oily substance secreted by sebaceous glands). Most of the pores from which sebum arises are also *hair* follicles.

Porphyria

Any of a group of uncommon and usually inherited disorders caused by the accumulation in the body of substances called porphyrins. Sufferers often have a rash or skin blistering brought on by sunlight and may have abdominal pain and nervous system disturbances from certain drugs.

CAUSES AND TYPES

Porphyrins are chemicals with a complex structure that are formed in the body during the manufacture of heme—a component of *hemoglobin* (the oxygen-carrying pigment in the blood).

The porphyrias result from blocks in the chemical processes by which heme is formed, resulting in the accumulation of porphyrins. Such blocks are the results of deficiencies of various *enzymes* in the body; these deficiencies are inherited in an autosomal dominant pattern (see *Genetic disorders*). Porphyria due to poisoning is also known.

Six types of porphyria are recognized—acute intermittent porphyria, variegate porphyria, and porphyria cutanea tarda (the more common types); and hereditary coproporphyria, protoporphyria, and congenital erythropoietic porphyria (all rare).

INCIDENCE

The incidence of each varies throughout the world. The combined prevalence in Canada is unknown, but is probably about one affected person per 10,000 to 50,000 population.

SYMPTOMS AND SIGNS

The different types of porphyria have different features.

ACUTE INTERMITTENT PORPHYRIA This type usually first appears in early adulthood with attacks of abdominal pain, which may mimic appendicitis. Limb cramps, muscle weakness, and psychiatric disturbances are common. There are no skin symptoms, but the patient's urine turns red when left to stand. A large number of drugs are known to precipitate attacks, including barbiturate drugs, phenytoin, oral contraceptives, and tetracyclines.

VARIEGATE PORPHYRIA This type is similar in many respects to acute intermittent porphyria, but with blistering of sun-exposed skin. Attacks may be brought on by the same drugs that precipitate acute intermittent porphyria.

PORPHYRIA CUTANEA TARDA This type also causes blistering of sun-exposed skin, but no abdominal or nervous system disturbance. Wounds are characteristically slow to heal. The urine is sometimes pink or brown. Many cases are precipitated by liver disease, including alcoholic liver disease.

HEREDITARY COPROPORPHYRIA This type of porphyria is similar to acute intermittent porphyria, with additional skin symptoms in some sufferers.

PROTOPORPHYRIA This type usually causes mild skin symptoms after exposure to sunlight.

CONGENITAL ERYTHROPOIETIC PORPHYRIA This type is extremely rare; it is characterized by red discoloration of urine and teeth, excessive hair growth, severe skin blistering and ulceration, and hemolytic *anemia*. Death may occur in childhood.

DIAGNOSIS AND TREATMENT

The porphyrias are diagnosed by finding abnormal levels of porphyrins in the urine and feces. More specific tests are available for some types.

Treatment is difficult. Avoiding exposure to sunlight and/or to precipitating drugs is the most important measure. Attacks of acute intermittent porphyria, variegate porphyria, and hereditary coproporphyria can sometimes be helped by administration of glucose or of hematin, which is chemically related to heme. Porphyria cutanea tarda can be helped by the removal of blood through a vein (*venesection*).

Portal hypertension

Increased blood pressure in the portal vein, a large blood vessel that carries blood from the stomach, intestine, and spleen to the liver. The pressure in the veins of the upper stomach and lower esophagus is raised, causing them to widen (a condition known as *esophageal varices*) and sometimes to rupture. In addition, fluid is forced from the overloaded portal vein, resulting in *ascites*, an accumulation of fluid in the abdomen.

CAUSES

The most common cause of portal hypertension is the liver disease *cirrhosis*, in which scarring and regenerative tissue in the organ obstruct the portal vein. Another cause is *thrombosis* (abnormal blood clotting) in the vein. This may occur shortly after birth or later in life, when it is usually the result of narrowing of the vein by cirrhosis, compression of the vein by enlarged lymph nodes, or inflammation resulting from an infection. Portal hypertension may also be caused by narrowing of the vein from birth.

Rarely, portal hypertension is due to an abnormal connection between the portal vein and an artery (*arteriovenous fistula*), usually as a result of injury. Portal hypertension can also be caused by increased blood flow from the spleen if disease has caused this organ to enlarge; this is a common cause in the tropics.

SYMPTOMS AND SIGNS

If the veins in the esophagus and stomach rupture, this causes massive recurrent vomiting of blood and the passing of black feces. Ascites results in abdominal swelling and discomfort and sometimes difficulty in breathing.

DIAGNOSIS

Portal hypertension is usually diagnosed from the patient's symptoms and signs. The cause can be determined by examining the liver and surrounding blood vessels by means of *ultrasound scanning* and X-ray examination of the blood vessels (see *Angiography*).

TREATMENT AND OUTLOOK

Bleeding from ruptured blood vessels is stopped by sclerotherapy, which comprises the injection of a sclerosant (hardening) solution into or around the veins. This induces inflammation, subsequent scarring, and consequent thickening of the vessels' walls so that the veins are blocked off. Ascites is controlled by restriction of dietary sodium chloride (salt) and by *diuretic drugs*, which increase overall urine production.

In some cases, an operation known as a *shunt* may be carried out to divert blood from the portal vein to some other blood vessel, thus relieving the high pressure.

P

PORTAL HYPERTENSION

The most common cause of this condition is liver cirrhosis or some other obstruction to blood flow through the liver. The portal vein becomes congested with blood, and back pressure develops through the system of veins that join the portal vein.

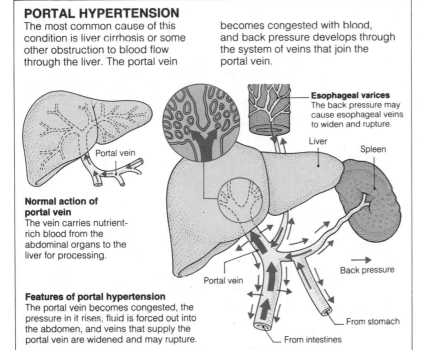

Esophageal varices
The back pressure may cause esophageal veins to widen and rupture.

Liver

Spleen

Portal vein

Back pressure

From stomach

From intestines

Normal action of portal vein
The vein carries nutrient-rich blood from the abdominal organs to the liver for processing.

Features of portal hypertension
The portal vein becomes congested, the pressure in it rises, fluid is forced out into the abdomen, and veins that supply the portal vein are widened and may rupture.

The outlook depends on how successfully the underlying cause of this condition can be treated.

Port-wine stain

A purple-red birthmark that is level with the skin's surface. A port-wine stain is a permanent and often unsightly type of *hemangioma*. Cosmetic treatment by laser surgery may be possible in some cases.

Positron emission tomography

See *PET scanning.*

Postcoital contraception

See *Contraception, postcoital.*

Posterior

Relating to the back of the body. In human anatomy, the term is synonymous with *dorsal.*

Postmaturity

A condition in which a *pregnancy* persists for longer than 42 weeks; the average length of a normal pregnancy is 40 weeks from the first day of the last menstrual period (see *Gestation*). Postmaturity may be due to a family tendency to prolonged pregnancy, or it may be an indication that the head is bigger than the mother's pelvis and that the baby is unable to descend properly (see *Engagement*). Many obstetricians attempt to avoid postmaturity by *induction of labor* as the pregnancy nears 42 weeks' gestation.

COMPLICATIONS
Because the postmature baby is larger than average and the bones of the baby's skull are harder and thus mold less readily, postmaturity is associated with a prolonged labor.

The major risk of postmaturity is fetal death and consequent stillbirth; the risk of this occurring doubles by the 43rd week of pregnancy and trebles by the 44th week as compared to the normal 40-week pregnancy. This increase in fetal death rate is in part a consequence of diminished placental efficiency that causes the fetus to be starved of nutrients and oxygen.

Postmature infants tend to have dry skin which cracks and peels and may be more susceptible to infection.

Postmortem examination

Another term for an *autopsy.*

Postmyocardial infarction syndrome

Another name for *Dressler's syndrome.*

Postnasal drip

A watery or sticky discharge from the back of the *nose* into the *nasopharynx* (the uppermost part of the throat, behind the nose). As the fluid trickles down the throat, it may cause a cough, hoarseness, or the sensation that a foreign body is present. Postnasal drip is usually caused by *rhinitis* (inflammation of the mucous membrane in the nose); treatment is of this underlying cause.

Postnatal care

Care of the mother after *childbirth* until about six weeks after delivery.

After delivery the mother's temperature, pulse, and blood pressure are monitored, especially after a *cesarean section* or if there have been any complications, such as *preeclampsia* or bleeding.

The length of stay in hospital depends on whether or not there have been any complications. Women used to remain in hospital for up to a week after delivery, but nowadays the length of stay after a straightforward delivery may be only 48 hours or even less. During the hospital stay, a daily check is made for any signs of *puerperal sepsis* (infection of the genital tract after childbirth), including inspection of the *lochia* (vaginal discharge after childbirth). If the woman had an *episiotomy* or tears around the vagina, the wounds are checked daily.

The woman is encouraged to walk as soon as possible after delivery to reduce the risk of *thrombosis* (abnormal blood clotting). If necessary, help is given with feeding techniques (see *Bottle-feeding; Breast-feeding*). There may also be instruction on various abdominal and *pelvic floor exercises.*

A final postnatal checkup usually takes place about six weeks after delivery. The obstetrician or family practitioner checks the woman's blood pressure and weight, examines the uterus and bladder to make sure they are in the correct position, and ensures that any wounds are healing properly. Advice on *contraception* may also be given.

Postnatal depression

Depression in a woman after *childbirth*. Postnatal depression is probably caused by a combination of sudden hormonal changes and a variety of psychological and environmental factors. Postnatal depression ranges from an extremely common and short-lived attack of mild depression ("baby blues") to a depressive psychosis in which the woman is very severely depressed and requires admission to hospital to prevent harm to herself or her baby.

P

MILD DEPRESSION

Probably more than two thirds of mothers have the "blues," which usually start about four to five days after childbirth. The woman feels miserable, discouraged, irritable, sometimes mentally confused, and may cry easily. Apart from hormonal changes, psychological factors may play a role, including a sense of anticlimax after the birth or an overwhelming sense of responsibility for the baby's care. With reassurance and support from family and friends, the depression usually passes in two or three days.

MORE SEVERE DEPRESSION

In about 10 to 15 percent of women the depression is more marked and persists for weeks. There may be a constant feeling of tiredness, difficulty in sleeping, loss of appetite, and restlessness. This type of postnatal depression seems more likely to develop if the woman has a strained relationship with her partner, has no support from her family, has financial or other worries, or has a *personality disorder*. At particular risk are women who suffered from depression or anxiety during the pregnancy, first-time mothers, and single parents. In many cases, however, no risk factors are present. The condition usually clears up of its own accord or responds to *antidepressant drugs*.

DEPRESSIVE PSYCHOSIS

This severe form of postnatal depression follows about one in 1,000 pregnancies and usually starts two to three weeks after childbirth. Depressive psychosis is marked by severe mental confusion, feelings of worthlessness, threats of suicide or of harm to the baby, and sometimes *delusions*. The woman's moods may change rapidly. Treatment requires admission to hospital, sensitive counseling, and possibly *family therapy*. Antidepressant drugs are often necessary.

Postpartum depression

See *Postnatal depression*.

Postpartum hemorrhage

Excessive blood loss after *childbirth*. Postpartum hemorrhage occurs in about 2 percent of all births. It is more common after a long labor, after a multiple birth, or if the woman required general anesthesia. Before the development of *blood transfusion*, postpartum hemorrhage was a common cause of maternal death.

CAUSES

Most cases of postpartum hemorrhage occur immediately after delivery (primary postpartum hemorrhage) and are due to excessive bleeding from the site where the placenta was attached to the uterus. Such bleeding may be caused by failure of the uterus to contract efficiently after delivery or by the retention of placental tissue within the uterus.

Postpartum hemorrhage immediately after delivery may also be caused by tears anywhere along the birth canal. Tearing is more likely to occur during a *forceps delivery* or a *breech delivery*. In some cases, postpartum hemorrhage occurs because the mother has a *bleeding disorder*.

Occasionally, it occurs with pain and fever between five and 10 days after delivery (secondary postpartum hemorrhage). In these cases, the cause is usually infection of a retained fragment of placenta.

TREATMENT

A blood transfusion may be given to replace lost blood, and emergency treatment may be needed for *shock*. Other treatment depends on the cause of the hemorrhage. Any retained placental tissue may need to be removed under general anesthetic, an injection of *ergometrine* may be given to stimulate uterine contractions, and any lacerations in the vagina or on the cervix are sutured (stitched). *Antibiotic drugs* are used to treat infection.

Post-traumatic stress disorder

A specific form of *anxiety* that comes on after a stressful or frightening event. Common causes include natural disasters (such as earthquakes), violence, *rape*, torture, and serious physical injury. The condition may also result from military combat, when it is sometimes known as battle fatigue or shell shock.

The symptoms include recurring memories or dreams of the event, a sense of personal isolation, and disturbed sleep and concentration. There may be a deadening of feelings, or irritability and painful feelings of guilt, sometimes building up to form a true depressive illness (see *Depression*). Symptoms may begin immediately after the trauma or may develop many months later. The symptoms are made worse by any reminder of the traumatic experience.

Most people recover given time, emotional support, and counseling. However, prolonged physical deprivation (such as that experienced in a concentration camp) may scar people psychologically for life.

Postural drainage

A technique that enables a person whose lungs are clogged with sputum (phlegm) or other secretions to drain them. The person lies in such a way that the secretions drain by gravity into the trachea (windpipe), from where they are coughed up. Postural drainage is used to treat disorders in which stagnant secretions have become infected (as in chest infections in people suffering from chronic *bronchitis*, *bronchiectasis*, and *cystic fibrosis*).

Postural drainage is sometimes done in association with chest clapping (in which another person gently strikes the chest) intended to loosen sticky secretions.

HOW IT IS DONE

The affected person lies on a bed and each lobe of the lung is drained in turn by the adoption of different postures. The different postures are achieved by lying supine, prone, or on each side; by raising the foot of the bed by varying amounts; and by the use of pillows to elevate different parts of the body. At the same time, the affected person loosens lung secretions by "huffing" (breathing out forcibly) and by raising and lowering the elbows, and sometimes by a helper clapping his or her cupped hand on the affected person's chest wall. A mechanical *vibrator* is sometimes applied to the chest.

Postural hypotension

See *Hypotension*.

Posture

The relative position of different parts of the body at rest or during movement. Good posture consists of efficiently balancing the body weight around the body's center of gravity in the lower spine and pelvis. It is dependent on the shape of the *spine* and on balanced contraction of *muscles* around the spine and in each limb. Maintaining good posture helps prevent neck pain and *back pain*.

Many people have bad posture as the result of habit, such as sitting slumped in a chair or standing with the shoulders and back hunched. *Obesity* increases the likelihood of bad posture because it increases the strain on muscles. Poor posture may also be caused by neurological disorders (such as *Parkinson's disease*), by muscle disorders (such as *muscular dystrophy*), or by disorders of the joints or bones (such as *ankylosing spondylitis*).

Post-viral fatigue syndrome

See *Myalgic encephalomyelitis*.

P

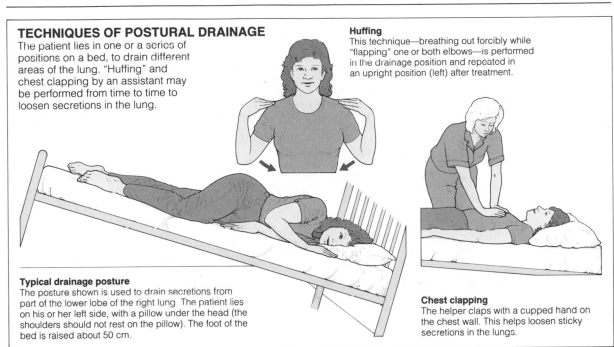

TECHNIQUES OF POSTURAL DRAINAGE

The patient lies in one or a series of positions on a bed, to drain different areas of the lung. "Huffing" and chest clapping by an assistant may be performed from time to time to loosen secretions in the lung.

Huffing
This technique—breathing out forcibly while "flapping" one or both elbows—is performed in the drainage position and repeated in an upright position (left) after treatment.

Typical drainage posture
The posture shown is used to drain secretions from part of the lower lobe of the right lung. The patient lies on his or her left side, with a pillow under the head (the shoulders should not rest on the pillow). The foot of the bed is raised about 50 cm.

Chest clapping
The helper claps with a cupped hand on the chest wall. This helps loosen sticky secretions in the lungs.

Potassium

A mineral which, in combination with *sodium* and *calcium*, maintains normal heart rhythm, regulates the body's water balance, and is responsible for the conduction of nerve impulses and the contraction of muscles.

The body of an average-sized person contains about 140 g of potassium, mainly contained inside the cells. Almost all foods contain potassium, so dietary deficiency is rare. Particularly rich sources include lean meat, whole grains, green leafy vegetables, beans, and many fruits (especially bananas and oranges).

POTASSIUM DEFICIENCY

A low level of potassium in the blood (called hypokalemia) usually occurs as a result of *gastroenteritis* or some other disorder of the digestive tract that causes loss of gastrointestinal fluids through diarrhea and/or vomiting. Children are especially vulnerable to this type of potassium loss.

Other potential causes of hypokalemia include prolonged treatment with *diuretic drugs* or *corticosteroid drugs*; overuse of *laxative drugs*; *diabetes mellitus*; *Cushing's syndrome* (overproduction of corticosteroid hormones by the adrenal cortex); *aldosteronism* (overproduction of the hormone aldosterone by the adrenal cortex); certain kidney diseases; excessive intake of coffee or alcohol; and extremely profuse sweating.

Mild hypokalemia causes fatigue, drowsiness, dizziness, and muscle weakness. In more severe cases, there may be abnormalities of heart rhythm and paralysis of the muscles.

POTASSIUM EXCESS

Much less common than hypokalemia is an excess of potassium in the blood, a condition called hyperkalemia. This may be caused by excessive amounts of potassium, usually in the form of supplements to correct hypokalemia; by severe *kidney failure*; by *Addison's disease*; or by prolonged treatment with potassium-sparing diuretic drugs.

The effects of hyperkalemia include numbness and tingling, muscle paralysis, heart rhythm disturbances, and, in severe cases, *heart failure*.

Potassium permanganate

A drug that has an *antiseptic* and *astringent* effect, useful in the treatment of *dermatitis* (skin inflammation). Potassium permanganate is sometimes applied on a dressing, may be placed in water as a soak, or may be applied directly to the skin. It can occasionally cause irritation and can stain the skin and clothing.

Potency

The ability of a man to perform *sexual intercourse*; or the strength of a *drug* assessed from its ability to cause certain desired effects.

Potential years of life lost (PYLL)

A new way to measure how much any given cause of death shortens lifespan. One year of potential life lost is counted for each year a person dies prematurely, usually before the age of 75. This system places greater weight on diseases such as prematurity, childhood leukemias, and accidents than on diseases of old age, since one child dying in infancy accounts for 75 PYLL, while it would take five people dying at 60 to produce 75 PYLL. (See *Accidental death; Mortality*.)

Pott's fracture

A combined fracture and dislocation of the *ankle* caused by excessive or violent twisting. In a Pott's fracture, the fibula (the outer of the two bones of the lower leg) is broken just above the ankle, and the tibia (shin) also breaks or the ligaments tear, resulting in dislocation.

Treatment consists of manipulating the bones back into position under general anesthetic, followed by immobilization of the foot, ankle, and lower leg in a *cast* for between eight and 10 weeks. Sometimes metal screws are inserted to hold the bone fragments in place.

Severe fracture dislocations may result in stiffness of the ankle, and increase the likelihood of *osteoarthritis* developing in later life.

P

817

Poultice

A warm pack consisting of a soft, moist substance (such as *kaolin*) spread between layers of soft fabric. Poultices were once widely used for reducing local pain or inflammation, for bringing boils to a head, and for improving local circulation.

Pox

Any of various infectious diseases characterized by blistery skin eruptions (for example chickenpox, cowpox, or smallpox). Pox was formerly a common term for *syphilis* and is still sometimes used as a slang word for this disease.

Praziquantel

An *anthelmintic drug* used to treat *tapeworm infestation*. Adverse effects may include dizziness, drowsiness and, if the digestive system is upset, nausea, vomiting, and abdominal pain.

Prazosin

A *vasodilator drug* used in the treatment of *hypertension* (high blood pressure). Prazosin is usually given with a *diuretic drug* and sometimes with other antihypertensive drugs.

Prazosin is also used to treat *heart failure* (reduced pumping efficiency) and *Raynaud's phenomenon* (a circulatory disorder).

Prazosin may cause dizziness and fainting by lowering the blood pressure too fast or too much. Other possible adverse effects are nausea, headache, and dry mouth.

Precancerous

A term applied to any condition in which *cancer* has a tendency to develop. There are three types of such conditions. In the first, there are no tumors present but the condition is known to carry an increased risk of cancer. Examples include *ulcerative colitis* (which carries an increased risk of malignant tumors of the colon or rectum) and *Down's syndrome* (which carries an increased risk of *leukemia*).

In the second type, there are benign tumors that tend to become malignant themselves, such as colonic polyps, or are associated with the development of malignant tumors elsewhere in the body. Examples of this type include *neurofibromatosis* (von Recklinghausen's disease), in which there are large numbers of tumors on the nerves, any of which may become malignant; and *tuberous sclerosis*, in which cancer may develop in the brain, the back of the eye, and various endocrine glands.

The third type comprises disorders that have chronic, sometimes inflammatory or irregular features from the beginning, but which do not always become fully malignant. Disorders within this group include cervical dysplasia (see *Cervix, cancer of*); *leukoplakia* of the mouth (see *Mouth cancer*); and papillomas of the bladder (see *Bladder tumors*).

Predisposing factors

Factors that lead to increased susceptibility to a disease. For example, predisposing factors that make a person more likely to have *coronary artery disease* are a family history of the disease, tobacco smoking, high blood pressure, high lipid (fat) levels in the blood, being overweight, lack of regular exercise, and mental stress.

Prednisolone

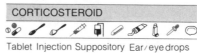

CORTICOSTEROID
Tablet Injection Suppository Ear/eye drops
Prescription sometimes needed

A *corticosteroid drug* used to reduce inflammation and improve symptoms in a variety of disorders, including *eczema, conjunctivitis, iritis, ulcerative colitis, rheumatoid arthritis*, and *asthma*.

Prednisolone is also used in the treatment of blood disorders, such as *thrombocytopenia* and *leukemia*.

High doses or prolonged treatment may cause adverse effects typical of corticosteroid drugs, such as facial rounding, *acne, hypertension, osteoporosis, peptic ulcer*, and *diabetes mellitus*.

Prednisone

A *corticosteroid drug* used to reduce inflammation and improve symptoms in a variety of disorders, including *rheumatoid arthritis, ulcerative colitis* and severe *asthma*.

Other disorders that are occasionally treated with prednisone include *Addison's disease* and blood disorders, such as *leukemia*. Prednisone is also used to prevent organ rejection after *transplant surgery*.

Large doses taken over a prolonged period may cause adverse effects typical of other corticosteroid drugs.

Preeclampsia

A serious condition in which *hypertension* (high blood pressure), *edema* (accumulation of fluid in tissues), and *proteinuria* (protein in the urine) develop in a woman in the second half of pregnancy. Additional symptoms may include headache, nausea and vomiting, abdominal pain, and visual disturbances. The condition is sometimes known as preeclamptic toxemia or PET.

Preeclampsia affects about 7 percent of pregnancies. It is more common in first pregnancies and in women aged under 25 or over 35; it is also more common if *diabetes mellitus*, hypertension, or kidney disease is present. Untreated preeclampsia may lead to *eclampsia*, which is characterized by seizures; eclampsia may cause maternal or fetal death.

TREATMENT

For mild cases of preeclampsia, the woman is confined to bed, and *antihypertensive drugs* may be used to reduce blood pressure. If the woman is close to term or if eclampsia is imminent, *induction of labor* or a *cesarean section* may be necessary.

Pregnancy

The period from conception to birth. Pregnancy begins with conception, the *fertilization* of an ovum (egg) by a sperm, and the subsequent implantation of the fertilized egg. The egg develops into the *placenta* and *embryo*, and later into the *fetus*. Most fertilized eggs implant into the uterus. However, very occasionally, an egg implants into an abnormal site, such as a fallopian tube, resulting in an *ectopic pregnancy*, which may develop into an emergency situation. (See illustrated boxes on the facing page and on page 820.)

WEIGHT GAIN DURING PREGNANCY

The average increase in pregnancy is 12.7 kg—70 percent of it occurring during the last 20 weeks. At term, the typical fetus weighs 3.4 kg and the placenta and fluid together weigh another 1.4 kg. The remaining weight is largely due to water retention and increased fat stores. Within six weeks of delivery, most women return to their prepregnancy weight.

STAYING WELL

Provided the pregnancy is desired and the woman takes care of herself and has *prenatal care*, there is no reason for her not to feel completely healthy during pregnancy.

A balanced and nutritious diet is important. Appetite will increase, but pregnant women should avoid filling up on high-calorie snacks that are low in nutritional value. It is better to eat frequent, smaller meals. Many physicians prescribe *folic acid* and *iron* supplements during pregnancy.

P

Tobacco smoking and *alcohol* should be avoided throughout pregnancy, and no other drug should be taken except under medical supervision (see *Pregnancy, drugs in*).

Exercise can be continued during pregnancy but strenuous exertion and potentially dangerous sports are generally best avoided.

Sexual intercourse can continue throughout pregnancy (unless there is bleeding or if the waters break). Adopting different positions may make intercourse more comfortable. Libido may decrease during early and late pregnancy, but many women enjoy sex throughout pregnancy.

PROBLEMS DURING PREGNANCY

In addition to the expected nausea and tiredness, some women experience other minor problems. The symptoms may be troublesome but generally disappear after delivery.

During pregnancy, food passes through the intestine more slowly, which enables more nutrients to be absorbed for the fetus, but which also tends to cause *constipation*. *Hemorrhoids* are fairly common during late pregnancy, as is *heartburn* due to *acid reflux*. The gums may become spongy and bleed easily. *Pica* (a craving to eat substances other than foods, such as clay or coal) is fairly common.

Swollen ankles are common during the second half of pregnancy, especially during the evening. *Varicose veins* may appear in the later months in susceptible women. Leg cramps, backache, and breathlessness are also common during late pregnancy. Pigmentation tends to increase and may cause *chloasma* (commonly called the mask of pregnancy).

Urinary tract infections are more common during pregnancy, and stress incontinence (see *Incontinence, urinary*) may occur, especially during the later weeks. Vaginal *candidiasis* (thrush) is also more common when a woman is pregnant.

STAGES AND FEATURES OF PREGNANCY

Pregnancy typically lasts 40 weeks, counted from the first day of the pregnant woman's last menstrual period, and is conventionally divided into three trimesters, each lasting three months. For the first eight weeks following conception, the developing baby is called an embryo; thereafter, it is known as a fetus. It is during the early part of pregnancy (first trimester) that the growing baby is most vulnerable to damage.

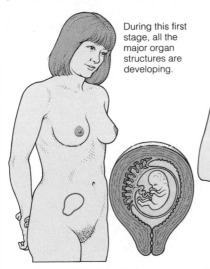

During this first stage, all the major organ structures are developing.

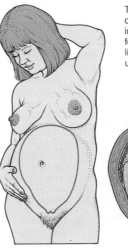

The fetus, now with features that are recognizably human, grows rapidly in size.

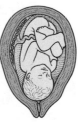

The fetal organs mature in preparation for birth and life outside the uterus.

First trimester (0 to 12 weeks)
The first sign of pregnancy is usually the absence of a menstrual period, though some women have breakthrough bleeding. The breasts start to swell and may become tender as the mammary glands develop to prepare for *breast-feeding*. The nipples start to enlarge and the veins over the surface of the breasts become more prominent. A supportive bra should be worn.

Nausea and vomiting are common, are often worse in the morning, and usually persist for six to eight weeks (see *Vomiting in pregnancy*). Urine is passed more frequently and there is often a creamy white discharge from the vagina. Many women feel unusually tired during the early weeks. Some notice a metallic taste in the mouth or a craving for certain foods. Weight begins to increase.

Second trimester (13 to 28 weeks)
From 16 weeks, the enlarging uterus is easily felt and the woman begins to look noticeably pregnant. The nipples enlarge and darken, and skin pigmentation may deepen. Some women may feel warm and flushed. Appetite tends to increase and weight rises rapidly. Facial features tend to become heavier. By 22 weeks (usually between the 18th and 20th weeks), most pregnant women have felt the baby moving around (sometimes called "quickening").

During the second trimester, nausea and frequency of urination diminish, and the woman may feel generally better and more energetic than during the early weeks. The heart rate increases, as does the volume of blood pumped by the heart, to allow the fetus to develop properly. These changes put an extra strain on the heart of women who have preexisting heart disease.

Third trimester (29 to 40 weeks)
In some women, stretch marks develop on the abdomen, breasts, and thighs. A dark line may appear running from the umbilicus to the pubic hair. *Colostrum* can be expressed from the nipples.

Minor problems are common. Many women become hot and sweat easily, as body temperature rises slightly. More rest may be needed at this stage, though many women find it difficult to find a comfortable position. *Braxton Hicks' contractions* may get stronger.

The baby's head engages (drops down low into the pelvis) around the 36th week in a first pregnancy, but not until a few weeks later in subsequent pregnancies. This "lightening" may relieve pressure on the upper abdomen and on breathing, but increases pressure on the bladder and may result in more vaginal discharge.

P

Women may find that their moods are more changeable. They may also feel more lethargic than usual, may experience bouts of depression, may be easily annoyed or angered, and may be prone to bouts of crying. On the other hand, some women feel more content during pregnancy.

For complications of pregnancy, see *Antepartum hemorrhage; Diabetic pregnancy; Miscarriage; Polyhydramnios; Preeclampsia; Prematurity; Rh incompatibility; Vomiting in pregnancy.* (See also *Childbirth; Fetal heart monitoring; Pregnancy, multiple*).

Pregnancy, drugs in
Drugs taken during *pregnancy* may pass from the mother through the placenta to the baby. Although only a few drugs have been proved to cause harm to a developing baby, no drug should be considered completely safe, especially during early pregnancy. For this reason, a pregnant woman should not take any drug (including over-the-counter drugs) without first consulting her physician.

Drug treatment during pregnancy is usually prescribed only if the potential benefits of treatment outweigh any risk to the baby. Treatment for long-term conditions, such as *epilepsy* or *diabetes mellitus*, is continued during pregnancy but drug therapy may require modification (sometimes even before conception if a woman plans to become pregnant).

Problems in a developing baby may also be caused if a pregnant woman drinks alcohol (see *Alcohol* and pregnancy box), smokes (see *Tobacco smoking*), or takes drugs of abuse.

POSSIBLE ADVERSE EFFECTS
Drugs taken during the first three months of pregnancy may interfere with the normal formation of the baby's organs, causing *birth defects*.

Drugs taken later in pregnancy may slow the rate at which the baby grows, causing a low birthweight. Or they may damage specific fetal tissue—for example, developing teeth may be damaged by *tetracycline drugs*.

Drugs taken toward the end of pregnancy or during labor and delivery (see *Childbirth* pain relief box) may cause problems for the newborn baby. Narcotic analgesics, for example, may cause breathing difficulty.

Drug abuse during pregnancy can cause serious problems. The babies of women who use *heroin* during pregnancy tend to have a low birthweight and have a higher death rate than normal during the first few weeks after birth. These babies may suffer withdrawal symptoms, such as feeding and sleeping difficulties, trembling, and seizures. Babies born to women who are intravenous drug abusers have a high risk of being infected with *HIV*, the *AIDS* virus.

Pregnancy, false
An uncommon psychological disorder, medically known as pseudocyesis, in which a woman has the physical signs of pregnancy, including morning sickness, amenorrhea (lack of periods), breast enlargement, and abdominal swelling. Although the results of *pregnancy tests* prove negative and the fetal heart cannot

P

EFFECTS OF HORMONES DURING PREGNANCY

A pregnant woman undergoes many changes that enable her to maintain the pregnancy, nourish the baby, and prepare for breast-feeding.

These adaptations are brought about by increased levels of the female sex hormones *estrogen* and *progesterone*, and by the action of two other

hormones, human chorionic gonadotropin (HCG) and human placental lactogen (HPL), produced only by the placenta.

TYPICAL RESULTS

Progesterone	Decreases the excitability of smooth muscle, thereby helping to prevent uterine contractions and premature labor. Induces constipation and esophageal acid reflux as a result of its effects on smooth muscle. Increases body temperature. Affects mood. Increases breathing rate.	**Estrogens**	Are important for the development of the reproductive system and breasts. Stimulate growth of the uterine muscle to enable the powerful contractions of labor. Increase vaginal secretions. Increase the size of the nipples and help the development of milk glands in the breasts. Increase the production of protein, which is essential for healthy growth of the woman and fetus. Alter collagen and other substances to allow body tissues to soften and stretch in preparation for labor. Relax ligaments and joints. May cause sciatica and backache, and may also contribute to the formation of varicose veins as a result of their effects on body tissue.
Human placental lactogen (HPL)	Increases energy production necessary for fetal development. Causes enlargement of breasts and development of milk glands. Induces temporary diabetes mellitus (gestational diabetes) in susceptible women as a result of its effects on metabolism.		
Human chorionic gonadotropin (HCG)	Increases energy production necessary for fetal development. Induces gestational diabetes in susceptible women.	**Melanocyte-stimulating hormone (MSH)**	Stimulates pigmentation (in combination with estrogens), particularly of the nipples. May also produce chloasma (darkening of the facial skin).

be heard during examination, the woman remains quite convinced that she is pregnant.

Many women with pseudocyesis are childless or approaching the *menopause* and have an intense desire to have children. Treatment of pseudocyesis may involve *counseling* or *psychotherapy*. (See also *Conversion disorder*.)

Pregnancy, multiple

The presence of more than one fetus in the uterus. Multiple pregnancy can occur if two or more ova (eggs) are released from the ovary and fertilized at the same time. It can also result if a single fertilized ovum divides at an early stage of development. Today, most pregnancies in which there are three or more babies result from the use of *fertility drugs*.

INCIDENCE

Twins occur in about one in 80 pregnancies, triplets in about one in 8,000, and quadruplets in about one in 73,000 pregnancies. Multiple pregnancies are more common in women who are successfully treated with fertility drugs or if a number of already fertilized ova are implanted during *in vitro fertilization*.

DIAGNOSIS AND TREATMENT

During the woman's prenatal examination, the physician may be able to feel more than one fetus, and may find that the abdomen is larger than expected for the duration of gestation.

The physician may also be able to hear more than one fetal heartbeat when listening through a stethoscope. *Ultrasound scanning* may be used to confirm the diagnosis.

The woman is advised to rest during pregnancy and to increase her protein intake. *Iron* and *folic acid* tablets are usually recommended.

COMPLICATIONS

Hypertension (high blood pressure), *polyhydramnios*, *postpartum hemorrhage*, and *malpresentation* occur more frequently in a multiple pregnancy. *Prematurity* is a common complication, and the weight of each baby is usually less than that of a single baby. Cesarean section is necessary more often than in single pregnancies.

Pregnancy tests

Tests on urine or blood performed to determine whether or not a woman is pregnant; some can be performed at home. Pregnancy tests check for the presence of human chorionic gonadotropin (see *Gonadotropin, human chorionic*), produced by the placenta.

HOW IT IS DONE

Urine tests are used most often. Most can detect pregnancy from about two weeks after a missed period, although some of the newer tests can detect pregnancy within a few days of a missed period. The test is usually performed on an early morning midstream urine specimen (because urine is most concentrated at this time).

Urine tests are about 97 percent accurate if the result is positive and about 80 percent accurate if the result is negative. If the result is negative and there is no menstrual period within about a week, the pregnancy test should be repeated.

Blood tests are normally used only when a very early diagnosis of pregnancy is needed. Blood tests measure the level of human chorionic gonadotropin in the blood by a laboratory technique called *immunoassay*. This produces a result from within nine to 12 days of conception but is more expensive to perform.

Premature ejaculation

See *Ejaculation, disorders of*.

Prematurity

Birth of a baby before 37 weeks' *gestation*. A premature labor carries little risk for the mother, but the premature infant may be less than sufficiently developed to cope with independent life and needs special care.

Prematurity was once a major cause of infant mortality, but improved medical techniques have dramatically increased survival rates for premature babies in developed countries. Approximately 5 to 10 percent of babies are born prematurely.

CAUSES

Some 40 percent of all premature deliveries occur for no known reason. The remainder are due to conditions affecting the mother, the fetus, or the placenta.

Preeclampsia is the most common maternal cause of premature labor. Other maternal causes include *hypertension* (high blood pressure), long-standing kidney disease, *diabetes mellitus*, and heart disease. Women who have any of these conditions carry an increased tendency to go into labor prematurely, although some mothers tend to deliver prematurely for no apparent reason. However, more commonly, the pregnancy is curtailed early by *cesarean section* or *induction of labor* by the obstetrician to avoid further risk to mother and baby.

Similarly, *antepartum hemorrhage*, which may be caused by separation of the *placenta* from the uterus before the baby is born, may result in premature labor due to the irritant effect of blood within the uterus. Antepartum hemorrhage sometimes makes induction of labor necessary. Other common causes of premature labor are intrauterine infection or premature rupture of membranes.

MULTIPLE PREGNANCY

About one pregnancy in 80 is multiple (e.g., twins or triplets). The rate is highest among women in their 30s. Problems arise more often in multiple pregnancies than in single pregnancies. For example, twins are much more likely than single babies to be born prematurely.

Placenta
Amniotic fluid
Fetal limb
Fetal heads
Division between amniotic sacs
Wall of uterus

Ultrasound scan revealing twins
Ultrasound scanning of the woman's uterus can reveal twins within the first several weeks of pregnancy. Here, two fetal heads, a limb that belongs to the fetus on the right, and the membrane that divides the two amniotic sacs can be seen.

P

PREGNANCY TEST KIT

Just one of the many types of pregnancy test kit is shown. No kit is 100 percent accurate. Whether a test indicates pregnancy or gives a negative result despite a missed period, it is wise to consult a physician for confirmation.

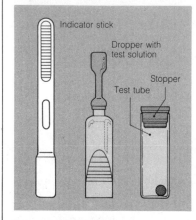

Components of test kit
The kit has three main parts—a dropper tube containing a test solution, a test tube with stopper, and an indicator stick.

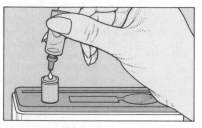

1 The end of the dropper tube is squeezed gently to introduce the test solution into the test tube, which is held upright in a stand provided.

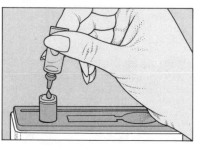

3 Five drops of urine are added to the solution in the test tube. The stopper is put in the test tube, the contents are shaken, and the stopper is removed.

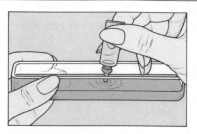

2 The lid of the test kit is used to collect a urine sample early in the morning. Some urine is drawn up into the dropper tube by squeezing and releasing.

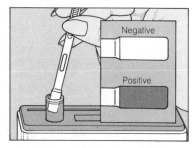

4 The indicator stick is placed in the test tube. The result can be read after 30 minutes. If the end of the stick changes color, it signifies a pregnancy.

The most common fetal cause of prematurity is multiple pregnancy (see *Pregnancy, multiple*), a state which accounts for approximately 15 percent of all premature births. Multiple pregnancy may cause problems in the mother that make cesarean section or induction of labor necessary, or it may cause excessive stretching of the uterus, which stimulates contractions and leads to premature labor. A similar mechanism may occur with *polyhydramnios* (excessive amniotic fluid) or if the woman's uterine cavity is smaller than normal.

PREVENTION
If labor begins prematurely, the obstetrician may in some cases attempt to stop labor by administering a drug (such as ritodrine, isoxsuprine, salbutamol, or turbutaline) that has the effect of inhibiting contractions of the uterus.

THE PREMATURE INFANT
The premature infant is not only smaller than a full-term baby but has a characteristic physical appearance—the infant lacks subcutaneous fat, is covered with downy hair called lanugo, and has a very thin, gelatinous skin.

The baby's internal organs are also immature and less than completely developed, making it necessary for the baby to be monitored in a special hospital environment until he or she has developed sufficiently to sustain independent life.

The major complication for a premature infant is *respiratory distress syndrome*, which results from lung immaturity. Other organs, particularly the liver, may also be immature, leading to increased risk of brain hemorrhage, *jaundice*, and *hypoglycemia* (low blood sugar). A premature baby has a limited ability to suck and to maintain body temperature. Additionally, the immune system is poorly developed.

TREATMENT
Premature infants are usually nursed in a special baby unit that provides intensive care. The baby is placed in an *incubator*, which provides warmth and allows easy observation. Other special care may include artificial *ventilation* to assist breathing, artificial feeding through a stomach tube or into a vein, and treatment with *antibiotic drugs* and *iron* and *vitamin supplements*. The baby is usually kept in hospital until he or she reaches a weight of at least 2.25 kg, is growing satisfactorily, and is capable of feeding well.

OUTLOOK
The survival chances of a premature baby increase with the length of the pregnancy. With modern techniques, some infants now survive even if they are born as early as 23 weeks' gestation and when weighing less than 1 kg, but this remains exceptional. Of babies born at 28 weeks' gestation and given specialist care, approximately 80 percent survive. Most premature babies catch up with full-term babies before the end of their first year.

Premedication
The term applied to drugs given, often by injection, between one and two hours before an operation to prepare a person for surgery. Premedication usually contains a narcotic *analgesic drug* (painkiller) to help relieve pain and anxiety and to reduce the dose of anesthetic that will be needed to produce unconsciousness (see *Anesthesia, general*). An *anticholinergic drug* is often also included because it reduces secretions in the airways and also protects the heart.

Premenstrual syndrome
The combination of various physical and emotional symptoms that occurs in women the week or two before

P

PREMATURITY

A premature baby may need to be nursed in an incubator where the temperature and humidity are carefully controlled and the baby can be closely observed. If breathing difficulties develop, they may be treated by artificial ventilation. Very small babies cannot suck so they must be fed intravenously or via a tube passed into the stomach. If jaundice develops, it may be treated by *phototherapy* (light therapy), which breaks up the bilirubin that causes the yellow discoloration of the skin.

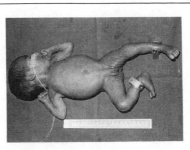

Premature infant
This baby girl was born several weeks prematurely. She is being fed via a flexible tube that passes through the nose and esophagus into the stomach.

FEATURES AND COMPLICATIONS OF PREMATURITY

Physical features	Complications
Low birth weight (often less than 2.5 kg)	Increased risk of birth injury
Small size	Respiratory distress syndrome
Relatively large head and hands	Recurrent episodes of breathing stoppage
Thin, smooth, shiny skin	Jaundice
Veins visible under the skin	Infection
Little fat under the skin	Poor temperature control
Wizened, wrinkled features	Anemia
Soft, flexible ear cartilage	Hypoglycemia (low blood sugar level) and other disturbances of body chemicals
Short toenails (but normal length fingernails)	Rickets
Downy (lanugo) hair	Increased bleeding tendency
Reduced vernix (greasy substance that covers the newborn)	Brain hemorrhage
Protuberant abdomen	Necrotizing enterocolitis (severe intestinal inflammation that may lead to death of intestinal tissue)
Enlarged clitoris (girls)	
Small scrotum (boys)	
Feeble, whining cry	
Irregular breathing	
Poor sucking and swallowing ability	
Tendency to regurgitate	

menstruation. Premenstrual syndrome (PMS) begins at or after *ovulation* and continues until the onset of menstruation. PMS affects more than 90 percent of fertile women at some time in their lives and in some women is so severe that work and social relationships are seriously disrupted.

CAUSES

Many theories exist for the cause of PMS. Hormonal changes that occur throughout the menstrual cycle clearly influence PMS, but an imbalance between estrogen and progesterone levels has not been consistently found. Similarly, deficiencies of *vitamin E*, pyridoxine (see *Vitamin B complex*), *magnesium*, or *prostaglandins* have been suggested but not confirmed.

SYMPTOMS AND SIGNS

The most common emotional symptoms of PMS are irritability, tension, depression, and fatigue. Physical symptoms include breast tenderness, fluid retention, headache, backache, and lower abdominal pain.

TREATMENT

No single method of treatment has proved completely successful. Treatments that may relieve specific symptoms include relaxation techniques to relieve anxiety and tension; *diuretic drugs* to relieve fluid retention; and dietary changes during the latter half of the menstrual cycle (such as avoidance of salt, caffeine, and chocolate). Taking pyridoxine (vitamin B_6) or evening primrose oil may help some women with breast symptoms, irritability, and depression. *Oral contraceptives* can relieve symptoms by eliminating the normal menstrual cycle. Progesterone supplements are widely used but do not help all women.

Premenstrual tension

See *Premenstrual syndrome.*

Premolar

One of eight permanent grinding *teeth*, two in the upper and two in the lower jaw on each side of the mouth, located between the canines and molars. (See also *Eruption of teeth; Permanent teeth.*)

Prenatal care

Care of a pregnant woman and her unborn baby throughout pregnancy with the aim of making sure both are healthy at delivery. Such care involves regular tests on the woman and the fetus to detect disease, defects, or potential hazards, and advising the woman on general aspects of pregnancy, such as diet and exercise.

FIRST VISIT

A woman should see her family physician or obstetrician as soon as she believes she is pregnant. The physician will take a medical history and examine the woman to confirm that she is pregnant and to check her general health. A vaginal examination is usually carried out to check that the reproductive organs and pelvis are normal and to confirm the estimated date of delivery, which is calculated from the first day of the woman's last period.

The first of a series of screening tests to detect any abnormalities in the woman or baby may be carried out at this visit (see the prenatal screening procedures chart on the following page). Some of these tests, such as *ultrasound scanning* to detect any gross abnormality, usually need to be carried out only once; others, such as *blood tests* or *urinalysis* to detect *anemia* or *diabetes mellitus* in the woman, may be performed at periodic intervals throughout the pregnancy.

The woman is also given advice about diet and told to avoid smoking (which can stunt the baby's growth) or drinking alcohol (which can result in *fetal alcohol syndrome*).

SUBSEQUENT VISITS

If there are no problems, the woman visits the physician every month until the 28th week, then every two weeks until the 36th week, and then weekly until the delivery date, which, on average, is the 40th week from the first day of the mother's last menstrual period. If the pregnancy is a high-risk one—for example, if the woman is over 35 years old or is suffering from *hypertension* or diabetes (see *Diabetic pregnancy*)—or if problems develop,

P

visits will be more frequent and, in some cases, the woman may need to be admitted to hospital for closer observation.

At each visit, as well as undergoing the tests detailed in the chart, the woman is weighed, her blood pressure is taken, and the size of the uterus is estimated to confirm that the baby is growing well.

After the 32nd week, the position of the baby in the uterus (whether it is head-down as it should be) is determined, and the degree of engagement (how far the baby's head has descended into the woman's pelvis) is regularly recorded. The woman is also asked about the baby's movements; frequent, pronounced movements usually indicate that the baby is active and healthy.

PREPARATION FOR CHILDBIRTH CLASSES
Childbirth preparation classes are given in hospitals, health centers, community meeting places, or private homes. Such classes aim to provide information on all aspects of pregnancy, labor, and delivery, including advice on exercise, diet, and sexual activity. The woman learns what happens during labor and the different types of pain relief available during it; she may also learn breathing exercises. (See also *Childbirth, natural.*)

Prenatal screening
Tests carried out during pregnancy to check for abnormalities, disorders or infections in the woman or her unborn baby (see illustrated chart).

Prepuce
See *Foreskin.*

Presbycusis
The progressive loss of *hearing* that occurs with age. Presbycusis is a form of sensorineural *deafness* (degeneration of the hair cells and nerve fibers in the inner ear), which makes sounds less clear and tones, especially higher tones, less audible.

SYMPTOMS AND CAUSES
People with presbycusis often have difficulty in understanding speech and are usually unable to hear well in the presence of background noise. The severity and progression of the condition vary considerably from person to person (some people who are 80 have far better hearing than others who are only 60).

The natural process of presbycusis may be exacerbated by exposure to high *noise* levels, by diminished blood supply to the inner ear due to an

PRENATAL SCREENING PROCEDURES

When performed	Procedure	Reason for procedure
First visit	Blood tests	To check the woman's *blood group* and, sometimes, to check for presence of *hepatitis B* virus which might be transmitted to the baby.
	Cervical smear test (Pap smear)	To test for an early cancer of the cervix (if a test has not been performed recently).
First visit and throughout the pregnancy	Blood tests	To check for *anemia* in the woman and, in women with RH-negative blood groups, to look for the presence of Rhesus antibodies.
	Urine test	To check for *proteinuria*, which could indicate a *urinary tract infection* or *preeclampsia*.
	Blood and urine test	To check for *diabetes mellitus*.
	Blood pressure check	To screen for *hypertension*, which interferes with blood supply to the placenta and is a sign of preeclampsia.
First visit and after any infection	Blood tests	To screen for immunity to *rubella*, which can cause defects in the baby, and for *syphilis* and other possible infections.
First 12 weeks	Chorionic villus sampling	May be performed if there is a risk of certain genetic (inherited) disorders being passed on.
16 to 18 weeks	Ultrasound scanning	Is carried out to date the pregnancy accurately and to detect any abnormalities present in the fetus.
	Amniocentesis	Carried out on older women and those who have children with *spina bifida* or *Down's syndrome* to detect possible abnormalities in the fetus.
	Blood test	In some cases, the amount of *alpha-fetoprotein* in the blood is tested to determine whether the baby has spina bifida.
	Fetoscopy and fetal blood sampling	In some cases, these are carried out if there is doubt about the normality of the baby.
High-risk or overdue pregnancies	Blood and urine tests	May be administered to assess placental function and well-being of the fetus.
	Electronic fetal monitoring	To check on the fetal heartbeat.
	Ultrasound scanning	Extra scans may be recommended to assess fetal growth and development, the location of the placenta, and the amount of amniotic fluid.

arterial disease such as *atherosclerosis*, and by toxic damage to the inner ear from certain drugs, such as *aminoglycoside drugs*.

TREATMENT

Hearing aids can help most people, except for those with a poor ability to discriminate between speech sounds (who therefore have difficulty in understanding what is being said). A person speaking to someone with presbycusis should remember to speak slowly and clearly. It is also recommended to speak loudly, unless the person with presbycusis is wearing a hearing aid.

Presbyopia

The progressive loss of the power of *accommodation* for near vision. The focusing power of the eyes weakens with age until, after about the age of 65, little focusing power remains. Presbyopia is usually noticed around the age of 45 when the eyes cannot accommodate within normal reading distance. Large print can still be seen, but it may be difficult to bring small print into focus unless it is read at arm's length.

Simple reading *glasses* with convex lenses are used to correct presbyopia. Glasses may need to be changed four to five times over the course of about 20 years, until all the focusing is eventually being done by the glasses.

Prescription

An instruction written by a physician that directs a pharmacist to dispense a particular drug in a specific dose. A prescription also details how often the drug must be taken, how much is to be dispensed, and any other relevant facts. Drugs that require a prescription (prescription medicines) are available only on the authorization of a physician because they may be dangerous, habit-forming, or used to treat a disease that needs to be monitored. All prescriptions must bear the name and address of the patient and the physician's signature. The pharmacist keeps a record of all prescriptions dispensed.

Preservative

A substance that inhibits the growth of bacteria, yeasts, and molds and so protects foods from putrefying and fermenting. Examples of preservatives include sulfur dioxide, benzoic acid, salt, sugar, and nitrites. Fat preservatives are termed antioxidants because they inhibit oxidation. (See also *Food additives*.)

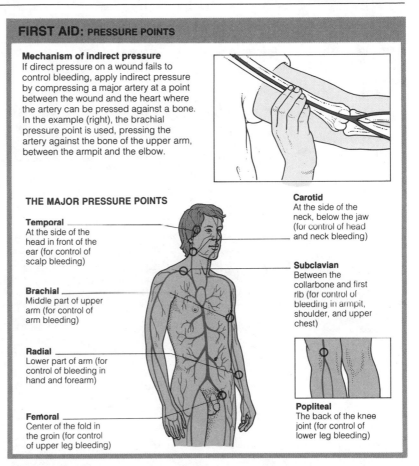

FIRST AID: PRESSURE POINTS

Mechanism of indirect pressure
If direct pressure on a wound fails to control bleeding, apply indirect pressure by compressing a major artery at a point between the wound and the heart where the artery can be pressed against a bone. In the example (right), the brachial pressure point is used, pressing the artery against the bone of the upper arm, between the armpit and the elbow.

THE MAJOR PRESSURE POINTS

Temporal
At the side of the head in front of the ear (for control of scalp bleeding)

Brachial
Middle part of upper arm (for control of arm bleeding)

Radial
Lower part of arm (for control of bleeding in hand and forearm)

Femoral
Center of the fold in the groin (for control of upper leg bleeding)

Carotid
At the side of the neck, below the jaw (for control of head and neck bleeding)

Subclavian
Between the collarbone and first rib (for control of bleeding in armpit, shoulder, and upper chest)

Popliteal
The back of the knee joint (for control of lower leg bleeding)

Pressure points

Places on the body where arteries lie near the surface and where pressure can be applied to limit severe arterial *bleeding*. Application of pressure at these points will not stop venous bleeding

Arterial bleeding can be identified because blood from arteries is bright red and is pumped out in regular spurts as the heart beats. To stop bleeding, pressure is applied by hand to compress the appropriate artery against the underlying bone. (See illustrated box.)

Pressure sores

A common name for *bedsores*, the decubitus ulcers that develop on the skin of patients who are bedridden, unconscious, or immobile.

Prevalence

The number of cases of a disease at any one time in a defined population; often expressed as the number of cases per 100,000 people. Prevalence is useful to express the frequency of diseases that have a gradual onset and last a relatively long time. (See also *Incidence*; Prevalence table.)

Preventive dentistry

An aspect of *dentistry* concerned with the prevention of tooth decay and gum disease rather than their treatment. Preventive dentistry consists of encouraging the practice of good *oral hygiene* and a reduced intake of sugary foods, *fluoride* treatment to strengthen tooth enamel, and *scaling* to remove any accumulated dental *plaque* and *calculus* from the teeth.

Preventive medicine

The branch of medicine that deals with the prevention of disease by public health measures, such as the provision of pure water supplies; by health education to discourage smoking and excess alcohol consumption, to promote exercise, and to advise on a prudent diet; by specific preventive measures, such as immunization against infectious diseases; and by screening programs to detect dis-

P

PREVALENCE OF VARIOUS CHRONIC CONDITIONS IN CANADA

Prevalence (Number of people with the condition per 100,000 population)	Categorization	Examples
More than 25,000	Extremely common	Male pattern baldness Errors of refraction
5,000 to 25,000	Very common	Hypertension (high blood pressure) Osteoarthritis
1,000 to 5,000	Common	Chronic bronchitis Diabetes mellitus (all types) Impaired vision Impaired hearing Rheumatoid arthritis
200 to 1,000	Fairly common	Epilepsy Parkinson's disease Schizophrenia
50 to 200	Uncommon	Ankylosing spondylitis Down's syndrome Multiple sclerosis Ulcerative colitis
5 to 50	Rare	Autism Crohn's disease Cystic fibrosis
Less than 5	Very rare	Albinism Galactosemia

P

eases such as cancer of the cervix or breast, hypertension (high blood pressure), glaucoma, and tuberculosis, before they cause symptoms.

Most of the increase in the world's population during the 19th century was due to improvements in public health, particularly improvements in the overall standard of nutrition, and the provision of pure water supplies and proper sanitation. Today, these measures remain the priorities of preventive medicine in developing countries, and, along with a program of immunization in childhood, have been targeted as major objectives by the World Health Organization.

However, in developed countries, the primary objective is to persuade the adult population to adopt a healthier life-style. In Canada, many deaths in adults before the age of 65 are preventable, being due to accidents and/or linked to such factors as smoking, an unhealthy diet, excessive drinking, and insufficient exercise. Adoption of a healthier life-style, the

wider use of screening for cancers, and measures to reduce accidents could lead to substantial improvements in health.

Priapism

Persistent, painful *erection* of the *penis* without sexual arousal. Priapism is a dangerous condition that requires emergency treatment.

CAUSES
Priapism occurs because blood fails to drain from the spongy tissue of the penis, keeping the penis erect. Possible causes include damage to nerves that control the supply of blood to the penis; a blood disease that causes partial clotting of blood in the penis; and, rarely, blockage of the normal outflow of blood from the penis as a result of an infection (such as *prostatitis* or *urethritis*).

TREATMENT
Urgent treatment is needed because of the risk of permanent damage to the penis. Treatment may involve *spinal anesthesia* (injection of local anes-

thetic into the spinal canal) or withdrawal of blood from the penis through a wide-bore needle.

Prickly heat

An irritating skin rash that is associated with profuse sweating. The medical name for prickly heat, miliaria rubra, literally means "red millet seeds." This term describes the multiple tiny, red, itchy spots that cover the mildly inflamed affected areas of skin. Prickly heat is accompanied by aggravating, prickling sensations. The irritation tends to affect sites on the body where sweat collects, particularly the waist, upper trunk, armpits, and the sides of the elbows.

A milder variety (miliaria crystallina) produces clear, shiny, fluid-filled blisters that tend to dry up quickly without treatment.

CAUSES
The mechanism by which prickly heat is caused is not fully understood, but unevaporated sweat is known to be an important factor. The skin becomes unhealthy and waterlogged. Sweat ducts become blocked with debris and eventually leak sweat into the skin. Sleep is often possible only in cool surroundings, and lack of sleep combined with the intense irritation of the rash can make the sufferer irritable.

TREATMENT AND PREVENTION
Prickly heat does not occur when people live and work in air-conditioned buildings. If these are not available, frequent cool showers and sponging the affected areas relieve the itching, although ordinary soap should not be used on affected areas. Application of *calamine* lotion and dusting powder can further relieve the discomfort. Clothing should be clean, starch-free, and loose-fitting to help the evaporation of sweat. The chances of developing prickly heat are much reduced by slow acclimatization to hot weather. If the sweating has occurred because of fever, *antipyretic drugs* (fever-reducing drugs), such as ASA or acetaminophen, may help.

Primaquine

A drug used in the treatment of vivax and ovale *malaria*. Primaquine is often given after prophylactic treatment with *chloroquine* has failed to prevent the infection. Primaquine is not effective in preventing a malaria attack but kills the parasites in the liver.

Adverse effects include nausea, vomiting, and abdominal pain. In people with *G6PD deficiency*, primaquine may cause hemolytic *anemia*.

Primary

A term applied to a disease that has originated within the organ or tissue affected, and is not derived from any other cause or source. Primary liver cancer, for example, is the result of some cancer-producing change in liver cells. Secondary liver cancer results from the spread of cancer cells from another part of the body.

The term primary is also applied to the first of several diseases to affect a tissue or organ in turn. For example, when a viral infection of the lungs is succeeded by a bacterial infection, the viral infection is called primary and the bacterial infection is termed secondary. Primary is also used to mean "of unknown cause."

Primary teeth

The first teeth (also known as deciduous, or milk, teeth), which usually start to appear at the age of 6 months and are gradually replaced by the permanent teeth from the age of about 6 years.

There are 20 primary teeth, 10 in each jaw. Each set of 10 consists of four incisors (biting teeth) at the front, flanked by two canines (eye teeth), with four molars (grinding teeth) at the back. (See also *Eruption of teeth; Teeth; Teething*.)

Primidone

An *anticonvulsant drug* used in the treatment of *epilepsy* and, occasionally, *tremor*. Primidone is usually prescribed with another anticonvulsant. Adverse effects include drowsiness, clumsiness, and dizziness.

Probenecid

A drug used in the long-term treatment of *gout* which reduces the level of uric acid in the body by increasing the amount excreted in the urine.

Probenecid also slows the excretion of some *antibiotic drugs* (such as *penicillin drugs* and *cephalosporin drugs*) from the kidneys and is therefore occasionally prescribed with these drugs to boost their effects.

Probenecid may cause nausea and vomiting. It also increases the risk of kidney stones in some people.

Probucol

A *lipid-lowering drug*. Probucol is often prescribed with other lipid-lowering drugs to boost their effect. Treatment is usually monitored by blood tests.

Possible adverse effects include diarrhea, flatulence, pain in the abdomen, and, rarely, dizziness.

Procainamide

An *antiarrhythmic drug* used in the treatment of certain types of *tachycardia* (abnormally rapid heartbeat): for example, ventricular *arrhythmias* that occur after a *myocardial infarction* (heart attack).

Procainamide may cause nausea, vomiting, loss of appetite, and, rarely, confusion. Prolonged treatment may induce *lupus erythematosus*, causing fever, joint pain, swelling, and rash.

Procaine

A local anesthetic (see *Anesthesia, local*) used before surgical or dental treatment and, occasionally, during childbirth. Procaine has largely been replaced by drugs that are quicker to take effect or are longer-acting.

Occasionally, procaine causes an allergic reaction, with a rash or swelling of the face, lips, mouth, or throat. Rare adverse effects of this drug include anxiety, drowsiness, or tinnitus (ringing in the ears).

Procarbazine

An *anticancer drug* particularly useful in the treatment of *lymphomas*. Procarbazine is also used to treat brain tumors and certain cancers of the skin, lungs, and bone marrow.

In addition to the adverse effects typical of anticancer drugs, procarbazine may cause a sudden rise in blood pressure if taken with certain foods or drinks (e.g., cheese and red wine).

Prochlorperazine

A *phenothiazine*-type *antipsychotic drug*. Prochlorperazine is used to relieve the symptoms of certain psychiatric disorders, including *schizophrenia* and *mania*. In smaller doses, it is also used as an *antiemetic drug* to relieve nausea and vomiting.

Prochlorperazine may cause involuntary movements of the face and limbs, lethargy, dry mouth, blurred vision, and dizziness.

Procidentia

A medical term for severe *prolapse* (displacement of an organ from its normal position in the body), usually of the uterus.

Proctalgia fugax

A severe cramping pain in the *rectum* unconnected with any disease. Proctalgia fugax may be due to muscle spasm, sometimes associated with stress or anxiety. The pain, which may occur at any time, is of short duration and subsides of its own accord.

Proctitis

Inflammation of the *rectum*, causing soreness, bleeding, and sometimes a discharge of mucus and pus. Proctitis commonly occurs with inflammation of the colon as a feature of *ulcerative colitis*, *Crohn's disease*, or *dysentery*. In cases where inflammation is confined to the rectum, the cause is often unknown. However, especially in male homosexuals, proctitis is sometimes due to *gonorrhea* or another sexually transmitted disease. Rare causes of proctitis include *tuberculosis*, *amebiasis*, *schistosomiasis*, injury, certain drugs, allergy, or radiation injury.

DIAGNOSIS AND TREATMENT
The diagnosis is made by *proctoscopy* (inspection of the rectum with a viewing instrument). A *biopsy* (removal of a small sample of tissue for laboratory analysis) is sometimes required to determine the exact cause of the rectal inflammation.

Successful treatment of any underlying cause usually clears the problem. *Corticosteroid drugs*, in the form of suppositories or enemas, may relieve symptoms, especially in cases of ulcerative colitis or Crohn's disease.

Proctoscopy

Examination of the *anus* and *rectum* by means of a proctoscope (a rigid viewing instrument) inserted through the anus. A short, flexible sigmoidoscope (see *Sigmoidoscopy*) is sometimes used and is more comfortable for the person being examined.

Procyclidine

An *anticholinergic drug* used in the treatment of *Parkinson's disease*. Procyclidine reduces excessive salivation and muscle rigidity and may improve tremor. Possible adverse effects include dry mouth and blurred vision.

Prodrome

An early warning symptom of illness. For example, a *migraine* headache may be preceded by pins and needles in the hands or feet or by an *aura* of visual symptoms. Awareness of a prodrome may enable a migraine headache sufferer to use certain preventive medicines that are far less effective once a headache is established.

Progeria

Premature aging. There are two distinct forms of progeria, both of which are extremely rare.

In Hutchinson-Gilford syndrome, aging starts around the age of 4, and by 10 or 12 the affected child has all the external features of old age, including gray hair, baldness, and loss of fat, resulting in thin limbs and sagging skin on the trunk and face. There are also internal degenerative changes, such as widespread *atherosclerosis* (narrowing of the arteries by fatty deposits). Death usually occurs at puberty, most commonly from coronary artery disease.

Werner's syndrome, or adult progeria, starts in adolescence or early adult life and follows the same rapid progression as the juvenile form.

The cause of progeria is unknown, although victims' cells show only a few generations of cell division before they stop reproducing.

Progesterone hormone

A female sex hormone essential for the healthy functioning of the female reproductive system. Progesterone is produced in the *ovaries* during the second half of the menstrual cycle (see *Menstruation*) and by the placenta during *pregnancy*. Small amounts of progesterone are also produced in the adrenal glands and testes.

Following *ovulation*, increased production of progesterone causes the endometrium (lining of the uterus) to thicken in preparation for the implantation of a fertilized egg. If fertilization does not take place, the production of progesterone and also of *estrogen hormones* falls, resulting in shedding of the uterine lining and the unfertilized egg in the monthly period.

During pregnancy, progesterone is produced by the placenta and causes changes in the mother's body—for example, it contributes to breast changes. Progesterone also passes into the developing baby's circulation, where it is converted in the adrenal glands to *corticosteroid hormones*. At the end of pregnancy, a fall in the level of progesterone helps initiate labor.

Other effects of progesterone produce changes in the cervix and vagina during the menstrual cycle, increased deposition of fat, and increased *sebum* production by glands in the skin.

Progestogen drugs

COMMON DRUGS

Dydrogesterone Levonorgestrel
Medroxyprogesterone Norethindrone
Progesterone

A group of drugs similar to *progesterone hormone*, which includes both natural progesterone and synthetic progesterone derivatives.

WHY THEY ARE USED

Progestogen drugs are used in *oral contraceptives*, either on their own (in the minipill) or with *estrogen drugs* (in combined and phased pills). Such drugs work by making the cervical mucus impenetrable to sperm, altering the lining of the uterus so that it prevents the implantation of a fertilized egg, and reducing the production of *gonadotropin hormones*, which may prevent eggs from ripening in either of the ovaries.

Progestogen drugs are also prescribed, sometimes with estrogen drugs, to treat menstrual problems (see *Menstruation, disorders of*).

In *hormone replacement therapy*, a progestogen drug is used in combination with an estrogen drug to reduce the risk of cancer of the uterus (see *Uterus, cancer of*), which may occur if estrogens alone are taken over a long period of time. The progesterone induces the monthly shedding of the uterine lining.

Progestogen drugs are used also to treat *premenstrual syndrome, endometriosis* (a disorder in which fragments of tissue that normally lines the uterus occur elsewhere in the pelvic cavity), and *hypogonadism* (underdevelopment of the ovaries). Progestogen drugs are sometimes effective as *anticancer drugs* in the treatment of certain types of cancers (such as uterine endometrial cancer) that are sensitive to progesterone hormones.

POSSIBLE ADVERSE EFFECTS

Adverse effects include weight gain, *edema* (accumulation of fluid in tissues), loss of appetite, headache, dizziness, rash, irregular periods, breast tenderness, and, less commonly, *ovarian cysts*.

Prognathism

Abnormal protrusion of the lower jaw or both jaws. If the condition interferes with biting and chewing (see *Malocclusion*) or is disfiguring, *orthognathic surgery* may be performed.

Prognosis

A medical assessment of the probable course and outcome of a disease. It is based on the recorded history of the disease (e.g., 90 percent of people with small cell carcinoma of the lung die within five years of the condition's developing), the physician's own experience of treating the disease, and the patient's general condition and age. However, every prognosis is no more than an informed guess, and any patient may prove it wrong.

Progressive

A term used to describe a condition that becomes more severe and/or extensive over time; for example, in progressive muscular atrophy (a type of *motor neuron disease*), weakness and muscle wasting usually begin in the hands, gradually spread to the arms, shoulders, and legs, and eventually affect the entire body.

Progressive muscular atrophy

A type of *motor neuron disease* in which the muscles of the hands, arms, and legs become weak and wasted and twitch involuntarily. This is a progressively debilitating condition which eventually spreads to other muscles in the body.

Proguanil

An antimalarial drug used in the prevention of *malaria*. Travelers visiting parts of the world where there is a risk of malaria need to start taking proguanil at least 24 hours before leaving home and continue taking it for at least four weeks after returning from the journey.

In some countries, the malaria parasite has become resistant to proguanil, and another antimalarial drug, such as *chloroquine*, should be taken in combination with proguanil to ensure adequate protection.

Proguanil rarely causes adverse effects. Indigestion, nausea, or vomiting may occur but usually disappears as treatment continues.

Prolactin

A *hormone* produced by the *pituitary gland*. Prolactin, acting with certain other hormones, stimulates the growth and development of the mammary glands (see *Breast*). Secretion of prolactin is increased during *pregnancy*, and helps to initiate and maintain milk production for *breastfeeding*. (See also *Prolactinoma*.)

Prolactinoma

A benign tumor of the *pituitary gland* that causes overproduction of the hormone *prolactin*. In a woman, a prolactinoma may result in *galactorrhea* (breast secretion at any time other than a few days before childbirth or during breast-feeding), *amenorrhea* (absence of periods), or *infertility*. In a man, a prolactinoma may cause *impotence* and *gynecomastia* (breast enlargement). In either sex, it may cause headaches, *diabetes insipidus*, and, if it presses on the optic nerves, gradual loss of the outer field of vision.

P

The condition is diagnosed from blood tests to measure prolactin levels, and from *CT scanning* or *MRI* of the brain. Treatment may consist of removal of the tumor, *radiation therapy*, or the drug *bromocriptine*, which inhibits prolactin secretion.

Prolapse
Displacement of part or all of an organ or tissue from its normal position. Common structures that prolapse include the uterus (see *Uterus, prolapse of*) and intervertebral disks (see *Disk prolapse*).

Promazine
A *phenothiazine*-type *antipsychotic drug* used as a sedative, especially in the elderly, and valuable in treating nausea and vomiting.

Possible adverse effects of promazine include abnormal movements of the face and limbs, drowsiness, lethargy, dry mouth, constipation, and blurred vision. Long-term treatment may cause *parkinsonism*.

Promethazine
An *antihistamine drug* used to relieve itching in a variety of skin conditions, including *urticaria* (hives) and *eczema*. Promethazine is also used as an *antiemetic drug* to relieve nausea and vomiting caused by *motion sickness* and *Meniere's disease*.

Promethazine has a sedative effect and is therefore sometimes used as a *premedication* (drug used to prepare a person for surgery) and as a short-term sleeping drug for children. Occasionally, promethazine is given to produce sedation during *childbirth*.

Possible adverse effects of promethazine include dry mouth, blurred vision, and drowsiness.

Pronation
The act of turning the body to a prone (facedown) position, or the hand to a palm backward position. The opposite movements are called *supination*.

Propantheline
An *antispasmodic drug* used in the treatment of *irritable bowel syndrome* and forms of urinary *incontinence*.

Possible adverse effects include dry mouth, blurred vision, and abnormal retention of urine.

Prophylactic
A drug, procedure, or piece of equipment used to prevent disease; the term prophylactic is also sometimes used to refer to a *condom*.

Propoxyphene
A weak narcotic analgesic suitable for treatment of mild or moderate pain. Because propoxyphene has a long duration of action, it may be more convenient for relief of chronic pain than other mild analgesics. Side effects are dizziness and nausea. If patients take the drug over long periods, there is a danger of physical dependence.

Propranolol
A *beta-blocker drug* used to treat *hypertension* (high blood pressure), *angina pectoris* (chest pain due to inadequate blood supply to the heart muscle), and cardiac *arrhythmias* (irregularities of the heartbeat). It is also used occasionally to reduce the risk of further damage to the heart after *myocardial infarction* (heart attack).

Propranolol is used to relieve symptoms of *hyperthyroidism* (overactivity of the thyroid gland), the palpitations, sweating, and tremors of *anxiety*, and to prevent attacks of *migraine*.

Possible adverse effects are typical of other beta-blocker drugs.

Proprietary
A term to describe a drug patented for production by one company. The patent protects the drug's name, ingredients, and process of manufacture.

Proprioception
The body's internal system for collecting information about its position relative to the outside world and the state of contraction of its muscles. This is achieved by means of sensory nerve endings within the muscles, tendons, joints, and sensory hair cells in the balance organ of the inner ear. These structures are called proprioceptors (literally "one's own sensors").

Information from the proprioceptors passes to the spinal cord and brain and is used to make adjustments in the state of contraction of muscles so that posture and balance are maintained. During movement, there is a continuous feedback of information to the brain from the proprioceptors and from the eyes. This helps ensure that actions are smooth and coordinated.

Proptosis
A term for protrusion, particularly of the eyeball (see *Exophthalmos*).

Propylthiouracil
A drug used to treat *hyperthyroidism* (overactivity of the thyroid gland) or to control symptoms of hyperthyroidism in preparation for a *thyroidectomy*

(removal of the thyroid gland). Unless an operation is planned, treatment with propylthiouracil is given for at least a year.

Possible adverse effects include itching, headache, rash, and joint pain. Propylthiouracil may reduce the production of white blood cells by the bone marrow and thus increase the risk of infection.

Prostaglandin
One of a group of *fatty acids* that is made naturally in the body and that acts in a similar way to *hormones*. Prostaglandins are divided into broad groups according to their chemical structure. They were first discovered in semen but are now known to occur in many different body tissues, including the uterus, brain, and kidneys. Some prostaglandins are prepared synthetically for use as drugs (see *Prostaglandin drugs*).

EFFECTS
Prostaglandins produce a wide range of effects on the body, including causing pain and inflammation in damaged tissue, protecting the lining of the stomach and duodenum against ulceration, and stimulating contractions in labor (see box below).

EFFECTS OF SOME PROSTAGLANDINS

Type	Effect
PGA_1	Lowers blood pressure. May protect against peptic ulcer
PGD_2	Causes inflammation
PGE_1	Stimulates contractions of the uterus. Lowers blood pressure. Reduces stickiness of platelets in blood
PGE_2	Causes inflammation. Widens airways. Increases stickiness of platelets in blood. Stimulates contractions of the uterus. Protects against peptic ulcer
PGF_2	Stimulates contractions of the uterus. Narrows airways
PGG_2	Causes inflammation
PGI_2	Reduces stickiness of platelets in blood

Certain drugs counteract the effects of prostaglandins within the body. *Nonsteroidal anti-inflammatory drugs* (NSAIDs), *ASA,* and *corticosteroid drugs* relieve pain and inflammation by reducing prostaglandin production in tissues. Taken long-term, however, NSAIDs and ASA may increase the risk of a *peptic ulcer,* in part by reducing production of prostaglandins that protect the stomach lining.

Prostaglandin drugs

Synthetically produced *prostaglandins* which have many therapeutic uses.

One, dinoprostone, is used to stimulate uterine contractions for *induction of labor* at full term, after a fetal death, or to induce a late abortion (see *Abortion, induced*).

Alprostadil is an E_1 prostaglandin used to treat newborn infants awaiting surgery for certain types of congenital heart disease. It is also being investigated for use in the treatment of *Raynaud's disease.*

Other prostaglandin drugs are under investigation for use in a variety of disorders, including *peptic ulcer.*

Prostate, cancer of

A malignant growth arising in the outer zone of the *prostate gland.* It is one of the most common cancers in men; about 9,000 cases are diagnosed in Canada each year. Prostate cancer sometimes develops in middle age but most often occurs in the elderly. While its precise cause is unknown, the hormone *testosterone* appears to be involved.

SYMPTOMS AND SIGNS

Symptoms may be caused by enlargement of the prostate (see *Prostate, enlarged*) and include difficulty in starting to pass urine, poor flow of urine, and increased frequency of urination. There may be no urinary symptoms, however, and the first evidence of the disease may be pain in the bones from secondary growths of the cancer. When the tumor causes difficulty in passing urine, the flow of urine may eventually cease completely either because the urethra is totally blocked or because the cancer has spread to the bladder and ureters. In advanced cases, pain may be caused by involvement of nerves within the pelvis or by spread (metastasis) of cancer to bones anywhere in the body.

DIAGNOSIS

Cancer of the prostate is usually diagnosed at a *rectal examination* in which the physician feels the prostate

through the rectum; a diseased gland feels hard and knobby. The diagnosis may be confirmed by *ultrasound scanning, urography,* and prostatic biopsy (the removal of a sample of tissue for microscopic analysis). Blood tests and a bone scan may be performed to assess the extent to which a cancer has spread.

TREATMENT

Treatment may be by *prostatectomy* (surgical removal of the prostate) or *radiation therapy;* if the disease has spread to other parts of the body, patients may be helped by reducing the level of testosterone. This may be done by *orchiectomy* (surgical removal of the testes), by giving *estrogen drugs,* antiandrogens (drugs which block the action of testosterone) or by giving drugs that block release of the pituitary hormone that regulates the release of testosterone.

OUTLOOK

When the growth is discovered at an early stage, the outlook is very good. However, if the cancer has spread outside the prostate gland and does not respond to hormone treatment, the prognosis is poor.

Prostatectomy

An operation to remove part or all of the *prostate gland.* Prostatectomy is usually performed when enlargement of the gland is causing obstruction to the flow of urine (see *Prostate, enlarged*). The operation may also be performed to treat cancer of the prostate (see *Prostate, cancer of*) or, occasionally, prostatitis.

HOW IT IS DONE

The most common method is transurethral prostatectomy, which is performed during *cystoscopy.* If the prostate gland is very enlarged, retropubic prostatectomy may be performed (see illustrated box).

RECOVERY PERIOD

In rare cases, bleeding after the operation is severe, and *blood transfusions* are required. Blood clots that may form within the bladder can be washed out through the catheter inserted during the operation.

Following removal of the catheter, urination may initially be frequent and sometimes painful; in some cases, there is mild incontinence for a few weeks. Patients are encouraged to drink large amounts of fluid to help to wash out the remaining blood in the urine.

The hospital stay is about four or five days for transurethral prostatectomy and about eight to 10 days for

the retropubic operation. After several weeks, patients may resume all activities, including intercourse.

OUTLOOK

Uncommonly, prostatectomy affects potency or sexual sensation. In most cases, the operation causes sterility because semen is expelled backward into the bladder during orgasm instead of being ejaculated via the penis (a condition known as retrograde ejaculation). Seminal fluid in the bladder is not harmful and is excreted in the urine.

Prostate, enlarged

An increase in the size of the inner zone of the *prostate gland,* also known as benign prostatic hypertrophy. The condition is most common in men over 50. The cause is unknown.

SYMPTOMS AND SIGNS

Symptoms usually develop gradually as the enlarging prostate compresses and distorts the urethra. The flow of urine is obstructed; there is difficulty in starting to pass urine, and the stream of urine is weak.

Initially the bladder muscle becomes overdeveloped to force urine through the obstructed urethra. Eventually the bladder is unable to expel all the urine (see *Urinary retention*) and becomes distended, causing abdominal swelling.

There may be *incontinence* due to overflow of small quantities of urine, and the bladder may become overactive, resulting in frequency of urination (see *Urination, frequent*). This is a sign of bladder muscle failure and usually means surgery is needed.

Severe abdominal pain and the ability to pass only a few drops of urine require immediate treatment.

DIAGNOSIS

Enlargement of the prostate can be detected during a *rectal examination* (in which the physician inserts a gloved finger into the rectum). The physician also feels the abdomen for signs of bladder distention.

A sample of urine may be tested for infection and a blood test performed to provide a measurement of kidney function. *Ultrasound scanning, urography,* and a recording of the strength of urine flow may be performed to give additional information about the severity of the obstruction and any effects elsewhere in the urinary system, especially the kidneys.

TREATMENT

Mild symptoms of prostatic enlargement do not require treatment. If symptoms are more severe, the usual

P

PROSTATECTOMY—REMOVAL OF THE PROSTATE GLAND

Of the two possible methods of removal shown, the transurethral method is the most commonly used.

It avoids the disadvantages of an abdominal incision and usually permits a shorter stay in hospital.

The retropubic method may be necessary if the prostate is very enlarged or if a cancer is suspected.

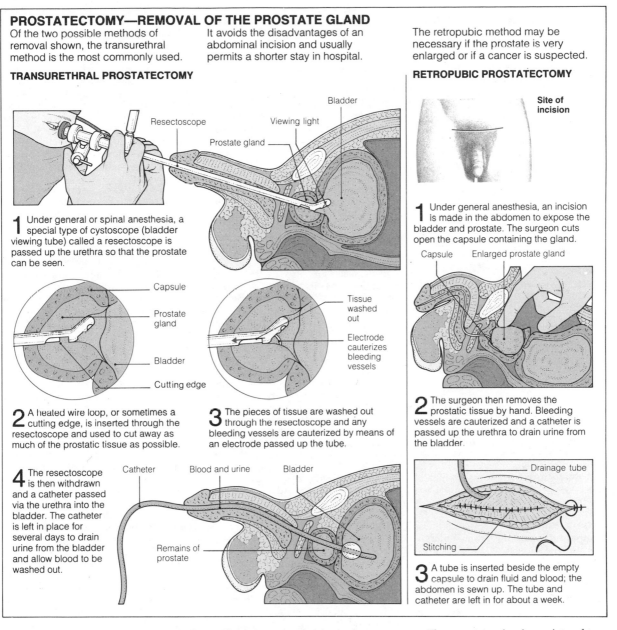

TRANSURETHRAL PROSTATECTOMY

1 Under general or spinal anesthesia, a special type of cystoscope (bladder viewing tube) called a resectoscope is passed up the urethra so that the prostate can be seen.

2 A heated wire loop, or sometimes a cutting edge, is inserted through the resectoscope and used to cut away as much of the prostatic tissue as possible.

3 The pieces of tissue are washed out through the resectoscope and any bleeding vessels are cauterized by means of an electrode passed up the tube.

4 The resectoscope is then withdrawn and a catheter passed via the urethra into the bladder. The catheter is left in place for several days to drain urine from the bladder and allow blood to be washed out.

RETROPUBIC PROSTATECTOMY

1 Under general anesthesia, an incision is made in the abdomen to expose the bladder and prostate. The surgeon cuts open the capsule containing the gland.

2 The surgeon then removes the prostatic tissue by hand. Bleeding vessels are cauterized and a catheter is passed up the urethra to drain urine from the bladder.

3 A tube is inserted beside the empty capsule to drain fluid and blood; the abdomen is sewn up. The tube and catheter are left in for about a week.

treatment is *prostatectomy* (removal of the prostate gland). Retention of urine is treated initially by urinary *catheterization* and then by prostatectomy. If surgery is considered too dangerous because of age or ill health, a catheter may be kept in place permanently.

Prostate gland

A solid, chestnut-shaped organ surrounding the first part of the urethra in the male. The prostate gland is situated immediately under the bladder and in front of the rectum.

The prostate gland produces secretions that form part of the seminal fluid during *ejaculation*. The ejaculatory ducts from the seminal vesicles pass through the prostate gland to enter the urethra.

The prostate gland weighs only a few grams at birth. Enlargement to adult size starts at puberty from the effect of *androgen hormones* and stops at around the age of 20, when it reaches its adult weight of about 20 g. In most men, the prostate begins to enlarge further after the age of 50.

The prostate gland consists of two main zones: an inner zone (which produces secretions responsible for keeping the lining of the urethra moist) and an outer zone (which produces seminal secretions).

DISORDERS
Prostatic problems very rarely occur before the age of 30. *Prostatitis* (inflammation of the prostate) is usually caused by bacterial infection and may be sexually transmitted. It usually affects men in their 30s and 40s, but can occur later in life.

LOCATION OF PROSTATE GLAND

Located under the bladder and in front of the rectum, the prostate gland secretes substances into the semen as the fluid passes through ducts leading from the seminal vesicles into the urethra.

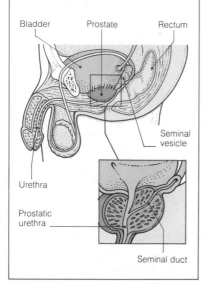

Bladder   Prostate   Rectum

Seminal vesicle

Urethra

Prostatic urethra

Seminal duct

Enlargement of the prostate (see *Prostate, enlarged*) usually affects men over 50 and may interfere with urination by compressing the urethra.

Cancer of the prostate (see *Prostate, cancer of*) is common in old age and may cause symptoms similar to those caused by enlargement of the prostate gland.

Prostatism

Symptoms resulting from enlargement of the prostate gland (see *Prostate, enlarged*).

Prostatitis

Inflammation of the *prostate gland*, usually affecting men between the ages of 30 and 50.

Prostatitis is often caused by a bacterial infection that has spread from the urethra. The infection may or may not be sexually transmitted. Presence of a urinary catheter increases the risk of prostatitis.

SYMPTOMS AND SIGNS

Prostatitis causes pain when passing urine and increased frequency of urination; it sometimes causes fever and a discharge from the penis. There may be pain in the lower abdomen, around the rectum, and in the lower back, and blood in the urine.

DIAGNOSIS AND TREATMENT

The physician performs a *rectal examination* by inserting a gloved finger into the rectum; the gland will be tender and enlarged. To investigate the cause of infection, tests are carried out on a urine sample and on urethral secretions obtained after massaging the prostate gland.

Treatment is with *antibiotic drugs*. Despite treatment, the condition may be slow to clear up and tends to recur.

Prosthesis

An artificial replacement for a missing or diseased part of the body. Examples of prostheses used to restore normal function include false legs or arms fitted after amputation (see *Limb, artificial*) or artificial heart valves used to replace valves damaged by disease (see *Heart valve surgery*).

Prostheses are also used for cosmetic reasons. Examples include a breast prosthesis fitted after *mastectomy* (removal of a breast) and glass eyes inserted following removal of diseased eyes (see *Eye, artificial*).

Prosthetics, dental

The branch of *dentistry* concerned with the replacement of missing teeth and their supporting structures. Prosthetics includes three basic kinds of replacement—partial or complete *dentures* (which are easily removed for cleaning), semipermanent appliances such as overdentures (fittings that are attached over existing teeth), and permanent restorations such as crowns (see *Crown, dental*) and bridges (see *Bridge, dental*).

Proteins

Large molecules that consist of hundreds or thousands of *amino acids* linked (by peptide bonds) to form long chains, which are often folded in various ways. In addition to amino acids, proteins may contain other constituents such as sugars (glycoproteins) and lipids (lipoproteins).

There are two main types of proteins: fibrous and globular. Fibrous proteins are insoluble and form the structural basis of many body tissues, such as hair, skin, muscles, tendons, and cartilage. Globular proteins are soluble and include all *enzymes* (substances that promote biochemical reactions in the body), many *hormones* (such as growth hormone and prolactin) and various proteins in the blood, including *hemoglobin* and *antibodies*. In addition, the *chromosomes* in cell nuclei are formed of proteins linked with *nucleic acids*; proteins linked with lipids constitute a major part of cell membranes (see *Cell*).

PROTEINS AND DIET

Proteins are needed in the diet primarily to supply the body with amino acids. Ingested proteins are broken down in the *digestive system* to amino acids, which are then absorbed and rebuilt into new body proteins (see *Protein synthesis*). Proteins are the only major foodstuff that contains nitrogen. The balance between dietary intake of protein and the excretion of breakdown products from the body (mainly *urea* in the urine) can be followed by measuring the nitrogen intake and the nitrogen output. (See also *Nutrition*.)

Protein synthesis

The formation of *protein* molecules inside cells through the linking of much smaller substances called *amino acids*. Because proteins provide many of the structural components and the *enzymes* that promote biochemical reactions in the body, their manufacture—in the correct numbers and order—is essential to all aspects of development and growth.

Different cells manufacture a different range of proteins. The instructions for their manufacture are held by the hereditary material—the *genes*, which consist of *DNA* (deoxyribonucleic acid)—within the nucleus of the cell. Protein synthesis starts with a gene (a particular length of DNA) acting as a template for the manufacture of a strand of a substance called messenger *RNA*. Like DNA, RNA is a *nucleic acid* and consists of a string of building blocks called nucleotide bases. There are four different types of nucleotide bases; their sequence in the strand of messenger RNA provides the coded instructions (the *genetic code*) for making a particular protein.

The strand of messenger RNA passes out of the cell nucleus, where it is then decoded (see diagram) to form a polypeptide chain (string of amino acids). Several polypeptide chains may be manufactured and combine to form one protein molecule.

The rate of protein synthesis is regulated through adjustments in the amount of the relevant messenger RNA formed within the cell nucleus. Highly complex mechanisms exist for "blocking" or "unblocking" the copying of DNA by messenger RNA; this ensures that the cell makes the right type of proteins, in the right quantities, and at the right time.

STEPS IN PROTEIN SYNTHESIS

Proteins consist of one or more subunits called polypeptides. These are formed, within cells, from building blocks called amino acids, which are provided to each cell as raw materials. The instructions for making polypeptides are encoded in the DNA within the cell nucleus.

1 To make a specific protein or polypeptide, the relevant section of DNA (or *gene*) in a cell nucleus is used as a template to make a strand of a substance called messenger RNA. Like DNA, this consists of a string of substances called nucleotide bases.

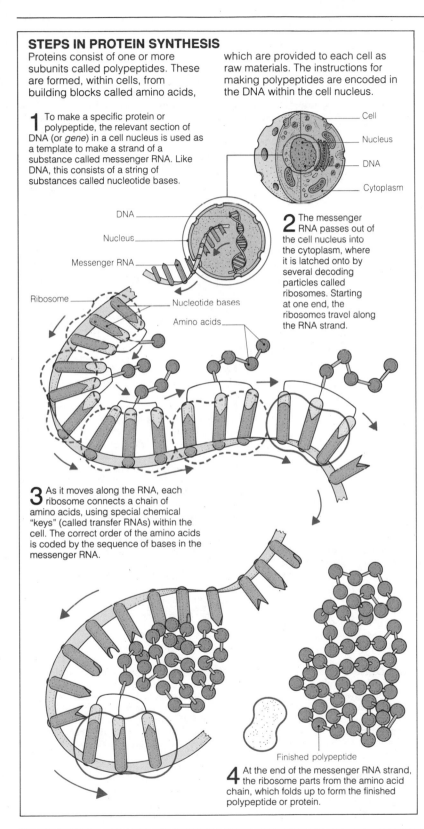

2 The messenger RNA passes out of the cell nucleus into the cytoplasm, where it is latched onto by several decoding particles called ribosomes. Starting at one end, the ribosomes travel along the RNA strand.

3 As it moves along the RNA, each ribosome connects a chain of amino acids, using special chemical "keys" (called transfer RNAs) within the cell. The correct order of the amino acids is coded by the sequence of bases in the messenger RNA.

4 At the end of the messenger RNA strand, the ribosome parts from the amino acid chain, which folds up to form the finished polypeptide or protein.

Finished polypeptide

Labels: Cell, Nucleus, DNA, Cytoplasm, DNA, Nucleus, Messenger RNA, Ribosome, Nucleotide bases, Amino acids

Proteinuria

The passage of increased amounts of *protein* in the *urine*. Proteinuria may result from damage to the glomeruli (filtering units in the *kidney*), allowing proteins to leak from the blood into the urine (see *Glomerulonephritis*). Proteinuria may also result from *urinary tract infection* and from damage to the kidney tubules that prevents the normal reabsorption of protein from the patient's urine.

Increased protein in the urine may also occur because of a generalized disorder (such as *multiple myeloma*) that causes an increase in the level of protein in the blood.

Proteinuria rarely causes any symptoms, although the urine may appear frothy. The condition is usually discovered during a routine *urine test* or during investigation of an underlying disorder.

Protoplasm

An obsolescent term for the entire contents of a cell, including the cytoplasm and organelles, such as the nucleus. Today, the word protoplasm has largely been replaced by specific terms for the individual cell components (see *Cell*).

Protozoa

 The simplest, most primitive type of animal; each protozoon consists of a single cell. All types of protozoa are of microscopic size but are bigger than bacteria. The more advanced types are capable of excretion, respiration, and engulfing food particles; they move around through jellylike movements or the use of whiplike or hairlike attachments called flagella. Some are parasites of larger animals during various stages of their life-cycle.

About 30 different types of protozoa are troublesome parasites of humans. Included among them are the organisms responsible for *amebiasis* and *giardiasis* (intestinal infections that cause diarrhea); the sexually transmitted infection *trichomoniasis*; and the insect-borne tropical diseases *malaria, sleeping sickness,* and *leishmaniasis* and *toxoplasmosis* (acquired from cats).

Protriptyline

An *antidepressant drug*. Protriptyline is especially useful in treating *narcolepsy* or *depression* accompanied by lethargy and tiredness, because it is less likely than other antidepressants to cause drowsiness.

P

Possible adverse effects include palpitations, anxiety, insomnia, and a rash aggravated by sunlight.

Provincial health plans

Insured health care services, which the provinces are responsible for administering and delivering. Each province has a health plan that conforms to the requirements of the *Canada Health Act* and the Medical Care Act of 1966. (See *Medicare*.)

Proximal

A term describing a part of the body that is nearer to a central point of reference, such as the trunk. The hip joint is proximal to the knee; the knuckle is proximal to the fingernail. The opposite of proximal is *distal*.

Prurigo

Thickening and itching of the *skin* due to repeated scratching.

Pruritis

The medical term for *itching*. It is used, for example, in pruritus ani, which is the medical term for itching of the skin around the anus, and pruritus vulvae, which is the term for itching of the external genital area in women.

Pseud-/pseudo-

Prefixes that mean false, as in pseudocyesis (a false pregnancy).

Pseudarthrosis

A term meaning false joint which is used to describe an operation in which the ends of two opposing bones within a joint are removed and a piece of tissue (usually muscle) is fixed between the resulting gap to act as a cushion. This procedure is used to restore mobility and reduce pain when a hip *arthroplasty* (joint-replacement operation) has failed. Pseudarthrosis results in shortening of the affected leg and instability of the joint. A walking aid is usually required.

The term pseudarthrosis also describes a rare condition in children in which congenital abnormality of the bone of the lower half of the tibia (shin) leads to spontaneous fracture without injury. Treatment of this condition consists of inserting a nail through the bone ends and applying a *bone graft*. If the bone ends fail to unite, amputation of the leg, followed by the fitting of an artificial limb, may be necessary.

Pseudocyesis

See *Pregnancy, false*.

Pseudodementia

A form of severe *depression* in elderly people that mimics *dementia*. Features of both illnesses include intellectual impairment and loss of memory. Nearly one in 10 of those initially thought to be suffering from dementia may turn out to have a depressive illness. Unlike dementia, depression is treatable; many people respond well to *antidepressant drugs*.

Pseudoephedrine

A *decongestant drug* used to relieve *nasal congestion*. Pseudoephedrine is an ingredient in a variety of cough and cold remedies.

High doses may cause anxiety, nausea, dizziness, and, occasionally, hypertension (high blood pressure), headache, and palpitations.

Pseudoepidemic

An outbreak of an illness in a community or in an institution (such as a school) that has no detectable physical cause but is thought to be due to a form of *hysteria*. Typically, the symptoms are vague and mild—headache and a general feeling of sickness—and are induced by group suggestibility combined with anxiety provoked by contact with somebody who already has the symptoms.

Pseudogout

A form of *arthritis* that results from the deposition of calcium pyrophosphate crystals in a joint. The underlying cause of pseudogout is unknown; in rare cases, it is a complication of *diabetes mellitus, hyperparathyroidism*, and *hemochromatosis*.

Symptoms include intermittent attacks of arthritis similar to *gout*. Pseudogout can be distinguished from gout only by examining a sample of the joint fluid under a microscope to identify the crystals, which are different from the urate crystals found in gout. Treatment is with *nonsteroidal anti-inflammatory drugs* (NSAIDs).

Pseudohermaphroditism

A *congenital* abnormality in which the external genitalia resemble those of the opposite sex. Thus, a female pseudohermaphrodite may have an enlarged clitoris resembling a penis and enlarged labia resembling a scrotum. Conversely, a male may have a very small penis and a divided scrotum resembling labia.

In pseudohermaphroditism, an affected person has only ovarian or testicular tissue. This condition thus differs from true *hermaphroditism*, in which an affected person has both. (See also *Sex determination*.)

Psilocybin

An alkaloid present in some types of mushrooms, especially in *PSILOCYBE MEXICANA*. It is a powerful *hallucinogenic drug* with properties similar to those of *LSD*.

Psittacosis

A rare illness resembling *influenza* that is caused by a microorganism, *CHLAMYDIA PSITTACI*, and is spread to humans from birds or poultry.

The infection is contracted by inhaling dust contaminated by the droppings of infected birds. Most cases occur among poultry farmers, pigeon owners, and people working in pet shops, although anyone who acquires a pet parrot is at slight risk.

The illness in birds is occasionally serious or even fatal, but often causes no more than lethargy.

Human illness is extremely variable in its features, the most common symptoms being fever, severe headache, and cough, which develop a week or more after exposure to infected birds. Other symptoms include muscle pains, sore throat, nosebleed, lethargy, and depression. In some severe cases, there is also breathing difficulty.

The cause of the condition is often suspected from the patient's occupation; it is diagnosed by finding *antibodies* (proteins with a defense role) specific to the causative organism in the patient's blood.

Treatment with *tetracycline drugs* is usually effective. Without treatment, the illness may continue for several weeks or months before subsiding. Psittacosis may occasionally be fatal if unrecognized and thus not treated.

Psoas muscle

A muscle that bends the hip upward toward the chest. It is composed of two parts (psoas major and psoas minor) which originate from the lower spine. The lower end of psoas minor is attached to the margin of the pelvis; the lower end of psoas major is joined to the bony prominence just below the neck of the femur (thigh bone).

A rare disorder of the psoas muscle is an *abscess* (collection of pus), which develops as a complication of *osteomyelitis* (bone infection) of the spine, usually caused by *tuberculosis*.

P

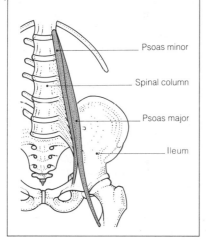

LOCATION OF PSOAS MUSCLE
The muscle has two parts—major and minor. The psoas major acts to flex the hip (bend it up toward the trunk) and rotates the thigh inward. The psoas minor acts to bend the spine down toward the pelvis.

Psoas minor

Spinal column

Psoas major

Ileum

Psoralen drugs

Drugs containing chemicals called psoralens, which occur in certain plants (such as buttercups) and are present in some perfumes. When absorbed into the skin, psoralens react with *ultraviolet light* to cause darkening or inflammation of the skin. They may be taken by mouth or applied directly to the affected skin.

WHY THEY ARE USED
Psoralen drugs may be used to treat *psoriasis* (a disorder characterized by a scaly rash) and *vitiligo* (a disorder in which patches of skin lose color).

HOW THEY WORK
Psoralen drugs are used in conjunction with ultraviolet light (a combination that is known as PUVA) as a form of *phototherapy*. This treatment stimulates the production of skin pigment and, in psoriasis, additionally slows the rate at which skin cells grow and multiply.

POSSIBLE ADVERSE EFFECTS
Overexposure to ultraviolet light during psoralen treatment or too high a dose of a psoralen drug may cause redness and blistering of the skin, thus worsening the original condition. Psoralens in perfumes may cause a rash when the skin is exposed to ultraviolet light (see *Photosensitivity*). The use of psoralens in suntanning preparations is prohibited in some countries because these chemicals can cause *sunburn*.

Psoriasis

A common skin disease characterized by thickened patches of inflamed, red skin, often covered by silvery scales. Although psoriasis does not usually cause itching, the affected area may be so extensive that great physical discomfort and social embarrassment may result.

CAUSES AND INCIDENCE
The exact cause of psoriasis is not known but it tends to run in families. Psoriasis occurs in about 2 percent of people in North America and Europe and is probably less common in black people and Asians. It affects men and women equally. Psoriasis usually appears between the ages of 10 and 30, but infants occasionally suffer from the condition and it may also sometimes develop in old age.

The underlying abnormality in psoriasis is that new skin cells are produced about 10 times faster than normal. As a result, live cells accumulate and form characteristic thickened patches covered with dead skin.

Psoriasis tends to recur in attacks of varying severity; attacks may be triggered by a number of factors, such as emotional stress, skin damage, and physical illness.

The skin eruption is sometimes accompanied by a painful swelling and stiffness of the joints, which can be very disabling (see *Arthritis*).

TYPES
The disease has different forms, which may need different treatment.

DISCOID OR "PLAQUE" PSORIASIS In this, the most common form, patches appear on the trunk and limbs, particularly the elbows and knees, and on the scalp. In addition, the nails may become pitted, thickened, or separated from their beds.

GUTTATE PSORIASIS This form occurs most frequently in children. It consists of numerous small patches that develop rapidly over a wide area of skin, often after a sore throat.

PUSTULAR PSORIASIS This form is characterized by small pustules, which may occur all over the body or be confined to localized areas.

TREATMENT
Mild psoriasis may be helped by moderate exposure to sunlight or an ultraviolet lamp (see *Phototherapy*) and use of an emollient (soothing cream). Moderate attacks are usually treated with an ointment containing *coal tar* or *dithranol*. Other methods of treating psoriasis include *corticosteroid drugs*, *PUVA* (a type of phototherapy), and other drugs, such as *methotrexate*.

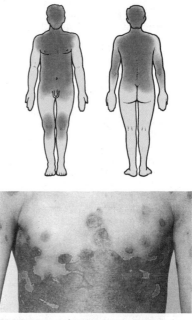

Distribution and appearance of psoriasis
The knees, elbows, scalp, trunk, and back are common sites for psoriasis. The usual appearance is of patches of thickened skin covered by dry, silvery, adherent scales.

Accompanying arthritis is treated with *nonsteroidal anti-inflammatory drugs* (NSAIDs), *antirheumatic drugs*, or methotrexate.

OUTLOOK
For most people, psoriasis is a long-term condition with no permanent cure, although individual attacks can be completely relieved with appropriate treatment.

Psych-

A prefix meaning mental processes or activities, as in psychology.

Psyche

A term meaning mind (as opposed to body) derived from the ancient Greek for soul or spirit. The most influential description is provided by Freud's *psychoanalytic theory*, which treats the psyche as an organ of the body that is divided into the conscious and unconscious, each with its own functions.

Psychedelic drugs

Drugs, many of which are illicit, that may produce hallucinations, also known as *hallucinogenic drugs*.

Psychiatric hospital

There are about 15 provincially funded hospitals in Canada for the treatment of mental disorders. In contrast to the mental hospitals of 40 years ago, in which the retarded, the homeless, and the elderly were confined along with the mentally ill, modern psychiatric hospitals stress rapid evaluation, treatment, and discharge of patients either to their homes or to community-based care facilities. Many general hospitals have short-term psychiatric treatment facilities, and psychiatric hospitals generally include short-term or day care facilities.

Improvements can be attributed in part to *antipsychotic drugs*, and in part to psychiatric social workers, psychiatric nurses, rehabilitation counselors, psychologists, and other professionals who evaluate patients in the social context and help place them back in the community.

Psychiatry

The branch of medicine concerned with the study, prevention, and treatment of mental illness and emotional and behavioral problems. In this it differs from *psychology*, which is concerned with normal mental processes and behavior.

Psychiatry is broad in scope; it approaches the understanding and treatment of mental problems from psychological, social, and physical aspects. Some psychiatrists emphasize that major mental illness is due to genetic and biochemical factors, while psychoanalytically oriented psychiatrists believe that environmental experiences are still the major cause of mental illness. Psychiatrists usually conduct examinations of physical and mental state, and trace the patient's personal and family history to seek the cause of the problem. Laboratory investigations and drug treatments have played an increasingly important role in modern psychiatry.

Within psychiatry there are a number of subspecialties, including child and adolescent psychiatry, community psychiatry (concerned with care of the mentally ill outside psychiatric hospitals), forensic psychiatry (dealing with legal issues, such as rape), neuropsychiatry (relating to brain disorders with mental symptoms), psychiatry of the elderly, and psychiatry of mental handicap (concerned with the psychiatric needs of people with learning disabilities).

Treatment methods in psychiatry may include the use of medication, counseling or *psychotherapy* (individually or in groups), *psychoanalysis*, or *behavior therapy*.

Psychoanalysis

A treatment for psychiatric disorders based on *psychoanalytic theory*. The system was developed by Sigmund Freud at the beginning of the 20th century as a result of treating, under hypnosis, patients who were supposedly suffering from hysteria. Freud believed that mental disorders were a result of the failure of normal emotional development during childhood. By encouraging the patient to reenact these years and to verbalize any problems (past or present), Freud believed that important information would emerge from the unconscious mind; the cause of any internal strife would be uncovered and resolved, and the illness would be cured.

Psychoanalysts may have had previous training in various disciplines, including medicine, social work, or psychology, before beginning their training as a psychoanalyst, which usually involves their undergoing analysis themselves.

WHY IT IS DONE

Psychoanalysis can help people with *neurosis* and *personality disorders*. A modified psychoanalytic approach has also been used to treat *psychosis* (when medication is often an important adjunct). Psychoanalysis aims to help the patient understand his or her emotional development and to help the person make appropriate adjustments in particular situations.

HOW IT IS DONE

The treatment involves interviews between a trained analyst and the patient, each lasting perhaps an hour, repeated up to six times a week and continuing for an indefinite period, usually for several years.

Traditionally, the patient lies on a couch with the analyst behind and out of sight. Some therapists prefer to face the patient, who sits in a chair. In dealing with psychotic patients, the structure and reality of face-to-face contact with the psychiatrist is an extremely important element.

The patient is encouraged to talk as freely as possible about his or her life history and any problems that may have occurred in the past or are currently causing concern. This stream of talk is one of free association, with one word or idea leading to another without conscious control so that any repressed material has the opportunity to surface. The analyst interprets these associations in the light of psychoanalytic theory, paying particular attention to areas of resistance that may contain clues to the person's problem. This leads to different trains of thought, more experiences relived, and sometimes exposure of reasons for symptoms.

Psychoanalysis relies on a number of other key processes. A very close relationship develops with the analyst, who eventually comes to be associated in the patient's mind with important people in his or her history (for example, father, mother, brother, or sister). This experience is called *transference*.

Interpretation of the patient's dreams is another important aspect of the treatment. It is believed that material normally repressed comes to the surface while the patient dreams, usually in the form of symbolic representations (see *Dream analysis*).

The patient is often reluctant to accept the analyst's interpretations and may introduce *defense mechanisms* (such as denial) to cope with the unfolding explanation of his or her behavior. This reaction is a defense against the anxiety that is stimulated as these repressed conflicts break through into consciousness. Understanding the self-destructive patterns of living is an essential aspect of psychoanalytic treatment.

Psychoanalytic theory

A system of ideas developed by Sigmund Freud early in this century that explains the development of personality and behavior in terms of unconscious wishes and conflicts.

Psychoanalytic theory has undergone considerable distillation by psychoanalysts over the years. However, its basic concepts and the use of *psychoanalysis* (therapy based on the concepts of psychoanalytic theory) dominated psychiatry until recently.

KEY FEATURES OF FREUDIAN THEORY

Freud placed great emphasis on the importance of sexuality (in its broadest sense) in psychological development. His theory postulates that, during the first 18 months, an infant passes through three phases—oral, anal, and genital—each representing the area of the body to which the child devotes attention at a particular age. After these phases, the child is able to direct attention to people outside himself or herself. Sexual attraction to the parent of the opposite sex develops with consequent desire to eliminate the other parent, who prevents fulfillment of the desire—this is called the *Oedipus complex*.

By the age of 5 or 6, sexual feelings become latent, but reemerge at *puberty*. At this time, psychological and emotional problems may occur if the individual has not developed normally through the successive stages and has become fixed at a primitive level (see *Fixation*). Problems may also occur if the Oedipus complex has not been successfully dealt with.

Less specifically sexual aspects of psychological development are seen as depending on the interaction among the three parts that make up the personality—the id, ego, and superego. The id is the basic component that guides the individual unconsciously and instinctively toward pleasure; the ego mediates, by conscious reasoning, between internal desires and the reality of the outside world; the superego is also a controlling force but is unconscious, being derived from moral and social standards indoctrinated by parents and other authorities.

It is thought that mental disorders result if conflict between the three aspects of personality cannot be satisfactorily resolved. Freud believed that under normal circumstances tension is dealt with by (among other *defense mechanisms*) repression (in which painful or unacceptable thoughts or memories are kept out of consciousness) and sublimation (in which emotional drives that cannot openly be expressed are channeled into an acceptable activity, such as sport). These normally healthy unconscious processes can become harmful if they occur inappropriately or in excess.

MODERN DEVELOPMENTS

Psychoanalysis has progressed since Freud. In general, modern psychoanalysis is based on the observation that emotional problems for the most part are the result of troubled childhood experiences in the family. The pre-Oedipal problems that are caused by difficulties in the early mother-child relationship are probably even more important than later Oedipal conflicts. Such conflicts may form the basis of later neurotic or psychotic disturbances.

It is necessary for the child to separate from the mother to become an individual and comprehend reality. A healthy mother and father help the child to become an individual. Conflict-ridden parents distort reality and program patterns of disturbed self-destructive behavior. Psychoanalysis in practice attempts to bring to light these unconscious conflicts with the parent (which have led to distortions of reality). The aim is to free the individual from the past and help him or her become a real person in the present. The relationship and interaction between physician and patient is an essential part of this process.

As the biological basis for psychiatric problems becomes ever more apparent, psychoanalytic theory is decreasing in its influence.

Psychodrama

An adjunct to *psychotherapy* in which the patient acts out certain roles or incidents. These may relate to people closely involved with the patient or may concern situations that he or she finds particularly stressful. The aims of psychodrama are to bring out hidden concerns and to allow a person's disturbing feelings to be expressed. Psychodrama is often carried out with a partner or in a group of patients; music, dance, and mime are also commonly utilized.

Psychogenic

A symptom or disorder that originates from psychological or emotional problems and is not produced or caused by any physical illness.

Psychology

The scientific study of mental processes. Psychology deals with all internal aspects of the mind, such as *memory*, feelings, *thought*, and *perception*, as well as external manifestations, such as *speech* and behavior. Psychology is also concerned with *intelligence, learning*, and *personality* development. Methods employed in psychology include direct experiments, observations, surveys, study of personal histories, and special tests (such as *intelligence tests* and *personality tests*).

Psychologists make an important contribution to the diagnosis and treatment of mental and emotional problems. They play a major part in the use of behavior therapy, counseling, and in the treatment of behavioral disorders affecting people with a mental handicap. However, because psychologists are not medically qualified, they are not able to prescribe drugs.

Within psychology, a number of different approaches are used. Neuropsychology attempts to relate human behavior to brain and body functions. Behavioral psychology studies the ways in which people react to events and learn to adapt accordingly. Cognitive psychology concentrates on thought processes and is based on the theory that what a person thinks about his or her behavior is of equal importance to the behavior itself. Psychoanalytic psychology stresses the role of the unconscious and of childhood experiences (see *Psychoanalytic theory*).

There are many specialized areas within the science. Educational psychologists study learning and intelligence; clinical psychologists are concerned with emotional and behavioral problems; social and industrial psychologists consider the effects of work and the environment on behavior; and experimental psychologists concentrate on research into new ways of understanding mental events. The emergence of developmental psychology as a specialist area is due to the work of the Swiss psychologist Jean Piaget, who noted that a child's intellectual development passes through certain stages—from simple motor skills to logical and abstract thought.

Psychometry

The measurement of psychological functions. Psychometry includes statistical assessment of intelligence and personality (see *Intelligence tests; Personality tests*) as well as numerous methods of testing specific aptitudes, such as memory, logic, concentration, and speed of response. The design of such measurements has become increasingly sophisticated, but the validity of some tests (i.e., whether they measure what they are supposed to measure) is less certain.

Psychoneurosis

A term now used interchangeably with *neurosis*. Neurosis originally referred to any disorder of the nerves; psychoneurosis specifically described nervous disorders associated with psychological symptoms.

Psychopathology

The study of abnormal mental processes. There are presently two main approaches in psychopathology—the descriptive and the psychoanalytic.

Descriptive psychopathology aims to record, as objectively as possible, the symptoms that make up a diagnosis of mental illness. It is particularly concerned with abnormality of *thought*, with mood disturbances, and with the various forms of *hallucination* and *delusion*. The ability to recognize such symptoms when interviewing patients is an important part of the psychiatrist's job.

P

The psychoanalytic approach is concerned with the unconscious feelings and motives of the individual.

Psychopathy

An outdated term for an *antisocial personality disorder*.

Psychopharmacology

The study of drugs that affect mental states. Since the early 1950s, more effective medications for a range of mental illness have been developed. Particular advances have occurred in the treatment of psychotic illnesses, with the development of *antipsychotic drugs* and *antidepressant drugs*. *Antianxiety drugs* have proved to be extremely effective in relieving symptoms in neurotic illness, although the dangers of dependence have been recognized recently.

Psychosexual disorders

A range of conditions related to sexual function. Psychosexual disorders are assumed to stem from psychological problems, although some (e.g., *impotence*) may also be caused by physical injury or illness. Psychosexual disorders include *transsexualism* (a sense that one's anatomical sex is inappropriate), *psychosexual dysfunction* (interference with the normal process of sexual response), and sexual behavior in which intercourse between consenting adults is not the final aim (see *Deviation, sexual*).

Psychosexual dysfunction

A disorder in which there is interference with the normal process of sexual response in the absence of any known organic cause. Psychosexual dysfunctions are very common in both men and women. They usually start in early adult life, often disappearing spontaneously with experience and increased confidence.

The main dysfunctions affecting men are lack of sexual desire (see *Sexual desire, inhibited*), *impotence*, and premature ejaculation (see *Ejaculation, disorders of*); those affecting women are lack of sexual desire, painful intercourse (see *Intercourse, painful*), *vaginismus*, and lack of orgasm (see *Orgasm, lack of*).

Most psychosexual problems start in early adult life. Some are associated with certain personality traits, including *anxiety* and obsessiveness. Unpleasant early experiences, such as sexual interference in childhood or problems with one's first sexual encounters, are especially likely to

inhibit later sexual performance. Unrealistic ideas about normal sexual behavior or a strict upbringing may also increase the likelihood of sexual problems. Many different kinds of feelings and conflicts (basically nonsexual) can be expressed sexually or can interfere with normal modes of sexual expression.

Psychosexual dysfunctions are common and not usually evidence of serious illness. About 80 percent of people respond well to *sex therapy*.

Psychosis

A severe mental disorder in which the individual loses contact with reality. Psychosis contrasts with *neurosis*, which describes the milder group of mental illnesses. Neurotic individuals generally know they are ill, but psychotic illness so disturbs the ability to think, perceive, and judge clearly that sufferers often do not realize they are unwell. Psychosis is what people commonly think of as "madness."

TYPES

Three main forms of psychosis are generally recognized: *schizophrenia*, *manic-depressive illness*, and organic brain syndrome (see *Brain syndrome, organic*). However, the symptoms overlap and there is considerable debate about whether each is truly a separate category.

Paranoid illness (see *Paranoia*) is sometimes regarded as a fourth form of psychosis, but many psychiatrists see it as a distinctive disorder.

SYMPTOMS

The main feature of psychotic symptoms is that they may lead the person to view life in a distorted way. Symptoms include *delusions*, *hallucinations*, *thought disorders*, loss of *affect* (emotion), *mania*, and *depression*.

CAUSES

It is highly likely that the cause is due to a disorder of brain function.

Research is centered on the role of *neurotransmitters* (chemicals released by nerve endings), such as *dopamine*, and on the importance of the limbic system and frontal lobes of the brain. As yet, no specific physical abnormality that might be isolated by a blood test or X ray has been clearly related to psychosis. However, a new form of brain imaging, *PET scanning*, may reveal the causes of these disorders.

TREATMENT AND OUTLOOK

Antipsychotic drugs are usually very effective in controlling symptoms. Treatment may need to be long-term, but many sufferers are able to lead normal working lives. In many cases,

more extensive rehabilitation is needed, as is continual support for many years.

Psychosomatic

A term used to describe physical disorders that seem to have been caused, or worsened, by psychological factors. Just as a physical reaction (such as crying) may be due to emotion, so it is presumed that worries or unpleasant events can cause physical illness.

For a disorder to be labeled psychosomatic, the psychological factor and physical effect must be closely connected in time and repeatedly related. This is because many chronic illnesses constantly vary in severity, regardless of a person's psychological state, and because there is a tendency to assume that an event was stressful just because a person has become ill.

Common examples of conditions that may fit the psychosomatic label are headache, breathlessness, nausea, *asthma*, *irritable bowel syndrome*, *peptic ulcer*, and certain types of *eczema*. (See also *Somatization disorder*.)

Psychosurgery

Any operation on the brain carried out as a treatment for serious mental illness. Psychosurgery is performed only as a last resort to treat severe mental illnesses that have not responded to other forms of treatment.

TYPES

Prefrontal *lobotomy* was once the most widely used form of psychosurgery, but there were often harmful side effects and this procedure has now been largely replaced by other operations which are safer.

The most commonly performed operations today are forms of *stereotaxic surgery*. In these procedures, a small hole is drilled in the skull above one temple. A diathermy probe is inserted and, under X-ray control, guided to specific areas of the brain, where small cuts are made in nerve fibers. Stereotaxic procedures are most often carried out to provide relief from severe *depression* or *anxiety* or to treat disabling *obsessive-compulsive disorder*.

Performed less often are the more complex, "open" operations, in which a complete portion of the skull is cut through and lifted up to expose the brain so that specific areas can be removed. Parts of the temporal lobe are cut out to treat *temporal lobe epilepsy*. In rare cases, complete lobes have been removed to treat violent or aggressive behavior.

P

Psychosurgery has produced good results in some people, enabling those who would otherwise be chronically disabled to lead more useful lives. However, the operations tend to have inconsistent and unpredictable results, and can produce adverse changes in personality and intellect. They remain a controversial form of treatment for psychiatric illness.

Psychotherapy
The treatment of mental and emotional problems by psychological methods. In psychotherapy, the patient talks to a therapist about symptoms and problems and establishes a therapeutic relationship with the therapist.

Any person who uses psychotherapy as a formal method of treatment can be called a psychotherapist. Many psychotherapists have no medical background, but certain personal characteristics are deemed especially important, notably empathy (the ability to understand what a patient is feeling), genuineness (the therapist appears to mean what he or she says), and warmth. The psychotherapist also requires sufficient maturity and experience to be able to cope with the demanding task of dealing with the mental and emotional problems of his or her patients.

WHY IT IS DONE
Psychotherapy is used to help people suffering from *neurosis* or *personality disorders*, as well as individuals with specific personal problems. The aim is to help patients learn about themselves, develop new insights into past and present relationships, and change fixed patterns of behavior.

HOW IT IS DONE
Treatment varies according to the approach used. *Counseling* is the simplest form of psychotherapy, consisting of advice and psychological support. At the opposite end of the spectrum is *psychoanalysis*, which attempts to explore the deep unconscious feelings and early childhood experiences of the individual (see *Freudian theory; Jungian theory*).

Dynamic psychotherapy is based on psychoanalytic principles. The therapist tries to understand and interpret the patient's unconscious messages (without the benefit of formal psychoanalysis) so that the individual can develop a better understanding of his or her underlying feelings and cope with them more effectively.

A course of treatment may be brief, consisting of two or three sessions, or it may extend over many years, depending on the particular problems involved. It may vary in intensity from a simple, supportive approach during a difficult period to an in-depth analysis aimed at reconstructing the personality.

Psychotherapy may involve one person, a couple (see *Marital counseling*), a family (see *Family therapy*), or a group (see *Group therapy*).

Psychotropic drugs
Drugs that have an effect on the mind. Psychotropic drugs thus include *hallucinogenic drugs, sedative drugs, sleeping drugs, tranquilizer drugs*, and *antipsychotic drugs*.

Psyllium
A bulk-forming *laxative drug* used in the treatment of *constipation, diverticular disease*, and *irritable bowel syndrome*. Psyllium is also given to increase the firmness of bowel movements in a person with an *ileostomy*.

Adverse effects include bloating, excess gas, and abdominal pain.

Pterygium
A wing-shaped thickening of the *conjunctiva* (the transparent membrane covering the white of the eye and the inside of the eyelids). Pterygium extends from either side of the eye, across the margin of the cornea toward its center. The condition is attributed to prolonged exposure to bright sunlight and is common in tropical areas. Unless vision is notably affected, no treatment is necessary, but if the extension is threatening the sufferer's vision, the pterygium should be surgically removed. Occasionally, a prominent pterygium may be removed simply because it causes discomfort. If a pterygium recurs, further treatment may be necessary.

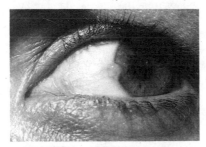
Appearance of pterygium
The conjunctiva has extended beyond the white of the eye to encroach on the cornea (transparent front part of the eye).

Ptomaine poisoning
An obsolete term for *food poisoning* now known to be caused not by ptomaines—chemical compounds present in decaying foodstuffs—but by bacteria or bacterial poisons.

Ptosis
Drooping of the upper eyelid. The condition may be *congenital* or it may occur later in life, either spontaneously or as a result of injury or disease, such as *myasthenia gravis*. Ptosis is usually due to a weakness of the levator muscle of the upper lid or to interference with the nerve supply to the muscle.

Severe congenital ptosis, in which the drooping lid covers the pupil, should be surgically corrected to avoid the development of *amblyopia* (failure of visual development).

Acquired ptosis without obvious cause may be a sign of a neurological disease, such as a *brain tumor* or a cerebral *aneurysm*, and should be investigated by a physician.

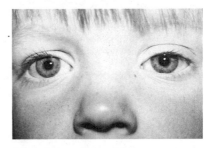
Congenital ptosis in a child
This condition, present from birth, should be corrected surgically to prevent any disturbance of visual development.

Ptyalism
See *Salivation, excessive*.

Puberty
The period when secondary sexual characteristics develop and the sexual organs mature, allowing reproduction to become possible. Puberty is the term used for the physical changes that underlie the emotional changes of *adolescence*.

Puberty usually occurs between the ages of 10 and 15 in both sexes; it is initiated by the *pituitary gland* producing hormones (known as *gonadotropins*) that stimulate the *ovaries* to increase secretion of *estrogen hormones* and the *testes* to increase secretion of *testosterone*. It is not known what triggers this action by the pituitary gland, but the primary change probably occurs in the part of the brain

P

called the hypothalamus, which controls the pituitary by producing "releasing" and "inhibitory" factors.

Puberty is accompanied by a significant growth spurt and increase in weight. Body weight may double during this period, due primarily to muscle growth in boys and increased fat in girls. The growth spurt occurs later in boys.

PUBERTY IN GIRLS

The first sign of puberty in girls is usually breast budding, which occurs around the age of 11; in about one third of girls, pubic hair appears first. The rate of growth of the two breasts may be unequal but any difference usually disappears by the time full maturity is reached. The first menstrual period usually does not occur for a year or more after the start of puberty, by which time pubic and underarm hair are in the fully developed adult pattern.

Other secondary sexual characteristics, such as the wider pelvis and the female distribution of fat, develop progressively during this period. Puberty is considered to be complete when menstrual periods occur at regular, predictable intervals.

The age at which menstruation starts has decreased during the past century, probably because of a general improvement in nutrition and living standards, but is now stable. Strenuous sports or other hard physical activity (such as ballet) and debilitating disease can also delay the onset of menstrual periods.

PUBERTY IN BOYS

In boys, puberty is heralded by a sudden increase in the rate of growth of the testes and scrotum, followed by the appearance of pubic and facial hair. The penis begins to grow around the age of 13 and reaches its adult size about two years later. However, there is a wide range of variation so that, at the age of 14, some boys may be sexually mature while others still have immature genitals.

The body's increased secretion of testosterone stimulates sperm production and causes the prostate gland and seminal vesicles to mature. It leads to the development of the typical male distribution of hair on the face, chest, and abdomen. The larynx enlarges and the vocal cords become longer and thicker, causing the pitch of the voice to drop.

ABNORMAL PUBERTY

Extremely rarely there are instances in which the normal events of puberty occur at a very young age, sometimes

CHANGES OF PUBERTY

There is considerable variation in the age of onset of puberty, but girls, on average, undergo puberty earlier than boys. The entire process takes about three to four years to complete. In addition to the sex-specific changes, height and weight both increase rapidly.

10 to 12   15 to 16   12 to 14   15 to 18

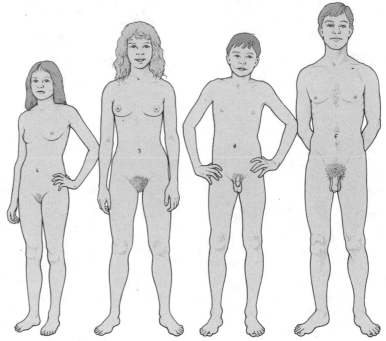

Girls
Puberty most often starts between the ages of 10 and 12 in girls. Major changes include growth of breasts and pubic hair, widening of the hips, enlargement of the uterus, and the onset of menstruation.

Boys
The main changes are enlargement of the sex organs, widening of the shoulders, deepening of the voice, and the growth of facial and pubic hair. The onset is usually between the ages of 12 and 14.

within the first five years of life; the youngest mother on record gave birth to a healthy baby at the age of 5 years 8 months. Precocious sexual development can occur in either sex. In boys, it may be caused by virilizing hormones from the adrenal gland or by a cyst or tumor in the hypothalamus.

Pubes

The pubic hair or its area of growth.

Pubic lice

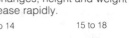 Small, wingless insects that live in the pubic hair and feed on blood. Also called crab lice or crabs (because of their crablike claws, which they use to grasp hair), they are usually spread by sexual contact. The scientific name for pubic lice is *PHTHIRUS PUBIS*.

Each louse has a flattened body, up to 2 mm across, and can be seen with the naked eye. The females lay minute eggs (called nits) on the hair, where they hatch about eight days later.

Both lice and eggs are visible in the pubic hair. On hairy men the lice may also be found in hair around the anus, on the legs, and on the trunk, and occasionally even in facial hair. The bites sometimes cause itching. Pubic lice can infest children, usually by transmission from parents. In children, lice may attach to the eyelids.

An insecticide lotion containing lindane (gamma benzene hexachloride) or benzyl benzoate kills the lice and eggs soon after application. An infested person's sexual partner should also be treated; clothes and bedding should be washed in water hotter than 60°C before use.

P

Public health

A branch of medicine which arose in the 19th century as physicians became aware of the importance of the provision of pure water supplies and safe systems for the disposal of sewage. The medical pioneers in this field instigated the construction of reservoirs and of water and sewage systems. They also turned their attention to working conditions in factories and mines. Measures to control infectious diseases were studied and introduced along with improvements in the care of women during pregnancy and of children in the first few years of life. There were also programs to improve nutrition and provide immunization against infectious diseases.

Today, the functions of public health are covered by many different people and agencies, such as medical officers of health and government departments.

Pudenda

A term for the external *genitalia*.

Pudendal block

A type of *nerve block* used during childbirth to provide pain relief for a *forceps delivery*. A local anesthetic (see *Anesthesia, local*) is injected into either side of the vagina near the pudendal nerve, which passes under the bony prominences on each side of the lower pelvis. The lower part of the vagina becomes insensitive to pain within about five minutes.

Puerperal sepsis

Infection that originates in the genital tract within 10 days after childbirth, miscarriage, or abortion. Puerperal sepsis is rare, occurring in between 1 and 3 percent of pregnancies. Infection usually starts in the vagina and spreads to the uterus.

CAUSES

Infection may be caused by bacteria that normally inhabit the vagina but usually cause harm only if the woman's resistance is low or if placental tissue has been retained in the genital tract. Puerperal sepsis may also be caused by bacteria entering the genital tract from other parts of the body or from outside.

SYMPTOMS AND TREATMENT

The main symptoms are fever, offensive-smelling *lochia* (vaginal discharge after childbirth), headache, chills, and pain in the lower abdomen. If infection spreads to the fallopian tubes (see *Salpingitis*), the tubes may become blocked and cause *infertility*. Further spread of infection may lead to *peritonitis* and *septicemia*, which may quite rapidly be fatal unless emergency treatment is given.

Treatment includes *antibiotic drugs* and the removal of any remaining placental tissue.

Puerperium

The period of time following *childbirth* during which the woman's uterus and genitals return to their state before the pregnancy.

Pulmonary

Pertaining to the *lungs*. For example, the pulmonary artery is the blood vessel that carries blood from the heart to the lungs.

Pulmonary edema

Accumulation of fluid in the *lungs*. Pulmonary edema is usually due to left-sided *heart failure*, which results in a back-pressure of fluid in the lungs. Pulmonary edema may also be due to chest infection, inhalation of irritant gases (such as sulfur dioxide and chlorine), or to any of the causes of generalized *edema*.

SYMPTOMS AND SIGNS

The main symptom is breathlessness, which may be very severe. The breathlessness is usually worse when the sufferer lies flat (a symptom known as orthopnea), and may cause him or her to suddenly waken during the night. There is also a cough that produces frothy sputum, which may be stained pink. Breathing may cause a bubbling sound, or may be wheezy (a condition sometimes called cardiac asthma). Crackling sounds in the patient's chest can be heard through a stethoscope.

DIAGNOSIS AND TREATMENT

Pulmonary edema is diagnosed by *physical examination*. A *chest X ray* will clearly indicate the presence of fluid in the lungs.

Treatment with *diuretic drugs* is usually effective. In severe cases, these drugs may need to be given by injection. Other treatment may include the administration of *morphine, oxygen therapy*, and *aminophylline*. In rare cases, artificial *ventilation* may be necessary.

Pulmonary embolism

Obstruction of the pulmonary artery or one of its branches in the *lung* by an *embolus*, usually a blood clot that originated in a vein in the leg or pelvis as a complication of deep vein thrombosis (see *Thrombosis, deep vein*). If the embolus is large enough to block the main pulmonary artery leading from the heart to the lungs, or if there are many clots, the condition is life-threatening. Pulmonary embolism affects about twice as many women as men; recent surgery, pregnancy, and immobility increase the risk.

PULMONARY EMBOLISM

This condition results when one or more emboli (fragments of material) break off from a blood clot in a vein and are carried, via the heart, to the lungs. The effects depend on the size and numbers of emboli and on the general health of the person's lungs and heart.

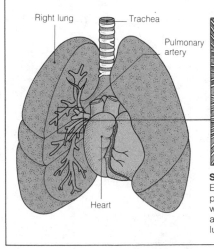

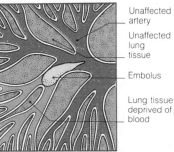

Site of obstruction
Emboli are carried into the lungs by the pulmonary artery. Most of them lodge within one of the larger or medium-sized arteries and partially deprive a section of lung tissue of blood.

SYMPTOMS

Symptoms depend partly on the size of the embolus. A massive embolus that blocks the main pulmonary artery can cause sudden death. Smaller emboli may cause severe shortness of breath, a rapid pulse, dizziness due to low blood pressure, sharp chest pain that is worse when breathing, and coughing up of blood. Small pulmonary emboli may produce no symptoms, but, if they are recurrent, they may eventually lead to *pulmonary hypertension* (increased pressure of blood flow in the lungs).

DIAGNOSIS

Investigation of the lung may include a *chest X ray*, *radionuclide scanning*, and pulmonary *angiography*. An *ECG* may show changes in the electrical activity of the heart, and *venography* helps determine the source of the embolus.

TREATMENT

Treatment depends on the size and severity of the embolus. A small embolus gradually dissolves but there is a risk of more emboli developing. *Anticoagulant drugs* (such as heparin and warfarin) are given to reduce the clotting ability of the blood and to reduce the chance of more clots occurring. *Thrombolytic drugs* may hasten the process of clot dissolution. If the embolus is very large, an emergency operation may be necessary in order to remove it.

Pulmonary fibrosis

Scarring and thickening of lung tissue, usually as a result of previous lung inflammation, such as *pneumonia* or *tuberculosis*. Pulmonary fibrosis may occur throughout both lungs (see *Interstitial pulmonary fibrosis*) or may affect only part of one lung.

Shortness of breath is a common symptom. Diagnosis is confirmed by *chest X ray*. Treatment depends on the underlying cause, but the fibrosis may be irreversible.

Pulmonary function tests

A group of procedures used to evaluate the function of the *lungs* and to confirm the presence of some lung disorders. Pulmonary function tests are also performed before any major operation on the lungs, such as *lobectomy* (removal of a lobe of the lung), to ensure that the person will not be disabled by the reduction in his or her lung capacity.

Spirometry and measurement of lung volume are performed to detect any restriction of normal lung expansion or to detect obstruction of air flow. A *peak flow meter* is used to assess the degree of *bronchospasm* (narrowing of the airways), while a test of *blood gases* (measurement of the concentration of oxygen and carbon dioxide in the blood) demonstrates the efficiency of the gas exchange in the alveoli in the lungs.

Another test of lung function (diffusing capacity) shows the efficiency of the lungs in absorbing gas into the bloodstream. This is done by measuring the volume of carbon monoxide breathed out after a low concentration of the gas has been inhaled.

Pulmonary hypertension

A disorder in which the blood pressure in the arteries supplying the lungs is abnormally high. Pulmonary hypertension develops in response to an increased resistance to blood flow through the lungs. To maintain an adequate blood flow, the right side of the heart, which pumps blood to the lungs, must contract more vigorously than was necessary before. This causes an enlargement of the heart's muscle wall. Eventually, right-sided *heart failure* may develop.

Several conditions can lead to increased resistance to blood flow through the lungs. The most important is an inadequate supply of oxygen to the lungs' small air sacs, which may be due, for example, to chronic *bronchitis*. Lack of oxygen causes the small branches of the arteries in the lungs to constrict (narrow) and to thicken their muscular walls, thus causing a permanent increase in resistance.

Other causes of the condition are *pulmonary embolism* (in which a blood clot blocks off one or several arteries in the lungs), *interstitial pulmonary fibrosis* (thickening and scarring of lung tissue, which can have many causes of its own) and some types of congenital heart disease (see *Heart disease, congenital*).

Primary pulmonary hypertension is the term used to describe cases in which the cause is not known.

SYMPTOMS AND SIGNS

As long as the enlargement and strengthening of the right side of the heart is sufficient to maintain a normal blood circulation, the patient will have little indication that there may be problems ahead. But, with the onset of *heart failure* as the right side of the heart falters and fails to meet its work load, a number of symptoms develop. Such symptoms include enlargement of veins in the neck, enlargement of the liver, and generalized *edema* (swelling due to fluid in tissues).

TREATMENT

Treatment is directed at the underlying disorder (if known) and to the relief of the effects of right-sided heart failure. *Diuretic drugs* may be valuable in relieving edema, and sometimes *oxygen therapy* is useful.

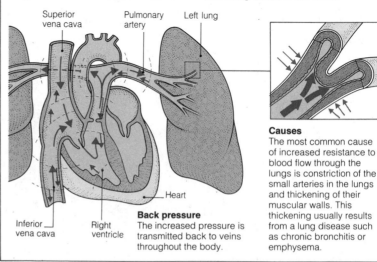

PULMONARY HYPERTENSION

In this condition, there is increased resistance to blood flow through the lungs (red arrows), usually due to lung disease. The result is a rise in pressure in the pulmonary artery, the right side of the heart (gray lines and arrows), and in the veins that bring blood to the heart.

Superior vena cava

Pulmonary artery

Left lung

Heart

Inferior vena cava

Right ventricle

Back pressure
The increased pressure is transmitted back to veins throughout the body.

Causes
The most common cause of increased resistance to blood flow through the lungs is constriction of the small arteries in the lungs and thickening of their muscular walls. This thickening usually results from a lung disease such as chronic bronchitis or emphysema.

P

Pulmonary insufficiency

A defect of the pulmonary valve at the exit of the ventricle (lower, pumping chamber) on the right side of the *heart*. The valve fails to close properly after each contraction of the ventricle, allowing blood pumped out of the chamber to leak back again.

Pulmonary insufficiency is a rare type of heart valve defect. When it does occur, it is usually the result of *rheumatic fever, endocarditis,* or severe *pulmonary hypertension* (raised pressure in the pulmonary artery). Pulmonary insufficiency may cause a heart *murmur* that is audible through a stethoscope.

Usually the condition is of little significance. When accompanied by pulmonary hypertension, the eventual result may be right-sided *heart failure*. In such cases, treatment is usually of the pulmonary hypertension rather than an attempt to repair or replace the defective valve.

Pulmonary stenosis

A *heart* condition in which the outflow of blood from the ventricle (lower, pumping chamber) on the right side of the heart is obstructed. With pulmonary stenosis, the heart must work much harder than normal to pump blood to the lungs.

The obstruction may be caused by narrowing of the pulmonary valve at the exit of the chamber, by narrowing of the pulmonary artery (large blood vessel beyond the valve) that carries blood to the lungs, or by narrowing of the upper part of the ventricle itself.

CAUSES AND INCIDENCE
Pulmonary stenosis is nearly always congenital (present from birth). About one baby in 8,000 is born with the defect alone or as part of a more complex set of heart defects, called the *tetralogy of Fallot.* Very rarely, pulmonary stenosis develops later in life, usually due to *rheumatic fever.*

SYMPTOMS
In severe cases, a newborn baby's heart begins to enlarge as soon as breathing is established. If the blood supply to the lungs is inadequate, the baby becomes breathless, and damming of blood behind the valve may lead to swelling of the liver and abdomen due to *heart failure.* The baby also may not suck. This is an emergency that can often be helped by surgery.

In less severe cases (which are more common), symptoms may not appear until the child gets older and becomes more active. The main symptom is breathlessness. Marks resembling *chilblains* may appear on the cheeks, hands, and feet as a result of the slower circulation. In mild cases there are no symptoms, and the condition is detected only when a physician discovers a heart *murmur.*

When pulmonary stenosis exists with other types of heart defect, such as a *septal defect* (hole in the heart), some deoxygenated blood bypasses the lungs and goes back into the general circulation, leading to *cyanosis* (blue-purple skin coloration).

Pulmonary stenosis acquired in later life may lead to the symptoms of heart failure.

DIAGNOSIS
A *chest X ray* may show enlargement of the heart. *ECG* (measurement of the electrical activity of the heart), *echocardiography,* and Doppler *ultrasound* techniques (imaging of the heart using sound waves) can help diagnose the severity of the narrowing.

TREATMENT
In some cases, a *balloon catheter* is used to relieve the narrowing without the need to open the chest. Alternatively, *heart valve surgery* or other types of *open heart surgery* are often successful.

Pulp cavity

The hollow space which contains dental pulp. (See *Pulp, dental.*)

Pulp, dental

The soft tissue in the middle of each tooth (see *Teeth*). The dental pulp has a rich supply of blood vessels and contains nerves that respond to heat, cold, pressure, and pain.

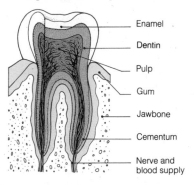

Location of the dental pulp
The pulp forms the soft core at the center of a tooth. If tooth decay reaches as far as the pulp, the latter degenerates rapidly and must be removed to save the tooth.

Pulpectomy

The complete removal of the pulp of a tooth (the soft tissue in the middle of the tooth that contains blood vessels and nerves). A pulpectomy operation is part of *root-canal treatment.*

Pulpotomy

Removal of the coronal part of the pulp of a tooth (the soft tissue in the middle of the tooth that contains blood vessels and nerves). The procedure is undertaken when the pulp has become inflamed, usually as a result of bacterial infection.

The infection is most commonly the result of extensive dental *caries* (tooth decay) or of a dental fracture (see *Fracture, dental*) that exposes the pulp. Successful pulpotomy prevents further degeneration of the pulp remaining in the tooth.

HOW IT IS DONE
Under a local anesthetic, the dentist removes the damaged pulp and covers the wound with a dressing that encourages it to heal. The gap in the overlying dentin and enamel is then sealed (see *Restoration, dental*). If the treatment is unsuccessful, *root-canal treatment* may be required.

Pulse

The rhythmic expansion and contraction of an artery as blood is forced through it, pumped by the *heart.*

The pulse is usually checked during the course of a *physical examination* because it can give clues to the patient's state of health or illness. It is detected by pressing one or more fingers or thumb against the skin over an artery, usually at the wrist, although it

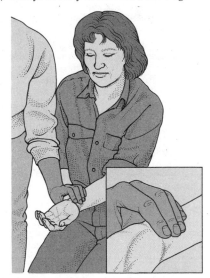

Taking the pulse
Two fingertips are pressed against the wrist just below the base of the thumb to feel the pulse in the radial artery.

843

can also easily be felt in the neck or the groin. The pulse is sometimes easily visible at the temple or in the neck.

The pulse can be described in terms of its rate (number of expansions per minute), its rhythm, strength, and whether the blood vessel feels hard or soft. The rate is easily determined by counting the beats in a set period (minimum 15 to 20 seconds) and multiplying to give the beats per minute. The pulse rate usually corresponds to the *heart rate*, which varies according to the person's state of relaxation or physical activity.

Abnormally high or low rates, or abnormal rhythms, may be a sign of a heart disorder (see *Arrhythmia, cardiac*). When the heart is beating very fast, some of its beats may be too weak to be detectable in the pulse, effectively making the pulse rate slower than the heart rate.

If the pulse feels weak, it may be a sign of *heart failure, shock,* or an obstruction to the blood circulation. A weak or absent pulse in one or both legs is a sign of *peripheral vascular disease.* The vessel wall should feel soft when the pulse is felt; a wall that feels hard may be a sign of *arteriosclerosis.*

Pump, infusion
A machine for the administration of a continuous, controlled amount of a drug or other fluid through a needle which may be inserted into a vein or under the skin.

An infusion pump consists of a small battery-powered pump that controls the flow of fluid from a syringe into the needle. The pump, which is strapped to the patient, is preprogrammed to deliver the fluid at a constant rate. If required, it can also be programmed to deliver additional amounts of medication or other fluid at scheduled times.

Infusion pumps are commonly used to administer morphine and other drugs to patients suffering from cancer. They are also used to give insulin to patients who have diabetes mellitus (see *Pump, insulin*; see also *Intravenous infusion*).

Pump, insulin
A type of infusion pump (see *Pump, infusion*) used to administer a continuous dose of insulin to some patients with *diabetes mellitus.* The needle is inserted under the skin, usually in the patient's upper arm or abdominal wall. The rate of insulin flow is adjusted so that the level of blood glucose (sugar) is constant.

Punchdrunk
A condition characterized by slurred speech, impaired concentration, and slowed thought processes. It occurs as a result of brain damage caused by several episodes of brief loss of consciousness due to head injury. The name comes from the high incidence of the condition in boxers.

Pupil
The circular opening in the center of the *iris.* In bright conditions, the pupil constricts (narrows) in order to reduce the amount of light admitted to the *eye*; in dim light, the pupil dilates (widens) to allow more light to reach the retina. Constriction and dilation are controlled by muscles in the iris.

Several drugs affect the size of the pupil. For example, *atropine* eye drops dilate the pupil and *pilocarpine* eye drops constrict it.

DISORDERS
The pupil may be congenitally small, irregular in shape, or displaced to one side; there may also be a coloboma (a missing segment or fissure in the iris).

Adie's pupil is a condition in which the affected pupil is larger than the other pupil, with poor constriction

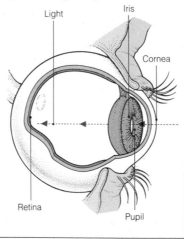

LOCATION OF THE PUPIL
The pupil is the circular opening in the center of the iris. It can be widened or narrowed by muscles in the iris to adjust the amount of light entering the eye.

Light

Iris

Cornea

Retina

Pupil

in response to light and slow dilation in the dark.

In Argyll Robertson pupil, usually caused by *syphilis*, the pupil is small and irregular, and does not constrict in response to light but does so when an effort at *accommodation* is made.

The pupil is often affected by injury to the iris. This may produce permanent dilation of the pupil or distortion of its shape.

Purgative
A term for a *laxative drug.*

Purine
Any of a group of nitrogen-containing compounds synthesized in the body or produced by the digestion of certain proteins. Increased levels of purine can cause *hyperuricemia* (a raised level of uric acid in the blood), which may lead to *gout*. Foods high in purine include sardines, liver, kidneys, legumes, and poultry. Purine is also present in other substances, including caffeine and theophylline.

Purpura
Any of a group of disorders characterized by purplish or reddish-brown areas or spots of discoloration, visible through the skin, and caused by bleeding within underlying tissues. Purpura also refers to the discolored areas themselves, which can range from the size of a pinhead to 2.5 cm or so in diameter. The smaller bleeding points are sometimes called *petechiae*; larger, darker areas of discoloration are called ecchymoses or bruises.

TYPES AND CAUSES
There are many different types and causes of purpura.

Common purpura, also often called senile purpura, is the most common of all bleeding disorders, affecting for the most part middle-aged or elderly women. Large discolored areas appear on the thighs or the back of the hands and forearms. These are caused by thinning of the tissues supporting blood vessels beneath the skin, which as a result rupture easily. Bleeding may also be visible under the membrane that lines the mouth.

Schönlein-Henoch purpura (also called anaphylactoid purpura) is caused by inflammation of blood vessels beneath the skin, sometimes as a result of an allergic reaction. Similar changes may occur in patches within the gastrointestinal tract.

Purpura can also occur as a result of a lack of platelets in the blood—a condition called *thrombocytopenia.* Platelets are the small blood cells that play a crucial role in clotting. A lack of platelets may occur as a result of a disease of the bone marrow (such as *leukemia* or aplastic *anemia*), as a side effect of certain drugs or excessive radiation, or for no apparent reason.

P

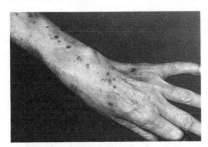

Appearance of senile purpura
This common condition of middle to old age is caused by thinning of the tissues that support blood vessels beneath the skin.

Other types of purpura include that seen in *scurvy* and in forms of the condition caused by damage to blood vessels by certain infections, *autoimmune disorders*, *septicemia* (blood poisoning), or biochemical disturbances such as uremia (see *Kidney failure*).

DIAGNOSIS
Purpura is investigated by a physician studying the signs and symptoms and by a full examination and testing of the blood, including *blood-clotting tests*. The state of the blood platelets is of primary interest. It is essential for the physician to determine exactly the type and cause of the purpura, because treatment depends on the specific type.

TREATMENT
Common purpura may be helped by estrogen *hormone replacement therapy*. Other types may be helped by *corticosteroid drugs* or *immunosuppressant drugs*. In severe cases, *plasmapheresis* (removal of blood, replacement of plasma, and retransfusion) has been effective. Platelet deficiency is treated according to the cause. In some cases, transfusions of platelets must be given.

Autoimmune thrombocytopenia (sometimes called idiopathic thrombocytopenic purpura) is usually treated with corticosteroid drugs or by a splenectomy, which is a surgical removal of the *spleen*.

Purulent

A term that means containing, producing, or consisting of *pus*.

Pus

A pale yellow or green, creamy fluid found at the site of bacterial infection. Pus is composed of millions of dead white blood cells, partly digested tissue, dead and living bacteria, as well as minute quantities of other substances. A collection of pus within solid tissue is called an *abscess*.

Among the main pus-forming organisms are streptococci, pneumococci, and *ESCHERICHIA COLI*. Many bacteria produce a distinctive type of pus—for example, *PSEUDOMONAS AERUGINOSA* produces pus with a bluish tinge.

Pustule

A small *skin* blister containing pus. Pustules may occur in a hair follicle or elsewhere in the skin, and may or may not be the result of infection; the pustules in *acne* are noninfective. A *stye* is a pustule at the root of an eyelash.

PUVA

A type of *phototherapy* used to treat certain skin conditions, especially *psoriasis*. PUVA combines the use of a *psoralen drug*, which sensitizes the skin to sunlight, and a controlled dose of long-wavelength *ultraviolet light*. The abbreviation stands for psoralens and ultraviolet A.

Pyelitis

See *Pyelonephritis*.

Pyelography

A procedure for taking X-ray pictures of the body's urinary system. (See *Urography*.)

Pyelolithotomy

An operation performed to remove a *calculus* (stone) from the kidney. The surgeon approaches the kidney via a longitudinal incision to the right or left of the spine, the junction between the kidney and ureter is cut open, and the calculus is removed with forceps.

Pyelolithotomy is being replaced by *lithotripsy* using ultrasonic waves to break up the stones.

Pyelonephritis

Inflammation of the *kidney*, usually caused by a bacterial infection. Pyelonephritis may be acute, taking the form of a sudden attack, or chronic, in which repeated or inadequately treated attacks may cause permanent damage to the kidney.

ACUTE PYELONEPHRITIS
Acute pyelonephritis is more common in women and more likely to occur during pregnancy. It usually results when bacteria causing *cystitis* spread up to the kidney.

Symptoms include a high fever, chills, and back pain. Treatment consists of *antibiotic drugs*, which may need to be given by intravenous infusion in severe cases. *Septicemia* (blood poisoning) is a possible complication.

CHRONIC PYELONEPHRITIS
Chronic pyelonephritis often starts in childhood. The condition is usually caused by reflux (backflow) of urine from the bladder into one of the ureters, often because the child has a congenital abnormality of the valve that is found where the ureter enters the bladder.

Persistent reflux of urine causes repeated kidney infection, leading, in some children, to inflammation and scarring, which may cause permanent kidney damage. Children in whom recurrent urinary tract infections develop require testing by a physician. Micturating *cystourethrography* may be among techniques used to help identify the presence of reflux so that the underlying abnormality can be corrected surgically.

Possible complications arising from chronic pyelonephritis include *hypertension* (high blood pressure) and *kidney failure*.

Pyloric stenosis

Narrowing of the pylorus (the lower outlet from the stomach) that obstructs the passage of food into the duodenum (the first part of the small intestine). Pyloric stenosis occurs in babies and in adults.

PYLORIC STENOSIS IN INFANTS
In infantile pyloric stenosis, the muscle surrounding the outlet from the stomach is abnormally thickened, as shown in the enlarged drawing (below). The condition occurs more often in male than female babies and tends to run in families—infants of a woman who was affected with pyloric stenosis as a baby are liable to develop it.

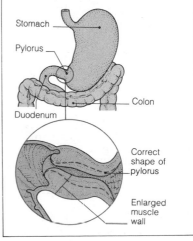

Stomach

Pylorus

Duodenum

Colon

Correct shape of pylorus

Enlarged muscle wall

P

CAUSES AND INCIDENCE

In infants, the condition is caused by a thickening of the pyloric muscle, which occurs, for unknown reasons, soon after birth; about one in every 4,000 babies is affected.

In adults, the narrowing is usually the result of scarring caused by a *peptic ulcer* or of a malignant tumor of the lower stomach (see *Stomach cancer*).

SYMPTOMS AND DIAGNOSIS

Three to four weeks after birth, an affected infant starts projectile vomiting (profuse, forceful vomiting in which the stomach contents may be ejected a distance of several metres) after feeding. Adults with the disorder vomit undigested food several hours after a meal.

In an infant, a physician can feel the thickened muscle through the abdominal wall, but a barium meal (see *Barium X-ray examinations*) may be required to confirm the diagnosis.

In adults, pyloric stenosis is diagnosed by a barium meal and *gastroscopy* (examination of the stomach with a flexible viewing instrument).

TREATMENT

Infant pyloric stenosis is sometimes treated with drugs. However, in most cases the only satisfactory treatment is pyloromyotomy: under general anesthetic, the abdomen is opened and the obstruction relieved simply by making an incision along the length of the thickened muscle.

In adults, surgery is necessary to correct the underlying cause.

Pyloroplasty

An operation in which the pylorus (the outlet from the stomach) is widened to ensure the free passage of food into the intestine. Pyloroplasty may be performed as part of the surgical treatment for a *peptic ulcer*; it prevents tightening of the pyloric muscles following *vagotomy* (cutting of the vagus nerve to reduce stomach acid production).

HOW IT IS DONE

While the patient is under general anesthesia, a lengthwise incision is made across the pylorus. The beginning and end of the incision are pushed inward till they meet, and the opening, which is now at a right angle to the original incision, is sewn up. This creates an extra wide passage for the movement of food.

Pyo-

A prefix that denotes a relationship to pus. The prefix py- is also used, as in pyuria, pus in the urine.

Pyoderma gangrenosum

A rare condition characterized by ulcers, usually on the legs, that turn into hard, painful areas surrounded by discolored skin. Pyoderma gangrenosum occurs as a rare complication in *ulcerative colitis*.

Pyrantel

An *anthelmintic drug* used to treat intestinal *worm infestations*. A single dose of pyrantel is usually sufficient to eradicate the worms. Possible adverse effects include nausea, loss of appetite, and abdominal pain.

Pyrazinamide

A drug sometimes used to treat *tuberculosis*. Possible adverse effects are nausea and an increased risk of gout. There may also be liver damage, resulting in loss of appetite and jaundice.

Pyrexia

A medical term for *fever*.

Pyridostigmine

A drug used to improve muscle strength in *myasthenia gravis*. Pyridostigmine is not curative. In the initial stages of treatment, the drug should be taken under the close supervision of a physician.

Pyridoxine

Vitamin B_6, one of the B group of vitamins (see *Vitamin B complex*).

Dietary deficiency of this vitamin is very rare but can be induced by various drugs; deficiency causes *neuritis* (nerve inflammation).

Large doses of pyridoxine (50 to 100 mg per day) are sometimes used to treat *premenstrual syndrome* but the results of this treatment are not conclusive.

Pyrimethamine

A drug used to prevent and treat attacks caused by certain strains of *malaria* parasite and also to treat *toxoplasmosis*. Pyrimethamine is usually given in combination with a *sulfonamide drug* or *dapsone*.

Possible adverse effects include loss of appetite, vomiting, and, rarely, rash. Long-term use may reduce blood cell production by the bone marrow, causing *anemia*, abnormal bleeding, or increased susceptibility to infection. Because of the risk of blood disorders during prolonged use, regular blood counts are made and vitamin supplements are given, especially to pregnant women.

Pyrogen

A substance that produces *fever*. The term is usually applied to proteins that are released by white blood cells in response to bacterial or viral infections. These proteins act on the temperature-controlling center within the brain, causing it to raise body temperature. The word pyrogen is also sometimes used to refer to chemicals released by microorganisms—such as bacterial *endotoxins*—which have a similar temperature-raising effect.

Pyromania

A persistent impulse to start fires. The typical person with pyromania becomes fascinated with fires as a child, obtains relief of tension (or even pleasure) from setting fire to something and watching it burn, and has no other motive (such as money) for doing so. The disorder is more often diagnosed in males, and may be associated with a low IQ, alcohol abuse, and sometimes a *psychosexual disorder* (some people seem to be sexually aroused by fires). Pyromania is often difficult to treat; imprisonment is not unusual.

Pyuria

The presence of white blood cells (pus cells) in the *urine*. Pyuria is usually an indication of infection and inflammation in the *kidney* or *urinary tract*.

Microscopic examination and *culture* of the urine are performed to look for a causative microorganism so that appropriate *antibiotic drugs* may be given. In some cases, pyuria occurs when no microorganisms are present and may indicate inflammation of the kidney due to another cause.

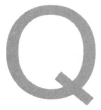

Q fever

An uncommon illness with symptoms similar to those of *influenza*. Q fever occurs throughout the world.

The causative organism, COXIELLA BURNETTI, is a type of *rickettsia* harbored by farm animals. It occurs in the urine, feces, milk, flesh, and placentas of infected animals. In dry areas, Q fever may be contracted by inhaling dust contaminated with feces, urine, or birth products. It may rarely be spread by tick bites.

About 20 days after infection, the illness begins suddenly with a high fever (which may persist for up to two weeks), severe headache, muscle and chest pain, and cough. During the second week, a form of pneumonia develops. The patient then usually recovers. In some cases, however, the disease is prolonged; *hepatitis* develops in one third of these and some suffer *endocarditis*. In less than 1 percent of cases, the illness is fatal.

A diagnosis of Q fever may be confirmed by a *blood test*. Treatment is with *antibiotic drugs*. An effective vaccine is available for people at risk of catching the disease.

Quackery

A false claim by someone to have both the ability and experience to diagnose and treat disease.

Quadriceps muscle

A muscle with four distinct parts that is located at the front of the thigh, and which straightens the knee.

DISORDERS

The most common disorder of the quadriceps is a *hematoma* (a collection of blood) caused by a direct blow. Bruising may follow a few days later. In rare cases, bone forms within the hematoma, restricting movement.

Sudden stretching of the leg may tear the muscle, especially in middle-aged or elderly people. Any knee disorder that brings on pain or swelling, limiting full extension of the leg, causes the quadriceps muscle to begin wasting away within 48 hours,

LOCATION OF THE QUADRICEPS MUSCLE
One upper end attaches to the pelvis; the other two ends attach to the femur. The lower ends merge into a tendon that surrounds the patella and attaches to the tibia.

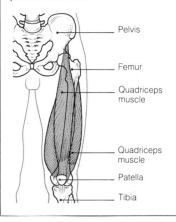

making the knee feel as though it is giving way when weight is placed on the affected leg.

Quadriparesis

Muscle weakness in all four limbs and the trunk. (See also *Quadriplegia*.)

Quadriplegia

Paralysis of all four limbs and the trunk. Quadriplegia may be caused by damage to the *spinal cord* in the neck region. The condition results in loss of feeling and power in the affected parts. (See also *Paraplegia*.)

Quarantine

Isolation of a person or persons recently exposed to a serious infectious disease. The aim is to prevent the spread of a disease by an infected, but symptomless, person.

The term quarantine comes from the Italian phrase *una quarantina* (about 40). In the past, ship's crews had to stay at sea for 40 days after leaving a port where an epidemic illness, such as *cholera*, *smallpox*, or *plague*, was raging. Later, the 40 days was reduced to a period that corresponded more closely to the *incubation period* of the disease involved.

Today, the reduced incidence of serious infectious diseases and the widespread availability of *immunization* against many of them make quarantine procedures rarely necessary. In some cases, quarantine has been replaced by compulsory vaccination

for travel between certain countries. The contacts of people with highly infectious diseases (such as pneumonic *plague*) may have restrictions placed on their travel in addition to being given preventive immunization. The principal remaining quarantine regulations in Canada apply to birds and other animals.

Quickening

The stage of *pregnancy* when the movements of the fetus are first felt by the pregnant woman. Quickening usually occurs between 16 and 20 weeks of gestation.

Quinacrine

Developed during World War II to treat malaria, quinacrine is now used to treat *giardiasis*. The drug is prone to cause nausea and vomiting, and is likely to cause a yellow discoloration of the skin and urine. This effect is harmless.

Quinidine

An *antiarrhythmic drug* used to treat irregular or abnormally fast heartbeat. Quinidine may cause nausea, vomiting, diarrhea, and, occasionally, a dangerous drop in blood pressure or a worsening of the *arrhythmia*. A few people develop blurred vision, ringing in the ears, vertigo, headache, and hot flashes.

Quinine

The oldest drug treatment for *malaria*. Quinine is now used mainly to treat strains of the disease that are resistant to other antimalarial drugs. Large doses are needed and there is a high risk of adverse effects, including headache, nausea, hearing loss, ringing in the ears, and blurred vision.

Quinine is commonly prescribed to help prevent painful leg cramps.

Quinsy

An abscess around the tonsil, usually occurring as a complication of *tonsillitis*. The infection causes a painful throat, high temperature, headache, impaired speech, dribbling, and swollen, tender lymph nodes in the neck. Trismus (difficulty in opening the mouth) is often present. The uvula (the protuberance that hangs down from the soft palate at the back of the mouth) is displaced to the unaffected side of the throat.

Antibiotic drugs taken at an early stage sometimes clear up the infection. Otherwise, the abscess requires surgical incision and drainage.

R

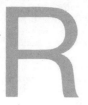

Rabies

An acute viral infection of the nervous system, formerly known as hydrophobia. Rabies primarily affects animals, but it can be transmitted from a rabid animal to a human by a bite or by a lick over a break in the skin. The causative virus, present in the animal's saliva, travels from the wound along nerve pathways to the brain, where it causes inflammation resulting in delirium, painful muscle spasms in the throat, and other severe symptoms. Once symptoms develop, rabies in humans is usually fatal.

CAUSES AND INCIDENCE

The geographical distribution of rabies and of some important animal species affected is shown on the map below. Most human cases result from a bite by a rabid dog. However, the possibility of rabies must be considered whenever any mammal (domestic or wild) bites a human in a country where the virus is present.

In Canada, foxes and skunks are most often carriers of rabies although the virus can infect almost any animal. At times the incidence of rabies rises in the animal populations of certain areas, yet human cases are extremely rare. Worldwide, there are an estimated 15,000 cases of rabies in humans each year.

SYMPTOMS AND SIGNS

The incubation period between a bite and the appearance of symptoms is between nine days and many months (the average is four to eight weeks), depending largely on the site of the bite. The first symptoms are slight fever, headache, and loss of appetite, leading to restlessness, hyperactivity, disorientation, and, in some cases, seizures. Often the victim is intensely thirsty, but attempts to drink induce violent, painful spasms in the throat (hence the term hydrophobia). Eye and facial muscles may become paralyzed. Coma and death follow three to 20 days after the onset of symptoms.

TREATMENT

Once symptoms appear they are treated with sedative drugs and *analgesic drugs* (painkillers). A very small number of people with established rabies are reported to have survived as a result of intensive care aimed at maintaining breathing and the action of the heart. However, the main emphasis must be on preventing the disease.

PREVENTION

Any animal bite should be thoroughly cleansed (see *Bites, animal*). Medical opinion should be sought immediately on whether post-exposure *immunization* is necessary. If there is a risk of rabies, passive immunization is given with human rabies *immune globulin* (ready-made *antibodies* against the rabies virus), and rabies vaccine is given by a course of injections lasting several weeks. Passive immunization is not given to people who have been vaccinated before exposure. Today's vaccines have milder side effects than those used before 1970.

Every attempt should be made to capture and confine the biting animal. If it appears rabid, it should be killed and its brain examined. If no evidence of rabies infection can be found or if a healthy animal remains symptom-free after 10 days, treatment of the bitten person is stopped.

If immunization is given within two days of the bite, rabies is almost always prevented. The chances of prevention decrease with delay, but immunization can still be effective even weeks or months after a bite.

Rachitic

A term used to describe bony or other abnormalities associated with *rickets* (a bone disease produced by a deficiency of vitamin D). Rachitic is also used to refer to people or populations that are particularly afflicted by rickets.

Rad

A unit of absorbed dose of ionizing radiation (see *Radiation* units box). Rad is an acronym for radiation absorbed dose.

Radial nerve

A branch of the *brachial plexus*. The radial nerve is one of the main nerves of the arm, running down its full length into the hand. The radial nerve controls muscles which straighten the wrist so that the back of the hand is in line with the forearm. The radial nerve also conveys sensation from the back of the forearm; from the thumb, second, and third fingers; and from an area at the base of the thumb.

GEOGRAPHICAL DISTRIBUTION OF RABIES

In most rabies-affected areas, the disease circulates mainly among wild animals. Some of the principal animal "reservoirs" of rabies are shown on the right, but other mammals may also be affected—for example, raccoons and bats in North America. Most human cases result from the bite of a rabid dog. The dog may have acquired the virus through contact with a wild animal, but, in some areas, such as the Far East, stray dogs are themselves principal carriers. Vaccinating dogs can largely prevent rabies in humans. A few countries (mainly islands) are rabies-free.

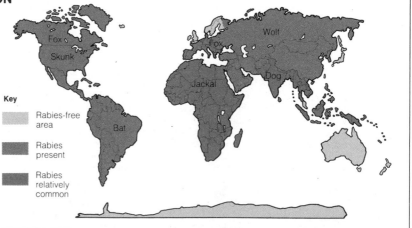

Key

- Rabies-free area
- Rabies present
- Rabies relatively common

DISORDERS

The radial nerve winds around the shaft of the humerus (upper-arm bone) and so may be damaged by a fracture of this bone. The nerve may also be damaged by persistent pressure on the armpit (e.g., from a crutch). Such damage may result in *wristdrop* (inability to straighten the wrist) and numbness in the areas of skin supplied by the radial nerve.

Radiation

The emission of energy in the form of waves or particles. There are two main types of radiation—ionizing and non-ionizing. Ionizing radiation is capable of forcibly ejecting one or more of the electrons which orbit the nucleus of an atom, thereby creating an entity called an *ion* that has an electrical charge and is capable of chemical combination with other ions. When ionization occurs in the atoms of molecules that play an important role in the body, it can lead to biological damage.

Nonionizing radiation has a different effect on molecules. It tends to cause excitation of the molecules' constituent atoms (somewhat like shaking them) but it does not impart enough energy to the atoms to displace electrons and form ions.

IONIZING RADIATION

There are three types of ionizing radiation—*X rays*, gamma rays, and particle radiation.

X rays are electromagnetic waves (i.e., they are part of the same continuous spectrum—the electromagnetic spectrum—that includes radio waves, *infrared* radiation, visible light, *ultraviolet light*, and gamma rays) of very short wavelength and very high frequency. They are produced by special electrical machines (X-ray generators). X rays have no mass and no electrical charge; their penetrating power depends on their energy, which, in turn, depends on the voltage used to generate them. X rays generated at a few tens of thousands of volts can penetrate only a few millimetres of tissue, whereas those generated at about 100,000 volts are just energetic enough to pass completely through the body and produce X-ray images. X rays used in *radiation therapy* are generated at several million volts and are sufficiently energetic to destroy deep-seated tumors. They can also destroy other tissues in their path.

Gamma rays have almost identical properties to X rays. The principal difference between the two is that gamma rays are produced by the

RADIATION UNITS

Becquerel	The SI unit of radioactivity. One becquerel (symbol Bq) is defined as one disintegration (or other nuclear transformation) per second. Although the number of becquerels is a measure of how strongly	radioactive a particular source is, it takes no account of the different effects of different types of radiation on tissue; for medical purposes, the sievert is generally more useful.
Gray	The SI unit of absorbed dose of ionizing radiation, the gray (symbol Gy) has superseded the rad. One gray is defined as an energy	absorption of 1 joule per kilogram of irradiated material. One gray is equivalent to 100 rads.
Rad	An acronym for radiation absorbed dose, the rad is a unit of absorbed dose of ionizing radiation. One rad is equal to an energy absorption of 100 ergs (an erg is a unit of work or	energy) per gram of irradiated material. The rad has been superseded by the gray (the corresponding SI unit); 1 rad is equivalent to 0.01 grays.
Rem	An acronym for roentgen equivalent man, the rem is the absorbed dose of ionizing radiation that produces the same biological effect as 1 rad of X rays or gamma rays. The rem was introduced as a result of the observation that some types of ionizing radiation, such as neutrons, produce a greater biological effect for an equivalent amount of absorbed energy than X rays or gamma rays. In short, the rem is a measure of the biological effectiveness of irradiation. For X rays and gamma rays, the rem is	equal to the rad. For other types of radiation, the number of rems equals the number of rads multiplied by a special factor (called the quality factor or relative biological effectiveness) that depends on the type of radiation involved. The rem has been superseded by the sievert in the SI system of units; 1 rem is equivalent to 0.01 sieverts.
Sievert	The SI unit of equivalent absorbed dose of ionizing radiation, the sievert (symbol Sv) has superseded the rem. One sievert is the absorbed dose of radiation that	produces the same biological effect as 1 gray of X rays or gamma rays. One sievert is equivalent to 100 rems.

Measurement of radiation levels

In the SI system (the internationally agreed system of units), three main units are used to measure radiation levels—the becquerel, the gray, and the sievert. These three units are defined above, along with two other radiation units (the rad and rem) that have now been largely superseded but are still occasionally used for some purposes.

spontaneous decay of radioactive materials rather than by a machine. They tend to have shorter wavelengths and higher frequencies (and thus greater energies) than X rays, although there is some overlap between the two.

Particle radiation—unlike X rays and gamma rays—has mass and may also have electrical charge. It represents parts of atoms, such as electrons (beta particles, which have a negative electrical charge and a very small mass), protons (positively charged particles, each with a mass about 1,800 times that of an electron), or neutrons (particles with the same mass as protons but no electrical charge). It also represents the nuclei of small atoms such as helium (helium nuclei are also known as alpha particles), or even larger atomic nuclei. Particle radiation may be produced during the decay of radioactive atoms or by machines.

SOURCES OF IONIZING RADIATION

Ionizing radiation may originate from natural or man-made sources.

One natural source is cosmic rays, which come from remote parts of the universe as well as from the sun and contribute about 14 percent of the total radiation exposure in the Canadian population. These rays consist largely of very high-energy protons, along

R

with a few atomic nuclei (principally helium nuclei). Cosmic rays are highly energetic and not only can irradiate people on the Earth's surface, but also can pass through many metres of soil and rock. The amount of cosmic rays an individual receives depends on the altitude at which he or she lives. A person who is living at an altitude of about 2,000 m, for example, receives more than twice the annual radiation dose of cosmic rays received by a person living at sea level.

Secondary radiation is generated in the upper atmosphere from cosmic rays and consists mainly of gamma rays and high-energy electrons. The annual dose from such secondary radiation varies with latitude, being greatest at the Earth's poles and least at the equator.

The other principal natural source of radiation is radioactivity. Many minerals contain unstable atomic nuclei that spontaneously disintegrate (a process known as radioactive decay), thereby emitting alpha or beta particles and/or gamma rays. The naturally occurring radioactive isotope potassium 40 (isotopes are varieties of an element that are chemically identical but differ in some physical properties) is the principal source of radiation from within the body. Many other natural materials are radioactive and, in some areas, *radon* from soil, rocks, and/or building materials is a major contributor to the annual radiation dose.

Medical X rays—used to diagnose and/or treat numerous diseases and disorders—are the greatest artificial source of radiation to which the general public is exposed. Radioactive isotopes, also used in diagnosis and treatment, are another medical source of radiation (see *Radionuclide scanning*). Radioisotopes that emit gamma rays are most commonly used (although particle-emitting radioisotopes are also employed); the types selected are usually short-lived to reduce the dose to the patient. In Canada, the average yearly radiation dose from medical sources is about 20 percent of the total dose of radiation from all sources.

Nuclear reactors are not only potential sources of direct radiation (such as gamma rays and neutrons, which are normally absorbed by thick shielding to prevent them from escaping into the environment), but are also prolific producers of radioactive isotopes. *Uranium* is the most commonly used fuel, often enriched so that it contains

more of the fissionable isotope uranium 235 than is present in natural uranium ores. In the reactor it undergoes fission (splitting), thereby producing heat and leaving behind a wide variety of radioactive isotopes. Radioisotopes of iodine, ruthenium, tellurium, and cesium are among those produced in the greatest amounts, although others of greater biological importance, such as *strontium* isotopes, are also produced. In fast-breeder reactors, *plutonium* is used as the main fuel; uranium 238 is the source from which additional plutonium fuel is made.

Nuclear weapons, including atomic bombs of the types used at Hiroshima and at Nagasaki (in which either uranium or plutonium undergoes rapid fission) and hydrogen bombs (which combine nuclear fission and fusion) are intense sources of man-made radiation. However, except for the relatively small battlefield weapons and the "radiation-enhanced" weapon (the so-called neutron bomb), the lethal effects from direct irradiation occur only comparatively near the point of explosion, whereas the lethal effects of blast and heat extend over a considerably larger area.

NONIONIZING RADIATION

The most widespread type of nonionizing radiation is ultraviolet light, a component of sunlight (although much is absorbed by the atmosphere); it is also produced by sunlamps. This type of radiation can penetrate only superficial layers of body tissue but it causes damage to the RNA (ribonucleic acid) and DNA (deoxyribonucleic acid) molecules in cells, which may lead to skin cancer.

Microwave ovens cook food by means of radio-frequency electromagnetic radiation, which can also heat body tissues and thereby damage them. This type of injury is unlikely to occur because modern appliances are shielded to prevent microwaves from escaping; they also have safety cutoffs to stop radiation emission when the door is opened. Radio and television transmissions are harmless forms of electromagnetic radiation.

The other types of nonionizing radiation to which people are subjected are magnetic fields and *ultrasound*. Weak magnetic fields are generated around all wires carrying electricity, and strong fields are used in medicine for *MRI* (magnetic resonance imaging). The effects of such fields are currently being studied, but

there is no evidence that they are harmful. Ultrasound (inaudible high-frequency sound waves) is used in medicine for diagnosis and treatment. Its effects depend on the power used and the duration of exposure. The low power levels and relatively short durations used in medicine are harmless, but exposure to ultrasound at high power levels and/or for a long time may damage tissue. (See also *Radiation hazards; Radiation sickness*.)

Radiation hazards

Hazards from *radiation* may arise from exposure to external sources of radiation (such as *X rays* or gamma rays) or from the effects of radioactive materials taken into the body. The effects of radiation depend on the dose received, the duration of exposure, and how critical are the organs exposed.

Some forms of radiation damage occur when the total radiation dose exceeds a certain threshold, usually 1 sievert or more (see *Radiation* units box). Examples of such damage include radiation *dermatitis, cataracts*, failure of various organs (which may not occur until many years after exposure), or *radiation sickness*.

In the case of other radiation effects, the severity of damage does not depend upon the specific radiation dose, but the risk that damage will occur increases with increasing doses. *Cancer* is the major example of this type of radiation damage, and is initiated by the mutagenic effect of high-energy radiation. A *mutation* is a change in the genetic material of living cells. Radioactive leaks from nuclear reactors can cause a rise in mutation rates that affects large numbers of people. This may lead to an increase in various cancers, such as forms of *leukemia*, to *birth defects* in succeeding generations, and to hereditary diseases. Cancer usually develops years after exposure, typically five to 15 years for leukemia, and 40 years or longer for skin, lung, breast, and other cancers.

The International Commission on Radiological Protection has concluded that the total risk factor for death from radiation-induced cancers is about one in 100 per sievert of radiation absorbed. The risk of genetic damage producing a hereditary disorder within the first two generations following irradiation of either parent is also thought to be about one in 100 per sievert, and the additional risk to subsequent generations is thought to be the same.

AVOIDING RADIATION DAMAGE

Radiation damage can be controlled by limiting the exposure of individuals. It is particularly important for people exposed to radiation in the course of their work to have their exposure closely monitored to ensure that it does not exceed what are considered to be safe limits, and that their cumulative radiation exposure is kept below the threshold dose. Younger people and those of reproductive age should have their reproductive organs shielded when having X rays or *radiation therapy*.

Despite some adverse publicity, there is no evidence of any radiation hazards associated with visual display terminals (VDTs) or with the *irradiation of food*. VDTs do not emit significant amounts of penetrating radiation, and food which has been irradiated does not itself become radioactive.

Radiation sickness

The term applied to the acute effects of ionizing *radiation* on the whole, or a major part, of the body when the dose is greater than about 1 gray (1 Gy) of X rays or gamma rays, or 1 sievert (1 Sv) of other types of radiation (see *Radiation* units box).

SYMPTOMS

The effect of exposure to radiation depends critically on the dose and the length of time exposure is maintained. Acute exposures of more than 30 to 100 Gy cause the rapid onset of nausea, vomiting (which may be repeated and severe), anxiety, and disorientation. Within a few hours, the victim usually loses consciousness and dies due to direct damage to the nervous system from the radiation, and to edema (accumulation of fluid) of the brain; these effects are known as the central nervous system syndrome.

People who have received radiation doses of 10 to 30 Gy also experience an early onset of nausea and vomiting, which tend to start within about two hours of exposure but disappear a few hours later. However, such individuals invariably die within four to 14 days of exposure as a result of radiation damage to the gastrointestinal tract—which causes severe and frequently bloody diarrhea (known as the gastrointestinal syndrome)—and overwhelming infection due to radiation damage to the *immune system*.

At doses of 1 to 10 Gy, transient nausea and occasional vomiting may occur, but these early symptoms usually disappear rapidly and are often followed by a two- to three-week period of relative well-being. However, by the end of this period, the effects of radiation damage to the bone marrow and immune system begin to appear, with repeated infections (which may be fatal unless treated with antibiotic drugs), and petechiae (pinpoint spots of bleeding under the skin). Some victims may be treated successfully by a *bone marrow transplant* or by isolation in a sterile environment until their own bone marrow recovers.

Radiation damage to other tissues, such as the skin and lining of the respiratory tract, may cause complications. Total body doses of less than 2 Gy are unlikely to be fatal to an otherwise healthy adult, but few survive doses of more than 6 Gy.

Radiation therapy

Treatment of *cancer*, and occasionally other diseases, by X rays or other sources of radioactivity. Sources of this kind produce ionizing *radiation*, which, as it passes through the diseased tissue, destroys or slows down the development of abnormal cells. Provided the correct dosage of radiation is given, normal cells suffer little or no long-term damage. Transient side effects that develop during treatment are, however, a reflection of acute damage to normal tissue.

Radiation therapy has various applications in the treatment of cancer. For example, it may be used on its own in an attempt to destroy all the abnormal cells in various types of cancer, such as cancer of the larynx (see *Larynx, cancer of*), *basal cell carcinoma* and *squamous cell carcinoma* (two types of skin cancer), cancer of the cervix (see *Cervix, cancer of*), *Hodgkin's disease* (a cancer of lymphoid tissue), and *leukemia*.

Radiation therapy may also be used in conjuction with other forms of cancer treatment. For example, it is often used after surgical excision of a malignant tumor (such as in the treatment of *breast cancer*) to destroy any remaining tumor cells.

A further use of radiation therapy is to reduce the size of a tumor in order to relieve the symptoms of a cancer that is too far advanced to be curable. Such *palliative* treatment may be directed, for example, at relieving obstruction to swallowing caused by an esophageal tumor (see *Esophagus, cancer of*), relieving pain caused by *bone cancer*, and relieving headaches or paralysis caused by a *brain tumor*.

If the benefits of destroying diseased tissue far outweigh the risk of damage to healthy tissue, radiation therapy may be used to treat nonmalignant diseases. A common example is use of radioactive iodine to destroy part of an overactive thyroid gland that is producing severe symptoms (see *Thyrotoxicosis*).

HOW IT IS DONE

Some of the main techniques of radiation therapy are shown in the illustrated box on page 852. Radiation is usually passed through the diseased tissues by X rays (or sometimes electrons) produced by a machine called a linear accelerator. This device has largely supplanted earlier apparatus containing radioactive cobalt, which has the drawback of producing ionizing radiation that is both less intense than the radiation of X rays and incapable of being shut off.

Some malignant tumors are not treated by radiation from an external source, but by the insertion of radioactive material directly into the growth itself or the surrounding tissue (see *Interstitial radiation therapy*) or alternatively into a body cavity (see *Intracavitary therapy*). Both procedures require an anesthetic.

Radiation used to treat thyrotoxicosis is given in the form of a liquid containing radioactive iodine. The patient drinks the liquid through a straw, and the radioactive iodine concentrates in the thyroid gland.

COMPLICATIONS

Radiation therapy may produce unpleasant side effects, including fatigue, nausea and vomiting (for which *antiemetic drugs* may be prescribed), and loss of hair from irradiated areas. Rarely, there may be reddening and blistering of the skin, which can be alleviated by *corticosteroid drugs*.

RESULTS

Radiation therapy cures most cancers of the larynx or skin. The cure rate for other types of cancer varies depending on how early the treatment is begun, but the cure rate can be 80 percent or higher.

Radical surgery

Extensive surgery aimed at eliminating a major disease by removing all affected tissue and any surrounding tissue that might be diseased.

In the past, radical surgery was commonly performed in an attempt to cure cancer. Radical *mastectomy* performed to treat *breast cancer*, for example, involved removing the

R

USE OF RADIATION THERAPY

Before treatment, calculations are made of the doses of radiation needed and of the directions from which the rays should be aimed. The areas of the patient's body to be targeted are marked directly on the patient or on a plastic coat that he or she wears. The treatment is usually performed on an outpatient basis, with the patient receiving treatment several times a week.

Radiation therapy machine in use

The patient lies on a table under the machine in a room designed to prevent radiation leakage. A radiation oncology technologist operates the machine, which sends X rays, in the predetermined directions and amounts, through the diseased area of the patient's body. The procedure causes no discomfort and usually lasts just a few minutes.

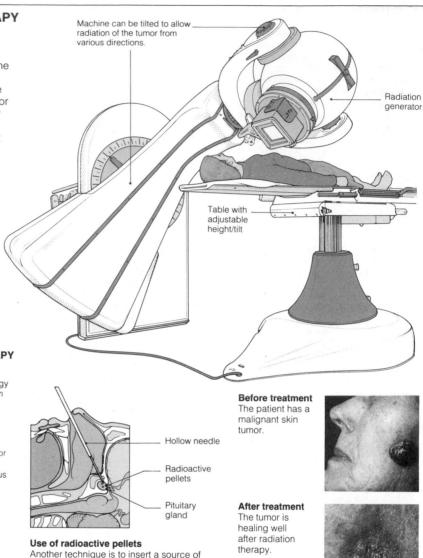

Machine can be tilted to allow radiation of the tumor from various directions.

Radiation generator

Table with adjustable height/tilt

EXAMPLES OF RADIATION THERAPY

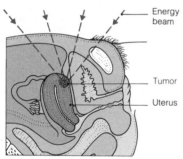

Energy beam

Tumor

Uterus

Rays from different directions
By aiming relatively low-energy rays coming from many directions at a tumor, a large enough dose is achieved in the locality of the tumor to destroy it. Tissues through which the rays pass are unharmed.

Hollow needle

Radioactive pellets

Pituitary gland

Use of radioactive pellets
Another technique is to insert a source of radiation, in the form of tiny radioactive pellets, directly into the tumor via a hollow needle. Pituitary tumors are sometimes treated in this way.

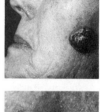

Before treatment
The patient has a malignant skin tumor.

After treatment
The tumor is healing well after radiation therapy.

---

entire affected breast, along with chest muscles, underarm lymph nodes, and other tissue. Such operations are rarely performed today.

Amputation, which is usually performed to prevent the spread of *gangrene* (tissue death), is another form of radical surgery.

Radiculopathy

Damage to the nerve roots that enter or leave the *spinal cord*. Radiculopathy may be caused by *disk prolapse*, spinal *arthritis*, thickening of the meninges (the membranes that cover the brain and spinal cord), and sometimes *diabetes mellitus* or ingestion of heavy metals, such as lead.

Symptoms of radiculopathy are severe pain and, occasionally, loss of feeling in the area supplied by the affected nerves, and weakness, paralysis, and wasting of muscles supplied by the nerves. Treatment is of the underlying cause if possible; otherwise, symptoms may be relieved by *analgesic drugs* (painkillers), *physiotherapy*, or, in some cases, surgery.

Radioactivity

The emission of alpha particles or beta particles and/or gamma rays that occurs when the nuclei of certain unstable substances spontaneously disintegrate. Natural radioactivity is due to the disintegration of naturally occurring radioactive substances, such as uranium ores. However, most elements can be induced to become radioactive by bombarding them with high-energy particles (such as neutrons)—so-called artificial radioactivity. (See also *Radiation*.)

Radiography

The use of *radiation* to obtain images of parts of the body. Technologists prepare patients for *X-ray* examinations, take and develop X-ray pictures, and assist with other *imaging techniques*.

X-ray technologists also assist radiologists in performing specialized X-ray examinations, such as contrast-medium studies, and carrying out other imaging techniques, such as *radionuclide scanning, ultrasound scanning*, and *MRI*. (See also *Radiology*.)

Radioimmunoassay

A very sensitive laboratory technique that employs radioactive isotopes to measure the concentration of specific proteins in a person's blood.

Proteins that can be detected by radioimmunoassay now include hormones, parts of microorganisms, and antibodies formed against microorganisms or allergy-producing substances. (See *Immunoassay*.)

Radioisotope scanning

A diagnostic process, which is based on *radiation* emissions. (See *Radionuclide scanning*.)

Radiology

The medical specialty that uses *X rays, ultrasound, MRI* (magnetic resonance imaging), and *radionuclide scanning* for investigation, diagnosis, and treatment. In general, a radiologist (a physician who is specially trained and certified in the use of imaging techniques) is seen only on referral from another physician. Other specialists may also employ radionuclide (radioisotope) scanning for purposes of diagnosis and treatment.

Radiological methods can provide images of almost any organ, system, or part of the body in a *noninvasive* way so that diagnoses can be made and treatment planned or monitored frequently without the patient's needing to undergo exploratory surgery.

Radiological techniques also enable instruments (such as needles and catheters) to be accurately guided into different parts of the body both for diagnosis and, increasingly, for treatment. This subspecialty is known as interventional radiology.

Radiolucent

Almost transparent to *radiation*, especially to X rays and gamma rays. Objects that are entirely transparent to radiation are termed radiotransparent. Objects that are not transparent to radiation are termed *radiopaque*.

RADIONUCLIDE SCANNING

In this imaging technique, a radionuclide is introduced into the body, where it is taken up in different amounts by different tissues. The radiation emitted by the tissues that take up the radionuclide is then detected by a gamma camera. The radionuclides used may be radioactive varieties of elements that occur naturally in the body (e.g., iodine) or synthetic radioactive elements (e.g., technetium).

Radionuclide scan of the heart
This image shows radionuclide-labeled red blood cells in the heart. The lower dark area is the left ventricle of the heart.

Gamma camera — Nuclear medicine technologist — Patient

Radionuclide scanning

A diagnostic technique based on the detection of *radiation* emitted by radioactive substances (radionuclides) in the body. Different radionuclides are taken up in greater concentrations by different types of tissue. For example, the thyroid gland takes up more radioactive iodine than other parts of the body. The images provided by radionuclide scanning reflect the functioning of an organ better than other techniques, although they provide less anatomical detail.

HOW IT WORKS

A radionuclide substance is swallowed or injected into the bloodstream and accumulates in the target organ. Radiation in the form of gamma rays (similar to X rays but of shorter wavelength) is emitted from the organ and detected by an instrument known as a gamma camera. The camera contains a scintillation crystal that reacts to gamma rays by emitting minute quantities of light (photons). These are used to produce an image that can be displayed on a screen or in digital (numerical) form.

Using a principle similar to *CT scanning*, cross-sectional images ("slices") can be constructed by a computer from radiation detected by a gamma camera that rotates around the patient. This specialized form of radionuclide scanning is known as SPECT (single photon emission computed tomography). It is also possible to create moving images with a computer by recording a series of images immediately following the administration of the radionuclide.

WHY IT IS DONE

Radionuclide scanning can detect certain disorders earlier than other imaging techniques because changes in the functioning of an organ often occur before the structure is affected. For example, infection of bone results in increased activity of bone cells, resulting in radionuclide being taken up in greater amounts by diseased bone before structural changes show on conventional X rays.

The technique is also useful for detecting disorders that affect only function (some thyroid disorders, for example).

R

Moving images can provide information on functions such as blood flow, the movement of the heart walls, urine flow through the kidneys, and bile flow through the liver.

RISKS

Radionuclide scanning is a safe procedure. It requires only minute doses of radiation and, because the radionuclide is ingested or administered by intravenous injection, it also avoids the risks associated with some X-ray procedures in which a radiopaque contrast medium is administered by inserting a catheter into the organ (as in cardiac *catheterization* and coronary *angiography*). Moreover, unlike radiopaque contrast media, radionuclides carry virtually no risk to the patient of toxicity or hypersensitivity.

OUTLOOK

Advances in radionuclide scanning depend on the continuing development of radionuclides specific to certain tissues. The fact that monoclonal antibodies (see *Antibody, monoclonal*) can now be produced for use against almost any antigen means that it should be possible to target almost any tissue. Experiments that use labeled antitumor monoclonal antibodies to assess tumor spread and recurrence may further enhance this procedure's usefulness.

Radiopaque

Blocking the passage of *radiation*, especially *X rays* and gamma rays. Many body tissues, with the notable exception of bones, are *radiolucent* (almost transparent to X rays). For some types of diagnostic X-ray imaging, it is therefore necessary to introduce special radiopaque substances into the body to make organs stand out more clearly. In intravenous *urography*, for example, radiopaque iodine compounds are excreted by the kidney into the lower urinary tract to make the structures clearly visible on X-ray photographs.

Radium

A rare radioactive metallic element which does not occur naturally in its pure form but is present as various compounds in *uranium* ores, such as pitchblende and carnotite. Radium has four naturally occurring isotopes (varieties of the element that are chemically identical but differ in some physical properties). In order of decreasing abundance they are radium 226, radium 228, radium 224, and radium 223. Artificial radium isotopes have also been produced.

The most important isotope is radium 226, which is produced by the decay of naturally radioactive elements of the uranium series. It is relatively long-lived (with a *half-life* of about 1,600 years), and itself decays to form the gas *radon*, which then decays further to form other, solid, radioactive decay products. During these decay stages, *radiation* is emitted in the form of alpha and beta particles and gamma rays. Radium 226 was formerly used to treat tumors but it has now been superseded by other radioisotopes, such as cobalt 60 and cesium 137.

The use of radium in some luminous paints was discontinued after it was discovered that the radium caused leukemia and bone tumors in those using the paint.

Radius

The shorter of the two long bones of the forearm; the other is the *ulna*. The radius is the bone on the thumb side of the arm.

The shaft of the radius has a broad base that articulates with the lower end of the ulna and with the upper bones of the wrist. The disk-shaped head of the radius, which is smaller than the base, articulates with the lower end of the *humerus* (the bone of the upper arm) to form part of the elbow joint.

The radius takes most of the strain when weight is placed on the wrist and is a common site of fractures (see *Colles' fracture; Radius, fracture of*). A fall or blow may sometimes cause

---

LOCATION OF THE RADIUS
The radius is the bone on the outside of the forearm with the palm facing forward, or on the inside with the palm facing backward.

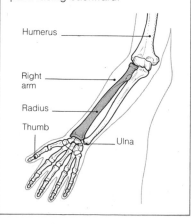

Humerus

Right arm

Radius

Thumb

Ulna

---

dislocation of the radius from the elbow joint along with fracture of the ulna, a condition that is known as *Monteggia's fracture*.

Radius, fracture of

A common type of fracture that may affect the lower end, upper end, or shaft of the *radius* (the shorter of the two long bones in the forearm).

Fracture of the radius just above the wrist is the most common of all fractures in people over 40. It is usually caused by falling on the palm of an outstretched hand, resulting in backward displacement of the wrist and hand (see *Colles' fracture*).

Fracture of the disk-shaped head of the bone just below the elbow joint is one of the most common fractures in young adults. Treatment in such cases consists of removing any blood clot via a syringe and then immobilizing the forearm (bent at a right angle to the upper arm) and the elbow in a plaster *cast* to allow the fracture to heal. If the head of the bone is crushed or splintered, it may need to be removed surgically before the cast is applied. Early movement of the healing arm should be encouraged.

Fracture of the shaft of the radius often results in displacement of the bone ends. An operation is usually required to reposition the bone ends and fix them together with wires or plates and screws. In some cases, however, the bones can be externally manipulated back into position. Once the bones have been repositioned, the limb is immobilized by the use of a plaster cast.

Radon

A colorless, odorless, tasteless, radioactive gaseous element that is produced by the radioactive decay of *radium*.

Radon has three naturally occurring isotopes (varieties of the element that are chemically identical but which differ in some physical properties)—radon 219, radon 220, and radon 222. Each of these is short-lived (radon 219 has a *half-life* of about four seconds, radon 220 of about 51 seconds, and radon 222 of about 3.8 days).

These isotopes disintegrate—with the emission of *radiation* (in the form of alpha particles)—to form solid radioactive materials known as radon daughters, which themselves emit alpha and beta particles and gamma rays. In addition to radon's naturally occurring radioisotopes, several artificial ones have been produced.

R

The parent sources of radon occur naturally in many materials, such as soil, rocks, and building materials, and the gas is continually released into the atmosphere. As a result, radon makes the largest single contribution (about 40 percent) to the total radiation exposure of the Canadian population. This fact has led some researchers to suggest that radon may be a significant causative factor in some cases of cancer (particularly lung cancer). However, this claim has not been demonstrated in the general population. Workers in certain specialized mining industries, such as uranium, fluorspar, and hematite mining (in which radon gas is encountered) have an increased risk of lung cancer.

Ranitidine

An *ulcer-healing drug* belonging to the *H2-receptor antagonist* group. It is used to prevent and treat *peptic ulcers* and to treat *esophagitis*. Possible side effects include headache, skin rash, nausea, constipation, and lethargy.

Ranula

A cyst in the floor of the mouth which produces a translucent bluish swelling. Ranulas probably arise from damaged *salivary glands*. Treatment is by surgical removal.

Rape

Sexual intercourse with an unwilling partner, which is achieved by the use or the threat of force or violence and against the victim's will, or without the victim's consent. In Canada, rape has been dropped from the Criminal Code in favor of aggravated sexual assault.

Society, the police, and the courts have in the last decade attempted to do more for rape victims and there is today a greater understanding of the traumatic effects that the act can have on the victim. Studies have clarified the nature of rape, revealing that, contrary to popular belief, it most often occurs between people who know each other, is not always accompanied by physical violence, and is not provoked by the victim.

INCIDENCE

Recent years have seen a considerable increase in reported sexual assaults. It is difficult to know whether this reflects a genuine increase in incidence or a greater willingness on the part of victims to report the crime. Nevertheless, it is still one of the least reported of all crimes. It is estimated that the majority of sexual assaults is unreported due to the victim's shame, fear of being disbelieved, fear of family rejection, fear of reprisal by the rapist, or fear of the publicity and trauma associated with going through a trial.

MOTIVES

Rape is a violent act motivated by a need to dominate the victim. The rapist may use forcible sex as one of many forms of abusive, dehumanizing behavior, being motivated by a profound hostility toward women.

Rape is rarely sexually motivated; it is an act of dominance, anger and hostility, rather than one of passion. There is evidence of a link between alcohol abuse and rape.

About 20 percent of rapists are reconvicted of sexual offenses; up to 80 percent subsequently commit other crimes and may have a long history of violent crime.

EFFECTS

The rape victim may suffer a variety of physical injuries, usually as a result of beating or choking. Severe injury to the genitals is rare, but there may be swelling of the labia, bruising of the vaginal walls or cervix, and, occasionally, tearing of the anus or the perineum (the area between the genitals and the anus).

Even in the absence of physical injury, the psychological effects of rape are often severe, including significant *anxiety*, *depression*, or *posttraumatic stress disorder*. Nightmares or daytime flashbacks of the event may also occur.

FORENSIC TESTS

The physician examining a rape victim performs a physical examination, noting signs of bruising or injury, particularly to the genital area. The examination includes visual inspection of the vaginal canal. A woman is usually present to support the victim.

For laboratory analysis, the physician collects swabs from any suspected bite marks, from soiled areas of the body, and from the vagina, anus, or throat; fingernail scrapings or clippings; and any torn-out strands of hair from the head or pubic region. Such specimens allow comparisons to be made with samples taken from suspects.

Clothing worn by the victim at the time of the assault is also retained for forensic examination.

TREATMENT

Physical injuries are treated as required. Postcoital contraception (see *Contraception, postcoital*) may be prescribed. Treatment for *sexually transmitted disease* may be required in some cases.

In the treatment of psychological trauma, rape crisis counseling can be highly beneficial. In some cases, psychiatric support may also be needed. Many victims are now helped by rape support groups organized locally in most urban communities.

Rash

A group of spots or an area of red, inflamed skin. A rash is usually temporary and only rarely is a sign of a serious underlying problem. It may be accompanied by itching or fever.

TYPES

A rash may be localized (affecting only a small area of the skin) or generalized (covering the entire body). Physicians also describe rashes according to the type of spots present.

A blistering rash may be either bullous, consisting of large blisters, or vesicular, consisting of small blisters. A pustular rash is made up of pus-filled blisters.

A macular rash consists of spots that are level with the surrounding skin and discernible from it only by a difference in color or texture.

Nodular and papular rashes are composed of small, raised bumps, which may or may not be the same color as the surrounding skin.

CAUSES

A rash is the main sign of many childhood infectious diseases (such as *chickenpox* and *scarlet fever*) and of many other infections, ranging from ringworm (see *Tinea*) to *typhus*.

Rashes are a feature of many *skin disorders*, such as *eczema* and *psoriasis*. A rash may also indicate an underlying medical problem. Examples of such rashes include the purple-red spots characteristic of *purpura* (a bleeding disorder); the rash of *scurvy* or *pellagra*, caused by vitamin deficiency; and the rashes appearing in systemic *lupus erythematosus* and other *autoimmune disorders*.

The rashes of *urticaria* (hives) or of contact *dermatitis* may be caused by an allergic reaction to something that has been eaten or with which the skin has come in contact. Drug reactions, particularly to *antibiotic drugs* and *barbiturate drugs*, are also a common cause.

DIAGNOSIS AND TREATMENT

The physician makes a diagnosis based on the appearance and distribution of the rash, the presence of any accompanying symptoms, and the possibility of allergy (e.g., to drugs).

R

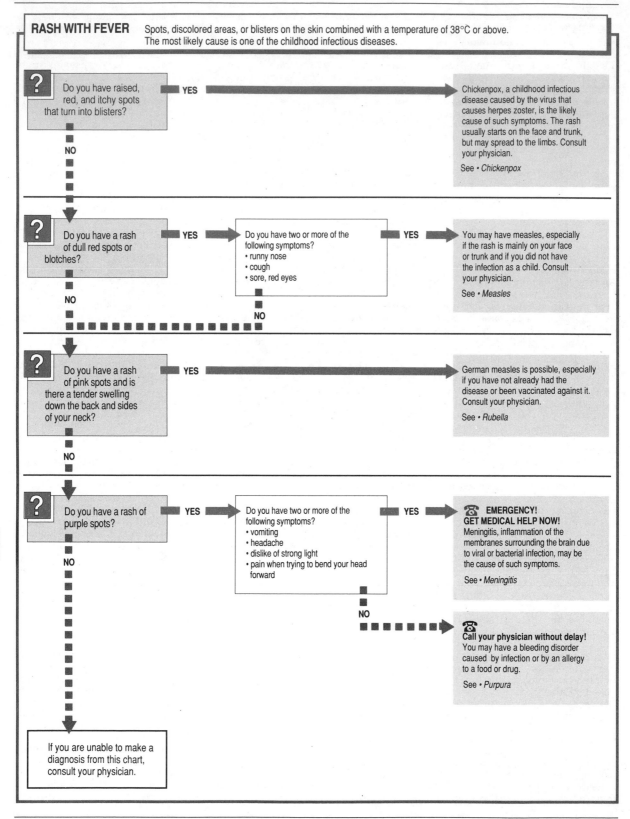

RASH WITH FEVER Spots, discolored areas, or blisters on the skin combined with a temperature of 38°C or above. The most likely cause is one of the childhood infectious diseases.

? Do you have raised, red, and itchy spots that turn into blisters?

YES → Chickenpox, a childhood infectious disease caused by the virus that causes herpes zoster, is the likely cause of such symptoms. The rash usually starts on the face and trunk, but may spread to the limbs. Consult your physician.

See • *Chickenpox*

NO

? Do you have a rash of dull red spots or blotches?

YES → Do you have two or more of the following symptoms?
• runny nose
• cough
• sore, red eyes

YES → You may have measles, especially if the rash is mainly on your face or trunk and if you did not have the infection as a child. Consult your physician.

See • *Measles*

NO

NO

? Do you have a rash of pink spots and is there a tender swelling down the back and sides of your neck?

YES → German measles is possible, especially if you have not already had the disease or been vaccinated against it. Consult your physician.

See • *Rubella*

NO

? Do you have a rash of purple spots?

YES → Do you have two or more of the following symptoms?
• vomiting
• headache
• dislike of strong light
• pain when trying to bend your head forward

YES → ☎ **EMERGENCY!**
GET MEDICAL HELP NOW!
Meningitis, inflammation of the membranes surrounding the brain due to viral or bacterial infection, may be the cause of such symptoms.

See • *Meningitis*

NO

NO → ☎
Call your physician without delay!
You may have a bleeding disorder caused by infection or by an allergy to a food or drug.

See • *Purpura*

If you are unable to make a diagnosis from this chart, consult your physician.

R

RASH WITH ITCHING   Itchy spots or discolored and/or raised areas of itchy skin.

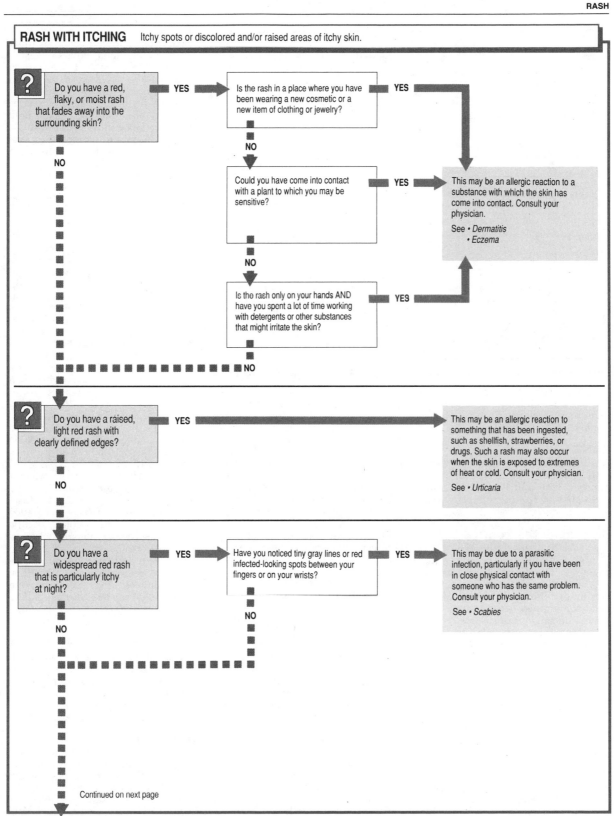

Do you have a red, flaky, or moist rash that fades away into the surrounding skin?

YES → Is the rash in a place where you have been wearing a new cosmetic or a new item of clothing or jewelry?

YES →

NO ↓

Could you have come into contact with a plant to which you may be sensitive?

YES →

NO ↓

Is the rash only on your hands AND have you spent a lot of time working with detergents or other substances that might irritate the skin?

YES →

NO

This may be an allergic reaction to a substance with which the skin has come into contact. Consult your physician.

See • *Dermatitis*
    • *Eczema*

NO ↓

Do you have a raised, light red rash with clearly defined edges?

YES →

This may be an allergic reaction to something that has been ingested, such as shellfish, strawberries, or drugs. Such a rash may also occur when the skin is exposed to extremes of heat or cold. Consult your physician.

See • *Urticaria*

NO ↓

Do you have a widespread red rash that is particularly itchy at night?

YES → Have you noticed tiny gray lines or red infected-looking spots between your fingers or on your wrists?

YES →

NO

This may be due to a parasitic infection, particularly if you have been in close physical contact with someone who has the same problem. Consult your physician.

See • *Scabies*

NO

Continued on next page

R

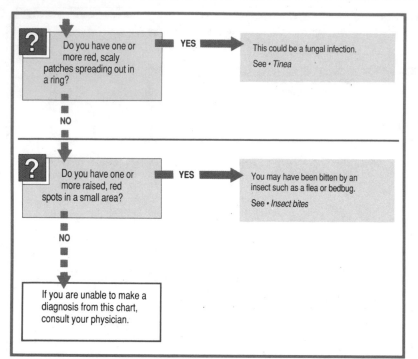

Do you have one or more red, scaly patches spreading out in a ring? — **YES** → This could be a fungal infection.
See • *Tinea*

NO

Do you have one or more raised, red spots in a small area? — **YES** → You may have been bitten by an insect such as a flea or bedbug.
See • *Insect bites*

NO

If you are unable to make a diagnosis from this chart, consult your physician.

Any underlying cause is treated if possible. An itching rash may be relieved by a soothing lotion, such as *calamine*, or an *antihistamine drug*.

RAST

An abbreviation for radioallergosorbent test. RAST is a type of radio-immunoassay and is used to detect antibodies to specific allergens. (See *Immunoassay*.)

Rats, diseases from

Rats are shy but potentially aggressive rodents that live close to human habitation; in many cities they outnumber humans. Rats damage and contaminate crops and food stores and can spread disease.

Various microorganisms harbored by rats can cause illness if spread to people. The organisms responsible for *plague* and one type of *typhus* are transmitted to humans by the bites of rat fleas. *Leptospirosis* (Weil's disease) is caused by contact with anything contaminated by rat's urine.

Rat-bite fever is a rare infection, transmitted directly by a rat bite. Either of two types of bacterium may be responsible. Symptoms may include inflammation at the site of the bite and affecting nearby lymph nodes and vessels, bouts of fever, a rash, and, in one type, painful joint inflam-mation. Antibiotic drugs are effective in treating either type of infection.

Rabies can be transmitted by the bites of infected rats in some parts of the world. *Lassa fever*, another danger-ous viral disease, may be contracted from the urine of infected rats in West Africa. Other diseases that can also be transmitted by infected rats in some areas are the viral infection lympho-cytic chorio-meningitis, and the bacte-rial infection *tularemia*.

Effective control of urban rat popu-lations is important in the prevention of rat-borne epidemic diseases.

Raynaud's disease

A disorder of the blood vessels in which exposure to cold causes the small arteries that supply the fingers and toes to contract suddenly. This action cuts off blood flow to the digits, which become pale. The fingers, usually on both hands, are more often affected than the toes. Young women are the most commonly affected.

When the symptoms develop with no known cause, the disorder is called Raynaud's disease. When symptoms are secondary to some other condi-tion, the disorder is termed *Raynaud's phenomenon*, and there may be more serious long-term consequences.

SYMPTOMS AND SIGNS
On exposure to cold, the digits turn white because of lack of blood. As sluggish blood flow returns, the digits become blue; when they are warmed and normal blood flow is reestab-lished, they turn red. During an attack, there is often a feeling of tingling, numbness, or burning.

In rare cases, the walls of the arter-ies gradually thicken, permanently reducing blood flow and eventually leading to painful ulceration or even to *gangrene* (tissue death) at the tips of the affected digits.

DIAGNOSIS AND TREATMENT
The condition is diagnosed from the patient's history. A person with Ray-naud's disease should keep the hands and feet as warm as possible. Ciga-rette smokers should stop smoking because smoking further constricts the arteries. *Vasodilator drugs* may be prescribed to relax the walls of the blood vessels. *Sympathectomy* (an op-eration in which the nerves that con-trol the diameter of the arteries are cut) has been tried in severe cases.

Raynaud's phenomenon

A circulatory disorder affecting the fingers and toes that shares the mechanism, symptoms, and signs of *Raynaud's disease* but results from a known underlying disorder.

Possible causes of Raynaud's phe-nomenon include arterial diseases (such as *Buerger's disease, atherosclero-sis, embolism,* and *thrombosis*); connec-tive tissue diseases (such as *rheumatoid arthritis, scleroderma,* and systemic *lupus erythematosus*); and various drugs (such as *ergotamine, methyser-gide,* and *beta-blocker drugs*). Raynaud's phenomenon is a recognized occupa-tional disorder of people who use pneumatic drills, chain saws, or other vibrating machinery; it is sometimes seen in typists, pianists, and others whose fingers suffer repeated trauma.

Treatment is the same as for Ray-naud's disease, along with treatment of the underlying disorder.

Reagent

A general term for any chemical sub-stance that takes part in a chemical reaction. The term usually refers to a chemical (or mixture of chemicals) used in chemical analysis or employed to detect a biological substance.

Receding chin

Underdevelopment of the lower *jaw*. The condition can be corrected by facio-maxillary *cosmetic surgery* in one of three ways—lengthening each side of the jaw by inserting a wedge of bone into it, increasing the bulk of the

R

bone at the front of the chin by a bone graft, or implanting a plastic bone-substitute at the front of the chin.

Receptor

A general term for any sensory nerve cell—that is, one that converts stimuli into nerve impulses.

The term receptor is also used to refer to a specific area on the surface of a cell with a characteristic chemical and physical structure. Many of the natural body chemicals must bind to receptors on cells in order to exert their effects. For example, the hormone epinephrine binds to three different types of receptors (called alpha-, $beta_1$-, and $beta_2$-receptors) which are found on the cells of organs such as the heart and lungs.

Recombinant DNA

A section of *DNA* (genetic material) from one organism that has been artificially spliced into the existing DNA of another organism, often a viral or bacterial cell.

An example of the use of recombinant DNA is the addition of a DNA section containing the genetic code for a hormone such as insulin. If the recipient cell can be encouraged to replicate, large amounts of the hormone can be obtained. (See also *Genetic engineering*.)

Reconstructive surgery

An operation performed in order to improve body functions or appearance. (See *Arterial reconstructive surgery*; *Plastic surgery*.)

Recovery position

The correct position in which to place a casualty who is breathing, and who has *not* a broken neck or spine, while awaiting the arrival of medical help (see first aid box, p. 861).

Rectal bleeding

The passage of blood from the *rectum* or *anus*. Such blood may originate in the rectum or anus, or may come from higher in the gastrointestinal tract. The blood may be mixed with feces, on the surface of feces, or passed separately. Blood passed in this way may range in color from bright red to dark brown or black. The passage of blood may or may not be accompanied by pain. Rectal bleeding requires investigation by a physician.

TYPES OF RECEPTOR

Stimuli are detected by the free endings of sensory nerve cells or by special structures forming the endings of these cells. These respond to specific stimuli (such as light of a certain wavelength) and send a signal indicating the presence of the stimulus to the spinal cord and/or the brain.

Cell surface or chemical receptors (right) are tiny structures on the outer surface of a cell. They allow certain chemicals to bind to the cell and trigger some change within it.

Skin receptors
The skin contains many types of receptor that respond to stimuli such as pressure, cold, heat, and hair movement, allowing the sensations of touch, temperature, and pain. They include such structures as pacinian corpuscles and Merkel's disks and are all special types of nerve cell ending.

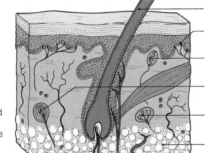

- Hair shaft
- Merkel's disk
- Meissner's corpuscle
- Pacinian corpuscle
- Organ of Ruffini
- Subcutaneous fat

Receptors in tongue
Each taste bud (below) consists of many receptor cells. Each has surface receptors that respond to chemicals in food.

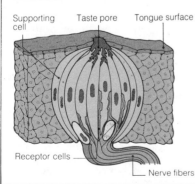

Supporting cell — Taste pore — Tongue surface
Receptor cells — Nerve fibers

Receptors in eye
The retina, located at the back of the eye, contains receptor cells, called rods and cones, which are responsive to light.

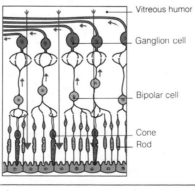

- Vitreous humor
- Ganglion cell
- Bipolar cell
- Cone
- Rod

HOW CELL SURFACE OR CHEMICAL RECEPTORS WORK
Most cells have many surface receptors (only one is shown below). Their existence allows the activity of the cell to be influenced from outside.

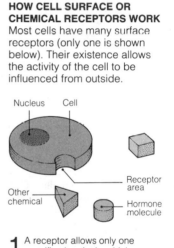

Nucleus — Cell
Other chemical — Receptor area — Hormone molecule

1 A receptor allows only one specific chemical—which may be a hormone or a neurotransmitter substance—to bind to it. The chemical must have a configuration that "fits" the receptor.

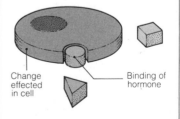

Change effected in cell — Binding of hormone

2 The binding of chemical to receptor alters the outer cell membrane and triggers a change—such as contraction by a muscle cell or increased activity in an enzyme-producing cell.

R

RECOMBINANT DNA AND GENETICALLY ENGINEERED INSULIN

Genetic engineering can force bacteria to produce human insulin. The insulin gene is obtained (by removing it from human DNA, then purifying it) and spliced into the DNA of a bacterium, causing it to produce human insulin. The bacterium is then cultured for large-scale insulin extraction.

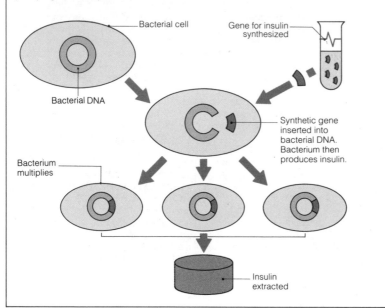

Bacterial cell

Bacterial DNA

Gene for insulin synthesized

Synthetic gene inserted into bacterial DNA. Bacterium then produces insulin.

Bacterium multiplies

Insulin extracted

CAUSES

The type of bleeding often gives a clue to its origin. *Hemorrhoids* are the most common cause of rectal bleeding in the form of small amounts of bright red blood found on the surface of the feces or on toilet paper. *Anal fissure, anal fistula, proctitis,* or *rectal prolapse* may also cause this type of bleeding.

Some disorders of the colon, such as *diverticular disease,* may cause dark red feces. Cancer of the colon (see *Colon, cancer of*), cancer of the rectum (see *Rectum, cancer of*), or polyps can also cause bleeding. Bloody diarrhea may be due to *ulcerative colitis, amebiasis,* or *shigellosis.*

Bleeding high in the digestive tract, usually from a *peptic ulcer,* may cause *melena* (black, tarry feces).

The physician may be able to make a diagnosis from a *rectal examination. Proctoscopy, sigmoidoscopy, colonoscopy,* and air-contrast *barium X-ray examination* may also be performed.

Rectal examination

Examination of the *anus* and *rectum,* performed to assess symptoms and to check for the presence of tumors of the rectum or *prostate gland.*

A rectal examination is performed as a part of a general *physical examination,* or when a person reports abdominal pain, pelvic pain, or a change in bowel habits. A rectal examination may also be performed if a man complains of urological symptoms and, sometimes (in addition to a pelvic examination), if a woman has gynecological problems.

The patient usually lies on his or her left side, with the knees bent toward the chest. The physician inserts a gloved, lubricated finger into the rectum to feel for any tenderness or abnormalities, such as ulcers or growths, and to examine the prostate or cervix, which can be felt through the rectum.

Rectal prolapse

Protrusion outside the *anus* of the lining of the *rectum,* usually brought on by straining to defecate. The condition causes discomfort, a discharge of mucus, and rectal bleeding.

In infants and young children, prolapse is usually temporary. In elderly people it tends to be permanent because of weakening of the tissues that support the *perineum* (the area between the anus and the external genitals). Rectal prolapse may occur with prolapsing *hemorrhoids.* If the rectal prolapse is large, leakage of feces may occur.

In younger people, a fiber-rich diet may be all that is necessary to cure the condition. Surgery is sometimes performed, and especially on older people; the operation is not always successful, however.

Rectocele

A bulging inward and downward of the back wall of the *vagina* as the *rectum* pushes against weakened tissues in the vaginal wall. A rectocele is usually associated with a *cystocele* (protrusion of the bladder into the front wall of the vagina) or prolapsed uterus (see *Uterus, prolapse of*).

Depending on its size, a rectocele may cause no symptoms or may lead to constipation by interfering with muscle contraction in the rectum.

Exercises to strengthen the muscles of the pelvic floor may help relieve symptoms (see *Pelvic floor exercises*). If they do not, an operation may be recommended to tighten the tissues at the back of the vagina to improve support for the rectum.

Rectum

A short, muscular tube that forms the lowest part of the large intestine and connects it to the *anus.*

STRUCTURE

Like all of the colon, the very first part of the rectum consists of four layers—the outermost serous layer; the muscular layer; the submucous layer; and the innermost mucous layer, which lubricates the rectum. There is no serous layer in the last 8 to 10 cm of the rectum.

FUNCTION

The rectum collects feces that have formed in the alimentary tract. Pressure on the wall of the rectum causes nerve impulses to pass to the brain; the urge to defecate occurs when feces distend (stretch) the rectum, although defecation may be voluntarily delayed.

DISORDERS

In rare cases, a baby is born with no rectum or anus (see *Anus, imperforate*).

The rectum may also be affected by various diseases and disorders. These include inflammation (see *Proctitis*), *polyps* (grapelike growths), familial *polyposis* (a condition characterized by numerous polyps that usually become cancerous), and cancer (see *Rectum, cancer of*).

FIRST AID: THE RECOVERY POSITION

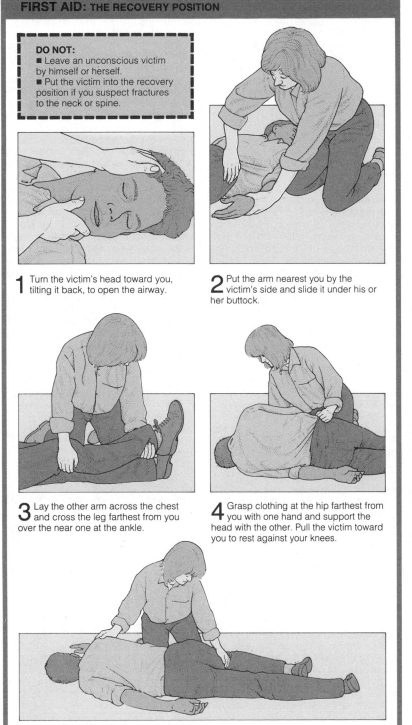

DO NOT:
- Leave an unconscious victim by himself or herself.
- Put the victim into the recovery position if you suspect fractures to the neck or spine.

1 Turn the victim's head toward you, tilting it back, to open the airway.

2 Put the arm nearest you by the victim's side and slide it under his or her buttock.

3 Lay the other arm across the chest and cross the leg farthest from you over the near one at the ankle.

4 Grasp clothing at the hip farthest from you with one hand and support the head with the other. Pull the victim toward you to rest against your knees.

5 Bend the uppermost arm and leg to support the body and stop the victim from rolling onto his or her face. The other arm should now be free. Readjust the head to make sure it is tilted well back and check to see if the airway is clear.

The rectum can become obstructed as a result of narrowing caused by *radiation therapy*, by *granuloma inguinale* (a sexually transmitted disease), or by a pelvic infection. In rare instances, an ulcer develops in the rectum, causing bleeding and discharge. Bleeding and discharge may also result from injury to the rectum caused by anal intercourse or the insertion of foreign objects into the rectum.

Rectal prolapse occurs when the lining of the rectum protrudes outside the anus. In a *rectocele*, the rectum and rear wall of the vagina bulge downward into the vagina.

Rectal disorders are usually diagnosed by physical examination (see *Rectal examination*) and by examination with a viewing instrument (see *Proctoscopy*; *Sigmoidoscopy*).

Rectum, cancer of

A malignant tumor in the muscular tube that forms the last part of the large intestine.

CAUSES AND INCIDENCE

The cause of cancer of the *rectum* is unknown, but dietary factors and genetic factors are thought to play a part in its development, as in cancer of the colon (see *Colon, cancer of*). Certain diseases of the colon (e.g., familial *polyposis* and *ulcerative colitis*) increase the risk of colorectal cancer (cancer of the colon and/or rectum).

Colorectal cancer is responsible for about 11 percent of all cancer deaths in Canada. Rectal cancer accounts for between one quarter and one third of tumors of the large intestine; it is more common in people who are between the ages of 50 and 70.

SYMPTOMS

The earliest symptom may be *rectal bleeding* during defecation. There may also be a change in bowel habits—diarrhea or constipation—and a sensation of incomplete emptying of the bowel. Later, pain may occur. Untreated, the cancer eventually may cause severe bleeding and pain and block the intestine, preventing the passage of feces. It may also spread to other organs in the pelvis and to other sites, such as the liver.

DIAGNOSIS

A physician can often detect rectal cancer by a *rectal examination*. The diagnosis is confirmed by *proctoscopy* or *sigmoidoscopy* (examination of the rectum with a rigid or flexible viewing instrument) and *biopsy* (removal of a sample of tissue for microscopic analysis).

R

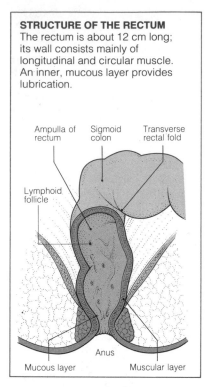

STRUCTURE OF THE RECTUM
The rectum is about 12 cm long; its wall consists mainly of longitudinal and circular muscle. An inner, mucous layer provides lubrication.

Ampulla of rectum

Sigmoid colon

Transverse rectal fold

Lymphoid follicle

Anus

Mucous layer

Muscular layer

TREATMENT
In most cases surgery is performed. If the tumor is in the uppermost part of the rectum, the abdomen is opened, the upper rectum and descending colon are removed, and the two ends are sewn together. To promote healing, a temporary *colostomy* (which diverts feces through a surgical opening in the abdomen) may be performed.

If the growth is in the lower rectum, the surgeon performs an operation called an abdomino-perineal resection, in which the abdomen is opened, the colon is cut through above the rectum, an incision is made around the anus, and the entire rectum and anus are removed. The wound is closed and, because there is no longer any outlet for the feces, a permanent colostomy is created.

Patients who have undergone surgery are examined at regular intervals to ensure that the tumor has not reappeared or spread elsewhere.

In elderly or debilitated people unable to undergo major surgery, *diathermy* (the application of high-frequency electric current) may be used to destroy the surface of the tumor and control local symptoms. Other forms of treatment when surgery is not possible are *radiation therapy* and, less often, *anticancer drugs*.

OUTLOOK
The long-term outlook for patients with cancer of the rectum depends on how far the tumor has spread before treatment takes place. About 50 percent of all people operated on for rectal cancer are alive three years later and almost 40 percent 10 years later. Survival rates are considerably higher when the disease is treated early.

Red eye
Another name for *conjunctivitis*.

Reducing
See *Weight reduction*.

Reduction
The process of manipulating a displaced part of the body back to its original position. Reduction may be carried out to realign fractured bone ends (see *Fracture*), to replace a dislocated joint in its socket (see *Dislocation, joint*), or to treat an abdominal *hernia* by pushing the protruding intestine back through the abdominal wall.

Referred pain
Pain felt in a part of the body at some distance from its cause. Referred pain occurs because some apparently remote parts of the body are served by the same nerve or the same nerve root (group of nerves that joins the spinal cord at one point). Nerve impulses that reach the brain from one of these areas may be misinterpreted as coming from another.

Common examples of referred pain are the pain down the inside of the left arm caused by *angina pectoris* or *myocardial infarction*; the pain felt in the tip of the shoulder from irritation of the diaphragm; the pain felt in a testis when the ureter is stretched by a urinary tract *calculus*; and the pain felt in the leg or foot from compression in the spine by a *disk prolapse*.

Reflex
An action that occurs automatically and predictably in response to a particular stimulus, independent of the will of the individual. Both the sensing of the stimulus and initiation of the action are carried out by components of the *nervous system*.

In the simplest reflex, a sensory nerve cell, perhaps at the skin surface, reacts to a stimulus such as heat or pressure. The sensory cell sends a signal along its nerve fiber to the central nervous system (brain and spinal cord). There, the end of the fiber connects to another nerve cell, which becomes stimulated in turn. Activity in this second cell then causes a muscle to contract or a gland to increase its secretory activity. The passage of the nerve signal from original sensation to final action is called a reflex arc.

Sometimes the reflex is more complicated. Sensory signals may be sent from thousands of sensory receptors to groups of nerve cells within the central nervous system. Complex analysis of these signals may occur before responses are made.

Many reflexes are inborn, including those that control basic body functions. Examples include shivering automatically in response to cold, increased breathing in response to a rise in carbon dioxide in the blood, and contraction of the bladder to expel urine after it has filled beyond a certain point. The part of the nervous system concerned with these processes is called the *autonomic nervous system*. Parts of the *brain stem* and the *hypothalamus* in the forebrain are processing centers for the autonomic nervous system. Some autonomic system reflexes are under partial voluntary (willed) control—emptying of the bladder can be voluntarily delayed for example. Ultimately, however, reflex is stronger than will.

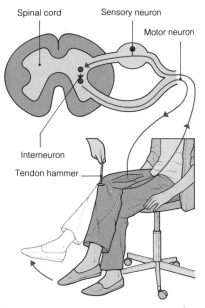

Spinal cord

Sensory neuron

Motor neuron

Interneuron

Tendon hammer

Simple knee-jerk reflex
A tap with a rubber hammer just below the kneecap stretches a tendon of one of the thigh muscles. A signal passes via a sensory neuron (nerve cell) to the spinal cord, activating a motor neuron, which contracts the muscle, jerking the lower leg upward.

Some inborn reflexes occur only in babies (see *Reflex, primitive*). An example is the grasp reflex when an adult's finger is placed in the palm.

A physical examination usually includes testing several simple, inborn reflexes, such as the knee jerk, plantar reflex (curling of the toes in response to irritation of the sole of the foot), and constriction of the pupil in response to light. Changes in these reflexes may indicate damage to the nervous system. A full neurological examination also includes the testing of various other reflexes.

The examination of vital reflexes controlled by the brain stem is the basis for diagnosing *brain death*.

CONDITIONED REFLEXES
Reflexes that are acquired as a result of experience rather than being inborn are called conditioned reflexes. They result from the formation of new pathways and connections within the nervous system during life. The process by which these reflexes are acquired is called *conditioning*. One type, operant conditioning, is a particularly important process in *learning*. Once a satisfactory response to a new situation has been discovered (often by a process of trial and error) and repeated several times, it is eventually automatically elicited by that situation or stimulus and thus becomes a sort of reflex. For example, a person walking home from work may follow a familiar route without needing to make any conscious effort to do so.

Reflexology
A form of *alternative medicine* in which the practitioner massages parts of the patient's feet in an attempt to cure disorders affecting other parts of the body.

Reflex, primitive
An automatic movement in response to a stimulus that is present in newborn infants but disappears during the first few months after birth. Primitive reflexes are believed to represent actions that may have been important for survival in earlier stages of human evolution.

Because some of these reflexes can give an indication of the condition of an infant's *nervous system*, they are tested by the pediatrician (a specialist in diseases of children) at the first examinations after birth. Any abnormality of the primitive reflexes may indicate a disorder of the nervous system. Their persistence beyond the

TYPES OF PRIMITIVE REFLEX

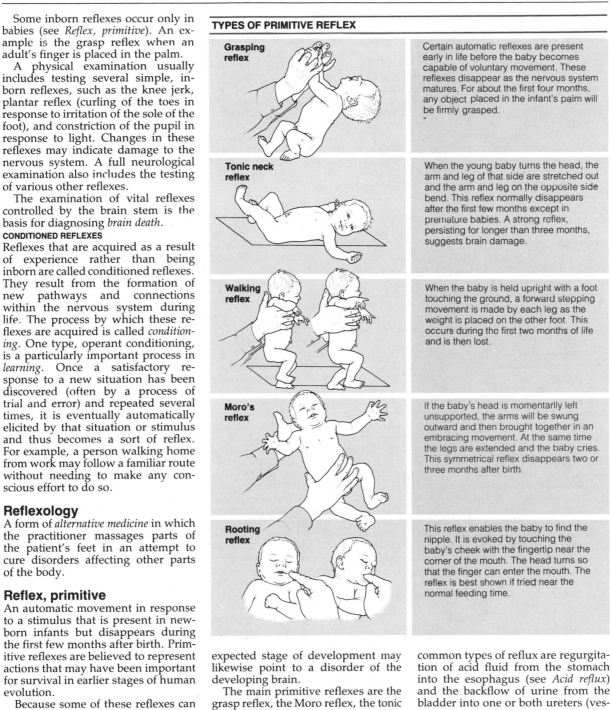

Grasping reflex
Certain automatic reflexes are present early in life before the baby becomes capable of voluntary movement. These reflexes disappear as the nervous system matures. For about the first four months, any object placed in the infant's palm will be firmly grasped.

Tonic neck reflex
When the young baby turns the head, the arm and leg of that side are stretched out and the arm and leg on the opposite side bend. This reflex normally disappears after the first few months except in premature babies. A strong reflex, persisting for longer than three months, suggests brain damage.

Walking reflex
When the baby is held upright with a foot touching the ground, a forward stepping movement is made by each leg as the weight is placed on the other foot. This occurs during the first two months of life and is then lost.

Moro's reflex
If the baby's head is momentarily left unsupported, the arms will be swung outward and then brought together in an embracing movement. At the same time the legs are extended and the baby cries. This symmetrical reflex disappears two or three months after birth.

Rooting reflex
This reflex enables the baby to find the nipple. It is evoked by touching the baby's cheek with the fingertip near the corner of the mouth. The head turns so that the finger can enter the mouth. The reflex is best shown if tried near the normal feeding time.

expected stage of development may likewise point to a disorder of the developing brain.

The main primitive reflexes are the grasp reflex, the Moro reflex, the tonic neck reflex, the walking or stepping reflex, and the rooting reflex (see illustrated box above).

Reflux
An abnormal backflow of fluid in a body passage due to failure of the passage's exit to close fully. The most common types of reflux are regurgitation of acid fluid from the stomach into the esophagus (see *Acid reflux*) and the backflow of urine from the bladder into one or both ureters (vesico-ureteric reflux). Persistent reflux of urine may lead to kidney damage (see *Nephropathy*).

Refraction
The bending of light rays as they pass from one substance to another. In the *eye*, refraction provides the mecha-

R

nism by which an image is focused on the retina, thereby permitting *vision*. The term is also used to describe the testing of the eye to determine whether there is any refractive error, such as *myopia*, *hypermetropia*, or *astigmatism* (see *Vision tests*).

Regenerative cell therapy

A treatment that claims to revitalize the skin. One technique involves the injection of preparations made from a mixture of animals' endocrine glands. Similar claims concerning revitalization have been made for skin creams containing sex hormones or animals' placentas. There is no evidence that any of these treatments works.

Regression

A term used in *psychoanalytic theory* to describe the process of returning to a childhood level of behavior. Sigmund Freud suggested that human beings progress psychologically through various stages of development from infancy to adulthood. Although disturbed adults may be superficially mature, they may be unconsciously fixated at an earlier level of development. When such people are frustrated or under stress, they undergo regression to immature forms of behavior, such as thumb-sucking or exposing the genitals. (See also *Fixation*.)

Regurgitation

A backflow of fluid. In medicine, the term is commonly used to describe the return of swallowed food or drink from the stomach into the esophagus and mouth. The term *acid reflux* is used to describe the backflow of acid juices from the stomach. Regurgitation of milk is very common in babies after feeding, when small amounts of milk are brought up with wind.

The term regurgitation is also used medically to describe the backflow of blood through a *heart valve* that does not close fully because of a disorder, such as *mitral insufficiency* or *aortic insufficiency*. (See also *Reflux*.)

Rehabilitation

Treatment aimed at enabling a person to live an independent life following injury (such as *spinal injury*), illness (such as a *stroke*), *alcohol dependence*, or *drug dependence*. Treatment may include *physiotherapy*, *occupational therapy*, and *psychotherapy*, depending on the problem.

Rehabilitation is often carried out in special centers, some of which are residential. In rehabilitation centers, people from different specialties work together to assess the severity of an individual's *disability* or dependence and develop a tailor-made treatment program. Industrial rehabilitation centers provide job retraining for people who are unable to return to their previous employment. Drug and alcohol rehabilitation centers help people through the period of withdrawal from the substance they have been addicted to, and also provide psychological support to reduce the risk of relapse.

Rehydration therapy

The treatment of *dehydration* by the administration of fluids and salts by mouth (oral rehydration) or by *intravenous infusion*. The amount of fluid necessary depends both on the person's age and weight, and on the degree of dehydration.

In mild dehydration (which occurs in many young children with *diarrhea*) rehydration can usually be carried out with solutions given by mouth. Oral rehydration preparations are available commercially in liquid form, or in powder or tablet form to be added to water. The simplest solutions contain only water, sodium chloride, and glucose; others may include potassium and sodium bicarbonate. Any unused solution should be discarded after 24 hours.

If commercial preparations are not available, a home-made oral rehydration solution may be prepared by adding one level teaspoon of salt and eight level teaspoons of sugar to one litre of boiled water.

In severe dehydration, or if the patient is unable to take fluids by mouth because of nausea or vomiting, an intravenous infusion of saline (sodium chloride) solution, glucose solution, or a combination of both, sometimes supplemented with potassium chloride, may be given in hospital. Additional treatment may be necessary depending on the underlying condition.

Reimplantation, dental

Replacement of a *tooth* in its socket after an accident so that it can become reattached to supporting tissues. Most commonly, it is a front tooth.

The dentist rinses the tooth in a sterile solution, replaces it in the socket, and maintains it with a splint (see *Splinting, dental*), often for several weeks. Successful reimplantation relies on replacing the tooth soon after the accident (ideally within 30 minutes). The outlook also depends on the age of the patient (the younger the better). Keeping the tooth moist and sterile (e.g., with saliva) also increases the chances of success.

Reiter's syndrome

A condition in which there is a combination of *urethritis*, *arthritis* and *conjunctivitis*. There may also be *uveitis*. Reiter's syndrome is more common in men than in women; it is the most common cause of arthritis in young men.

CAUSES AND INCIDENCE

The syndrome usually develops after *nonspecific urethritis*, affecting about 2 percent of men with this disorder. It may also occur after an attack of bacillary *dysentery*.

Yet although induced by infection, Reiter's syndrome results from an immunological response and usually develops only in people with a genetic predisposition. About 80 percent of people with the syndrome have the HLA-B27 tissue-type (see *Histocompatibility antigens*).

SYMPTOMS AND SIGNS

Reiter's syndrome usually starts with a urethral discharge followed by conjunctivitis and then arthritis. The arthritis seldom affects more than one or two joints and is often associated with fever and malaise. The affected joints, usually the knee or ankle, are warm, painful, and stiff. Inflammation persists for periods varying from a few days to several months. Tendons and ligaments (especially the Achilles tendon) may become inflamed, as may fibrous tissue in the soles of the feet. Skin rashes are common.

DIAGNOSIS AND TREATMENT

Diagnosis and treatment are based on the symptoms. *Analgesic drugs* and *nonsteroidal anti-inflammatory drugs* relieve pain and inflammation but may have to be taken for a long period. Antibiotic drugs are of no value in treating the arthritis.

OUTLOOK

Relapses occur in about one third of cases, especially after further episodes of nonspecific urethritis.

Rejection

An *immune response* aimed at destroying organisms or substances that the body's adaptive *immune system* recognizes as foreign. Rejection commonly refers to the nonacceptance by the immune system of tissues grafted or of organs transplanted into the body from other sources.

In an attempt to forestall rejection, as close a match as possible is made between the tissues of the donor and the recipient (see *Tissue-typing*). In addition, *immunosuppressant drugs*, such as *azathioprine*, *corticosteroid drugs*, and *cyclosporine*, are given to the recipients of organ transplants to suppress rejection by damping down the activity of the immune system. (See also *Grafting; Transplant surgery*.)

Relapse
The recurrence of a disease after an apparent recovery, or the return of symptoms after a *remission*.

Relapsing fever
An illness caused by infection with spirochetes (spiral-shaped bacteria) transmitted to humans by ticks or lice and characterized by high fever. Relapsing fever occurs in many parts of the world but not in Canada.

SYMPTOMS AND SIGNS
Relapsing fever starts with a sudden high fever—up to 40°C—accompanied by shivering, headache, muscle pains, nausea, and vomiting. The symptoms persist for three to six days, culminating in a crisis, with a risk of collapse and death. The affected person then apparently recovers but, some seven to 10 days later, suffers another attack. In tick-borne fever, several of these relapses, each progressively milder, are common.

DIAGNOSIS AND TREATMENT
A *blood smear* reveals the presence of the causative spirochetes. Relapsing fever can be effectively treated with *antibiotic drugs*.

Relaxation techniques
Methods of consciously releasing muscular tension to achieve a state of mental calm. Relaxation techniques can be useful on their own or in conjunction with other forms of therapy.

WHY THEY ARE USED
Relaxation techniques can assist people suffering from *anxiety* symptoms, can help to reduce *hypertension* (high blood pressure), and are a useful means of relieving the stress caused by a busy job or personal problems. They are taught to pregnant women to help them cope with the pain of labor (see *Childbirth, natural*).

TYPES
Active relaxation consists of tensing and then relaxing all the muscles in the body in turn, usually starting with the head and moving down to the feet. Passive relaxation may also be used. This involves clearing the mind of everything else in order to concentrate on a single phrase or sound. Control of the breathing rate (see *Breathing exercises*) is emphasized in both techniques. This helps prevent *hyperventilation* which often worsens anxiety. Taped instructions or *biofeedback training* may help reinforce learning. Once mastered, the techniques can be put into practice in potentially stressful situations.

Traditional methods of concentration, such as *yoga* and *meditation*, employ similar techniques.

Rem
A unit of equivalent absorbed dose of ionizing radiation (see *Radiation* units box). Rem is an acronym for roentgen equivalent man.

Remission
A temporary disappearance or reduction in the severity of the symptoms of a disease, or the period during which this occurs.

Remissions occur in many long-term diseases; the most notable example is *multiple sclerosis*, which typically follows a pattern of alternating remissions and *relapses*. In this disease remissions may initially last for months or even years, but usually become progressively shorter and may eventually become so short as to disappear completely.

Renal
A term meaning related to the *kidney*.

Renal biopsy
See *Kidney biopsy*.

Renal cell carcinoma
The most common type of kidney cancer (see *Kidney cancer*).

Renal colic
Spasms of severe pain on one side of the back, usually caused by a kidney stone (see *Calculus, urinary tract*).

The pain of renal colic occurs when kidney stones start to pass down the *ureter*. Stones in the ureter cause a severe pain that extends down to the groin. Sharp intermittent spasms, each usually lasting several minutes, are superimposed on a background of continuous dull pain. There may also be nausea, vomiting, sweating, and blood in the urine.

Renal colic is usually treated with bed rest, plenty of fluids, and injections of an *analgesic drug* (painkiller), such as *meperidine*.

Renal failure
See *Kidney failure*.

Renal transplant
See *Kidney transplant*.

Renal tubular acidosis
A condition in which the kidneys are unable to excrete normal amounts of acid generated by the body's *metabolism* (internal chemistry). In renal tubular acidosis, the blood is more acidic than normal and the urine is less acidic than normal.

The cause of renal tubular acidosis is often unknown. Possible causes include kidney damage due to disease, drugs, or a genetic disorder.

Problems that may result from renal tubular acidosis include *osteomalacia* (softening of the bones), kidney stones (see *Calculus, urinary tract*), *nephrocalcinosis* (calcification of the kidney), and hypokalemia (an abnormally low level of *potassium* in the blood).

Renal tubular acidosis may be treated with sodium bicarbonate (to counteract the blood acidity) and potassium supplements.

Renin
An *enzyme* involved in the regulation of *blood pressure*. When blood pressure falls, the kidneys release renin, which converts an inactive substance called angiotensinogen to the protein *angiotensin I* (also inactive). This protein is then rapidly converted to an active form, angiotensin II, which constricts (narrows) blood vessels and so increases blood pressure. In addition, angiotensin II stimulates the release of the hormone *aldosterone*, which causes the kidneys to retain sodium in the body, thereby helping to increase blood pressure.

Blood pressure can be lowered by drugs that affect the renin-angiotensin system, e.g., *beta-blocker drugs*, which inhibit the production of renin, and *ACE inhibitor drugs* (angiotensin-converting enzyme inhibitor drugs), which interfere with the conversion of angiotensin I to angiotensin II.

Renography
A technique used to measure *kidney* function. Renography is performed quickly and painlessly, and utilizes only a small dose of radiation.

A radioactive substance—either hippuran or pentetic acid—is injected into the bloodstream and passes through the kidney into the urine. Radiation counts are taken contin-

R

uously during the procedure. The information is recorded graphically as a renogram (a curve of counts per second against time). Both kidneys are examined simultaneously so that a comparison can be made of their function.

Renography is used when obstruction to the passage of urine is suspected. Normally, the radiation count rate increases rapidly for about 30 seconds after injection, rises more slowly for about five minutes, and then decreases as the radioactive substance passes into the bladder. If obstruction is present, the radioactive substance accumulates in the kidney and the count rate continues to rise, producing a differently shaped renogram. (See also *Kidney imaging*.)

Repetitive strain injury
See *Overuse injury*.

Reproduction, sexual
The process of producing a new generation to continue the existence of a species by the fusion of two cells from different individuals; this is achieved in humans by the fusion of one *sperm* and one *ovum*. This fusion, called *fertilization*, is achieved by *sexual intercourse* or *artificial insemination*.

Reproductive system, female
The organs that enable a woman to ovulate (see *Ovulation*), to have *sexual intercourse*, to nourish a fertilized *ovum* until it has developed into a full-grown *fetus*, and to give birth (see *Childbirth*). With the exception of the *vulva* (external genitalia), the female reproductive organs lie within the pelvic cavity.

Ova are released at monthly intervals from the *ovaries*, two small egg-shaped glands. The ovaries also secrete female sex hormones (see *Estrogen hormones*; *Progesterone hormone*), which control the reproductive cycle. Adjacent to each ovary is a *fallopian tube*, which carries ova to the *uterus*, a hollow, pear-shaped organ between the bladder and the rectum. If, on its journey along the fallopian tube, an ovum is successfully penetrated by a sperm, *fertilization* takes place.

Sperm travel upward through the *cervix* and uterus on their journey to the fallopian tubes. The cervix projects into the top of the *vagina*, a muscular passage which forms the lower part of the birth canal and receives ejaculated sperm during sexual intercourse. Surrounding and protecting the opening of the vagina are the fleshy folds of the vulva.

The normal functioning of the female reproductive system begins at *puberty* with the onset of *menstruation*; the potential for reproduction ends at the time of the *menopause*.

Reproductive system, male
The organs that enable a man to have *sexual intercourse* and to fertilize ova (eggs) with *sperm*.

Sperm and male sex hormones (see *Androgen hormones*) are produced in the *testes*, a pair of ovoid glands suspended in a pouch called the *scrotum*. From each testis, sperm pass into an *epididymis*, a long coiled tube situated behind the testis, where they slowly mature and are stored.

Shortly before *ejaculation*, sperm are propelled from the epididymis into a long duct called the *vas deferens*. The vas deferens then carries the sperm to the seminal vesicles, a pair of sacs that lie behind the bladder. These sacs produce seminal fluid, which is added to the sperm. It is this combination that produces *semen*.

Semen travels from the vesicles along two ducts to the urethra, a tube that acts as a passage for urine and for semen. The ducts pass through the *prostate gland*, a chestnut-shaped organ which lies beneath the bladder and surrounds the upper urethra. The prostate produces secretions that are added to the semen.

At *orgasm*, semen is ejaculated from the urethra through the erect *penis*, which during sexual intercourse is placed in the woman's vagina.

Resection
Surgical removal of all or part of a diseased or injured organ or structure. An anterior resection is an operation that removes part of the colon as a treatment for cancer.

Reserpine
An *antihypertensive drug*, derived from a tropical plant, used alone or with a *diuretic drug* in the treatment of *hypertension* (high blood pressure).

Possible adverse effects of reserpine include nasal congestion, dry mouth, *bradycardia* (slow heartbeat), depression, lethargy, and nightmares.

Resident physician
A physician undergoing specialized training in a hospital or medical center, usually after completing internship. (See also *Intern*.)

Resistance
In medical usage, the word resistance has several different meanings.

A resistance to the flow of blood is exerted by the blood vessel walls. This resistance increases as the diameter of blood vessels decreases, whether due to normal physiological processes or to narrowing as a result of disease. An increased resistance leads to a rise in blood pressure.

In *psychoanalysis*, resistance refers to the blocking off from consciousness of repressed material (such as memories or emotions). The psychoanalyst helps the patient to overcome this resistance.

FEMALE REPRODUCTIVE SYSTEM
Each month an ovum from one ovary is carried along the fallopian tube. If fertilized, it begins to divide and implants into the lining of the uterus to develop into an embryo. At birth, the baby is forced out via the cervix, the usually narrow passage that forms the neck of the uterus.

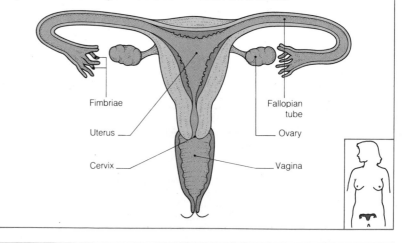

Fimbriae

Uterus

Cervix

Fallopian tube

Ovary

Vagina

MALE REPRODUCTIVE SYSTEM

Sperm made in the testis pass via the vas deferens to the seminal vesicle. Secretions from the prostate increase the volume of the semen, which is ejaculated from the penis via the urethra during orgasm.

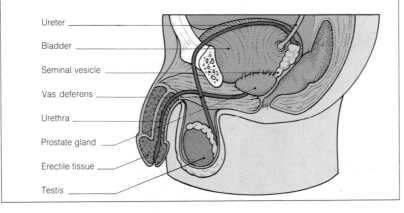

Ureter
Bladder
Seminal vesicle
Vas deferens
Urethra
Prostate gland
Erectile tissue
Testis

Resistance may also refer to an ability to withstand attack from noxious agents (such as poisons, irritants, or microorganisms). A person's resistance to infection is called *immunity*. The degree of immunity varies according to age, nutritional status, general health, the integrity of the person's *immune system*, and previous exposure to infective organisms.

DRUG RESISTANCE

The term drug resistance refers to the ability of some microorganisms to withstand attack from previously effective drugs. Certain bacteria have acquired *genes* (units of hereditary material) that confer protection against specific *antibiotic drugs*. Overuse of these antibiotics encourages the multiplication and spread of the resistant strains, which include some varieties of the organisms responsible for *gonorrhea*, *typhoid fever*, *salmonella* poisoning, *shigellosis* (bacterial dysentery), and other serious infections. Some strains of the parasites that cause *malaria* have become resistant to chloroquine, an important antimalarial drug.

When any dangerous infectious disease can no longer be treated with established remedies, the situation is potentially serious. The development of new drugs has, to date, largely kept pace with the threat. Strategies to prevent the emergence of new resistant strains have included the cyclical use of different antibiotic drugs to treat particular types of infection in hospitals. Physicians now try to avoid the indiscriminate prescription of antibiotics, which encourages the emergence of resistance.

Resorption, dental

Loss of substance from *teeth*. Resorption of a tooth may be external (affecting the surface of the root) or internal (affecting the wall of the pulp cavity).

CAUSES AND INCIDENCE

External resorption of tooth roots, which causes the teeth to become loose, is part of the process by which *primary teeth* are shed. It is thought to be activated by pressure from the underlying *permanent teeth* as they erupt (see *Eruption of teeth*).

Some degree of external resorption, affecting the roots, occurs in most adults as part of the aging process. External resorption may also be caused by injury to a tooth, periapical *periodontitis* (inflammation of tissues around the root tip), or pressure from an *orthodontic appliance*, a tumor, or an impacted tooth (see *Impaction, dental*). Completely impacted teeth occasionally undergo resorption of both the crown and the root.

Internal resorption is a rare form of tooth resorption that occurs in about 1 percent of adults. The cause is unknown. The condition sometimes spreads outward from the pulp cavity.

DIAGNOSIS AND TREATMENT

Resorption is usually detected from *dental X rays*. Treatment of external resorption is of the underlying cause (such as removing an impacted tooth). Internal resorption can usually be successfully halted by *root canal treatment*.

Respiration

A term for the processes by which oxygen reaches body cells and is utilized by them in *metabolism*, and by which carbon dioxide is eliminated.

The various stages in respiration are described in the illustrated box on page 869. (See also *Respiratory system*.)

Respirator

See *Ventilator*.

Respiratory arrest

Sudden cessation of *breathing*. Respiratory arrest results from any process that severely depresses the function of the respiratory center in the brain. Causes include prolonged *seizures*, an overdose of *narcotic drugs*, *cardiac arrest*, *electrical injury*, serious *head injury*, *stroke*, or *respiratory failure*.

Respiratory arrest leads to *anoxia* (lack of oxygen to tissues) and, if untreated, to cardiac arrest, brain damage, coma, and death. These effects may occur within a few minutes. The victim should be given *artificial respiration* or placed on a *ventilator* without delay. The underlying cause is treated if possible.

Respiratory distress syndrome

A lung disorder that causes difficulty in breathing. Respiratory distress syndrome results in a life-threatening deficiency of oxygen in the blood. The condition affects premature babies or may occur later in life.

CAUSES AND INCIDENCE

In premature babies, respiratory distress syndrome occurs because the lungs are insufficiently mature to cope with independent breathing. The syndrome occurs because of a deficiency of surfactant, a group of chemicals that normally open or keep open the *alveoli* (tiny air sacs) in the lungs.

In adults, the condition affects people whose lungs have been damaged by disease or injury. The disorder is caused by a stiffening of lung tissue and an increase of fluid in the tissue between the alveoli. The many possible causes include severe *pneumonia*; inhalation of vomit, an irritant gas (such as smoke or chlorine), or a high concentration of oxygen; *drowning*; an overdose of a *narcotic drug*, such as heroin or morphine; certain *autoimmune disorders*, and *septicemia* (blood poisoning).

SYMPTOMS AND SIGNS

The condition starts with an increase in breathing rate. Breathing then becomes labored and more rapid. Babies with respiratory distress syndrome make grunting noises and draw in the wall of the chest when they breathe. If the condition worsens, progressive deoxygenation of

R

the blood makes the sufferer turn blue. Without treatment, death may eventually result.

DIAGNOSIS AND TREATMENT

Respiratory distress syndrome is confirmed by listening to the lung with a stethoscope, by a *chest X ray*, and by analysis of *blood gases*. In some cases, other tests may also be needed.

Patients are treated in an *intensive-care* unit. In the early stages, humidified oxygen is given by mask. If the condition does not worsen, this may be the only treatment required and is continued until the patient recovers. If respiratory distress increases, an *endotracheal tube* is inserted through the nose or mouth; breathing is then maintained by a *ventilator*. Any underlying cause is treated if possible.

OUTLOOK

Respiratory distress is the most common cause of death in premature babies, but with modern intensive care the survival rate for newborn babies with respiratory distress syndrome approaches 90 percent. For adults with respiratory distress syndrome, the survival rate is between 25 and 50 percent. Some survivors of respiratory distress syndrome are left with permanent lung damage.

Respiratory failure

A condition in which there is a buildup of carbon dioxide and a fall in the level of oxygen in the blood (see *Hypoxia*). Respiratory failure may be caused by any disorder that disrupts the normal transfer of gases in the blood, including lung disorders (such as *emphysema*, severe *asthma*, or chronic *bronchitis*). Respiratory failure may also be due to damage to the respiratory center in the brain from an overdose of *narcotic drugs*.

Symptoms include breathlessness, cough, cyanosis (blue discoloration of the skin), an increased respiratory rate, or, less commonly, a reduced respiratory rate.

Respiratory failure usually requires *oxygen therapy*, in which a carefully controlled dose of oxygen is given. In severe cases, the patient must be placed on a *ventilator*. The underlying cause is also treated.

Respiratory function tests

See *Pulmonary function tests*.

Respiratory system

The organs responsible for carrying oxygen from the air to the bloodstream and expelling the waste product carbon dioxide.

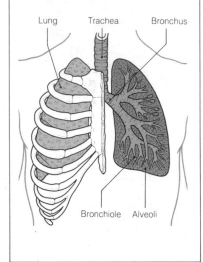

LOCATION OF THE RESPIRATORY SYSTEM
The system includes the upper air passages, lungs, and the muscles that control breathing.

Lung   Trachea   Bronchus

Bronchiole   Alveoli

Air passes from the *nose* or *mouth*, via various respiratory passages, to millions of balloonlike sacs, the *alveoli*, in the *lungs*. Oxygen in the inhaled air passes through the thin walls of the alveoli into the bloodstream, and carbon dioxide passes from the blood into the alveoli to be breathed out (see *Respiration* box).

Air is inhaled and exhaled by the action of the chest muscles and *diaphragm* (see *Breathing*).

DISORDERS

Disorders of the respiratory system can affect the air passages (causing obstruction of the passage of air into or out of the lungs) or can affect the lung tissues (resulting in a poor exchange of oxygen and carbon dioxide). The functioning of the respiratory system can also be impaired by disorders, such as *poliomyelitis*, that affect the chest muscles and diaphragm and make inflation of the lungs difficult. (See also *Respiratory tract infection*.)

Respiratory tract infection

Infection of the breathing passages, which extend from the nose to the alveoli. Most of these illnesses, which are classified as upper or lower respiratory tract infections, are caused by viruses or bacteria.

Upper respiratory tract infections affect the nose, throat, sinuses, and larynx. They are among the most com-

mon of all illnesses, especially in early childhood. The most familiar upper respiratory tract infections are the common *cold*, *pharyngitis*, *tonsillitis*, *sinusitis*, *laryngitis*, and *croup*.

Lower respiratory tract infections, which affect the trachea, bronchi, and lungs, include acute *bronchitis*, acute *bronchiolitis*, and *pneumonia*.

Restless legs

A syndrome characterized by unpleasant tickling, burning, prickling, or aching sensations in the muscles of the legs. Symptoms tend to come on at night in bed, although prolonged sitting sometimes triggers the discomfort; relief may be obtained only by movement, such as walking.

Restless legs affects as much as 15 percent of the population, although many cases are very mild. The condition tends to run in families and is most common in middle-aged women, in people who consume large amounts of caffeine, in smokers, and during pregnancy. It often develops in people with *rheumatoid arthritis*.

The exact cause is unknown; there is no apparent nerve, muscle, or circulatory problem. There is no single cure; some patients benefit from cooling the legs, others from warming them. Treatment with certain drugs, including *levodopa* and *calcium channel blockers* (such as nifedipine) has been found to be effective in some patients.

Restoration, dental

The process of reconstructing part of a tooth that has been damaged by disease or injury. Restoration also refers to the material or substitute part used to rebuild the tooth.

Small areas are usually repaired by first removing the decayed or diseased area and then *filling* the tooth with an inactive material. For more extensive repairs, it may be necessary to fit a dental *inlay* or a *crown*. These are constructed outside the mouth and then cemented into place.

For repairing chipped front teeth the dentist may use a *bonding* technique, in which the surface of the tooth is etched with an acid solution. This makes the teeth more receptive to the plastic or porcelain material, which is attached to the surface.

Restricted growth

See *Short stature*.

Resuscitation

See *Artificial respiration; Cardiopulmonary resuscitation*.

R

RESPIRATION

The function of respiration is to provide the energy needed by body cells. Cells obtain this energy mainly by metabolizing glucose with oxygen, and so they require a constant supply of oxygen. In addition, the waste products of the metabolic process—mainly carbon dioxide—must be carried away from the cells.

Respiration includes the breathing of air into the lungs, the transfer of oxygen from the air to the blood, the transport of oxygen in the blood to the body cells, the metabolism of glucose with oxygen in the cells, and the transport of carbon dioxide to the lungs to be breathed out.

During exercise, respiration increases to compensate for higher energy demands by muscle cells.

1 Air, containing oxygen, is breathed into the lungs and enters the alveoli (tiny air sacs). Oxygen diffuses from the air into the blood vessels surrounding the alveoli.

2 The oxygen-saturated blood passes from the lungs via the pulmonary veins to the left side of the heart.

3 From the left side of the heart, the oxygenated blood is pumped via the aorta to the body tissues. The oxygen is carried within the blood by red cells.

4 As the blood passes through tissue capillaries, it gives up oxygen (and nutrients such as glucose) to the body tissues and cells and picks up the waste products of cellular respiration—carbon dioxide and water.

5 Within body cells, glucose and oxygen take part in a complex series of reactions, which provides energy to power the cells. During this cellular respiration (left), glucose is converted to carbon dioxide and water.

6 Carbon dioxide is carried back in the blood to the heart, then to the lungs, where it diffuses into the alveoli and is breathed out of the body.

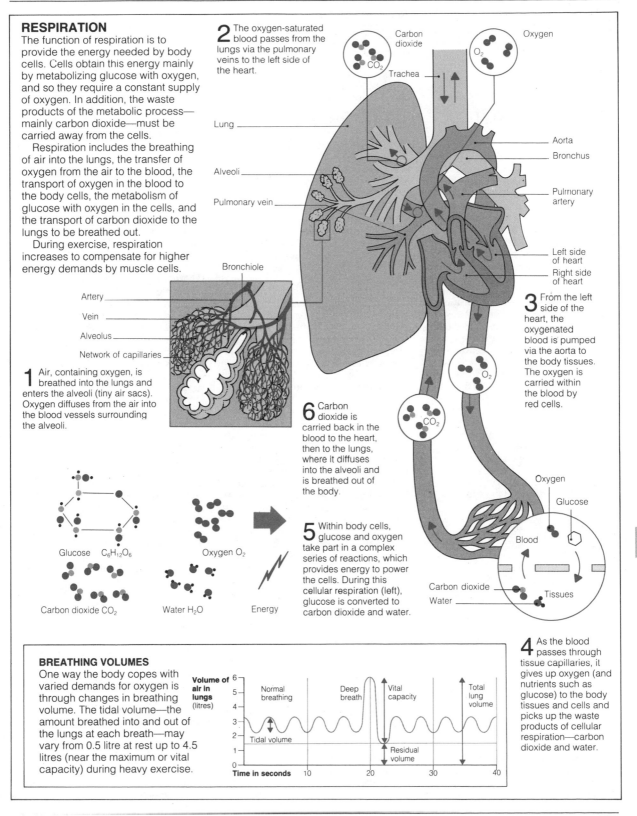

Carbon dioxide CO_2

Trachea

Oxygen O_2

Lung

Alveoli

Pulmonary vein

Bronchiole

Artery

Vein

Alveolus

Network of capillaries

Aorta

Bronchus

Pulmonary artery

Left side of heart

Right side of heart

Glucose $C_6H_{12}O_6$

Oxygen O_2

Carbon dioxide CO_2

Water H_2O

Energy

Oxygen

Glucose

Blood

Carbon dioxide

Water

Tissues

BREATHING VOLUMES

One way the body copes with varied demands for oxygen is through changes in breathing volume. The tidal volume—the amount breathed into and out of the lungs at each breath—may vary from 0.5 litre at rest up to 4.5 litres (near the maximum or vital capacity) during heavy exercise.

Volume of air in lungs (litres)

Normal breathing

Tidal volume

Deep breath

Vital capacity

Residual volume

Total lung volume

Time in seconds   10   20   30   40

R

Retardation
See *Mental retardation*.

Reticular formation
A network of nerve cells scattered throughout the *brain stem*.

Reticulosarcoma
A term for non-Hodgkin's lymphoma (see *Lymphoma, non-Hodgkin's*).

Retina
The light-sensitive membranous layer that lines the inside of the back of the *eye*, on which images are cast by the *cornea* and *lens*. The retina contains specialized nerve cells (the rods and cones) that convert light energy into nerve impulses. The retina also contains a network of connecting and integrating cells, some with very long fibers, that convey these impulses back along the *optic nerve* to the *brain*.

The rods are exceptionally sensitive, responding to very dim light. Cones are less sensitive but are responsible for *color vision*, producing impulses that vary in strength.

Near the center of the retina is the fovea. Here, retinal blood vessels are absent and the light-sensitive cells (almost all cones) are packed so that vision in this area has the highest resolution. (See also *Retina* disorders box.)

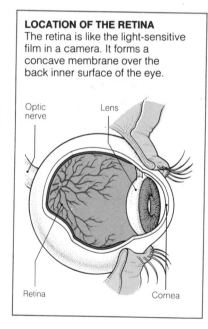

LOCATION OF THE RETINA
The retina is like the light-sensitive film in a camera. It forms a concave membrane over the back inner surface of the eye.

Optic nerve

Lens

Retina

Cornea

Retinal artery occlusion
Blockage of an artery supplying blood to the *retina*, affecting either the main retinal artery or one of its branches.

Retinal artery occlusion is most commonly caused by *thrombosis* (abnormal blood clot formation) or *embolism* (a condition in which a clot or fatty deposit is carried by the blood from another area). If the main artery is blocked long enough, the affected eye will become permanently blind. If a small branch is blocked, loss of part of the field of vision will occur.

Retinal detachment
Separation of the *retina* (the light-sensitive inner layer) from the outer layers at the back of the *eye*.

CAUSES
Retinal detachment may follow major injury to the eye, but in most cases the disorder occurs spontaneously. Detachment of the retina is usually preceded by a *retinal tear* (split in the retina), which may be due to natural degeneration or to the pulling away of the retina as a consequence of the contraction of strands in the vitreous humor. As a result of the tear, vitreous fluid collects between the retina and the underlying *choroid* layer, thus separating them.

Detachment is more common in highly myopic (nearsighted) people, who have thinned retinas with areas of degeneration, and in people who have had *cataract surgery*.

SYMPTOMS AND SIGNS
Retinal detachment is painless and the symptoms are exclusively visual. The first indication is the appearance of bright flashes of light, seen at the edge of the field of vision and accompanied by *floaters*. The flashes are caused by strong stimulation of the light-sensitive cells as the tear occurs, and the floaters by the release of blood or pigment into the vitreous humor.

These symptoms do not always occur; the affected person may be unaware of the detachment until a black "drape" obscures vision. This drape descends in a lower detachment, ascends in an upper detachment, enters from the right in a left detachment, and so on.

TREATMENT
Retinal detachment requires prompt medical attention. An ophthalmologist must be consulted before the macula (the site of central vision) becomes detached. Once detachment has occurred, it may not be possible to restore normal central vision.

In the case of an upper detachment (ascending drape), there is a risk that the accumulating fluid will gravitate downward and strip off the macula; it is therefore safer for the sufferer to lie flat on his or her back. In the case of a lower detachment (descending drape), an upright posture is unlikely to promote any extension of the detachment.

Treatment usually involves surgical repair of the underlying retinal tear. A soft silicone rubber sponge may be sewn in place on the outside of the *sclera* (outer layer of the eye) overlying the detachment. The sponge indents the sclera and leads to absorption of the fluid under the retina, causing the retina to settle back into place. The retina is then fixed in place by cryopexy (the application of extreme cold) or *diathermy* (the application of heat), which causes an inflammatory adhesiveness of the underlying tissues. If the macula has not been detached, the results can be excellent.

Retinal hemorrhage
Bleeding into the *retina* (the light-sensitive inner layer at the back of the eye) from one or more blood vessels. Retinal hemorrhage may be caused by *diabetes mellitus*, which leads to the formation of abnormal, small blood vessels which are fragile and bleed easily. Retinal hemorrhages also occur in *hypertension* (high blood pressure) and *retinal vein occlusion* (blockage of one of the veins that drain blood from the retina).

When the macula (the site of central vision) is involved, vision is severely impaired. Peripheral hemorrhages may pass unnoticed and may be detected only when the eye is examined with an ophthalmoscope.

Retinal tear
The development of a split in the *retina* (the light-sensitive inner layer at the back of the eye), usually caused by degeneration. Retinal tear is more common in people with severe *myopia* (nearsightedness). A retinal tear may also be caused by severe injury to the eye, especially a penetrating injury. *Retinal detachment* usually follows a retinal tear.

If a retinal tear is found before there is any secondary retinal detachment, the hole should be sealed by *laser treatment* or cryopexy (the application of extreme cold).

Retinal vein occlusion
Blockage of a vein carrying blood away from the *retina*, affecting either the main retinal vein or one of its branches. Retinal vein occlusion usually results from *thrombosis* (abnormal blood clot formation) in the

R

affected vein or an embolus carried from another area. The condition is more common in people who have *glaucoma* and usually causes disturbance of vision. Retinal vein occlusion may also cause glaucoma and can result in complete blindness.

Retinitis
Inflammation affecting the *retina*. (See also *Retinopathy*.)

Retinitis pigmentosa
A degeneration of the rods and cones of the *retina* (the light-sensitive inner layer) at the back of both eyes. Retinitis pigmentosa usually has a genetic basis, but seldom appears before a person reaches adolescence and may not appear until middle age.

The first symptom of retinitis pigmentosa is usually an awareness that vision in dim light is very poor (night blindness). Testing of the *visual field* shows a ring-shaped area of blindness which, over the course of years, gradually extends to destroy an increasing area of the field.

The cones in the macula (the site of central vision) seem more resistant than the peripherally placed rods, so central vision is retained, often for many years. Progression and severity are variable.

DISORDERS OF THE RETINA

Despite its small size, the retina is subject to a wide variety of disorders, many of which seriously affect the vision or, in some cases, produce blindness.

CONGENITAL AND GENETIC DISORDERS
Color blindness (see *Color vision deficiency*), an abnormality of retinal cones (color receptors in the retina), usually has a genetic basis. Hereditary degenerative disorders of the macula may appear at any age, leading to serious impairment of central vision. Other degenerative disorders of the retina with a genetic basis include *Tay-Sachs disease* and *retinitis pigmentosa*.

Retrolental fibroplasia may result from exposure of a premature baby to excessive oxygen concentration, which causes abnormalities in the retinal vessels.

INFECTION
Toxoplasmosis is an infection of the retina, acquired before birth and recurring later in life, with progressive damage to the retina.

TOXOCARA CANIS is a parasitic worm whose larvae may lodge in the retina and cause severe retinal destruction, producing a white mass resembling a tumor (see *Toxocariasis*). *Onchocerciasis*, an infestation by a tropical worm, may cause severe retinal damage. Bacterial and fungal infections elsewhere in the body can be carried by the blood to the retina. People whose immune systems are impaired are more susceptible to viral infections of the retina.

TUMORS
Retinoblastoma is a malignant tumor that usually appears in the first three years of life. The affected eye may have visual loss and a visible whiteness in the pupil; *squint* often develops. The tendency to this cancer can be inherited. Secondary malignant tumors, spreading to the eye from primary tumors elsewhere in the body, can occur. A variety of benign tumors occur in the retina. Malignant melanoma can arise from the *choroid* (the layer beneath the retina).

INJURY
The retina may be torn or detached due to severe penetrating or blunt (nonpenetrating) injury (see *Retinal detachment*; *Retinal tear*). Permanent damage may be caused by a retinal burn, sometimes caused by looking directly at an eclipse of the sun.

METABOLIC DISORDERS
Diabetes mellitus may cause *retinopathy*, with fluid leakage and hemorrhage into the retina and with the growth of new, fragile blood vessels on the retinal surface, which bleed readily. Hemorrhage into the vitreous humor may occur from blood vessels, and fibrous tissue can grow forward onto the humor in cases of "proliferative" retinopathy. This is a major cause of permanent loss of vision.

IMPAIRED BLOOD SUPPLY
Retinal vein occlusion (or *retinal artery occlusion*), a common cause of blindness, results from blockage of the central vein or artery of the retina. Hypertensive retinopathy is damage to the retina caused by high blood pressure, which leads to narrowing and *atherosclerosis* of the retinal arteries, which may both lead to retinal damage.

POISONS
A combination of heavy tobacco smoking, heavy alcohol intake, and poor nutrition may lead to visual loss. Vitamin deficiency in combination with lead poisoning may cause visual loss. *Methanol* causes widespread and permanent destruction of certain retinal tissues, leading to blindness.

DRUGS
Many drugs can damage the retina, such as *chloroquine*, used in large doses over a long period for the treatment of conditions such as rheumatoid arthritis, and *phenothiazine drugs*, used in the treatment of psychiatric disorders.

OTHER DISORDERS
Age-related *macular degeneration*, causing progressive loss of vision, is common in older people. Retinal detachment often occurs in the absence of injury and may be more common in people with severe *myopia* (nearsightedness).

INVESTIGATION
Retinal disorders are investigated by checking the visual acuity and the visual fields (see *Vision tests*). After dilating the pupils with drops, the retinas are inspected by means of a direct or indirect *ophthalmoscope*. Fluorescein can be injected into a vein, where it is carried by the blood to outline the retinal vessels. Electrophysiological tests can also be carried out to study certain ocular diseases. *Ultrasound* testing can be used to study tumors in or under the retina.

R

An examination of the retinas by ophthalmoscopy shows numerous masses of branching black pigment, distributed in areas corresponding to the extent of visual loss. Affected individuals or the parents of an affected child should seek *genetic counseling*.

Retinoblastoma

A *cancer* of the *retina* (the light-sensitive inner layer at the back of the eye) that affects babies and infants.

An affected eye may be blind, commonly causing a *squint* to develop, which is often the first indication of a retinoblastoma. The tumor may also show itself as a visible whiteness in the pupil. Without early treatment, retinoblastoma can spread from the eye to the orbit (eye socket) and along the *optic nerve* to the brain.

Retinoblastoma occurs in approximately one baby in 20,000. The tendency to develop retinoblastoma has a genetic basis. All the cells of people with this cancer lack part of one of the *chromosomes* in pair number 13. People belonging to families in which there is a tendency to retinoblastoma should seek *genetic counseling*. Infants from affected families should be given regular eye examinations, beginning shortly after birth.

The tumor is treated by surgical removal of the affected eye, or by *radiation therapy*. If both eyes are affected, then the eye with the larger tumor may be removed and the other eye given radiation therapy.

Retinoids

See *Vitamin A*.

Retinol

The principal form of *vitamin A* found in the body.

Retinopathy

Disease of the *retina*, usually resulting from either *diabetes mellitus* or alternatively from persistent *hypertension* (high blood pressure).

Diabetic retinopathy is characterized by tiny aneurysms (balloonlike swellings) of the capillaries (tiny blood vessels) in the retina, leakage of fluid from the capillaries, and hemorrhage (bleeding) into the retina. New abnormal blood vessels, which are fragile and bleed readily, grow on the retinal surface. Hemorrhage into the vitreous humor may occur, and fibrous tissue can grow forward into the vitreous humor. Advanced diabetic retinopathy is a major cause of permanent visual loss.

Hypertensive retinopathy is characterized by narrowing of the retinal arteries. Areas of retina may be destroyed, and hemorrhage and white deposits may occur in the retina. (See also *Retrolental fibroplasia*.)

Retractor

A surgical instrument used to hold an incision open or to hold back surrounding tissue so that the surgeon has free access to the underlying area being operated on. Some retractors are held by the nurse or an assisting physician; self-retaining retractors have a locking device that keeps them in position without support.

Retrobulbar neuritis

A form of *optic neuritis* in which the inflammation affects the optic nerve behind the eyeball.

Retrolental fibroplasia

Also called retinopathy of *prematurity*, a condition that mainly affects the eyes of premature infants.

Retrolental fibroplasia is usually caused by giving high concentrations of oxygen to premature infants who have a very low birthweight. Excess oxygen causes immature tissues, including those at the margin of the *retina* (the light-sensitive inner layer at the back of the eye), to shut down their blood vessels. When normal oxygen concentrations are resumed, affected retinal tissues sometimes send out strands of new vessels and fibrous scar tissue into the vitreous humor behind the lens. This process may interfere seriously with vision and lead to *retinal detachment*.

Babies with retrolental fibroplasia may be given *laser treatment*.

Retroperitoneal fibrosis

Inflammation and scarring of tissues at the back of the abdominal cavity. Retroperitoneal fibrosis often causes obstruction of the *ureters*, blocking the flow of urine from the kidneys. In severe cases, this obstruction results in *kidney failure*.

Most cases of retroperitoneal fibrosis occur in middle-aged men and are of unknown cause. In some cases, the condition is caused by long-term treatment with *methysergide* (a drug used to treat *migraine*).

Retrosternal pain

Pain in the central region of the chest, in the area of the sternum (breastbone). The most serious cause of retrosternal pain is a *myocardial infarc-*

tion (heart attack). More commonly, pain in this region is due to irritation of the *esophagus* or to *angina pectoris*. (See also *Chest pain*.)

Rett's syndrome

A recently discovered *brain* disorder that only affects girls. This rare condition was first described in the 1960s by an Austrian, Andreas Rett, but became medically recognized only during the 1980s. Rett's syndrome affects about one in every 15,000 female babies born and is thought to be caused by a *genetic disorder*.

The health and development of an affected baby appear normal until symptoms occur, usually when the child is 12 to 18 months old. Skills that had been acquired, such as walking and talking, gradually disappear and the girl becomes progressively handicapped and may show signs of *autism*. Odd, repetitive writhing movements of the hands and limbs are characteristic of the condition, and there are often inappropriate outbursts of crying or laughter.

There is no cure for Rett's syndrome; sufferers need constant care and attention because of the level of handicap. Parents of an affected child should receive *genetic counseling*.

Reye's syndrome

A rare disorder characterized by brain and liver damage following an upper *respiratory tract infection*, *chickenpox*, or *influenza*. Reye's syndrome is almost entirely confined to children under the age of 15.

CAUSES

Evidence suggests that Reye's syndrome is often (but not invariably) related to taking *ASA* for a viral infection. Physicians now recommend that children should be given *acetaminophen* instead of ASA.

Reye's syndrome develops as the child is recovering from the infection and starts with uncontrollable vomiting, often with lethargy, memory loss, disorientation, or delirium. Swelling of the brain may cause seizures, deepening coma, disturbances in heart rhythm, and cessation of breathing. Jaundice in Reye's syndrome indicates severe damage to the liver.

Swelling of the brain is controlled by *corticosteroid drugs* and by intravenous infusions of *mannitol*. *Dialysis* or *blood transfusions* may be carried out to correct the changes in blood chemistry caused by damage to the liver. If breathing stops, the patient is placed on a *ventilator*.

R

OUTLOOK

With increasing knowledge of the condition, the death rate from Reye's syndrome has dropped dramatically from about 60 percent to around 10 percent. The outlook is worse for those who have seizures, lapse into deep coma, and stop breathing. Patients who survive a serious attack may suffer brain damage.

Rhabdomyolysis

Destruction of *muscle* tissue accompanied by the release of *myoglobin* (the oxygen-carrying red muscle pigment) into the blood.

The most common cause of rhabdomyolysis is a severe, crushing muscle injury (see *Crush syndrome*). Other causes include *polymyositis* (a viral infection of muscles) and, rarely, excessive physical exercise.

Rhabdomyolysis usually causes temporary paralysis or weakness of the affected muscle. Except in cases of severe injury, an affected muscle usually regenerates and the condition clears up without treatment.

Rhabdomyosarcoma

A very rare, malignant tumor of *muscle*. Rhabdomyosarcoma may develop during infancy, usually affecting the throat, bladder, prostate gland, or vagina, or it may occur in old age, when it commonly affects a large muscle in the arm or leg. The tumor grows rapidly and spreads to other tissues. Treatment is by surgical removal, combined with *radiation therapy* and *anticancer drugs*.

Rh$_o$ (D) immune globulin

See *Anti-D (Rh$_o$) immune globulin*.

Rheumatic fever

A disease that causes inflammation in various tissues throughout the body. Inflammation of the *joints* is a major feature, but this is less serious in the long term than the risk of permanent heart damage. In some cases, the nervous system is also affected.

Rheumatic fever is now rare in most developed countries, but is still a common and significant cause of heart disease in the poorer countries of Asia and Africa. Children between the ages of 5 and 15 are the group that is most commonly affected by rheumatic fever.

CAUSES

Rheumatic fever always follows a throat infection with certain strains of streptococcal bacteria. It is not caused by the presence of the bacteria in the affected tissues but is generally believed to be some form of *autoimmune disorder* (one in which the body's immune system attacks its own tissues) induced by streptococci. The development of rheumatic fever can usually be prevented by prompt treatment of streptococcal throat infections with *antibiotic drugs*.

SYMPTOMS AND SIGNS

The disease causes fever with pain, inflammation, and swelling of one or more of the larger joints. As one joint improves, symptoms tend to develop in another, although several joints may be affected simultaneously.

If damage to the heart occurs, it develops insidiously; there may be no symptoms until some years later. The heart may be affected in various ways, the most common and most serious being a thickening and scarring of the *heart valves*, leading to narrowing and/or leaking of valves (see *Mitral insufficiency*; *Mitral stenosis*). These effects on the heart are permanent and progressive.

Involvement of the nervous system may cause *Sydenham's chorea*, in which there are irregular, uncontrollable, aimless, jerky movements, and usually some emotional upset. Rheumatic fever may also cause nodules beneath the skin and a rash.

DIAGNOSIS

There are no specific tests for rheumatic fever, but tests may be performed to look for *antibodies* directed against streptococci. The diagnosis may be suspected when arthritis moves from joint to joint, but in other instances the condition may be discovered only after the development of later heart damage, causing *heart failure* or a heart *murmur*.

TREATMENT

As soon as the diagnosis of acute rheumatic fever is made, a *penicillin drug* is used to eradicate streptococci. *ASA* or other salicylate drugs are used to control the joint pain and inflammation and to try to minimize heart damage. In some cases, *corticosteroid drugs* may be needed. Sedatives and tranquilizers are helpful in the treatment of Sydenham's chorea.

If heart valve damage occurs, *heart valve surgery* may be needed.

OUTLOOK

The outlook depends on the degree to which the heart has been affected and on whether recurrences can be avoided. The use of penicillin, taken daily for many months or years, may be necessary to prevent further infection with streptococci.

Rheumatism

A popular term for any disorder that causes pain and stiffness in *muscles* and *joints*, including minor aches and twinges as well as disorders such as *rheumatoid arthritis*, *osteoarthritis*, and *polymyalgia rheumatica*.

Rheumatoid arthritis

A type of *arthritis* (joint inflammation) in which the joints of the fingers, wrists, toes, or other joints in the body become painful, swollen, stiff, and, in severe cases, deformed. The disease usually takes the form of recurrent moderate attacks. The frequency of attacks, the number of affected joints, and the severity of symptoms are variable. Rheumatoid arthritis is medically distinct from *osteoarthritis*.

CAUSES AND INCIDENCE

Rheumatoid arthritis is an *autoimmune disorder* (one in which the *immune system* attacks the body's own tissues). The disease usually starts in early adulthood or middle age but can also develop in children (see *Rheumatoid arthritis, juvenile*) or the elderly.

Rheumatoid arthritis occurs worldwide and affects 1 to 2 percent of the population. It affects two to three times more women than men.

SYMPTOMS AND SIGNS

The onset of the disease is usually gradual, with mild fever and generalized aches and pains preceding specific joint symptoms. In some cases, joint inflammation develops suddenly.

Affected joints become swollen, red, warm, painful, and stiff. Structures around the joint may also become inflamed, resulting in weakness of the ligaments, tendons, and surrounding muscles. The finger joints are the most commonly affected, resulting in a weak grip. *Raynaud's phenomenon* (a condition in which the fingers turn white on exposure to cold) may occur. Swelling of the wrist may cause *carpal tunnel syndrome* (tingling and pain in the fingers caused by pressure on the median nerve). *Tenosynovitis* (inflamed painful tendon sheaths) also sometimes develops in the wrist. Rheumatoid arthritis affecting the feet may cause pain in the toes, arches, and ankles. Other parts of the body sometimes affected by rheumatoid arthritis include the shoulders, knees, and neck joints. Early morning stiffness is common, and sufferers may require help with getting out of bed and dressing.

Soft nodules sometimes develop beneath the skin, especially in areas

RHEUMATOID ARTHRITIS

One of the most serious forms of joint disease, rheumatoid arthritis may occur as a single episode or a succession of progressively severe attacks. It results from a disturbance in the body's defenses against infection, causing these defenses to attack various body tissues. In the worst cases, joints are completely destroyed, but modern treatment has reduced the incidence of severe disability.

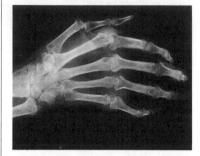

X ray of the hand in rheumatoid arthritis
Note the destructive changes in the joints and the way the finger bones curve away from the thumb side of the hand.

Affected joints
Rheumatoid arthritis can affect virtually any joint, but especially the fingers, wrists, shoulders, knees, hips, and spinal joints in the neck.

Disease progression
The synovium (membrane lining the capsule of an affected joint) becomes inflamed and thickened (right). Later, inflammation may spread to the cartilage and bone.

Bone

Inflamed synovium

Cartilage

Capsule

TREATMENT OF RHEUMATOID ARTHRITIS

Drug treatment
may include antirheumatic drugs to slow the progress of the disease, nonsteroidal anti-inflammatory drugs to relieve joint pain, and immunosuppressants to dampen the activity of the immune system.

Occupational therapy
can help people who are disabled by rheumatoid arthritis. Sufferers are shown how to cope with everyday tasks, provided with aids for use in the home, and taught principles of joint protection.

Prostheses
Many joints, such as the hip, can now be replaced with substitutes made from hard-wearing metal and plastic materials. Prostheses may be the only satisfactory solution if a joint becomes seriously damaged.

Physiotherapy
aids in the relief of pain and stiffness and helps sufferers to regain use of affected joints and muscles. The physician or physiotherapist may recommend removable splints to relieve pain in the hands and wrists.

TREATMENT

Depending on individual requirements, rheumatoid arthritis may be treated by drugs, *physiotherapy*, *occupational therapy*, or surgery.

Nonsteroidal anti-inflammatory drugs (NSAIDs) may be used to relieve joint pain and stiffness. *Antirheumatic drugs*, such as *gold* or *penicillamine*, may be used to arrest or slow the progress of the disease. *Immunosuppressant drugs*, such as *corticosteroid drugs* or *azathioprine*, are given to suppress the body's immune system if antirheumatic drugs fail to control the disorder or if they produce severe side effects. Corticosteroid drugs may be injected into affected joints to provide local pain relief.

Physiotherapy often plays an important part in the treatment of people with rheumatoid arthritis. Exercising in a warm hydrotherapy pool can lessen muscle spasm and joint stiffness. In some cases, removable splints can be extremely helpful in reducing pain in the hands and wrists. The use of insoles and, if necessary, special surgical shoes can help to relieve pain in the feet.

People disabled by rheumatoid arthritis can also be helped by *occupational therapy*. The occupational therapist can advise sufferers on how to cope with everyday tasks, and can recommend various dressing and household aids (see the illustrated box on physical aids for the disabled that accompanies the *Disability* entry). Severely disabled sufferers may be provided with a *wheelchair*.

In severe cases, surgery may be performed to replace destroyed joints—hip or knee for example—with artificial substitutes (see *Arthroplasty*).

As yet there is no evidence that special diets play any significant role in relieving the symptoms of rheumatoid arthritis, but a normal diet supplemented by fish or fish oils may be more beneficial than one without. *Acupuncture* may relieve pain, but it has no effect on the course of the disease.

COMPLICATIONS

Severe rheumatoid arthritis may have complications affecting various parts of the body. The covering of the heart may become inflamed, causing *pericarditis*. The small blood vessels may be affected, resulting in poor circulation and the development of ulcers on the hands and feet. Involvement of the lungs may lead to *pleural effusion* or to *pulmonary fibrosis*. The eyes and mouth may become dry (see *Sjögren's*

subjected to physical stress. Some sufferers develop *bursitis*, in which the fluid-filled sac around a joint becomes inflamed. When the knee is affected, a fluid-filled swelling known as a *Baker's cyst* may develop behind it. Many sufferers feel fatigued, partly as a result of the *anemia* that usually accompanies the disease. The diagnosis is based on the patient's condition and medical history, on *X rays* of affected joints, and on *blood tests* (including a check for specific antibodies known as rheumatoid factor). If rheumatoid factor is absent from a person who otherwise appears to have rheumatoid arthritis, the condition is known as seronegative rheumatoid arthritis.

R

syndrome). The lymph nodes may become enlarged, producing tender swellings in the neck, armpit, and groin. The spleen sometimes becomes enlarged, resulting in *hypersplenism* (overactivity of the spleen); the combination of rheumatoid arthritis and hypersplenism is known as Felty's syndrome.

OUTLOOK

Most sufferers must take drugs for the rest of their lives, but effective control of symptoms often allows a near-normal level of activity. Modern methods of treatment have reduced the incidence and severity of deformity and disability.

Rheumatoid arthritis, juvenile

A rare form of *arthritis* (joint inflammation) that affects children. Juvenile arthritis occurs more often in girls than in boys, and most commonly starts between the ages of 2 and 4 years or around puberty.

TYPES AND SYMPTOMS

There are three main types of juvenile rheumatoid arthritis.

Still's disease, also called systemic onset juvenile arthritis, starts with an illness in which there is fever, rash, enlarged lymph nodes, abdominal pain, and weight loss. These symptoms last for several weeks, and the joint pain, swelling, and stiffness may not begin for several months.

The other two main types are characterized mainly by joint symptoms. Polyarticular juvenile arthritis causes pain, swelling, and stiffness in many joints. Pauciarticular juvenile arthritis affects four or fewer joints.

DIAGNOSIS

Diagnosis is based on the symptoms and signs and the exclusion of other disorders that can cause joint symptoms in children. This would include various bacterial infections, rheumatic fever, Crohn's disease, ulcerative colitis, hemophilia, sickle cell anemia, and leukemia, and the physician would first rule these out as sources of the problem. Blood tests may help identify the cause of the arthritis. Juvenile rheumatoid arthritis is not diagnosed unless the condition persists for longer than three months.

COMPLICATIONS

Possible complications include short stature, *anemia*, *pleurisy*, *pericarditis* (inflammation of the outer lining of the heart), and enlargement of the liver and spleen. *Uveitis* (inflammation of the iris and the surrounding muscles in the eye) may develop and, if untreated, may damage vision.

Rarely, *amyloidosis* (deposition of a starchy substance in body organs) may occur; if the kidney is involved, *kidney failure* may develop.

TREATMENT

Joint pain and stiffness may be relieved by *ASA*, *nonsteroidal anti-inflammatory drugs*, and, in very severe cases, *antirheumatic drugs* (such as gold, penicillamine, chloroquine, or azathioprine) or *corticosteroid drugs*.

Removable splints may be worn during the day to rest acutely inflamed joints and at night to reduce the risk of deformities. *Physiotherapy* reduces the risk of muscle wasting and contractures (deformities due to shrinkage of tissue). Excessive physical exercise should be avoided lest joints be subjected to too much stress. Special shoes should be worn to reduce the risk of foot deformity.

OUTLOOK

In most children the arthritis disappears after several years. However, some are left with joint deformity.

Rheumatoid spondylitis

See *Ankylosing spondylitis*.

Rheumatology

The branch of medicine concerned with the causes, development, diagnosis, and treatment of diseases that affect the *joints*, *muscles*, and *connective tissue*. Rheumatologists use a variety of investigative techniques, ranging from X rays of joints to tests of muscle function and blood analysis. Treatment is similarly varied, including drug treatment with anti-inflammatory drugs or analgesic drugs, and physiotherapy.

Rh incompatibility

A mismatch between the blood of a pregnant woman and that of her baby with respect to the Rhesus (Rh) *blood group*. In certain circumstances, this mismatch can lead to *hemolytic disease of the newborn*.

In the past, hemolytic disease of the newborn was a common cause of stillbirth and of hydrops fetalis, a severe and often fatal condition in the newborn resulting from the destruction of fetal blood cells. Hemolytic disease of the newborn due to Rh sensitization is now becoming rare. This is primarily due to the use of *anti-D(Rh_o) immune globulin* to prevent Rh sensitization.

CAUSE

Rh incompatibility results from exposure of a Rh-negative woman to Rh-positive blood. The Rh system (first identified in rhesus monkeys) is based on the presence or absence in the blood of several factors, of which the most important is a substance known as D antigen. The blood of people who are Rh positive contains D antigen whereas the blood of people who are Rh negative does not. Whether an individual has a positive or negative blood type is determined by *genes* (i.e., it is an inherited trait).

Rh incompatibility can arise only when a woman's blood is Rh negative and her baby's blood is Rh positive. This can happen only if the baby's father's blood is also Rh positive. There are usually no problems during a woman's first pregnancy with a baby whose blood is Rh positive. However, as shown in the diagram, the baby may sensitize the woman to Rh-positive blood; if she has a subsequent

R

HOW Rh INCOMPATIBILITY OCCURS

Without preventive treatment, an Rh-negative woman who is exposed to D antigen (a substance present only in Rh-positive blood) may develop antibodies that will attack the red blood cells of any future Rh-positive babies.

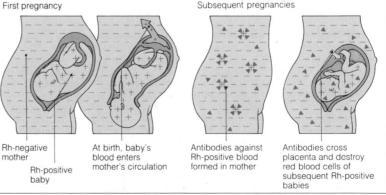

First pregnancy

Rh-negative mother

Rh-positive baby

At birth, baby's blood enters mother's circulation

Subsequent pregnancies

Antibodies against Rh-positive blood formed in mother

Antibodies cross placenta and destroy red blood cells of subsequent Rh-positive babies

pregnancy with an Rh-positive baby, there is a risk of hemolytic disease of the newborn. A woman whose blood is Rh negative can also be sensitized if she is mistakenly given a transfusion of Rh-positive blood.

INCIDENCE

Among white people, about one person in six has Rh-negative blood; in about one pregnancy in 11, the mother's blood is Rh negative and the baby's blood is Rh positive. Rh incompatibility is less common in black and Oriental families than in white families because of a comparative rarity of the Rh-negative blood group in people who are not white.

TREATMENT AND PREVENTION

An injection of anti-D(Rh$_o$) immune globulin is given to Rh-negative women soon after the birth of an Rh-positive baby. The injection contains antibodies to Rh factor, which destroy any of the baby's blood cells that may have entered the woman before they have a chance to sensitize her. When given within 72 hours of delivery, the injection prevents Rh sensitization in 99 percent of cases.

Anti-D(Rh$_o$) immune globulin is also given to Rh-negative women after any miscarriage, induced abortion, amniocentesis, or other procedure that might result in exposure of the mother to the fetal blood cells.

If a woman has Rh-negative blood, she is tested for the presence of Rh antibodies at her first prenatal visit and also at subsequent visits. The management of the pregnancy and birth, if antibodies are present and there is a risk to the baby, is as described under *Hemolytic disease of the newborn*.

Rhinitis

Inflammation of the *mucous membrane* that lines the *nose*, usually manifested by some combination of nasal obstruction, nasal discharge, sneezing, and facial pressure or pain.

TYPES

VIRAL RHINITIS This type is a feature of the common cold (see *Cold, common*) and may lead to *sinusitis*.

ALLERGIC RHINITIS Rhinitis due to allergy (see *Rhinitis, allergic*), also known as hay fever, may be seasonal (usually caused by pollens) or occur throughout the year (usually caused by house dust, molds, or pets). Allergic rhinitis most commonly occurs with vasomotor rhinitis.

VASOMOTOR RHINITIS This may be intermittent or continual. The nose becomes too responsive to stimuli, such

as pollutants (e.g., tobacco smoke), changes or extremes in temperature or humidity, some foods, some medicines, or certain emotions. Vasomotor rhinitis is common in pregnancy and in those taking combined *oral contraceptives* or other *estrogen drugs*.

HYPERTROPHIC RHINITIS This type of rhinitis, characterized by thickening of the nasal mucous membrane and chronic congestion of the nasal veins, can be caused by repeated nasal infections. Hypertrophic rhinitis results in constant stuffiness and sometimes impairment of the sense of smell. In severe cases, treatment may involve surgical removal or shrinkage of part of the swollen tissue.

ATROPHIC RHINITIS This wasting of the mucous membrane can result from aging, from chronic bacterial infections, or from extensive nasal surgery. Other features of atrophic rhinitis include persistent nasal infection, a discharge that dries to a crust, loss of smell, and an unpleasant odor. Treatment is with *antibiotic drugs* and sometimes with *estrogen drugs*.

Rhinitis, allergic

Inflammation of the *mucous membrane* that lines the *nose* due to *allergy* to pollen, dust, or other airborne substances. Allergic rhinitis, also known as hay fever, causes sneezing, a runny nose, and nasal congestion.

CAUSES

In some people, the inhalation of particles of certain harmless substances provokes an exaggerated response by the *immune system*, which forms *antibodies* against them. These otherwise harmless substances, known as allergens, also trigger the release of *histamine* and other chemicals that cause inflammation and fluid production in the lining of the nose and nasal *sinuses* (air cavities around the nose). The most common of the allergens that cause allergic rhinitis are tree, grass, and weed pollens; molds; animal skin scales, hair, or feathers; house dust; and house-dust mites.

Pollen-induced allergic rhinitis is seasonal. Tree pollens are most prevalent in spring, grass pollens in summer, and weed pollens in summer and autumn. Sufferers are worst affected on days when the pollen count is high—that is, during hot and windy weather, especially in heavily vegetated, low-lying areas.

People affected by household allergens, such as dust, tend to have less severe symptoms but are affected throughout the year.

INCIDENCE

Allergic rhinitis is a common complaint, affecting as many as 5 to 10 percent of the population. It is more common in people who have other allergies, such as *asthma* or *eczema*; like these disorders, it has a tendency to run in families. The condition usually develops before the age of 30 and affects more women than men.

SYMPTOMS AND SIGNS

Exposure to the allergen produces an itching sensation in the nose, palate, throat, and eyes. This is followed by sneezing, stuffiness, a runny nose, and, usually, watering eyes. The eyes may also be affected by *conjunctivitis*, which makes them red and sore.

PREVENTION

Skin tests help identify the allergen responsible for the disorder. Once the allergen is known, exposure should be avoided or kept to a minimum, although this is difficult when the cause is pollens.

TREATMENT

For mild attacks of allergic rhinitis, occasional use of a *decongestant drug* in the form of a spray or drops may clear up symptoms, but use for more than three or four days can make the condition worse. Many sufferers are helped by taking *antihistamine drugs*, which reduce itching and some degree of nasal congestion and runny nose, but may cause drowsiness.

Allergic rhinitis may also be treated with *corticosteroid drugs*, which are available in nasal preparations, if prescribed by your physician.

The drug sodium cromoglycate, inhaled regularly throughout the pollen season, may help prevent attacks by blocking the allergic response. Long-term relief of symptoms can sometimes follow desensitization to a particular pollen allergen by a course of injections (see *Hyposensitization*).

Rhinophyma

Bulbous deformity and redness of the *nose* occurring almost exclusively in elderly men. Rhinophyma is a complication of severe *rosacea* (a skin disorder of the nose and cheeks). The tissue of the nose thickens, small blood vessels enlarge, and the sebaceous glands become overactive, making the nose excessively oily.

Rhinophyma can be remedied by an operation. Under a general anesthetic, the swollen tissue is cut away until the nose is restored to a satisfactory shape. Skin grafting is not necessary because the remaining tissue rapidly regenerates.

R

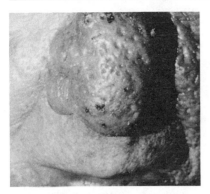

Example of rhinophyma
This disfiguring condition is remedied by paring away the excess tissue. The skin soon regenerates after treatment.

Rhinoplasty

An operation that alters the structure of the *nose* to improve its appearance or to correct a deformity caused by injury or disease.

Under either a local or a general anesthetic, incisions are made within the nose (to avoid visible scars). The septum (the vertical wall of cartilage and bone that divides the nose) may be altered if breathing passages are blocked. The cartilage and bone of the nasal structure are then reshaped; occasionally, a bone or cartilage graft is used. The nose is finally splinted in position for about 10 days.

Rhinoplasty usually causes considerable bruising and swelling, and the results may not be clearly visible for weeks or months. Rare complications include recurrent nosebleeds due to persistent crusting at the incision sites and breathing difficulty due to narrowing of the nasal passages.

Rhinorrhea

The discharge of watery mucus from the nose, usually due to *rhinitis*. Rarely, the discharge consists of cerebrospinal fluid due to a head injury.

Rh isoimmunization

The development of antibodies formed against Rh-positive blood in a person who has Rh-negative blood. (See *Hemolytic disease of the newborn; Rh incompatibility*.)

Rhythm method

See *Contraception, natural methods of*.

Rib

Any of the flat, curved bones that form a framework for the chest and a protective cage around the heart, lungs, and other underlying organs.

There are 12 pairs of ribs, each joined at the back of the rib cage to a vertebra in the spine. Their arrangement is shown in the illustrated box. Between the ribs, and attached to them, are thin sheets of muscle that help to expand and relax the chest during breathing. The intercostal spaces between the ribs also contain nerves and blood vessels.

DISORDERS
The ribs can easily be fractured by a fall or blow (see *Rib, fracture of*).

A rib is one of the more common sites for a benign *bone tumor* or for a *metastasis* (a secondary malignant tumor that has spread from cancer elsewhere in the body).

In rare cases a person is born with one or more extra ribs lying above the uppermost normal rib. Known as *cervical ribs*, the additional ribs may press on nerves supplying the arm or cause other problems.

Ribavirin

A recently introduced *antiviral drug*, also known as tribavirin, that is used in the treatment of infants and children with viral *bronchiolitis* caused by respiratory syncytial virus. Ribavirin is administered by aerosol inhalation or by means of a nebulizer. Adverse effects of the drug are rare.

Clinical trials have shown that ribavirin is also effective against a wide variety of other viral infections, including herpes simplex, hepatitis, and several strains of influenza.

Rib, fracture of

Fracture of a *rib* is usually caused by a fall or blow. It may also be caused by minor stress on the rib cage, such as that produced by prolonged coughing or even laughing.

The fracture causes severe pain that is made worse by deep breathing, and tenderness and swelling of the overlying tissue. The diagnosis is confirmed by *X rays*. Pain is relieved by *analgesic drugs* (painkillers) or, occasionally, by an injection of a long-acting, local anesthetic.

Most rib fractures are undisplaced (i.e., the bone ends remain in alignment) and usually heal easily without specific treatment. Strapping is rarely used because it increases the risk of *pneumonia*. Instead, the patient is encouraged to take deep breaths while holding the injured side.

ANATOMY OF THE RIBS

There are seven true ribs attached to the sternum, three false ribs, each attached to a rib above, and two floating ribs on each side. When the ribs are pulled up by the intercostal muscles (between the ribs), they expand the chest, drawing air into the lungs. The front ends of the true ribs are linked to the sternum by cartilages.

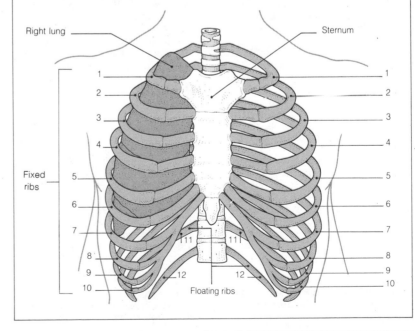

Right lung
Sternum
Fixed ribs
Floating ribs

R

A fracture that is displaced or splintered may pierce a lung, thereby causing lung collapse (see *Pneumothorax*). Multiple rib fractures can result in *flail chest* (a type of chest injury in which part of the chest wall moves in the direction opposite to normal during breathing).

Riboflavin

The chemical name of vitamin B_2 (see *Vitamin B complex*).

Rickets

A disease caused by nutritional deficiency that causes deformity of the skeleton during childhood. In rickets, *bones* become deformed because inadequate amounts of *calcium* and *phosphate* are incorporated into them as they grow. A similar deficiency of calcium and phosphate in the bones of adults results in *osteomalacia*.

CAUSES AND INCIDENCE

The most common cause of rickets is deficiency of *vitamin D*, which is vital for the absorption of calcium from the intestines into the blood and for its incorporation into bone. Vitamin D is found in fat-containing animal substances, such as oily fish, butter, egg yolk, liver, and fish liver oils. There are also small amounts in human and animal milk. Vitamin D is also made in the body through the action of sunlight on the skin.

Rickets occurs primarily in poor countries and in communities where babies (and mothers) receive inadequate vitamin D in the diet and also do not get enough sunlight. Breast milk alone cannot provide all a baby's needs for vitamin D, so a breast-fed baby who gets little sun should be given vitamin D supplements.

Rickets is now rare in developed countries, where vitamin D supplements are often given to infants; where the vitamin is added to margarine, and where most children and babies eat a varied diet and get adequate exposure to the sun. The disorder is seen only in vulnerable groups, such as premature babies and some food faddists who avoid foods rich in vitamin D.

Rickets occasionally develops as a complication of a digestive disorder that causes *malabsorption* (failure to absorb nutrients from the intestines). Rickets may also occur in certain rare forms of kidney and liver disease and in children undergoing long-term therapy with types of *anticonvulsant drugs* that interfere with the action of vitamin D.

SYMPTOMS AND SIGNS

The most striking feature of advanced rickets is deformity of the bones, especially of the legs and spine. Typically, there is bowing of the legs and, in infants, flattening of the head as a result of the softness of the skull. Infants with rickets often sleep poorly and show delay in crawling and walking. Other features include *kyphoscoliosis* (spinal curvature), a tendency to *fractures*, and enlargement of the wrists, ankles, and ends of the ribs. There may also be pelvic pain and muscle weakness.

DIAGNOSIS AND TREATMENT

Rickets is diagnosed from the child's physical appearance and from the results of *X rays* and *blood tests*.

Rickets due to dietary deficiency is treated with vitamin D supplements, which can restore normal bone growth; in most cases, bone deformities disappear as the child continues to grow. Rickets that occurs as a complication of another disorder, such as malabsorption or kidney disease, is treated according to the cause.

Rickettsia

A type of parasitic microorganism. Rickettsiae resemble small *bacteria* but, like viruses, they are able to multiply only by invading the cells of another life form.

Rickettsiae are primarily parasites of the arthropods (insects and insect-like animals), such as lice, fleas, ticks, and mites. Such arthropods sometimes transmit rickettsiae to the blood of larger animals (such as rodents, dogs, or humans) in their saliva via bites or in their feces via a small break in the skin. Human diseases caused by different types of rickettsiae include *Q fever*, *Rocky Mountain spotted fever*, and the various forms of *typhus*.

Rifampin

An *antibacterial drug* that is used mainly in the treatment of *tuberculosis* and also to treat *leprosy*, *endocarditis*, and *osteomyelitis*. Rifampin is usually prescribed with other antibacterial drugs because some strains of bacteria quickly develop *resistance* if rifampin is used alone.

The drug causes harmless, orange-red discoloration of the urine, saliva, and other body secretions. Other possible effects include muscle pain, nausea, vomiting, diarrhea, jaundice, flulike symptoms, rash, and itching. This drug interferes with the action of oral contraceptives.

Rigidity

Increased tone in one or more *muscles*, which causes them to feel tight; the affected part of the body becomes stiff and inflexible.

Causes of rigidity include injury to a muscle, arthritis affecting a nearby joint, a neurological disorder, such as Parkinson's disease, or stroke. Rigidity of the abdominal muscles is a sign of *peritonitis*. (See also *Spasticity*.)

Rigor

A violent attack of shivering, often associated with a fever. Rigor may also refer to stiffness or rigidity of body tissues, as in *rigor mortis*.

Rigor mortis

The stiffening of *muscles* that occurs after *death*. Rigor mortis starts some three to four hours after death and is usually complete after about 12 hours; the stiffness then gradually disappears over the next 48 to 60 hours. The greater the amount of physical exertion before death, the sooner rigor mortis begins. Similarly, the sooner rigor mortis begins, the sooner it passes. These facts have important medicolegal implications and, along with other factors, are used to assess the time of death, a factor in matters as divergent—and as critical—as solving a crime or settling an estate.

Ringing in the ears

See *Tinnitus*.

Ringworm

A popular name for certain types of fungal skin infections (commonly of the feet, groin, scalp, nails, or trunk). Ringworm is marked by ring-shaped, reddened, scaly, or blistery patches on the skin. (See *Tinea*.)

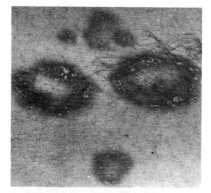

Patch of ringworm
The name arises from the tendency for certain skin fungus infections to spread uniformly outward, leaving normal skin inside the ring.

Ritodrine

A drug used to prevent or delay premature labor (see *Prematurity*) by relaxing the muscles of the uterus. Possible side effects of ritodrine include tremor, palpitations, nausea, vomiting, chest pain, breathlessness, and hot flashes.

River blindness

See *Onchocerciasis*.

RNA

The abbreviation for ribonucleic acid. RNA is one of the two substances that carry the inherited, coded genetic instructions in cells. The other such substance is deoxyribonucleic acid (*DNA*).

In all animal and plant cells, it is DNA that holds a permanent record of the instructions; RNA helps decode the instructions. In some viruses, however, the instructions for viral multiplication are held by RNA. (See also *Nucleic acids; Protein synthesis*.)

Rocky Mountain spotted fever

A rare, infectious disease causing fever and a rash with spots that spread over the body, darken, enlarge, and bleed. The disease was originally recognized in the Rocky Mountain states of the US but also occurs elsewhere in North and South America. Rocky Mountain spotted fever is caused by a rickettsia (a microorganism similar to a bacterium) and is transmitted from rabbits and other small mammals by tick bites.

The diagnosis can be confirmed by laboratory tests on blood and by tissue samples. Treatment with *chloramphenicol* or *tetracycline* usually cures the disease.

Rodent ulcer

A common name for *basal cell carcinoma*; a type of skin cancer.

Roentgenography

See *Radiology; X rays*.

Role-playing

The acting out of a role (the pattern of behavior expected of an individual in a given social situation). The conscious adoption of different roles can be a useful technique for learning about oneself, other people, or particular situations.

The phrase "sick role" describes the type of passive behavior expected and allowed of a patient; people with social or emotional problems may unconsciously adopt this role as a means of escaping from social obligations and of gaining the sympathy and understanding of others.

Root canal treatment

A dental procedure performed to save a tooth in which the pulp (the living tissue within a tooth) has died or become untreatably diseased, usually as the result of extensive dental *caries*.

X rays are taken to establish the length of the pulp cavity. Root canal treatment may be performed after administration of a local anesthetic. To prevent infection, a *rubber dam* (a small sheet of rubber) is used to isolate the tooth from the saliva.

ROOT CANAL TREATMENT

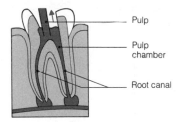

1 A hole is drilled into the crown to remove all material from the pulp chamber. The root canals are then slightly enlarged and shaped with fine-tipped instruments. The procedure is usually monitored by X rays.

Pulp
Pulp chamber
Root canal

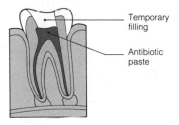

2 The cavity is washed out, and antibiotic paste and a temporary filling are packed into it. Some days later, the filling is removed and the canals are checked for sterility.

Temporary filling
Antibiotic paste

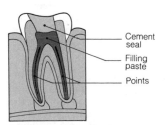

3 When no infection can be detected, the cavity is filled with a sealing paste and/or tapering solid "points" made of gutta-percha resin mixed with zinc and bismuth oxides. The roots are then sealed with cement.

Cement seal
Filling paste
Points

The main steps in root canal treatment are shown in the illustrations, including removal of the pulp, sealing with a temporary filling, checking for infection, and the final filling and sealing of the tooth.

COMPLICATIONS

If the pulp cavity has not been filled completely, bacteria may enter, leading to apical *periodontitis* (inflammation of the tissues around the root tips). It may then be necessary to make an opening in the gum and bone overlying the affected root to allow pus to drain. In some cases, an apicectomy (removal of a small portion of the root tip) and filling of the area with amalgam may be necessary.

RESULTS

Teeth whose pulp cavities have been filled may function well for as long as normal teeth. Treated teeth may, however, turn slightly gray; if a tooth is unsightly, its appearance can be restored by bonding (see *Bonding, dental*), by the fitting of an artificial crown (see *Crown, dental*), or by bleaching (see *Bleaching, dental*).

Rorschach test

A psychological test based on the assessment of a person's responses to a standardized set of inkblot pictures. The test was devised by the Swiss psychiatrist Hermann Rorschach early in the 20th century. It was intended to reveal an individual's attitudes, conflicts, and emotions but is now rarely used. (See also *Personality tests*.)

Rosacea

A chronic *skin* disorder in which the nose and cheeks are abnormally red. The cause of the disorder is usually unknown, but in some cases it results from overuse of *corticosteroid* creams in the treatment of other skin disorders. Rosacea affects about one in 500 people and is most common among middle-aged women.

Rosacea usually begins with temporary flushing, often after drinking a hot beverage or alcohol, eating spicy food, or entering a hot environment. It may then develop into permanent redness of the skin, sometimes accompanied by pustules resembling those of *acne*. In some elderly men, rosacea leads to *rhinophyma* (bulbous swelling of the nose).

TREATMENT

A lengthy course of the antibiotic drug *tetracycline* usually suppresses symptoms but does not cure the disorder. Rosacea tends to recur for five to 10 years and then disappears.

R

Roseola infantum

A common infectious disease that mainly affects children between the ages of 6 months and 2 years. Roseola infantum is probably caused by a virus and is characterized by the abrupt onset of irritability and fever. The temperature may rise as high as 40.5°C. However, on the fourth or fifth day, it drops suddenly back to normal. At about the same time, a rash appears on the trunk, often spreading quickly to the neck, face, and limbs. The rash rarely lasts longer than a day or two. Other symptoms may include a sore throat and enlargement of lymph nodes in the neck.

Occasionally, a child may have a febrile convulsion (see *Convulsion, febrile*) during the course of the fever, but the disease has no serious effects. The only specific treatment is to keep the child cool (by tepid sponging if necessary) and by giving *acetaminophen* to reduce the fever.

Rotator cuff

A reinforcing structure around the shoulder joint composed of four muscle tendons that merge with the fibrous capsule enclosing the joint.

The rotator cuff may be torn as the result of a fall. A partial tear may cause *painful arc syndrome* (pain when the arm is lifted in a certain arc away from the body). A complete tear seriously limits the ability to raise the arm and, in cases of severe disability, may require surgical repair.

Roughage

See *Fiber, dietary*.

Roundworms

Also known as nematodes, a class of elongated, cylindrical worms that are the main parasites of humans. In many cases, the adult worms inhabit the human intestines, usually without causing symptoms unless there is a large number of worms.

Sometimes, passage of worm larvae through various parts of the body is the main cause of symptoms. Most types of roundworm infestation are relatively easily treated with *anthelmintic drugs*.

In temperate areas, such as Canada, the only common type of roundworm disease is *pinworm infestation* (which mainly affects children). *Ascariasis, whipworm infestation, trichinosis,* and *toxocariasis* occasionally occur, although they often cause no symptoms. Some people return from abroad with *hookworm infestation*. In tropical countries, roundworm diseases are quite common; they include those mentioned and *strongyloidiasis, guinea worm disease,* and different types of *filariasis*. A diet containing raw fish may lead to infestation with the worms that cause anisakiasis or eustrongyloidiasis.

Royal College of Physicians and Surgeons of Canada

The organization that examines and certifies *medical specialists* for practice.

Rubber dam

A rubber sheet used to isolate one or more teeth during certain dental procedures. The dam acts as a barrier against saliva and prevents the inhalation of debris or small instruments. To fit a dam, the dentist punches small holes in the sheet for the teeth to protrude, and secures the sheet with clamps and a frame.

Rubefacient

A substance that causes redness of the skin by increasing blood flow to the area. Rubefacients are sometimes included in ointments used to relieve muscular aches and pains. They work by producing counterirritation (i.e., they cause a less unpleasant sensation that diverts attention from the original pain). Methyl salicylate, menthol, camphor, and turpentine are all examples of rubefacients.

Rubella

A viral infection, also known as German measles (although the similarities with measles are few). Rubella causes a trivial illness in children and a slightly more troublesome one in adults. It is serious only when it affects a woman in the early months of pregnancy, when there is a chance that the virus will infect the fetus and cause any of a range of severe birth defects, known as rubella syndrome.

CAUSES AND INCIDENCE

Apart from mother-to-baby transmission, the rubella virus is spread from person to person in airborne droplets. Symptoms develop after an incubation period of two to three weeks.

Once common worldwide, rubella is now much less prevalent in most developed countries as a result of *immunization* programs. A combined vaccine against measles, mumps, and rubella (see *MMR vaccination*) has been developed for infants.

SYMPTOMS AND COMPLICATIONS

The infection usually occurs in children aged between 6 and 12, and is almost invariably mild. A rash appears on the face, spreads to the

DISEASES CAUSED BY ROUNDWORMS (NEMATODES)

Disease	Adult length	Distribution	How acquired
Ascariasis (common roundworm)	15–38 cm	Worldwide	By swallowing worm eggs that have contaminated food or fingers
Enterobiasis (pinworm)	0.2–1.5 cm	Worldwide	By swallowing worm eggs that have contaminated fingers
Trichuriasis (whipworm)	2.5–5 cm	Worldwide	By swallowing worm eggs that have contaminated food or fingers
Ancylostomiasis (hookworm)	1.5 cm	Tropics	By penetration of skin of feet by worm larvae in soil
Strongyloidiasis	0.2 cm	Tropics	By penetration of skin of feet by worm larvae in soil
Toxocariasis	Several cm	Worldwide	By swallowing worm eggs from dirt or dog feces
Trichinosis (porkworm)	0.1 cm	Worldwide	By eating undercooked pork containing encysted worm larvae
Filariasis	2–50 cm	Tropics	By mosquito and other insect bites

trunk and limbs, persists for a few days, then disappears. There may be a slight fever and enlargement of lymph nodes at the back of the neck. In some cases, the entire infection passes unnoticed. In adolescents and adults, there may be more marked symptoms, such as headache before the rash appears and a more pronounced fever. The virus may be transmitted to others from a few days before the symptoms appear until one day after they disappear. Polyarthritis (inflammation affecting several joints) is an occasional, short-lived complication, starting after the rash has faded.

CONGENITAL INFECTION

Rubella is a risk to the unborn baby only if the mother is infected during the first four months of pregnancy. The earlier in pregnancy that infection occurs, the more likely the infant is to be affected, and the more serious the abnormalities tend to be. In very early pregnancy, miscarriage may occur.

An affected infant may have one or many defects. The most common abnormalities, in order of frequency, are *deafness*, congenital *heart disease*, *mental retardation*, *cataract* and other eye disorders, *purpura*, *cerebral palsy*, and bone abnormalities. About 20 percent of affected babies die in early infancy. An affected infant continues to harbor the virus and may infect others via his or her urine, feces, and saliva for a year or more after birth.

DIAGNOSIS AND TREATMENT

Rubella is easily confused with other viral infections, *scarlet fever*, and *drug* reactions, which may produce similar symptoms. Rubella can be positively diagnosed only by laboratory isolation of the virus from a throat swab or by tests to look for *antibodies* to the virus in the blood. There is no specific treatment for rubella. *Acetaminophen* can be given to reduce fever. Treatment of rubella syndrome depends on the particular defects present.

PREVENTION

Rubella vaccine provides effective, long-lasting immunity to the disease; it is now given in the MMR vaccine to all babies at about 15 months of age. Reactions to the vaccine are usually negligible. Rubella infection itself also provides immunity.

Any woman who may become pregnant and is unsure whether or not she has been immunized or has had rubella should have her immune status checked. If she is not immune, vaccination should be performed.

A nonimmune pregnant woman must avoid contact with anyone who

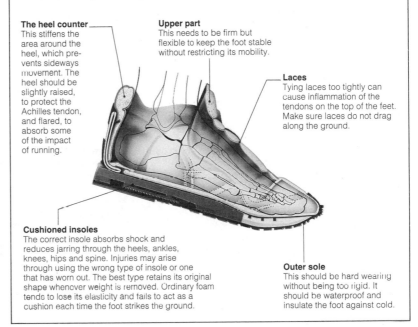
has rubella; if such contact occurs, she should immediately seek a physician's advice. Passive immunization by *immune globulin injection* may help prevent infection of the fetus.

Rubeola

Another name for *measles*.

Running injuries

Disorders resulting from the effects on the body of jogging or running. Such injuries are common but most could be prevented by taking simple precautions. Running injuries most commonly affect the feet and legs.

TYPES

Common types of running injury include *tendinitis* (inflammation of a tendon); *stress fracture* of the tibia (shin), the fibula (the other long bone in the lower leg), or a bone in the foot; and plantar *fasciitis* (inflammation of tissue in the sole of the foot).

Sprinters commonly suffer from tearing of the *hamstring muscles* at the back of the thigh. Long-distance runners are more likely to suffer back pain due to jarring of the spine, tibial *compartment syndrome* (painful cramp in the lower leg caused by muscle compression), or *shin splints* (pain along the inner edge of the tibia).

PREVENTION

Shoes should fit snugly to provide stability but should not cramp the foot; insoles are needed to cushion the jarring force on the legs and spine. Shoes should not be allowed to become worn, because this can cause abnormal positioning of the foot during running, leading to foot strain.

Before running, warming-up exercises should be performed to reduce the risk of injury. Beginners should run short distances at first, and experienced runners should keep their running within sensible bounds. Running should be done in an upright posture, with trunk, neck, and arms relaxed. Long periods of running uphill, downhill, or along the side of a slope should be avoided as they increase stress on the ankle and knee.

Rupture

A common term for a *hernia*, especially an abdominal hernia.

R

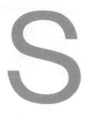

S

Sac

A baglike organ or body structure. For example, the amniotic sac is the thin, membranous, fluid-filled bag that surrounds the fetus.

Saccharin

An *artificial sweetener*.

Sacralgia

Pain in the *sacrum* (the triangular spinal bone below the lumbar *vertebrae*) caused by pressure on a spinal nerve in this area. Sacralgia is usually the result of a *disk prolapse*. In rare cases, it may be due to *bone cancer*. (See also *Back pain*.)

Sacralization

Fusion of the fifth (lowest) lumbar *vertebra* with the upper part of the *sacrum* (the triangular spinal bone below the lumbar vertebrae).

Sacralization may be present at birth, in which case it usually produces no symptoms and is discovered only when an X ray of the back is taken for some other reason.

A surgical procedure to produce sacralization may be performed to treat a *disk prolapse*, or a condition called *spondylolisthesis*, in which a vertebra is displaced over the one below it. (See also *Spinal fusion*.)

Sacroiliac joint

One of a pair of rigid *joints* between each side of the *sacrum* (the triangular spinal bone below the lumbar *vertebrae*) and each *ilium* (the largest of the bones that form the outer walls of the *pelvis*). The bony surfaces within the joint are lined with cartilage and have a small amount of synovial fluid between them. Strong ligaments between the sacrum and ilium permit only minimal movement at the joint.

The sacroiliac joint may be strained, usually as a result of childbirth or of overstriding when running. Such strains produce pain in the lower back and buttocks. The sacroiliac joint may also become inflamed, a condition called *sacroiliitis*.

Sacroiliitis

Inflammation of a *sacroiliac joint* (one of a pair of joints between each side of the *sacrum* and each *ilium*).

Sacroiliitis can be caused by *ankylosing spondylitis*, *rheumatoid arthritis*, *Reiter's syndrome*, or the form of arthritis that occurs with *psoriasis*. In rare cases, sacroiliitis is caused by an infection spread through the bloodstream from elsewhere in the body.

The principal symptom of sacroiliitis is pain in the lower back, buttocks, groin, and back of the thigh. The pain may be accompanied by fever and malaise if the underlying cause is an infection. If the cause is ankylosing spondylitis, pain may be accompanied by stiffness in the back and hips, which is worse after rest and alleviated by exercise.

Sacroiliitis is diagnosed by *X rays*, *blood tests*, and, sometimes, scans (see *Bone imaging*). If infection is suspected, fluid may be removed from the joint and examined for microorganisms. Treatment is with *nonsteroidal anti-inflammatory drugs* or, if the joint is infected, with *antibiotic drugs*.

Sacrum

The large triangular bone in the lower spine. The sacrum's broad upper part articulates with the fifth (lowest) lumbar *vertebra*, and its narrow lower part with the *coccyx*. The sides of the sacrum are connected by the *sacroiliac*

STRUCTURE OF THE SACROILIAC JOINT

The joint forms an interface between the sacrum at the back of the pelvis and the ilium (hip bone) on each side of the body.

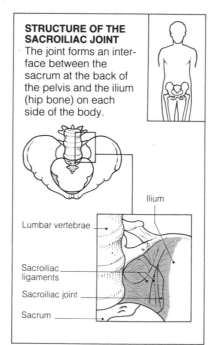

Ilium

Lumbar vertebrae

Sacroiliac ligaments

Sacroiliac joint

Sacrum

STRUCTURE OF THE SACRUM

The sacrum consists of five vertebrae (spinal bones) that are fused together to form a single solid structure.

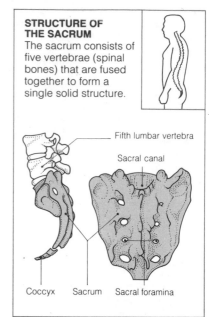

Fifth lumbar vertebra

Sacral canal

Coccyx   Sacrum   Sacral foramina

---

joints to each ilium (the largest of the bones that form the *pelvis*). The sacrum thus sits like a wedge in the center of the back of the pelvis.

DISORDERS

The sacrum is a strong bone and is only rarely fractured. If a fracture does occur, it is usually a result of a fall or of a powerful direct blow to the bone.

Other disorders affecting the sacrum include: *sacralgia* (pain in the sacrum, sometimes due to a *disk prolapse*); *spondylolisthesis*, in which the fifth lumbar vertebra slips over the sacrum; and *sacralization*, in which the sacrum is fused to the fifth lumbar vertebra. (See also *Bone* disorders box; *Spine* disorders box.)

Sadism

Pleasure, particularly sexual pleasure, derived from the infliction of suffering or pain on others. Sadism often refers specifically to the attainment of *orgasm* through hurting, humiliating, or torturing someone else. The term is derived from the name of the French writer the Marquis de Sade.

Sadism is more common in men than in women and may be accompanied by *masochism* (a desire to be abused). Sadistic activities include beating, whipping, and tying a victim up, perhaps also with verbal abuse. *Rape* often has a sadistic basis, but the genuinely sadistic murderer is rare. It is very unusual for sadists to seek help from a psychiatrist. (See also *Sadomasochism*.)

Sadomasochism

Sexual arousal caused by inflicting pain (*sadism*) or by receiving abuse (*masochism*). Sadism and masochism may be combined in an individual, although one trait usually predominates. The sadomasochist is generally male and may practice other sexual *deviations*, such as *fetishism*.

Sadomasochistic literature is a common form of pornography. The practice of sadomasochism may be more widespread than is generally known; biting is a common sex practice. In a broad sense, any relationship in which there is one very dominant and one submissive partner can be said to have sadomasochistic elements.

SADS

The abbreviation for *seasonal affective disorder syndrome*.

Safe period

See *Contraception, natural methods of.*

Safe sex

A term used to describe preventive measures taken to reduce the risk of acquiring a sexually transmitted disease. Safe sex has been publicized recently because of the spread of *HIV* infection, but the same principles apply to reducing the risks of contracting other sexually transmitted diseases (STDs), such as gonorrhea, genital herpes (see *Herpes, genital*), and hepatitis B (see *Hepatitis, viral*).

Sexual intercourse is completely safe only if you and your partner are monogamous (have not had sex with anyone else) and neither you nor your partner has an STD. To reduce the risk of acquiring AIDS, casual sex and sex with multiple partners should be avoided. People with a higher risk of carrying HIV include: intravenous drug abusers; homosexual and bisexual men; prostitutes; promiscuous men or women; people who received transfusions of blood products before the screening of blood for HIV was introduced (e.g., hemophiliacs); and people from areas where there is a very high incidence of HIV infection (e.g., Central Africa and Haiti).

Known methods of transmitting HIV include vaginal intercourse, anal intercourse, oral sex, sharing sex aids such as vibrators, and any sexual activity that causes bleeding in the vagina or anus. Sex during menstruation is particularly dangerous if the woman is a carrier. Any sexual practice that involves contact with urine or feces also poses a risk.

The virus is thought not to be transmitted during dry kissing, cuddling, caressing, massage, or mutual masturbation (provided the skin is not broken and no semen is ejaculated into or onto the partner's body).

To reduce the risk of acquiring AIDS or any other sexually transmitted disease, a condom should be used. If a condom fails to prevent transmission, the cause is most likely to be incorrect use, although condoms do occasionally tear or split, especially during anal intercourse.

Saint Vitus' dance

An outdated term for the disorder now called *Sydenham's chorea*.

Salbutamol

A *bronchodilator drug* used in the treatment of *asthma*, chronic *bronchitis*, and *emphysema*. Because salbutamol also relaxes the muscles in the wall of the uterus, it is also occasionally used in the prevention of premature labor.

Salicylate drugs

A group of drugs with an anti-inflammatory, antipyretic (fever-reducing), and mild analgesic (painkilling) action. *ASA* (acetylsalicylic acid), *benorylate*, and *sodium salicylate* are examples of salicylate drugs.

Overdose of drugs in this group causes salicylate poisoning, characterized by hyperventilation (overbreathing), tinnitus (ringing in the ears), deafness, sweating, abnormal bleeding, biochemical disturbances, and, in severe cases, convulsions and coma.

Salicylic acid

A *keratolytic drug* (a drug that loosens and removes the tough outer layer of the skin). Salicylic acid is used to treat skin disorders, including *dermatitis*, *eczema*, *psoriasis*, *dandruff*, *ichthyosis*, *acne*, *warts*, and callosities (see *Callus, skin*). Salicylic acid is also sometimes used to treat *fungal infections*.

Salicyclic acid may cause inflammation and skin *ulcers* if used over a long period or applied to a large area.

Saline

A term meaning salty, or referring to a solution of salt (sodium chloride). Solutions with the same concentration of salt as body fluids are known as normal, or physiological, saline.

HOW TO USE A CONDOM

Using a condom is not a guarantee against transmission of HIV (the AIDS virus) or other sexually transmitted disease, but it does reduce the risks. Whether a condom is used to prevent disease transmission or to prevent conception, it should be used in conjunction with a spermicide preparation.

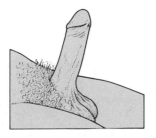 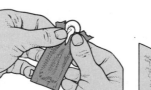 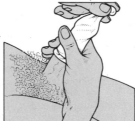 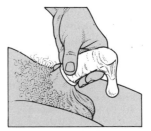

1 The penis should be fully erect before the condom is put on. The condom should be in place before any vaginal or anal penetration by the penis and before oral sex.

2 Manufacturers are required to meet standards set by Health and Welfare Canada. Do not use a condom that has no teat or is beyond its expiry date.

3 The teat-end should be squeezed free of air and the condom unrolled fully over the penis. Do not stretch the condom tightly; a tight condom is more likely to burst.

4 The penis should be withdrawn soon after ejaculation. During withdrawal, the base of the condom should be held to prevent spilling the semen.

Normal saline may be given in large amounts by *intravenous infusion* to replace body fluids in cases of dehydration; it is sometimes used in small quantities to dissolve drugs for injection. Normal saline is included in contact lens solutions, which have a close resemblance to natural tears.

Saliva

The watery, slightly alkaline fluid secreted into the mouth by the *salivary glands* and the *mucous membranes* that line the mouth.

Saliva contains the digestive enzyme amylase, which helps break down carbohydrates (see *Digestive system*). Saliva also keeps the mouth moist, lubricates food to aid swallowing, and makes it possible to taste food (taste buds are stimulated only by dissolved substances).

In addition to amylase, saliva contains minerals (such as sodium, potassium, and calcium), various proteins, mucin (the principal constituent of mucus), urea, white blood cells, and debris from the lining of the mouth.

Salivary glands

Three pairs of glands that secrete *saliva*, via ducts, into the mouth.

The largest pair, the *parotid glands*, lies over the angle of the jaw on each side, just below and in front of the ears; the ducts of these glands run forward and inward to open inside the cheeks.

The sublingual glands are situated in the floor of the front of the mouth, where they form a low ridge on each side of the frenulum (the central band of tissue that attaches the underside of the tongue to the floor of the mouth). This ridge has a row of small openings through which saliva is secreted.

The submandibular glands lie toward the back of the mouth close to the sides of the jaw. Their ducts run forward to open under the tongue on two small swellings, one on each side of the frenulum.

DISORDERS
Among the most common salivary gland disorders is infection of the parotid glands with the *mumps* virus. Another important disorder is the formation of *calculi* (stones) in a duct or within the substance of a gland. A stone in a duct causes a swelling that enlarges during eating because of damming of the flow of saliva; it may also be painful. Surgical removal of a stone in a duct is straightforward, but a stone in a gland itself may necessitate removal of the entire gland.

ANATOMY OF THE SALIVARY GLANDS
Each gland consists of thousands of saliva-secreting sacs. Tiny ducts carry the saliva into the main ducts leading to the mouth.

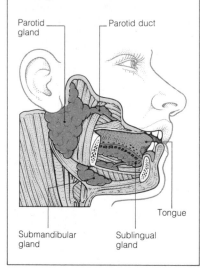

Parotid gland

Parotid duct

Tongue

Submandibular gland

Sublingual gland

Occasionally, the parotid glands are affected by *sarcoidosis*, which may cause considerable swelling. In rare cases, sarcoidosis also affects the facial nerve lying near the gland, which may result in *facial palsy*.

If *oral hygiene* is poor, the salivary glands may become infected by bacteria spreading from the mouth, which can lead to the development of an abscess in the affected glands.

Tumors of the salivary glands are rare, except for a type of parotid tumor which is usually slow-growing, painless, and benign (but which may rarely become malignant).

Insufficient secretion of saliva, causing a dry mouth (see *Mouth, dry*), may result from *dehydration* or *Sjögren's syndrome*. Certain drugs also decrease salivation as a side effect. (See also *Salivation, excessive*.)

Salivation, excessive

The production of too much *saliva*, sometimes known as ptyalism. Excessive salivation sometimes occurs during pregnancy. It also occurs in a wide variety of disorders.

Excessive salivation commonly occurs in conditions affecting the mouth, including irritation of the inside of the mouth (caused by jagged teeth or ill-fitting *dentures*), dental *caries*, *toothache*, *gingivitis* (inflammation of the gums), *mouth ulcers*, or any type of painful mouth injury. Digestive tract disorders, such as *esophagitis* (inflammation of the esophagus) and *peptic ulcer*, are other possible causes of this symptom.

Excessive salivation may also be caused by a variety of conditions affecting the nervous system, such as *Parkinson's disease, rabies, mercury poisoning*, and overactivity of the parasympathetic division of the *autonomic nervous system* (which controls the salivary glands), usually due to disease or drugs.

In some cases, excessive salivation can be relieved by *anticholinergic drugs*.

Salmonella infections

Infections caused by any of the SALMONELLA group of bacteria. One type of salmonella causes *typhoid fever*; others commonly cause bacterial *food poisoning*. Infants, the elderly, and people who are debilitated are the most likely to be affected.

The reported incidence of food poisoning due to salmonella has increased during the past decade. The commonest sources of infection are chicken meat and eggs.

SYMPTOMS
Between 12 and 20 hours after infection, malaise, headache, nausea, abdominal pain, and diarrhea and sometimes fever may develop. The illness rarely lasts longer than three days. *Dehydration* and *septicemia* may occur in the elderly or the very young.

DIAGNOSIS AND TREATMENT
Diagnosis is confirmed by laboratory tests that show the causative organism in the stools.

Treatment consists mainly of *rehydration therapy* to replace lost fluids. No solid food should be eaten during the first 24 hours of the illness. In severe cases and in babies, fluid replacement by *intravenous infusion* may be necessary. Salmonella food poisoning is treated with *antibiotic drugs* only if the infection has spread into the bloodstream.

PREVENTION
General food hygiene practices should be observed (see *Food poisoning*). People who have had salmonella food poisoning should take particular care with personal hygiene because they may continue to excrete salmonella bacteria in their feces for as long as six months after infection.

In general, it is advisable to avoid foods that contain raw egg (such as home-made mayonnaise, mousses, and ice cream) that might possibly be contaminated. Salmonella organisms are not killed by light cooking, and eggs should therefore always be well cooked.

Salpingectomy

Surgical removal of one or both *fallopian tubes*. Salpingectomy may be performed if the tube has become infected (see *Salpingitis*), as a method of contraception (see *Sterilization, female*), or to treat an *ectopic pregnancy*. (See also *Salpingo-oophorectomy*.)

Salpingitis

Inflammation of a *fallopian tube* (the tube that runs from the ovary to the top of the uterus), commonly caused by infection spreading upward from the vagina, cervix, or uterus.

CAUSES AND INCIDENCE

Salpingitis may be a result of a *chlamydial infection* or a bacterial infection, especially *gonorrhea*. Although salpingitis usually results from a sexually transmitted disease, it may also follow childbirth, miscarriage, or induced abortion. Other causes include *peritonitis* (inflammation of the abdominal lining), or, rarely, a blood-borne infection, such as *tuberculosis*.

SYMPTOMS AND SIGNS

Symptoms and signs include severe abdominal pain, and fever. The abdomen is very tender and the sufferer is usually most comfortable lying on her back with her legs bent. Vaginal examination is painful.

DIAGNOSIS

The presence of infection may be confirmed by a blood test showing a high number of white blood cells. A culture of a swab sample of the vaginal discharge allows identification of the causative microorganism. *Laparoscopy* (examination of the inside of the abdominal cavity with a viewing instrument) may be performed to confirm the diagnosis and to exclude the possibility of *ectopic pregnancy* or *appendicitis*, which can cause similar symptoms.

COMPLICATIONS

Pus may collect within the fallopian tube itself (a condition known as pyosalpinx), sometimes followed by the collection of fluid within the tube (a condition known as hydrosalpinx). A pelvic *abscess* (a collection of pus within the pelvic cavity) sometimes develops.

Occasionally, salpingitis persists despite treatment and causes a variety of symptoms, for example persistent back pain that is worse before menstruation, frequent heavy periods, and pain during intercourse. If the infection damages the inside of the fallopian tubes, ova may be unable to pass the blockage, resulting in *infertility* or an increased risk of an ectopic pregnancy.

TREATMENT

Treatment includes bed rest, fluids, *analgesic drugs* (painkillers), and *antibiotic drugs*. Surgery is performed to drain a pyosalpinx, hydrosalpinx, or pelvic abscess. If infection persists despite treatment with antibiotics, the damaged tubes may be removed, sometimes with the uterus and most of the ovary. (See also *Salpingectomy*; *Salpingo-oophorectomy*.)

Salpingography

See *Hysterosalpingography*.

Salpingo-oophorectomy

Removal of one or both *fallopian tubes* and *ovaries*. Salpingo-oophorectomy may be performed to treat persistent *salpingitis* (inflammation of the fallopian tubes) or certain types of benign *ovarian cyst*. It may also be performed together with a *hysterectomy* (removal of the uterus) to treat cancer of the ovary (see *Ovary, cancer of*) or cancer of the uterus (see *Uterus, cancer of*).

Salpingo-oophorectomy is carried out under a general anesthetic. Removal of the fallopian tube or tubes is a brief, straightforward procedure and the recovery period is short and usually problem-free.

Salt

Any compound of an acid and a base. Popularly, the term usually refers specifically to one such compound: common table salt, known chemically as sodium chloride (see *Sodium*). The term salt may also be applied to any chemical salt or to a mixture of salts used medicinally, such as magnesium sulfate. (See also *Saline*.)

Salve

A term for a healing, soothing, often medicated ointment.

Sandfly bites

Bites of sandflies, which are small, delicate, long-legged flies, about 3 mm long, found in most warm parts of the world. Sandflies can breed in a variety of habitats, including sand, forests, and city rubble.

In some parts of the world, sandflies are harmless, but in other regions sandfly bites can transmit disease to humans. In tropical and subtropical regions sandfly bites may transmit various forms of *leishmaniasis*. In parts of the Mediterranean and Asia, they may transmit the virus responsible for sandfly fever, an influenzalike illness of short duration. In the western Andes, sandfly bites may transmit bartonellosis, causing either joint pain and fever, or a rash, depending on the form of the disease.

Sandflies bite mainly after dusk. In areas where they are numerous, the best protection is to use insect repellents and to wear clothing that covers the arms and legs and is snug at the wrists and ankles (see *Insect bites*).

Sanitary protection

Articles used to protect clothing from bloodstains during *menstruation*. Disposable sanitary napkins or tampons are available in different absorbencies.

Sarcoidosis

A rare disease of unknown cause in which there is inflammation of tissues throughout the body, especially in the lymph nodes, lungs, skin, eyes, and liver. The disorder occurs mainly in young adults.

SYMPTOMS AND SIGNS

Sarcoidosis may cause a variety of symptoms, including fever, generalized aches, painful joints, arthritis, and painful and bloodshot eyes. Sarcoidosis may also cause enlargement of lymph nodes in the neck and elsewhere, breathlessness, *erythema nodosum* (purplish swellings on the legs), a purplish rash on the face, and areas of numbness. In some cases, there are no symptoms.

Possible complications include *hypercalcemia* (an abnormally high calcium level in the blood), which may damage the kidneys, and *pulmonary fibrosis* (scarring and thickening of the lung tissues).

DIAGNOSIS AND TREATMENT

A diagnosis may be suggested by a *chest X ray* that shows enlarged lymph nodes or diffuse shadowing, and by the characteristic rash. A biopsy of the lung, skin, lymph nodes, or liver confirms the diagnosis.

In many cases, no treatment is required. About 90 percent of patients recover completely within two years, with or without treatment, but the remaining 10 percent develop a persistent, chronic form of the disease.

Corticosteroid drugs are prescribed to treat persistent fever or persistent erythema nodosum, to prevent blindness in an affected eye, and to reduce the risk of permanent lung damage. *Chloroquine* is sometimes used to treat skin abnormalities.

S

Sarcoma

A cancer of *connective tissue* (material that surrounds body structures and holds them together). Types of sarcoma include *osteosarcoma* (arising in bone), *chondrosarcoma* (arising in cartilage), *Kaposi's sarcoma* (common in *AIDS* victims), and *fibrosarcoma*.

Saturated fats

See *Fats and oils*; *Nutrition*.

Scab

A crust that forms on the skin or on a mucous membrane at the site of a healing wound or infected area. A scab is composed of fibrin (a blood protein involved in clotting) and serum (the fluid part of blood) that has leaked from the wound and dried, along with skin scales, pus, and other debris. A similar term is eschar, used in relation to burns.

Scabies

 A skin infestation caused by the mite *SARCOPTES SCABIEI*, which burrows into the skin, where it lays eggs. Scabies is highly contagious during close physical contact. The disorder is most common in infants, children, young adults, or in people who are institutionalized.

SYMPTOMS
The mite's burrows can be seen on the skin as tiny, gray, scaly swellings, usually between the fingers, on the wrists and genitals, and in the armpits. Later, reddish lumps may appear on the limbs and trunk. The infestation causes intense itching, particularly at night, and scratching results in the formation of scabs and sores.

TREATMENT
The condition is treated by applying an insecticide lotion, such as *lindane* (also called gamma benzene hexachloride) to all skin below the sufferer's head. The lotion usually kills the mites, but itching may persist for up to two weeks. All sexual contacts and all members of the affected person's household (even if they show no signs of infestation) should be treated simultaneously.

Scald

A *burn* caused by hot liquid or steam.

Scaling, dental

Removal of dental *calculus* (a hard, chalky deposit) from the teeth, performed to prevent or treat *periodontal disease* (disorders of the gums and other tissues supporting the teeth).

Scaling is carried out with an instrument called a scaler. This may have a sharp, scraping edge or be an ultrasonic model with a tip that vibrates at high speed to chip away the deposit. After scaling, the teeth are usually polished with a mild abrasive paste and motorized buffers.

Scalp

The skin of the head, and its underlying tissue layers, that is normally covered with hair.

Scalp skin differs from other areas of skin in several ways: it is tougher than other skin, and is attached to an underlying sheet of muscle (called the epicranius) that extends from the eyebrows, over the top of the head, to the nape of the neck. This muscle sheet is only loosely attached to the skull, making it comparatively easy for areas of scalp to be torn off (e.g., as a result of catching the hair in machinery). Because the scalp is richly supplied with blood vessels, scalp wounds bleed profusely.

The scalp may be affected by a variety of hair or skin disorders. The most common are *dandruff*; hair loss, particularly in men (see *Alopecia*); *sebaceous cysts*; *psoriasis*; fungal infections, such as ringworm (see *Tinea*); and parasitic infestations, such as *lice*. *Cradle cap*, a harmless form of seborrheic *dermatitis* in which greasy, crusty patches appear on the scalp, is common in infants.

Scalpel

A surgical knife for cutting tissue. Scalpels with steel blades are most commonly used, but sharper, diamond or ruby blades are used for some types of surgery, such as for some eye operations.

Scanning techniques

Methods of producing images of body organs by techniques that record, process, and analyze sound waves, radio waves, or X rays that pass through or are generated by body tissues.

The most widely used scanning technique in medicine is *ultrasound scanning*, in which inaudible, ultra-high-frequency sound waves are passed into the region being examined. These sound waves are reflected more strongly by some structures than others, and the pattern of reflections is detected by one or more transducers and displayed on a screen. Ultrasound was originally developed for the detection of submarines beneath the sea and was first

used for medical diagnosis by a Scottish physician in the 1950s. In the past 20 years it has been refined and developed to examine the developing fetus and also the heart, liver, kidney, and other organs.

CT scanning uses X rays to measure variations in the density of the organ being examined; it compiles an image or picture by computer analysis.

Radionuclide scanning involves the injection into the body of radioactive substances which are taken up in different amounts by different organs. Radioactive iodine, for example, becomes concentrated in the thyroid gland. A radioactivity detector, such as a gamma camera, is positioned near the organ under study, and the pattern of radiation being emitted is recorded and displayed on a screen.

MRI (magnetic resonance imaging) uses a powerful electromagnet to align the nuclei of atoms of hydrogen, phosphorus, or other elements in the body. The nuclei are then knocked out of position by radio waves; in realigning themselves with the magnetic field, the nuclei produce a radio signal that can be detected and transformed into a computer-generated image.

PET scanning (positron emission tomography) is based on the detection of positively charged particles that are emitted by radioactively labeled substances introduced into the body. A computer is used to build up a three-dimensional image that reflects the chemical activity of the tissue that is being studied.

Scaphoid

One of the *wrist* bones. The scaphoid is the outermost bone on the thumb side of the hand in the proximal row of carpals (the row of wrist bones nearest the elbow).

A fracture of the scaphoid is one of the most common wrist injuries, usually occurring as a result of a fall on an outstretched hand. A characteristic symptom of this injury is tenderness in the space between the two prominent tendons at the base of the thumb on the back of the hand. This symptom may be a more positive indication of a scaphoid fracture than an X ray. Treatment consists of immobilizing the wrist in a *cast*.

An undiagnosed, untreated scaphoid fracture may not heal, which can lead to *osteoarthritis* or, in some cases, to necrosis (death) of part of the bone. These complications may result in persistent pain in the wrist and restriction of its movement.

S

Scapula

The anatomical name for the shoulder blade. The scapula is a flat, triangular bone situated over the back of the upper ribs. On its rear surface is a prominent spine (which can be felt under the skin) that runs diagonally upward and outward to a bony prominence (called the acromion) at the shoulder tip.

The acromion articulates with the end of the *clavicle* (collarbone) to form the *acromioclavicular joint*. Just below the acromion is a socket (called the glenoid cavity) into which the head of the humerus (upper-arm bone) fits to form the shoulder joint.

FUNCTION

The scapula serves as an attachment for certain muscles and tendons of the arm, neck, chest, and back, and is involved with movements of the arm and shoulder.

Because the scapula is well padded with muscle, great force is required to fracture it. Treatment of a fracture consists of putting the shoulder in a *sling* until the fracture has healed. *Physiotherapy* may be needed to restore movement to the joint.

Scar

Any mark left on damaged tissue after it has healed. Scar tissue forms not only on the skin but on all internal wounds—for example, after a muscle tear or at sites where surgery has been performed.

The body repairs a wound, ulcer, or other lesion by increasing the production of the tough, fibrous protein *collagen* at the site of the damage. This helps form new *connective tissue*, which covers the area of the lesion. If the edges of an incision are brought together when healing takes place, the resultant scar is narrow and pale; if the edges are left apart, the scar is more extensive (see *Healing*).

ABNORMAL SCARS

The term hypertrophic scar is used to describe a large, unsightly scar that sometimes develops at the site of an infected wound. Some people have a family tendency to develop hypertrophic scars for no apparent reason.

A *keloid* is a large, irregularly shaped scar that continues to grow in size as the body continues to produce extra collagen after a wound has healed; this type of scar is more common in black people than in white people.

Adhesions are areas of scar tissue that form between unconnected parts of internal organs; they are a potential complication of intestinal surgery.

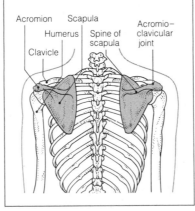

LOCATION OF THE SCAPULAE
The two scapulae are the prominent wing-shaped bones in the upper back. They facilitate many arm and shoulder actions.

Acromion   Scapula
Humerus   Spine of   Acromio-
              scapula   clavicular
Clavicle   joint

Scarlatina

Another name for *scarlet fever*.

Scarlet fever

An infectious disease, more common in childhood, that is caused by a strain of streptococcal bacteria. Characterized by a sore throat, fever, and rash, scarlet fever is far less common and far less dangerous than formerly.

CAUSES AND SYMPTOMS

The bacteria are spread in droplets coughed or breathed into the air. After an incubation period of usually two to four but sometimes up to seven days, a sore throat, headache, and fever develop. A rash soon appears, caused by a *toxin* released by the bacteria. The rash begins as a mass of tiny red spots on the neck and upper trunk and spreads rapidly. The face is flushed (except for an area around the mouth) and a white coating with red spots may develop on the tongue (called "strawberry tongue"). After a few days this coating comes off to reveal a bright red appearance. Soon the fever subsides, the rash fades, and there may be some skin peeling, especially on the hands and feet.

As with other types of sore throat caused by streptococci (see *Strep throat*), there is a risk of *rheumatic fever* or *glomerulonephritis* (inflammation of the filtering units in the kidneys) if the infection is not treated promptly.

DIAGNOSIS AND TREATMENT

The physician diagnoses scarlet fever from the symptoms and signs and, if necessary, by *culture* of the bacteria from a throat swab.

Treatment is with *antibiotic drugs*, usually penicillin (or erythromycin if the patient is allergic to penicillin). Treatment usually leads to a rapid recovery. During the illness, the patient should rest, drink plenty of fluids, and be given *acetaminophen* to relieve discomfort and reduce fever. Some physicians take throat swabs from contacts (such as members of the family) to exclude infection, or may give them a short course of penicillin.

Schistosome

A type of fluke (flattened worm). Three types of schistosomes are parasites of humans, causing different forms of the tropical disease *schistosomiasis*.

Schistosomiasis

A parasitic disease, also known as bilharziasis, that occurs in most tropical countries and afflicts more than 200 million people worldwide.

CAUSES AND INCIDENCE

The disease is caused by any of three species of flukes called schistosomes and is acquired from bathing or wading in infested lakes, rivers, and irrigation systems. Forms of schistosome (cercariae) can penetrate the bather's skin and develop within the body into adult flukes (see life-cycle diagram overleaf). Eggs produced by the adult females provoke inflammatory reactions, which in turn may cause symptoms.

The infestation causes bleeding, ulceration, and *fibrosis* (scar tissue formation) in the bladder or intestinal walls; infestation may also cause inflammation and fibrosis in other organs, such as the liver.

SYMPTOMS

Symptoms vary considerably. Some infested people have no symptoms, others become severely ill and suffer serious complications.

The first symptom is usually tingling and an itchy rash where the cercariae have penetrated the skin. Many weeks later, when the adults start producing eggs, an influenzalike illness may develop. Sometimes severe, the illness is marked by high fever, chills, aching, and pains. Subsequent symptoms may include blood in the urine or feces, abdominal or low back pain, and enlargement of the liver or spleen or both.

Complications of long-term infestation with the schistosome parasite may include liver *cirrhosis*, *bladder tumors*, and *kidney failure*.

S

DIAGNOSIS

The diagnosis is made from a special blood test for *antibodies* to the parasites (see *Immunoassay*), and from microscopic examination of a sample of the victim's urine or feces to detect the presence of eggs.

TREATMENT

Since the early 1980s, the treatment of schistosomiasis has been revolutionized by use of *praziquantel*, a single dose of which kills the flukes and thus prevents, or limits, damage to internal organs.

PREVENTION

Since no vaccine is available against the disease, visitors to areas where schistosomiasis is present (i.e., much of the tropics) should avoid wading or bathing in any lake, river, or irrigation system.

Control of the disease rests on the provision and the regular use by the population of latrines in order to avoid contamination of inland water. The Chinese and others have achieved some success through measures directed toward eradicating freshwater snails and through imposing strict sanitary regulations.

Schizoid personality disorder

Inability to relate socially to other people. People with this trait, which is apparent from childhood, are often described as "loners" and have few, if any, friends. They are markedly eccentric, seem to lack warmth or concern for others, and may be vague and apparently detached from normal day-to-day activities.

Schizophrenia develops in about 10 percent of people who are diagnosed as having a schizoid personality. However, not all people with schizophrenia initially have schizoid personalities. Although the social and employment prospects for schizoid people are severely impaired, some people with schizoid personality disorder do succeed in socially isolated occupations.

Schizophrenia

A general term for a group of psychotic illnesses characterized by disturbances in thinking, emotional reaction, and behavior. Schizophrenia is sometimes incorrectly called "split personality." The disorder should not be confused with *multiple personality*.

Schizophrenia is a disabling illness with a prolonged course that almost always results in chronic ill health and some degree of personality change.

PREVALENCE

Schizophrenia is the most common form of psychotic illness, with a markedly consistent prevalence rate throughout the world of just under 1 percent. For reasons that are not understood, schizophrenia is more common in certain geographical areas and in inner-city populations. Onset is usually between the ages of 15 and 30, being, on average, five years later in females than in males; otherwise, the sexes are affected equally.

CAUSES

Inheritance has been shown to play a role in the development of schizophrenia. First-degree relatives (i.e., parents, children, or siblings) of people with schizophrenia have a 10 percent chance of the illness; more distant relatives have a lower risk. If a person has two parents with schizophrenia or an identical twin with the disorder, he or she has an approximately one in two chance of developing schizophrenia. However, factors other than genetics must also play a part or schizophrenia would inevitably develop in both twins.

Biological studies have shown that certain brain disorders, such as *temporal lobe epilepsy*, *brain tumors*, and *encephalitis*, tend to be related to schizophrenic symptoms. Brain imaging techniques, especially *CT scanning* and *PET scanning*, have revealed abnormalities of structure and function in the brains of people suffering from schizophrenia. It has also been demonstrated that certain drugs, such as *amphetamine drugs*, can cause a schizophrenic illness, and that drugs that block the action of *dopamine* often relieve schizophrenic symptoms.

It seems likely that schizophrenia is possibly worsened by stress in the individual's personal life.

SYMPTOMS

Schizophrenia may begin insidiously, with the individual becoming slowly more withdrawn and introverted, and losing his or her drive and motivation. The change may not be noticed for months or years, until it becomes apparent that the individual is suffering from *delusions* (false ideas that do not respond to reasoned argument) or *hallucinations* (a sensory experience in the absence of an external stimulus). In other cases, the illness comes on more suddenly, usually in response to some external stress.

S

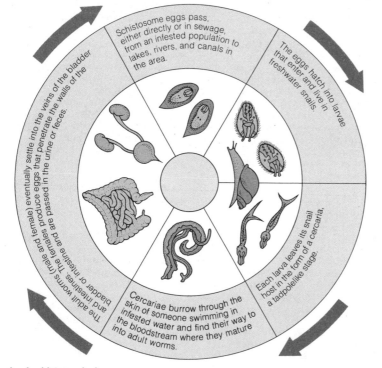

Schistosome eggs pass, either directly or in sewage, from an infested population to lakes, rivers, and canals in the area.

The eggs hatch into larvae that enter and live in freshwater snails.

Each larva leaves its snail host in the form of a cercaria, a tadpolelike stage.

Cercariae burrow through the skin of someone swimming in infested water and find their way to the bloodstream where they mature into adult worms.

The adult worms (male and female) eventually settle into the veins of the bladder and intestines. The females produce eggs that penetrate the walls of the bladder or intestines. The eggs are passed in the urine or feces.

Cycle of schistosomiasis
The disease affects a large proportion of the population in some parts of the world, such as the Nile valley in Egypt. Many methods have been tried to break the cycle of the disease in affected areas, with varying success. Methods used have included strict sanitary regulations and measures to eradicate freshwater snails.

Delusions may take a variety of forms, ranging from single ideas, such as the belief that one is Jesus Christ or Napoleon, to elaborate delusional systems in which special significance is attached to everyday objects or events. In paranoid schizophrenia, the illness is dominated by delusions of grandeur, persecution, or jealousy.

Hallucinations frequently are experienced as voices that comment on behavior or thoughts, occasionally in the form of conversations in which the sufferer is referred to as he or she. This type of auditory third person hallucination occurs exclusively in schizophrenia. True visual hallucinations are rare in Western cultures, but distortions of visual perception do occur; faces or objects may look sharper or change shape. Bodily sensations, such as tingling, are common.

Most schizophrenics also suffer from a variety of thought disorders, which impair concentration or clear thinking. Sufferers describe their thoughts as being blocked or inserted into or withdrawn from their minds by some outside force. They may also feel that their thoughts are being broadcast to others.

Disordered thinking is reflected in muddled and disjointed speech. Disturbance of association results in the schizophrenic jumping from one subject to another, seemingly unrelated, one. Inability to think in abstractions often leads to bizarre responses to questions. For example, when a girl was asked why she was turning in a circle, she said she felt she was in a knot and was trying to unravel herself. In some cases, speech disintegrates, becoming a "word salad" of odd phrases, *neologisms* (made-up words), and detached syllables.

In a rare form of schizophrenia, catatonia may occur. Sufferers of catatonic schizophrenia adopt prolonged rigid postures or engage in outbursts of repeated movement.

Symptoms of *manic-depressive illness* may accompany schizophrenia, especially in the early stages. However, as the illness progresses, emotions usually become severely blunted, there is increasing detachment from other people, and there is a loss of interest in hobbies or occupations. Behavior becomes more eccentric and self-neglect is common.

DIAGNOSIS
For a diagnosis of schizophrenia to be made, the individual must have continuous signs of a profound break with reality and evidence of fragmentation (disorganization) of the personality for at least six months during some time in his or her life. This six-month period must include at least one phase when there are symptoms of hallucinations, delusions, or marked thought disorders.

TREATMENT
The main form of treatment consists of *antipsychotic drugs*, such as *chlorpromazine*, which reduce the symptoms and make the person more amenable to *psychotherapy*. Some antipsychotic drugs can be given as long-acting *depot injections*.

Drug treatment is effective in suppressing the more obvious symptoms of schizophrenia, such as hallucinations, in most victims. However, such treatment may cause certain unpleasant side effects, particularly *dyskinesia* (abnormal muscular movements) and tremor.

Schizophrenics may be treated initially in hospital; once the major symptoms are controlled, most sufferers return to the community. Adequate provision of day centers, suitable housing, and vocational opportunities can help to control symptoms, to improve the sufferer's self-reliance, to prevent relapse, and to reduce the stigma attached to mental illness. If the patient is to live at home, the family needs to be provided with support and guidance, since some schizophrenics may be difficult to live with. A certain number relapse, especially if they do not take their medication regularly.

OUTLOOK
Although some 10 percent of the people who develop schizophrenia remain severely impaired for life, the majority can return to varying degrees of independence. About 30 percent will return to normal lives and occupations.

The particular form of the illness is important in determining the outlook. Individuals who have schizophrenia combined with manic-depressive symptoms often recover fully, as do many with catatonia. Paranoid schizophrenics, because of the preservation of their personalities, are often able to function well, albeit as somewhat eccentric members of the community. Schizophrenia that comes on slowly, starting around puberty, often causes significant impairment.

Although drugs have improved the outlook for most schizophrenics, inadequate community care frequently results in relapse, neglect, vagrancy, or imprisonment.

Schönlein-Henoch purpura
A disorder, primarily of young children, due to inflammation of the smaller blood vessels of the skin, joints, kidneys and intestines. The most prominent features are raised purplish rash on the buttocks and backs of the arms and legs. Since the condition often follows an infection, it is thought to be a form of allergy. Recovery occurs without specific treatment, although recurrence is possible.

Sciatica
Pain that radiates along the *sciatic nerve*. The pain usually affects the buttock and thigh, but sometimes extends down the leg to the foot. In severe cases, the pain may be accompanied by numbness and/or weakness in the affected area.

CAUSES
The most common cause of sciatica is a prolapsed intervertebral disk pressing on a spinal root of the nerve (see *Disk prolapse*). Less commonly, it may be caused by pressure on the nerve from a tumor, abscess, or blood clot, from local muscle spasm, or simply from sitting in an awkward position. Any disorder that involves nerves (such as certain infections, *diabetes mellitus*, or *alcohol dependence*) may affect the sciatic nerve and lead to the development of sciatica.

TREATMENT AND OUTLOOK
Treatment is directed toward the underlying cause, but in many cases the cause is not identified. Thus, treatment consists of measures to relieve the pain, including taking *analgesic drugs* (painkillers) and resting in bed. With such treatment, the pain usually disappears within a few days. In severe cases of sciatica, the pain may persist for several weeks. The condition tends to recur.

Sciatic nerve
The main nerve in each leg and the largest nerve in the body. Each sciatic nerve is a branch of the sacral plexus (nerve network) in the pelvis, and is formed from several lumbar and sacral *spinal nerves*. From the sacral plexus, the sciatic nerve passes below the sacroiliac joint (at the back of the pelvis, near the sacrum) and backward to the buttock, from where it passes behind the hip joint and runs down the back of the thigh. Above the back of the knee, the sciatic nerve divides into two main branches, known as the tibial nerve and the common peroneal nerve.

S

LOCATION OF THE SCIATIC NERVE

The diagram below shows the nerve in a cutaway of the right thigh and knee, as seen from behind.

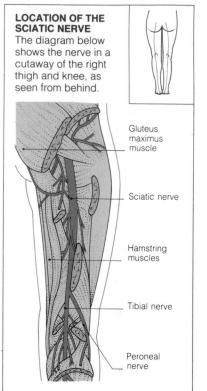

Gluteus maximus muscle

Sciatic nerve

Hamstring muscles

Tibial nerve

Peroneal nerve

The sciatic nerve supplies the hip joint, many of the thigh muscles, and the skin on the back of the thigh. The tibial and peroneal branches supply the knee and ankle joints, all the muscles of the lower leg and foot, and most of the skin below the knee.

DISORDERS

Probably the most common disorder of the sciatic nerve is *sciatica*, which is often caused by a prolapsed intervertebral disk pressing on a spinal root of the nerve (see *Disk prolapse*). The upper part of the nerve may also be damaged by dislocation of the hip joint, which, in severe cases, may result in paralysis of muscles below the knee and widespread numbness of the skin in that part of the body.

Damage to the peroneal nerve, often due to a fracture of the upper *fibula* (the outer bone of the lower leg), may produce *footdrop* and numbness of the skin at the side of the lower leg and back of the foot.

The tibial nerve is deeply buried in body tissues and is thus rarely injured. However, this nerve is sometimes damaged by dislocation of the knee, which may cause paralysis of the lower leg and foot, and numbness in the sole of the foot.

Scintigraphy

A less common, alternative name for *radionuclide scanning*.

Scirrhous

A medical term meaning hard and fibrous. The word is usually applied to malignant tumors that have dense, fibrous tissue within them.

Sclera

The white outer coat of the *eye*, visible through the transparent *conjunctiva*. The sclera is composed of dense, fibrous tissue formed from *collagen*, which is strong and protects the inner structures of the eye from injury. The sclera may, however, be penetrated by sharp objects.

Disease of the sclera is uncommon, but *scleritis* (inflammation of the sclera) may occur, usually with a *collagen disease*, such as *rheumatoid arthritis*. The healthy sclera sometimes shows a blue tinge from the underlying *choroid*. If the sclera is exceptionally thin, which occurs in *osteogenesis imperfecta*, this blue appearance is pronounced.

Scleritis

Inflammation of the *sclera* (the white outer coat of the *eye*). Scleritis usually accompanies a *collagen disease*, such as *rheumatoid arthritis*. It also occurs in *herpes zoster* ophthalmicus and in Wegener's granulomatosis. Scleritis may lead to areas of local thinning and possible perforation of the sclera.

Scleritis is usually persistent, but often responds well to eye drops containing a *corticosteroid drug*. In severe cases, corticosteroids may increase the risk of perforation.

Scleroderma

A rare condition, also known as systemic sclerosis, that can affect many organs and tissues in the body, particularly the skin, arteries, kidneys, lungs, heart, gastrointestinal tract, and joints. Scleroderma is an *autoimmune disorder* (in which the body's immune system attacks its own tissues). Scleroderma is twice as common in women as in men and is most likely to appear between the ages of 40 and 60.

SYMPTOMS AND SIGNS

The number and the severity of symptoms vary dramatically. The most common symptom is *Raynaud's phenomenon* (in which the fingers or toes become white and painful on exposure to cold); this phenomenon may be present for many years without any other symptoms.

LOCATION OF THE SCLERA

The sclera is about 0.5 mm thick and is continuous with the cornea at the front of the eye. The sclera is extremely tough and protects the inner structures of the eye.

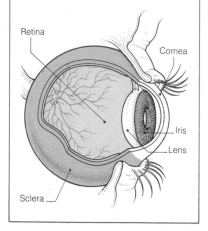

Retina

Cornea

Iris

Lens

Sclera

Also common are changes in the skin, especially of the face and fingers, which becomes shiny, tight, and thickened. There is often puckering around the mouth, giving the sufferer a characteristic masklike appearance. The pulled skin often leads to difficulty in performing certain maneuvers, such as bending the fingers or opening the mouth.

In some people, other parts of the body are affected, leading to problems such as difficulty in swallowing, shortness of breath, palpitations, high blood pressure, joint pain, stiffness, and muscle weakness.

There are wide variations from person to person in the degree to which different parts of the body are involved and the rate at which the disease progresses. Progression of scleroderma is often rapid in the first few years and then slows down or even stops. In a small number of people, degeneration is rapid, and leads usually to death from *heart failure*, *respiratory failure*, or *kidney failure*.

DIAGNOSIS AND TREATMENT

A physical examination is usually sufficient to confirm the diagnosis, but a blood test and a skin *biopsy* (removal of a sample of tissue for microscopic examination) may be performed.

There is no cure for scleroderma, but treatment can relieve symptoms and associated problems. *Vasodilator drugs* and avoiding exposure to cold can relieve Raynaud's phenomenon. *Physiotherapy* may be recommended

S

for joint problems. *Antihypertensive drugs* may be given to treat high blood pressure and *dialysis* may be used to treat kidney failure. *Corticosteroid drugs* are sometimes prescribed if the muscles are involved, but may not be effective.

Scleromalacia

Softening of the *sclera* (the white outer coat of the *eye*). Scleromalacia is commonly a complication of *scleritis* (inflammation of the sclera), especially when scleritis is caused by *rheumatoid arthritis*.

Scleromalacia perforans is a rare, severe form of the condition in which the entire thickness of sclera is involved; the underlying *choroid* layer of the eye bulges through and sometimes perforates the sclera.

Sclerosis

A medical term for hardening of a body tissue. The term is usually used to refer to hardening of blood vessels, as in *arteriosclerosis* (hardening of arteries), or to hardening of nerve tissue due to deposition of abnormal connective tissue, which occurs in the later stages of *multiple sclerosis*.

Sclerotherapy

A method of treating *varicose veins* (swollen, tortuous veins), especially in the legs. *Hemorrhoids* (varicose veins in the anus) and *esophageal varices* (swollen veins at the bottom of the esophagus) are also sometimes treated in this way.

In sclerotherapy, the affected vein is injected with a strongly irritant solution (called a sclerosant). This causes inflammation in the lining of the vein, leading to fibrosis (scar tissue formation), and the eventual obliteration of the vein.

Scoliosis

A deformity in which the *spine* is bent to one side. The thoracic (chest) or lumbar (lower back) regions are the most commonly affected.

TYPES AND CAUSES

Scoliosis usually starts in childhood or adolescence and becomes progressively more marked until the age at which growth stops. In many such cases, another part of the spine curves toward the opposite side of the body to compensate for the scoliotic curvature, and resulting in the spine becoming S-shaped. The cause of juvenile scoliosis is unknown; if the condition is not corrected, it may lead to severe deformity.

More rarely, scoliosis develops as a result of a congenital abnormality of the vertebrae (the spinal bones), *poliomyelitis* that has weakened the spinal muscles on one side of the body, or tilting of the pelvis due to one leg being shorter than the other. Occasionally, a spinal injury (such as a *disk prolapse* or ligament sprain) causes temporary scoliosis. In such cases, the spinal curvature appears suddenly and is accompanied by back pain and *sciatica*.

DIAGNOSIS AND TREATMENT

Scoliosis is diagnosed by a physical examination of the spine, hips, and legs, along with X rays of the spine.

If the cause of the condition is known, treatment is directed toward that cause (e.g., bed rest for a disk prolapse or wearing an orthopedic shoe with a raised heel to correct a pelvic tilt due to unequal leg lengths).

Scoliosis of unknown cause may not require treatment if the curvature is slight. However, regular measurement of the spine is necessary to assess the progression of the condition. If the scoliosis seems to be worsening—or if the curvature is already marked—it may be treated by immobilization of the spine in a hinged plaster jacket or adjustable metal brace, followed by surgery and bone grafting to fuse the affected spinal vertebrae in a straight line (see *Spinal fusion*). A steel rod with hooks may be used to keep the spine straight until the bones become fused.

Scopolamine

An *anticholinergic* drug that has an *antispasmodic* effect on the intestine and bladder. Scopolamine is also used to treat motion sickness and as a premedication, because it dries up secretions in the *pharynx* and respiratory tract. It can cause a number of side effects, including drowsiness and blurred vision.

Scorpion stings

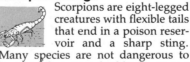 Scorpions are eight-legged creatures with flexible tails that end in a poison reservoir and a sharp sting. Many species are not dangerous to humans, but some highly venomous species of scorpion are found in North Africa, South America, the southern US, Mexico, parts of the Caribbean, and India.

SYMPTOMS

The effects of many scorpion stings are little worse than a bee sting, with mild to moderate pain and tin-

gling or burning at the site of the puncture wound. With more dangerous species, there may be sweating, restlessness, diarrhea, and vomiting (caused by stimulation of the *autonomic nervous system*) in addition to severe pain. The venom may also affect the rhythm and strength of the heart's contractions. Fatalities are uncommon in adults; young children and the elderly are at greater risk.

TREATMENT

Any person stung by a scorpion should seek immediate medical attention. If pain is the only symptom, mild *analgesic drugs* (painkillers) and cold compresses may be all that is needed. In severe cases, local anesthetics and powerful painkillers may be required as well as an *antivenin*.

Scotoma

An area of abnormal vision within the *visual field*.

Screening

The testing of apparently healthy people with the aim of detecting disease at an early, treatable stage. The ideal screening test is reliable, with a low rate of false-positive results (in which the results of the test are positive even though the people tested do not in fact have the disease) and a low rate of false-negative results (in which the results of the test are negative even though the people tested have the disease). An ideal test is also inexpensive, simple, and acceptable to people, causing neither discomfort nor danger. For a screening test to be of practical use, people found to have the disease must benefit from early diagnosis. For example, screening for unsuspected diabetes is of no use since there is no evidence that the late complications of the disease are lessened by diagnosis before symptoms develop. (See also *Cancer screening*.)

Scrofula

Tuberculosis of the lymph nodes in the neck, often those just beneath the angle of the jaw. Scrofula was once a common disorder, usually caused by drinking contaminated milk. Abscesses would form in the lymph nodes and, after bursting through the skin, leave scars on the neck.

Today scrofula is rare in developed countries. It occasionally develops in Asian or African immigrants in whom the infection has spread from tuberculosis elsewhere in the body. Antituberculous drugs clear up the condition in most cases.

S

Scrotum

The pouch that hangs behind the penis and contains the *testes*. The scrotum consists of an outer layer of thin, wrinkled skin over a layer of muscle-containing tissue.

Swelling of the scrotum may be caused by an inguinal *hernia*, a swelling of one of the testes, a *hydrocele* (fluid in the sac around one of the testes), or by edema (accumulation of fluid) in severe *heart failure*.

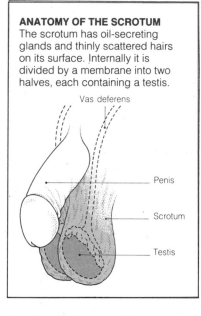

ANATOMY OF THE SCROTUM
The scrotum has oil-secreting glands and thinly scattered hairs on its surface. Internally it is divided by a membrane into two halves, each containing a testis.

Vas deferens

Penis

Scrotum

Testis

Scuba-diving medicine

A minor medical specialty concerned with the physiological hazards of underwater diving with self-contained underwater breathing apparatus (SCUBA).

THE MAIN HAZARDS
Most diving hazards stem from the increase in pressure with depth. At a depth of 10 m, the total pressure is twice the surface pressure. At 30 m, it is four times the surface pressure.

MECHANICAL EFFECTS OF PRESSURE CHANGE
During descent, divers must introduce gas into their middle ear cavities and facial sinuses to prevent damage as the pressure mounts. This mounting pressure is what airline passengers also experience during descent and repressurization (see *Barotrauma*).

Whatever depth they attain, divers must be supplied with breathing mixtures at a pressure equal to the external water pressure. Thus, at 30 m, a diver breathes gas at four times the surface pressure. During ascent, gas in the lungs expands and can rupture

the lung tissues if the diver panics and holds his or her breath—a serious condition known as pulmonary barotrauma (burst lung). Symptoms may include coughing up blood, inability to pass urine, breathing difficulties, and unconsciousness.

TOXIC EFFECTS OF GASES Amateur divers breathe compressed air, which consists mainly of nitrogen and oxygen. These gases are harmless at surface pressures but become toxic at high pressure. Nitrogen impairs the nervous system when air is breathed at depth, causing slowed mental functioning and other symptoms that mimic alcohol intoxication (a condition known as nitrogen narcosis); regulations in most provinces allow commercial divers using air to go no deeper than 50 m. Oxygen becomes toxic when air is breathed at increased pressure, when it can cause convulsions or lung damage.

To attain greater depths without risking nitrogen and oxygen poisoning, professional divers use gas mixtures other than air. A typical mixture consists of helium, with only small amounts of oxygen and nitrogen; the helium is relatively nontoxic.

THE BENDS At depth, divers accumulate in their tissues excess quantities of any inert gas they are breathing (nitrogen, if air is being breathed). If pressure is released too quickly (i.e., the diver ascends too fast) and if a large amount of gas has accumulated because the diver remained at depth for too long, this gas can no longer be held in solution in the tissues and may form bubbles in tissues and in the circulation, causing *decompression sickness*.

OTHER HAZARDS Additional hazards include *hypothermia* (dangerous chilling) due to immersion in cold water, bites or stings from marine animals, and risk of *drowning*.

ACCIDENT PREVENTION AND TREATMENT
Anyone taking up scuba diving should first have a medical checkup and thorough training at a recognized diving school.

Pressure-related accidents, such as burst lung and decompression sickness, are treated by recompression of

HYPERBARIC CHAMBER FOR DIVING ACCIDENTS
Divers suffering from the bends or other pressure-related accidents are often treated in a hyperbaric chamber. The patient is usually accompanied in the chamber by a nurse, a technician, or a physician.

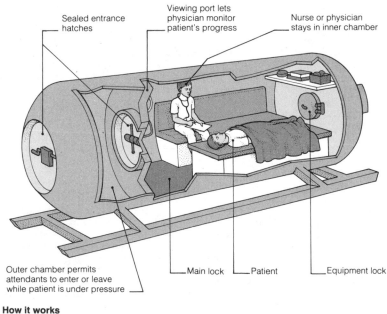

Sealed entrance hatches

Viewing port lets physician monitor patient's progress

Nurse or physician stays in inner chamber

Outer chamber permits attendants to enter or leave while patient is under pressure

Main lock

Patient

Equipment lock

How it works
A gas mixture (usually air) is pumped into the chamber. As pressure increases, bubbles (pockets of gas) in the diver's tissues are reabsorbed, and symptoms disappear. Once all symptoms have gone, the pressure is slowly released.

the diver in a special pressure chamber (known as a hyperbaric chamber) so that any bubbles or pockets of gas in the blood or tissues are reabsorbed. This is followed by slow release of the pressure.

Treatment of other accidents (such as hypothermia and near drowning) is as for nondivers.

Scurvy

A disease caused by inadequate intake of *vitamin C*. Scurvy is rare today in developed countries as a result of increased consumption of fresh fruit and vegetables. Body stores of vitamin C give protection against scurvy for about three months.

CAUSES AND SYMPTOMS

Inadequate supplies of vitamin C disturb the body's normal production of *collagen*, which is a protein in *connective tissue* (material that surrounds body structures and holds them together). Collagen continues to be produced in scurvy but is unstable, causing weakness of small blood vessels and poor healing in wounds. Hemorrhages may occur anywhere in the body. They are most obvious in the skin, where they result in widespread bruising. Bleeding from the gums and loosening of the teeth are common; bleeding into muscles and joints also occurs in scurvy, causing considerable pain.

Scurvy is especially serious in children because bleeding into the membranes surrounding the long bones may cause separation of the growing ends of the bones and interference with growth. Major, and sometimes fatal, hemorrhages into and around the brain can occur.

Scurvy is often associated with other vitamin deficiencies, and *anemia* is common.

PREVENTION AND TREATMENT

A modest intake of fruit (particularly citrus fruit) and vegetables provides the body with sufficient vitamin C to prevent scurvy. Other minor sources are milk, liver, and kidneys.

Scurvy is treated with large doses of vitamin C. Bleeding stops in 24 hours, healing resumes, and muscle and bone pain quickly disappear.

Sealants, dental

Plastic materials applied to the chewing surfaces of the back *teeth* to help prevent decay. The molars and premolars have minute surface grooves in which food debris and bacteria can collect and cause decay (see *Caries, dental*). Sealing the teeth stops harmful material from getting into the grooves. Sealants are of most benefit to children and should be applied as soon as possible after the permanent teeth have erupted.

Teeth to be sealed often require no drilling or anesthesia. The tooth surface must be acid-etched to roughen it so that the sealant will adhere better (see *Bonding, dental*). The semiliquid sealant is then applied and is usually hardened by directing a narrow beam of ultraviolet light at the treated tooth for a few seconds.

Some dental sealants are premixed with a chemical activator that causes them to set.

Seasickness

A type of *motion sickness*.

Seasonal affective disorder syndrome

A form of *depression* in which mood changes occur with the seasons. The name seasonal affective disorder syndrome, often abbreviated to SADS, was first used in the 1980s but the disorder is probably as old as man himself. Alternative names are seasonal affective disorder (SAD) and winter depression.

SYMPTOMS

Sufferers from SADS become depressed in the autumn and winter of most years, and then get better in the spring. As many as one person in 20 may be affected to some extent.

Several research studies have shown that people who usually become depressed in the dark cold months of winter may prevent the onset of symptoms by exposing themselves to bright light for two to four hours each morning. The mechanism by which exposure to light has its effects remains unknown.

Sebaceous cyst

A nonspecific term for a large, smooth nodule under the skin (also called a wen if it occurs on the scalp). The most common sites of sebaceous cysts are the scalp, face, ear, and genitals. The cysts contain a smooth, yellow, cheesy material.

Although harmless, sebaceous cysts may grow very large and sometimes become infected by bacteria, in which case they are painful. Large cysts or cysts that have been infected should be removed under local anesthetic. The physician makes a small incision in the skin and removes the cyst. If the entire cyst wall is removed, recurrence is rare.

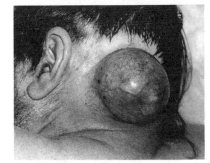

Massive sebaceous cyst
Cysts rarely grow as large as this one, located on the back of the neck. Sebaceous cysts are easily removed surgically.

Sebaceous glands

Minute glands in the *skin* that secrete a lubricating substance that is called *sebum*. Sebaceous glands either open into hair follicles or discharge directly onto the surface of the skin. Sebaceous glands are particularly numerous on the scalp, face, and around the anus, but they do not occur at all on the palms of the hands or on the soles of the feet. The production of sebum by the sebaceous glands is partly controlled by *androgen hormones* (male sex hormones).

Disorders of the sebaceous glands may lead to *seborrhea* or *acne* vulgaris.

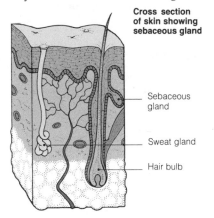

Cross section of skin showing sebaceous gland

Sebaceous gland

Sweat gland

Hair bulb

Seborrhea

Excessive secretion of *sebum*, causing increased oiliness of the face and a greasy scalp. The exact cause is uncertain, although *androgen hormones* (male sex hormones) are known to play a part. Common in adolescent boys, seborrhea usually improves in adulthood. People with seborrhea are more likely than average to have other skin conditions, particularly seborrheic *dermatitis* and *acne* vulgaris.

S

Seborrheic dermatitis
See *Dermatitis*.

Sebum
The oily secretion produced by the *sebaceous glands* of the *skin*. Composed of fats and waxes, sebum lubricates the skin, keeps it supple, and protects it from becoming sodden when immersed in water or cracked when exposed to a dry atmosphere. Sebum also protects the skin from invasion by bacteria and fungi.

Oversecretion of sebum, called *seborrhea*, causes a greasy skin, and may lead to seborrheic *dermatitis* or *acne* vulgaris.

Secobarbital
A barbiturate drug with actions similar to others of this family, but with more rapid onset and shorter duration of action. Because it is likely to be habit-forming, it is rarely prescribed.

Secondary
A term applied to a disease or disorder that results from or follows another disease (which is called the *primary* disease). For example, secondary *hypertension* (high blood pressure) occurs as a result of some underlying primary disorder, such as a hormonal problem or kidney disease.

The term secondary is also used to refer to a *metastasis* (a malignant tumor that has spread from a primary cancer elsewhere).

Secretion
The manufacture and release by a cell, gland, or organ of chemical substances (such as *enzymes* or *hormones*) that are needed for metabolic processes elsewhere in the body. In contrast, *excretion* is the production and release of waste products. The term secretion is also used to refer to the secreted substances themselves.

The secretions of *exocrine glands* (e.g., the salivary glands) are carried away in ducts; the secretions of *endocrine glands* (e.g., the thyroid) are released directly into the bloodstream.

Security object
A significant item, such as a special blanket, an old garment, or a favorite soft toy, that provides comfort and reassurance to a young child. In many cases, a child settles down to sleep more easily if his or her security object is near. Some children are unable to sleep without their security objects.

Sometimes referred to as transitional objects, these items represent to the child something part way between a person and a thing. The child may become deeply attached to the object and may become highly distressed if an attempt is made to remove it.

Security objects are often important during the toddler stage and may be used for several years. Most children grow out of the need for such an item by the time they are about 7 or 8 years old, but close attachments to special toys may persist. There is no evidence that security objects are in any way harmful. (See also *Thumb-sucking*.)

Sedation
The use of a drug to calm a person. Sedation is used to reduce excessive *anxiety* and occasionally to control dangerously aggressive behavior. It may also be used as part of *premedication* to produce relaxation before an operation or before an uncomfortable procedure such as *gastroscopy*. (See also *Sleeping drugs*.)

Sedative drugs
A group of drugs used to produce *sedation* (calmness). Sedative drugs include *sleeping drugs*, *antianxiety drugs*, *antipsychotic drugs*, and some *antidepressant drugs*. A sedative drug is often included in a *premedication* (drug given to prepare a person for surgery).

Seizure
A sudden episode of uncontrolled electrical activity in the *brain*. Recurrent seizures are called *epilepsy*. Seizures may be partial or generalized.

In a partial seizure, abnormal electrical activity remains confined to one area of the brain. The affected person may experience tingling or twitching of only a small area of the face, body, or an extremity. Other possible symptoms include *hallucinations*, intense feelings of fear, or *déjà vu*.

In a generalized seizure, abnormal electrical activity spreads throughout the brain. This causes loss of consciousness and features of a grand mal, petit mal, or less common form of generalized seizure.

Seizures may be caused by many different neurological or medical problems, including *head injury*, *stroke*, *brain tumor*, infection, metabolic disturbances, withdrawal symptoms in *alcohol dependence*, or a hereditary intolerance of alcohol. Whatever the cause, treatment with *anticonvulsant drugs* can control or at least reduce the number of seizures.

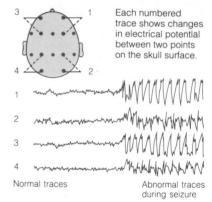

Each numbered trace shows changes in electrical potential between two points on the skull surface.

Normal traces   Abnormal traces during seizure

EEG changes during a seizure
The traces are recordings of electrical activity in a patient's brain, obtained from electrodes placed at various locations on the scalp and linked to an EEG machine. They show the change in activity at the onset of a seizure.

Selegiline
An *antiparkinson drug* that acts by slowing down the depletion of *dopamine*, a *neurotransmitter* important in coordinating movements. Selegiline has relatively few side effects, and can be given in the earliest stages of parkinsonism. It can also be useful in more advanced cases, to enhance the effects of *levodopa*.

Selenium
A *trace element* which may help to preserve the elasticity of body tissues. The richest dietary sources are meat, fish, whole grains, and dairy products. The selenium content of vegetables depends on the amount of the mineral in the soil.

DEFICIENCY AND EXCESS
Neither deficiency nor excess of selenium usually has any effect on health.

Excessive intake as a result of taking supplements, occupational exposure, or, rarely, eating vegetables grown in soil with an abnormally high selenium content (as is found in some intensively irrigated areas) may cause a smell of garlic in the breath and urine, and red-orange discoloration or loss of the hair and nails. Some selenium compounds may irritate the skin or, if inhaled, the respiratory tract.

Claims that the selenium content of the diet may influence the risk of developing heart disease have not been substantiated.

MEDICAL USES
Selenium is a constituent of some *multivitamin* and *mineral* preparations. Selenium sulphide is used in some antidandruff shampoos.

S

Self-help organizations

Self-help or mutual aid organizations in medical care are usually started by patients or relatives of those who suffer from specific diseases, disabilities, addictions, or emotional problems. The groups may provide individuals with information, emotional support, and even financial assistance. Some are also active in raising funds for research and in improving public relations and promoting legislation for their cause.

Self-image

An individual's view of his or her own personality and abilities. It is argued that neurotic disorders may stem from incongruity between self-image and how others see one, as, for example, in an *inferiority complex*. *Psychotherapy* treats neurosis by bringing about a change in the person's perception of the self. Cognitive therapy attempts to improve self-image by changing negative thoughts about oneself.

Self-injury

The act of deliberately injuring oneself. Self-mutilation most often occurs in young adults with *personality disorders*, many of whom are also drug or alcohol abusers, and is three times more common in women.

Self-mutilation usually takes the form of cutting the wrists or burning the forearms with cigarettes. The reasons often given by self-mutilators for their behavior include aggressive impulses, relief of tension, and sadomasochistic fantasies. Some self-mutilators have had a violent upbringing. In people with a learning disability or a mental handicap, such behavior may be a means of gaining attention or avoiding specific situations or demands.

More unusual forms of self-harm, such as gouging out the eyes or mutilating the genitals, are almost always due to *psychosis*. Self-destructive biting is a feature of Lesch-Nyhan syndrome, a rare *metabolic disorder* causing mental retardation.

Semen

Fluid produced by the male on *ejaculation*. Semen is composed of fluid from the seminal vesicles (which produce the greatest part of the semen volume), fluid from the *prostate gland* and Cowper's glands, and *sperm*.

An important constituent of the fluid from the seminal vesicles is fructose (a sugar), which stimulates the sperm to become mobile. The concentration of fructose, the production of sperm, and the volume of the semen is dependent on the presence of the male sex hormone *testosterone*.

Seminal fluid analysis is a procedure performed as part of the investigation of male *infertility*.

Semen analysis

A method of determining the concentration, shape, and motility (ability to move) of sperm. Semen analysis is important in the investigation of male *infertility*. It is also performed some weeks after *vasectomy* (male sterilization) to ensure that the semen no longer contains sperm.

The specimen is produced by masturbation and should be as fresh as possible. The volume of semen is measured and the specimen examined under the microscope.

Normal semen contains from 20 million to 200 million sperm per millilitre. Semen analysis may show *oligospermia* (a deficiency in the number of sperm) or *azoospermia* (a complete absence of sperm), altered shape, or diminished motility.

Semen, blood in the

A condition in which a small amount of blood is present in the *semen*. Blood in the semen, known medically as hemospermia, is nearly always harmless. The blood, which is usually seen as a darkish stain in the semen at *ejaculation*, usually comes from small blood vessels in the region of the prostate gland or seminal vesicles. In the majority of cases, no cause is found.

Seminoma

See *Testis, cancer of*.

Senile dementia

See *Dementia*.

Senility

A term meaning old age or, more commonly, the changes in mental ability caused by old age. Many people over 70 suffer from a mild degree of impaired memory and reduced ability to concentrate. This does not mean that the person is developing senile *dementia*; indeed, only 5 percent of elderly people become demented. The incidence of dementia does rise with age, but even in those over 80, four out of five retain their mental faculties. Mental performance may also be affected by *confusion* due to physical disease or by depressive illness (see *Depression*), both of which become more common with increasing age.

Senna

A *laxative drug* obtained from the leaves and pods of the Arabian shrubs *CASSIA ACUTIFOLIA* and *CASSIA ANGUSTIFOLIA*. Senna stimulates bowel contraction and is used to treat severe *constipation*; it may color the urine yellow-brown or red.

Sensation

A feeling or impression (such as a sound, odor, touch sensation, or hunger) that has entered consciousness. The senses are the faculties by which information about the external environment and about the body's internal state is collected and brought to the *central nervous system* (the *brain* and *spinal cord*).

SENSORY RECEPTORS

Information is collected by millions of microscopic structures called *receptors*. Receptors are found throughout the body in the skin, muscles, and joints, in the internal organs, in the walls of blood vessels, and in special sense organs, such as the *eye* and inner *ear*. Receptors are attuned to a particular stimulus, such as light of a particular wavelength, chemical molecules of a certain shape, vibration, or temperature. They fire (send an electrical signal) when excited.

Some receptors are the terminals (free nerve endings) of long nerve cell fibers, others are specialized cells that connect to such fibers. When a receptor fires, a signal passes along the appropriate nerve fiber to the spinal cord and/or brain. The principal pathways and destinations of sensory information entering the brain are shown in the diagram. Only a proportion of this information reaches the *sensory cortex* of the brain and is consciously perceived.

THE SPECIAL SENSES

The special senses include *vision*, *hearing*, *taste*, and *smell*. The receptor cells for these senses are collected into special organs—the retina in the eyes, the auditory apparatus in the ears, the taste buds in the *tongue*, and the apparatus for smell in the *nose*. Information from these organs passes directly to the brain via *cranial nerves*. Much of the information passes to the cerebral cortex, although some goes to other areas of the brain (e.g., from the eyes to the *cerebellum*, where it is used to help maintain balance).

INTERNAL AND TOUCH SENSES

These senses include the pain, proprioception (position), pressure, and temperature sensations. Propriocep-

S

tion relies on receptors in the muscles and joints to provide information on the position in space of parts of the body. Pain is one of the most primitive senses; it warns of noxious stimuli through receptors both at the skin surface and internally.

Many different types of receptors are found in the skin. Some are sensitive to pressure, others to the movement of hairs, others to variations of temperature. Skin receptors are made up of the terminals of nerve fibers, which are wrapped around the roots of hairs, formed into disks, or surrounded by a series of membranes to form onionlike structures (called pacinian corpuscles). Different patterns of stimulation of these receptors give rise to such sensations as pain, tickling, firm or light pressure, heat or cold. Certain skin areas (the lips, palms of the hands, and genitals) have a particularly high concentration of receptors.

Most of the signals from these receptors pass, via the cranial or *spinal nerves* and tracts in the brain or spinal cord, to the *thalamus* and then to two regions of the sensory cortex called the somatosensory cortices. Sensations perceived at certain points within these regions correspond to the parts of the body from which the signals originated. Much larger areas of cortex are devoted to sensations originating from the hands and lips than from less sensitive parts.

Sensation, abnormal

Unpleasant, dulled, or otherwise altered *sensations* without obvious stimulus (e.g., a burning sensation when there is no source of heat). Abnormal sensations result from damage to, or pressure on, sensory nerve pathways.

TYPES

Numbness and *pins and needles* are common abnormal sensations, sometimes combined with *pain* and sometimes occurring with sensations of coldness or burning. *Neuralgia* is characterized by pain with a stabbing, brief, repetitive quality.

More unusual abnormal sensations include a feeling that fluid is trickling down the skin, that part of the body is being constricted by a tight band, or that insects are crawling over the skin (a sensation known as formication).

The special senses can also be impaired or altered by damage to the relevant sensory apparatus or nerve tracts (see *Deafness*; *Smell*; *Tinnitus*; *Vision, disorders of*).

CAUSES

Neuropathy (damage to peripheral nerves) from thiamine deficiency in alcoholics, from *diabetes mellitus*, or from heavy metal (such as lead) poisoning is a common cause of abnormal sensation. The sufferer may complain of tingling or a feeling of walking on cottonwool. The peripheral nerves may also be damaged or irritated by infections such as *herpes zoster* (shingles) or by a tumor pressing on a nerve, often causing severe pain. *Spinal injury*, *head injury*, *stroke*, and *multiple sclerosis* are other causes of disruption to nerve pathways in the *brain* or *spinal cord*.

Damage to the *thalamus* (a relay station for sensory pathways in the center of the brain) can produce particularly unpleasant results, such as a spreading sensation resembling an electric shock that occurs after a simple pinprick. Damage to the parietal lobe in the brain can also have unfortunate consequences such as loss of the ability to locate or recognize objects by touch.

DIAGNOSIS

Many tests (including tests of sensation, testing of *reflexes*, *blood tests*, *urinalysis*, and *CT scanning* or *angiography*) may be required in order to discover the cause of abnormal sensation.

TREATMENT

Pressure on or damage to nerves can sometimes be relieved by surgery or by dietary or other treatments to remove or treat the underlying cause. In other cases, severe intractable pain or other abnormal sensation can be relieved only by cutting the relevant sensory nerve fibers or by giving injections to block chemically the transmission of signals along them.

Senses

See *Sensation*.

PRINCIPAL SENSORY PATHWAYS INTO THE BRAIN

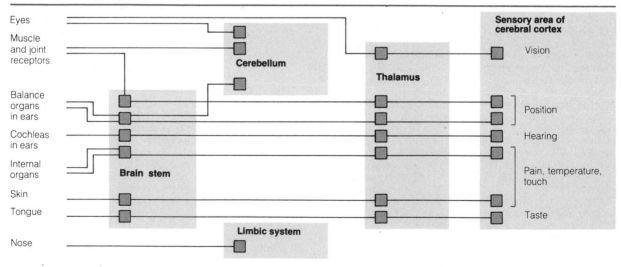

Destinations of sensory information
Some of the information entering the brain passes via the brain stem and/or thalamus to the cerebral cortex (outer surface of the brain), where sensations are perceived. Other information does not lead to conscious sensation. This includes certain data about body posture, processed in the cerebellum, and about internal body functioning, processed in the brain stem.

Sensitization

The initial exposure of a person to an allergen or other substance recognized as foreign by the body's *immune system*, which leads to an immune response. On subsequent exposures to the same substance, there is a much stronger and faster immune reaction. This forms the basis of *allergy* and other types of *hypersensitivity* reaction.

Sensory cortex

A region of the outer part of the *cerebrum* (the main mass of the *brain*) in which sensory information comes to consciousness. The sensory cortex contains several layers of linked *neurons* with complex interconnections.

Pressure, pain, and temperature sensations from the skin, muscles, joints, and internal organs, and taste sensations are perceived in regions of the parietal lobe (upper side part of the cerebrum) on both sides of the brain. These regions are called the somatosensory cortices. Light, color, and other visual sensations are perceived in the occipital lobes at the back of the cerebrum; sounds are perceived in the temporal lobes at the sides.

Sensory deprivation

Removing the normal sights, sounds, and physical feelings from a person. Sensory deprivation can produce a variety of mental changes, demonstrated by studies in which volunteers lie immobile in bed (or in a bath of warm water) wearing masks and gloves in a sound-deadened room. After long periods, reported effects generally include feelings of unreality, difficulty in thinking, and *hallucinations*; *EEG* recordings show a slowing of brain activity.

Prisoners kept in solitary confinement experience similar symptoms, and infants deprived of the companionship and presence of others tend to be disturbed in later life. (See also *Bonding*; *Emotional deprivation*.)

Separation anxiety

The feelings of distress that a young child experiences when parted from his or her parents or home. Separation anxiety is a normal aspect of infant behavior which increases in intensity until about 2 years of age, but is often minimal by the age of 3 or 4. When threatened with separation, the child usually reacts by crying, clinging to the parent, and demanding to be cuddled. Such signs are indicative of *bonding*, which is considered essential to a child's emotional development.

NEUROLOGICAL SENSORY TESTING

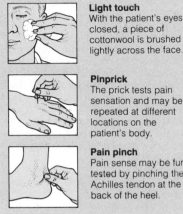

Light touch
With the patient's eyes closed, a piece of cottonwool is brushed lightly across the face.

Pinprick
The prick tests pain sensation and may be repeated at different locations on the patient's body.

Pain pinch
Pain sense may be further tested by pinching the Achilles tendon at the back of the heel.

Vibration
A vibrating tuning fork is held against a prominent bone, such as the ankle bone or mastoid bone.

Position sense
The patient, with eyes closed, tells in which direction his or her finger is moved.

Two-point discrimination
Measures the ability to distinguish two pinpricks from a single prick.

Standard tests
When examining a patient's nervous system, a physician usually includes several standard tests of touch, position, pain, and vibration senses, such as those above.

Separation anxiety disorder is a childhood illness in which the reaction to separation is greater than that expected for the child's level of development. The anxiety may manifest itself in the form of headaches, nausea, toothaches, dizziness, or difficulty in sleeping. When separated from the family, the child may worry that he or she will never be reunited with the parents or that they will be killed. Some children refuse to visit friends or to attend school. Separation anxiety disorder may be a feature of *depression*.

Sepsis

Infection of a wound or body tissues with bacteria that leads to the formation of *pus* or to the multiplication of the bacteria in the blood. If the blood becomes infected with bacteria that the *immune system* can prevent from multiplying excessively or can eradicate entirely, the condition is known as *bacteremia*. However, if bacteria that form *toxins* are present in the blood in large numbers and are multiplying rapidly, the condition is called *septicemia* (blood poisoning). (See also *Septic shock*.)

Septal defect

A *heart* abnormality, developed before birth, in which there is a hole in the septum (partition) between the left and right sides of the heart. Commonly known as a hole in the heart, septal defect varies in its effects according to its size and position.

TYPES
When the hole is in the septum separating the two ventricles (lower chambers of the heart), the abnormality is known as a ventricular septal defect; when it is in the septum between the two atria (upper chambers), it is called an atrial septal defect. In both types, the hole allows some of the freshly oxygenated blood in the left half of the heart (which supplies tissues throughout the body and which is under higher pressure) to flow into the right half, mix with deoxygenated blood, and recirculate through the lungs. If the hole is large, the misdirection of blood results in excessive blood flow through the lungs, with increased pressure in the pulmonary circulation and breathing difficulties.

Some children are born with both atrial and ventricular septal defects; either type may be accompanied by one or more other heart abnormalities and/or other congenital defects.

The precise cause of septal defects is unknown in most cases. (For information on factors influencing the development of congenital heart abnormalities, see *Heart disease, congenital*, and *Birth defects*.)

Ventricular septal defects are the most common type of congenital heart abnormality, occurring in about 25 percent of all cases of congenital heart disease and affecting about 200 babies in every 100,000. Atrial septal defects are less common, affecting about 60 babies per 100,000.

S

SYMPTOMS AND SIGNS

A small defect of either kind produces little or no effect. With a large ventricular hole, *heart failure* may develop six to eight weeks after birth, causing breathlessness, feeding difficulties, pallor, and sweating. With large atrial defects, however, heart failure may not develop for many years or may not develop at all although there may be some fatigue on exertion.

With both types of defect, *pulmonary hypertension* (high blood pressure in the arteries supplying the lungs) may develop. This is more likely, and occurs at an earlier age, if there is a large ventricular defect.

With a ventricular defect there is also a slight risk that *endocarditis* (inflammation of the lining of the heart) may develop; in atrial septal defect, *atrial fibrillation* (rapid, irregular beating of the atria) may occur in patients who are 30 years or older.

DIAGNOSIS

The diagnosis is based on hearing a heart *murmur* (a type of abnormal heart sound made by turbulent blood flow) through a stethoscope, followed by a *chest X ray* and an *ECG*. The diagnosis can be confirmed by Doppler *echocardiography*.

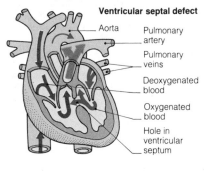

Ventricular septal defect

Aorta — Pulmonary artery

Pulmonary veins

Deoxygenated blood

Oxygenated blood

Hole in ventricular septum

Atrial septal defect

Aorta — Pulmonary artery

Hole in atrial septum

Oxygenated blood

Deoxygenated blood

Two types of septal defect
In both cases, oxygenated blood is forced from the left to the right side of the heart through the hole in the septum. Too much blood passes to the lungs (via the pulmonary artery) and too little to the body tissues (via the aorta).

TREATMENT

Atrial septal defects are repaired surgically if they cause symptoms or if examination and tests suggest that complications may develop.

As the child grows, small ventricular holes often become smaller, or even close, on their own. If a large ventricular defect is causing heart failure, it is treated with *diuretic drugs* and with *digitalis drugs*. If the hole does not close spontaneously, it may be repaired by *open heart surgery*, usually before the child reaches school age. The operation has a very high success rate.

OUTLOOK

Modern surgery is so effective in dealing with large septal defects that it enables most affected people to lead normal lives.

Septicemia

Rapid multiplication of bacteria and the presence of bacterial *toxins* in the blood, a condition commonly known as blood poisoning. As distinct from *bacteremia* (in which bacteria are present in the blood but do not always multiply), septicemia is always a serious, and potentially life-threatening, condition.

CAUSES

Septicemia usually arises through escape of bacteria from a focus of infection somewhere in the body (such as a *urinary tract infection*, *gastroenteritis*, *pneumonia*, *meningitis* or an *abscess*). Septicemia is more likely in people whose natural resistance to infection has been lowered by an *immunodeficiency disorder* or by *immunosuppressant drugs*, allowing the bacteria to multiply unchecked. Septicemia is also more likely to develop in drug addicts who use contaminated needles, and in people who have *cancer*, *diabetes mellitus*, or other debilitating diseases.

SYMPTOMS AND SIGNS

A person with septicemia develops a high fever, chills, rapid breathing, headache, and, in many cases, clouding of consciousness. Skin rashes or jaundice may occur. In some cases, the hands are unusually warm. In many cases, especially when large amounts of toxins are produced by the circulating bacteria, the sufferer passes into a state of *septic shock*, a life-threatening condition.

DIAGNOSIS AND TREATMENT

A diagnosis of septicemia can be confirmed, and the infective bacteria identified, by growing a *culture* of the organisms from a blood sample.

Treatment is started as soon as septicemia is suspected. Glucose and/or saline are administered by *intravenous infusion*, and *antibiotic drugs* are given intravenously by infusion or injection. Tests are performed to identify the original site of infection if this is not apparent. Surgery may be necessary in some cases to remove infected material.

Provided the infection is recognized and treated promptly before the development of septic shock, most patients make a full recovery.

Septic shock

A highly dangerous condition in which there is tissue damage and a dramatic drop in blood pressure as a result of *septicemia* (the multiplication of bacteria and the presence of bacterial *toxins* in the blood).

In many cases, the toxins are the main cause of trouble because they can damage cells and tissues throughout the body, promote clotting of blood in the smallest blood vessels, and seriously interfere with the normal blood circulation. Damage occurs especially to tissues in the kidneys, heart, and lungs. The toxins may cause leakage of fluid from blood vessels and a reduction of the ability of the vessels to constrict, leading to a drop in blood pressure.

CAUSES AND INCIDENCE

Septic shock is most common in people with debilitating disorders, such as *diabetes mellitus*, *cancer*, or liver *cirrhosis*, who also have a focus of infection somewhere in the body (often the intestines or urinary tract) that has led to septicemia. Progression to septic shock is especially likely in people who have an *immunodeficiency disorder*, in people taking *immunosuppressant drugs*, or in people given prolonged and inappropriate treatment with *antibiotic drugs*. Newborn infants with septicemia are also particularly susceptible to septic shock.

SYMPTOMS AND SIGNS

The symptoms vary with the extent and site of major tissue damage. Broadly, they are the same as in septicemia, with additional symptoms including cold hands and feet, often with *cyanosis* (blue-purple coloration) due to slowed blood flow, a weak, rapid pulse, and markedly reduced blood pressure. There may be vomiting and diarrhea. A poor output of urine may indicate that damage to the kidneys is occurring and that there is a risk of *kidney failure*. *Heart failure* and abnormal bleeding may also develop.

TREATMENT

Septic shock requires immediate treatment, including the use of *antibiotic drugs* and sometimes surgery to remove the focus of infection. Rapid fluid replacement by transfusion and the maintenance of urine flow to prevent the effects of kidney failure are other essential procedures. Measures are also taken to raise the blood pressure and to promote better blood supply to tissues. These measures include *intravenous infusions* and *oxygen therapy*.

Despite treatment, septic shock remains a serious condition; survival rates are no better than 50 percent.

Septum

A thin dividing wall within or between parts of the body. (The nasal septum is the sheet of cartilage and bone that separates the nostrils.)

Sequela

A condition that results from or follows a disease, a disorder, or an injury. The term is usually used in its plural form (sequelae) to refer to the complications of a disease. For example, the sequelae of a common cold may include *bronchitis*, *sinusitis*, and *otitis media* (inflammation of the middle ear).

Sequestration

A portion of diseased or dead tissue separated from, or joined abnormally to, surrounding healthy tissue. The term usually refers to a complication of *osteomyelitis* (bone infection) in which part of a bone dies and becomes separated from healthy bone.

The term sequestration may also refer to a rare congenital abnormality of the lungs in which part of a lobe is not directly connected to a bronchus (airway) but may be connected to surrounding alveoli (air sacs).

Serology

A branch of laboratory medicine concerned with analysis of the contents of blood *serum* (the clear fluid that separates from clotted blood).

Various serological techniques are extremely useful in the diagnosis of infectious diseases. If a person has been exposed to a particular infectious organism, *antibodies* (proteins with a role in immunity) directed specifically against the organism appear in that person's serum some days after exposure. The presence or absence of particular antibodies in the blood can be detected by various laboratory techniques, including *immunoassay* techniques, such as the *ELISA test* and *radioimmunoassay*. The absence of specific antibodies may enable a physician to exclude a particular infection as the cause of an illness; a rising level of antibodies may give good evidence that a particular infection is present.

Serological techniques are also used to identify the *antigens* (foreign proteins) of infectious organisms by studying the reaction between the antigens (obtained by *culture* of a specimen taken from a patient) and serum samples known to contain certain antibodies. A series of tests may be carried out in which the unknown antigen is added to test tubes containing various *antiserum* preparations which contain specific antibodies; a positive reaction is sometimes revealed by a color change.

In addition to devising and carrying out diagnostic tests, serologists may be involved in developing antisera for passive *immunization*.

Serologists may also test blood samples for various genetically determined protein markers, including substances that determine *blood groups*. Such tests can help resolve paternity suits (see *Paternity testing*) or cases in which blood left at the scene of a crime can be compared with blood taken from suspects.

Serotonin

A substance found in many tissues, particularly blood platelets, the lining of the digestive tract, and the brain. Serotonin has a variety of effects in the body. It is released from platelets at the site of bleeding, where it constricts small blood vessels, thus reducing blood loss. In the digestive tract, it inhibits gastric secretion and stimulates smooth (involuntary) muscles in the intestinal wall. In the brain, it acts as a *neurotransmitter* (a chemical involved in the transmission of nerve impulses between nerve cells). Serotonin is thought to be involved in controlling states of consciousness and mood; its action in the brain is disrupted by certain hallucinogenic drugs, notably *LSD*.

Serum

The clear fluid that separates from *blood* when it clots. Serum does not contain blood cells or fibrinogen (the protein in blood that helps form clots). It does contain salts, glucose, and other proteins, including various *antibodies* formed by the body's *immune system* to protect against infection.

Serum prepared from the blood of a person (or animal) who has been infected with a microorganism usually contains antibodies that can protect against that organism if the serum is injected into someone else. This is called an *antiserum*, and its use forms the basis of passive *immunization*.

Serum sickness

A short-lived illness that may develop about 10 days after injection with an *antiserum* of animal origin (e.g., equine antirabies serum, which is obtained from horses). Serum sickness is a type of *hypersensitivity* reaction similar to an allergic reaction; comparable reactions can occur after taking certain drugs.

CAUSES

Antisera are preparations obtained from human or animal blood that contains specific *antibodies* (substances with a role in immunity). Antisera are sometimes given to protect against dangerous infections. When an antiserum is prepared from animal blood, a protein in the serum may be misidentified by the body's *immune system* as a potentially harmful *antigen* (foreign protein). In serum sickness, the immune system produces antibodies that combine with the antigen to form particles called immune complexes. These are deposited in various tissues, stimulate more immune reactions, and lead to inflammation and symptoms.

Certain drugs can cause a similar response, although the drug molecules probably combine with a protein in the blood or tissues before they are misidentified as antigens. *Penicillin drugs* are the most important drugs capable of causing serum sickness.

Serum sickness is different from *anaphylactic shock*, another type of hypersensitivity reaction that can also develop in response to antisera, drugs, and other substances. Anaphylactic shock is a more severe, immediate reaction.

SYMPTOMS AND TREATMENT

Symptoms appear a week or two after exposure to the antiserum or drug. There may be an itchy rash, joint pain, fever, and enlarged lymph nodes. In severe cases, a state similar to *shock*, with low blood pressure, develops. Symptoms usually clear up within a few days, provided, in the case of a drug, that its use is stopped.

Soothing lotions can help relieve itching. The physician may prescribe a *nonsteroidal anti-inflammatory drug* to relieve joint pain and an *antihistamine*

S

drug to shorten the duration of the reaction. In severe cases, a *corticosteroid drug* may be prescribed.

People who have had serum sickness or anaphylactic shock should note the name of the injection or drug to which they are sensitive. A note should also be included in their medical records to warn health care personnel against future use of the drug.

Sex
Another term for gender and a commonly used term for *sexual intercourse*.

Sex change
Radical surgical procedures, usually combined with sex hormone therapy, that alter a person's anatomical gender. Sex-change operations are performed either on transsexuals (see *Transsexualism*) or on people whose external sex organs are neither completely male nor completely female (see *Genitalia, ambiguous*).

WHY IT IS DONE
Sex change operations on transsexuals are performed to give the person a physical appearance that he or she believes coincides with his or her psychological *gender identity*.

Sex change operations on people with ambiguous genitalia are performed to modify or improve the anatomical appearance and thus provide a more defined sexual identity.

HOW IT IS DONE
TRANSSEXUALS Sex change involves a series of major operations on the genitourinary tract which are carried out after hormone therapy and extensive counseling.

The male-to-female sex change is the more common procedure. Prosthetic breasts may be implanted to augment breast growth that has been induced by hormone therapy. An operation removes the erectile tissue of the penis and repositions the urethra. The skin of the penis is used to make the lining for a vagina, which is created in the *perineum*. The testes are removed and the skin of the scrotum is used to make the labia.

In the female-to-male sex change, a mastectomy is performed to remove the breasts. Afterward, removal of the uterus and ovaries is carried out. This may be followed by constructing a penis. The female-to-male operation has less satisfactory results than the male-to-female operation.

AMBIGUOUS GENITALIA Operations are usually carried out in infancy. Babies with ambiguous genitalia are assigned a sex as soon as possible after birth,

given appropriate surgical and hormonal treatment, and reared as a member of the assigned sex.

Operations on adults who have ambiguous genitalia are uncommon today. In general, they are similar to those performed on transsexuals, with variations depending on the specific anatomical problems.

OUTLOOK
The degree to which transsexuals adjust to their new gender varies. Some make a complete adjustment but others are left with serious psychological problems. Hormone therapy may need to be continued for life to maintain secondary sexual characteristics such as body shape and hair distribution. Female transsexuals can have intercourse but cannot conceive. Males cannot impregnate or ejaculate; they achieve an erection only with mechanical aids (e.g., *penile implants*).

Sex chromosomes
A pair of *chromosomes* that determines an individual's sex. All the cells in a person's body (except for egg or sperm cells) contain a pair of sex chromosomes together with 22 other pairs of chromosomes known as autosomes. In women, the sex chromosomes are of similar appearance and are called X chromosomes. In men, one sex chromosome is an X and the other, a smaller one, a Y. Thus, the normal sex chromosome complement for women is XX, and for men, XY.

FUNCTION
Like all chromosomes, the X and Y chromosomes exert their effects in the body through the activities of their constituent *genes*. These genes contain the coded instructions for chemical processes within cells and for aspects of growth and development within the body as a whole.

The X and Y chromosomes differ in one fundamental way. Genes on the Y chromosome are concerned solely with *sex determination*. Their presence ensures a male, their absence a female. The X chromosome, occurring in both sexes, contains many genes vital to general development and functioning. Absence of the X chromosome is incompatible with life.

The presence of a single X chromosome and 22 pairs of autosomes in the nuclei of ordinary body cells appears to provide the blueprint for general body functioning and development, which seems to have an underlying female pattern. This can be seen in

people with *Turner's syndrome*, who have only one sex chromosome, an X. Although full female sexual characteristics never develop, these people are unmistakably female in appearance and identity. Full female sexual characteristics develop only in the presence of a second X chromosome. Addition of a Y chromosome converts the female to the male pattern.

Sex determination
The factors that determine biological sex. The underlying determinants are the *sex chromosomes* in a person's cells—two X chromosomes in females, and one X and one Y chromosome in males. During early life in the embryo, these chromosomes cause the development of different gonads (primary sex organs)—the testes in males and the ovaries in females. In males, the testes then produce hormones that cause the development of a male reproductive tract, including a penis. In females, absence of these male hormones leads to a different pattern of development, with the formation of fallopian tubes, uterus, and vagina. At *puberty*, another surge of hormones from the gonads leads to the development of secondary *sexual characteristics*, such as facial hair in males and breasts in females.

Defects can arise in this process, leading, in some cases, to ambiguous sex. Some people acquire an abnormal complement of sex chromosomes (see *Chromosomal abnormalities*) and all the characteristics of one sex do not develop. In some female fetuses, a metabolic defect causes production of large amounts of male hormones (see *Adrenal hyperplasia, congenital*), causing masculinization of the female genitals (such as enlargement of the clitoris to form an appendage resembling a penis). Conversely, in some male fetuses, male hormones are not produced or they are produced but fail to cause masculinization; the child's genitals are feminized to some degree (the extreme case of this is called *testicular feminization syndrome*). Finally, there are very rare cases of true *hermaphroditism*, in which a child is born with both testicular and ovarian tissue and may have both a vagina and a penis. These ambiguities are different from *transsexualism*, in which a person's biological sex is not in doubt, although it conflicts with his or her psychological disposition.

When an infant is born with ambiguous genitalia, the cause of the ambiguity is investigated and the child is

S

assigned the sex believed to offer the best chance for a healthy life. The decision depends on the possibilities for establishing one sex or another through hormonal and/or surgical treatment. In most cases, a satisfactory male or female appearance and sexual capacity can be achieved. The ability to have children can also be achieved in some cases.

Sex hormones

Hormones that control the development of primary and secondary sexual characteristics and regulate various sex-related functions in the body, such as the menstrual cycle and the production of eggs or sperm. There are three main types of sex hormones—*androgen hormones* (male sex hormones), *estrogen hormones* (female sex hormones), and *progesterone hormone* (which has the specialized function of preparing for and maintaining *pregnancy*).

Sex-linked Inheritance

The process by which a trait or a disorder determined by the *sex chromosomes* in a person's cells, or by the *genes* carried on those chromosomes, is passed to the next generation.

Most people carry two sex chromosomes in their cells. Disorders caused by an abnormal number of sex chromosomes include *Turner's syndrome* (which affects females only and is caused by a missing X chromosome) and *Klinefelter's syndrome* (which affects males only and is caused by one or more extra X chromosomes).

Most other sex-linked traits or disorders are caused by recessive genes on the X chromosome (see *Genetic disorders*). In females, recessive genes for traits or disorders carried on the X chromosome are usually masked by a normal gene on the other X chromosome; males have only a single X chromosome, so no such masking takes place. As a result, X-linked traits or disorders affect many more males than females. Examples of such conditions include *hemophilia*, Duchenne *muscular dystrophy*, and *color vision deficiency*.

Sex therapy

Counseling for and treatment of *psychosexual dysfunction* (sexual difficulties not due to a physical cause). Sex therapy is usually undertaken in conjunction with *marital counseling*.

It is estimated that at least 50 percent of couples experience some form of sexual problem at some stage in their relationships; in most cases, the problem is psychological in origin. Sex therapy can help by changing the general attitude of one or both partners toward sex, by increasing each person's understanding of his or her sexual needs and those of the partner, and by teaching techniques to deal with specific problems. Both partners usually attend the therapy sessions, but individual sex therapy or group therapy may also be useful.

TECHNIQUES

In the sensate-focus technique, the couple explores pleasurable, relaxed, sensual rather than sexual, bodily sensations. The goal of this technique is to reduce anxiety about sexual performance and to increase individual awareness of how to give and receive pleasure for at least 15 minutes.

The most common sexual problem in men is premature ejaculation (see *Ejaculation, disorders of*). Two preventive techniques are taught. One is the squeeze technique (see illustration). The other technique requires both partners to stop thrusting a moment before ejaculation is imminent. In either case, once the man has achieved control over the ejaculatory reflex, sexual activity is resumed. The techniques can be repeated as many times as required. They can easily be learned and are highly successful.

A woman who rarely or never experiences orgasm (see *Orgasm, lack of*) or who has *vaginismus* (spasm of the vaginal muscles, preventing intercourse) may be treated individually,

---

THE SQUEEZE TECHNIQUE
This technique is used for treating and preventing premature ejaculation in men.

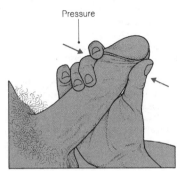

Pressure

Method
Either partner squeezes the penis when the man is about to ejaculate, pressing just beneath the glans (head of the penis) using the thumb and two fingers.

---

with her partner, or at group therapy sessions. The woman is encouraged to come to terms with her sexuality. She is taught to perform exercises for relaxing and tightening the pelvic muscles (see *Pelvic floor exercises*) and to stimulate the clitoris to achieve orgasm through masturbation as a preliminary to intercourse.

RESULTS

Sex therapy has proved successful for many sexual problems, with particularly effective results in treating vaginismus, premature ejaculation, lack of orgasm, impotence, and failure to consummate marriage.

Sexual abuse

The subjection of a person to sexual activity that has caused or is likely to cause physical or psychological harm. The victims of sexual abuse are most commonly children or women. The perpetrator is usually an adult male and the activity may be heterosexual or homosexual.

Many episodes are unreported or are unrecognized for lengthy periods. The causes are badly understood but may be indicative of sexual deviation or of sexual problems in the man.

Forms of sexual abuse range from abnormally affectionate relationships within a family (see *Incest*) to extremely violent sexual assaults, and include the sexual exploitation of children and adolescents who live in or are exposed to an unacceptable sexual environment. When physical sexual abuse of a child is suspected, it is important that the child should be interviewed and examined by a trained physician who is experienced in sexual abuse cases. (See also *Child abuse*; *Rape*.)

Sexual characteristics, secondary

Physical features appearing at *puberty* that indicate the onset of adult reproductive life.

In girls, the earliest secondary sexual characteristic is enlargement of the nipples and breasts. Shortly afterward, pubic and underarm hair appears, while body fat increases around the hips, stomach, and tops of the thighs to produce the female body shape.

In boys, enlargement of the testes is the first change, followed by thinning of the skin of the scrotum and enlargement of the penis. Pubic, facial, axillary, and other body hair appears, the voice deepens, and muscle bulk and bone size increase.

S

Sexual desire, inhibited

Lack of sexual desire or of the ability to become physically aroused during sexual activity (see *Sexual intercourse*). Either form of the condition may be physical or psychological.

CAUSES

LACK OF DESIRE A high proportion of women and some men experience loss of sexual desire at some point in their lives. Common physical causes include fatigue, ill health, and vaginal tenderness after childbirth. Certain drugs can also reduce sexual desire, including sleeping pills, antidepressants, antihypertensives, oral contraceptives, and alcohol. Psychological factors include *depression*, anxiety, severe stress, an unsatisfactory relationship with the sexual partner, grief at the death of a sexual partner, an unwanted pregnancy, an abortion, or a traumatic sexual experience such as *rape* or *incest*.

LACK OF PHYSICAL AROUSAL It is rare for a woman or a man to be incapable of physical sexual arousal. The most common reason for failure is poor or insensitive sexual technique on the part of the partner, although hostility, anxiety, guilt about the sex act, or fear of sexual inadequacy may contribute to the problem. In some cases, an individual may simply be unable to respond to a particular partner but be capable of responding to another, making the sexual problem selective rather than general.

TREATMENT

Problems that have a psychological basis or that are caused by the partner's sexual technique can often be successfully treated by *sex therapy* or *marital counseling*. Sexual problems with a physical or chemical cause often improve once the underlying condition is resolved.

Sexual deviation

See *Deviation, sexual*.

Sexual dysfunction

See *Psychosexual dysfunction*.

Sexual intercourse

A term sometimes used to describe a variety of sexual activities, but more commonly used to refer specifically to the act during which a man inserts his penis into a woman's vagina.

Sexual intercourse provides pleasurable sensations that may result in *orgasm* for one or both partners. The *ejaculation* of *semen* into the woman's reproductive tract is the usual means by which *fertilization* is achieved.

Couples bring many variations to the sexual act in terms of emotions, positions, and techniques used. However, for most couples, kissing, tenderness, and foreplay precede penetration. During sexual intercourse, a series of physiological responses occurs.

PHASES OF INTERCOURSE

Physiologically, intercourse can be divided into four phases—arousal, a plateau phase, orgasm, and resolution (see illustrated box opposite).

DISORDERS

Problems with intercourse may have physical or psychological origins. (See *Intercourse, painful; Psychosexual dysfunction; Sexual problems*.)

Sexuality

A general term for the capacity, behavior patterns, impulses, emotions, and sensations connected with reproduction and the use of the sex organs. In biology, sex refers specifically to the anatomical differences between male and female.

Heterosexuality is sexuality directed toward the anatomically opposite sex; in *homosexuality* the attraction is toward the same sex. The term *bisexuality* refers to people who experience sexual attraction to members of either sex. (See also *Gender identity*.)

Sexually transmitted diseases

Infections transmitted primarily, but not exclusively, by sexual intercourse.

HISTORY AND INCIDENCE

Also known as venereal diseases, sexually transmitted diseases (STDs) are acquired more often by people who have many sex partners. Some of the major STDs are also transmitted by blood and thus occur in drug addicts who share needles.

Until about 25 years ago, STDs were thought to be limited to *syphilis, gonorrhea, chancroid,* and *lymphogranuloma venereum*. Today, however, these four diseases account for only about 10 percent of all STDs seen in STD clinics. Other conditions also reported by STD clinics now include *chlamydial infections, trichomoniasis,* genital herpes (see *Herpes, genital*), *molluscum contagiosum, scabies, pubic lice,* genital warts (see *Warts, genital*), HIV infection and *AIDS*. Some other diseases, including viral *hepatitis* and *candidiasis*, can also be transmitted by sexual intercourse but are not always STDs.

During World War II, STDs became more prevalent and then declined when the introduction of penicillin provided a cure for syphilis and gonorrhea. In the 1960s and 1970s, however, STDs increased again with the introduction of oral contraception. The pill led not only to women having more sex partners, but also to fewer couples using barrier contraceptives, such as condoms, which provide some protection against infection.

In the 1970s, it was recognized that so-called *nonspecific urethritis* was usually due to chlamydia. By the early 1980s a diagnosis of nonspecific urethritis and nonspecific genital infection was being made in about 25 percent of patients visiting STD clinics; in nearly 50 percent of these, careful laboratory testing gave evidence of chlamydial infection.

Throughout the 1970s and the early 1980s, most patients with an STD could expect a rapid cure with an antibiotic drug. In the late 1970s, however, it became apparent that certain STDs (notably herpes and hepatitis B) could not be cured by drugs and that herpes could become chronic and hepatitis could be fatal.

With the recognition of AIDS in 1982, STDs became a threat to life. Promiscuous sex is now a high-risk activity worldwide.

DIAGNOSIS AND TREATMENT

Diagnosis and treatment are given at special STD clinics or from specialists in genitourinary medicine. The physician determines which STDs are present (there may be more than one) and then assesses the sensitivity of the infection to various antibiotics. Once drugs have relieved the symptoms, tests are performed to ensure that the patient is no longer infectious.

PREVENTION AND OUTLOOK

To prevent transmitting infection, all recent sexual partners should be traced, examined, and, when necessary, treated. The confidential tracing and treatment of contacts is an essential part of the management of STDs (see *Contact tracing*).

The incidence of most STDs (excluding AIDS) fell in the mid-1980s. But a rise in penicillin-resistant gonorrhea in some countries in 1988 suggests that the pattern could change again, particularly if people fail to practice *safe sex* techniques.

Sexual problems

Any of a wide variety of difficulties associated with sexual performance or behavior. A sexual problem may be perceived by both partners in a relationship, by one partner who is affected by a disorder that lies primarily with the other, or by a person

S

SEXUAL INTERCOURSE

The term sexual intercourse usually refers to the act during which the male's penis is inserted into the female's vagina. However, some people use the term more broadly to refer to a much wider range of sexual activity. Physiologically, intercourse falls into four main stages—arousal (which generally includes a period of foreplay), a plateau (during which penetration usually occurs), orgasm, and resolution. The duration of each stage of intercourse varies.

Arousal in men
Sexual thoughts, the sight and feel of his partner's body, and foreplay may sexually arouse a man. Blood enters the penis so that it becomes firm and erect.

Plateau phase in men
Vaginal penetration usually takes place during this phase and thrusting movements begin. The penis reaches maximum size and the testes elevate.

Orgasm in men
Muscular contractions in the ducts connecting the testes, prostate, and penis force semen out of the penis, accompanied by intensely pleasurable sensations.

Resolution in men
The penis returns to half its fully erect size and the testes descend.

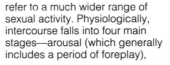

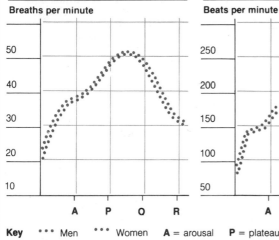

Seminal vesicle
Prostate gland
Urethra
Vas deferens
Clitoris
Vulva
Uterus
Glans
Vagina
Penis
Testis

Arousal in women
Similar factors lead to arousal in women as in men, though foreplay may be more important. The clitoris lengthens, the vagina enlarges, and its walls secrete a lubricating fluid.

Plateau phase in women
Muscular contractions in the walls of the vagina help grip the penis. The uterus rises, and the clitoris may pull back beneath its hood of skin.

Orgasm in women
The walls of the outer part of the vagina contract rhythmically and strongly several times and an intense sensual feeling spreads from the clitoris and throughout the body.

Resolution in women
The clitoris subsides and, more gradually, the vagina relaxes and the uterus falls.

BREATHING RATE
Breaths per minute

50
40
30
20
10

A   P   O   R

HEART RATE
Beats per minute

250
200
150
100
50

A   P   O   R

BLOOD PRESSURE
Millimetres of mercury (mm Hg)

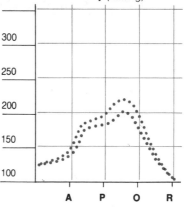

300
250
200
150
100

A   P   O   R

Key ••• Men   ••• Women   **A** = arousal   **P** = plateau   **O** = orgasm   **R** = resolution

Breathing rate
Both men and women breathe faster and louder as sexual excitement builds. The rate rises gradually, peaking at about twice the normal rate at orgasm.

Heart rate
Intercourse provides vigorous exercise for the heart. The heart rate increases rapidly during arousal, peaks as high as 200 beats per minute at orgasm, then drops.

Blood pressure
Systolic blood pressure rises in a similar pattern to the heart rate, peaking at orgasm. The rise may be more marked in men than in women.

S

INCIDENCE OF GONORRHEA IN CANADA

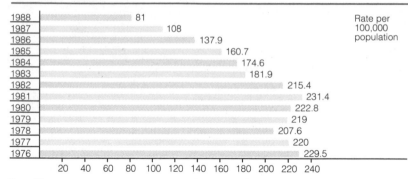

Year	Rate
1988	81
1987	108
1986	137.9
1985	160.7
1984	174.6
1983	181.9
1982	215.4
1981	231.4
1980	222.8
1979	219
1978	207.6
1977	220
1976	229.5

Rate per 100,000 population

20 40 60 80 100 120 140 160 180 200 220 240

Gonorrhea
There has been a steady decline in the incidence of gonorrhea since the early 1980s. It remains, however, one of the more common sexually transmitted diseases.

INCIDENCE OF SYPHILIS* IN CANADA

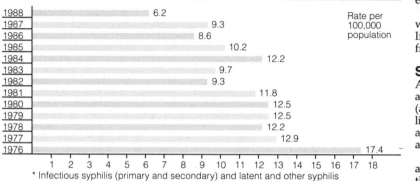

Year	Rate
1988	6.2
1987	9.3
1986	8.6
1985	10.2
1984	12.2
1983	9.7
1982	9.3
1981	11.8
1980	12.5
1979	12.5
1978	12.2
1977	12.9
1976	17.4

Rate per 100,000 population

1 2 3 4 5 6 7 8 9 10 11 12 13 14 15 16 17 18
* Infectious syphilis (primary and secondary) and latent and other syphilis

Syphilis
The decline in the incidence of syphilis since the late 1970s reflects changes in sexual behavior among male homosexuals as a result of the appearance of AIDS.

AIDS IN CANADA (CASES BY YEAR OF DIAGNOSIS)

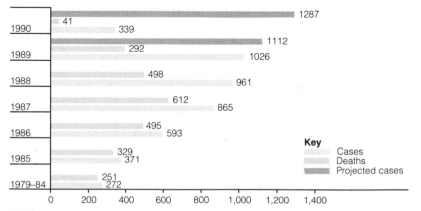

Year		
1990	41 / 339	1287
1989	292	1112 / 1026
1988	498	961
1987	612	865
1986	495 / 593	
1985	329 / 371	
1979–84	251 / 272	

0 200 400 600 800 1,000 1,200 1,400

Key
Cases
Deaths
Projected cases

AIDS
The graph shows the cumulative total number of cases of AIDS reported in Canada up to September 1990. It is estimated that there are at least 25 times as many people infected with the AIDS virus (i.e., who are HIV-positive) as there are with full-blown AIDS. Up to mid-1989, homosexual or bisexual men accounted for about 80 percent of AIDS cases, and about half of all those who had developed full-blown AIDS had died.

S

worried about his or her own sexual identity or behavior. Many sexual problems are psychological in origin (see *Deviation, sexual*; *Psychosexual dysfunction*; *Transvestism*).

Sometimes, sexual problems are due to organic disease, such as a disorder affecting blood flow or a hormonal problem. Disorders of the sexual organs may cause pain during intercourse (see *Intercourse, painful*). Sexual performance can be affected by certain drugs, such as *alcohol*, *antihypertensive drugs*, and *oral contraceptives*.

People with disabilities may have difficulty achieving gratification because of mobility problems or because the disabled person may be avoided sexually. The mentally handicapped may not show normal control over their sexual behavior, because of poor education and social skills.

Many sexual problems disappear when the underlying cause is treated. In other cases, people may benefit from sex education and counseling.

Sézary syndrome
A rare condition in which there is an abnormal overgrowth of *lymphocytes* (a type of white blood cell) in the skin, liver, spleen, and lymph nodes. Sézary syndrome mainly affects middle-aged and elderly people.

The first symptom is the appearance of red, scaly patches on the skin that spread to form a severe, itchy and flaking rash. There may also be an accumulation of fluid beneath the skin, baldness, and distorted nail growth. Sézary syndrome is sometimes associated with *leukemia*.

Treatment includes *anticancer drugs* and *radiation therapy*.

Shellfish poisoning
See *Food poisoning*.

Shell shock
See *Post-traumatic stress disorder*.

Shigellosis
An acute infection of the intestine by bacteria belonging to the genus Shigella. Also known as bacillary dysentery, shigellosis causes diarrhea and abdominal pain.

CAUSES AND INCIDENCE
The source of infection is the feces of infected people. The causative bacteria may be spread by an infected person failing to wash the hands after defecation and then handling food, by flies in areas of poor sanitation, or the lack of safe, clean water.

Endemic in some countries, shigellosis occurs in isolated outbreaks in Canada, where up to 2,000 cases are reported annually. It is particularly prevalent in children 1 to 4 years of age and in institutions for the elderly and the mentally ill.

SYMPTOMS AND SIGNS

The disease usually starts suddenly, with watery diarrhea, abdominal pain, nausea, vomiting, generalized aches, and fever. After a few days, the need to defecate becomes frequent and urgent, and small, watery feces containing pus and blood are passed. Persistent diarrhea may cause *dehydration*, especially in babies and older people. Occasionally, *toxemia* (the presence of bacterial poisons in the blood) develops, resulting in a high fever. The illness usually subsides after a week or so, but in severe cases may last several weeks. Death is rare, usually occurring only in dehydrated babies and older people.

DIAGNOSIS AND TREATMENT

The diagnosis is confirmed by growing a *culture* of the causative bacteria from a sample of feces.

Hospital treatment may be necessary in severe cases; people with mild infections should stay at home, where precautions should be taken to prevent the spread of infection. Dehydration is treated by *rehydration therapy*. *Antibiotic drugs* may be prescribed.

Shingles

See *Herpes zoster*.

Shin splints

A condition characterized by pain in the front and sides of the lower leg that develops or worsens during exercise. There may also be tenderness over the shin and edema (accumulation of fluid in tissues) of the surrounding area. Shin splints are a common problem in runners.

CAUSES

Shin splints may be caused by various disorders, including *compartment syndrome* (buildup of pressure in a muscle that may sometimes result from exercise), *tendinitis* (inflammation of a tendon), *myositis* (inflammation of a muscle), a muscle tear, or *periostitis* (inflammation of the outer layer of a bone).

DIAGNOSIS AND TREATMENT

Diagnosis is based on the symptoms, along with an *X ray* or a radionuclide bone scan (see *Bone imaging*) to exclude the possibility of a *stress fracture* of the tibia (shin bone), which produces similar symptoms.

In most cases, shin splints clear up after a week or two of rest. However, if the pain is severe or recurrent, other treatment may be necessary, such as a course of *nonsteroidal anti-inflammatory drugs* or *corticosteroid drugs*; infrequently, a surgical operation is performed to alleviate excessive pressure in a muscle. Some people benefit from *physiotherapy* including exercises to stretch and strengthen the legs.

Shivering

Involuntary trembling of the entire body caused by the rapid contraction and relaxation of muscles. Shivering is the body's normal automatic response to cold; it also occurs in association with fever.

When the body becomes cold, temperature-sensitive nerve cells in the *hypothalamus* (part of the brain) act as a thermostat, initiating the shivering reflex. This causes muscles to contract, generating heat. Shivering caused by cold usually disappears as soon as the body is warmed.

Shivering during fever is caused by the release of certain substances by the white blood cells. These substances effectively "reset" the thermostat at a higher point, causing the body to shiver when it needs to lose, rather than retain, heat. The trigger for this release is usually an infection, but fever also occurs in some metabolic, autoimmune, and malignant diseases, and as a side effect of certain drugs.

Shock

A dangerous reduction of blood flow throughout the body tissues which, if untreated, may lead to collapse, coma, and death.

Shock in this sense is physiological shock—different from the state of anxiety or mental distress that may follow a physically or emotionally traumatic experience (see *Post-traumatic stress disorder*). Reduced blood pressure is, in most cases, a major factor in causing physiological shock and is one of its main features.

CAUSES

Shock is a common accompaniment to severe injury or illness.

The condition may develop in any situation in which a person's blood volume is reduced (through blood or fluid loss), in which blood vessels are abnormally widened, in which the heart's action is weak, in which blood flow is obstructed, or through a combination of these factors.

Causes include severe *bleeding* or *burns*, persistent *vomiting* or *diarrhea*, *myocardial infarction* (heart attack), *pulmonary embolism* (blockage of blood flow to the lungs), *peritonitis* (inflammation of the abdominal cavity), *spinal injury*, and some types of *poisoning*. *Septic shock* results from bacteria multiplying in the blood and releasing toxins. *Anaphylactic shock* is a type of severe *hypersensitivity* or allergic reaction to an injected substance, such as insect venom or a drug. Shock is made worse by pain and anxiety. Symptoms

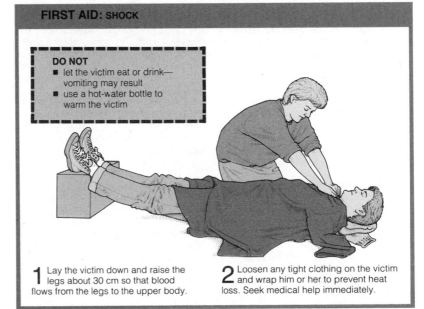

FIRST AID: SHOCK

DO NOT
- let the victim eat or drink— vomiting may result
- use a hot-water bottle to warm the victim

1 Lay the victim down and raise the legs about 30 cm so that blood flows from the legs to the upper body.

2 Loosen any tight clothing on the victim and wrap him or her to prevent heat loss. Seek medical help immediately.

S

include rapid, shallow breathing; cold, clammy skin; rapid, weak pulse; dizziness; weakness; and fainting.

TREATMENT
First aid for shock after an injury includes measures to arrest bleeding (see *Bleeding, treatment of*), maintenance of an open airway, keeping the victim flat, reducing heat loss with blankets, and reassurance. A physician or ambulance should be called immediately, and no food or drink should be given.

Emergency treatment in hospital involves an *intravenous infusion* of fluid or a blood transfusion, *oxygen therapy*, and, if necessary, *morphine* or similar powerful painkillers. Further treatment depends on the underlying cause. (See also *Shock, electric; Toxic shock syndrome*.)

Shock, electric

The sensation caused by an electric current passing through the body, and its effects. A mild shock may produce a sense of having been slightly shaken. A current of sufficient size and duration can cause loss of consciousness, cardiac arrest (cessation of the heartbeat), respiratory arrest, burns, and tissue damage. (See also *Electrical injury*.)

Shock therapy

The use of electricity or other agents to produce a sudden and severe disturbance in the nervous system as a means of treating mental illness, particularly severe *depression*. The mechanism of action is unknown.

Only *ECT* (electroconvulsive therapy) is regularly used today. Insulin coma therapy (in which coma was induced by repeated injections of insulin) was a form of shock therapy used in the 1940s and 1950s; it was abandoned because of the risk of permanent, severe brain damage. Another earlier method, involving the use of drugs to stimulate the nervous system, was abandoned because patients often suffered fractures and other injuries due to violent seizures.

Short stature

A height significantly below the lower limit of the normal range for a person's age. Short stature is also called dwarfism or, sometimes, restricted growth.

Poor linear growth may be apparent from birth, may become evident in early or mid-childhood, or may begin at *puberty* if sex hormone production is defective.

CAUSES
There are many causes of short stature, although sometimes no cause is found. Short stature in children is often due to hereditary factors or to slow bone growth. In most cases, growth eventually speeds up, resulting in normal height.

Less commonly, short stature is due to a specific disorder. It may be caused by bone disease, as in untreated *rickets* or *achondroplasia* (a hereditary disorder in which the ends of the limb bones do not grow fully, resulting in disproportionately short limbs).

Certain disorders of the *endocrine system* will cause delayed growth. Examples are deficiency of *growth hormone*, and *hypothyroidism* (thyroid hormone deficiency), which also affects brain development. In these conditions, the ends of the long bones and the small bones of the hands and feet develop slowly, resulting in delayed bone age (see *Age*).

Emotional deprivation, common in abused or neglected children, chronic malnutrition (undernourishment), and untreated infections, such as *tuberculosis*, may also result in poor growth. Children with such conditions show a *failure to thrive* and are also underweight. *Malabsorption* (impaired absorption of important nutrients, such as protein, trace elements, and vitamins, from the intestine) can also limit growth. Causes include untreated *cystic fibrosis* and *celiac disease*.

Certain chromosomal disorders are responsible for short stature. In *Down's syndrome*, there is some stunting and in *Turner's syndrome*, the pubertal growth spurt is absent.

Other causes of restricted growth in children include the prolonged use of certain drugs, particularly *corticosteroid drugs* and *anticancer drugs*. Severe respiratory disease and congenital heart disease, in which the supply of oxygen to growing tissues is insufficient, also cause short stature unless they are treated.

INVESTIGATION
The physician takes into account the parents' height and looks for signs of any possible underlying disease.

Most importantly, the child's growth rate is determined by means of regular measurements of height plotted on a chart. If the growth rate is normal, it indicates that the child's short stature is probably due to heredity or to temporary slow skeletal development. Slow growth rate suggests that short stature has an abnor-

mal cause. A sudden drop in growth rate can indicate the onset of disease, such as an endocrine disorder affecting the thyroid gland.

Other tests may include *X rays* to determine bone age and *blood tests* to measure hormone levels.

TREATMENT
Any underlying disorder is treated as appropriate; for example, thyroxine is given if hypothyroidism is diagnosed. Growth hormone is given not only for growth hormone deficiency but may also be used to treat short stature due to disorders such as Turner's syndrome. Growth hormone is sometimes given in combination with the anabolic steroid oxandrolone. (See also *Growth, childhood*.)

Shoulder

The area of the body where the arm attaches to the trunk. The rounded bony surface at the front of the shoulder is the upper part of the *humerus* (upper-arm bone); the bony surfaces that form the top and back of the shoulder are parts of the *scapula* (shoulder blade). The *clavicle* (collarbone) articulates with the acromion (the bony prominence at the outer top part of the scapula) at the *acromioclavicular joint* and extends across the top of the chest to the *sternum* (breastbone), to which it is attached at the sternoclavicular joint.

Just below the acromion, on the outer wall of the scapula, is a socket

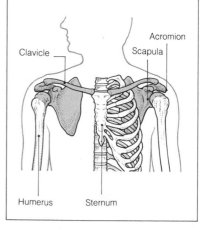

STRUCTURE OF THE SHOULDER
Three bones meet at the shoulder—the scapula (shoulder blade), clavicle (collarbone), and humerus (upper-arm bone). The shoulder is an example of a ball-and-socket joint.

Clavicle

Acromion

Scapula

Humerus

Sternum

S

(called the glenoid cavity) into which the head of the humerus fits to form the shoulder joint. A *bursa* (fluid-filled sac) under the acromion reduces friction at the joint. The shoulder joint is a ball-and-socket joint with a wide range of movement produced by part of the *biceps muscle*, several small muscles that make up the *rotator cuff*, various muscles in the chest wall, and the *deltoid* muscle (the muscle at the top of the upper arm and shoulder).

DISORDERS

Shoulder injuries are relatively common, including dislocation of the shoulder joint (see *Shoulder, dislocation of*) or of the acromioclavicular joint, and *fractures* of the clavicle or of the upper part of the humerus. Fractures of the scapula are less common.

The shoulder joint may be affected by any joint disorder, including *arthritis* and *bursitis* (inflammation of a bursa). In severe cases, a joint disorder may lead to *frozen shoulder* (a condition in which movements at the joint are extremely restricted). Movement of the shoulder may also be painful and/or restricted as a result of *tendinitis* (inflammation of a tendon) affecting the tendons of the shoulder muscles. Inflammation of a tendon or a bursa around a shoulder joint can cause *painful arc syndrome*, in which pain occurs while raising the arm to the side of the body. (See also *Bone* disorders box; *Joint*.)

Shoulder blade

The common name for the *scapula*.

Shoulder, dislocation of

Displacement of the head of the humerus (upper-arm bone) out of the shoulder joint. The most common type of dislocation is a forward and downward displacement, caused by a fall onto an outstretched hand or onto the shoulder itself. A backward dislocation may occur as a result of a powerful direct blow to the front of the shoulder or as a result of violent twisting of the upper arm, such as that caused by an electric shock or a seizure. Either type of dislocation may be accompanied by a fracture, usually of the humerus (see *Humerus, fracture of*).

The main symptom is pain in the shoulder and upper arm that is made worse by movement. A forward dislocation often produces obvious deformity of the shoulder; a backward dislocation usually does not.

A dislocation is diagnosed by *X rays*, which also reveal whether there is an accompanying fracture.

DISLOCATION OF SHOULDER
In this injury, the rounded head of the humerus (upper-arm bone) has been forced out of its socket just beneath the acromion (tip of the shoulder blade).

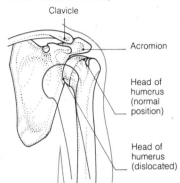

Forward dislocation of left shoulder
A forward and downward dislocation, as shown above, is the most common type.

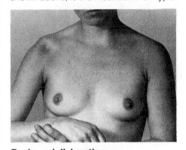

Backward dislocation
A pit can be seen in this woman's right shoulder where the head of the humerus is normally situated.

TREATMENT

Treatment is by reduction (maneuvering the head of the humerus back into the joint socket), which is usually performed under anesthesia. After reduction, X rays are taken to ensure the head of the humerus has been correctly repositioned; the shoulder is then immobilized in a sling for about three weeks. When the humerus has been fractured, treatment is usually the same, although the arm may require a longer period of immobilization.

COMPLICATIONS

A dislocation may damage nerves, causing weakness and numbness in the shoulder. Such nerve damage is usually temporary, with full recovery occurring within two to three months. Occasionally, a dislocation damages one of the arteries in the upper arm, causing pain and discoloration of the arm and the hand. In severe cases, *arterial reconstructive surgery* may be necessary.

A violent dislocation may damage the muscles that support the shoulder, making the joint susceptible to recurrent dislocation after only minor injuries. Such cases can often be successfully treated by surgery to tighten one of the supporting muscles.

Shoulder-hand syndrome

Pain and stiffness affecting one shoulder and the hand on the same side of the body; the affected hand may also become hot, sweaty, and swollen. The condition is also known as reflex sympathetic dystrophy. Because of the pain and stiffness, the arm cannot be used properly and the arm muscles may wither as a result of lack of use (see *Sudeck's atrophy*).

The precise cause of shoulder-hand syndrome is unknown, but the condition may occur as a complication of *myocardial infarction* (heart attack), *stroke*, *herpes zoster* (shingles), or a burn or other injury to the shoulder.

In most cases, recovery occurs within about two years. This period may be shortened by *physiotherapy* and treatment with *corticosteroid drugs*. In rare cases, a cervical *sympathectomy* (severing of nerves of the sympathetic nervous system on one side of the neck) is performed.

Shunt

An abnormal or surgically created passage between two normally unconnected parts. The term shunt is usually used to refer to a passage created to relieve abnormal fluid pressure around the brain in *hydrocephalus* or to relieve pressure in the portal veins in *portal hypertension*.

An *arteriovenous fistula* is a shunt between an artery and a vein, which may be created artificially to provide easy access to the bloodstream in people undergoing *dialysis*.

SHUNT FOR HYDROCEPHALUS

The shunt for hydrocephalus consists of two catheters and a valve to prevent backflow. The first catheter is inserted through the skull to drain fluid from the ventricles of the brain. The second is passed into another body cavity, usually the abdominal cavity or the right atrium of the heart, where the excess fluid is absorbed.

This procedure will need to be repeated several times during the first 10 years to replace the catheter as the child grows. In some cases, the shunt may become blocked or infected.

S

SHUNT FOR PORTAL HYPERTENSION

Various surgical procedures may be used to reduce pressure in the portal system (the veins that carry blood from the digestive organs and spleen to the liver) and thus reduce the risk of bleeding from *esophageal varices*. Shunts are made by creating a direct link between the portal system and the vena cava. Shunt operations prevent bleeding but do not improve liver function and, in fact, may worsen it. The operation itself carries a fairly high mortality that is related to the severity of the disease. Although bleeding is controlled, it is questionable whether survival is prolonged.

Shy-Drager syndrome

A rare degenerative condition that causes progressive damage to the *autonomic nervous system*. The cause of Shy-Drager syndrome is unknown. The condition begins gradually, affecting people between the ages of 60 and 70, and occurs more commonly in men than in women.

The main symptoms are postural *hypotension* (dizziness and fainting when getting up or after standing still for a long time), urinary incontinence, reduced ability to sweat, impotence, and *parkinsonism* (muscle tremor, rigidity, and slow movements). The condition worsens over several years, leading to disability and sometimes to premature death.

Although there is no cure and no means of slowing the inevitable degeneration, many of the symptoms, particularly the parkinsonism and low blood pressure, can be relieved by drug treatment.

SIADH

An abbreviation for syndrome of inappropriate antidiuretic hormone (secretion). SIADH is a condition in which there is excessive production of *ADH* (antidiuretic hormone), resulting in retention of water and a low level of sodium in the body.

CAUSES

SIADH may be associated with various underlying disorders. These include: cancers, such as small cell carcinoma of the lung (see *Lung cancer*), cancer of the pancreas (see *Pancreas, cancer of*), or *Hodgkin's disease*; certain lung diseases, such as *pneumonia* or chronic obstructive lung disease (see *Lung disease, chronic obstructive*); or brain disorders, such as *encephalitis*, a brain hemorrhage, or brain damage that results in the pituitary gland's overproducing ADH. Certain drugs,

such as chlorpropamide or *oxytocin*, may increase ADH production and lead to SIADH.

SYMPTOMS AND DIAGNOSIS

The symptoms of SIADH include weakness, tiredness, and confusion. The condition is diagnosed from the symptoms and from the results of tests that measure the level of ADH in the blood and compare the concentrations of sodium in the blood and in the urine.

TREATMENT

Treatment includes restriction of water intake, *diuretic drugs* to increase water loss, and saline infusions to increase the concentration of sodium in the body. However, these measures treat only the symptoms; the underlying cause must be treated successfully to bring about a cure.

Siamese twins

Two babies that are born physically joined, also known as conjoined *twins*. The name Siamese twins comes from the first recorded pair, Chang and Eng, who were born in Thailand (formerly Siam) in 1811 and lived for 63 years joined at the hip.

Siamese twins are essentially an identical set of twins that fail to separate completely, and thus grow independently, during development from a single fertilized egg. The cause is unknown.

Siamese twins range from two well-developed individuals, connected only by skin and superficial tissue, to a person with only one extra body part (such as an extra leg) as evidence of the second twin. Between these extremes are Siamese twins with two heads and two trunks joined at the waist but with only two legs.

In some cases one of the twins is very small and poorly developed. There are instances too where the internal organs and brains of Siamese twins may be separate, or some or all of these organs may be shared.

TREATMENT

If the twins survive birth, and if each one is sufficiently developed to function independently, complete separation by surgery may be possible.

Sibling rivalry

A term that describes the intense competition that sometimes occurs between siblings (brothers and/or sisters). It may occur, for example, after the birth of a new baby, when an older sibling constantly seeks to command the parents' attention. Feelings of rivalry may persist through life.

Sick building syndrome

A collection of symptoms sometimes reported by people who work in modern office buildings; the symptoms include loss of energy, headaches, and dry, itching eyes, nose, and throat.

The cause of the syndrome is unknown, although it has been attributed to air conditioning, passive exposure to tobacco smoke, loss of natural ventilation and light, and psychological factors, especially frustration at being unable to control physical conditions (e.g., temperature and ventilation) in the working environment. Less convincingly, it has been attributed to fluorescent lighting.

Treatment using environmental agents, such as ionizers, has been unsuccessful. Modification of the working environment may be the best solution.

Sickle cell anemia

 An inherited blood disease that occurs primarily in black people and, less commonly, in people of Mediterranean origin. In sickle cell anemia, the red cells are abnormal, resulting in a chronic, very severe form of *anemia* (reduced oxygen carrying capacity of the blood).

CAUSE

The red cells of affected people contain an abnormal type of *hemoglobin* (oxygen-carrying pigment) called hemoglobin S. In the blood capillaries, where there is less oxygen in the blood, the deficiency of oxygen causes hemoglobin S to crystallize, distorting the red cells into a sickle shape. This makes the cells fragile and easily destroyed, leading to hemolytic anemia. The abnormal cells are also unable to pass easily through tiny blood vessels, and this difficulty causes intermittent blockage of the blood supply to various organs, causing sickle cell crises.

Sickle cell anemia occurs in people who have inherited hemoglobin S from both their parents. If hemoglobin S is inherited from one parent, the person has sickle cell trait and is usually free of symptoms. If two such carriers have a child, there is a one in four chance that the child will have sickle cell anemia, a two in four chance that the child will have sickle cell trait, and a one in four chance that the child will have neither.

PREVALENCE

About one in 10 people of black origin carries the gene for the sickle cell trait.

S

The prevalence of sickle cell anemia within the black community is estimated at between 1 in 100 and 1 in 200.

SYMPTOMS AND SIGNS

The symptoms of sickle cell anemia usually first appear after the age of 6 months. Chronic hemolytic anemia causes its victims to suffer fatigue, headaches, shortness of breath on exertion, pallor, and *jaundice*.

Sickle cell crises are sometimes brought on by an infection, cold weather, or dehydration (caused, for example, by prolonged vomiting and diarrhea), but may also occur for no apparent reason. The crises start suddenly, and attack or damage various parts of the body. The sufferer may experience pains (especially in the bones), blood in the urine (from kidney damage), or damage to the lungs or intestines. The brain may also be affected, leading to *seizures*, a *stroke*, or unconsciousness.

In some children, the spleen enlarges and traps red cells at a particularly high rate, causing a severe, life-threatening form of anemia. From adolescence onward, the spleen usually shrivels and ceases to function; as a result, affected people are at risk of developing *septicemia* (blood poisoning) if they are infected by certain types of bacteria, especially pneumococci.

Children with sickle cell anemia have an increased risk of pneumococcal *pneumonia*. There is also an increased risk of *gallstones*.

DIAGNOSIS

The diagnosis is made from examination of a specially treated *blood smear* for the presence of sickle-shaped red cells and from *electrophoresis* to check for the presence of hemoglobin S.

TREATMENT

There is no cure for sickle cell anemia. Chronic hemolytic anemia is treated with a lifelong course of *folic acid* supplements. Affected children should be immunized against pneumococcal infection, and people who have sickle cell anemia may be advised to take a *penicillin drug* to guard against septicemia.

Because sickle cell crises can be life-threatening, they require prompt treatment. *Intravenous infusions* of fluids are given for dehydration, *antibiotic drugs* are given to treat and prevent infections, *oxygen therapy* is carried out to increase blood oxygenation, and *analgesic drugs* are given to relieve severe pain.

If a severe crisis does not respond to the above measures, an exchange *blood transfusion* may be performed to effect a temporary replacement of hemoglobin S. This may be done regularly for people who suffer frequent severe crises. Exchange transfusions may also be carried out during pregnancy to reduce the risk of a crisis (with possibly fatal consequences for mother and child) and before surgery, since anesthesia presents a hazard to people who have sickle cell anemia (and, to a lesser degree, to those with sickle cell trait).

OUTLOOK

Until about 30 years ago, sickle cell anemia usually proved fatal in childhood. Today, although the mortality is still high in those under 5 years old, improving methods of treatment have enabled more sufferers to survive into adulthood. Some sufferers are now having children.

Black people, and the close relatives of anyone with sickle cell anemia, who do not know whether they carry the sickle cell gene are advised to find out by having a blood test. A couple, both of whom have sickle cell anemia and/or trait, should obtain *genetic counseling* before starting a family. Tests can be performed in early pregnancy to determine whether a fetus has inherited a double dose of the sickle cell gene and thus will have sickle cell anemia.

Sick sinus syndrome

Abnormal function of the sinoatrial node (the heart's pacemaker) that leads to episodes of *bradycardia* (slow heart rate), alternating bradycardia and *tachycardia* (fast heart rate), or very short episodes of *cardiac arrest* (complete stoppage of the heartbeat). The most common cause of sick sinus syndrome is *coronary artery disease*, but the condition can also be caused by a *cardiomyopathy*.

Symptoms include light-headedness, dizziness, fainting, and, occasionally, palpitations (awareness of the heartbeat).

The diagnosis is confirmed by a 24-hour *ECG* recording. Treatment is usually by *antiarrhythmic drugs* and the fitting of an artificial *pacemaker*.

Side effect

A reaction or consequence of medication or therapy that is additional to the desired effect. The term usually (although not always) refers to an unwanted or adverse effect. It is not usually applied to the toxic effects produced by a drug overdose, but to a secondary effect of a normal dose.

A side effect may occur if the desired effect of therapy continues beyond the desired limits, such as when bleeding results from treatment with *anticoagulant drugs*. Alternatively, the side effect may be completely unrelated to the aim of therapy, such as when drowsiness results from *antihistamine drugs* prescribed to alleviate allergic *rhinitis* (hay fever). However, an unwanted side effect in one circumstance may be a desired effect in another (drowsiness is the desired effect when antihistamines are used as sedatives).

Side effects that can be expected from the known actions of a particular drug and that can occur in most patients taking that drug are known as type I side effects. Type II side effects occur in only a minority of patients and are usually unpredictable —until the physician discovers the connection between a particular drug and a patient's idiosyncratic response to it. Type II effects may be caused, for example, by a genetic disorder (such as the lack of a specific enzyme that usually inactivates the drug) or by an allergic reaction. Common type II side effects include a rash, swelling of the face, or jaundice. The occurrence of a type II side effect usually necessitates withdrawal of the drug.

Siderosis

Any of a variety of conditions in which there is too much *iron* in the body. Excess iron in the blood or tissues without associated damage is usually called *hemosiderosis*.

SIDS

An abbreviation for *sudden infant death syndrome*.

Sievert

The SI unit of equivalent absorbed dose of ionizing radiation (see *Radiation* units box).

Sight

See *Vision*.

Sight, partial

Loss of vision short of total *blindness*. Partial sight may involve a loss of *visual acuity*, of *visual field*, or of both.

Sigmoid colon

Also known as the pelvic colon, the S-shaped part of the *colon* in the lower abdomen which extends from the brim of the pelvis, usually down to the third segment of the *sacrum* (the triangular bone in the lower spine).

S

The sigmoid colon is connected to the descending colon above and the rectum below.

Sigmoidoscopy

Examination of the *rectum* and the *sigmoid colon* (last parts of the large intestine) with a viewing instrument called a sigmoidoscope or proctosigmoidoscope. Sigmoidoscopy is a form of *endoscopy*.

WHY IT IS DONE

Sigmoidoscopy is performed to investigate symptoms relating to the lower gastrointestinal tract, such as bleeding from the rectum or lower colon, and to look for evidence of disorders, such as polyps (small benign growths), *ulcerative colitis*, or cancer (see *Colon, cancer of*). Attachments on the end of the sigmoidoscope allow a *biopsy* (removal of a small sample of tissue for analysis) to be performed if necessary.

HOW IT IS DONE

Sigmoidoscopy is sometimes performed as a follow-up to a *rectal examination*, in which the physician examines the rectum with a gloved finger. Sigmoidoscopy may also be preceded by *proctoscopy* (an examination of the anal canal and rectum with a viewing instrument).

The procedure involved, along with a typical view through a sigmoidoscope, is shown in the illustrated box.

Sign

An objective indication of a disease or disorder (e.g., *jaundice*) that is observed or detected by a physician as opposed to a *symptom* (e.g., pain), which is noticed by the patient.

Silicone

Any of a specific group of silicon compounds. Silicones are defined as polymeric (long-chain), organic (carbon-containing) compounds of silicon and oxygen. They exist and are used medically in the form of oils, greases, plastics, or rubbers.

Synthetic silicones are widely used as implants in *cosmetic surgery* because they are resistant to body fluids, permeable to oxygen, and are not rejected by the body. Silicone oil in a silicone rubber bag is used in breast reconstruction or breast enlargement (see *Mammoplasty*).

Silicosis

A lung disease caused by the inhalation of dusts containing silica—a common mineral found in sand, quartz, and various types of rock. (See *Pneumoconiosis*.)

PROCEDURE FOR SIGMOIDOSCOPY

This is an outpatient procedure taking less than half an hour and needing no anesthetic. Either a rigid or a flexible endoscope (viewing tube) may be used. An *enema* may be given beforehand. The patient lies on the left side with knees drawn up. The entry of the lubricated instrument causes little discomfort.

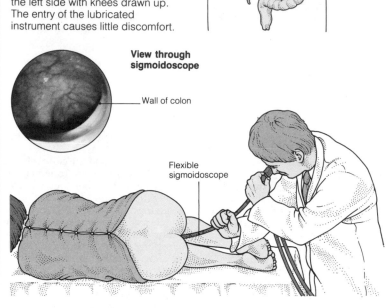

Transverse colon

Small intestine

Sigmoid colon

View through sigmoidoscope

Wall of colon

Flexible sigmoidoscope

Value of sigmoidoscopy

If the bowel is properly cleared of feces beforehand and distended by air pumped in through the instrument, a good view of the lining of the rectum and lower colon may be obtained. This area is often affected by benign growths, ulcers, or cancer. Direct observation of disorders allows early diagnosis and treatment.

Silver nitrate

An *astringent* occasionally used to treat inflamed or infected burns and wounds. Silver nitrate is also applied to the cervix (neck of the womb) to reduce bleeding from *cervical erosion*. In some countries, silver nitrate is used to prevent neonatal *ophthalmitis* (conjunctivitis in the newborn).

The application of silver nitrate may cause irritation or pain. If used on the skin for long periods silver nitrate can cause blue-black discoloration.

Silver sulfadiazine

An *antibacterial* agent that can be applied as a cream to prevent infections in burns. The silver in the drug contributes to its antibacterial action, and it is effective against a wide range of bacteria and yeasts. Its most common adverse effect is a skin irritation that may be difficult to distinguish from the burn itself.

Simethicone

Included as an antifoaming agent in many medications for the relief of gas and indigestion. (See *Antacid drugs*.)

Sinew

A common nonmedical term for a *tendon*, a tough fibrous cord that joins a muscle to a bone.

Singer's nodes

Small, grayish-white lumps or nodules that develop on the vocal cords as the result of constant voice strain. Singer's nodes occur in singers, teachers, politicians, and other people who use their voices excessively, causing hoarseness or loss of voice.

A *biopsy* (removal of a sample of tissue for microscopic examination) may exclude the possibility of there being a malignant tumor (see *Larynx, cancer of*). In acute cases, treatment consists of resting the voice. In

S

chronic cases, surgical removal of the nodes may be necessary. People who develop singer's nodes may benefit from voice training.

Sinoatrial node

The natural pacemaker of the *heart*. The sinoatrial node consists of a cluster of specialized muscle cells within the wall of the right atrium (upper chamber) of the heart. Without any external influence, these cells emit electrical impulses at a rate of 100 per minute, which initiate the contractions (beats) of the heart. Various hormones and nervous system activities can affect the node, causing it to emit impulses at a different rate, thus slowing down or speeding up the heart. (See also *Heart rate.*)

Sinus

A cavity within a bone, in particular one of the air-filled spaces, lined with mucous membrane, in the bones surrounding the nose (see *Sinus, facial,* and illustrated box overleaf).

The term sinus also refers to any wide channel that contains blood, such as the venous sinuses in the outermost covering of the brain.

Sinus is also a term for an abnormal, often infected, tract.

Sinus bradycardia

A slow, but regular, heart rate (less than 60 beats per minute). Sinus bradycardia is caused by reduced electrical activity in the sinoatrial node (the heart's pacemaker). Unlike *heart block,* there is no impairment to the transmission of electrical impulses through the heart. Sinus bradycardia is normal in athletes and in people who exercise regularly; it can be achieved by relaxation techniques.

Sinus bradycardia may also be caused by *hypothyroidism,* by a *myocardial infarction* (heart attack), or by taking certain drugs, such as *beta-blocker drugs* or *digoxin.*

Sinus, facial

Any of the air-filled cavities, lined with mucous membrane, in the bones surrounding the nose. The facial sinuses comprise: the two frontal sinuses in the frontal bone of the forehead just above the eyebrows; the two maxillary sinuses in the cheek bones; the two ethmoidal sinuses, which are honeycomblike cavities in bones that lie between the nasal cavity and the eye sockets; and the sphenoidal sinuses, which are a collection of air spaces in the large, winged bone

LOCATION AND FUNCTION OF THE SINOATRIAL NODE

The sinoatrial (SA) node is a small mass of muscle cells in the right atrium of the heart. It sends out impulses at an inherent rate of over 100 impulses per minute. External control by the vagus nerve reduces the rate to about 70 per minute. Other mechanisms also affect the rate.

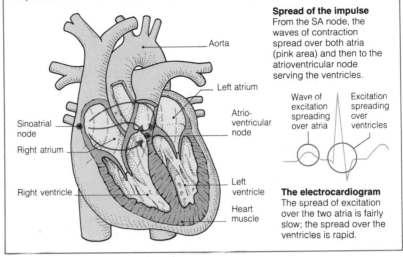

Aorta

Left atrium

Atrio-ventricular node

Sinoatrial node

Right atrium

Right ventricle

Left ventricle

Heart muscle

Spread of the impulse
From the SA node, the waves of contraction spread over both atria (pink area) and then to the atrioventricular node serving the ventricles.

Wave of excitation spreading over atria

Excitation spreading over ventricles

The electrocardiogram
The spread of excitation over the two atria is fairly slow; the spread over the ventricles is rapid.

behind the nose that forms the central part of the base of the skull. Mucus drains from each sinus along a narrow channel that opens into the nose.

Infection, usually spreading from the nose, may cause *sinusitis* (inflammation of the lining of the sinuses).

Sinusitis

Inflammation of the membrane lining the facial *sinuses* (the air-filled cavities in the bones surrounding the nose) caused by infection. The maxillary sinuses, in the cheek bones, and the ethmoidal sinuses, between the eyes, are the most commonly affected.

CAUSES

Most sinusitis is caused by infection spreading to the sinuses from the nose along the narrow passages that drain mucus from the sinuses into the nose. The disorder is usually the result of a bacterial infection that develops as a complication of a viral infection, such as the common *cold.* Less commonly, infection may arise from an abscess in an upper tooth (see *Abscess, dental*), from infected water being forced into the sinuses when a person jumps feet first into water without covering the nose, or from a severe facial injury.

INCIDENCE

Sinusitis is an extremely common disorder. Many people suffer an attack after every common cold. It seems that once the tendency to sinus infection is established, recurrence is more likely with each cold.

SYMPTOMS AND SIGNS

Sinusitis usually causes a feeling of tension or fullness in the affected area and sometimes a throbbing ache. It may also result in fever, a stuffy nose, and loss of the sense of smell.

A common complication is the formation of pus in the affected sinuses. Rare complications include orbital cellulitis (see *Orbit*), *osteomyelitis,* and *meningitis.*

DIAGNOSIS AND TREATMENT

X rays are sometimes taken to determine the location and extent of the disorder; a *culture* may be grown from a lavage (washing) of the maxillary sinus to identify the infective bacteria.

Antibiotic drugs are given immediately to combat the infection, but the antibiotic chosen may be changed after the result of a culture is known. Use of nose drops or a spray containing a *decongestant drug* restores drainage of the sinuses by reducing inflammation of the mucous membranes. Steam inhalations moisten the secretions and are helpful in removing them. If sinusitis persists despite this treatment, surgical drainage of the affected sinuses may be performed.

Sinus tachycardia

A fast, but regular, heart rate (more than 100 beats per minute). Sinus tachycardia is caused by increased electrical activity in the sinoatrial node (the heart's pacemaker). Such a heartbeat is normal during sudden stressful

S

LOCATION AND FUNCTION OF THE SINUSES

The air spaces, or sinuses, in the skull bones lighten the skull and improve the resonance of the voice. The sinuses surround the nose and are lined with mucous membrane. Mucus produced by this membrane drains into the nasal cavity via narrow channels.

Cross section through skull

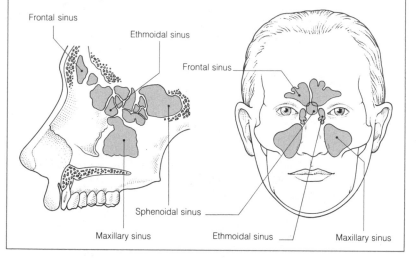

Frontal sinus
Ethmoidal sinus
Frontal sinus
Sphenoidal sinus
Maxillary sinus
Ethmoidal sinus
Maxillary sinus

or anxious moments. It is also normal during exercise and for a short time afterward. Persistent sinus tachycardia at rest may be caused by fever, *hyperthyroidism*, and other disorders. (See also *Tachycardia*.)

Situs inversus

An unusual condition in which the internal organs are situated in the mirror image of their normal positions. No treatment is required unless there is an associated abnormality of any of the organs, in which case surgery may be necessary. (See also *Dextrocardia*.)

Sjögren's syndrome

A condition in which the eyes and mouth become excessively dry. The nasal cavity, throat and vagina may also be affected. Sjögren's syndrome tends to occur with certain *autoimmune disorders*, such as *rheumatoid arthritis* or systemic *lupus erythematosus*. The exact cause is unknown. However, because the autoimmune disorder upsets the body's defense system, it begins to destroy the glands that produce lubricating secretions.

About 90 percent of sufferers are women—mostly middle-aged and often postmenopausal.

The most characteristic and troublesome feature of the condition is *keratoconjunctivitis sicca* (dry eye), which causes itching and burning of the eyes

and a sense that there is a foreign body under the eyelid. Artificial tears can be used to moisten the eye. Lack of saliva leads to an increased risk of dental *caries*; good oral hygiene and dental care are therefore essential. A water-soluble lubricating jelly may be used to facilitate sexual intercourse.

Skeleton

The average human adult skeleton has 213 *bones* (counting each of the nine fused *vertebrae* of the *sacrum* and *coccyx* as individual bones) joined with *ligaments* and *tendons* to form a protective and supportive framework for the attached muscles and underlying soft tissues of the body. In some people, however, there may be a variation in the number of vertebrae or there may be additional small bones (called sesamoids) in tendons around the joints.

STRUCTURE

The skeleton consists of two main parts, known as the axial and appendicular skeletons.

The axial skeleton comprises the *skull*, *spine*, *ribs*, and *sternum* (breastbone). Together, they have a total of 87 bones: 29 in the skull (including the *hyoid* bone and three pairs of auditory *ossicles*); 33 in the spine (seven cervical, 12 thoracic, and five lumbar vertebrae, the five fused vertebrae of the sacrum, and the four

fused vertebrae of the coccyx); and 25 in the chest (12 pairs of ribs and the sternum).

The appendicular skeleton consists of the two limb girdles (the *shoulder* and *pelvis*) and their attached limb bones. The appendicular skeleton includes 126 bones, 64 in the shoulders and upper limbs and 62 in the pelvis and lower limbs. There are two bones in each shoulder: the *clavicle* (collarbone) and *scapula* (shoulder blade); three in each arm—the *humerus* (upper-arm bone) and the *radius* and *ulna* (forearm bones); eight carpals in each *wrist*; five *metacarpals* in each palm; and 14 *phalanges* in the digits of each hand (two in each thumb and three in each finger).

The pelvic girdle consists of two innominate (hip) bones. There are 30 bones in each of the lower limbs: a *femur* (thigh bone), *patella* (kneecap), and *tibia* and *fibula* (lower leg bones) in each leg; seven tarsals in the *ankle*, heel (see *Calcaneus*), and back part of the foot; five *metatarsals* in the middle of each foot; and 14 phalanges in the toes (two in each big toe and three in each other toe).

There are only minor differences between the skeletons of men and women. In general, men's bones tend to be slightly larger and heavier than the corresponding bones in women; the female pelvic cavity is wider than that of the male to facilitate childbirth.

The individual bones of the skeleton are connected by three types of *joints*, which differ in the amount of mobility they permit.

FUNCTION

The skeleton plays an indispensable role in movement by providing a strong, stable but mobile framework on which the muscles can act. In effect, it consists of a series of independently movable internal levers on which the muscles can pull to move different parts of the body.

The skeleton also supports and protects body organs, notably the brain and spinal cord, which are encased in the skull and spine, and the heart and lungs, which are protected by the ribs. The ribs also make breathing possible by supporting the chest cavity so that the lungs are not compressed, and by helping in the breathing movements.

The skeleton is not an inert frame, however. It is an active organ that produces blood cells (formed in bone marrow) and acts as a reservoir for minerals such as calcium, which can be drawn on, if required, by other parts of the body.

S

BONES OF THE SKELETON

There are two main parts to the skeleton—the axial and appendicular skeletons (shown below). Some parts, such as the skull and pelvis, consist of several fused or associated bones. The skeleton is not merely an inert framework that supports and protects organs and makes movement possible; the bones are active living structures that constantly produce blood cells and interchange minerals with the blood.

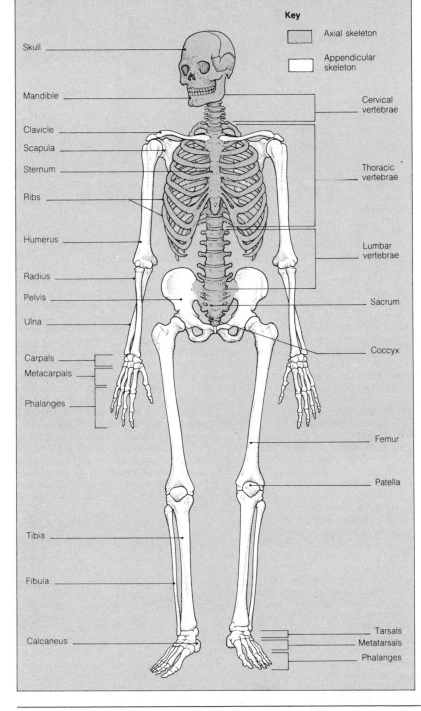

Key

Axial skeleton

Appendicular skeleton

Skull
Mandible
Clavicle
Scapula
Sternum
Ribs
Humerus
Radius
Pelvis
Ulna
Carpals
Metacarpals
Phalanges
Tibia
Fibula
Calcaneus

Cervical vertebrae
Thoracic vertebrae
Lumbar vertebrae
Sacrum
Coccyx
Femur
Patella
Tarsals
Metatarsals
Phalanges

Skin

The outermost covering of body tissue, which protects the internal organs from the environment. The skin is the largest organ in the body. Its cells are continually being replaced as they are lost by wear and tear.

STRUCTURE

The skin consists of a thin outer layer (the epidermis) and a thicker inner layer (the dermis). Beneath the dermis is the subcutaneous tissue, which contains fat. The *hair* and *nails* are extensions of the skin and are composed mainly of *keratin*, which is the main constituent of the outermost part of the epidermis.

EPIDERMIS The epidermis is made up of flat cells that resemble paving stones when viewed under the microscope. Its thickness varies depending on the part of the body, being thickest on the soles and palms and very thin on the eyelids. It is generally thicker in men than in women and normally becomes thinner with age.

The outermost part of the epidermis is composed of dead cells, which form a tough, horny, protective coating. As these dead cells are worn away, they are replaced. The new cells are produced by rapidly dividing living cells in the innermost part of the epidermis. Between the outer and inner parts is a transitional region that consists of both living and dead cells.

Most of the cells in the epidermis are specialized to produce keratin, a hard protein substance that is the main constituent of the tough, outermost part. Some of the cells produce the protective pigment *melanin*, which determines skin color.

DERMIS The dermis is composed of connective tissue interspersed with various specialized structures, such as hair follicles, *sweat glands*, and *sebaceous glands* (glands that produce an oily substance called *sebum*). The dermis also contains blood vessels, lymph vessels, and nerves.

FUNCTION

The skin's most important function is a protective one. It acts as the main barrier between the environment and the internal organs of the body, shielding them from injury, the harmful rays of sunlight, and invasion from infective agents, such as bacteria.

The skin is a sensory organ containing many cells that are sensitive to touch, temperature, pain, pressure, and itching. It also plays a role in keeping body temperature constant. When the body is hot, the sweat glands cool it by producing perspira-

S

tion and the blood vessels in the dermis dilate (widen) to dissipate heat; if the body gets cold, the blood vessels in the skin constrict (narrow), which conserves the body's heat.

The epidermis contains a unique fatty substance that makes the skin waterproof—thus making it possible to sit in a bath without soaking up the water like a sponge. The outer epidermis also has an effective water-holding capacity, which contributes to its elasticity and serves to maintain the body balance of fluid and electrolytes. If the water content drops below a certain level, the skin becomes cracked, reducing its efficiency as a barrier.

Skin allergy
Many substances can provoke an allergic reaction through direct contact with the skin of a susceptible person. However, the substance first must have sensitized the person's *immune system* during a previous contact. If the skin reaction is truly allergic, the causative substance produces symptoms only in susceptible people. Many substances (fiberglass spicules, for example) are irritant by nature, rather than allergenic, and can affect anyone.

There are two main types of allergic skin reaction. Contact allergic *dermatitis* consists of red, itchy patches, which may blister or form crusts. The patches correspond to the area of contact with the causative substance and develop between a few hours and two days after contact. Substances that can produce such a reaction include adhesives, elastic, nickel in jewelry, some plants, some cosmetics, and chromium salts used in hat and shoe manufacture.

Contact *urticaria* (red, itchy, raised areas on the skin) may develop within a few minutes to half an hour after skin contact with some medications, chemicals, plants, insect saliva (from a bite), and foods such as shellfish. Urticaria can also be a symptom of an allergic reaction to something eaten, but the majority of cases are probably not allergic in origin. Many drugs can cause skin eruptions, some of which resemble urticaria, but not all of them are allergic in nature.

Atopic *eczema* is an itchy skin condition which is most common in babies and children, particularly those with a family history of allergic-type illnesses such as asthma. Atopic eczema does not seem to be caused by skin contact with an allergen, but in some cases may be the result of a food allergy.

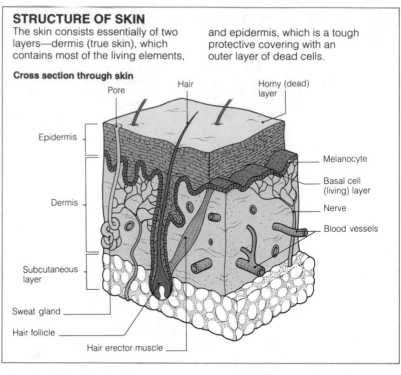

STRUCTURE OF SKIN
The skin consists essentially of two layers—dermis (true skin), which contains most of the living elements, and epidermis, which is a tough protective covering with an outer layer of dead cells.

Cross section through skin

Pore
Hair
Horny (dead) layer
Epidermis
Dermis
Subcutaneous layer
Sweat gland
Hair follicle
Hair erector muscle
Melanocyte
Basal cell (living) layer
Nerve
Blood vessels

In many skin allergies, the causative substance is obvious and contact with it should be minimized. In other cases, it may be difficult to know which ingredient (e.g., of a cosmetic) is the cause of allergy. The causative agent may be discovered only through exhaustive tests in which the skin is challenged by exposure to various suspected substances (see *Skin tests*).

Skin biopsy
Removal of a portion of diseased skin for laboratory analysis. Skin *biopsy* may be performed when *skin cancer* is suspected or to confirm the diagnosis of certain skin disorders, such as *pemphigus* or *dermatomyositis*.

Under local anesthesia, the skin is removed with a *scalpel* or a *curet*. When a highly malignant condition, such as *melanoma*, is suspected, all of the affected area is cut away, together with the skin around and beneath it. Otherwise, only a small portion of skin is removed. The wound usually requires minimal stitching and leaves little or no scar.

Skin cancer
A malignant tumor in the *skin*. Skin cancer is one of the most common forms of cancer.

Basal cell carcinoma, *squamous cell carcinoma*, and malignant *melanoma* are common forms of skin cancer related to long-term exposure to sunlight. *Bowen's disease*, a rare skin disorder that can become cancerous, may also be related to sunlight exposure. Less common types of skin cancer include *Paget's disease of the nipple* and *mycosis fungoides*; both produce inflammation similar to that of eczema. *Kaposi's sarcoma* is a type of skin cancer commonly found in patients with *AIDS* (although elderly patients may have Kaposi's sarcoma and not have AIDS).

Even though most skin cancers can be easily cured if treated at an early stage of the disease, many people die because they delay seeking treatment, especially from squamous cell carcinoma and malignant mela-

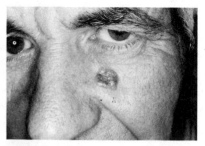

Basal cell carcinoma
This is the most common form of skin cancer. Also called rodent ulcer, it develops most commonly on the face.

S

noma. All changed or new skin growths should be seen by a physician.

Skin flap

A surgical technique in which a section of *skin* and underlying tissue, sometimes including muscle, is moved to cover an area from which skin and deeper tissue have been lost or damaged through injury, disease, or surgery.

WHY IT IS DONE

Unlike a *skin graft*, a flap retains its blood supply—either by remaining attached at one end to the donor site or through reattachment of its blood vessels to vessels at the new site. A flap is therefore useful for covering an area, such as exposed bone or tendon, that has lost its blood supply and on which a graft would not "take." Flaps are also used for regions that require thick covering to protect them (e.g., bony prominences like the hip). Because flaps are less likely to contract than skin grafts, they are useful for releasing tension from scarred areas. Skin flaps may be preferable to grafts because healing is more reliable and cosmetic results better.

HOW IT IS DONE

When the area to be covered is relatively small and there is sufficient skin near by, the flap may be left attached at one end and moved by stretching, rotating, or transposing it. Otherwise, the flap is removed from another area of the body and its vessels are attached to new arteries and veins at the site of the graft using microsurgical techniques (see illustrated box). The area left bare by cutting the flap is closed with stitches or, if necessary, by a skin graft. (See also *Microsurgery*.)

Skin graft

A technique used in plastic surgery to repair areas of lost or damaged *skin*. A piece of healthy skin is detached from one part of the body and transferred to the affected area. New cells grow from the graft and cover the damaged area with fresh skin.

Skin taken from an identical twin can be used for a graft, but skin from another person or an animal is soon rejected by the recipient's body (although it may provide useful temporary cover).

WHY IT IS DONE

A skin graft is performed because the area is too large to be repaired by stitching or because natural healing would result in scarring that might be unsightly or restrict movement.

TECHNIQUE FOR MOVING A SKIN FLAP

A flap of skin and underlying tissue can be moved to a new site to replace lost tissue; if its blood supply is maintained, the flap will adhere well. Microsurgery to rejoin blood vessels facilitates the technique.

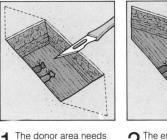

1 The donor area needs a good blood supply if muscle is also to be taken.

The ends of the donor area need to be tapered to allow satisfactory closure.

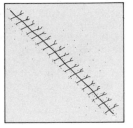

3 The skin may have to be undercut and freed before the wound is closed.

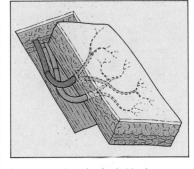

An artery and a vein of suitable size must be available at the recipient site to be joined to blood vessels in the flap.

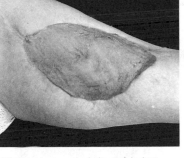

Skin flaps are particularly useful when there has been extensive loss of deep tissue. The results are usually excellent.

HOW IT IS DONE

Most grafts are performed by removing skin from the donor site and transferring it to the recipient site. There are two basic types of skin graft: split-thickness and full-thickness (see illustrated box overleaf). In some cases, underlying muscle is removed with the full thickness of skin (see *Skin flap*).

All grafts leave scars. Full-thickness grafts yield more natural color and texture, and contrast less than split-thickness grafts. However, full-thickness grafts are less likely to "take."

Skin infections

See *Skin* disorders box.

Skin peeling, chemical

A cosmetic operation to remove freckles, acne scars, delicate wrinkles, or other surface skin blemishes. A paste containing phenol (carbolic acid) or some other caustic agent is applied to the skin, left for a half hour, and then scraped off. The outer layers of the skin peel away with the paste.

Because of *photosensitivity*, the raw area must not be exposed to sunlight until new skin layers have fully grown. Permanent discoloration of the skin is common; it may be improved by wearing makeup.

Skin tag

A small, brown or flesh-colored, protruding flap of skin usually occurring spontaneously, but caused occasionally by unsatisfactory healing of a wound. Anal tags often occur as a complication of *anal fissures* or hemorrhoids. Skin tags can usually be removed easily by a physician.

Skin tests

Procedures for determining the body's reaction to various substances by injecting a small quantity of the substance underneath the skin or by applying it to the skin.

Patch tests are widely used in the diagnosis of contact allergic *dermatitis* (a type of skin allergy). Various suspected substances are applied by

S

means of adhesive patches to the skin. After a specific period of time, the patches are removed and the reactions observed. If one substance has caused reddening or blistering, the person is probably allergic to the substance and should try to avoid it in the future.

Substances injected under the skin may help identify allergens responsible for *asthma*, allergic *rhinitis* (hay fever), or other allergic-type illnesses, even though skin symptoms are not one of the primary features of these conditions. The tests may also be used to test immunity to certain infectious diseases (such as in the *tuberculin test*).

Skin tumors

A growth on or in the *skin* that may be cancerous (see *Skin cancer*) or benign (noncancerous).

Very common types of benign skin tumors include *keratoses* (wartlike growths caused by overproduction of keratin) and squamous *papillomas* (small, raised, sometimes stalked growths). Other benign skin tumors include *sebaceous cysts*, cutaneous *horns* (hard protrusions from the skin), *keratoacanthomas* (rapidly growing, flesh-colored nodules), and *hemangiomas* (birthmarks formed by a collection of blood vessels in the skin).

Skull

The bony skeleton of the head. The skull encases and protects the brain, houses organs of the special senses, provides points of attachment for muscles, and helps form the first parts of the respiratory and digestive tracts. Many of the bones are hollow, reducing the weight of the skull and adding to the resonance of the voice.

STRUCTURE

The arrangement of the bones in the skull is shown in the illustrated box on page 918. All the skull bones, except the mandible, are fixed to each other by immovable joints called sutures. The mandible articulates with the temporal bones at the freely movable temporomandibular joints.

Closely associated with, but not strictly part of, the skull are the hyoid (a small bone at the back of the tongue) and the auditory ossicles (the three tiny bones in each middle ear). The skull's cavities include the cranial cavity (which houses the brain), the nasal cavity (involved in smell and breathing), and the orbits (which house the eyeballs and their associated muscles). Part of the mouth is also formed by the skull.

TYPES OF SKIN GRAFT

The two main types of skin graft are split-thickness (in which less than the full thickness of skin is removed from the donor site) and full-thickness. There are advantages to each of these types.

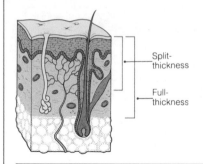
Split-thickness
Full-thickness

Split-thickness graft
When large areas need to be covered, such as after burns, split-thickness grafts are used and the donor sites are left to regenerate, which they do in a few days. Such sites can be repeatedly harvested.

Full-thickness graft
Full-thickness skin grafts are usually preferred for the face because they more closely match the appearance of normal skin. However, donor sites are limited and must be sutured (stitched).

HOW A FULL-THICKNESS GRAFT IS DONE

Most skin grafts are performed under general anesthesia. Full-thickness grafts are easily cut with a scalpel. Subcutaneous fat is avoided and any bleeding at the recipient site prevented.

1 Skin for a full-thickness graft is often taken from behind the ear.

2 The graft must be larger than the area to be covered, to allow for shrinkage.

3 Precise fitting and firm pressure are needed to ensure there is a satisfactory "take."

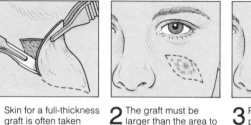
Dermatome
Scalpel

Instruments
Split-skin grafts are cut, usually from the abdomen or thigh, with an instrument called a dermatome. If necessary, the skin can be expanded into a trellislike mesh on the donor site.

Several of the skull bones, notably the maxillas, sphenoid bone, frontal bone, and ethmoid bone, contain *sinuses* (air-filled spaces); these sinuses are called the paranasal sinuses. In addition, there are spaces in the temporal bones that house the structures of the middle and inner ear.

In the cranium, there are many holes for the passage of nerves and blood vessels. Passing through are the *cranial nerves* (which supply most of the sensory structures and muscles of the head and neck) and blood vessels, such as the *carotid arteries* and *jugular veins* (which carry blood to and

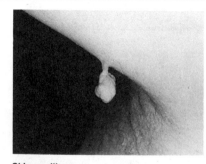

Skin papilloma
This harmless type of tumor is common in elderly people. It can easily be snipped off (and the base cauterized) by a physician.

S

DISORDERS OF THE SKIN

The skin is the largest and most vulnerable organ of the body. Although skin conditions are seldom life-threatening, many can be severely debilitating and cause psychological problems.

CONGENITAL DISORDERS

A *birthmark* is a type of *nevus* (pigmented skin blemish) present from birth. Nevi include moles, freckles, and *hemangiomas*, such as port-wine stains and strawberry marks.

INFECTION AND INFLAMMATION

Viral infections of the skin include *cold sores*, *warts*, *chickenpox*, *molluscum contagiosum*, and *herpes zoster* (shingles). Bacterial infections include *boils*, *cellulitis*, *erysipelas*, and *impetigo*. Fungal infections, such as *tinea*, cause *athlete's foot* and ringworm.

Inflammation of the skin occurs in *dermatitis* and *eczema*; it may be caused by an allergic reaction to a substance (such as nickel), a detergent, a plant, or a drug. *Psoriasis* is a common and persistent skin disease of unknown cause that consists of large, red patches with silvery, scaly surfaces. *Prickly heat* is an irritating rash that is caused by blockage of the sweat glands.

TUMORS

Benign (noncancerous) tumors of the skin are extremely common; these include seborrheic *keratoses* and most types of nevi. *Bowen's disease* is a skin disorder that may slowly become cancerous. Three common forms of skin cancer are *basal cell carcinoma*, *squamous cell carcinoma*, and malignant melanoma (see *Melanoma, malignant*). Less common skin cancers include *Paget's disease of the nipple*, *mycosis fungoides*, and *Kaposi's sarcoma*.

INJURY

The skin is vulnerable to many minor injuries, including cuts and bites (see *Bites, animal*; *Insect bites*) as well as more serious *wounds*. *Burns* can be among the most serious of all skin injuries and may cause extensive scarring or death.

HORMONAL DISORDERS

Acne is partly related to the action of androgens (male sex hormones) on the sebaceous glands; it is common among adolescents.

NUTRITIONAL DISORDERS

Deficiency of vitamins A, B, and C can cause *rashes* and other problems.

IMPAIRED BLOOD SUPPLY

Leg ulcers, which are particularly common in the elderly, may be caused by poor blood flow to the skin as a result of *atherosclerosis*, by poor drainage of blood through *varicose veins*, or by the leg swelling associated with heart failure.

DRUGS

Many drugs, including antibiotics, barbiturates, and sulfonamides, may cause a rash. Some cause *urticaria* (hives), others cause *eczema* or a measleslike rash, and some cause *photosensitivity*.

RADIATION

All forms of radiation are potentially damaging to the skin. Overexposure to sunlight (ultraviolet radiation) causes premature aging of the skin and increases the risk of skin cancer (see *Sunlight, adverse effects of*). High doses of other forms of radiation, such as X rays, may cause severe injury to the skin and may lead to cancer.

AUTOIMMUNE DISORDERS

These disorders include *lupus erythematosus*, a disorder that may affect the skin alone or the skin and other organs; *vitiligo*, characterized by pure white patches and caused by destruction of the skin's pigment cells; *dermatomyositis*, characterized by a specific skin rash and muscle weakness; *morphea* and *scleroderma*, in which there is progressive hardening of the skin and other tissues; and *pemphigoid* and *pemphigus*, in which large blisters develop on the skin.

OTHER DISORDERS

A *keloid* is an abnormally large and protruding *scar* caused by the continuing production of scar tissue long after healing would usually be complete. *Striae* (stretch marks) often develop during pregnancy and may also develop as a side effect of treatment with *corticosteroid drugs*.

Erythema simply means redness and has many possible causes. *Purpura* is a condition in which blood leaks into tissues, giving rise to *petechiae* (tiny pinpoints of blood) or larger bruises.

Xanthelasma are yellowish patches that tend to occur on the eyelids; they are a result of the deposition of cholesterol.

INVESTIGATION

Most skin disorders can be diagnosed from their physical characteristics. A *skin biopsy* (removal of a tissue sample for microscopic analysis) may also be performed, usually to aid in the diagnosis of a skin problem or to exclude skin cancer.

---

from the brain). The largest of the holes, called the foramen magnum, is situated in the occipital bone (which forms part of the base and back of the cranium); this hole allows the brain stem to enter the spinal canal, where it continues as the spinal cord.

The skull rests on the first cervical vertebra, called the atlas, which is a ring-shaped bone that articulates with the occipital bone and permits nodding movements of the head. Turning the head is a function of the joint between the atlas and the second cervical vertebra, called the axis. The occipital bone, atlas, and axis are connected by numerous small muscles.

DISORDERS

The skull may be affected by any bone disorder (see *Bone* disorders box) that involves the skeleton, such as *Paget's disease*, but the most common disorder is injury. A blow to the head may cause a fracture (see *Skull, fracture of*), which may result in damage to the brain, and, if a foramen is involved, in damage to a blood vessel or cranial nerve. (See also *Head injury*.)

Skull, fracture of

A break in one or more of the bones of the *skull* caused by injury to the head. A fracture of the skull may be either a closed (or simple) fracture, in which there is no displacement of the broken pieces, or an open (or depressed) fracture, in which displacement of the bone fragments occurs.

Because the skull is extremely strong, most skull fractures are closed and cause no complications. However, severe injury to the head may result in an open fracture in which the bone fragments are displaced, usually inward. In this case, the blood vessels in the *meninges* (the membranes that cover the brain) may be ruptured, resulting in an *extradural hemorrhage* (bleeding into the space between the skull and the outer membrane) or a *subdural hemorrhage* (bleeding into the space between the outer and middle membranes). The resultant blood clot may press on and displace brain tissue. Less commonly, all the meninges may be torn, and the brain itself may be damaged.

SYMPTOMS AND SIGNS

The degree of brain injury does not always correlate with the degree of skull damage. Some injuries cause a skull fracture but little or no brain damage. Other injuries cause severe brain damage even though there is no fracture of the skull.

The symptoms and signs of skull fractures (see *Head injury*) depend mainly on the degree of brain damage sustained. Leakage of cerebrospinal fluid (the liquid that bathes the brain and spinal cord) through the nose or ears indicates rupture of the meninges by a fracture of the base of the skull.

DIAGNOSIS

Any person who has suffered a significant blow to the head—particularly a blow that has caused unconsciousness, even if only for a very brief period—should consult a physician without delay, even if there are no symptoms. If the physician suspects a hemorrhage, *CT scanning* may be performed.

TREATMENT

A person with a closed fracture is hospitalized and observed closely for 12 to 24 hours for signs of complications. If no signs develop, treatment is generally not necessary because the fracture usually heals by itself.

An open fracture often requires treatment by a neurosurgeon. A hemorrhage may necessitate a *craniotomy* to drain the blood and repair damaged vessels. When deeply depressed fractures have penetrated the meninges and brain tissue, an operation is performed to raise or remove the pieces of fractured bone and repair the damaged tissue. After such an operation, there may be some degree of skull distortion.

Antibiotic drugs are given for all open fractures because of the risk of infection of the meninges (see *Meningitis*) or of the brain itself (see *Encephalitis*).

Skull X ray

A technique for providing images of the *skull*.

WHY IT IS DONE

X rays of the skull are usually taken after a *head injury* to look for a fracture (see *Skull, fracture of*) or to locate any foreign bodies in the soft tissues within the skull.

A skull X ray that appears normal does not rule out the possibility that the victim has suffered significant brain injury. If such an injury is suspected, or if a skull fracture is found, *CT scanning* of the brain is also performed.

Skull X rays are useful in the evaluation of a variety of conditions that affect the bones of the skull, such as *pituitary tumors* or metabolic disorders (e.g., *hyperparathyroidism*), and in the evaluation of tumors that have spread to the skull bones.

HOW IT IS DONE

X rays of the skull are taken from different angles by a technician. Depending on the number of views taken, the procedure usually takes about 20 minutes. The X-ray films are interpreted by a radiologist.

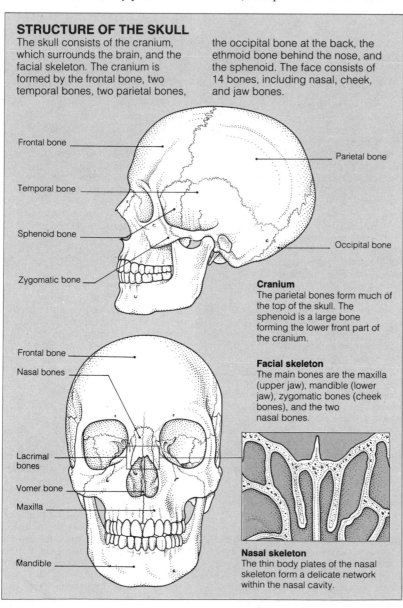

STRUCTURE OF THE SKULL

The skull consists of the cranium, which surrounds the brain, and the facial skeleton. The cranium is formed by the frontal bone, two temporal bones, two parietal bones, the occipital bone at the back, the ethmoid bone behind the nose, and the sphenoid. The face consists of 14 bones, including nasal, cheek, and jaw bones.

Frontal bone

Temporal bone

Sphenoid bone

Zygomatic bone

Parietal bone

Occipital bone

Cranium
The parietal bones form much of the top of the skull. The sphenoid is a large bone forming the lower front part of the cranium.

Facial skeleton
The main bones are the maxilla (upper jaw), mandible (lower jaw), zygomatic bones (cheek bones), and the two nasal bones.

Frontal bone

Nasal bones

Lacrimal bones

Vomer bone

Maxilla

Mandible

Nasal skeleton
The thin body plates of the nasal skeleton form a delicate network within the nasal cavity.

S

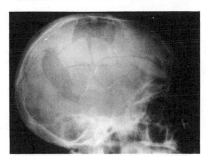

Multiple skull fracture
This side-view X ray shows the cranium smashed into several pieces. Some pieces have been surgically removed.

SLE

The abbreviation for the disorder systemic *lupus erythematosus*.

Sleep

The natural state of lowered consciousness and reduced *metabolism*. Sleep takes up about one third of an average person's life.

PHYSIOLOGY

EEG recordings of the electrical impulses produced by the brain during sleep show that there are two distinct types of sleep, known as REM (rapid eye movement) and NREM (nonrapid eye movement) sleep. These two types alternate in cycles lasting roughly 90 minutes throughout the sleep period. NREM sleep, which accounts for the major part of sleep, starts with drowsiness; brain waves become increasingly deeper and slower until brain activity and metabolism fall to their lowest level. Dreams are infrequent.

In REM sleep, the brain suddenly becomes more electrically active (with a wave pattern resembling that of an awake person) and its temperature and blood flow increase. The eyes move rapidly and *dreaming* occurs. REM sleep, also known as paradoxical sleep, periodically interrupts NREM sleep. The first REM period usually takes place 90 to 100 minutes after the onset of sleep and lasts about five to 10 minutes. REM sleep periods increase in length as sleep continues; the last of a night's four or five REM sleep periods may last about an hour. REM sleep occupies about one half of sleep time in babies and about one fifth of sleep time in adults.

FUNCTIONS OF SLEEP

Sleep is a fundamental human need, as is shown by the detrimental effects of *sleep deprivation*. However, it is not understood exactly in what way sleep is beneficial, or why a few, extremely rare individuals sleep very little yet suffer no ill effects. Apart from the obvious theory that the brain and metabolic processes require periodic rest to function efficiently, it has been suggested that dreaming is necessary to enable the brain to sort out information gathered during waking hours.

SLEEP REQUIREMENTS

The need for sleep decreases with age. A 1-year-old baby requires about 14 hours of sleep a day, a child of 5 about 12 hours, and adults about seven to eight hours. However, these amounts can vary from person to person: some adults need to sleep 10 hours or more a day, while others function efficiently on half that amount or less.

As people age, their ability to sustain sleep generally declines. Elderly people tend to sleep less than younger adults at night but doze more during the day.

SLEEP DISORDERS

Sleep disorders are divided into four main categories: difficulty in falling asleep or in remaining asleep (see *Insomnia*); difficulty in staying awake (see *Narcolepsy*; *Sleep apnea*); disruption in the sleeping/waking cycle (see *Jet lag*); and other problems that interfere with sleep (see *Bed-wetting*; *Night terrors*; *Sleepwalking*).

Sleep apnea

Episodes of temporary cessation of breathing, lasting 10 seconds or longer, which occur during *sleep*.

People with sleep apnea may not be aware of having any problem during the night, but they may be excessively sleepy during the day, with poor memory and difficulty in concentrating. This can interfere with work and social activities and, in children, with school performance.

SLEEP PATTERNS

The brain does not rest when a person is sleeping, but there is some reorganization of activity within it.

EEGs (electroencephalograms) and other recordings reveal cyclical patterns to this activity.

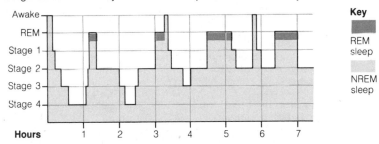

Key
REM sleep
NREM sleep

Phases of sleep
There are two types of sleep, REM (rapid eye movement) and NREM (nonrapid eye movement). They can be distinguished by the presence or absence of REMs and by EEGs or other recordings. The chart shows how a sleeper passes in cycles between the four stages of NREM sleep during the night, with bursts of REM sleep.

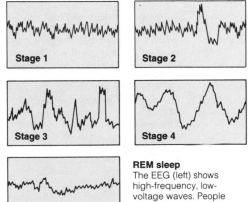

Stage 1

Stage 2

Stage 3

Stage 4

REM sleep

REM sleep
The EEG (left) shows high-frequency, low-voltage waves. People awakened during REM sleep often report dreams.

NREM sleep
This is sometimes called orthodox sleep; in adults it makes up about 80 percent of the sleeping pattern. It has four stages of progressively greater "depth" of sleep, characterized by EEG waves (left) of increasingly larger voltage (amplitude) and lower frequency (number of waves per second). People awakened during NREM sleep often report they were "thinking" about everyday matters but rarely report dreams.

S

Severe sleep apnea is a potentially serious condition, because it may result in *hypertension* (high blood pressure), *heart failure* (reduced pumping efficiency), *myocardial infarction* (heart attack), or *stroke*.

Sleep apnea may be classified as obstructive, central, or mixed.

OBSTRUCTIVE SLEEP APNEA This is the most common type and may affect anyone. As many as one in 100 men between the ages of 30 and 50 may have the condition. The typical sufferer is overweight and a heavy snorer. People with obstructive sleep apnea who are very obese and excessively sleepy are said to have *pickwickian syndrome*. Obstructive sleep apnea has been linked with some instances of *sudden infant death syndrome*.

The most common cause of obstructive sleep apnea is overrelaxation of the muscles of the soft *palate* in the *pharynx* (throat). The muscles sag and obstruct the passage of air during sleep. Obstruction to the passage of air may also be caused by enlarged *tonsils* or *adenoids*, or by an abnormally large tongue or small jaw.

In all cases, the obstruction to air movement usually causes loud snoring. If a complete obstruction occurs, breathing stops. Failure to breathe triggers the brain to restart breathing, and as breathing recommences, a gasp is produced and the person may waken briefly.

CENTRAL SLEEP APNEA In this form, breathing stops because the diaphragm and chest muscles temporarily cease to work, probably as a result of a disturbance in the brain's control of breathing. Causes include paralysis of the *diaphragm* muscles, and disorders of the *brain stem*. Snoring is not a predominant feature.

MIXED SLEEP APNEA This is a combined form of sleep apnea. Usually, there is a short period of central sleep apnea, followed by a longer period of obstructive sleep apnea.

TREATMENT
People who are overweight should attempt to lose weight. Alcohol and sleeping drugs should be avoided, as both interfere with the mechanism of breathing and may aggravate sleep apnea. Tricyclic *antidepressant drugs* may help in milder cases. Some patients with severe sleep apnea benefit from treatment with continuous positive airway pressure (CPAP). In CPAP, air from a compressor is forced into the airway via a mask worn over the nose. Nighttime artificial *ventilation* may be needed.

In some cases, surgical treatment is necessary to relieve obstruction. *Tonsillectomy* (removal of the tonsils), *adenoidectomy* (removal of the adenoids), or *tracheostomy* (creation of an opening into the windpipe, allowing air to flow directly to the lungs) may be performed, depending on the cause of the problem. An operation called uvulo-palato-pharyngoplasty (UPPP) to shorten the soft palate may be recommended in extreme cases.

Sleep deprivation
An insufficient amount of *sleep*. Studies of sleep-deprived volunteers have shown that irritability and a shortened attention span may occur after a night in which there was less than three hours' sleep.

After longer periods without sleep, individuals become increasingly unable to concentrate and their performance of tasks deteriorates as they continually slip into short periods of "microsleep." People with epilepsy are more prone to *seizures* after sleep deprivation. Three days or more without sleep may lead to visual and auditory *hallucinations* and, in some cases, to *paranoia*.

Sleep deprivation has been employed as a form of torture, in order to extract confessions, and as a brainwashing technique.

Sleeping drugs

COMMON DRUGS
Benzodiazepines
Flurazepam Temazepam Triazolam
Others
Chloral hydrate
Dichloralphenazone
Promethazine

A group of drugs used in the treatment of *insomnia*. Sleeping drugs include *benzodiazepine drugs*, the drugs most commonly used for this particular problem, *antihistamine drugs*, *antidepressant drugs*, and *chloral hydrate*.

WHY THEY ARE USED
Sleeping drugs may be given to reestablish the habit of sleeping, usually after self-help measures (for example, taking a warm bath or drinking hot milk before going to bed) have not worked. These drugs promote sleep by reducing the activity of nerve cells within the brain.

HOW THEY ARE USED
Sleeping drugs should always be taken in the smallest effective dose for the shortest period of time. In general,

they should be taken for no longer than three weeks and, preferably, not every night. Sleeping drugs may cause drowsiness, unsteadiness, and impaired concentration on waking. These effects can be hazardous to the elderly, who are prone to falls, and they can affect a person's ability to drive or to operate machinery.

Long-term use of sleeping drugs may induce *tolerance* (needing a higher dose to have the same effect) and *dependence* (which produces withdrawal symptoms when the person stops taking the drug).

Sleeping sickness
A serious infectious disease of tropical Africa caused by the protozoan (single-celled) parasite TRYPANOSOMA BRUCEI. The disease is also known as African trypanosomiasis.

There are two forms. One, occurring in West and Central Africa, is spread primarily from person to person. The other occurs in East Africa and mainly affects wild animals, but is occasionally transmitted to humans. Both forms are spread by the bites of tsetse flies, which transmit the protozoa to people and animals. Within humans, the parasites multiply and spread to the bloodstream, lymph nodes, heart, and brain.

SYMPTOMS AND SIGNS
With both forms of sleeping sickness, a painful nodule develops at the site of the tsetse fly bite.

In the West African form, the disease then takes a slow course, with bouts of fever and lymph node enlargement. After months or years, spread to the brain occurs, causing headaches, confusion, and, eventually, severe lassitude. The victim may become completely inactive, have drooping eyelids, and a vacant expression. Without treatment, coma and death follow.

The East African form runs a faster course. A severe fever develops within a few weeks of infection, and effects on the heart may be fatal before the disease has spread to the brain.

DIAGNOSIS AND TREATMENT
Microscopic examination of the blood, lymph fluid withdrawn from a lymph node, or cerebrospinal fluid obtained by a *lumbar puncture* reveals the presence of the parasites.

Drugs are effective against the parasites but may cause severe side effects. In most cases, a complete cure can be achieved, although there may be residual brain damage if the infection has already spread to the brain.

S

CYCLE OF SLEEPING SICKNESS

The life cycle of the trypanosomes that cause sleeping sickness is shown. They multiply in a person's blood and lymph vessels and may spread to the brain or heart with serious effects.

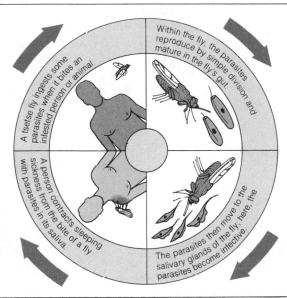

A tsetse fly ingests some parasites when it bites an infested person or animal.

Within the fly, the parasites reproduce by simple division and mature in the fly's gut.

The parasites then move to the salivary glands of the fly; here, the parasites become infective.

A person contracts sleeping sickness from the bite of a fly with parasites in its saliva.

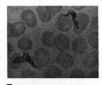

Trypanosomes
The parasites are shown here in blood.

PREVENTION

Sleeping sickness is controlled by eradication measures directed against the tsetse fly. Nevertheless, tens of thousands of Africans—and some visitors to safari parks—still contract the disease each year.

To avoid sleeping sickness, visitors to rural parts of Africa should take measures to protect themselves against tsetse fly bites (see *Insect bites*).

Sleep paralysis

The sensation of being unable to move at the moment of going to sleep or when waking up. The experience may be accompanied by *hallucinations*, which often are frightening. Sleep paralysis most often occurs in people with *narcolepsy*, but occasionally affects otherwise healthy people. Although alarming, the sensation rarely lasts for more than a few seconds. (See also *Cataplexy*.)

Sleep terror

See *Night terror*.

Sleepwalking

Walking while asleep, also known as somnambulism. Sleepwalking occurs during NREM (nonrapid eye movement) *sleep*, or during arousal from this type of sleep, and does not represent the acting out of dreams. Some people show a regular tendency to sleepwalk.

Usually a sleepwalker calmly gets out of bed, wanders around aimlessly for a few minutes, and then goes back to bed. Sometimes sleepwalking arises from a *night terror*, in which case the sleepwalker's behavior is more frantic and may involve shrieking or thrashing. He or she sometimes talks (usually simple words or phrases) during the sleepwalk, urinates in an inappropriate place, or gets into the wrong bed. Waking the sleepwalker is difficult and unnecessary; steer him or her gently back to bed. Take precautions, such as blocking off the stairs, to avoid injury.

Sleepwalking in children is seldom associated with psychological problems, although it may be aggravated by anxiety, and tends to disappear naturally with age. Sleepwalking in adults may be related to anxiety, or may be associated with use of sleeping pills, especially in the elderly.

Slimming

See *Weight reduction*.

Sling

A device used to immobilize, support, or elevate an arm. A sling is usually made from a triangular *bandage*, although an emergency sling can be created from a belt, tie, or scarf.

An arm sling may be used as a first aid measure to support the arm following a fracture, sprain, or other injury (see illustrated box overleaf). A sling may also be used after an operation on the hand or arm, or if the arm is infected.

An elevation sling is a type of sling that is used to hold the hand in a well-raised position to control bleeding or to prevent movement of the arm and shoulder if the clavicle (collarbone) is broken or the shoulder dislocated. This type of sling is applied in a similar fashion to an arm sling, except that the victim's arm is placed across the chest with the fingers nearly touching the opposite shoulder.

Slipped disk

See *Disk prolapse*.

Slipped femoral epiphysis

See *Femoral epiphysis, slipped*.

Slit lamp

An illuminated microscope that is used to examine the internal structures of the front part of the eye. The use of special lenses allows the slit lamp to be used to examine the retina. (See also *Eye, examination of*.)

Slough

Dead tissue that has been shed from its original site. Examples of sloughing include the loss of dead skin cells from the skin's surface and the shedding of the lining of the uterus during menstruation. Sloughing also occurs as part of the healing process.

Slow virus diseases

A group of diseases of the central nervous system (brain and spinal cord) that occur many months or even years after infection with a virus. The diseases take a slow course in which there is gradual widespread destruction of nerve tissue. This causes progressive loss of brain function and, at present, a fatal outcome.

Slow virus diseases in humans include *Creutzfeldt-Jakob syndrome*, *kuru*, possibly a form of *Alzheimer's disease*, subacute sclerosing panencephalitis (a complication of measles), and possibly the brain disease that occurs in some people infected with *HIV*.

Slow virus diseases in animals include scrapie, which has been known in sheep for many years, and bovine spongiform encephalopathy (BSE) in cows, which is a new disease transmitted in feedstuffs containing contaminated sheep and cattle nervous tissue. These diseases are unlikely to be transmitted to humans.

Small cell carcinoma

The most dangerous and rapidly spreading form of *lung cancer*. Also called oat cell carcinoma, this type of tumor accounts for about 25 percent

S

FIRST AID: ARM SLING

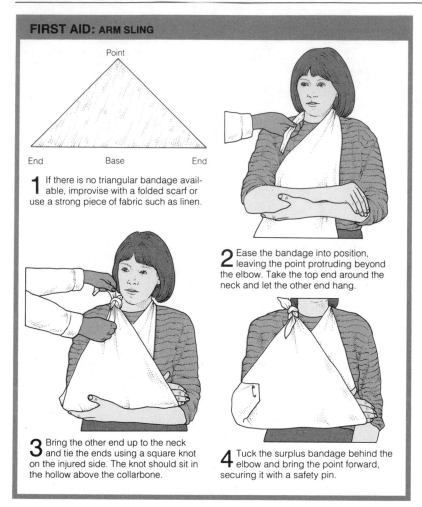

1 If there is no triangular bandage available, improvise with a folded scarf or use a strong piece of fabric such as linen.

2 Ease the bandage into position, leaving the point protruding beyond the elbow. Take the top end around the neck and let the other end hang.

3 Bring the other end up to the neck and tie the ends using a square knot on the injured side. The knot should sit in the hollow above the collarbone.

4 Tuck the surplus bandage behind the elbow and bring the point forward, securing it with a safety pin.

S

of lung cancers. Most small cell carcinomas reach an inoperable stage by the time a diagnosis is made. The extension of a life by surgery is achieved in about 10 percent of cases, but, even in these people, the outlook is poor. Spread to other parts of the body is almost inevitable.

Treatment is usually with *anticancer drugs* with or without *radiation therapy*. *Bone marrow transplants* are also currently being tried.

Smallpox

A highly infectious viral disease, common in the 19th century and before, with the distinction of having been totally eradicated by a successful worldwide vaccination campaign. The World Health Organization declared smallpox extinct in 1980.

Smallpox was transmitted from person to person; it was characterized by an illness resembling influenza and a rash that spread over the body and eventually developed into pus-filled blisters. The blisters became crusted and would sometimes leave deeply pitted scars. Complications included blindness, pneumonia, and kidney damage. There was no effective treatment for the disease, which killed up to 40 percent of its victims.

Eradication was achieved through the cooperative international use of a highly effective vaccine. Eradication was possible because smallpox affected only humans, cases of infection were easily recognized, and victims of the disease were infectious to others only for a short time. These characteristics are shared by some other diseases (e.g., measles, another possible candidate for eradication).

Smallpox vaccination certificates are no longer required for travel abroad, and most countries have discontinued vaccination because there is no longer any risk of the disease and because there is a risk of encephalitis from the vaccine. The virus responsible for smallpox is still maintained at a few research laboratories.

Smear

A specimen for microscopic examination prepared by spreading a thin film of cells onto a glass slide. A common use is in the *cervical smear test*.

Smegma

An accumulation of sebaceous gland secretions beneath the foreskin in an uncircumcised male, usually as a result of poor hygiene.

Fungal or bacterial infection of smegma may cause *balanitis* (inflammation of the glans). In a child with *phimosis* (tight foreskin), smegma occasionally hardens into a small stone, known as a smegma pearl. The higher incidence of cancer of the penis in uncircumcised men who smoke may be due to the build-up of cancer-inducing substances in the smegma.

An uncircumcised man should wash his penis daily with the foreskin retracted to prevent an accumulation of smegma.

Smell

One of the five senses. The mechanisms by which smell is perceived are shown in the illustrated box.

DISORDERS

Disturbance of the sense of smell may consist of anosmia (loss of smell, which may be complete or partial, temporary or permanent) or dysosmia (abnormal smell perception). The senses of smell and *taste* are closely connected, so disturbances of smell usually result in disturbances of taste.

Temporary partial anosmia frequently results from inflammation of the nasal mucous membrane, as in the common *cold*, *influenza*, and several forms of *rhinitis*, notably allergic rhinitis (hay fever). Cigarette smoking may also cause anosmia. In hypertrophic rhinitis, the mucous membrane thickens, burying and sometimes distorting the olfactory nerve endings, which may cause permanent anosmia unless the condition is treated. In atrophic rhinitis, the nerve endings waste away, causing some degree of permanent anosmia; there is also a foul-smelling discharge that may overpower other odors.

The olfactory nerves can be torn in a head injury. If both nerves are torn, complete permanent anosmia results;

during recovery from less severe damage, dysosmia, in the form of illusory bad smells, may occur.

Rarely, anosmia is caused by a *meningioma* (tumor of the meninges, the membranes that surround the brain) or a tumor behind the nose (see *Nasopharynx, cancer of*).

Dysosmia, in the form of illusory, unpleasant odors, may occur as a feature of various psychological disorders, such as *depression* or *schizophrenia*. The condition may also occur in some forms of *epilepsy* and during "drying out" periods in severe *alcohol*

dependence. A person with dysosmia may believe the source of the smell is his or her own body and, despite reassurance to the contrary, will not be convinced otherwise. As a result, the victim may wash excessively and tend to avoid others. (See also *Sensation*.)

Smelling salts

A preparation of *ammonia* that causes a person to withdraw from the pungent substance. Smelling salts were in the past commonly used to prevent fainting or to revive a person who had fainted.

Smoking

See *Tobacco smoking*.

Snails and disease

Snails act as host to various types of parasitic flukes (flattened, wormlike animals), which, at different stages in their own life cycles, infest people. These flukes include *liver flukes* and the parasites responsible for *schistosomiasis* and various other tropical diseases. Control of snail populations can be an important factor in combating these diseases.

THE SENSE OF SMELL

The smell receptors are specialized nerve cell endings situated in a small patch of mucous membrane lining the roof of the nose. The axons (fibers) of these sensory cells pass up through tiny perforations in the overlying bone to enter the two elongated olfactory bulbs lying on top of the bone. These bulbs are swellings at the ends of the olfactory nerves; the nerves contain millions of nerve fibers and enter the brain on its lower surface. The olfactory nerves carry sensory information to smell centers situated within the brain.

Smell centers
The centers in the brain concerned with smell include parts of the limbic system and frontal lobes.

Olfactory bulbs
Here, the receptor cell fibers are linked to the nerves that run into the brain.

Nasal cavity
In the nose, hairlike projections from the smell receptor cells lie in the mucous membrane layer.

Labels: Olfactory nerve, Olfactory bulb, Nasal hairs

Labels: Limbic system, Nerve pathway, Frontal lobe, Olfactory bulb

Physiological basis of smell
The receptor cell bodies are swollen at their lower ends; each one gives off several cilia that extend down to the surface of the mucous membrane. The cilia contain the receptor sites at which stimulation by the molecules of odorous substances gives rise to nerve impulses passing up to the brain. We know that we are able to distinguish several thousand different odors, but the exact basis of this high degree of specificity is uncertain. No microscopic difference can be detected among different receptors.

Labels: Olfactory bulb, Axon, Lamina cribrosa, Receptor cell, Supporting cell, Cilia

Probable mechanism
The smell process is probably based on a physical "fit" between the odor molecules and the receptor sites. For example, the receptors on some cells may fit only with ether molecules, others with molecules of

Labels: Cilia, Receptor sites, Layer of mucus, Odor molecules, Ether, Garlic, Bleach

bleach. The molecules must dissolve in the mucus before they can stimulate the receptors. The sensitivity of the system is remarkable; as few as four molecules can give a recognizable smell.

S

Snakebites

There are only three kinds of venomous snakes in Canada, and they are restricted to small, southern sections of the country. All venomous bites in Canada, and nearly all those in the United States, are caused by pit vipers. These snakes, which belong to the crotalid family, include the copperhead, water moccasin (cottonmouth) and the many varieties of rattlesnake. The three types in Canada are the Pacific rattlesnake, found in the dry interior valleys of British Columbia, the prairie rattlesnake, in the southern parts of Alberta and Saskatchewan, and the massasauga rattlesnake, which occurs mainly around Ontario's Georgian Bay, but also in a band along the shores of Lakes Huron and Erie. Although people can be bitten by other snakes outside these regions, there is no danger of the bites being poisonous.

The only other venomous snake native to North America is the coral snake, found in the southern US. It belongs to a group of snakes called the elapids, which includes the cobras, kraits, and mambas of Africa and Asia. They are decorated with alternating bands of black and bright colors, which are mimicked by other, nonvenomous species.

Worldwide, hundreds of thousands of people are bitten by snakes every year; cobra bites alone account for 10,000 deaths in India each year.

EFFECTS OF A BITE

Most bites are by nonpoisonous species, and even in bites by poisonous snakes, frequently no venom is injected, so the chance of death or serious injury from a bite is relatively small. The bite of a nonvenomous snake is a minor wound, but harmful bacteria from the snake's mouth may be left behind. The effects of a venomous bite vary considerably depending on the species of snake, the amount of venom injected, and the age and health of the victim.

Rattlesnakes and other pit vipers have a pair of long fangs that make two distinct puncture wounds in the skin. If venom is injected (and often it is not), there is an immediate burning pain at the site of the wound and swelling of the bitten limb. Over the next 20 minutes the pain increases in severity and the victim becomes dizzy, nauseated, pale, and sweaty. Blood pressure falls and there is an increase in heart rate. Thirst, headache, and a pins and needles sensation are other common symptoms.

The venom may prevent the blood from clotting, causing bleeding and widespread tissue destruction around the wound, bruises beneath the skin and bleeding into the urine or from the mouth, rectum, or vagina.

Coral snakes and other elapids have tiny fangs that leave marks little different from other teeth. They may chew the skin, making several wounds. A bite from a coral snake usually causes little pain or swelling. The venom primarily affects the nervous system. Serious symptoms can develop within 10 minutes, but may be delayed by up to eight hours. They include drooping eyelids, slurred speech, and double vision. The victim becomes drowsy or delirious and may have convulsions. Eventually, if treatment is not given, respiratory paralysis causes death.

TREATMENT

Any person accompanying a victim of a snakebite should calmly offer reassurance. If the snake was a pit viper and there is no burning pain or rapid swelling, probably no venom was injected and the bite is not an emergency. Even if venom was injected, it travels very slowly by drainage through the lymphatic system, not the bloodstream, and this takes hours. As fear abates, some of the "symptoms" may disappear.

Given that most victims in southern Canada will be near a road and medical help, the current recommendations for first aid are simple. Slow the spread of the poison by keeping the injured limb low and immobile. Allow the victim to move as little as possible while transporting him or her to a medical facility. Do not apply a tourniquet.

Older advice to make a cut over each fang puncture and suck out the poison has fallen into disfavor; it has never been proven that the methods work, and the techniques are dangerous if done improperly.

For all bites, whether venomous or not, antibiotics and injections of tetanus antitoxin are given to prevent bacterial infection or tetanus. If there are signs that venom was injected by a pit viper, the victim is given an *antivenin* effective against all types of pit viper bites. For coral snakes, another *antivenin* is available.

In the most severe cases, kidney dialysis to treat renal failure or artificial ventilation to overcome respiratory paralysis may be required; the outlook for victims who receive prompt medical care is excellent.

AVOIDING SNAKEBITES

Anyone working, camping, or walking in areas known to be inhabited by venomous snakes should take these precautions: wear long pants and boots; keep to cleared tracks when hiking through the brush; if moving large rocks or logs, investigate with a stick. Snakes bite in self-defense; leave them alone.

Sneezing

The involuntary, convulsive expulsion of air through the nose and mouth as a result of irritation of the upper respiratory tract. The irritation may be caused by inflammation of the tract, which occurs in the common *cold*, *influenza*, and allergic *rhinitis* (hay fever); by the presence of mucus; or by inhaling an irritant substance, such as dust or pepper.

Snellen's chart

A standard method of measuring *visual acuity* used during *vision tests*. The Snellen's chart bears several rows of letters of standard sizes, which are progressively smaller from top to bottom. The chart is set at a distance of 6 metres (20 feet) from the patient. With one eye covered, the patient is asked to read as far down the chart as possible. The procedure is repeated with the other eye.

Normal vision (6/6 or 20/20 vision) requires that all the letters in a line near the bottom of the chart be read correctly by the patient. If the person being tested can read only the letters twice as large as those on the 6/6 line (which a normal eye would be able to read at 12 metres, or 40 feet), the acuity is said to be 6/12, or 20/40.

Snoring

Noisy breathing through the open mouth during sleep, produced by vibrations of the soft palate. Snoring is usually caused by some condition that hinders breathing through the nose, such as a common *cold*, allergic *rhinitis*, or enlarged *adenoids*. Snoring is more common when a person is sleeping on his or her back because in this position the lower jaw tends to drop open. In some cases, snoring alternates with *sleep apnea* (temporary cessation of breathing).

Snoring can sometimes be prevented by sewing an object into the nightclothes near the small of the back, thus making it uncomfortable to sleep on the back. Removal of enlarged adenoids will usually cure the condition in children.

S

Snow blindness

Actinic keratopathy due to exposure to sunlight shining over snow. The risk is highest at high latitudes in the spring, but skiers and hikers should always protect their eyes when the sun is shining in the winter.

Snuff

A preparation of powdered *tobacco* (often with other substances) for inhalation into the nose. Snuff is addictive because it contains *nicotine*, irritating to the nasal lining, which may become abnormally thin and inflamed, and carcinogenic, causing an increased risk of cancer of the nose and throat.

Snuffles

A general term for nasal obstruction, especially in infants suffering from an upper *respiratory tract infection*.

Social skills training

An aspect of behavior modification by which individuals are encouraged to improve their ability to communicate with others.

Social skills training is an important part of *rehabilitation* for people who have chronic psychiatric and psychological disorders, including *schizophrenia* and *alcohol dependence*, and for people with *mental retardation*.

Role-playing is a commonly used technique in social skills training. During role-play, the person being helped and his or her trainer simulate various social situations, particularly those in which the person feels inadequate or lacks self-assertion. The person is shown how to respond in particular situations, is given a chance to practice, and is told how he or she is performing, sometimes with the aid of a video recording. Early stages of training may be followed by practice in groups and by trial outings—for example, to a café or shop.

Social skills training is undertaken by psychologists or by other professionals, such as teachers or psychiatric nurses, under their guidance.

Sociopathy

An outdated term for *antisocial personality disorder*.

Sodium

A *mineral* that helps regulate the body's water balance, helps maintain normal heart rhythm, and is involved in the conduction of nerve impulses and the contraction of muscles.

The body of an average-sized person contains about 55 g of sodium.

The level of sodium in the blood is controlled by the kidneys, which eliminate any excess of the mineral via the urine.

Almost all foods contain sodium naturally or as an ingredient added during processing or cooking. The principal forms of sodium in food are sodium chloride (table salt) and sodium bicarbonate (baking soda). Apart from table salt, the main dietary sources of sodium are processed foods, cheese, breads and cereals, and smoked, pickled, or cured meats and fish. Pickles and snack foods contain large amounts; sodium is also present in water treated with water softeners.

DEFICIENCY

Because most foods contain sodium, deficiency is very rare. In fact, most Western diets contain too much sodium. Whereas many nutritionists suggest a daily intake of only 0.5 to 3 g, the average consumption is 3 to 7 g per day. There is no official recommended daily intake.

Sodium deficiency is usually the result of excessive loss of the mineral through persistent diarrhea or vomiting, through profuse sweating, or through prolonged or excessive treatment with *diuretic drugs*. In rare cases, deficiency is due to *cystic fibrosis*, underactivity of the *adrenal glands*, or certain kidney disorders.

Symptoms of deficiency include tiredness, weakness, muscle cramps, and dizziness. In severe cases, there may be a drop in blood pressure, leading to confusion, fainting, and palpitations. Treatment consists of taking sodium supplements. In very hot conditions, sodium supplements may help prevent *heat disorders* by compensating for sodium lost through heavy sweating.

EXCESS

Excessive sodium intake is thought to be a contributory factor in the high incidence of *hypertension* (high blood pressure) in Western countries. In people whose blood pressure is already raised, excessive sodium may increase the risk of heart disease, *stroke*, and kidney damage. Another adverse effect of excessive use is fluid retention, which, in severe cases, may cause dizziness and swelling of the patient's legs.

Sodium aurothiomalate

A preparation of *gold*, which is given by injection.

Sodium bicarbonate

An over-the-counter *antacid drug* used to relieve *indigestion, heartburn*, and pain caused by a *peptic ulcer*.

Sodium bicarbonate often causes belching and abdominal discomfort. Long-term use may cause swollen ankles, muscle cramps, tiredness, weakness, nausea, and vomiting. Sodium bicarbonate should not be taken by people with *heart failure* or a history of kidney disease.

Sodium cromoglycate

A drug used to treat some types of *asthma*, allergic *rhinitis* (hay fever), allergic *conjunctivitis*, and *food allergy*.

WHY IT IS USED

Sodium cromoglycate is commonly given by *inhaler* to prevent attacks of mild to moderate asthma in children. It is also prescribed for allergic asthma in adults and for asthma induced by exercise or cold air. Sodium cromoglycate has a slow onset of action, taking up to four weeks of regular treatment to produce its antiasthmatic effect. Use of this drug sometimes permits a reduction in the dosage of other drugs taken to relieve attacks. Sodium cromoglycate is not an effective treatment for an acute asthmatic attack.

Taken in the form of a nasal spray, sodium cromoglycate is useful in treating allergic rhinitis. In the form of eye drops, it treats allergic conjunctivitis, and in the form of capsules it can help in some types of food allergy.

HOW IT WORKS

Sodium cromoglycate works by blocking the release of *histamine* (a chemical released into the body when an allergic reaction occurs).

POSSIBLE ADVERSE EFFECTS

Side effects are generally mild and rarely require treatment to be stopped. Coughing and wheezing on inhalation may be prevented by first using a sympathomimetic *bronchodilator drug*. Throat irritation can be avoided by rinsing the mouth with water after inhalation.

Sodium salicylate

An *analgesic drug* used to relieve minor musculoskeletal pain and to reduce inflammation. Sodium salicylate has the same possible adverse effects as *ASA* and other *salicylate drugs*.

Soft-tissue injury

Damage to one or more of the tissues that surround bones and joints (for example to a *ligament, tendon*, or *muscle*). Soft-tissue injuries include ligament *sprain*, *tendinitis* (inflammation of a tendon), and muscle *strain*. (See also *Sports injuries*.)

S

Soiling

Inappropriate passage of *feces* after the age at which bowel control is achieved (usually at about 3 or 4 years of age). The term is usually applied to the accidental passage of soft, unformed feces into the clothing. More than half of the children with this problem also wet the bed (see *Enuresis*).

Causes of soiling include slowness in developing bowel control, long-standing *constipation* (in which fecal liquid leaks around hard feces blocking the large intestine), poor *toilet training*, and psychological stress (caused, for example, by starting school). Soiling is usually distressing to the child, who may hide the messy clothes.

Soiling due to constipation usually responds to treatment. If there is no physical cause, the problem may pass after a discussion involving the child, the parents, and the physician; if not, *psychotherapy* may be used.

Encopresis is a form of soiling in which children deliberately pass feces in inappropriate places, such as in their clothing or behind furniture. Such children have no specific physical problem, but often refuse to use a potty or toilet. Encopresis usually improves with time and is rare after the age of 10.

Solar plexus

The largest network of autonomic nerves in the body (see *Autonomic nervous system*). Also known as the celiac plexus, the solar plexus is situated behind the stomach, where it surrounds the celiac artery and lies between the adrenal glands. The solar plexus incorporates branches of the *vagus nerve*, the most important component of the parasympathetic nervous system, and the splanchnic nerves. The solar plexus sends out branches to the stomach, intestines, and most other abdominal organs.

Solvent abuse

The practice of inhaling the intoxicating fumes given off by certain volatile liquids. Glue sniffing is the most common form of solvent abuse, but many other substances are used, especially those containing toluene or acetone. The usual method of inhalation is from a plastic bag containing the solvent, but sometimes aerosols are sprayed into the nose or mouth.

INCIDENCE
Solvent abuse is common among boys in poor urban areas. It is usually a group activity that is indulged in for no more than a few months. Solitary abuse over a longer period is frequently associated with delinquency and a disturbed family background.

EFFECTS
Inhalation of solvent fumes produces an effect similar to that of becoming drunk or getting high on drugs, sometimes including hallucinations. Solvent abuse can cause headache, vomiting, stupor, confusion, and coma. Occasionally, death occurs due to a direct toxic effect on the heart, a fall, choking on vomit, or asphyxiation by a clinging plastic bag.

Long-term harmful effects include erosion of the membrane lining the nose and throat, and damage to the kidneys, liver, and nervous system.

DIAGNOSIS
The signs of solvent abuse include intoxicated behavior, a flushed face, ulcers around the mouth, a smell of solvent, and personality changes, such as moodiness and nervousness.

TREATMENT
Solvent abusers should be warned of the serious risks to health. Professional counseling may be needed. Acute symptoms resulting from solvent abuse, such as vomiting or coma, require urgent medical attention.

Somatic

A term that means related to the body (soma), as opposed to the mind (psyche), or related to body cells, as opposed to germ cells (eggs and sperm). The term somatic also refers to the body wall, in contrast to visceral (referring to the internal organs).

Somatization disorder

A condition in which a person complains over a period of several years of various physical problems for which no physical cause can be found. The disorder, previously classified as *hysteria*, usually begins before the age of 30 and leads to numerous tests by many physicians. Unnecessary surgery and other treatments often result.

This disorder may be slightly more prevalent in women, many of whom have a family history of *antisocial personality disorder* in male relatives. Symptoms most commonly complained of are neurological (such as double vision, seizures, weakness), gynecological (painful menstruation, pain on intercourse), and gastrointestinal (abdominal pain, nausea). Associated features may include *anxiety* and *depression*, threats of *suicide*, and various forms of substance abuse.

Physical symptoms in this disorder are caused by underlying emotional conflicts, anxiety, and depression that the affected person is unable to confront and unconsciously displaces on to the body. It is thought that the sufferer finds it easier to view the problem as physical than rather face the emotional conflicts from which he or she is trying to escape. (See also *Conversion disorder*; *Hypochondriasis*.)

Somatotype

The physical build of an individual. Various attempts have been made to classify people according to body type and to identify corresponding personality traits.

In the 1920s, the German psychiatrist Ernst Kretschmer divided people into three types, each of which he thought was more prone to certain types of mental illness—asthenic (thin) types seemed more likely to have a schizoid personality or schizophrenia; pyknic (stocky) types were more prone to manic-depressive illness; athletic (muscular) types were not associated with any single disorder, but there was more delinquency within this group.

An American psychologist, W. H. Sheldon, working in the 1940s, believed that people did not fit into rigid categories of body type. Instead he identified three structural tendencies (each associated with certain personality traits), which everyone had in different proportions. These were endomorphic—a heavy physique, with poorly developed bones and muscles, associated with a sociable, loving personality; mesomorphic—strong, well-developed bones and muscles, paired with a physical, adventurous personality; and ectomorphic—a tall, thin physique, with light bones and muscles, linked with a restrained, self-conscious personality. Scientific support for such theories has not been convincing, and they have no application in medical care.

Somatrem

A preparation of human *growth hormone*. Somatrem is given to children to treat *short stature* caused by growth hormone deficiency.

Somnambulism

See *Sleepwalking*.

Sore

A term used to describe an ulcer, septic wound, or any disrupted area of the skin or mucous membranes.

S

BODY TYPES AND PERSONALITY

The idea that the features of the psyche (mind) are related to those of the soma (body) is not always borne out in practice. Even so, attempts have been made to relate the two (see below).

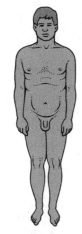

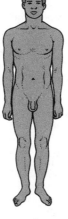

Endomorph
Tends to be sociable, easy-going, pleasure-loving, relaxed, and convivial.

Mesomorph
Is often physically active, strong, athletic, ready for action, and aggressive.

Ectomorph
Is more sensitive, self-conscious, restrained, introspective, and quiet.

The word sore is also used adjectivally to describe an area that is tender or painful.

Sore throat

A rough or raw feeling in the back of the throat that causes discomfort, especially when swallowing.

Sore throat is an extremely common symptom, which is usually caused by *pharyngitis*, and occasionally by *tonsillitis*. It may also be the first symptom of the common *cold*, *influenza*, *laryngitis*, infectious *mononucleosis*, and many childhood viral illnesses, including *chickenpox*, *measles*, and *mumps*.

Strep throat, a type of sore throat caused by infection with beta-hemolytic streptococcal bacteria, requires medical attention. Left untreated, strep throat may result in acute *glomerulonephritis* or *rheumatic fever*.

A sore throat can sometimes be relieved by gargling with salt water. Adults may benefit from taking ASA. If a sore throat persists for more than 48 hours or if a *rash* develops, a physician should be consulted.

Space medicine

A medical specialty concerned with the physiological and pathological effects of space flight. Space medicine is often linked with the specialty of *aviation medicine*.

During lift-off, there is a large upward acceleration that makes the astronaut feel many times heavier. There is also a tendency for blood to pool downward. To prevent loss of consciousness through blood draining from the brain, astronauts must lie in a reclining seat and wear a special suit that exerts pressure on certain parts of the body, thus maintaining blood flow to the head.

Once in stable orbit, the astronaut feels weightless. One effect of weightlessness is on the body's balance mechanisms. Initially, the brain may be unable to make sense of the lack of signals from the balance organ in the inner ear; one manifestation of this is *motion sickness*. Changes also occur in the cardiovascular system (heart and blood vessels) because, in the absence of weight, body fluids are redistributed toward the head. Other effects may include loss of bone and muscle tissue. Such effects could ultimately limit space travel, unless a means can be found to recreate "weight" within spacecraft.

Spasm

An involuntary, often powerful, contraction of a *muscle*. A spasm may affect one or more muscles and may occur once or more; pain is not necessarily an accompanying feature.

Examples of muscle spasms include *hiccups* (in which the diaphragm goes into spasm), muscle cramps (which often affect the muscles in the calves), and *tics* (which frequently affect the facial muscles).

Less commonly, a spasm may be the result of an abnormality in the central nervous system (brain and spinal cord) or a symptom of a muscle disorder. Spasms caused by disease of the nervous system include *myoclonus* and *chorea*. Conditions characterized by spasm include *trigeminal neuralgia* (which affects the muscles of the face and head), *tetany* (spasm caused by a drop of the calcium level in the blood), and *tetanus* (an infectious disease). Rare causes of widespread spasm are *rabies, strychnine poisoning*, and the bite of the black widow spider (see *Spider bites*).

Other types of muscle spasm include *bronchospasm* (contraction of muscles in the small airways of the lungs), which occurs in asthma, and vasospasm (tightening of the muscles in the walls of blood vessels), which occurs in Raynaud's disease.

Spasticity

Increased resistance to sudden stretching in a group of *muscles*, due to central nervous system or spinal cord damage. Spasticity can occur with or without *paralysis* or muscle weakness. In *cerebral palsy*, there is spasticity with paralysis.

Spastic paralysis

Inability to move a part of the body, accompanied by rigidity of the muscles. Causes of spastic paralysis include *stroke, cerebral palsy*, and *multiple sclerosis*. (See also *Paralysis*.)

Specific gravity

Also called relative density, the ratio of the *density* of a substance to that of water. Materials with a relative density of less than 1 are less dense ("lighter") than water; those with a relative density of more than 1 are denser ("heavier") than water. The specific gravity of urine shows if it has a large amount of material dissolved in it (near 1.030) or if it is almost water (near 1.010).

Specimen

A sample of tissue, body fluids (such as blood), waste products (such as urine), or an infective organism taken for the purpose of examination, identification, analysis, and/or diagnosis. The term specimen is also applied to a

S

sample of a tissue or an organism specially prepared for examination under a *microscope*. (See also *Blood tests*; *Urinalysis*.)

SPECT

The abbreviation for single photon emission computed tomography, a type of *radionuclide scanning*.

Spectacles

See *Glasses*.

Speculum

A device for holding open a body orifice (opening) to enable a physician to perform an examination. A speculum may be made of plastic or metal.

TYPES

There are many types of speculum designed for use on different parts of the body. The speculum used to examine the eardrum is funnel-shaped, with a narrow end inserted into the ear canal and a wide end attached to an *otoscope*. A nasal speculum is used to examine the inside of the nose. The speculum used to hold open the walls of the vagina during a pelvic examination may be shaped either like a duck's bill, with wide, smooth, curved edges and a self-retaining lock to hold it in position, or like a shoehorn bent at both ends at an angle of 90 degrees.

Speech

A system of sounds by which humans communicate.

LANGUAGE AND SPEECH

The terms "speech" and "language" are often used interchangeably, but have different meanings. Language is the representation of objects and ideas by strings of symbols, which form words. These symbols may be speech sounds, written characters, or hand signals. There are two main facets of language ability—understanding the meaning of words (comprehension) and generating words, in grammatical order, to express something meaningful (expression).

Speech is just one method by which language can be communicated to others. Writing and hand signals are others. Each method relies on sequences of muscle movements. Speech involves the muscles used in breathing, the larynx (voice box), tongue, palate, lips, jaw, and face.

LANGUAGE CENTERS

Language comprehension and expression take place in two areas of the cerebral cortex (the outer layer of the main mass of the brain) known as Wernicke's area and Broca's area. Both are in the dominant cerebral hemisphere (the left hemisphere in most people). In Wernicke's area, incoming messages (heard or read) are scanned and compared with information held in the memory to extract meaning. In Broca's area, words and sentences are composed from vocabulary and from grammatical rules stored in the memory.

SPEECH PRODUCTION

The movement sequences for speech sounds originate from two regions of the cerebral cortex on each side of the brain. These regions are linked to the center for language expression (Broca's area). The signals for movement pass down nerve pathways to the muscles controlling the larynx, tongue, and other parts involved in speech. The cerebellum (a region at the back of the brain) plays a part in coordinating these movements.

Air from the lungs is vibrated by opening and closing the vocal cords in the larynx. This produces a noise, which is amplified in the hollow cavities of the throat, nose, and sinuses. The sound of vibrated or nonvibrated air is modified by movements of the tongue, mouth, jaw, and lips to produce speech sounds. Vibrated air blown through top teeth resting on lower lips gives "v" or, if the air is not vibrated, "f." Consonants are produced mainly by contact between the tongue, roof of the mouth, teeth, and lips; vowels are produced by changing the shape of the mouth cavity.

LANGUAGE AND SPEECH DEVELOPMENT

Normal development of language and speech in a child depends on maturation of the nervous system and muscles, on the child's exploration of his or her environment, and on interaction with adults. Through play, the child acquires many concepts about different aspects of the world. From adults, the child acquires the verbal labels for objects and concepts that are needed for language development. Normal hearing is, therefore, essential. Language and speech are learned through listening to the speech of others and through monitoring one's own speech.

Stages in the development of language and speech in a child, with the significance of each, are shown in the accompanying table.

Speech disorders

Defects or disturbances can arise in various parts of the nervous system, muscles, and other apparatus involved in *speech*, leading to an inability to communicate effectively. Some of these disorders are, strictly, disturbances of language rather than of speech, since they result from an impaired ability to understand or to form words in the language centers of the brain, rather than from any fault of the apparatus of speech production. Most people with speech disorders can be helped by *speech therapy*.

DISORDERS OF LANGUAGE

Damage to the language centers of the brain (usually as a result of a *stroke*, *head injury*, or *brain tumor*) leads to disorders known as *aphasia* and *dysphasia*. Both children and adults can be affected. The ability to speak and write and/or to comprehend written or spoken words is impaired, depending on the site and extent of the damage.

Delayed development of language in a child is characterized by slowness to understand speech and/or slow growth in vocabulary and sentence structure. Delayed development has many causes, including hearing loss (see *Deafness*), lack of stimulation, or emotional disturbance (see *Developmental delay*). There are, however, considerable variations in speech development in children.

DISORDERS OF ARTICULATION

Articulation is the ability to produce speech sounds; a defect of articulation is sometimes referred to as *dysarthria*. Damage to nerves passing from the brain to muscles in the larynx (voice box), mouth, or lips can cause speech to be slurred, indistinct, slow, or nasal. The sources of such damage are similar to those that cause aphasia (including stroke, head injury, tumors, *multiple sclerosis*, *Parkinson's disease*) but the affected regions of the brain are different. Damage to the cerebellum, for example, produces a characteristic form of slurred speech. Structural abnormalities of the mouth, such as cleft palate (see *Cleft lip and palate*) and *malalignment* of the teeth, can also cause poor articulation.

Delayed development of articulation, characterized by an inability to make sounds at appropriate ages, may cause incomprehensible speech. Possible causes are hearing problems or slow maturation of the nervous system. Lisping and lalling (the mispronunciation of "r" as "l") result from poor tongue and lip control.

DISORDERS OF VOICE PRODUCTION

These disorders include hoarseness, harshness, inappropriate pitch or loudness of the voice, and abnormal

S

LANGUAGE AND SPEECH DEVELOPMENT IN CHILDHOOD

3 months	Period of babbling begins. The child produces strings of sounds for pleasure. Babbling is important in building sequences of muscle movements	that will be used later to produce meaningful speech sounds.
9 months	The child echoes the speech of others, but words are not yet used with meaning. By listening to and copying adults, the child learns that clusters of	sounds refer to specific objects, people, or situations.
12 to 18 months	The child begins to utter simple words with meaning, often accompanied by gestures. Examples include "bye-bye," "dog," "hot," and "daddy."	Single words are used, with vocabulary gradually increasing from two or three words initially.
18 to 24 months	The child begins to combine concepts to form two-word sentences (e.g., "Hello John" or "That hot!"). By the age of	2 years, the child may be using 100 or more different words.
2 to 3 years	The child's sentences become longer (e.g., "I like cake" or "Peter hit Mary"). He or she also begins to incorporate adjectives and adverbs into sentences (e.g., "That's daddy's old coat" or "I want lunch now").	By the age of 3 years, the average sentence length is four words. Most sounds have developed, with the possible exceptions of "th," "r," "j," "ch," and "sh."
3 years and older	More elaborate sentences with several nouns, verbs in past and future tenses, and linked phrases begin to be used (e.g., "We went to Amy's and we had milk and cookies" or "I think mummy went downstairs").	However, mistakes are often made (e.g., "What did you played?"), reflecting the child's linguistic immaturity. Language skills continue to develop throughout childhood.

nasal resonance. In many cases, the cause is a disorder affecting closure of the vocal cords (see *Larynx* disorders box). A voice that is pitched too high or low or that is too loud or soft may be caused by a hormonal or psychiatric disturbance or by severe hearing loss.

Abnormal nasal resonance is caused by too much air (hypernasality) or too little air (hyponasality) flowing through the nose during speech. Hypernasality may result from damage to the nerves supplying the palate (roof of the mouth) or be a result of cleft palate, and causes a deterioration in the intelligibility of speech. Hyponasality is caused by blockage to the nasal airways by congestion or excess mucus and has the sound of someone speaking with a cold. Nonfluent speech is marked by repetitions of single sounds or whole words and by interruptions in speech; the cause is not known (see *Stuttering*).

Speech therapy
A form of treatment that attempts to help people with any of a variety of communication problems.

WHY IT IS DONE
Any person with a disturbance of language or a disorder of articulation, voice production, or fluency of speech (see *Speech disorders*) may be helped by speech therapy. Such problems may occur as part of a broader problem, such as a physical *handicap*, *learning disability*, or *hearing loss*. Speech therapists work with all age groups.

HOW IT IS DONE
The therapist—a person trained in the causes, assessment, and treatment of speech and language problems—usually begins by finding out the case history from the client or from a relative or friend, asking how and when the difficulties developed. Relevant medical details are also sought from the client's physician if necessary.

The client may be asked to provide a sample of speech (which may be recorded) or of writing for detailed analysis. An examination of the physical structures of speech and a *hearing test* may be performed. The therapist may also assess language comprehension by observing the client's reaction to written or spoken requests.

After making an assessment, the therapist decides on the form of treatment, which usually has two parts. First, a program of exercises is started to improve a specific aspect of language ability or speech performance (e.g., a technique to improve speech fluency). Second, the therapist works with the people most involved with the client (family, teachers, or friends), explaining to them the nature of the difficulties and how they can help. The aim is to create a climate that will provide maximum opportunities for effective communication.

Sperm

The sex cell of the male, also known as spermatozoon (singular) or spermatozoa (plural), responsible for *fertilization* of the ovum of the female. Sperm are microscopically tiny, measuring 0.05 mm in length.

Sperm are produced within the seminiferous tubules of the *testes* by a process known as spermatogenesis. The production and development of sperm is dependent on the presence of the male sex hormone *testosterone* and of *gonadotropin hormones* produced by the *pituitary gland*. Sperm production commences at *puberty*.

The original cell from which a sperm develops contains 46 chromosomes, including the XY pair of male sex *chromosomes*. By a process of *cell division* known as *meiosis*, the number of chromosomes in the sperm is halved to 23, including either the X or the Y from the original pair of sex

S

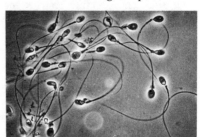

Human sperm magnified 350 times
Each sperm consists of a head that contains the hereditary material and a long, whiplike tail that propels it along.

chromosomes. This X or Y is responsible for determining the sex of an embryo that develops after fertilization of the ovum by the sperm (see *Sex determination*).

The final stage of spermatogenesis takes place in the *epididymis*, where each sperm grows a tail that will propel it through the woman's reproductive tract after *ejaculation* during *sexual intercourse*.

Spermatocele

A harmless cyst (fluid-filled swelling) of the *epididymis* (the tube that transmits sperm from the testis) containing fluid and sperm.

If a spermatocele grows to a large size or if it becomes uncomfortable, it is usually removed surgically. The operation is straightforward, but may result in an interruption of the passage of sperm through the epididymis, which may render the testis on the affected side infertile.

Spermatozoa

See *Sperm*.

Spermicides

Contraceptive preparations that kill *sperm*. Spermicides are available in the form of creams, gels, foams, and pessaries. They are usually recommended for use with a barrier device, such as a condom or diaphragm, to increase the contraceptive effect (see *Contraception, barrier methods of*).

Some spermicides, such as nonoxinol, may offer partial protection against the organisms that cause various *sexually transmitted diseases*, including *gonorrhea* and *AIDS*.

An uncommon possible adverse effect of spermicides is irritation of the genitals of either partner.

Sphenoid bone

The bat-shaped bone in the center of the base of the cranium (the part of the *skull* that encases the brain). The central body of the bone contains the sphenoidal sinus (air space) and, in the upper surface, a depression in which the *pituitary gland* is situated. The wings support part of the temporal lobe of the brain (see *Cerebrum*) and form part of the back and side walls of the orbits (eye sockets). Openings in the wings enable the optic and other cranial nerves to pass through.

Spherocytosis, hereditary

An inherited disorder so named because of the large number of unusually small, round, red blood cells (spherocytes) in the circulation. These cells have an abnormal membrane (outer envelope), which makes them fragile and causes them to have a much reduced life span because they are readily trapped, broken up, and consumed when blood passes through the *spleen*. At times, the rate of *hemolysis* (red cell destruction) exceeds the rate at which new cells can be made in the bone marrow, leading to *anemia* (reduced level of the oxygen-carrying pigment *hemoglobin* in the blood due to lack of red cells).

INCIDENCE
Hereditary spherocytosis is the most common form of inherited hemolytic anemia (see *Anemia, hemolytic*) in people of northern European extraction. About one person in 4,500 in Canada has the condition. The disorder is inherited in an autosomal dominant pattern (see *Genetic disorders*). Each of an affected person's children has a 50 percent chance of inheriting the defective gene responsible for the disease.

SYMPTOMS
Symptoms of anemia (e.g., tiredness, shortness of breath on exertion, and pallor) may develop. Other symptoms include *jaundice*, caused by the high rate of red blood cell destruction, and enlargement of the spleen.

Occasionally, there are crises (usually triggered when the patient acquires an infection) in which all symptoms worsen. *Gallstones*, which are caused by the high rate of red blood cell destruction, are a frequent complication.

DIAGNOSIS, AND TREATMENT
The diagnosis is made from the presence of spherocytes in the blood of someone with anemia and from tests to ascertain the structure of the red cell membrane.

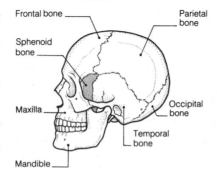

Location of the sphenoid bone
The sphenoid bone is a bat-shaped bone that lies in front of the temporal bones at the base of the skull.

The treatment is *splenectomy* (removal of the spleen). The red cells remain abnormally shaped, but the rate at which they are destroyed drops markedly, leading to a striking, and usually permanent, improvement in health. After removal of the spleen, susceptibility to certain bacterial infections increases, necessitating vaccination against pneumococcal infection as well as prompt treatment of infections with *antibiotic drugs*.

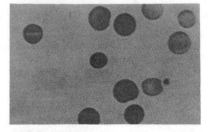

Spherocytes in blood
A person with hereditary spherocytosis has a large number of these unusually small, round, fragile, red cells in the blood.

Sphincter

A ring of muscle around a natural opening or passage that acts like a valve, regulating inflow or outflow. An example is the pyloric sphincter at the outlet of the stomach into the duodenum, which controls the stomach's outflow. Another example is the anal sphincter at the rectal outlet, which is partly under voluntary control and permits a voluntary decision on when to empty the bowel.

Sphincter, artificial

A surgically created valve or other device used to treat or prevent urinary or fecal *incontinence*.

An artificial urinary sphincter consists of an inflatable cuff that is inserted around the base of the bladder or upper part of the urethra. When inflated, the cuff prevents urine from leaking from the bladder. The patient deflates the cuff by using a pump, which is usually situated in the scrotum in males or adjacent to the labia in females.

An artificial sphincter to prevent fecal incontinence may be created after removal of the colon and rectum as an alternative to a conventional *ileostomy*. Creation of such a "continent ileostomy" involves using a loop of ileum to create a pouch in which bowel contents collect. Evacuation of feces is controlled by an artificial sphincter, surgically fashioned from a section of ileum.

A similar continent ileostomy may be provided for a person whose bladder has been removed because of cancer. In such cases, the ureters are joined to a segment of ileum that is formed into a pouch. This procedure is still considered experimental, as are other methods of continent *urinary diversion*.

Sphincterotomy

A surgical procedure that involves cutting the muscle that closes a body opening or that constricts the opening between body passages. In rare cases, sphincterotomy is performed on the anal sphincter to treat an *anal fissure*. It may also be performed on the ampulla of Vater (the opening of the common bile duct into the duodenum) to release an impacted *gallstone*.

Sphygmomanometer

An instrument for measuring blood pressure. A sphygmomanometer consists of a cuff with an inflatable bladder, which is wrapped around a person's upper arm, a rubber bulb to inflate the bladder, and a device that indicates the pressure of blood. This pressure device may consist of a calibrated glass column filled with mercury, a spring gauge and dial, or, in more modern instruments, a digital display. (For an explanation of how a sphygmomanometer is used, see *Blood pressure*.)

Spider bites

Nearly all spiders produce venom, which they inject, via a pair of fangs, to paralyze and kill their prey.

The hairy tarantula of southern Europe is relatively harmless, although its bite is painful. Spiders whose bites occasionally cause deaths in humans include the black widow spider and the brown recluse spider in North America, the banana spider in South America, and the redback spider and "funnel web" spider in Australia. *Antivenins* are available for these and many other dangerous spider bites.

Spider nevus

A discolored patch of skin in the form of a red, raised, pinhead-sized dot from which small blood vessels radiate. A spider nevus is the outward manifestation of a dilated arteriole (small artery) and its connecting capillaries.

Small numbers of spider nevi are common in children and pregnant

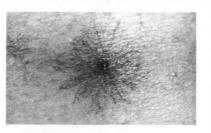

Typical spider nevus
The nevus consists of a tiny, red, raised dot from which widened blood capillaries radiate outward in all directions.

women. However, in larger quantities, spider nevi may be a sign of an underlying liver disease. (See also *Telangiectasia*.)

Spina bifida

A *congenital* defect in which part of one or more *vertebrae* fails to develop completely, leaving a portion of the *spinal cord* exposed. Spina bifida can occur anywhere on the spine but is most common in the lower back. The severity of the condition depends on how much nerve tissue is exposed.

CAUSES AND INCIDENCE
The cause of spina bifida remains unknown; it is thought that many factors are involved.

The incidence rate is highest among babies born to relatively young or to relatively old mothers. A woman who has had one affected child is 10 times more likely than average to have another affected child.

TYPES
There are four known distinct forms of spina bifida.

SPINA BIFIDA OCCULTA This is the most common and the least serious form. There is little external evidence of the defect apart from a dimple or a tuft of hair over the area of the underlying abnormality. Spina bifida occulta often goes completely unnoticed in otherwise healthy children, although occasionally there are accompanying abnormalities of the lower part of the spinal cord. Symptoms, which include leg weakness, cold and blue feet, and urinary incontinence, may be present from birth or may develop later in life.

MYELOCELE Also known as meningomyelocele, this is the most severe form of spina bifida. The nature of the defect is shown in the box overleaf.

A child with myelocele is usually severely handicapped. The legs are partly or completely paralyzed, with loss of sensation in all areas below the level of the defect; hip dis-

location and other leg deformities are common. *Hydrocephalus* (excess cerebrospinal fluid within the skull) is common and without treatment may result in brain damage. Associated abnormalities include *cerebral palsy*, *epilepsy*, *mental retardation*, and visual problems. Paralysis of the bladder leads to urinary incontinence or urinary retention, repeated urinary tract infections, and eventual kidney damage. The anus may be paralyzed, causing chronic constipation and leakage of feces.

MENINGOCELE This form is less severe than myelocele. The nature of the defect is shown in the box overleaf.

ENCEPHALOCELE This is a rare disorder, related to spina bifida, in which brain tissue protrudes through the skull. There is usually severe brain damage.

DIAGNOSIS
Closure of the vertebral canal usually occurs within four weeks of conception, meaning that meningomyelocele can often be diagnosed at an early stage in the pregnancy by *ultrasound scanning*. High levels of *alpha-fetoprotein* in the amniotic fluid or maternal blood may indicate spina bifida.

After birth, spina bifida is easy to recognize if there is a protruding sac. Spina bifida occulta can be diagnosed only by an *X ray* of the spine.

TREATMENT
In cases that are not severe, surgery may be performed to close the defect and thus prevent further damage to the spinal cord. Ideally, the operation should be performed in the first few days of life. If the abnormality is serious, surgery may allow the child to survive, although he or she may be severely handicapped physically and mentally. If hydrocephalus develops, a *shunt* (tube and valve mechanism) is inserted into the brain to relieve the buildup of fluid.

Urinary retention or urinary incontinence may be relieved by use of a catheter (see *Catheterization, urinary*), which is inserted into the bladder and changed every four to six weeks. Older children may be taught the technique of self-catheterization. *Laxative drugs* may be needed.

Physiotherapy encourages mobility and independence; for the more severely affected, wheelchairs and other walking aids may be required. Depending on the degree of disability, special schooling and training for employment may be needed.

PREVENTION
Parents who have had one child with spina bifida should undergo *genetic*

S

counseling if they are considering another pregnancy. During subsequent pregnancies the levels of alpha-fetoprotein in the blood and amniotic fluid are measured. Some research studies have suggested that vitamin supplements in early pregnancy may reduce the risk of spina bifida in the fetus.

Spinal accessory nerve
See *Accessory nerve*.

Spinal anesthesia
Injection of an anesthetic into the cerebrospinal fluid in the spinal canal in order to block *pain* sensations before they reach the *central nervous system* (brain and spinal cord). The main use of spinal anesthesia is during surgery on the lower abdomen and legs.

The procedure is performed by inserting a delicate needle between two vertebrae in the lower part of the spine (see *Lumbar puncture*) and introducing anesthetic into the cerebrospinal fluid surrounding the spinal cord and its terminal nerve roots. Because the nerves emerging from the spinal cord are bathed in cerebrospinal fluid, they absorb the anesthetic. The position of the injection and the subsequent controlled spread of the local anesthetic solution determine the area that is anesthetized.

After spinal anesthesia, a headache develops in between 1 and 5 percent of patients. (See also *Epidural anesthesia*.)

Spinal cord
A cylinder of *nerve* tissue, about 45 cm long and roughly the thickness of a finger, that runs down the central canal in the *spine*. The spinal cord is a downward extension of the *brain*. The spinal cord and brain can be considered parts of a single unit—the *central nervous system* (CNS).

STRUCTURE
At the core of the spinal cord is a region with a butterfly-shaped cross section, called the gray matter. This contains the cell bodies of neurons (nerve cells) along with glial (supporting) cells. Some of the nerve cells are motor neurons, whose axons (long, projecting fibers) pass out of the spinal cord in bundles within the *spinal nerves* and extend to glands or muscles in the trunk and limbs. Others are interneurons (nerve cells contained entirely within the central nervous system), which act to convey messages between other neurons. Also entering the gray matter are the axons

---

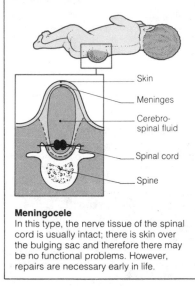
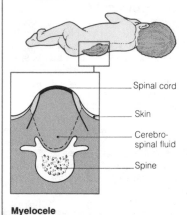
---

of sensory neurons, which have their cell bodies outside the spinal cord. These axons connect with the motor neurons or interneurons.

Surrounding the gray matter are areas of white matter, which consist of bundles of nerve cell axons running lengthwise through the cord.

Sprouting from the spinal cord on each side at regular intervals are two nerve bundles—the spinal nerve roots, which contain the fibers of motor and sensory nerve cells. These combine to form the spinal nerves, which emerge from the spine and are the communication cables between the spinal cord and all regions of the trunk and limbs.

The whole of the spinal cord is bathed in *cerebrospinal fluid* and surrounded by a protective sheath, a continuation of the *meninges* that protect the brain.

FUNCTION
The nerve tracts that make up the white matter of the spinal cord act mainly as highways for sensory information passing upward toward the brain (ascending tracts) or motor signals passing downward (descending tracts). However, the cord is also capable of handling some of the sensory information itself, and of providing appropriate motor responses without recourse to the brain. Many *reflex* actions (such as the knee jerk reflex) are controlled in this way by the spinal cord.

DISORDERS
The spinal cord may be injured as a result of trauma to the spine (see *Spinal injury*). Severing of an ascending or descending tract interrupts communication between the brain and parts of the body served from parts of the cord below the injury. This can lead to a variety of patterns of *paralysis* and/or loss of sensation, which are usually permanent because nerve cells and fibers within the cord do not regenerate. However, reflexes controlled by the spinal cord are usually maintained.

Pressure on the cord (e.g., by a blood clot, an abscess, or a tumor) can similarly affect movement and sensation. However, the effects of pressure can often be relieved by surgery.

Infections of the spinal cord (including *poliomyelitis*) are relatively rare but can cause serious damage. In *multiple sclerosis*, a degenerative disease, there is patchy loss of the insulating sheaths around nerve fibers.

S

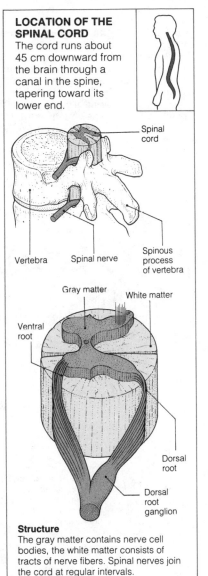

LOCATION OF THE SPINAL CORD
The cord runs about 45 cm downward from the brain through a canal in the spine, tapering toward its lower end.

Spinal cord

Vertebra   Spinal nerve   Spinous process of vertebra

Gray matter   White matter

Ventral root

Dorsal root

Dorsal root ganglion

Structure
The gray matter contains nerve cell bodies, the white matter consists of tracts of nerve fibers. Spinal nerves join the cord at regular intervals.

Spinal fusion
A major surgical procedure to join two or more adjacent *vertebrae*, the bones that make up the *spine*. Spinal fusion is performed if abnormal movement between adjacent vertebrae (as revealed by X *rays*) causes severe back pain or may damage the spinal cord. Such abnormal movement may be due to various spinal disorders, including *spondylolisthesis*, dislocated facet joints (the movable joints that connect vertebrae), *scoliosis*, *osteomyelitis*, a tumor or injury destroying one or more vertebrae, or *osteoarthritis* causing degeneration of spinal joints.

HOW IT IS DONE
Under general anesthesia, the affected vertebrae are exposed. *Arthrodesis* (joint fusion) is then carried out, sometimes together with a *bone graft*, using bone chips taken from the pelvis. While healing is in progress, the vertebrae are temporarily held together with a plate or screws.

The recovery period includes bed rest for up to six weeks. When mobility is resumed, the patient may initially need to wear a plaster *corset*. Full fusion takes up to six months.

Results are usually good, but fusing of the vertebrae may place greater strain on the rest of the spine and cause the patient more back pain. The potential gain must be weighed against the risks.

Spinal injury
Damage to the *spine* and sometimes to the *spinal cord*. Injury to the spinal cord may cause loss of sensation, and muscle weakness or *paralysis*.

CAUSES
Spinal injury is usually caused by one of three types of severe force: longitudinal compression, hinging, and shearing. Longitudinal compression, usually due to a fall from a height, crushes the *vertebrae* (spinal bones) lengthwise against each other. Hinging, which can occur in a whiplash injury suffered in a road traffic accident, subjects the spinal column to sudden, extreme bending movements. Shearing, which may occur when a person is knocked over by a motor vehicle, combines both hinging and rotational (twisting) forces.

Any of these forces can dislocate the vertebrae, fracture them, or rupture the *ligaments* that bind them together. In severe dislocations and fractures, the vertebrae, accumulated fluid, or a blood clot may press on the spinal cord, or the cord may be torn or even severed. In all of these cases the function of the spinal cord is impaired or destroyed. An unstable injury is one in which there is a possibility that vertebrae will shift and cause damage, possibly severing the spinal cord. Other injuries are called stable.

SYMPTOMS AND SIGNS
Damage to the vertebrae and ligaments usually causes severe pain and swelling of the affected area. Damage to the spinal cord results in loss of sensation and/or motor function below the site of injury. Injuries below the neck may cause *paraplegia* (weakness or paralysis of the legs and some-

times part of the trunk). Damage to the spinal cord in the neck may result in *quadriplegia* (weakness or paralysis of all four limbs and the trunk) or may be fatal. Weakness or paralysis is often accompanied by loss of bladder or bowel control, resulting in urinary or fecal incontinence or retention.

Pressure on the spinal cord may cause abnormalities of movement, such as muscle weakness or paralysis. It may also cause abnormalities of sensation, such as pain, tingling, or burning sensations.

DIAGNOSIS AND TREATMENT
After an accident in which a spinal injury may have occurred, the victim should be moved only by someone trained in all aspects of first aid. X *rays* of the spine are carried out to determine whether the spine has been injured and the extent of any damage.

In a stable injury, the patient must rest in bed until comfortable movement is possible; he or she may then need to wear an orthopedic *collar* or *corset* for support or to relieve pain in the injured area.

The priority in an unstable injury is to stabilize the affected bones. If they are dislocated, the surgeon usually manipulates them back into position under general anesthesia. Some unstable fractures are treated by skeletal *traction* to align the bone ends and hold them in position until healing occurs (which may take up to three months). Other unstable fractures require an operation to fasten the bone ends together permanently with a metal plate or wires.

Surgical repair of damaged nerve tracts in the spinal cord is not possible. Treatment is directed toward preventing the development of problems secondary to the main symptoms. For example, the patient is turned regularly in bed to prevent *bedsores* from forming as a result of immobility and lack of sensation in the skin. *Physiotherapy* is carried out to stop joints from locking and muscles from contracting as the result of paralysis. Retention of urine or feces may require *catheterization* or *enemas*.

OUTLOOK
Recovery is usually complete provided that the spinal cord has not been damaged, although there may be some residual pain and stiffness. When there has been pressure on the spinal cord, surgery to remove the source of the pressure can bring variable improvement in symptoms. Even when there is damage to the cord, some improvement may occur for up

S

to 12 months. In such cases, the patient's recovery can be aided by a program of *rehabilitation*. This may include forms of physiotherapy and *occupational therapy*, which can help morale and independence.

Spinal nerves

A set of 31 pairs of *nerves* that connect to the *spinal cord*.

The spinal nerves emerge in two rows from either side of the spinal cord and leave the *spine* through gaps between adjacent *vertebrae* (spinal bones). Because the spinal cord runs only two thirds of the way down the spinal canal, the lowest nine pairs of nerves must travel some distance down the canal before finally leaving the spine. These lowest nerves form a "spray" known as the cauda equina.

The distribution and branching of the spinal nerves ensure that all parts of the trunk, arms, and legs are supplied with a network of sensory and motor nerve twigs.

FUNCTION

Like all other nerves, spinal nerves consist of bundles of the axons (long fibers) of individual neurons (nerve cells). Some of these fibers carry information from sensory *receptors* in the skin, muscles, and elsewhere in the body toward the spinal cord; other motor fibers carry signals from the spinal cord to muscles and glands. Just before it connects to the spinal cord, each spinal nerve splits into two bundles, one of which carries only sensory fibers while the other carries only motor fibers. These bundles are sometimes called spinal nerve roots.

DISORDERS

Damage to the shock-absorbing disk of cartilage between two vertebrae sometimes leads to pressure on a spinal nerve root, causing pain (see *Disk prolapse*). Injury to a spinal nerve may lead to loss of sensation and movement in a part of the body. Damage or degeneration from such causes or from infection, *diabetes mellitus, vitamin deficiency*, or poisoning can lead to neurological symptoms such as pain, numbness, or twitching (see *Nerve injury; Neuropathy*).

Spinal tap

See *Lumbar puncture*.

Spine

The column of bones and cartilage that extends from the base of the skull to the pelvis, enclosing and protecting the *spinal cord* and supporting the trunk and head.

STRUCTURE AND FUNCTION

The spine is made up of 33 roughly cylindrical bones called *vertebrae*. Each pair of adjacent vertebrae is connected by a joint, called a facet joint, which both stabilizes the vertebral column and allows movement in it. Between each pair of vertebrae lies a disk-shaped pad of tough fibrous cartilage with a jellylike core (nucleus pulposus) called an intervertebral disk (see *Disk, intervertebral*). These disks cushion the vertebrae during movements such as running or jumping.

In a normal spine the cervical section curves forward, the thoracic section backward, the lumbar section forward (particularly in women), and the pelvic section backward.

The whole of the spine encloses the spinal cord, a column of nerve tracts running from the brain. Peripheral nerves (see *Peripheral nervous system*) branch off from the spinal cord to every part of the body, their roots passing between the vertebrae.

The vertebrae are bound together by two long, thick ligaments that

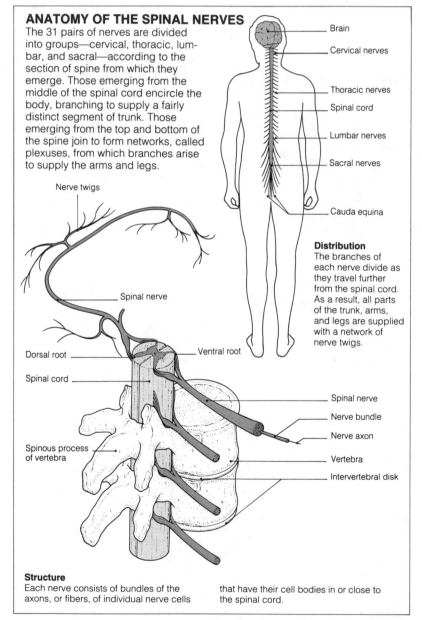

ANATOMY OF THE SPINAL NERVES

The 31 pairs of nerves are divided into groups—cervical, thoracic, lumbar, and sacral—according to the section of spine from which they emerge. Those emerging from the middle of the spinal cord encircle the body, branching to supply a fairly distinct segment of trunk. Those emerging from the top and bottom of the spine join to form networks, called plexuses, from which branches arise to supply the arms and legs.

Nerve twigs

Spinal nerve

Dorsal root

Spinal cord

Spinous process of vertebra

Ventral root

Brain

Cervical nerves

Thoracic nerves

Spinal cord

Lumbar nerves

Sacral nerves

Cauda equina

Distribution

The branches of each nerve divide as they travel further from the spinal cord. As a result, all parts of the trunk, arms, and legs are supplied with a network of nerve twigs.

Spinal nerve

Nerve bundle

Nerve axon

Vertebra

Intervertebral disk

Structure

Each nerve consists of bundles of the axons, or fibers, of individual nerve cells that have their cell bodies in or close to the spinal cord.

S

run the length of the spine, and by smaller ligaments between each of the vertebrae.

Several groups of *muscles* are attached to the vertebrae. These muscles control movements of the spine and also help to support it.

Spirochete

A spiral-shaped bacterium. Spirochetes cause *syphilis*, as well as *pinta* and *yaws* (which are both related to syphilis), *leptospirosis*, *relapsing fever*, and *Lyme disease*.

Spirometry

A *pulmonary function test* used to help diagnose or assess a *lung* disorder or to monitor treatment.

The procedure is shown in the illustrated box. The spirometer records the total volume of air breathed out, known as the forced vital capacity (FVC). It also records the volume of air breathed out in 1 second, known as the forced expiratory volume in 1 second (FEV_1).

In obstructive lung disease (such as *asthma*, *emphysema*, and chronic bronchitis), the FEV_1/FVC ratio is reduced because the airways are narrowed, thus slowing expiration. In a restrictive lung disease (such as *interstitial pulmonary fibrosis*), the FVC and FEV_1 are reduced almost equally with little change in the ratio.

Spironolactone

A potassium-sparing *diuretic drug*. Combined with thiazide or loop diuretics, it is given to treat *hypertension* (high blood pressure) and *edema* (accumulation of fluid in tissues).

Spironolactone may cause numbness, weakness, nausea, and vomiting. Less common adverse effects include diarrhea, lethargy, impotence, rash, and irregular menstruation in women. High doses of spironolactone may cause abnormal breast enlargement in men.

Spleen

An organ that removes and destroys worn-out red blood cells and helps fight infection. Weighing about 200 g, the spleen is a fist-sized, spongy, dark purple organ lying in the upper left abdomen behind the lower ribs.

STRUCTURE

The spleen is covered with a capsule from which many fibrous bands run inward to give the organ a spongelike structure. The spaces between the bands are filled with red blood cells, and with *lymphocytes* and *phagocytes* (cells that ingest other cells or foreign particles) which form part of the *lymphatic system*. Blood is supplied to the spleen by a large artery that branches extensively within the organ.

FUNCTION

One of the two main functions of the spleen is to control the quality of circulating red blood cells. It accomplishes this by removing and breaking down all worn-out red cells approximately 120 days after they have been produced in the *bone marrow* and by destroying other red cells that are

---

STRUCTURE OF THE SPINE

The spine is made up of a column of 33 roughly cylindrical bones called vertebrae. Running through the center of this bony structure is the spinal cord.

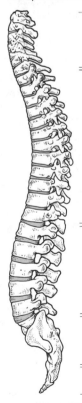

Cervical spine
Seven vertebrae, the topmost of which supports the skull.

Thoracic spine
Twelve vertebrae that run down the rear wall of the chest. A pair of ribs is attached to each vertebra.

Lumbar spine
Five vertebrae. This section is the one under the most pressure during lifting.

Sacrum
Five fused vertebrae.

Coccyx
Four fused vertebrae.

SPIROMETRY

This technique is used to assess certain lung conditions and the patient's response to treatment. It records the rate at which a patient exhales air from the lungs and the total volume exhaled.

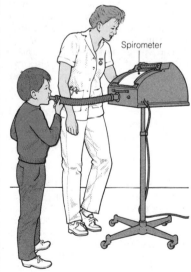

Spirometer

How it is done
The patient exhales forcibly through a mouthpiece into the spirometer. This causes the spirometer to produce a graph like those shown at right.

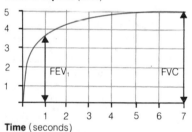

Volume expired (litres)

Time (seconds)

Normal
FEV_1 (forced expiratory volume in the first second) is the volume of air exhaled in the first second and is normally 70 to 80 percent of FVC (forced vital capacity), the total volume exhaled.

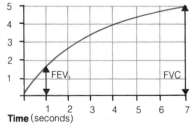

Volume expired (litres)

Time (seconds)

Asthma
A patient with asthma cannot exhale air as fast as normal, due to narrowing of the airways, so FEV_1 is reduced in comparison with FVC.

S

DISORDERS OF THE SPINE

Many disorders of the spine, despite their different causes, result in just one symptom—*back pain*.

CONGENITAL DISORDERS

Some children are born with a gap in the vertebrae that leaves part of the spinal cord exposed. This condition (*spina bifida*) may result in leg paralysis and incontinence.

INFECTION

Osteomyelitis (infection of bone and bone marrow) may in rare cases affect a vertebra, destroying both bone and disk. The most common cause is the spread of an infection, such as *tuberculosis*, from elsewhere in the body.

INFLAMMATION

In *ankylosing spondylitis*, and in some cases of *rheumatoid arthritis*, the joints in the spine become inflamed and later fuse, causing permanent stiffness. *Osteochondritis juvenilis* (inflammation of the growing area of bone in children and adolescents) can affect the vertebrae, when the disease may cause deformity of the spine.

INJURIES

Lifting heavy objects, twisting suddenly, or adopting bad posture can cause any of the following spinal injuries—a sprained ligament, torn muscle, *spondylolisthesis* (dislocated vertebrae), dislocated facet joint, or disk *prolapse* (rupture of the tough outer layer of the disk).

A direct blow, a fall from a height, or sudden twisting can result in fracture of one or more vertebrae. Overexercising the spine can have the same effect (see *Stress fracture*).

TUMORS

Tumors of the spine are usually malignant; in most cases, they have spread from cancer elsewhere in the body (see *Bone cancer*).

DEGENERATION

Osteoarthritis (degeneration of joint cartilage due to wear and tear) affects the joints in the spines of virtually everyone over 60, particularly people who do heavy manual work or people whose spines have already been affected by disease or injury.

Osteoporosis (thinning and softening of bone), which is most common in older women, can weaken the vertebrae. Under the weight of the trunk, the vertebrae may then fracture.

OTHER DISORDERS

In some people the spine becomes abnormally curved. The excessive curvature may be inward in the lower back (see *Lordosis*), outward in the upper back (see *Kyphosis*), or to one side (see *Scoliosis*). Causes include infection, osteoporosis, congenital spine disorder, and muscle disorders.

INVESTIGATION

Spinal disorders are investigated by *X rays*, *CT scanning*, and *myelography*. Other *bone imaging* techniques, including *MRI*, may sometimes be performed, as may other tests.

misshapen or defective. The spleen's other role is to help fight infection by producing some of the *antibodies*, phagocytes, and lymphocytes that help to neutralize and destroy invading microorganisms.

In the fetus, the spleen produces red blood cells. After birth, this function is taken over by the bone marrow. However, in certain diseases that affect red cell production in the bone marrow (such as *thalassemia*), the spleen may resume production.

Despite its functions, the spleen is not an essential organ. If it is removed, its activities are largely taken over by other parts of the lymphatic system, although the individual is more susceptible to infection.

DISORDERS

The spleen enlarges in many diseases. These include: infections, such as *malaria*, infectious *mononucleosis* (glandular fever), *schistosomiasis*, *tuberculosis*, and *typhoid fever*; blood disorders, such as *leukemia*, thalassemia, *sickle cell anemia* and other diseases that cause hemolytic *anemia*; and tumors of the spleen, such as *lymphomas* (tumors of lymphoid tissue which may develop in the spleen).

Enlargement of the spleen, which can often be felt as a swelling in the upper left abdomen, is sometimes accompanied by *hypersplenism* (overactivity of the spleen, which reduces the numbers of blood cells).

The spleen is sometimes ruptured by a severe blow to the abdomen, usually in a car crash or by a fall from a height. A rupture is much more likely if the spleen is enlarged or if overlying ribs are fractured. Rupture can cause severe bleeding, which may be fatal. For this reason, the injury requires an emergency operation to remove the spleen (see *Splenectomy*).

Splenectomy

Surgical removal of the *spleen*.

WHY IT IS DONE

Splenectomy is usually performed after the spleen has been seriously injured, causing severe hemorrhage. The organ is removed because it is difficult to repair and because, in an adult, its absence has virtually no known ill effects. Its function is largely taken over by other parts of the *lymphatic system* and by the *liver*.

In some cases, the spleen is removed to treat *hypersplenism* and certain types of anemia, such as hereditary *spherocytosis*. Splenectomy may be also performed during *laparotomy* (surgical exploration of the abdomen) as part of a process, known as staging, by which the extent of *Hodgkin's disease* is assessed.

HOW IT IS DONE

Under general anesthesia, a vertical or horizontal incision is made in the upper left abdomen, exposing the spleen. After attachments to other tissues have been cut and blood vessels leading into and out of the spleen have been clamped and severed, the organ is removed. The operation takes about an hour.

RECOVERY PERIOD AND OUTLOOK

Patients usually leave hospital six to 10 days after the operation. Complications, such as infection of the operation site, are rare.

In an adult, absence of the spleen slightly increases the risk of contracting infections; children become markedly more susceptible, particularly to pneumococcal *pneumonia*. A child who has undergone a splenectomy should be immunized with pneumococcal vaccine and given long-term *antibiotic drugs*. Healthy fragments of a

S

FIRST AID: SPLINTS

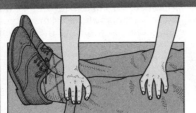

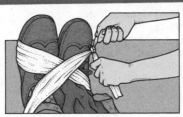

1 If help is coming, do not move the victim but support the limb by placing one hand above the fracture and the other below it.

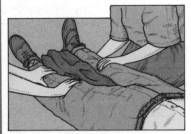

2 If the ambulance is delayed, or you must transport the victim yourself, immobilize the injured leg by using the uninjured leg as a splint. Place padding between the legs, especially between the knees and ankles. Gently bring the uninjured leg alongside the injured one. Another person should continue to support the injured limb until immobilization is complete. If it is essential to move the victim, a long, padded splint should also be placed along the outside of the injured leg.

3 Tie the victim's ankles and feet together with a figure-of-eight bandage (which should pass around the splint, if one is being used). Secure the bandage on the uninjured side. If the fracture is near the ankle, it may be necessary to modify the figure-of-eight bandage to avoid bandaging over the fracture site.

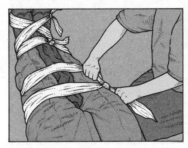

4 Tie other bandages around the knees, and above and below the fracture site. Do not bandage over the fracture site itself, and do not bandage below the fracture if it is near the ankle. If a splint is being used, also bandage around the upper thighs. Tie all knots on the uninjured side.

removed spleen are occasionally reimplanted in a child immediately after splenectomy; in some cases, these fragments regenerate to form an efficient new spleen.

Splint
A device used to immobilize part of the body. Splints may be made of acrylic, polyethylene foam, plaster of Paris, or aluminium. Ambulances may carry inflatable splints. In an emergency, a splint can be constructed from a piece of wood or a rolled-up newspaper secured to the injured part. (See also *Splinting*.)

Splinting
The application of a *splint*. Splinting is used as a first aid measure to prevent movement of a fractured limb or to immobilize a suspected fracture of the spine; this is especially important when the victim is being moved.

Splinting is sometimes required for leg fractures that are being treated by *traction*. Other uses include treatment of finger injuries, such as fracture or *baseball finger*, and of rheumatic disorders affecting the fingers, such as *tenosynovitis* (inflammation of tendon linings) and *rheumatoid arthritis*.

Splinting, dental
The mechanical joining of several teeth to hold them firmly in place while an injury heals or while *periodontal disease* is treated.

Splints may be used to secure teeth that have been fractured (see *Fracture, dental*) or loosened (see *Subluxated tooth*). They may also be used after a tooth has been reimplanted (see *Reimplantation, dental*). Occasionally, teeth loosened by periodontal disease may be splinted to adjacent, firmer teeth. Splints may also be required after *orthognathic surgery*.

Splints are fashioned directly in the mouth with materials such as wire, quick-setting plastic, and plastic crowns that can be bonded together. (See also *Wiring of the jaws*.)

Split personality
A term used to describe *multiple personality*, in which an individual has two or more personalities, each of which dominates at different times. It is also, incorrectly, used to describe *schizophrenia*, in which the sufferer's feelings and thoughts are not logically related to each other.

Spondylitis
Inflammation of the joints between the vertebrae in the *spine*. Spondylitis is usually caused by *osteoarthritis, rheumatoid arthritis*, or *ankylosing spondylitis*. In rare cases, it is due to a bacterial infection that has spread from elsewhere in the body.

Spondylolisthesis
The slipping forward (or occasionally backward) of a *vertebra* (spinal bone) over the one below it. A forward slippage of the fifth (lowest) lumbar vertebra over the top of the *sacrum* is the most common form of the condition, but it may also occur between the fourth and fifth lumbar vertebrae or between two cervical (neck) vertebrae.

CAUSES AND SYMPTOMS
Lumbar spondylolisthesis, which involves two lumbar vertebrae or the fifth lumbar vertebra and the sacrum, is usually due to *spondylolysis* (in which the bony arch of a lumbar vertebra is abnormally soft and thus liable to slip under stress) or to *osteoarthritis* of the spine (in which the joints between the vertebrae become worn and unstable).

The principal symptoms of lumbar spondylolisthesis include pain in the back that is worse when standing, and *sciatica*.

Cervical spondylolisthesis may be caused by a neck injury, congenital abnormality of the cervical spine, or *rheumatoid arthritis* (in which the supporting ligaments of the cervical spine are weakened or the joints between the vertebrae become worn). The main symptoms are pain and stiffness in the neck and, in severe cases, pain, numbness, or weakness in the sufferer's hands and arms.

DIAGNOSIS AND TREATMENT
Spondylolisthesis is diagnosed by *X rays* of the spine. Treatment may include *traction*, immobilization of the

S

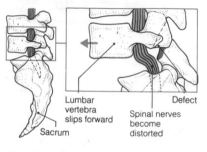

Lumbar
vertebra
slips forward
Sacrum

Defect

Spinal nerves
become
distorted

Normal spine   **Spondylolisthesis**

Lumbar spondylolisthesis
If the lowest lumbar vertebra slips forward
over the sacrum, it may distort or press on
spinal nerves, causing symptoms such as
backache or sciatica.

affected area in a plaster *corset* or
orthopedic *collar*, and *physiotherapy*. In
severe and rare cases in which there is
nerve compression damage or severe back pain, an operation to fuse
the affected vertebrae may be necessary (see *Spinal fusion*).

Spondylolysis
A disorder of the *spine* in which the
arch of the fifth (or, rarely, the fourth)
lumbar vertebra consists of relatively
soft fibrous tissue instead of normal
bone. As a result, the arch is weaker
than normal and is more likely to be
deformed or damaged under stress,
which may produce *spondylolisthesis*
(forward slippage of a vertebra over
the one below it). Otherwise, spondylolysis is usually symptomless.

Sponge, contraceptive
A disposable, circular piece of foam
impregnated with *spermicide* that is
inserted into the vagina as a method
of birth control. (See *Contraception,
barrier methods of*.)

Sporotrichosis
A chronic infection caused by the fungus SPOROTHRIX SCHENCKII, which
grows on moss and other plants. The
infection is most often contracted
through a skin wound; gardeners and
florists are particularly vulnerable. An
ulcer develops at the site of the wound
and is followed by the formation of
nodules (which can be seen as a chain
of protuberances beneath the skin) in
lymph channels around the site.
Potassium iodide solution taken by
mouth usually clears up the infection.
Rarely, in people whose resistance
to disease has been lowered, sporo-
trichosis spreads to the lungs, joints,
and various other parts of the body.

This condition may require prolonged
treatment with the *antifungal drug*
amphotericin.

Sports, drugs and
The use of drugs to improve athletic
performance has been universally
condemned by authorities because it
endangers the health of athletes and
gives drug users an unfair advantage.
Random urine tests to detect abuse are
performed in most sports during competition and at other times.
Certain drugs may be taken legiti-
mately by athletes for medical disorders, such as asthma or epilepsy.
Care should be taken, however, when
using a drug for the treatment of diarrhea, nasal congestion, or cough
because some common medications
contain substances prohibited in
sports.

TYPES OF DRUGS ABUSED
Four main types of drugs are abused
by athletes to enhance physical or
mental condition.
STIMULANTS Drugs of this group are
taken to prevent fatigue and to
increase self-confidence. However,
they also impair judgment and may
cause excessive aggression, which
increases the risk of injury to the user
or an opponent.
Stimulants, such as *amphetamine
drugs*, carry the risk of causing cardiac
arrhythmias (irregularities of the heartbeat); prolonged use may cause *heart
failure* (reduced pumping efficiency)
and increase the risk of a *brain hemorrhage*. Some cold and cough remedies
contain low doses of prohibited stimulant drugs and should be avoided
before competition.
Caffeine contained in coffee, tea, and
cola drinks, and available in tablets,
is another popular stimulant. Most
authorities only prohibit the use of
caffeine in high doses.
HORMONES Two types of hormone
drugs may be abused—anabolic
steroids (see *Steroids, anabolic*) and
growth hormone.
Anabolic steroids are substances
similar to the male sex hormone testosterone. These drugs are used
because they speed the recovery of
muscles after strenuous exercise. This
permits a more demanding training
schedule and causes an increase in
muscle bulk and strength. Anabolic
steroids are used primarily by weight-
lifters, by sprinters and athletes in
field events, and by bodybuilders.
Risks of abusing anabolic steroids
include liver damage, liver tumors,
and adrenal gland damage. In men

they may cause infertility and impotence; in women they may cause
virilization. If taken during childhood, anabolic steroids may cause
short stature by affecting the growing
areas of bones.
Growth hormone is abused to stimulate growth of muscle; it is likely to
cause *acromegaly* (excessive bone
growth leading to deformity of the
face, hands, and feet) and may cause
diabetes mellitus.
PAINKILLERS Only narcotic *analgesic
drugs* are prohibited but the use of any
painkiller (even a weak analgesic such
as acetaminophen) may aggravate an
injury. There is even the possibility
that use could lead to permanent
damage by allowing the individual
to participate with his or her pain
masked.
BETA-BLOCKER DRUGS *Beta-blocker drugs*
are taken to reduce tremor in sports in
which a steady hand is vital. Many
authorities now prohibit these drugs
in the absence of a specific medical
disorder that requires them.

Sports injuries
Any injury that arises during partici-
pation in sports. Most sports
injuries are not actually specific to
sports; they can also occur as a result
of other activities.
The wide range of sports injuries
includes *fractures*, *head injury* (including *concussion*), muscle *strain* or *compartment syndrome*, ligament *sprain*,
tendinitis (inflammation of a tendon)
or tendon rupture, joint *dislocation* or
joint *subluxation* (partial dislocation),
and injuries to a specific organ, such
as an *eye injury*.
Some injuries have a name that
includes a sports prefix, but most such
injuries can also be caused in ways
unrelated to sport. For example, *tennis
elbow* (painful inflammation around
the outside of the elbow) is a type of
overuse injury that may occur from
playing tennis, but more often results
from an activity such as sawing.
TREATMENT
Treatment of a sports injury depends
on the body part involved and the
severity of the damage. Recovery is
not complete until the damaged area
is free of pain during exercise. Exercises under the guidance of a sports
physician or physiotherapist may be
required to ensure full recovery of
movement, balance, and coordination
of the injured part and to restore
general fitness to reduce the likelihood of further injury. (See also
Sports medicine.)

S

Sports medicine

The branch of medicine concerned with assessment and improvement of *fitness* and the treatment and prevention of medical disorders related to sports. Physicians specializing in sports medicine give advice about exercises that improve endurance, strength, and flexibility; perform fitness tests; offer nutritional advice to improve performance; regulate the abuse of drugs by athletes (see *Sports, drugs and*); and provide on-site medical care at sporting events.

Preventive work in sports medicine includes advising the individual on footwear, clothing, and protective equipment to reduce the likelihood of injury, and on fluid requirements to prevent *dehydration*. In addition, the sports physician advises professional athletes on immunization requirements before competition abroad, and on coping with *jet lag* and changes in altitude and climate. In conjunction with a physiotherapist (see *Physiotherapy*), a sports physician diagnoses and treats *sports injuries*.

Spot

A general term for a small lump, mark, or inflamed area on the skin. Many different skin conditions produce particular types of spots, such as *blackheads, blisters, cysts, macules, nodules, papules, pustules,* and *scabs*. Spots may or may not be caused by infection. A collection of spots is known as a *rash*.

Spouse abuse

Repeated deliberate mental or physical injury inflicted by one spouse on the other, almost always by a man on a woman. In Canada, more than one woman in 10 is physically abused (this term includes battering and forced sexual relations) by her spouse usually over a long period of time. Because spouse abuse is usually kept a secret by both partners, much of it is not reported, and even less of it can be treated by psychiatrists and social agencies.

Men who abuse their spouses have usually learned domestic violence from their parents' behavior, are immature and have low self-esteem, which they bolster with "macho" behavior reinforced by their peer groups.

Women who submit to abuse do so for a number of reasons: threats of further abuse if they tell others, a feeling of personal inadequacy, a sense of guilt leading to the feeling that the violence may be justified, financial dependence, concern for the children, and underlying love for the partner. However, women who live with abusing men run a high risk of serious injury or death.

MANAGEMENT OF THE PROBLEM

Voluntary and provincially funded self-help groups such as Interval House offer a temporary respite for battered women and their children, legal advice, and marital counseling if the abuser is willing. This approach is probably the most hopeful for dealing with underlying or aggravating causes, such as alcohol or drug dependence, or morbid jealousy. The long-term solution to the problem probably lies in early detection of aggressors and their victims and widespread social disapproval of macho male behavior in a domestic setting.

Sprain

Tearing or stretching of the *ligaments* that hold together the bone ends in a *joint*, caused by a sudden pull. The fibrous capsule that encloses the joint may also be damaged. The most commonly sprained joint is the *ankle*, which is usually sprained as a result of "going over" on the outside of the foot so that the complete weight of the body is placed on the ankle.

A sprain causes painful swelling of the joint, which cannot be moved without increasing the pain. There may also be spasm (involuntary contraction) of surrounding muscles.

TREATMENT

An *X ray* of the joint is usually performed to exclude the possibility of a *fracture*. Treatment consists of applying an *ice pack* to reduce swelling, wrapping the joint with a compression bandage, resting it in a raised position until the pain and swelling begin to subside, and taking *analgesic drugs* (painkillers) to relieve pain. Once the joint is no longer painful, it should be gently exercised.

If ligaments are badly torn, *nonsteroidal anti-inflammatory drugs* may be prescribed to speed healing. In extremely severe cases, surgical repair may be necessary. (For first aid, see the illustrated box overleaf.)

Sprue

A disorder of the intestines that causes failure to absorb nutrients from food. There are two forms of sprue. One occurs mainly in tropical regions (see *Sprue, tropical*); the other, *celiac disease*, occurs more widely and is due to sensitivity to *gluten*.

Sprue, tropical

A disease characterized by chronic *malabsorption* (impaired absorption of nutrients from the diet by the small intestine) and consequent *malnutrition* and a type of anemia caused by deficiency of folic acid and vitamin B_{12} (see *Anemia, megaloblastic*).

As in *celiac disease*, villi (frondlike projections) on the lining of the intestine become flattened, decreasing their surface area and so reducing the absorption of nutrients.

CAUSE AND INCIDENCE

The cause of tropical sprue is unknown, but it may result from an infection of the intestine. The disease occurs in tropical regions, predominantly in India, the Far East, and the Caribbean.

SYMPTOMS

As well as megaloblastic anemia, symptoms include loss of appetite, weight loss, an inflamed mouth, sore tongue, and fatty diarrhea.

DIAGNOSIS AND TREATMENT

The diagnosis is confirmed by a *jejunal biopsy* (removal of a small sample of tissue from the upper small intestine for analysis). The disease responds well to treatment with *antibiotic drugs* and dietary supplements of folic acid, vitamin B_{12}, and, if necessary, other types of vitamins and minerals.

Sputum

Mucous material produced by the cells lining the respiratory tract. Also known as phlegm, sputum is released from glands in the walls of the bronchi (main airways in the lungs).

Sputum production may be increased by infection (see *Respiratory tract infection*), by an allergic reaction (see *Asthma*), or by inhalation of irritants, such as tobacco smoke (see *Cough, smoker's*). Sputum in the bronchi triggers a reflex *cough*.

The character of sputum varies. A bacterial infection usually causes yellow or green sputum, an allergic reaction usually produces colorless sputum, and *pulmonary edema* (fluid retention in the lungs) may result in frothy, pink sputum. *Hemoptysis* (blood in the sputum) may be caused by infection or *lung cancer*.

Laboratory tests on sputum include microscopic examination and analysis of a sputum *culture* to identify any bacteria that might be present.

Squamous cell carcinoma

One of the three most common types of skin cancer; the others are *basal cell carcinoma* and malignant *melanoma*.

S

939

FIRST AID: SPRAINS

WARNING
A severe sprain may be indistinguishable from a broken bone. If
in doubt, treat as a *fracture*.

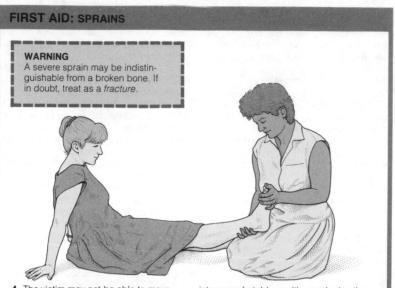

1 The victim may not be able to move the affected joint or stand up if the knee or ankle is injured. Help the victim into a comfortable position and raise the injured part of the body.

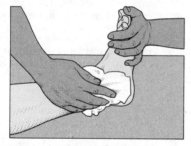

2 If the sprain is recent, apply a cold compress to the affected area and leave for about 30 minutes. This will reduce blood flow and swelling.

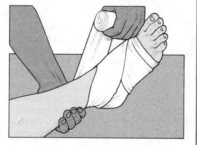

3 Cover the area with a layer of cotton wool and secure with a bandage. Make two turns around the foot, bring it across the top, and around the ankle.

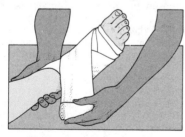

4 Continue figure-of-eight turns, with each turn of the bandage overlapping the previous turn by three quarters of its width.

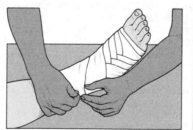

5 Bandage until the foot (not toes), ankle, and lower leg are covered. Secure the loose end. Seek medical aid—an X ray may be necessary.

CAUSES AND INCIDENCE

Squamous cell carcinoma arises from flattened, scalelike cells in the skin, usually in areas that have been exposed to strong sunlight for many years, where solar *keratoses* may have developed. This cancer is most common in pale-skinned, fair-haired people over the age of 60. The incidence is also higher than average in people whose work required them to handle or be exposed to certain substances, such as arsenic, tar, coal, paraffin, or heavy oils.

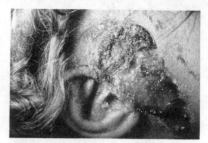

A squamous cell carcinoma
This tumor has spread slowly to cover much of the area in front of the patient's ear. It can be treated by radiation therapy.

SYMPTOMS AND SIGNS

The tumor starts as a small, firm, painless lump or patch (usually on the lip, ear, or back of the hand) and slowly enlarges, often resembling a wart or ulcer. Without treatment, the tumor may spread to other parts of the body and prove fatal. All suspicious skin areas should be reported to a physician.

DIAGNOSIS

The diagnosis is based on a skin *biopsy* (removal of a small sample of tissue for analysis).

TREATMENT

The tumor is either removed surgically or destroyed by *radiation therapy* or *cryosurgery* (application of extreme cold). Treatment with *anticancer drugs* may also be necessary.

Any person who has had a squamous cell carcinoma should limit his or her exposure to sunlight. A follow-up examination is required to check for recurrence.

Squint

A condition in which there is abnormal deviation of one eye in relation to the other. Squint, also known as strabismus, may be convergent, in which one eye is directed too far inward, or divergent, in which one eye is directed outward. Less commonly, one eye is directed upward or downward relative to the other eye (vertical strabismus).

CAUSES

Many young babies have a squint because the normal mechanism for aligning the two eyes has not yet developed. A squint that starts later in childhood usually results from a breakdown in the development of the mechanism for aligning the eyes; a common contributory factor in such cases is *hypermetropia* (farsightedness), which leads to excessive *accommodation* (adjustment of focus) and causes one eye to turn inward.

S

In children who are acquiring the capacity to see simultaneously with two eyes, squint causes double vision because the image in the squinting eye falls on the wrong part of the retina. To avoid such double vision, the brain suppresses the image from the deviating eye, eventually leading to *amblyopia* (reduced sharpness of vision).

In adults, squint may occur as a result of various disorders of the brain, of the nerves controlling the eye muscles, or of the eye muscles themselves. Squint in adults causes double vision, and may be a symptom of *stroke, diabetes mellitus, multiple sclerosis*, tumor, or *hyperthyroidism*. Treatment in children up to the age of about 6 or 7 years old may include covering the normal eye with a patch to force the child to use the weak eye. Such patching is designed to encourage normal vision to develop in the affected eye, by enabling the establishment of normal connections between the eye and the brain. Deviation of the squinting eye may be controlled by glasses and/or surgery.

Squint acquired later in life always requires medical investigation. Persistent double vision due to squint requires special prismatic glasses or surgery. Even if vision cannot be improved, surgery to improve appearance may be performed.

Stable

Unmoving, fixed, resistant to change, or in a state of equilibrium. A patient's condition is described as stable when it is neither deteriorating nor improving; a stable personality is one that is not susceptible to abnormal behavioral excesses or mental illness. In chemistry, a stable substance is one that is resistant to changes in its chemical composition or physical state, or is not radioactive.

Stage

A term used in medicine to refer to a phase in the course of a disease, particularly in the progression of *cancer*.

In assessing most types of cancer, a method known as staging is used to determine how far the cancer has progressed. The cancer is described in terms of how large the main tumor is, the degree to which it has invaded surrounding tissue, and the extent to which it has spread to lymph glands or other areas of the body. In *Hodgkin's disease*, staging also takes into account whether the lymph nodes on both sides of the diaphragm are affected, and whether the spleen is involved.

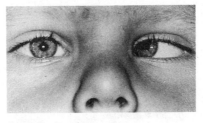

Convergent squint
This child has a convergent squint of the left eye—i.e., the left eye is directed too far inward (toward the nose).

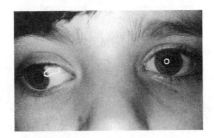

Divergent squint
This child has a divergent squint of the right eye—i.e., the right eye is directed too far outward (away from the nose).

Staging not only helps to assess outlook (in general, the more advanced the stage, the worse the outlook) but also the most appropriate treatment. For example, a cancer at a particular stage may respond better to *radiation therapy* than to surgery.

Staining

The process of dyeing specimens of cells, tissues, or microorganisms so that they are clearly visible or easily identifiable under a *microscope*. Staining is also sometimes carried out to detect or identify certain chemical substances in cells.

Before a specimen can be examined under a microscope, it must be preserved and then sliced or smeared extremely thinly. After these procedures, most specimens are almost transparent, so staining is necessary to make them easily visible.

One of the most commonly used staining techniques is the Papanicolaou stain test, which is used in *cytology* to allow the detection of cancerous and precancerous changes in cells.

Many different stains can be used to identify particular structures or products within cells. A very commonly used stain is hematoxylin and eosin, which is a double stain that colors nuclei blue and cytoplasm pink. Other stains may be used to identify a particular microorganism in tissues or to

clarify a diagnosis. A more recent development is the use of special fluorescent dyes that stain specific chemical constituents of cells or tissues; when illuminated with ultraviolet light, the stained constituents glow.

Another commonly used technique, known as immunoperoxidase staining, involves washing cells with a preparation containing specific types of *antibodies*. These antibodies become attached to specific cell components and chemicals. Tagging of the antibodies with a dye that can be seen under the microscope as red-brown enables the observer to identify certain components or chemicals if they are present within the cells.

Another example of a useful staining technique is *Gram's stain*, which is widely used to identify and differentiate between groups of bacteria.

Stammering

See *Stuttering*.

Stanford-Binet test

A type of *intelligence test*.

Stanozolol

A steroid drug (see *Steroids, anabolic*).

Stapedectomy

An operation on the *ear* to remove the *stapes* (the innermost of the three sound-conducting bones in the middle ear) and replace it with an artificial substitute. Stapedectomy is performed to treat *deafness* caused by *otosclerosis*, a disorder in which the base of the stapes becomes fixed by an overgrowth of spongy bone and can no longer move freely to transmit sound to the inner ear.

HOW IT IS DONE

The operation is performed under local or general anesthesia. An incision is made so that the eardrum can be folded forward to allow access to the middle ear. All or most of the stapes is then removed. One end of a plastic or metal prosthesis is inserted into the entrance to the inner ear, and the other end of the prosthesis is attached to the incus (the middle of the three sound-conducting bones in the middle ear). The eardrum is then sewn back in position.

OUTLOOK

Stapedectomy improves hearing considerably in more than 90 percent of cases. However, in about 1 percent of patients, hearing deteriorates or is lost altogether. Because of this risk, a stapedectomy is usually carried out on only one ear at a time.

S

Stapes

The innermost of the three auditory ossicles (the tiny, sound-conducting bones in the middle *ear*). The stapes, the Latin for stirrup (because of its shape), is the smallest bone in the body. Its head articulates with the incus (the middle auditory ossicle) and its base fits into the oval window in the wall of the inner ear.

In *otosclerosis*, the stapes becomes fixed by an overgrowth of bone and can no longer transmit sound to the inner ear. Hearing loss due to otosclerosis can be cured by an operation known as *stapedectomy*.

Staphylococcal infections

A group of infections caused by *bacteria* of the STAPHYLOCOCCUS genus. Staphylococci, which grow in grapelike clusters, are a common cause of skin infections but can also cause serious internal disorders.

Staphylococcal bacteria are present harmlessly on the skin of most people. If the bacteria become trapped within the skin by a blocked sweat or sebaceous gland, they may cause superficial skin infections, such as *pustules*, *boils*, *abscesses*, *styes*, or *carbuncles*. Infection of deeper tissues may result if the skin is broken (see *Wound infection*). In newborn babies, toxins released by bacteria on the skin can cause a severe, blistering rash called the scalded skin syndrome (see *Necrolysis, toxic epidermal*).

Staphylococcal bacteria are also harmlessly present in the membranes that line the nose and throat. When mucus is not cleared from the lungs, such as after a viral infection, organisms may accumulate in the lungs and cause *pneumonia*.

In menstruating women (particularly those using highly absorbent tampons), toxin-producing staphylococci may colonize the mucous membranes lining the vagina, causing *toxic shock syndrome*, a condition first recognized in the late 1970s. A different type of staphylococcus can cause *urinary tract infection*.

Sometimes staphylococci enter the bloodstream as a result of spread from a skin infection or as a result of introduction from a needle, leading to *septic shock*, infectious *arthritis*, *osteomyelitis*, or bacterial *endocarditis*.

Staphylococcal *food poisoning* is caused by ingestion of toxins produced by the bacteria. A common source of contamination is a pustule on the skin of a food handler.

Starch

See *Carbohydrates*.

Starvation

A condition caused by lack of food over a long period, resulting in weight loss, changes in *metabolism* (body chemistry), and extreme hunger. (See also *Anorexia nervosa; Fasting; Nutritional disorders*.)

Stasis

A slowing down or cessation of flow. For example, in venous stasis there is a reduction or stoppage of blood flow through one or more veins.

Statistics, medical

A science concerned with the collection and analysis of numerical data relating to medicine, and one with considerable impact on health care.

Information on the *incidence* and *prevalence* of various disorders and diseases, both in the general population and among certain groups of the population, is an important aspect of medical statistics. This science also covers such diverse topics as waiting times in outpatient clinics, infection rates after surgery, the frequency of side effects from drugs, and the evaluation of different types of treatment.

All medical research institutions today employ statisticians to advise on the design and interpretation of medical trials, and on the interpretation of data obtained from such trials. For example, when two treatments are to be compared—or when treatment is to be compared with not giving treatment—the statistician advises on such matters as the number of patients required in the trial to establish a valid conclusion, and on other matters, such as methodology, including how to allocate patients to various treatment groups, how frequently to take measurements of the outcomes of the treatments, and how to analyze the mathematical results. (See also *Statistics, vital*.)

Statistics, vital

Assessment of the health of a country's population, which relies on the collection of data on birth and death rates and on the causes of death (see *Mortality*). In most developed countries today, all deaths are certified (usually by a medical practitioner) and recorded in a national register. They are then classified by cause and analyzed according to factors such as age, sex, occupation, social class, and ethnic group.

Comparison of the vital statistics of different countries (or regions within a country) gives a measure of the relative health of their populations as a whole. A detailed comparison may also show variations between social classes or ethnic groups. (See also *Life expectancy; Statistics, medical*.)

Status asthmaticus

A severe and prolonged attack of *asthma*. Status asthmaticus is a serious and potentially life-threatening condition that requires urgent treatment.

Status epilepticus

Prolonged or repeated epileptic seizures without any recovery of consciousness between attacks. Status epilepticus is a medical emergency that may be fatal if not treated promptly. It is more likely to occur if *anticonvulsant drugs* are taken erratically or if they are withdrawn suddenly. (See *Epilepsy*.)

STDs

See *Sexually transmitted diseases*.

Steatorrhea

The presence of excessive fat in the feces. Steatorrhea causes diarrhea characterized by offensive-smelling, bulky, loose, greasy, pale-colored feces, which tend to float in the toilet and are difficult to flush away. Steatorrhea is a symptom of diseases that interfere with the breakdown and absorption of fat in the diet (notably *pancreatitis* and *celiac disease*) and of the removal of large segments of small intestine. Steatorrhea is also a side effect of some *lipid-lowering drugs*.

Stein-Leventhal syndrome

See *Ovary, polycystic*.

Stenosis

Narrowing of a duct, canal, passage, or tubular organ, such as a blood vessel or the intestine. *Aortic stenosis* is narrowing of the aortic valve opening from the left ventricle (lower chamber of the heart); *pyloric stenosis* is narrowing of the pylorus (the lower outlet from the stomach).

Stereotaxic surgery

Brain operations carried out by inserting delicate instruments through a surgically created hole in the skull and guiding them, with the aid of *X rays* or *CT scanning*, to a specific area.

WHY IT IS DONE
Stereotaxic procedures are used in the treatment of *pituitary tumors*, in which

S

the gland is cut out or a radio-active implant is inserted into the gland to destroy it.

Other uses include a brain *biopsy* (removal of a small sample of tissue for analysis), insertion of permanent stimulating wires to control otherwise intractable pain, and destruction of areas of the brain to treat disabling neurological disorders, such as severe *depression* (see *Psychosurgery*) or, in rare cases, *temporal lobe epilepsy*. Stereotaxic surgery is also occasionally used to treat people with *Parkinson's disease* in whom severe tremor has not responded to drugs.

HOW IT IS DONE
Under a general or local anesthetic, an adjustable metal frame is attached to the skull with screws. The area to be treated is located by X rays or CT scanning and the best position for inserting the instrument is calculated mathematically. The skull is then entered by means of a *burr hole* or *craniotomy*, and the angle of the frame is adjusted to hold and guide a hollow tube into the brain at the correct angle. The required instrument (a needle for biopsies, a scalpel or diathermy probe for cutting or destroying areas) is inserted through the tube and the operation performed; X rays or scans are taken during the procedure.

Sterility
The state either of being germ-free, or of permanent *infertility*.

Sterilization
A term that refers to the complete destruction or removal of living organisms or to any procedure that renders a person unable to reproduce (see *Sterilization, female; Vasectomy*).

The elimination of microorganisms is vitally important in preventing the spread of infection. It may be achieved by various physical or chemical means, such as by boiling, steaming, or autoclaving (steaming under high pressure); by irradiation with ultraviolet light, X rays, or gamma rays; or by applying *antiseptics* or *disinfectants*. Liquids can also be sterilized by passing them through extremely fine filters that trap microorganisms as tiny as viruses. Sometimes, more than one method is used (e.g., bed linen may be disinfected and then autoclaved).

Sterilization, female
A usually permanent method of *contraception* in which the fallopian tubes are sealed or cut to prevent a male's sperm from reaching the ova.

Sterilization is a common method of contraception; about 20,000 female sterilizations are carried out each year in Canada and nearly 10 percent of North American women 30 years or older have been sterilized.

WHY IT IS DONE
Women who have completed their families or who plan not to have children may choose to be sterilized to avoid the inconvenience or side effects of other methods of contraception. Sterilization may also be chosen by a woman in whom a pregnancy would be a serious threat to health, or in whom there is an unacceptably high risk of children being affected by a serious hereditary disease.

HOW IT IS DONE
The illustrated box shows common procedures for female sterilization, performed using *laparoscopy*.

Alternatively, the surgeon may work directly through a small incision just below the navel. Known as a minilaparotomy, this procedure is carried out in the first few weeks after a woman has given birth. In other cases, the fallopian tubes may be cut and tied off via an incision in the vagina. Alternatively, a hysteroscope (a type of *endoscope*) may be passed through the vagina and into the uterus; the exits of the fallopian tubes into the uterus are then plugged from the inside.

Surgical removal of the uterus (see *Hysterectomy*) or of the fallopian tubes and/or ovaries (see *Oophorectomy; Salpingectomy; Salpingo-oophorectomy*) to treat specific disorders also results in sterilization. These operations are performed through a larger abdominal incision and today are considered too drastic to be performed only for sterilization.

Female sterilization techniques may be performed on an outpatient basis but often the woman is admitted to hospital the day before laparoscopy and discharged the day after the operation.

FEMALE STERILIZATION
Laparoscopic sterilization (below) is the most common method. Both fallopian tubes must be cut, sealed, or otherwise obstructed so that eggs and sperm cannot meet for fertilization to occur.

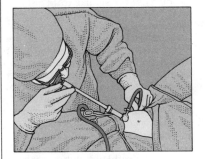

Laparoscopic sterilization
An endoscope (viewing tube) and an operating instrument are passed through separate small incisions in the abdomen.

Instruments
The trocar is a sharp-pointed inner stylus surrounded by a close-fitting tube, the cannula. The instrument can be passed through the abdominal wall. After insertion, the trocar is removed, leaving the hollow cannula in place. Other instruments are passed through the hollow cannula.

Cutting
A small loop of the fallopian tube may be drawn up, secured by a tight ligature, and then cut off.

Constriction
The loop is constricted by a tight band. Reversal is possible with this sterilization technique.

Clipping
A plastic or metal clip may be applied to obstruct egg passage. In theory, this method is also reversible.

Cautery
Electrocoagulation (diathermy) can be used to burn through, and thus seal, the fallopian tube.

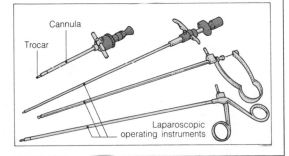

Cannula
Trocar
Laparoscopic operating instruments

S

OUTLOOK

Female sterilization has a very low failure rate (around 0.05 pregnancies per 100 women years of use—i.e., the number of pregnancies among 100 women using the method for one year). If pregnancy does occur after a sterilization operation, there is a greatly increased risk that it will be an *ectopic pregnancy*.

In some cases, microsurgical techniques may succeed in restoring fertility in a woman who has been sterilized; 70 to 75 percent of women who undergo such surgery later achieve pregnancy.

Sterilization, male

See *Vasectomy*.

Sternum

The anatomical name for the breastbone, the long, narrow, flat plate of bone that forms the central part of the front of the chest. The sternum consists of three main parts: an upper, triangular portion, called the manubrium; a long, narrow middle part, the body; and, at the lower end, a small, slightly flexible, leaf-shaped projection, the xiphoid process. The upper part of the manubrium articulates with the inner ends of the two *clavicles* (collarbones); attached to the sides of the manubrium and body are the seven pairs of costal cartilages that join the sternum to the *ribs*.

Between the manubrium and body is a type of joint known as a *symphysis*. This joint allows slight movement between these two parts of the sternum when the ribs rise and fall during breathing.

The sternum is very strong and requires great force to fracture it. The principal danger of such an injury is not the fracture itself, but the possibility that the broken bone may be driven inward and damage the heart (which lies behind the sternum).

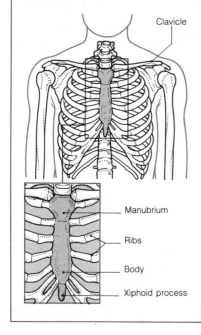

LOCATION OF THE STERNUM

The sternum, or breastbone, is joined to the ribs and clavicles by flexible couplings that allow the chest to move while breathing in and out.

Clavicle

Manubrium

Ribs

Body

Xiphoid process

Steroid drugs

A group of drugs that includes the *corticosteroid drugs*, which resemble hormones produced by the cortex *adrenal glands*, and the anabolic steroid drugs (see *Steroids, anabolic*), which have an effect similar to that of the male sex hormones.

Steroids, anabolic

COMMON DRUGS
Nandrolone Stanozolol

Drugs that have an anabolic (protein-building) effect similar to *testosterone* and other male sex hormones.

WHY THEY ARE USED

Anabolic steroids, by mimicking the anabolic effects of testosterone, build tissue, promote muscle recovery following injury, and help strengthen bones. They are given to treat some types of *anemia* and, occasionally, to treat postmenopausal women who have *osteoporosis*.

ABUSE

Anabolic steroids have been widely abused by athletes who wish to improve their strength and stamina. This practice has serious risks to health (see *Sports, drugs and*).

POSSIBLE ADVERSE EFFECTS

Adverse effects include acne, *edema*, damage to the liver, damage to the adrenal glands, infertility, impotence in men, and *virilization* in women.

Stethoscope

An instrument for listening to sounds in the body, particularly those made by the heart or lungs.

The standard stethoscope consists of a Y-shaped flexible plastic tube with an earpiece at the end of each arm of the Y, and a sound-detecting device at the base. One side of this device consists of a thin plastic diaphragm; the other side has a concave bell with a hole in its center. A physician presses the diaphragm against a patient's chest or back to hear high-pitched sounds. The concave bell side is placed gently against the skin to allow the physician to hear low-pitched sounds.

Stevens-Johnson syndrome

A rare skin condition characterized by severe blisters and bleeding in the mucous membranes of the lips, eyes, mouth, nasal passage, and genitals. Stevens-Johnson syndrome is a life-threatening form of *erythema multiforme*, and is believed in many cases to be caused by a *drug* reaction.

Sticky eye

A common description of one of the symptoms of *conjunctivitis* (inflammation of the conjunctival membrane) in which the eyelids tend to become stuck together with discharge.

Stiff neck

A very common symptom, usually due to spasm (involuntary contraction) in muscles at the side or the back of the neck.

In most cases, stiff neck occurs suddenly and for no apparent reason; the symptom is often first noticed upon waking. Stiff neck commonly occurs as a result of a minor neck injury—such as a ligament sprain or *subluxation* (partial dislocation) of a joint between neck vertebrae—that has passed unnoticed but has caused irritation of a nerve; this, in turn, leads to spasm of the neck muscles.

A stiff neck may also result from muscle spasm due to a *disk prolapse* or to a *whiplash injury*.

A relatively rare, but potentially serious, cause of a stiff neck is *meningi-*

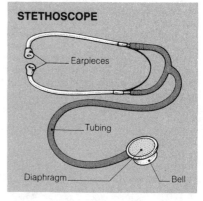

STETHOSCOPE

Earpieces

Tubing

Diaphragm

Bell

S

tis (infection of the membranes that surround the brain and spinal cord). In such cases, the stiffness is usually accompanied by headache, vomiting, fever, photophobia (abnormal sensitivity to light), and intense pain when bending the neck.

TREATMENT

Mild stiffness of the neck may be relieved by gentle massage, warming, and use of a *liniment*. Severe or persistent stiffness, or stiffness accompanied by symptoms suggestive of meningitis, requires medical attention. (See also *Torticollis*.)

Stiffness

A term used to refer to difficulty in moving a joint, to restriction of movement in a joint, or to difficulty in stretching a muscle.

Causes of joint stiffness include *arthritis* (inflammation of joint surfaces) and *bursitis* (inflammation of the joint lining). *Rheumatoid arthritis* characteristically causes severe joint stiffness for the first few hours after waking. Causes of muscle stiffness include *cramp* and *spasticity* (increased muscle rigidity).

Stilbestrol

See *Diethylstilbestrol*.

Stillbirth

Delivery of a dead fetus after the 28th week of *pregnancy*. Stillbirth is also called late fetal death. Stillbirths must be reported and the cause of death recorded on the death certificate.

INCIDENCE

The incidence of stillbirth has decreased dramatically in developed countries over the last 40 or 50 years and is now less than four per 1,000 live births in Canada.

As a general rule, stillbirths are more common in poor communities, among older women, and among women who do not receive good *prenatal care* and obstetric care.

CAUSES

The precise cause of stillbirth is unknown in at least one third of cases. Severely malformed babies, particularly those with *anencephaly*, *spina bifida*, or *hydrocephalus*, account for at least one fifth of stillbirths.

A maternal disorder, such as *antepartum hemorrhage*, *hypertension* (high blood pressure), or any other condition affecting the function of the *placenta*, may result in stillbirth, often because the fetus is deprived of oxygen. Another cause of stillbirth is severe *Rh incompatibility*.

Some infectious diseases (including *measles*, *chickenpox*, *influenza*, *toxoplasmosis*, *rubella*, *cytomegalovirus*, *herpes simplex*, *syphilis*, and *malaria*) may harm the fetus if contracted during pregnancy. In general, the more severe the infection, the greater the risk of stillbirth. A pregnant woman who is exposed to an infectious disease to which she is not immune should consult her physician.

PSYCHOLOGICAL EFFECTS

The bereaved parents usually experience a sense of loss that is just as intense as if any other loved person had died, and often they experience feelings of depression, guilt, anger, and inadequacy. Emotional support from friends, relatives, and self-help groups is useful, as is professional counseling.

Still's disease

See *Rheumatoid arthritis, juvenile*.

Stimulant drugs

COMMON DRUGS

Central nervous system stimulants
Caffeine Dexamphetamine

Respiratory stimulants
Ammophylline Nikethamide Theophylline

Drugs that increase nerve activity in the *brain* by initiating the release of *norepinephrine*, a type of *neurotransmitter* (chemical released from nerve endings).

TYPES

There are two main groups of stimulant drugs: central nervous system stimulants (including *amphetamine drugs*), which reduce drowsiness and increase alertness by their action on the reticular activating system in the *brain stem*; and respiratory stimulants (see *Analeptic drugs*), which act on the respiratory center in the brain stem.

WHY THEY ARE USED

Nerve stimulants are given to treat *narcolepsy* (excessive sleepiness). Paradoxically, they have also been found useful in the treatment of *hyperactivity* in children. Nerve stimulants also suppress the appetite but their use in the treatment of *obesity* is now rarely recommended.

Despite the risk of adverse effects, nerve stimulants are sometimes abused because they help prevent fatigue, increase alertness, and may improve self-confidence. Their use by athletes is widely condemned by physicians and prohibited by sports organizations (see *Sports, drugs and*).

POSSIBLE ADVERSE EFFECTS

Effects include shaking, sweating, palpitations, nervousness, sleeping problems, hallucinations, paranoid delusions, and seizures. Long-term use may lead to *tolerance* (the need for greater amounts to have the same effects) and *drug dependence* (withdrawal symptoms on stopping).

Stimulus

Anything that directly results in a change in the activities of the body as a whole or of any individual part (i.e., any agent or event that evokes a response). For example, the sight and smell of food stimulate salivation. Certain nerve cells (known collectively as *receptors*) are specialized to respond to specific stimuli. The rods and cones in the retina of the eye which respond to light are an example of such nerve cell specialization.

Stings

Stinging animals include scorpions and some insects (such as bees and wasps), jellyfish and related marine animals (such as anemones and corals), and some fish (such as stingrays). There are marked differences among these groups in the way the sting is delivered and its effects. (See *Insect stings*; *Jellyfish stings*; *Scorpion stings*; *Venomous bites and stings*.)

Nettles and some other plants carry tiny stinging hairs that hold an irritant liquid. These hairs penetrate and break off in the skin, causing release of the liquid, which has an immediate irritant effect that rarely lasts more than an hour or two. Washing the affected area and applying *calamine* lotion can provide relief. Contact with some other poisonous plants (see *Plants, poisonous*) may result in a more severe allergic reaction, sometimes requiring medical attention.

Stitch

A temporary, sudden, sharp pain in the abdomen or side that occurs during severe or unaccustomed exercise, usually running. The cause of a stitch is unknown.

Stitch is also the common name for a suture used to close a wound (see *Suturing*).

Stokes-Adams syndrome

Recurrent episodes of temporary loss of consciousness caused by insufficient blood flow from the heart to the brain. This deficient blood supply is due to irregularity of the heartbeat (see *Arrhythmia, cardiac*), which mark-

945

edly reduces the pumping efficiency of the heart, or to complete *heart block* (abnormally slow conduction of electrical impulses through the heart muscle), resulting in temporary cessation of the heartbeat.

SYMPTOMS AND TREATMENT
In a typical attack, the sufferer faints suddenly and turns blue if the period of unconsciousness is prolonged. The breathing rate increases and a very slow pulse can be felt. Occasionally, lack of oxygen supply to the brain may cause a *seizure* (convulsion).

In most cases, the heart soon starts beating again, the skin flushes, and consciousness is regained. If this fails to happen, *cardiopulmonary resuscitation* should be carried out promptly to prevent brain damage.

Most people with Stokes-Adams syndrome are fitted with a *pacemaker* to maintain normal heartbeat and prevent future attacks.

Stoma
A term meaning mouth or orifice. A surgically created stoma in the abdomen acts as an artificial anus. A temporary stoma may be used to divert feces from a healing wound in the intestine. A permanent stoma is created if part of the intestine has been removed. (See also *Colostomy*; *Ileostomy*.)

Stomach
A hollow, baglike organ of the *digestive system* which is connected to the esophagus and the duodenum (the first part of the small intestine). The stomach lies in the left side of the abdomen under the *diaphragm*.

STRUCTURE
The stomach is flexible, allowing it to expand when food is eaten; in an adult, the average capacity is about 1.5 litres. The stomach wall consists of layers of longitudinal and circular muscle, lined by special glandular cells that secrete gastric juice, and supplied by blood vessels and nerves. A strong muscle at the lower end of the stomach forms a ring called the pyloric sphincter that can close the outlet leading to the duodenum.

FUNCTION
Although the main function of the stomach is to continue the breakdown of food that is started in the mouth and completed in the small intestine, it also acts as a storage organ. If storage were not possible, food would have to be eaten every 20 minutes or so rather than only two or three times a day.

The sight and smell of food and the arrival of food in the stomach stimulate gastric secretion. The gastric juice secreted from the stomach lining contains pepsin (an enzyme that breaks down protein), hydrochloric acid (which kills bacteria taken in with the food and which creates the most suitable environment for the pepsin to work in), and intrinsic factor (which is essential for the absorption of vitamin B_{12} in the small intestine). The stomach lining also contains glands that secrete mucus, which helps provide a barrier to prevent the stomach from digesting itself.

The layers of muscle produce rhythmic contractions about every 20 seconds that churn the food and gastric juice; the combined effect of this movement and the action of the digestive juice convert the semisolid food into a creamy fluid. This process takes varying lengths of time, depending on the nature of the food. Generally, however, the richer the meal, the longer it takes to be emptied from the stomach. The partly digested food is squirted into the duodenum at regular intervals by the contractions of the stomach and by relaxation of the pyloric sphincter.

Stomachache
A common name for discomfort in the upper abdomen. (See *Indigestion*.)

Stomach cancer
A malignant tumor that arises from the lining of the *stomach*, also called gastric cancer.

CAUSES AND INCIDENCE
The cause of stomach cancer remains uncertain but evidence suggests that an environmental factor, probably diet, plays a part. Recent speculation has centered on an association between stomach cancer and eating quantities of salted, pickled, or smoked foods. Certain other factors, such as pernicious *anemia*, partial *gastrectomy*, and belonging to blood group A, seem to increase the risk of developing this cancer.

Stomach cancer rarely affects people under the age of 40 and is more common in men than in women. There is marked geographic variation—with a very high rate of 80 to 90 cases per 100,000 people in Japan compared with about 11 per 100,000 people annually in Canada, where it causes around 2,100 deaths a year. There has been a dramatic decrease in the worldwide incidence of stomach cancer over the past 50 years.

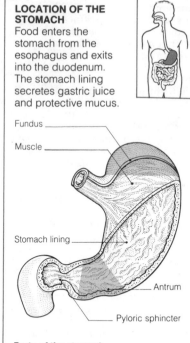

LOCATION OF THE STOMACH
Food enters the stomach from the esophagus and exits into the duodenum. The stomach lining secretes gastric juice and protective mucus.

Fundus
Muscle
Stomach lining
Antrum
Pyloric sphincter

Parts of the stomach
The fundus and antrum are two of the main parts of the stomach; the lower esophageal segment and pyloric sphincters control entry and exit of food.

SYMPTOMS AND SIGNS
The symptoms of stomach cancer (if any) are often indistinguishable from those of *peptic ulcer*. In the advanced stages, there is usually loss of appetite, the sensation that the stomach is filling up quickly, nausea and vomiting, and weight loss.

DIAGNOSIS AND TREATMENT
The condition is suggested by *barium X-ray examination* and confirmed by *gastroscopy* (examination of the stomach using a flexible viewing instrument). A *biopsy* (removal of a sample of tissue for microscopic examination) of the stomach lining may also be performed using a gastroscope.

The only effective treatment is total *gastrectomy*. However, only about 20 percent of patients are able to undergo such surgery; in the remainder, the tumor has spread too widely at the time of diagnosis. In inoperable, advanced cases, *radiation therapy* and *anticancer drugs* may be used.

OUTLOOK
If the cancer is detected at a very early stage (before it has spread beyond the stomach lining), a high cure rate is possible. In Japan, where mass

S

DISORDERS OF THE STOMACH

Disorders of the stomach have a variety of causes. Because the stomach is a reservoir, some disorders arise in the process of emptying its contents. Other problems relate to the stomach's role in the preparation of ingested food for digestion.

INFECTION

The large amount of hydrochloric acid secreted by the stomach protects the stomach from some infections by destroying many of the bacteria, viruses, and fungi that are taken in with food and drink. When the protective power is insufficient, a variety of gastrointestinal infections may occur.

TUMORS

Stomach cancer causes about 2,100 deaths annually in Canada. Early symptoms are often mistaken for *indigestion*, and diagnosis is often delayed until it is too late for a cure. Any change in the customary functioning of the digestive system is important, especially after the age of 50. A persistent feeling of fullness, or pain before or after meals, should never be ignored. Unexplained loss of appetite or frequent nausea should always be reported to a physician. A tumor in the upper part of the stomach, near the opening of the esophagus, can cause obstruction and difficulty in swallowing.

Sometimes a stomach tumor remains "silent" and the first signs are due to the appearance of secondary growths elsewhere in the body.

Benign (noncancerous) *polyps* can also develop in the stomach.

ULCERATION

The acid and other digestive juices secreted by the stomach sometimes attack the stomach lining. The healthy stomach is prevented from digesting itself mainly by the protective layer of mucus secreted by the lining and by the speed with which damaged surface cells are replaced by the deeper layers. Many influences can upset this delicate balance. One of the most important is excessive acid secretion. The resulting *peptic ulcers* are probably the most common serious stomach disorder. Peptic ulcers are sometimes caused by stress, or by severe injury, such as major burns, accidents, and after surgery and severe infections; often they occur for no apparent reason. The stomach lining can be damaged by large amounts of ASA or alcohol, sometimes causing *gastritis* (inflammation of the stomach lining). This may eventually lead to ulceration of the stomach lining.

AUTOIMMUNE DISORDERS

Pernicious anemia is caused by the failure of the stomach lining to produce intrinsic factor, a substance whose role is to facilitate the absorption of vitamin

B_{12} (itself necessary for red blood cell formation). Failure to produce the intrinsic factor occurs if there is atrophy of the stomach lining, which also causes failure of acid production. Tests that determine a person's ability to absorb vitamin B_{12} are important in the investigation of this condition. Pernicious anemia is usually due to an *autoimmune disorder*.

OTHER DISORDERS

Enlargement of the stomach may be caused when scarring from a chronic peptic ulcer occurs at the stomach outlet. It may also be a complication of *pyloric stenosis*, a rare but serious condition in which there is narrowing of the stomach outlet. Rarely, the stomach may become twisted and obstructed, a condition called *volvulus*.

INVESTIGATION

Stomach disorders are investigated primarily by *barium X-ray examinations* and/or *gastroscopy*. Occasionally, a *biopsy* (removal of a tissue sample for microscopic analysis) is performed.

---

screening by gastroscopy is performed, 85 percent of people are still alive five years after treatment by surgery. In advanced disease, however, the outlook is not good, with less than 10 percent of patients surviving for longer than five years.

Stomach imaging
See *Barium X-ray examinations.*

Stomach pump
See *Lavage, gastric.*

Stomach ulcer
A raw area in the stomach lining, also called a gastric ulcer. It is a type of *peptic ulcer.*

Stomatitis
Any form of inflammation or ulceration of the mouth. Examples include *mouth ulcers* and *cold sores.*

Stones
Small, hard collections of solid material within the body. Also called calculi, they are formed from substances that are present to excess in fluids such as urine or bile. (See *Calculus, urinary tract; Gallstones.*)

Stool
Another word for *feces.*

Stork mark
A small, flat, harmless, pinkish-red skin blemish found in 30 to 50 percent of newborn babies. Such marks, which are sometimes known as stork bites or salmon patches, are a type of *hemangioma* usually found around the eyes and at the nape of the neck. Stork marks around the eyes usually disappear within the first year; those at the base of the neck may persist indefinitely.

Strabismus
See *Squint.*

Strain
Tearing or stretching of *muscle* fibers as a result of suddenly pulling them too far. There is bleeding into the damaged area of muscle, causing pain, swelling, and muscle spasm; a bruise usually appears a few days after the injury. Muscle strain of the back is a common cause of nonspecific *back pain.* Strains are most common in athletes.

Treatment may include applying an *ice pack* to reduce swelling, use of *strapping* or a compression *bandage,* and resting an affected part (in a raised position if appropriate) for 48 hours. *Analgesic drugs* (painkillers) may also be taken to relieve pain. After the rest period, *physiotherapy* including stretching exercises should

S

be started to prevent possible shortening of the muscle due to the formation of scar tissue. In some cases, *nonsteroidal anti-inflammatory drugs* may be prescribed to speed healing.

The risk of muscle strain can be reduced by performing warm-up exercises before any sports activity.

Strangulation

The constriction, usually by twisting or compression, of a tube or passage in the body, blocking blood flow and interfering with the function of the affected organ. Strangulation may occur with a *hernia* or after twisting of the testis (see *Testis, torsion of*).

Strangulation is usually caused by herniation of part of the intestine, either inside the abdomen or externally as in an inguinal hernia, or by *volvulus* (twisting of a piece of intestine). The resulting intestinal obstruction requires an emergency operation (see *Intestine, obstruction of*).

Strangulation of the neck with the hands or with a ligature, such as a cord or scarf, may be deliberate or accidental. The main lethal effect arises from compression of the *jugular veins* in the neck.

This compression prevents blood from flowing out of the brain and head, where it stagnates and its oxygen content is quickly used up. In addition, compression of the *trachea* (windpipe) restricts breathing and impairs oxygenation of the blood. The victim's face becomes congested with blood, turning purple-blue in color. He or she loses consciousness and, some minutes later, brain damage and death occur from lack of oxygen.

Any constricting ligature must be removed as quickly as possible and medical help summoned. If the victim is not breathing, *artificial respiration* should be performed until an ambulance or physician arrives.

To prevent accidental strangulation, a child's environment should be kept free of potential ligatures—such as cords on toys or clothing, or dangerous restraining apparatus. Children should be discouraged from playing with lassos.

Strangury

A symptom characterized by a painful and frequent desire to empty the bladder, although only a few drops of urine can be passed. Causes of strangury include *prostatitis* (inflammation of the prostate gland), *cystitis*, bladder cancer (see *Bladder tumors*), and bladder stones (see *Calculus, urinary tract*).

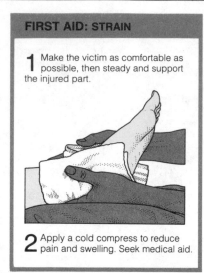

FIRST AID: STRAIN

1 Make the victim as comfortable as possible, then steady and support the injured part.

2 Apply a cold compress to reduce pain and swelling. Seek medical aid.

Strapping

The application of adhesive tape to part of the body to exert pressure and hold a structure in place.

Strapping is used to reduce pain and swelling caused by soft tissue injuries, such as *sprains* and *strains*. It may also be applied to joints to prevent injury due to excessive movement of the affected part, or to strengthen a joint that has been injured in order to help prevent recurrence of the injury.

Strawberry nevus

A bright red, raised spot which appears in early infancy. A strawberry nevus is a type of *hemangioma*.

Strep throat

A *streptococcal infection* of the *throat*. Strep throat is most common in children and is spread by droplets (containing the bacteria) coughed or breathed into the air.

In some people, the bacteria cause few or no symptoms, but a proportion suffer a sore throat, fever, general malaise, and enlarged lymph nodes in the neck. In some cases, toxins released by the bacteria lead to a rash, a condition known as *scarlet fever*.

DIAGNOSIS AND TREATMENT
The diagnosis is usually made by identifying the bacteria in a *culture* grown from a throat swab. The infection is treated with a *penicillin drug* or with another antibiotic drug if the person is allergic to penicillin.

An untreated strep throat infection may lead to the serious complications of *glomerulonephritis* (inflammation in the kidneys) and *rheumatic fever*.

Streptococcal infections

Types of infection caused by *bacteria* of the streptococcus group. Streptococci are spherical bacteria that grow in lines, like beads on a string; they are among the most common disease-causing bacteria in humans.

Certain types of streptococci are present harmlessly in most people's mouths and throats. If the bacteria gain access to the bloodstream (sometimes after dental treatment), they are usually destroyed. However, in some people with heart valve defects there is a risk that bacteria will settle in the heart to cause bacterial *endocarditis*. Another type of streptococcus is normally present harmlessly in the intestines but can spread to cause a *urinary tract infection*.

Other types of streptococci, known as hemolytic streptococci, cause *tonsillitis*, *strep throat*, *otitis media* (middle ear infection), *pneumonia*, *erysipelas*, or wound infections. Some hemolytic streptococcal infections may result in *scarlet fever*, and may also give rise to the serious complications of *rheumatic fever* and *glomerulonephritis*. These complications are prevented through prompt treatment with *antibiotic drugs* (usually penicillin).

People in whom rheumatic fever has developed are advised to take an antibiotic drug before, during, and after dental treatment and certain diagnostic and surgical procedures.

Streptokinase

A *thrombolytic drug* used to dissolve blood clots during a *myocardial infarction* (heart attack) or *pulmonary embolism*. A fast-acting agent, streptokinase is most effective in dissolving newly formed clots. Given by injection in the early stages of a myocardial infarction, streptokinase may limit the amount of damage that is caused to the heart muscle.

Treatment with streptokinase is strictly supervised because of the risk of allergic reaction or excessive bleeding. Adverse effects include rash, fever, wheezing, and cardiac *arrhythmias* (irregularities of the heartbeat).

Streptomycin

An *antibiotic drug* used to treat any of a number of uncommon infections, including *tularemia*, *plague*, *brucellosis*, and *glanders*. Streptomycin is sometimes given in conjunction with a *penicillin drug* to treat *endocarditis* (inflammation of the lining of the heart and heart valves).

S

Once used to treat a wide range of other infections, streptomycin has now been largely superseded by newer, more effective drugs with less serious side effects. Discovered in the 1940s, streptomycin was the first effective drug treatment for *tuberculosis*; it is still sometimes used to treat resistant strains of bacteria causing this disease.

POSSIBLE ADVERSE EFFECTS

Most seriously, streptomycin may damage nerves in the inner ear, disturbing balance and causing dizziness, ringing in the ears, and deafness. Other possible adverse effects include numbness of the face, tingling in the hands, headache, malaise, nausea, and vomiting.

Stress

Any interference that disturbs a person's healthy mental and physical well-being. A person may experience stress in response to a wide range of stimuli, including physical violence, internal conflicts, and significant life events (e.g., loss of a job, the death of a loved one, the birth of a baby, or divorce). Some people are more susceptible than others to stress-related health problems.

EFFECTS

When faced with a stressful situation, the body responds by increasing production of certain hormones, such as *cortisol* and *epinephrine*. These hormones lead to changes in heart rate, blood pressure, metabolism, and physical activity designed to improve overall performance. However, at a certain level, they disrupt an individual's ability to cope. Less than 20 percent of people are effective in the face of crises such as fires or floods.

Continued exposure to stress often leads to mental and physical symptoms, such as *anxiety* and *depression*, *indigestion*, palpitations, and muscular aches and pains. *Posttraumatic stress disorder* is a direct response to a specific stressful event. (See also *Relaxation techniques*.)

Stress fracture

A *fracture* that occurs as a result of repetitive jarring of a bone. Common sites include the metatarsal bones in the foot (see *March fracture*), the tibia or fibula (lower leg bones), the neck of the femur (thighbone), and the lumbar region of the spine. Stress fractures are most common among runners, particularly those who run on hard surfaces with inadequate footwear (see *Sports injuries*).

SYMPTOMS AND DIAGNOSIS

The main symptoms include pain and tenderness at the fracture site. Diagnosis is by *X rays*, although some stress fractures do not show up on X ray until they have started to heal. Occasionally, a radionuclide bone scan (see *Bone imaging*) may be performed to confirm the diagnosis.

Treatment consists of resting the affected area for four to six weeks. In some cases, it is also necessary to immobilize the fracture in a plaster *cast*. After recovery, modification of exercise routines and the use of suitably cushioned footwear may help to prevent a recurrence.

Stress ulcer

An acute *peptic ulcer* that sometimes develops after shock, serious burns, severe injuries, or during a major illness. Stress ulcers are usually multiple and are most common in the stomach; they differ from chronic peptic ulcers in that the raw area does not spread deep into the stomach lining.

The exact cause of stress ulcers is unknown. Treatment is primarily preventive; patients in intensive-care units are commonly given *antacid drugs* and/or *H_2-receptor antagonists*.

Stretcher

A frame covered with fabric that is used in first aid for carrying the sick, injured, or deceased. Many stretchers are available, including the standard stretcher, which consists of canvas stretched between two long poles on each side, and the trolley bed, a more sophisticated, adjustable stretcher on wheels carried in ambulances.

Stretchers can be improvised by passing two poles through holes made in the corners of canvas bags, or by rolling up poles in parallel sides of a strong rug· or blanket. An overcoat may also be used. Ideally, stretchers should be fairly rigid. The ends of a loaded stretcher should be lifted simultaneously. (See also illustrated box overleaf.)

Stretch mark

The common name for *stria*.

Stria

Commonly called a stretch mark, a line on the *skin* caused by thinning and loss of elasticity in the dermis (lower layer of the skin). Striae first appear as red, raised lines. Later they become purple, eventually flattening and fading to form shiny streaks.

Striae often develop on the hips and thighs during the adolescent growth spurt, especially in athletic girls. They are common in about 75 percent of pregnant women, and tend to occur on the breasts, the thighs, and the lower abdomen. Purple striae characteristically develop in people with *Cushing's syndrome*.

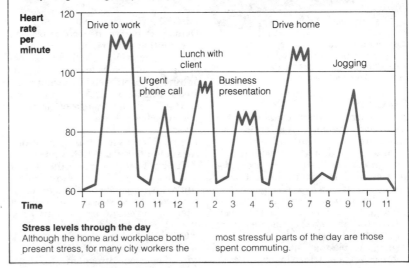

STRESS AND HEART RATE

The graph shows how a person's heart rate varies over a typical day. Exercise and stress both activate the body's "fight-or-flight" system and increase heart rate, but repeated alerting of the system without accompanying physical activity is probably harmful.

Stress levels through the day

Although the home and workplace both present stress, for many city workers the most stressful parts of the day are those spent commuting.

S

USING A STRETCHER

Stretchers are used to carry injured or seriously ill people to avoid the risk of further injury. Any type of stretcher should be fairly rigid and should always be tested for strength before use.

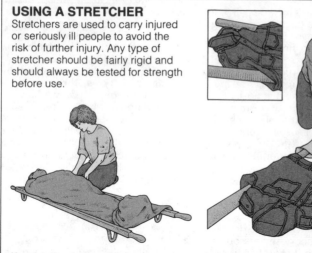

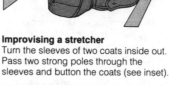

Keeping the victim warm
Place a blanket diagonally on the stretcher. Lift the victim carefully onto the blanket and tuck in the corners.

Improvising a stretcher
Turn the sleeves of two coats inside out. Pass two strong poles through the sleeves and button the coats (see inset).

Striae are possibly caused by an excess of *corticosteroid hormones*. These hormones are known to suppress fiber formation in the skin and to cause *collagen* in the skin to waste away. There is no effective means of prevention or treatment.

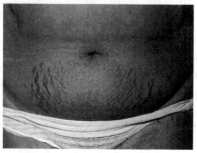

Appearance of striae
Commonly known as stretch marks, striae often develop on the abdomen, thighs, and breasts of pregnant women.

Stricture

Narrowing of a duct, canal, or other passage in the body. A stricture may result from infection and inflammation; damage to and subsequent formation of scar tissue in or around a passage; development of a tumor; spasm of muscles in a passage wall; or excessive growth of tissue around a passage, which occurs in *prostatism* when the enlarged prostate gland constricts the urethra (the passage between the bladder and outside). In some cases, a stricture is *congenital*.

Stridor

An abnormal breathing sound caused by narrowing or obstruction of the *larynx* or *trachea*.

Stridor is most common in young children. It usually occurs in *croup*, which is caused by a viral infection of the upper airways. A less common, but more serious, cause is the bacterial infection *epiglottitis*. Other causes of stridor include an inhaled *foreign body*, *hypocalcemia* (a low level of calcium in the blood), and certain disorders of the *larynx*, such as tumors, vocal cord paralysis, and laryngomalacia (softening of the cartilage of the larynx).

Stroke

Damage to part of the *brain* caused by interruption to its blood supply or by leakage of blood through the walls of blood vessels. Sensation, movement, or function controlled by the damaged area is impaired. Strokes can be fatal and are a leading cause of death in developed countries.

CAUSES
The main types and causes of stroke are shown in the illustrated box.

Certain factors increase the risk of having a stroke. The two most important are *hypertension* (high blood pressure), which weakens the walls of arteries, and *atherosclerosis* (narrowing of arteries by fatty deposits).

Other factors that increase the risk of a stroke include *atrial fibrillation* (a type of heartbeat irregularity), a dam-

aged *heart valve*, and a recent *myocardial infarction* (heart attack). All of these conditions can cause blood clots in the heart which may break off and migrate to the brain. *Polycythemia* (a raised level of red cells in the blood), *hyperlipidemia* (a high level of fatty substances in the blood), *diabetes mellitus*, and smoking also increase the risk of stroke by increasing the risk of hypertension and/or atherosclerosis. *Oral contraceptives* increase the risk of stroke in women under 50.

INCIDENCE
About 6,000 people in Canada die each year of *intracerebral hemorrhage* and about 14,000 die of *cerebral thrombosis*. The incidence, especially of thrombosis, rises steeply with age.

SYMPTOMS AND SIGNS
Damage to a specific area of the brain impairs bodily sensation, movement, or function controlled by that part of the brain. Some of the possible symptoms, signs and risk factors are shown in the illustrated box on the facing page. A stroke that affects the dominant cerebral hemisphere in the brain (usually the left hemisphere) may cause disturbance of language and speech (see *Aphasia*).

Movement on one side of the body is controlled by the cerebral hemisphere on the opposite side. Thus, damage to areas controlling movement in the right cerebral hemisphere results in weakness or paralysis on the left side of the body. Such one-sided weakness (*hemiparesis*) or paralysis (*hemiplegia*) is one of the most common effects of a serious stroke.

When symptoms last for less than 24 hours and are followed by full recovery, the episode is known as a *transient ischemic attack* (TIA). Such an attack, which usually lasts for only a few minutes, is a warning signal that a sufficient supply of blood is not reaching part of the brain.

About a third of major strokes are fatal, a third result in some disability, and a third have no lasting ill effects.

Possible complications of a major stroke include *pneumonia*, and the formation of blood clots in the veins of the leg (see *Thrombosis, deep vein*), which may travel to the artery supplying the lung to cause a potentially fatal *pulmonary embolism*.

DIAGNOSIS
If someone is thought to have had a stroke, a physician should be summoned immediately. The physician will assess whether hospital treatment is advisable or whether the patient is best kept at home.

S

TYPES AND CAUSES OF STROKE

Stroke may be caused by any of three mechanisms (below). Thrombosis and embolism both lead to cessation of the blood supply to part of the brain and thus to infarction (tissue death). Rupture of a blood vessel in or near the brain may cause an intracerebral hemorrhage or a subarachnoid hemorrhage. Any part of the brain may be affected by a stroke; accordingly, the symptoms vary considerably.

CEREBRAL THROMBOSIS

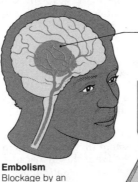

Area deprived of blood

Thrombus blocks artery

Thrombosis
Blockage by a thrombus (clot) that has built up on the wall of a brain artery accounts for 40 to 50 percent of strokes.

CEREBRAL EMBOLISM

Area deprived of blood

Embolus blocks artery

Embolism
Blockage by an embolus (usually a clot) swept into an artery in the brain accounts for 30 to 35 percent of strokes.

HEMORRHAGE

Area of bleeding

Burst artery

Bleeding
Rupture of a blood vessel and bleeding within or over the surface of the brain accounts for 20 to 25 percent of strokes.

Tissue death within the brain
The photograph (left) shows a vertical slice through the brain of someone who died of a stroke. A large region of tissue death (dark area), caused by bleeding and oxygen deprivation, can be seen on one side.

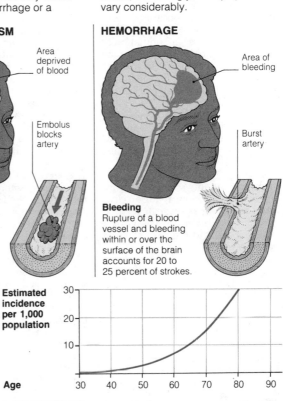

Estimated incidence per 1,000 population

Age

Incidence with age
Strokes are rare to uncommon under the age of 60, but thereafter the chances of one occurring increase rapidly.

SYMPTOMS

The symptoms of a stroke usually develop abruptly over minutes or hours, but occasionally over several days. Depending on the site, cause, and extent of damage, any or all of the symptoms shown on the right may be present, in any degree of severity. The more serious cases lead to rapid loss of consciousness, coma, and death or to severe physical or mental handicap, but some strokes cause barely noticeable symptoms.

Hemiplegia
Weakness or paralysis on one side of the body is one of the more common effects of a serious stroke.

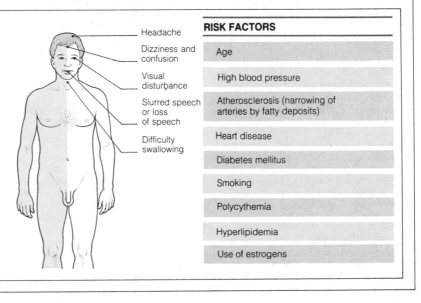

Headache

Dizziness and confusion

Visual disturbance

Slurred speech or loss of speech

Difficulty swallowing

RISK FACTORS

Age

High blood pressure

Atherosclerosis (narrowing of arteries by fatty deposits)

Heart disease

Diabetes mellitus

Smoking

Polycythemia

Hyperlipidemia

Use of estrogens

S

CT scanning of the brain may sometimes be performed to determine whether the symptoms are caused by a stroke or by some other disorder, such as a *brain tumor*, *brain abscess*, *subdural hemorrhage* (bleeding into the space between the outermost and middle membranes covering the brain), or *encephalitis* (inflammation of the brain). A *lumbar puncture* may occasionally be necessary to exclude the possibility of *meningitis* (inflammation of the membranes covering the brain and spinal cord).

To further examine the cause and extent of brain damage, investigations may include an *ECG*, *chest X rays*, *blood tests*, *angiography*, and, in specialist centers, *MRI*.

TREATMENT
In hospital, patients who are unconscious or semiconscious require a clear airway (breathing passages), feeding by means of *intravenous infusion* or a *nasogastric tube*, and regular changing of position to avoid *bedsores* or pneumonia. When a stroke has been caused by an embolism, *anticoagulant drugs* or, occasionally, *thrombolytic drugs* may be prescribed. In most cases, *ASA* is prescribed to reduce the risk of recurrence.

Every effort is made to restore any lost movement or sensation by *physiotherapy* and to remedy any speech disturbance by *speech therapy*.

OUTLOOK
About half of all patients recover more or less completely from their first stroke. Most people paralyzed by a stroke learn to walk again. Survivors left with some disability may require *occupational therapy* and aids in the home (see *Disability*). About 5 percent of patients require long-term institutional care.

Stroma
The tissue that forms the framework of an organ, as distinct from the functional tissue (called the *parenchyma*) and the fibrous outer layer that holds the organ together. For example, the stroma of the ovaries is the supporting tissue in which the ovarian follicles (the parenchyma) are embedded. The ovarian stroma consists of fibrous tissue, smooth muscle cells, spindle-shaped cells, and a rich supply of blood vessels.

Strongyloidiasis
An infestation of the intestines by a tiny parasitic worm, STRONGYLOIDES STERCORALIS, also called the threadworm. The disease is widespread in the tropics, especially the Far East. In Canada, it is occasionally found in refugees and in ex-servicemen who served in the Far East during World War II, but is otherwise rare.

Strongyloidiasis is contracted in affected areas by walking barefoot on soil contaminated with feces. Worm larvae penetrate the skin of the feet and then migrate, via the lungs and throat, to the small intestine. There they develop into adults, which burrow into the intestinal wall to produce larvae. Most larvae are passed in the feces, but some enter the skin around the anus to begin a new cycle. Thus, an infestation may persist in one person for more than 40 years.

SYMPTOMS
The larvae cause itching and raised red wheals where they pass through the skin. In the lungs they may cause *asthma* or *pneumonia*. Intestinal infestation may produce no symptoms but in cases of heavy infestation there may be discomfort, a swollen abdomen, and diarrhea. Occasionally, an infected person whose *immune system* is depressed dies of complications, such as *septicemia* or *meningitis*, many years after contracting the infection. Pneumonia may occur more readily in a person whose immune system has been compromised.

The disease is diagnosed from microscopic examination of a sample of feces and treated with an *anthelmintic drug*, usually *thiabendazole*.

Strontium
A metallic element which does not occur naturally in its pure form but is present in various compounds in certain minerals (notably strontianite and celestite), seawater, and marine plants. Strontium is also found in food and, although it is not essential to the body, it is metabolized in a manner similar to calcium and incorporated into bone.

In addition to strontium compounds, there are several radioisotopes (radioactive varieties) of the element, of which strontium 90 is medically the most important. This does not occur naturally, but is produced in relatively large amounts during nuclear fission reactions and is also present in the fallout from some nuclear bomb explosions. Strontium 90 emits *radiation* (in the form of beta particles) for a comparatively long time (the *half-life* of this radioisotope is about 28 years), and accumulates in bone, where the radiation may cause *leukemia* and/or *bone tumors*.

Other radioisotopes of strontium have also been used in medicine to diagnose and treat bone tumors.

Strychnine poisoning
Strychnine is an extremely poisonous chemical found in the seeds of STRYCHNOS species, a group of tropical trees and shrubs. Although once used as a tonic and general stimulant, strychnine is now no longer used in medicine. Its principal use today is as an ingredient in some rodent poisons; most cases of strychnine poisoning occur in children who accidentally eat such poisons. However, the extremely bitter taste of strychnine and its lack of easy availability make this form of poisoning rare.

The symptoms of poisoning begin soon after strychnine has been ingested. Initial symptoms include restlessness, stiffness of the face and neck, *photosensitivity* (increased sensitivity to light), and increased sensitivity of hearing, taste, and smell. These symptoms are followed by alternating episodes of seizures and floppiness. Eventually, death may occur from *respiratory arrest*.

The main objectives of treatment are to prevent seizures and to maintain breathing. The victim is given intravenous injections of a *tranquillizer drug* or a *barbiturate drug*, with a *muscle-relaxant drug* if necessary, which counteract the effects of strychnine and help prevent seizures. Breathing may be maintained by a *ventilator*. With prompt treatment, recovery usually occurs in about 24 hours.

Stuffy nose
See *Nasal congestion*.

Stump
The end portion of a limb that remains after *amputation*.

Stupor
A state of almost complete *unconsciousness* from which a person can be aroused only briefly and only by vigorous external stimulation. (See also *Coma*.)

Sturge-Weber syndrome
A rare, congenital condition that affects the skin and the brain. Characteristically, a large purple *hemangioma* (a birthmark caused by abnormal distribution of blood vessels) extends over one side of the face, including the eye. A similar malformation of blood vessels in the brain may cause some

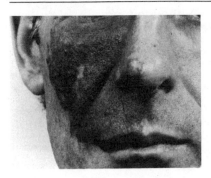

Appearance of Sturge-Weber syndrome
The characteristic flat, purple birthmark extends over the upper part of one side of this man's face.

weakness on the opposite side of the body, progressive *mental retardation*, and *epilepsy*. *Glaucoma* (increased pressure within the eyeball) may develop in the affected eye, leading to partial or complete loss of vision.

The birthmark can be disguised with masking creams; seizures can usually be controlled with *anticonvulsant drugs*. In severe cases, surgery on the affected part of the brain may need to be performed.

Stuttering

A speech disorder in which there is repeated hesitation and delay in uttering words, unusual prolongation of sounds, and repetition of word elements. Stuttering, also known as stammering, usually starts in childhood, beginning before the age of 8 in 90 percent of sufferers.

INCIDENCE

Stuttering occurs in about 1 percent of adults. Temporary stuttering is fairly common in children aged 2 to 4. About half the children whose stutter persists until the age of 5 will continue to stutter in adult life. Stuttering is more common in males, twins, and left-handed people.

SYMPTOMS

The words and sounds that cause problems vary from person to person. The severity of stuttering may be related to various circumstances. For example, some people find that stuttering is worse when they are anxious (such as during public speaking or when using the telephone), while others experience more difficulty when relaxed.

Problems rarely occur during singing or reading in unison (possibly because less communication is involved). Some people who stutter also have *tics* and *tremors*.

CAUSES

The cause of stuttering is uncertain, although the problem tends to run in families. Some researchers believe that stuttering is due to a subtle form of brain damage; others, however, regard stuttering as being primarily a psychological problem.

TREATMENT

Stuttering can often be improved by *speech therapy*. This may include teaching the affected person to give equal weight to each syllable, and use of electronic aids to mask the speaker's voice or to relay speech back to the speaker via headphones.

Stye

Also called a hordeolum, a small, pus-filled *abscess* near the eyelashes caused by infection.

If a stye is painful, applying warm compresses may help the pus to discharge. Use of an eye ointment containing an *antibiotic drug* can help to prevent a recurrence.

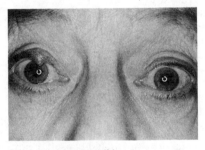

Stye on the upper eyelid
A stye most often forms near the inner corner of an eye but may develop at the base of any of the eyelashes.

Subacute

A medical term applied to a disease that runs a course in time between *acute* and *chronic*. In subacute *endocarditis*, for example, the disease may go undetected for many months during which time it causes severe damage to a heart valve.

Subarachnoid hemorrhage

A type of *brain hemorrhage* in which blood from a ruptured blood vessel spreads over the surface of the brain.

CAUSES AND INCIDENCE

The most common cause of subarachnoid hemorrhage is a burst *aneurysm* (balloonlike swelling of an artery), which commonly occurs on the circular arrangement of blood vessels at the base of the brain. Less commonly, subarachnoid hemorrhage is due to a ruptured *angioma* (abnormal proliferation of blood vessels within the brain). Bleeding takes place in the space between the arachnoid and the pia mater (the middle and the innermost of the three *meninges* that cover the brain). This space also contains *cerebrospinal fluid*, which becomes mixed with blood.

Subarachnoid hemorrhage usually occurs spontaneously, without any head injury, although it may follow unaccustomed physical exercise. Each year, about five to 10 people per 100,000 suffer a subarachnoid hemorrhage. This form of brain hemorrhage is less common than *intracerebral hemorrhage* (a form of *stroke*), in which bleeding occurs within the brain itself. Subarachnoid hemorrhage is particularly common in people aged between 35 and 60.

SYMPTOMS

An attack may cause immediate loss of consciousness or a sudden violent headache, often followed by loss of consciousness. If the person remains conscious, other symptoms such as *photophobia* (abnormal sensitivity to light), nausea, vomiting, drowsiness, and stiffness of the neck may develop. Unconscious patients may recover, but attacks during the ensuing days or weeks are common and often fatal.

The diagnosis is confirmed by *CT scanning* and by detection of large amounts of blood in the cerebrospinal fluid by *lumbar puncture*. The site of the burst blood vessel is investigated by *angiography* (X rays taken after the injection of a radiopaque substance into the bloodstream), which may not be performed until the patient's condition has stabilized.

TREATMENT

Treatment consists of general life-support procedures, bed rest, and measures aimed at reducing the risk of recurrence—principally, control of high blood pressure. In some cases, a burst aneurysm is surgically accessible. Angiomas can also sometimes be surgically removed, blocked off, or obliterated. Surgery is usually delayed for several weeks after the acute attack.

About one third of patients make a full recovery; another one sixth recover but have some residual disability, such as paralysis, mental deterioration, or epilepsy. The remaining patients (about half) die as a result of the initial or a recurrent attack.

Subclavian steal syndrome

Recurrent attacks of blurred or double vision, loss of coordination, or dizziness caused by reduced blood flow to

S

the base of the brain when one arm (usually the left) is moved. The underlying cause is narrowing of the major arteries that carry blood to the arms (usually due to *atherosclerosis*). The left subclavian artery is particularly affected. Blood supply to the affected arm is reduced but is sufficient provided the arm is kept at rest. When the arm is moved, its muscles require an increased amount of blood, which is diverted from the base of the brain.

A physician confirms the diagnosis by finding a weak pulse and low blood pressure in the affected arm. *Angiography* (X rays taken after the injection of a radiopaque substance into the bloodstream) establishes the site of the narrowed artery. Treatment is by *arterial reconstructive surgery*.

Subclinical

A medical term applied to a disorder that produces no symptoms or signs because it is so mild or because it is in the early stages of development. Although a subclinical disorder does not produce symptoms or signs, it may cause damage to organs.

Subconjunctival hemorrhage

Bleeding under the *conjunctiva* (transparent membrane covering the white of the eye). The small blood vessels of the conjunctiva are fragile, poorly supported, and frequently leak. Subconjunctival hemorrhage may occur spontaneously or after coughing or vomiting, which increases pressure in the veins. It is usually harmless and only rarely signals a serious disorder.

Subconjunctival blood disappears without treatment, usually within 10 to 14 days. Recurrences sometimes occur as a result of local weakness in a conjunctival blood vessel.

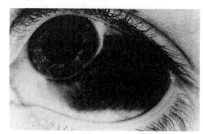

Subconjunctival hemorrhage
The bleeding causes a bright red area to appear in the white of the eye. This may look alarming but is usually harmless.

Subconscious

A term describing mental events (such as thoughts, ideas, or feelings) that one is temporarily unaware of but that

can be recalled under the right circumstances. In *psychoanalytic theory*, the subconscious refers to that part of the mind through which information passes on its way from the *unconscious* to the conscious mind.

Subcutaneous

A medical term meaning beneath the skin, as in a subcutaneous injection, one in which a drug is injected into the tissue under the skin.

Subdural hemorrhage

Bleeding into the space between the dura mater, the tough outer layer of the *meninges* (coverings of the brain) and the arachnoid (middle meningeal layer). The trapped blood slowly forms a large hematoma (enlarging blood clot) within the skull. The most common cause is torn veins on the inside of the dura mater following a blow to the head. Subdural hemorrhage most often affects elderly or alcoholic people who have fallen.

SYMPTOMS
The bleeding occurs slowly; it may be weeks or months before the hematoma enlarges sufficiently to cause symptoms by raising pressure within the skull and displacing and pressing on brain tissue. The symptoms, which tend to fluctuate, consist of headache, episodes of confusion and drowsiness, and the development of one-sided weakness or paralysis.

Any person in whom such symptoms develop should consult a physician immediately. Because the symptoms are similar to those of a *stroke*, it is important that mention be made of any *head injury* that occurred within the previous few months.

DIAGNOSIS AND TREATMENT
The diagnosis is confirmed, and the location of the hematoma investigated, by means of *angiography* (X rays taken after the injection of a radiopaque substance into the bloodstream) and *CT scanning*. Surgical treatment is by drilling burr holes into the skull (see *Craniotomy*), drainage of the blood clot, and repair of blood vessels, which usually allows a full recovery if carried out soon enough. (See also *Extradural hemorrhage*.)

Sublimation

The unconscious process by which primitive, unacceptable impulses are redirected into socially acceptable forms of behavior. Aggression, for example, may be channeled into sports. *Psychoanalytic theory* regards sublimation as a healthy process.

Subluxated tooth

A tooth displaced in its socket as the result of an accident. The upper front teeth are the most vulnerable. The tooth may be depressed deep into the gum, tilted backward or forward, and loosened. A dentist can usually manipulate a subluxated tooth back into position, after which it is usually immobilized with a splint (see *Splinting, dental*). If the tooth's blood vessels are torn and the pulp dies, the tooth requires *root-canal treatment*.

Subluxation

Incomplete *dislocation* of a *joint*—that is, displacement of the bony surfaces in a joint so that they no longer face each other exactly but remain in partial contact. In a dislocation, the joint surfaces are displaced so that there is total loss of contact between them. In general, a subluxation causes less damage to the joint and surrounding tissues than does a dislocation.

Normal
The diagram on the left shows the normal position of the bony surfaces in a simple joint, such as the joint in the middle of a finger.

Subluxation
In a subluxation, the surfaces of the bones are slightly displaced from their normal positions relative to each other but are still in contact.

Dislocation
Here, there is almost complete loss of contact between the bone surfaces and, in most cases, considerable damage to surrounding tissues.

Submucous resection

An operation to correct a deviated *nasal septum* (the central partition inside the nose) when this is causing breathing difficulty. Under a local or a general anesthetic, an incision is made in the mucous membrane covering the septum, and displaced cartilage and bone are then cut away. The membrane is closed with absorbable stitches, which do not require removal.

Subphrenic abscess

An *abscess* under the diaphragm, which is served by the *phrenic nerve*.

Substrate

A substance on which an *enzyme* acts. For example, the digestive enzyme amylase acts on the substrate starch (a polysaccharide) and breaks it down into smaller saccharide (sugar) units.

Sucking chest wound

An open wound in the chest wall through which air passes, causing the lung on that side to collapse (see *Lung, collapse of*). The mediastinum (central partition of the chest) may also shift to the other side, causing partial collapse of the other lung.

A sucking chest wound causes severe breathlessness and a life-threatening lack of oxygen. Emergency first aid treatment is vital. Cover the wound with your hand (or first cover it with a piece of airtight material, such as a plastic bag). It is essential that the wound is kept tightly sealed until medical attention is obtained.

Sucralfate

An *ulcer-healing drug* used to treat *peptic ulcer*. Sucralfate forms a protective barrier over the ulcerated stomach or duodenal lining and thus protects it from further attack by the digestive juices and allows an ulcer to heal.

Antacid drugs should not be taken within an hour of taking sucralfate as they may reduce its effectiveness.

Possible adverse effects include constipation and abdominal pain. Sucralfate may interfere with the absorption of certain drugs, such as *tetracycline drugs* and *digoxin*. In addition, prolonged treatment with sucralfate may impair the absorption of certain vitamins.

Suction

The removal of unwanted fluid or semifluid material from the body with a syringe and hollow needle or with an intestinal tube and a mechanical pump. Among the many uses of suction are: the clearing of secretions from the throats of newborn babies; clearing the throats of patients who have undergone an operation under general anesthesia; and the draining of blood and other fluids from the abdominal cavity during or after surgery.

Suction lipectomy

A cosmetic procedure used in *body contour surgery*.

Sudden death

See *Death, sudden*.

Sudden infant death syndrome

The sudden, unexpected death of an infant, which often cannot be explained even after an autopsy. Such deaths, also known as crib deaths, typically occur in apparently healthy babies who seem well when put to bed but are later found dead.

CAUSES AND INCIDENCE

In developed countries, sudden infant death syndrome (SIDS) is the most common form of death between the ages of 1 month and 1 year; three quarters of these occur in babies under 6 months old. SIDS is slightly more common among boys, among second children, and in winter. More deaths seem to occur between midnight and 9 a.m. and at weekends.

Much of the research has been focused on possible risk factors. These include: *prematurity* and low birth weight; bottle-feeding; cold weather; young, single mothers; smoking, drug addiction, or anemia in the mother; poor socioeconomic background; the death of a sibling as a result of SIDS; and so-called "near miss" infants who have been found near death and have been resuscitated just in time.

Most experts believe there is no single cause of SIDS. It seems probable that some babies die of a sudden overwhelming respiratory infection and others of undetected inborn errors of metabolism (see *Metabolism, inborn errors of*). Most deaths are thought to be caused by some abnormality in the breathing and heart rate. Abnormal breathing rhythms may be due to a fault in the brain stem, the lungs may have abnormally sensitive airway reflexes, or there may be an abnormality of surfactant (a substance that prevents the air sacs of the lungs from collapsing).

Even though most deaths seem to occur without warning, it is becoming clear that some babies may have been suffering from minor symptoms (such as a cold with a stuffy nose) for several days before death or have shown an inexplicable weight loss.

PREVENTION

Possible preventive measures include good *prenatal care*, avoidance of smoking and unnecessary taking of drugs during pregnancy, good obstetric care, breast-feeding, and close observation of the baby for several days after a minor illness.

Parents of a child who has died from SIDS and parents of "near miss" infants may be reassured by the use of an alarm that sounds if the baby stops breathing. However, there is no evidence that the use of alarms lowers the risk of death, and the number of false alarms that occurs may increase rather than allay the parental anxiety.

EFFECTS

The death of an infant from SIDS is a highly distressing experience.

Grief may manifest itself in a variety of ways, ranging from withdrawal and anger to physical symptoms. There may be feelings of intense guilt, and family relationships may be badly strained by misplaced blame and by severe and persistent grief. Parents may lose confidence in their ability to care properly for any other children. The family should be prepared for a visit from the police and the need for a postmortem examination of the baby. Siblings are also likely to be affected by the death; their grief may be expressed through nightmares, bedwetting, misbehavior, or regression to outgrown habits. Some siblings fear they will die in the same way.

Professionals, such as a family practitioner, a pediatrician, a social worker, or a minister, can provide support. Talking to other parents who have been through the same experience can provide great comfort.

Sudeck's atrophy

Swelling and loss of use of a hand or foot after a *fracture* or other injury.

Pain, swelling, and stiffness (especially in the joints) develop in the affected hand or foot about two months after the original injury, usually after the plaster cast has been removed. The nails may stop growing normally and hair on the affected limb may fall out. Despite physiotherapy and attempts to start using the hand or foot again, the pain, swelling, and stiffness persist.

The condition is diagnosed by *X rays*, which usually show thinning of the bones (see *Osteoporosis*). Treatment includes elevation of the affected hand or foot, gentle exercise, and *heat treatment*. Complete recovery is usual within about four months. However, if pain persists, a *nerve block* may be tried and, if the block is temporarily successful in relieving pain, *sympathectomy* (an operation to destroy nerve pathways) may be attempted. (See also *Shoulder-hand syndrome*.)

Suffocation

A condition in which there is a lack of oxygen due to an obstruction to the

S

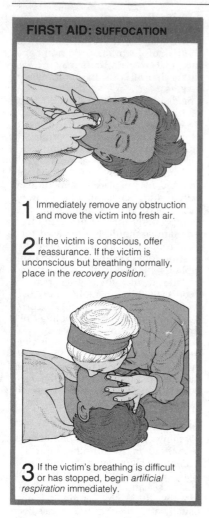

FIRST AID: SUFFOCATION

1 Immediately remove any obstruction and move the victim into fresh air.

2 If the victim is conscious, offer reassurance. If the victim is unconscious but breathing normally, place in the *recovery position*.

3 If the victim's breathing is difficult or has stopped, begin *artificial respiration* immediately.

passage of air into the lungs. Suffocation may be caused by blockage of the nose and mouth, by blockage of the pharynx or larynx, or by blockage of the trachea. (See also *Asphyxia; Choking; Strangulation*.)

Sugar
See *Carbohydrates*.

Suicide
The act of intentionally killing oneself. In Canada, about 3,600 suicides are reported each year.

CAUSES
Most people who commit suicide suffer from a psychiatric disorder such as *depression, schizophrenia* (particularly young men in the early stages of the disorder), *antisocial personality disorder*, or *alcohol dependence*. The act of suicide is triggered by a person's reaction to what seems an overwhelming problem—social isolation, recent death of a loved one, a broken home in childhood, serious physical illness, growing old, unemployment, financial problems, and drug abuse.

INCIDENCE
The incidence of suicide varies widely from country to country. Among the developed countries, Canada stands approximately in the middle with a rate of 14 per 100,000 per year. Recently, rates of suicide have been rising in the elderly, in people with chronic and incurable diseases, and in young native men (see *Depression*). Suicide is most common among divorced people, less common among the single and widowed, and least common among married people.

METHODS
In Canada, the most common reported methods of committing suicide are by hanging, strangulation or suffocation, with poisoning, usually by sleeping pills, a close second. Violent methods of suicide, such as shooting, are much commoner in men.

PREVENTION
One myth about suicide is that only people who are not serious about suicide talk about it beforehand. In fact, many people who commit suicide threaten repeatedly to take their own lives; relatives and friends should always take such threats seriously. Suicidal people usually feel desperately lonely, and the opportunity to talk to a sympathetic, understanding listener is sometimes enough to prevent the despairing act. Most Canadian cities have suicide prevention centers that provide a 24-hour telephone counseling service for suicidal people.

Following a suicide threat, family or friends should remove any obvious means of committing the act and should watch the person closely. The person's physician or psychiatrist should be consulted immediately so that appropriate treatment may be given. Hospitalization (or frequent sessions with a psychiatrist) may be necessary to provide enough support to help a suicidal person through a crisis period.

Suicide, attempted
Any deliberate act of self-harm that is or is believed to be life-threatening but that in effect proves nonfatal. Most attempted suicides, also known as parasuicides, are carried out in a setting that makes rescue possible. They must therefore be viewed as cries for help by people in extreme distress.

SUICIDE RATES (per 100,000 population, age standardized to world population)		
Country	**Year**	**Rate**
Hungary	1987	35.1
Finland	1986	22.6
Denmark	1986	21.7
Austria	1987	20.8
Switzerland	1987	18.5
France	1986	17.7
Belgium	1986	17.0
Luxembourg	1987	15.9
Czechoslovakia	1986	15.8
Japan	1987	15.3
Sweden	1986	14.9
Canada	1986	14.0
West Germany	1987	13.8
Norway	1986	12.1
Bulgaria	1986	12.0
Poland	1987	12.0
New Zealand	1986	11.5
Australia	1986	11.0
USA	1986	10.9
The Netherlands	1986	8.9
Portugal	1987	7.5
UK	1987	6.6
Italy	1985	6.1
Greece	1986	3.1

CAUSES AND INCIDENCE
People who attempt suicide constitute a sociologically different group from those who actually kill themselves (see *Suicide*), although there is some overlap between the two. Parasuicide is three times more common in women than in men and is most common in the 15 to 30 age group and in single and divorced people. The rate is highest among people with personality disorders, those who live in deprived urban areas, and those who have problems with alcohol or drugs. Common precipitating factors include an argument with a relative or sexual partner, the recent death of a loved one, financial worries, or severe loss of any kind that results in depression.

Suicide attempts far outnumber actual suicides and, since the 1950s, have become one of the primary reasons for hospital admission. The most common method used is to take an overdose of drugs, most often analgesic drugs (painkillers) or sleeping pills, often with alcohol.

TREATMENT AND PREVENTION
If someone is discovered to have taken a drug overdose, emergency help should be summoned; if the person is unconscious or not breathing, first aid measures should be carried out (see *Drug poisoning*). In other cases, appropriate measures depend on the victim's condition.

All suicide attempts should be treated seriously. Twenty to 30 percent of people who attempt suicide

S

repeat their attempt within a year, and 10 percent eventually kill themselves, especially socially isolated men with a physical or mental illness.

The basis of treatment is to provide support, to treat any underlying depression and to help the person to resolve the difficulties which precipitated the suicide attempt. In some cases, referral for psychiatric help may be necessary but in many cases, the family physician can provide the appropriate medical help.

Sulfacetamide

A *sulfonamide drug* which is used in the treatment of *conjunctivitis*. Sulfacetamide is also sometimes given to prevent infection after an eye injury or after the removal of a foreign body from the eye. Itching, redness, and swelling of the eyelids are occasionally caused by an allergic reaction.

Sulfamethoxazole

Sulfamethoxazole is a *sulfonamide drug* used to treat urinary tract and ear infections, and conjunctivitis. Combined with *trimethoprim* (another antibacterial drug), it is used for a wide variety of respiratory and urinary tract infections, *gastroenteritis*, and *gonorrhea*. It has a long duration of action. An adequate intake of fluid must be maintained to prevent formation of crystals in the urine. The commonest side effects are nausea and loss of appetite.

Sulfasalazine

A drug used to relieve inflammation in the intestinal disorders *ulcerative colitis* and *Crohn's disease*.

Sulfasalazine may cause nausea, vomiting, headache, abdominal pain, and loss of appetite. An allergic reaction, causing fever and rash, occasionally occurs. Prolonged treatment may cause *folic acid* deficiency, resulting in *anemia*.

Sulfinpyrazone

A drug used to treat *gout* (a type of arthritis associated with an excessive level of uric acid in the blood). Sulfinpyrazone does not relieve the symptoms of gout but does reduce the frequency of attacks.

Sulfinpyrazone is also given to reduce *hyperuricemia* (raised levels of uric acid in the blood) caused by certain drugs, such as thiazide *diuretic drugs* and some *anticancer drugs*. Sulfinpyrazone reduces the amount of uric acid in the blood by increasing the amount excreted in the urine.

POSSIBLE ADVERSE EFFECTS
Adverse effects of sulfinpyrazone include nausea, vomiting, headache, flushing, cloudy or bloodstained urine, rash, itching, wheezing, and breathlessness.

Sulfisoxazole

A *sulfa drug* used in treatment of lower urinary tract infections that involve the bladder but do not affect the kidneys. Sulfisoxazole is rapidly absorbed, and has a short duration of action. It needs to be taken four to six times per day. Side effects are nausea and loss of appetite.

Sulfonamide drugs

COMMON DRUGS

Sulfacetamide Sulfadiazine
Sulfamethoxazole Sulfisoxazole

A group of *antibacterial drugs*. Before the large-scale production of *penicillin drugs*, sulfonamide drugs were widely used to treat infectious diseases. Today, they are used mainly to treat urinary tract infections.

The combination drug *co-trimoxazole*, which contains the sulfonamide drug sulfamethoxazole and *trimethoprim*, is used to treat various infections, including *bronchitis*, certain types of *pneumonia*, skin infections, and infections of the middle ear.

Sulfur

A mineral that plays several important roles in the body. Sulfur is a constituent of vitamin B_1 (see *Vitamin B complex*) and of several essential *amino acids* (building blocks of proteins). In particular, sulfur is necessary for the manufacture of *collagen* (which helps to form bones, tendons, and connective tissue) and is a constituent of *keratin* (the chief component of the hair, skin, and nails).

MEDICAL USES
Sulfur is used in some ointments, creams, and skin preparations for the treatment of various skin disorders, including acne, dandruff, psoriasis, scabies, diaper rash, and certain fungal infections.

Sulindac

A *nonsteroidal anti-inflammatory drug* that reduces pain, stiffness, and inflammation. It is helpful in treatment of many forms of arthritis, including osteoarthritis, rheumatoid arthritis, and gout. Most common side effects are nausea, abdominal pain, and constipation.

Sunburn

Inflammation of the *skin* caused by overexposure to the sun. The *ultraviolet light* in sunlight may destroy cells in the outer layer of the skin and cause damage to tiny blood vessels beneath.

Sunburn is most common in fair-skinned people, whose skin produces only small amounts of the protective pigment *melanin*, and in people who attempt to acquire a tan too quickly in strong sunlight. The affected skin turns red and tender and may become blistered. Several days later the dead skin cells are shed by peeling. In severe cases, sunburn may be accompanied by symptoms of *sunstroke*—such as vomiting, fever, and collapse.

Repeated overexposure to sunlight can age the skin prematurely, producing yellowish, wrinkled skin through which tiny blood vessels may be seen. Overexposure can also increase the risk of *skin cancer*.

PREVENTION
Exposure to strong sunlight should be limited to no more than 15 minutes on the first day, particularly if the person has fair skin, and should be increased very gradually. This applies even if conditions are hazy. Until a tan is acquired, the skin should be covered or protected with a high protection factor *sunscreen*.

TREATMENT
Calamine lotion or a sunburn cream should be applied to soothe the burned skin, which should be protected from further exposure to the sun until healing takes place. *Analgesic drugs* (painkillers) may be needed to relieve tenderness. A person with severe sunburn should consult a physician, who may prescribe a cream containing a *corticosteroid drug* to relieve the symptoms. (See also *Sunlight, adverse effects of*.)

Sunlight, adverse effects of

Problems resulting from overexposure to the sun's rays. Some exposure to *ultraviolet light* from the sun is necessary for the body to produce *vitamin D*. Overexposure can have various harmful effects, particularly in fair-skinned people, who produce only small amounts of the protective skin pigment *melanin*.

Short-term overexposure causes *sunburn* and, in intense heat, can result in *heat exhaustion* or *heatstroke*. Repeated overexposure over a long period can cause premature aging of the skin and wartlike growths called solar *keratoses*. It also increases the risk of *skin cancer*.

S

Photosensitivity (abnormal sensitivity to sunlight) resulting in a skin rash may occur naturally or may be triggered by taking certain drugs. The condition may also occur in people who are suffering from systemic *lupus erythematosus* or *porphyria*.

Exposure to sunlight can also affect the eyes, causing irritation of the conjunctiva. More intense exposure may cause actinic *keratopathy* (damage to the cornea), sometimes called snowblindness. Symptoms include pain, watering and redness of the eyes, and photophobia; these usually clear up in a few days. Prolonged exposure to bright sunlight may cause the development of *pterygium* (a wing-shaped conjunctival thickening). Good sunglasses should be worn to avoid overexposing the eyes to sunlight.

Sunscreens

> **WARNING**
> Some suntanning preparations do not contain a sunscreen and therefore provide no protection against sunburn.

Preparations that protect the *skin* from the harmful effects of sunlight (see *Sunlight, adverse effects of*). Sunscreens are used mainly to prevent *sunburn*. They are also used to prevent rash caused by *photosensitivity* (abnormal sensitivity to sunlight).

Most sunscreens, including the very common para-aminobenzoic acid (PABA), work by absorbing ultraviolet rays. Some, such as titanium dioxide, reflect the sun's rays.

Sunscreen products may be labeled with a sun protection factor (SPF), the highest factor affording the greatest protection. Choice of product should depend on skin type (see box). A sunscreen with a lower SPF may be used once the skin is tanned. During prolonged sunbathing, sunscreens should be reapplied at regular intervals and also after swimming.

Some people are sensitive to sunscreen chemicals and develop a skin rash. This is most common with preparations containing PABA.

Sunstroke

The most common type of *heatstroke*. Sunstroke is usually brought on by overexposure to direct sun in a person who is unaccustomed to a hot climate. It is due to breakdown of the body's heat regulating mechanisms.

Suntan

Darkening of the *skin* after exposure to sunlight. Specialized cells in the outer layer of the skin respond to the *ultraviolet light* in sunlight by producing more of the protective pigment *melanin*. In dark-skinned people, this protective pigment is present in greater amounts. People who spend a lot of time in the sun are likely to experience premature wrinkling and run a greatly increased risk of *skin cancer*. (See also *Sunburn; Sunlight, adverse effects of*.)

Superego

The part of the personality, as described in *psychoanalytic theory*, that is responsible for maintaining an individual's standards of behavior. Popularly termed the "conscience," the superego arises as a result of a child's incorporating the ideals and moral views of those in authority (usually parents). The superego can create feelings of guilt and anxiety by criticizing the *ego* (the conscious "I") when the ego gives way to the impulses of the *id* (the pleasure-seeking part of the personality).

In psychoanalytic theory, an excessively strong superego is said to be the cause of severe, puritanical personality types and of *obsessive-compulsive behavior*. By contrast, failure to develop an appropriate superego leads to impulsive and immoral behavior. A harsh, self-punishing superego is said to result from childhood experience with a harsh parent.

Superficial

Situated near the surface, as in the superficial blood vessels (the capillaries that lie near the surface of the skin and play a part in regulating body temperature and in blushing).

Superinfection

A second *infection* that occurs during the course of an existing infection. The term usually refers to an infection by a microorganism that is resistant to drugs being used against the original infection.

The second microorganism may be a resistant strain of the first infection, an entirely different pathogen (disease-causing microorganism), or simply a member of the body's normal flora (microorganisms that are normally present in the body without producing ill effects). In this instance it has proliferated excessively because other microorganisms that normally keep it in check have been killed by drug therapy. For example, tetracycline therapy may result in superinfection of the mouth, vagina, and/or anus with the fungus that causes candidiasis (thrush).

Superiority complex

An exaggerated and unrealistic belief that one is better than other people. *Adlerian theory* suggests that a superiority complex develops in some people in response to the natural feelings of inferiority that everyone is born with. In more modern psychoanalytical theories, a superiority complex is considered to be a compensation for unconscious feelings of inadequacy or low self-esteem.

Supernumerary

A term meaning more than the normal number. For example, supernumerary nipples are additional nipples that develop along a line that extends from the armpit to the groin; these extra nipples are not usually associated with underlying glandular tissue. (See also *Supernumerary teeth*.)

Supernumerary teeth

One or more *teeth* in excess of the usual number (20 primary and 32 permanent). An extra tooth may be a duplicate of an existing tooth or it may have an abnormal shape and position (usually appearing as a small conical protrusion from the gum above the existing teeth in the upper front jaw).

Supernumerary teeth may interfere with the proper *eruption of teeth* and are therefore usually extracted.

RECOMMENDED MAXIMUM EXPOSURE TIMES USING SUNSCREENS

Protection factor	4	8	15
Skin type	**Maximum exposure time**		
Fair	10 minutes	40 to 80 minutes	1.5 to 2 hours
Medium	50 to 80 minutes	2 to 2.5 hours	5 to 5.5 hours
Dark	1.5 to 2 hours	3.5 to 4 hours	all day
Black	4 hours	all day	all day

S

Supination

The act of turning the body to a supine position (lying on the back with the face upward) or of turning the hand to a palm forward position. Movement in the opposite direction to supination is called *pronation*.

Suppository

A solid, cone- or bullet-shaped object containing a drug and an inert substance, usually derived from cocoa butter or another vegetable oil. The suppository is placed in the rectum and melts at body temperature, releasing the active ingredient.

Suppositories are used to treat rectal disorders, such as *hemorrhoids* or *proctitis*. They may also be used to soften feces and stimulate defecation. In addition, suppositories may be used to administer drugs into the general circulation via blood vessels in the rectum if vomiting is likely to prevent absorption after oral administration or if the drug would cause irritation of the stomach.

Drugs given by suppository include antifungal drugs, local anesthetics, corticosteroid drugs, nonsteroidal anti-inflammatory drugs, antibiotic drugs, and antiemetic drugs.

Suppuration

The formation or exudation of *pus*. Suppuration at the site of bacterial infection may result in the accumulation of pus, forming an *abscess* in solid tissue or forming a *boil* or *pustule* on the skin. Open sores often suppurate, especially if they are slow to heal, because the exposed underlying tissue tends to become repeatedly infected with bacteria.

Suprarenal glands

Another name for the *adrenal glands*.

Supraspinatus syndrome

See *Painful arc syndrome*.

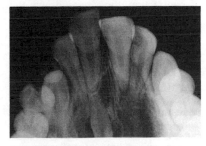

Supernumerary (extra) tooth
This X ray of the upper jaw shows a supernumerary incisor tooth on the roof of the mouth behind the normal incisors.

Supraventricular tachycardia

An abnormally fast but regular heart rate that occurs in episodes lasting for several hours or days. In most cases, the heart rate in supraventricular tachycardia is between 140 and 180 beats per minute, but in rare cases it may be as fast as 300 beats per minute.

Supraventricular tachycardia occurs when abnormal electrical impulses that arise in the atria (upper chambers) of the heart take control of the heartbeat from the *sinoatrial node* (the heart's own natural pacemaker). Symptoms may include palpitations, breathlessness, chest pain, or fainting (see *Stokes-Adams syndrome*).

Diagnosis of the condition is made by an *ECG* (electrocardiogram). An attack can sometimes be terminated by *Valsalva's maneuver* or by drinking cold water. Recurrent attacks are treated with *antiarrhythmic drugs*. Rarely, the condition may require treatment by applying an electric shock to the heart (see *Defibrillation*).

Surfactant

A substance that reduces surface tension; a wetting agent. Soaps, detergents, and emulsifiers are surfactants. Pulmonary surfactant is a substance secreted by the alveoli (air sacs) in the lungs that prevents them from collapsing during exhalation.

Surfer's nodules

Multiple *exostoses* (bony outgrowths) occurring on bones in the foot and on the tibial tubercle (the bony prominence below the knee at the top of the shin). Surfer's nodules are caused by the repeated banging of the surfboard against the knees and tops of the feet as the surfer kneels to paddle the board. They can be avoided by paddling in a lying position.

Surgery

The treatment of disease, injury, or other disorders by direct physical intervention, usually with instruments. The term is also used to denote those aspects of medical practice that deal with the study, diagnosis, and management of all disorders or injuries treated by operative surgery (as distinct from those treated by drugs, diet, or modification of life-style).

Operative surgery involves incision (cutting) into the skin or some other organ, inspection of tissues or organs, removal of diseased tissues or organs, relief of obstruction, replacement of structures in their normal position, redirection of body channels, trans-

plantation of tissues or complete organs, and implantation of mechanical or electronic devices.

Surgery may be minor or major. Minor operations are usually, but not always, performed under local anesthesia. Major operations are usually performed under general anesthesia, although local anesthesia is sometimes used.

Some surgeons, known as general surgeons, perform a variety of operations on almost all parts of the body. Other surgeons specialize in particular branches of surgery, such as orthopedic surgery, neurosurgery, obstetrics and gynecology, ophthalmology, gastrointestinal surgery, and plastic surgery. In recent years there has been an increasing trend toward further subspecialization; some surgeons now confine their practices to such narrow limits as surgery of the hand, the cornea, or the skin.

Surrogacy

The agreement by a woman to become pregnant and give birth to a child with the understanding that she will surrender the child after birth to the contractual parents. Surrogacy became publicized with the advent of *in vitro fertilization*, in which the egg and sperm are brought together in the laboratory. The fertilized egg can be transferred to the uterus of any woman who is at the appropriate stage of the menstrual cycle.

Another means of accomplishing surrogacy is through the *artificial insemination* of the surrogate mother with the contracting father's sperm.

The ethical and legal aspects of surrogacy have yet to be resolved here. Surrogacy for financial reward has been forbidden by law in some countries and would likely be deemed illegal in Canada.

Susceptibility

A total or partial vulnerability to an infection, disease, or disorder. In *AIDS*, the *immune system* is impaired and the sufferer is susceptible to a wide range of infections and diseases.

Suture

A type of *joint*, found only between the bones of the *skull*, in which the adjacent bones are mobile during birth but then become so closely and firmly joined by a thin layer of fibrous connective tissue that movement between them is impossible.

The term suture is also used to refer to a surgical stitch (see *Suturing*).

S

MOST COMMON OPERATIONS REQUIRING HOSPITALIZATION (rate per 100,000)

Men
Operation

Operation	Rate
Hernia repair	380
Prostatectomy	280
Reduction of fracture	250
Tonsillectomy/adenoidectomy	220
Spinal operations	140
Appendectomy	130
Removal of gallbladder	130
Coronary artery surgery	100

Rate   0   100   200   300   400   500

Women
Operation

Operation	Rate
Hysterectomy	470
Cesarean section	450
Dilatation and curettage	450
Removal of gallbladder	310
Breast surgery	260
Tonsillectomy/adenoidectomy	250
Reduction of fracture	210
Appendectomy	110

Rate   0   100   200   300   400   500

Admission to hospital
The chart shows only those operations that are done on patients who are admitted to hospital. Many minor operations, such as dental work, excision of skin lesions, and vasectomy, are done in physicians' offices or in hospital outpatient departments.

Suturing
The closing of a surgical incision or a wound by sutures (stitches) to promote healing.

MATERIALS USED
Various sterile materials can be used as sutures. These include: catgut (obtained from sheep intestines); linen, silk, or synthetic thread; and stainless steel wire.

Suture materials vary considerably in the length of time they retain their strength, the reaction they provoke in tissues, and the likelihood of their allowing minute pockets of infection to form. Certain materials, such as catgut, are absorbable (i.e., they eventually dissolve in the body). The choice of which material to use for an operation is made by the surgeon.

The thickness of sutures varies from almost 1 mm, used for the repair of major injuries, to a barely visible 0.01 mm, used for delicate eye and blood vessel surgery.

Most surgical needles are curved and have a point with a cutting edge. The needle is held in a tweezerlike instrument; larger needles may be held with the fingers.

HOW IT IS DONE
The method of suturing a typical incision and some alternative methods of skin closure are shown in the illustrated box, facing page. Deep incisions or wounds may need to be sutured at several levels to achieve full closure throughout the depth of tissue, thus preventing accumulation of blood in pockets below the surface.

Internal sutures, made of absorbable material, are left in place permanently. Skin sutures are removed by a painless procedure about one to two weeks after insertion.

Swab
A wad of absorbent material used in surgery or to obtain a sample of bacteria from an infected patient.

A surgical swab is commonly a folded piece of cotton gauze held in the hand or in a clamp. It is used to apply cleansing and antiseptic solutions to the skin before an incision is made and to soak up blood and other fluids during an operation. The swab often contains material opaque to X rays to enable it to be detected if it is accidentally left in the body, an occurrence that is usually prevented by a "swab count" made before the operation begins and again before the patient is stitched up.

A microbiological swab consists of a twist of cotton wool at the end of a thin stick, supplied in a sterile container. The swab is applied to an infected area of the body to absorb pus or mucus, from which a *culture* can be grown to identify infective microorganisms, such as bacteria.

Swallowing
The process by which food or liquid is conveyed from the mouth to the stomach via the esophagus. The first stage is voluntary (under conscious control), but is so familiar that little thought is given to it. Once food has been well chewed and mixed with saliva (which greatly facilitates swallowing), the tongue pushes it to the back of the mouth and the voluntary muscles in the palate push the food into the pharynx (throat).

The rest of the swallowing process is involuntary (automatic), brought about by a series of *reflexes*; once started, it is rapid, powerful, and difficult to stop. Entry of food into the pharynx causes the epiglottis (a flap of cartilage) to close over the larynx (voice box) leading to the trachea (windpipe). A sphincter (circular muscle) at the top of the esophagus relaxes, and the muscles of the pharynx seize the food and squeeze it in the form of a bolus (rounded lump) into the esophagus. Powerful waves of contraction then pass down the esophagus, propelling the food toward the stomach. Finally, the muscle at the entry to the stomach (the cardiac sphincter) relaxes and allows the bolus to pass.

Swallowing difficulty
A fairly common symptom with a wide variety of causes, known medically as dysphagia.

CAUSES
Temporary swallowing difficulty may be caused by a foreign object (such as a fish bone) lodging at the back of the throat or in the esophagus. Most

S

METHODS OF SUTURING

Suturing is carried out under a general or local anesthetic. The type of stitch used depends on the nature of the wound or incision (two types are shown below). In all cases the surgeon sews the wound edges together to produce minimal distortion of tissue.

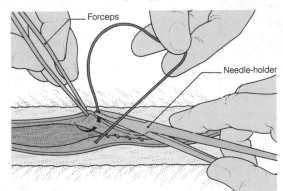

Forceps
Needle-holder

Technique
The surgeon grasps the edge of the wound with forceps held in one hand and, with the other hand, inserts the needle through the skin. In this illustration, the surgeon is shown using a needle-holder, which gives greater control for very fine stitches. In other cases, the needle may be held in the hand.

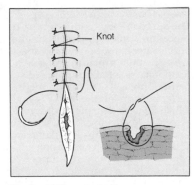

Knot

Standard interrupted sutures
The needle is passed into one skin edge, through the full depth of the wound, and out of the other skin edge. Each stitch is then knotted at the side.

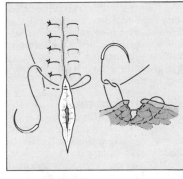

Mattress sutures
For deeper wounds, the needle is passed through the wound twice: first shallowly, close to the skin edges, and then more deeply, farther from the edges.

OTHER METHODS OF CLOSURE
Alternatives to suturing include removable staples and clips (staples are also used internally) and adhesive tape.

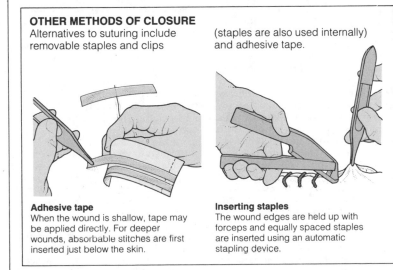

Adhesive tape
When the wound is shallow, tape may be applied directly. For deeper wounds, absorbable stitches are first inserted just below the skin.

Inserting staples
The wound edges are held up with forceps and equally spaced staples are inserted using an automatic stapling device.

foreign objects are able to pass on to the stomach, but a scratch in the lining of the throat or esophagus may cause discomfort. Swallowing difficulty may also result from insufficient production of saliva (see *Mouth, dry*).

Disorders of the esophagus that may disrupt normal swallowing include *esophageal spasm* (uncoordinated contractions of the esophagus), *esophageal stricture* (narrowing) caused by scarring or a tumor (see *Esophagus, cancer of*), *esophagitis* (inflammation), *achalasia* (abnormal contraction of the muscles at the lower end of the esophagus), or an *esophageal diverticulum* (an outward protrusion of part of the esophagus).

Esophageal atresia (closure or failure of the esophagus to open) can cause feeding problems in the newborn.

Difficulty in swallowing may also be caused by a nervous system disorder (e.g., *myasthenia gravis*, or *stroke*). It may also have a psychological cause, as in *globus hystericus*.

Pressure on the outside of the esophagus may obstruct the passage of food. Rarely, pressure is exerted by a *goiter*, an aortic *aneurysm*, or cancer of the bronchus (see *Lung cancer*).

DIAGNOSIS AND TREATMENT
Any person who experiences persistent swallowing difficulty should be examined without delay. Investigations may include *esophagoscopy* (examination of the esophagus with a viewing instrument) or barium swallow (see *Barium X-ray examinations*). Treatment depends on the cause.

Swamp fever
Another name for *leptospirosis*, an infectious disease caused by contact with water contaminated by rat's urine. The term has also been applied to *malaria* (swamps being a favorite breeding ground for mosquitoes).

Sweat glands
Minute structures deep within the *skin* that produce sweat. Each gland is made up of a coiled tube, in which the sweat is secreted, and a narrow passageway, which carries the sweat to the skin surface. The average person has about 3 million sweat glands.

TYPES
There are two types of sweat glands: eccrine and apocrine. Eccrine glands are the most common, especially on the palms and soles; these glands open directly to the skin surface. Apocrine glands, which develop at puberty, occur only in hairy areas, particularly the armpits, pubic region,

S

and around the anus. These glands produce cellular material as well as sweat, and open into a hair follicle before reaching the skin surface.

FUNCTION

Eccrine sweat is composed mainly of water (99 percent) and minute quantities of dissolved substances, including sodium chloride (salt).

The activity of the sweat glands is controlled by the *autonomic nervous system*. Usually the glands are stimulated to produce sweat to keep the body cool, in which case sweating is heaviest on the forehead, upper lip, neck, and chest. Sweating can also be caused by anxiety or fear, in which case sweat appears mainly on the palms and soles and in the armpits. Sweating also occurs with fevers.

Sweat is odorless until bacteria act upon it, producing *body odor*.

The most common problem affecting the sweat glands is *prickly heat*, an intensely irritating skin rash caused by blockage of the glands with debris and sweat. Less common disorders include *hyperhidrosis* (excessive sweating), *hypohidrosis* (reduced sweating), and abnormal or excessive skin odor.

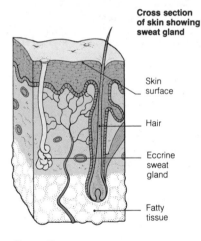

Cross section of skin showing sweat gland

- Skin surface
- Hair
- Eccrine sweat gland
- Fatty tissue

Sweating

The process by which the body cools itself. Sweating also occurs as a response to psychological stress or fear. (See *Heat disorders*; *Sweat glands*.)

Sweeteners, artificial

See *Artificial sweeteners*.

Swimmer's ear

A common name for *otitis externa*.

Sycosis vulgaris

Inflammation of the beard area, also called barbers' itch. The condition is caused by infection of the hair fol-

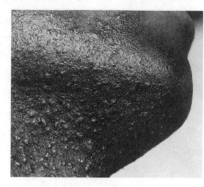

The characteristics of sycosis vulgaris
Sycosis vulgaris is caused by folliculitis (infection and inflammation of hair follicles) in the beard area. It tends to affect men with greasy skin, and may be persistent.

licles, usually with STAPHYLOCOCCUS AUREUS bacteria contracted from infected razors and towels. Pus-filled blisters or boils develop around the follicles, sometimes resulting in severe scarring unless they are treated. Treatment is usually with *antibiotic drugs*; growing a beard may help to prevent a recurrence.

Sydenham's chorea

A childhood disorder of the *central nervous system*, formerly called Saint Vitus' dance. The condition is characterized by involuntary (uncontrolled), irregular, jerky movements and usually follows an attack of *rheumatic fever*. Sydenham's chorea is rarely seen in Canada today but remains common in developing countries.

Restlessness and irritability usually precede the chorea, which affects the head, face, limbs, and fingers. The involuntary "fidgets" are random and unrepetitive. Voluntary (willed) movements are clumsy and the limbs are often floppy. Early signs are slurred speech and deteriorating handwriting.

Treatment is bed rest and *antibiotic drugs*. Sedation is sometimes necessary if the fidgeting is extreme. The condition usually clears up after two to three months and has no long-term adverse effects. Thereafter, the person may be given antibiotics before surgical or dental treatment to prevent possible heart complications.

Sympathectomy

An operation in which the ganglia (terminals) of sympathetic nerves are destroyed to interrupt the nerve pathway and thus improve blood supply to a limb or relieve chronic pain.

WHY IT IS DONE

The sympathetic nerves form part of the *autonomic nervous system* and control involuntary (automatic) activities in the body, including the widening and narrowing of blood vessels. In *peripheral vascular disease* (a disorder in which the blood vessels in the legs and sometimes in the arms become narrowed), stimulation from the sympathetic nerves produces spasms in the blood vessels that worsen the narrowing. Sympathectomy prevents these spasms from occurring and thus may improve blood supply to the affected area.

The sympathetic nerves also play an important part in producing the sensation of *pain*. In some cases of *causalgia* (a persistent severe pain usually caused by nerve injury), sympathectomy offers the only prospect of relieving the pain.

HOW IT IS DONE

The surgeon may first perform a trial procedure, injecting local anesthetic into the nerves supplying the affected area. If this provides considerable temporary relief of symptoms, a sympathectomy is usually performed.

Destruction of the nerve ganglia, which lie near the spinal cord, can be accomplished by injecting a sclerosing solution, which causes inflammation and subsequent degeneration of the nerves. Symptoms in the upper part of the body are controlled by an injection into the cervicodorsal sympathetic nerves at the base of the neck. To treat disorders of the lower part of the body, sclerosing solution is injected into the lumbar sympathetic nerves in the middle of the back.

Alternatively, nerve ganglia may be destroyed surgically while the patient is under general anesthesia. In a cervicodorsal sympathectomy, destruction of the ganglia is achieved through an incision made in the armpit; in a lumbar sympathectomy, the incision runs horizontally from the spine in the lower back almost to the navel.

In general, results depend on the disease for which the procedure is being performed. A sympathectomy performed to widen blood vessels has variable results. In controlling severe pain, however, the operation usually proves successful. Lumbar sympathectomy in men occasionally results in inability to ejaculate.

Sympathetic nervous system

One of the two divisions of the *autonomic nervous system*. In conjunction with the other division (the parasympathetic nervous system), this system controls many of the involuntary (automatic) activities of the glands, organs, and other parts of the body.

Sympatholytic drugs

A group of drugs that blocks the action of the *sympathetic nervous system*. Sympatholytic drugs include *beta-blocker drugs, guanethidine, hydralazine,* and *prazosin*. They work either by reducing the release of the stimulatory *neurotransmitter* norepinephrine from nerve endings, or by occupying the receptors that the neurotransmitters epinephrine and norepinephrine normally bind to, thereby preventing their normal actions.

Symphysis

An anatomical term for a type of *joint* in which two bones are firmly joined by tough, fibrous cartilage. Such joints occur between the bodies of the *vertebrae* (the bodies are the parts of the vertebrae that are separated by the intervertebral disks); between the two pubic bones at the front of the *pelvis;* and between the manubrium (upper part) and body (middle part) of the *sternum* (breastbone).

Symptom

An indication of a disease or disorder (such as pain) that is noticed by the sufferer. By contrast, the indications that a physician notes are called signs. The overall clinical picture, including both symptoms and signs, helps a physician to identify a particular disease.

Symptoms that prompt a person to obtain medical advice are known as presenting symptoms; such symptoms are not necessarily those that are the first to appear.

The distinction between symptoms and signs is not always clear. For example, fever is experienced by the patient and observed by the physician. Similarly, in *appendicitis,* pain is a key symptom; tenderness, which is pain felt only when pressure is applied, is a sign generally elicited by the physician, but which may also be elicited by the patient pressing on his or her own abdomen.

In some conditions, accurate recollection and precise description of symptoms are extremely important for an accurate diagnosis. For example, because physical signs are often absent in *angina pectoris,* diagnosis of this condition may depend almost entirely on the patient's description of the chest pain.

Symptothermal method

A contraceptive technique. See *Contraception, natural methods of.*

Synapse

A junctional connection between two *neurons* (nerve cells) across which a signal can pass. A single neuron may form thousands of these connections with adjacent nerve cells.

A typical neuron has one long fiber (axon) that projects from its cell body, and this splits into several smaller branches and twigs, each ending in a terminal that forms a synapse, usually close to the cell body of an adjacent neuron. At a synapse, the two neurons do not come directly into contact; their surface membranes are separated by a gap known as the synaptic cleft. When an electrical signal passes along a neuronal axon and reaches a synapse, it cannot bridge the cleft directly; instead, it causes the release of a chemical, called a *neurotransmitter.* The neurotransmitter travels across the synaptic cleft and is received at the surface membrane of the next neuron, where it changes the electrical potential of the membrane.

The axonal membrane from which the neurotransmitter is released is called the presynaptic membrane; the neuronal membrane at which it is received is called the postsynaptic membrane. Signals can be transmitted across a synapse in one direction only—from presynaptic to postsynaptic membrane.

A synapse may be excitatory or inhibitory. When a neurotransmitter passes across an excitatory synapse, the effect is to excite the postsynaptic membrane, making it more likely that the receptor neuron will "fire" and propagate an electrical impulse.

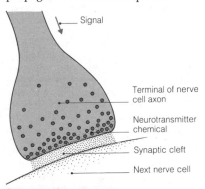

Structure of a synapse
When a signal arrives at the terminal of a nerve cell axon, it causes release of a neurotransmitter, which crosses the synaptic cleft and affects the next cell.

Most drugs that affect the *nervous system* work as a result of their effects on synapses. Such drugs may affect the release of neurotransmitters (e.g., *reserpine* and *amphetamine drugs*), or they may modify the effects of neurotransmitters on postsynaptic membranes (the mode of action of *atropine* and *beta-blocker drugs*).

Syncope

The medical term for *fainting.*

Syndactyly

A congenital (present at birth) defect in which two or more fingers or toes are joined. The toes are more frequently affected than the fingers.

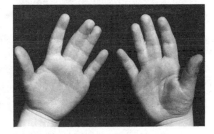

Syndactyly
In this case, the middle and ring fingers of both hands are partly joined. Sometimes, syndactyly occurs in association with other birth defects.

Syndactyly is often inherited and is more common in males than females. The condition is caused by incomplete development of the digits at the embryo stage, or by constriction of the digits by tissue within the uterus later in fetal development.

In mild cases of syndactyly, the affected fingers or toes are joined only by a web of skin. In more serious cases, the bones of adjacent digits are fused, as is the overlying skin, and there may be only one nail.

Treatment is usually by one or more operations during early childhood to separate the affected digits.

Syndrome

A group of symptoms and/or signs that, occurring together, constitutes a particular disorder. For example, *irritable bowel syndrome* is characterized by a combination of any or all of the following: intermittent pain in the lower abdomen (usually relieved by passing feces or wind), abdominal swelling, irregular bowel movements (often with a sense of incomplete evacuation of the bowel afterward), mucus in the feces, excessive wind, and worsening of symptoms after eating.

S

Synovectomy

Surgical removal of the *synovium* (thin membrane lining a joint capsule) to treat recurrent or persistent *synovitis* (inflammation of the synovium), usually in sufferers from severe *rheumatoid arthritis*. The operation is usually performed only if the condition is severely disabling and has not responded to injections of *corticosteroid drugs* or to the taking of *nonsteroidal anti-inflammatory drugs* or *antirheumatic drugs*.

The joint may be opened and the synovium cut away under general anesthesia, or the operation may be performed by means of *arthroscopy*. After the operation, the joint is kept mobile to inhibit scarring. Synovectomy is a temporary expedient that usually improves symptoms for no more than about two years; further surgery may then be required.

Synovitis

Inflammation of the *synovium* (thin membrane lining a joint capsule). The condition may be acute (of sudden onset and short duration), in which case it is usually caused by an attack of arthritis, injury, overuse of the joint, or infection; or chronic (recurrent or persistent), as in a disorder such as *rheumatoid arthritis*.

The inflammation causes the synovium to secrete an abnormal amount of lubricating fluid, which makes the joint swollen, painful, and often warm and red. To determine the cause of the condition, joint aspiration (removal of fluid from a joint) or a *biopsy* (removal of a sample of the synovium) may be required.

TREATMENT
Symptoms are relieved by rest, supporting the joint with a *splint* or *cast*, *analgesic drugs* (painkillers), *nonsteroidal anti-inflammatory drugs*, and, occasionally, an injection of a *corticosteroid drug*. Any causative infection is treated with *antibiotic drugs*.

Synovium

A thin membrane that lines the fibrous capsule surrounding a movable *joint*. The synovium also forms a sheath for certain tendons of the hands and feet, lining the fibrous or bony tunnels through which they glide. The membrane secretes synovial fluid, a clear, sticky liquid resembling egg white that lubricates the joint or the tendon. The synovium can become inflamed; in a joint lining this is known as *synovitis*, in a tendon sheath it is known as *tenosynovitis*.

LOCATION OF SYNOVIUM
Every movable joint is enclosed within a fibrous capsule. The inner lining of the capsule is known as the synovium.

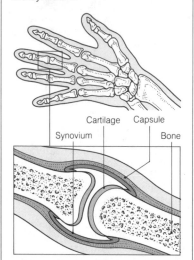

Cartilage   Capsule

Synovium   Bone

Function
The membrane secretes a thick fluid (synovial fluid) that lubricates the joint; the fluid may accumulate and cause pain if the joint is injured.

Syphilis

A *sexually transmitted disease* or *congenital* (present from birth) infection of worldwide distribution, first recorded as a major epidemic in Europe in the last decade of the 15th century following the return of Columbus from America. Today, infection is transmitted almost exclusively by sexual contact. The incidence of syphilis has fallen dramatically since the introduction of penicillin. About 300 new infections and 1,500 tertiary cases are reported in Canada each year.

Syphilis is caused by TREPONEMA PALLIDUM, a spirochete (spiral-shaped bacterium) that penetrates broken skin or *mucous membranes* in the genitalia, rectum, or mouth during sexual intercourse. Infection may also be acquired by kissing or by other intimate bodily contact with an infected person. The risk of infection during a single contact with an infected person is about 30 percent. After gaining access, the organism passes quickly by way of the bloodstream and lymphatic system to all parts of the body; within hours, the organism has spread beyond any hope of local treatment.

SYMPTOMS AND SIGNS
Untreated syphilis usually passes through the following stages.

PRIMARY The first symptom is a primary sore (chancre) that usually appears three to four weeks after contact. The chancre is a painless ulcer measuring less than 1 cm in diameter. It has a hard, wet base that is covered with serum teeming with spirochetes. The ulcer usually develops on the genitals but other possible sites include the anus, rectum, lips, throat, and, very rarely, the fingers. Often, the chancre is inconspicuous and may be missed. The lymph nodes connected with the area containing the chancre become painlessly enlarged and rubbery but are not tender. The chancre heals in four to eight weeks.

SECONDARY Six to 12 weeks after infection, the secondary stage begins. The most obvious feature is a skin rash, which may be transient, recurrent, or may last for months. In white people, the rash is conspicuous, with crops of pinkish or pale red, round spots; in black people, the rash is pigmented and appears darker than the normal skin color. The rash may be associated with extensive lymph node enlargement. Other possible symptoms include headache, aches and pains in the bones, loss of appetite, fever, and fatigue. Clumps of hair may fall out. Thickened, gray or pink patches (condylomata lata) may develop on moist areas of skin and are highly infectious. Meningitis may develop.

LATENT During this stage, which may last for a few years or may continue indefinitely, the infected person appears to be normal. A few untreated cases proceed to tertiary syphilis.

TERTIARY This stage usually starts within 10 years of infection, but may appear as early as three years or as late as 25 years afterward. The effects are varied. Tissue destruction, by a process called gumma formation, may involve the bones, palate, nasal septum, tongue, skin, or almost any organ of the body. Among the more serious effects are cardiovascular syphilis, which affects the aorta (the main artery of the body) and leads to aneurysm formation and heart valve disease; neurosyphilis, with progressive brain damage and general paralysis (formerly called general paralysis of the insane); and tabes dorsalis, which affects part of the spinal cord.

DIAGNOSIS
Primary syphilis can be readily diagnosed by finding active spirochetes during microscopic examination of a

---

S

smear taken from the chancre serum. Confirmation is given by blood tests, such as the Venereal Disease Research Laboratory (VDRL) test or a fluorescence test for antibodies to the organism. Secondary, latent, and tertiary syphilis give strongly positive results with these and similar tests. In cases of neurosyphilis, it may be necessary to perform these tests on a sample of *cerebrospinal fluid*.

TREATMENT

All forms of the disease are treated by a course of a *penicillin drug*. Although penicillin is, in general, very safe, the treatment of syphilis is not without danger. More than half of those treated suffer a severe reaction within six to 12 hours, caused by the body's response to the sudden killing of large numbers of spirochetes. Organ damage already caused by the disease cannot be reversed.

Promiscuous heterosexual or homosexual intercourse inevitably involves a risk of infection with syphilis. Infection can be avoided by maintaining monogamous relationships. Condoms offer some measure of protection but do not offer absolute protection (see *Safe sex*). People with syphilis are infectious in the primary and secondary stages but not in the latent and tertiary stages.

Syphilis, nonvenereal

A disease caused by the same organism that causes sexually transmitted *syphilis* but that is spread by different means, such as through broken skin and by sharing drinking vessels. Nonvenereal syphilis occurs mainly in the Middle East and Africa. Treatment is with a *penicillin drug*.

Syringe

An instrument for injecting fluid into, or withdrawing fluid from, a body cavity, blood vessel, or tissue. Most syringes consist of a barrel with a plunger at one end and, at the other, a nozzle to which a hollow needle can be attached. The barrel is calibrated to enable the correct dosage of medication to be given. Most modern syringes are disposable plastic instruments that are presterilized and packed in sealed bags.

Syringing of ears

A procedure for removing excessive *earwax* or, less commonly, a foreign body from the outer ear canal (see *Ear, foreign body in*). The physician first examines the ear to see if there is a condition (such as a perforated ear-

drum) that indicates syringing should not be performed. If there is no such indication, any hard wax may first require softening by putting drops of oil in the ear. The earwax is then washed out. Afterward, the canal is dried, sometimes using alcohol drops. Wax and other debris may be removed by suction or by small instruments.

Ear syringing may be uncomfortable. Sudden pain or dizziness may indicate a perforation of the eardrum and the need to stop the procedure.

Syringomyelia

A very rare, usually congenital (present from birth), condition in which a cavity forms in the *brain stem* (the low-

EAR SYRINGING
This procedure should be carried out by a physician or nurse; amateur attempts can damage the eardrum.

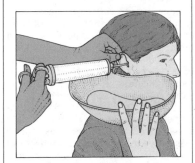

1 The nozzle of a large syringe is placed just inside the ear canal, which is straightened out by pulling the external ear upward and backward.

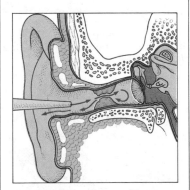

2 A jet of warm water or sodium bicarbonate solution is directed along the upper wall of the patient's ear canal in order to dislodge earwax or a foreign body.

est section of the brain) or at neck level in the *spinal cord*. The cavity gradually expands, filling with cerebrospinal fluid, eventually causing damage to nerve fibers.

The first symptoms usually appear in early adulthood. Affected persons are unable to feel pain or temperature changes in the neck, shoulders, arms, and hands, causing them to suffer injuries without realizing it. The muscles in the same region gradually become weak and wasted, and there is some loss of the sense of touch.

In advanced syringomyelia, there is spasticity (abnormal stiffness and rigidity) in the legs, nasal speech, and sometimes difficulty in swallowing. Many severely affected people are confined to wheelchairs.

No drug treatment is available. In some cases, surgical treatment to relieve pressure in the affected region (see *Decompression, spinal canal*) may arrest what is otherwise an inevitably progressive disease.

System

A group of interconnected or interdependent organs that perform a common function. For example, the parts of the *digestive system* (mouth, salivary glands, esophagus, stomach, intestines, gallbladder, pancreas, and liver) act together to ingest, break down and absorb food, and to excrete feces. The term system may also be applied to a method of classification, as in the ABO system for classifying *blood groups*.

Systemic

A term applied to something that affects the whole body rather than a specific part of it. For example, fever is a systemic symptom, whereas swelling is a localized symptom. The term systemic is also applied to the part of the blood circulation that supplies all parts of the body except the lungs.

Systemic lupus erythematosus

See *Lupus erythematosus*.

Systole

A period of muscular contraction of a chamber of the *heart* that alternates with a resting period, called *diastole*. With each *heartbeat*, the atria (upper chambers) contract first, squeezing blood into the ventricles (lower chambers); this is known as atrial systole. The ventricles then contract, pumping blood out of the heart into the arteries; this is known as ventricular systole.

S

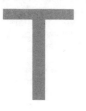

Tabes dorsalis

A complication of *syphilis*, once common but now rare, that affects the spinal cord, causing abnormalities of sensation, sharp pains, incoordination, and incontinence. Symptoms appear many years after infection.

Tachycardia

A heart rate of over 100 beats per minute in an adult. Most people have a rate of between 60 and 100 beats per minute, with an average of 72 to 78 beats. Tachycardia occurs in healthy people during exercise, when the heart is stimulated to work faster and thus increase blood flow to muscles. Tachycardia at rest may be caused by *fever, anxiety, hyperthyroidism, coronary artery disease* or any other cause of heart disease or heart failure, a high intake of *caffeine*, or treatment with an *anticholinergic drug* or some *decongestant drugs*. Types of tachycardia include *atrial fibrillation, sinus tachycardia, supraventricular tachycardia*, and *ventricular tachycardia*.

Symptoms of tachycardia may include *palpitations, breathlessness*, and light-headedness, depending on how fast the heart is beating and on how effectively it is pumping blood.

Tachypnea

An abnormally fast rate of *breathing*. Tachypnea may be caused by exercise, anxiety, a lung disorder (such as emphysema), or a cardiac disorder (such as heart failure).

T'ai chi

A Chinese exercise system based on a series of more than 100 postures between which many slow, continuous, ·deliberate movements occur. T'ai chi is characterized by outer movement and inner stillness; its purpose is to exercise the muscles and achieve integration of mind and body. Devotees believe that continuous flow of movement is important in performing the exercises because it prevents "blockage" of the internal flow of chi—the essential life energy.

Talipes

A *birth defect* in which the foot is twisted out of shape or position. There are many different varieties of talipes, all of which are commonly called clubfoot. The causes are not fully understood. Most cases are thought to be caused by pressure on the baby's feet from the mother's uterus during late pregnancy, but a genetic factor is also present (relatives of affected people have a higher incidence of the disorder).

The most common form of talipes is an equinovarus deformity, in which the heel is turned inward and the rest of the foot is bent downward and inward. In addition, the tibia (shin bone) may be twisted inward and there may also be underdevelopment of the muscles in the lower leg above the affected foot.

Talipes equinovarus is twice as common in boys as in girls. In about 50 percent of cases it affects both feet.

TREATMENT
Talipes equinovarus is treated by repeated manipulation of the foot and ankle, which should begin soon after birth. In some cases, a plaster *cast*, metal *splint*, or adhesive *strapping* may be needed to hold the foot in the corrected position. If manipulation and strapping are ineffective, an operation to cut the tight ligaments and tendons is performed and the foot is then immobilized in a plaster cast for at least three months. If treatment is not carried out before the age of 2, the foot cannot be restored to normal but function can be improved by lengthening a tendon or by transferring a tendon from one bone to another (see *Tendon transfer*).

Other types of talipes can usually be corrected by repeated stretching of the foot into a normal position. Occasionally, immobilization of the foot in a plaster cast is required.

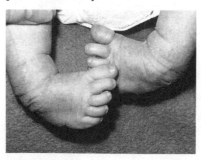

Talipes equinovarus
This birth defect affects about one baby in 900. Treatment is by gentle manipulation, repeated several times a day.

Tamoxifen

An *anticancer drug* used in the treatment of certain types of *breast cancer*. Tamoxifen is also sometimes effective in the treatment of other cancers, such as prostate cancer (see *Prostate, cancer of*).

In women of childbearing age, tamoxifen stimulates *ovulation* (egg release) and is therefore occasionally used as a treatment for certain types of *infertility*.

Tamoxifen works by blocking *estrogen hormone* receptors. It has fewer adverse effects than most anticancer drugs, but may cause hot flashes, nausea, vomiting, swollen ankles, and irregular vaginal bleeding.

Tampon

A plug of absorbent material, such as absorbent cotton, that is inserted into a wound or body opening to soak up blood or other secretions. The term is most commonly used to refer to a sanitary tampon inserted into the vagina to absorb menstrual blood.

Tamponade

Compression of the *heart*. Tamponade may occur in *pericarditis* (inflammation of the outer lining of the heart) due to the collection of fluid under the lining. Tamponade may also result from the collection of blood and blood clots around the heart after heart surgery or a penetrating chest injury.

Symptoms include breathlessness and, sometimes, collapse because the heart is unable to pump blood efficiently to the lungs and brain. The diagnosis is usually made by *echocardiography*.

Treatment involves immediate removal of any fluid that is pressing on the heart via a hollow needle guided through the chest wall. If blood clots are present, a *thoracotomy* is usually performed to open the chest wall and remove them.

Tan

See *Suntan*.

Tannin

Also known as tannic acid, an organic chemical that occurs in many plants, particularly in tea, oak apples, and the bark of oak, sumac, and mangrove trees.

Tannin has been used in medicine to stop bleeding, to control diarrhea, and as an antidote to plant poisons. It is no longer used therapeutically because more effective agents are available and because it can cause liver damage. Although tea contains significant amounts of tannin, drinking moderate amounts is unlikely to lead to liver damage. However, it may cause constipation.

Tantrum

An outburst of bad temper, common in toddlers, usually indicating frustration and anger. Tantrums occur in many children between the ages of 15 months and 4 years, but are especially likely in 2-year-olds.

During a tantrum, the child may scream, cry, yell, kick, bang the feet and fists, roll on the floor, go red in the face, spit, and bite. Some toddlers hold their breath during tantrums, sometimes turning blue and, in rare cases, momentarily losing consciousness (see *Breath-holding attacks*).

CAUSES

Tantrums occur at the age when a child starts to gain independence and becomes frustrated by restraints imposed by others, but is not yet able to express these feelings verbally. The outbursts are more likely when the child is tired, and are often brought on by a disagreement between child and parents. Tantrums may start with the birth of another baby, when the older child may believe that the baby is getting all the parents' attention.

Most children have occasional tantrums; frequent outbursts may indicate a *behavioral problem*, which may be due to emotional strain or a communication problem.

TREATMENT

Tantrums should be ignored as much as possible. An angry response will tend to make the child even more excited. Firm and consistent treatment is essential. A child's attention can often be diverted to a game or project. Most children grow out of tantrums when they develop the ability to describe their feelings.

If parents are unable to cope with tantrums, or if a child does not seem to be growing out of them, *child guidance* may be necessary.

Tapeworm infestation

 Tapeworms, also called cestodes, are ribbon-shaped parasitic worms that live in human or animal intestines. They are typically acquired by eating undercooked meat or fish. Each adult tapeworm bears suckers or hooks on its head, by which it attaches itself to the intestinal wall. The rest of the worm consists of a chain of flat segments.

CAUSES, TYPES, AND INCIDENCE

Tapeworms in humans have life cycles that usually also involve another animal host. A typical life cycle is shown in the illustrated box.

Three large types of tapeworm, acquired by eating undercooked, infected beef, pork, and fish, all have life cycles of this type. The adults may grow to 6 to 9 m long. All these tapeworms occur worldwide, but, in developed countries, infestations are largely prevented by measures such as adequate meat inspection and sanitary disposal of sewage. In Canada, tapeworm infections usually occur only in people infected abroad.

The much smaller dwarf tapeworm, which is only 2.5 cm long, has a different life cycle. An infested person may directly cause an infestation of someone else through accidental transfer of worm eggs from feces to fingers to mouth. The dwarf tapeworm is found worldwide, but especially in the tropics; it primarily affects children.

Humans may act as intermediate hosts to the larvae of a tapeworm for which dogs are the main host. The larvae grow and develop into cysts in the liver and lungs, a condition called *hydatid disease*.

SYMPTOMS

Despite their size, beef, pork, and fish tapeworms rarely cause symptoms, except mild abdominal discomfort or diarrhea. However, segments of the worm may detach and emerge through the anus or may appear in the feces. In rare cases, fish tapeworms cause *anemia*. Dwarf tapeworms can cause diarrhea and abdominal discomfort.

DIAGNOSIS AND TREATMENT

Tapeworm infestation is diagnosed from the presence of worm segments and/or eggs in the feces.

Infestations are treated by *anthelmintic drugs*, such as *niclosamide* and *praziquantel*, which effectively kill the tapeworms.

Treatment of pork tapeworms must be carried out carefully because there is a risk that worm eggs will be released and find their way back into the stomach. The patient may then accidentally become the host to the worm larvae, which burrow into the tissues and form cysts. This leads to a condition called cysticercosis, the symptoms of which may include muscle pains and convulsions.

Tarsalgia

Pain in the rear part of the foot, usually associated with *flatfeet*.

Tarsorrhaphy

An operation in which the upper and lower eyelids are sewn together.

WHY IT IS DONE

Tarsorrhaphy may be performed as part of the treatment of *corneal ulcer*. The eyelids act as a bandage to promote healing of the cornea. Tarsorrhaphy is commonly used to protect the corneas in people who cannot close their eyelids because of nerve or muscular disorders or scarring. Tar-

T

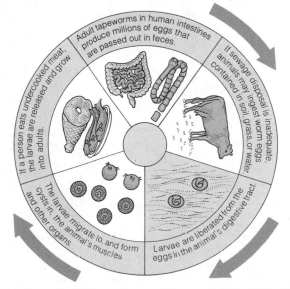

LIFE CYCLE OF TAPEWORM
Many tapeworms have life cycles in which the adult and larval worms infest different hosts. In the cycle on the right, the adult worms infest humans and the larvae infest cattle (called the intermediate hosts). Pigs and fish may also act as intermediate hosts to human tapeworms, and humans may act as intermediate hosts to dog and pig tapeworms.

Adult tapeworms in human intestines produce millions of eggs that are passed out in feces.

If sewage disposal is inadequate, animals may ingest worm eggs contained in soil, grass, or water.

Larvae are liberated from the eggs in the animal's digestive tract.

The larvae migrate to, and form cysts in, the animal's muscles and other organs.

If a person eats undercooked meat, the larvae are released and grow into adults.

sorrhaphy is also occasionally performed to protect the cornea in people with *exophthalmos*.

HOW IT IS DONE

A strip of tissue is removed from the upper and lower lid edges. The raw surfaces of the lids are then stitched together. By about two or three weeks after the operation, the eyelids have grown together and the stitches can be removed. After having allowed time for the original trouble to clear up, the eyelids are then cut apart and allowed to open.

Tartar

See *Calculus, dental*.

Taste

One of the five special senses. By itself, taste is a relatively crude sense, able to distinguish only between sweet, salty, sour, and bitter. In practice, however, many different flavors can be distinguished because of the combination of the sense of taste and the much more discriminating sense of *smell*. This combination explains why loss of the sense of smell (caused by a common cold, for example) also apparently causes loss of taste (see *Taste, loss of*). The full sensory appreciation of food also involves other factors, such as the appearance of food, which helps stimulate salivation, and

the consistency and temperature of the food. The structures on the tongue and the mechanisms involved in taste are shown in the illustrated box.

Taste, loss of

Loss of the sense of *taste*, usually occurring as a result of loss of the sense of *smell*, which contributes greatly to taste.

Loss of taste with loss also of smell is most often caused by inflammation of the nasal passages due, for example, to a common *cold*.

Loss of taste without loss of smell is relatively rare. A possible cause is any condition that results in a dry mouth

---

THE SENSE OF TASTE

Tastes are detected by special structures called taste buds, of which everyone has some 10,000, mainly on the tongue, with a few at the back of the throat and on the palate. These taste buds surround pores within papillae (protuberances) on the tongue surface and elsewhere. Four types of taste buds exist—sensitive to sweet, salty, sour, or bitter chemicals. All tastes are formed from a mixture of these four elements.

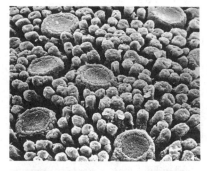

Fungiform papillae
These mushroom-shaped papillae occur in small numbers at random over the tongue surface, mainly in the middle.

Filiform papillae
These smaller peak-shaped protuberances occur in large numbers over all except the back of the tongue's upper surface, and on the palate.

Olfactory bulb

Tongue

Glosso-pharyngeal nerve

Vallate papillae

Taste pore

Taste buds

Vallate papillae

Filiform papillae

Fungiform papillae

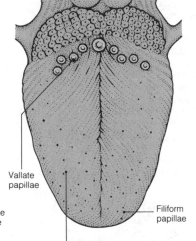

How a substance is tasted
Chemicals in food or drink dissolve in saliva and enter pores in the papillae on the tongue. Around these pores are groups of taste receptor cells—the taste buds. The chemicals stimulate hairs projecting from the receptor cells, causing signals to be sent from the cells along nerves to taste centers in the brain.

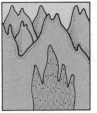

Magnified photograph of tongue surface
This photograph shows large (fungiform) and small (filiform) papillae. Taste buds are arranged around pores in the surface of the papillae.

Taste centers on the tongue
Taste buds sensitive to sweet, salty, sour, or bitter chemicals tend to be grouped into particular areas on the surface of the tongue.

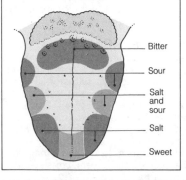

Bitter

Sour

Salt and sour

Salt

Sweet

T

(see *Mouth, dry*), because taste buds can detect the substances responsible for flavors only when those substances are dissolved in saliva.

Complete or partial loss of taste most commonly results from the natural degeneration of the taste buds with age. It may also result from damage to the taste buds themselves as a result of *stomatitis* (inflammation of the mouth), *mouth cancer, radiation therapy* to the mouth region (which also eliminates salivation by damaging the salivary glands), or the side effects of certain drugs.

In some cases, loss of taste is caused by damage to the cranial nerves that convey taste sensations to the brain. Nerve damage may occur as a result of a head injury, a tumor of the brain or of the cranial nerves associated with taste, or surgery on the head or neck. In these cases, loss of taste is usually accompanied by facial paralysis.

Disturbances of taste occur in some psychiatric disorders, usually taking the form of taste hallucinations rather than true loss of taste.

Tattooing

The introduction of permanent colors under the surface of the skin, usually to create a picture. Practiced for thousands of years, tattooing was originally used as a means of identification. Today it is almost always carried out for decorative purposes.

Tattooing, even by professionals, is potentially dangerous. If the tattooist does not follow strict sterile procedures, the viruses that cause *hepatitis* and *AIDS* may be transmitted through the needles used by the tattooist to introduce the dyes.

Removal of a tattoo is usually difficult and unsatisfactory: a scar almost always results. Small tattoos are best treated by complete removal of the colored area of skin and the stitching together of the edges of the wound. Larger tattooed areas can sometimes be removed by *dermabrasion* or by *laser treatment*.

Tay-Sachs disease

A serious inherited metabolic disorder that results in early death. Tay-Sachs disease is a type of inborn error of metabolism (see *Metabolism, inborn errors of*). It was formerly known as amaurotic familial idiocy.

CAUSES AND INCIDENCE
Tay-Sachs disease is caused by a deficiency of hexosaminidase A, a certain *enzyme* (a protein essential for regulating chemical reactions in the body). Deficiency results in a buildup of a harmful substance in the brain.

The disease is common among both Sephardic and Ashkenazi Jews. The incidence in these groups is around one in 2,500 births, 100 times higher than in other ethnic groups. The gene for Tay-Sachs disease is recessive (see *Genetic disorders*) and an Ashkenazi Jew or a Sephardic Jew has a one in 25 chance of carrying it. If two carriers marry, there is a one in four chance that they will have an affected child.

SYMPTOMS AND SIGNS
Signs of the illness, which usually appear after the first six months of life, are blindness, dementia, seizures, and paralysis. An exaggerated startle response to sound is an early sign. The disease progresses until the affected child dies, usually before reaching 4 years of age.

DIAGNOSIS
The diagnosis is based on the clinical history and physical examination; it is confirmed by enzyme analysis of a sample of white blood cells or a sample of skin tissue.

TREATMENT AND PREVENTION
There is no effective treatment for Tay-Sachs disease. Blood-testing programs for detecting carriers of the gene are well established in larger Canadian centers. Jewish couples in other locations should consult their family physician. Carriers and those with an affected child or relative should receive *genetic counseling* before starting a family or planning another pregnancy. If prenatal testing shows that a fetus is affected, the parents may choose to have an abortion and try again for a healthy child.

TB

An abbreviation for *tuberculosis*.

T cell

One of the two main classes of *lymphocytes* (a type of white blood cell). T cells play an important role in the body's *immune system*.

Tears

The salty, watery secretion produced by the lacrimal glands, part of the *lacrimal apparatus* of the *eye*. The tear film over the *cornea* and the *conjunctiva* consists of three layers: an inner, mucous layer secreted by glands in the conjunctiva; an intermediate layer of salt water; and an outer, oily layer secreted by the meibomian glands.

The principal function of tears is to keep the cornea and conjunctiva constantly moist. Moisture is essential to maintain transparency of the cornea and to prevent ulceration. By lubricating the surface of the eye, tears aid movement of the eyelid in blinking. Tears also wash away small foreign bodies and contain a natural antiseptic called lysozyme. Another function is their role in expressing emotion.

A deficiency in tear production causes *keratoconjunctivitis sicca* (dry eye). Excessive tear production may cause *watering eye*.

Tears, artificial

Preparations used to supplement inadequate production of tears in *keratoconjunctivitis sicca* and other conditions causing dryness of the eyes. To be effective, artificial tears must be applied at frequent intervals. Artificial tears may also be used to relieve discomfort caused by irritants.

Many preparations contain a preservative that can irritate the eyes. Contaminated preparations may cause serious eye infections.

Technetium

A radioactive metallic element. Technetium does not occur naturally either in its pure form or in compounds, but is produced during nuclear fission reactions. It was the first element to be made artificially (in 1937). Several isotopes (varieties of the element that are chemically identical but differ in some physical properties) have been synthesized, of which the most important medically is a form known as technetium 99m. This radioisotope, incorporated in various chemical substances, is used in *radionuclide scanning* of many of the body's organs, including the brain, heart, lungs, liver, kidneys, and bones.

Teeth

Hard bonelike projections set in the *jaws* and surrounded by the *gums*. The teeth are used for *mastication* (chewing), help people to speak clearly, and also give shape to the face.

Humans have two sets of teeth: the *primary teeth* (of which there are 20) and the *permanent teeth* (of which there are 32). The primary teeth usually erupt between the ages of 6 months and 3 years and start to be replaced by the permanent teeth at about the age of 6 (see *Eruption of teeth*). The arrangement of the teeth is shown in the illustrated box overleaf.

In some people, the teeth fail to grow in the correct relationship to each other, resulting in *malocclusion* (incorrect bite).

T

STRUCTURE AND ARRANGEMENT OF TEETH

At the heart of each tooth is the living pulp, which contains blood vessels and nerves. A hard substance called dentin surrounds the pulp. The part of the tooth above the gum, the crown, is covered by enamel. The roots of the tooth, which fit into sockets in the jawbone, are covered by a sensitive, bonelike material, the cementum. The periodontal ligament connects the cementum to the gums and to the jaw. It acts as a shock absorber and prevents jarring of the teeth and skull when food is being chewed.

Cross section

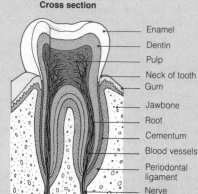

- Enamel
- Dentin
- Pulp
- Neck of tooth
- Gum
- Jawbone
- Root
- Cementum
- Blood vessels
- Periodontal ligament
- Nerve

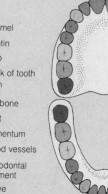

- Central and lateral incisors (7 to 9 years)
- First and second premolars (10 to 12 years)
- Second molars (11 to 13 years)
- Third molars (17+ years)
- First molars (6 to 7 years)
- Canines (12 to 14 years)

The permanent teeth
The illustration above shows the arrangement in the jaw of the permanent teeth—eight incisors, four canines, eight premolars, and 12 molars. The ages when these teeth erupt are indicated.

X ray of teeth
The panoramic X ray on the left shows all the teeth of the upper and lower jaw (there are no wisdom teeth) and their surrounding structures. The tooth roots, buried in the jawbones, can be clearly seen; several teeth have been filled.

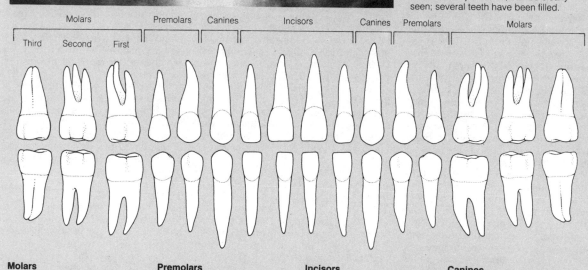

Molars — Third, Second, First | Premolars | Canines | Incisors | Canines | Premolars | Molars

Molars
The molars are large, strong teeth, efficient at grinding food. The third molars, or wisdom teeth, are the last to erupt; in some people, the wisdom teeth never appear.

Premolars
Also known as bicuspids, because of their two distinct edges, the premolars are concerned with grinding food. There are no premolars among the primary (milk) teeth.

Incisors
These teeth have a chisel-shaped, sharp cutting edge that is ideal for biting. The upper incisors overlap the lower incisors slightly when the jaws are closed.

Canines
The canines are sharp, pointed teeth, ideal for tearing food. They are larger and stronger than the incisors, with very long roots. The upper canines are often known as eye teeth.

Although the enamel that covers the crown of each tooth is the hardest substance in the body, it can be eroded when bacteria in the mouth break down carbohydrates in food (see *Caries, dental*). To help prevent decay, good *oral hygiene* is essential, consisting of daily *toothbrushing* and flossing (see *Floss, dental*).

Teeth, care of
See *Oral hygiene*.

Teething
The period when a baby cuts his or her first set of teeth. The primary teeth usually erupt between the ages of about 6 months and 3 years (see *Eruption of teeth*).

SYMPTOMS AND SIGNS

While teeth are erupting, a baby may be irritable, fretful, clinging, have difficulty in sleeping, and may cry more than usual. Extra saliva may be produced, resulting in dribbling, and the baby tends to chew on anything that he or she can hold.

Before a tooth comes through, the overlying gum may become red and swollen and the erupting tooth can be felt through the gum as a hard lump. When molars (back teeth) erupt, the cheek may feel warm and red on the affected side.

Teething should never be considered the cause of a very high temperature, vomiting, diarrhea, prolonged loss of appetite, earache, convulsions, cough, or diaper rash. These are symptoms of a disorder and a physician should be consulted.

TREATMENT

The baby should be given something firm to chew on, such as a piece of apple, or the swollen gum should be rubbed with a finger to ease the irritation. Painkilling dental creams or gels are available for rubbing on the gums.

Telangiectasia

An increase in the size of small blood vessels beneath the surface of an area of skin. Telangiectasia causes redness and an appearance sometimes called "broken veins." The condition is most common on the nose and cheeks. A localized form is the *spider nevus*.

Telangiectasia commonly results from heavy alcohol consumption over many years, or from the loss of supporting tissues in the skin due to overexposure to sunlight. Often, however, there is no obvious cause.

Less commonly, a connective tissue disease, such as systemic *lupus erythematosus* or *dermatomyositis*, is the cause. Telangiectasia may also be a feature of the facial redness of *rosacea*.

Appearance of telangiectasia
Although sometimes referred to as "broken veins," the blood vessels are in fact simply larger than usual.

Hereditary hemorrhagic telangiectasia is a rare disorder of the blood vessels in which frequent bleeding occurs from small, rounded patches of widened blood vessels around the mouth and nose or elsewhere in the skin or gastrointestinal tract. Frequent bleeding in hereditary hemorrhagic telangiectasia generally results in iron-deficiency *anemia*.

Telangiectasia is not usually a cause for concern. The only means of removal is electrodesiccation (electrical destruction of the upper layers of the skin) administered by a dermatologist. The procedure is successful only in some cases however.

Temazepam

A *benzodiazepine drug* used in the short-term treatment of *insomnia*.

Temperature

For the body to function optimally, its temperature must be maintained within narrow limits. The generally accepted figure for the average normal body temperature (measured in the mouth) is 37°C. However, in practice, body temperature varies not only among individuals, but also in the same person, being affected by factors such as exercise, sleep, eating and drinking, time of day (lowest at about 3 a.m. and highest at about 6 p.m.), and, in women, the stage of the menstrual cycle (lowest at menstruation and highest at ovulation). In most people, body temperature varies between 36.5°C and 37.2°C. The temperature is higher in the rectum (by about 0.3 to 0.4°C), and lower in the armpit (by about 0.2 to 0.3°C).

TEMPERATURE REGULATION

Body temperature is maintained within optimal limits by the *hypothalamus*, an area of the brain that acts like a thermostat, constantly monitoring blood temperature and automatically activating mechanisms to compensate for changes.

When body temperature falls, the hypothalamus sends nerve impulses to stimulate *shivering*, which generates heat by muscle activity, and to constrict blood vessels in the skin, which reduces heat loss. Conversely, when body temperature rises, the hypothalamus stimulates *sweating* and dilates (widens) blood vessels in the skin to increase heat loss.

A variety of factors—such as infections, certain disorders (notably those of the *thyroid gland*), unusual symptoms of a tumor, and overexposure to cold or extreme heat—may disrupt the body's heat-regulating system, resulting in *fever, heatstroke*, or, conversely, in *hypothermia*.

Temperature method

See *Contraception, natural methods of.*

Temporal arteritis

An uncommon disease of elderly people in which the walls of the arteries in the scalp that pass over the temples become inflamed. Other arteries in the head and neck may also be affected, as may the aorta (the large artery that carries oxygenated blood from the heart) and its main branches. The inflamed blood vessels become

---

TEMPORAL ARTERITIS
In this disorder, the temporal artery and other arteries in the head are inflamed. Early reporting of symptoms is vital, since, in untreated cases, there is a risk of sudden blindness.

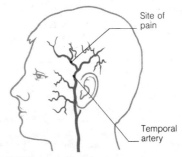

Telltale symptoms
If the temporal artery is inflamed, it is usually prominent and there is a persistent severe headache and scalp tenderness in the area shown.

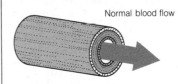

Normal artery
A normal artery has a smooth lining, and blood flow is sufficient to meet the needs of the tissues it supplies.

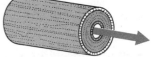

Inflamed artery
In arteritis, the walls of the artery become disrupted and thickened, and blood flow is markedly reduced.

narrowed, and blood flow through them is reduced. The disease is also known as giant cell arteritis.

CAUSES
The cause of temporal arteritis is unknown, but it is often associated with *polymyalgia rheumatica* (pain and stiffness in the muscles of the hips, thighs, shoulders, and neck). Nearly all sufferers are over 50 years old, and the disease affects more women than men.

SYMPTOMS AND SIGNS
The most common symptom is a headache, usually severe, on one or both sides of the head. The temporal artery (located at the side of the head above the earlobe) may be prominent and the scalp may be tender. In nearly 50 percent of sufferers, the ophthalmic arteries supplying the eyes may become affected, causing partial loss of vision or even sudden blindness. Other symptoms and signs include low fever, poor appetite, pain on chewing, and lethargy.

Involvement of the aorta or its main branches results in circulatory disorders, such as intermittent *claudication* (pain in the legs on walking) or *Raynaud's phenomenon* (pallor in the fingers on exposure to cold).

DIAGNOSIS AND TREATMENT
Early reporting of symptoms to a physician is essential because of the risk of blindness. The diagnosis is made by a *biopsy* (removal of a small sample of tissue for analysis) of the temporal artery and by *blood tests* to detect the presence of a raised *ESR* (erythrocyte sedimentation rate).

The disease responds rapidly to a *corticosteroid drug*, which is initially given in high doses to prevent blindness. Most people need to take the drug, at a reduced dosage, for one or two years. If the disease fails to respond to corticosteroid treatment, or if such treatment causes serious side effects, *immunosuppressant drugs* (such as azathioprine) may be given.

OUTLOOK
With treatment, the disease usually clears up within two years. Most people are not left with any lasting disability. However, if one or both eyes become blind before treatment has become effective, the blindness may be permanent.

Temporal lobe epilepsy

A form of *epilepsy* in which abnormal electrical discharges in the *brain* are confined to one temporal lobe (a localized region on the side of the brain). The seizures in temporal lobe epilepsy

---

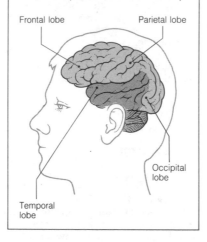

LOCATION OF THE TEMPORAL LOBE
The temporal lobe forms much of the lower side of each half of the cerebrum (main mass of the brain).

Frontal lobe

Parietal lobe

Occipital lobe

Temporal lobe

---

therefore differ from the generalized disturbances that occur in a grand mal seizure or petit mal (absence seizure).

CAUSE
In most cases there is an area of damage within one of the temporal lobes, which acts as a focus for the abnormal development of electrical discharges in attacks. Damage may be caused by a *birth injury, head injury, brain tumor, brain abscess,* or *stroke.* The temporal lobes are concerned with such functions as smell, taste, hearing, visual associations, and some aspects of memory. Abnormal electrical activity in a lobe may thus cause peculiarities in any of these functions.

SYMPTOMS AND SIGNS
People affected by temporal lobe epilepsy suffer dreamlike states that range from partial loss of awareness to total disregard. The person may have unpleasant hallucinations of smell or taste. Also common during attacks is the perception of an illusory scene or the phenomenon of *déjà vu.* There may also be facial grimacing, rotation of the head and eyes, and, often, sucking and chewing movements.

The affected person may perform tasks during the attack but have no memory of them afterward. An attack may last for minutes or hours before full consciousness returns.

In some cases, a temporal lobe seizure progresses to a generalized grand mal seizure.

DIAGNOSIS AND TREATMENT
The principles of investigation and drug treatment for temporal lobe epi-

---

lepsy are the same as for other types of epilepsy. Surgery to remove the part of the lobe containing the irritating focus for the attacks has been used with success in some cases. However, because of the possible effects on other important functions of the brain, such operations are performed only in severe cases that have not responded to drug treatment.

Temporomandibular joint

A *joint* connecting the mandible (lower *jaw* bone) to the temporal bone of the *skull* (see illustrated box).

Temporomandibular joint syndrome

Pain and other symptoms affecting the head, jaw, and face that are believed to result when the *temporomandibular joints* and the muscles and ligaments that control and support them do not work together correctly. This disorder is often known more simply as TMJ syndrome.

A common cause is spasm of the chewing muscles, often as a result of clenching or grinding the teeth due to emotional tension. An incorrect bite, which places additional stress on the muscles, may be a contributing factor.

Temporomandibular joint problems may also be caused by displacement of the joint as a result of jaw, head, or neck injuries. In rare cases, *osteoarthritis* is a cause.

LOCATION OF THE TEMPOROMANDIBULAR JOINT
The head of the mandible (jawbone) fits into a hollow on the underside of the temporal bone of the skull at the joint.

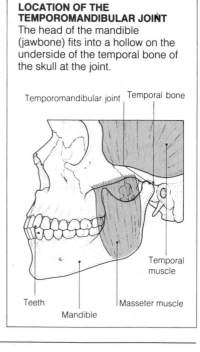

Temporomandibular joint   Temporal bone

Temporal muscle

Teeth

Mandible

Masseter muscle

T

Headaches, tenderness of the jaw muscles, and dull, aching facial pain with severe exacerbation in or around the ear are common symptoms of temporomandibular joint syndrome. Difficulty in opening the mouth, "locking" of the jaws, clicking noises as the mouth is opened or closed, or pain caused by opening the mouth wide or by chewing, if persistent, all together or individually, require careful medical diagnosis.

TREATMENT
In most cases, treatment is aimed at eliminating muscle spasm and relieving pain. This may be done by applying moist heat to the face, taking *muscle-relaxant drugs*, massaging the muscles, eating soft foods, or using a device that fits over the teeth at night to prevent clenching or grinding. *Counseling, biofeedback training,* and *relaxation exercises* may also help.

The bite may need to be adjusted by the use of a brace or other *orthodontic appliance*, or by occlusal adjustment (grinding down of specific teeth). In very severe cases, surgery on one or both jaw joints may be required.

Tenderness

Pain or abnormal sensitivity in a part of the body when it is pressed or touched. Tenderness experienced during palpation (medical examination by touch) is usually a sign of *inflammation*. For example, *appendicitis* (inflammation of the appendix) causes tenderness of the abdomen; *arthritis* (joint inflammation) causes tenderness around the affected joint. Tenderness is usually associated with swelling, redness, and warmth of the affected part.

Tendinitis

Inflammation of a *tendon*, usually caused by injury. Symptoms include pain, tenderness, and, occasionally, restricted movement of the muscle attached to the affected tendon. A common example is *painful arc syndrome*, which causes pain in the shoulder when the arm is raised between certain angles.

Treatment of tendinitis may include *nonsteroidal anti-inflammatory drugs* (NSAIDs), *ultrasound treatment*, or an injection of a *corticosteroid drug* around the tendon.

Tendolysis

An operation performed to free a *tendon* from *adhesions* (fibrous bands) that surround it and limit its free movement. Such adhesions are usually caused by *tenosynovitis* (inflammation of the inner lining of a tendon sheath).

Tendolysis consists of making a skin incision over the tendon and then splitting open its fibrous sheath. The adhesions are cut away from the tendon surface and the incisions in the sheath and the skin are stitched. Despite surgery, symptoms of tenosynovitis sometimes recur because adhesions form again.

Tendon

A fibrous cord that joins muscle to bone or muscle to muscle. Tendons are strong, flexible, but inelastic. Most are cylindrical; some, such as those attached to the flat muscles of the abdominal wall, consist of sheets of fibers known as aponeuroses.

Tendons are made up principally of bundles of collagen (a white, fibrous protein) and contain some blood vessels. The larger tendons (but not the aponeuroses) also have a nerve supply. Squeezing the tendon hard causes pain; stretching it triggers a *reflex* contraction of the adjoining muscle (e.g., the quadriceps jerk).

The tendons in the hands, wrists, and feet are enclosed in synovial sheaths (fibrous capsules) and bathed in a lubricating fluid secreted by the

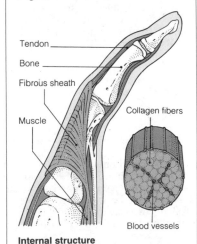

FINGER TENDONS
Finger bending and extension are controlled by tendons on either side of the finger; the tendons originate from forearm muscles.

Tendon
Bone
Fibrous sheath
Muscle
Collagen fibers
Blood vessels

Internal structure
A cross section of a tendon (above right) shows that it consists of numerous parallel bundles of collagen fibers together with some blood vessels.

lining of the sheath. These tendons require this additional protection because they do not move in a straight line and, without the fluid, might be subjected to excessive friction.

DISORDERS
Rupture of the *Achilles tendon* can occur during sprinting and jumping when sudden contraction of the calf muscles causes stretching of the tendon. Rupture of a tendon on the back of a finger, resulting in deformity of the fingertip, may be caused by a direct blow to the end of the finger (see *Baseball finger*). In many cases, however, because tendons are so strong, severe stress results in the pulling off of a piece of bone where the tendon is attached, rather than in tearing of the tendon itself.

The long tendon of the biceps muscle in the upper arm may become weakened as a result of repeated rubbing against the humerus (upper-arm bone) and may rupture under even moderate stress. Rupture of tendons in the hands can occur as a complication of *rheumatoid arthritis*.

Tendons in the hand are commonly severed by a deep cut; *tendon repair* using a tendon graft may be required. *Tendinitis*, inflammation of a tendon, may follow an injury. *Tenosynovitis*, inflammation of the inner lining of a tendon sheath, usually affects tendons in the hands and wrists and results from overuse. If the outer wall of a tendon sheath is inflamed, the gliding movement of the tendon through the sheath may be restricted, a condition called *tenovaginitis*.

Tendon release
See *Tendolysis*.

Tendon repair
An operation to join the cut or torn ends of a *tendon* or to replace a damaged tendon.

If the cut or torn ends can easily be brought together, they are stitched together with sutures. If the ends are widely separated or contained within a sheath, it may be necessary to insert a tendon graft. Tendons for grafting are taken from elsewhere in the body, usually the foot.

Tendon transfer
An operation to reposition a *tendon* so that it causes a muscle to perform a different function. Tendon transfer may be used to restore function impaired by a deformity, such as *talipes* (clubfoot), or by permanent muscle injury or paralysis.

T

To perform the transfer, the tendon is cut away from its original point of attachment and reattached elsewhere. Tendon transfer causes the muscle to which the tendon is attached to lie in a different position and thus to produce a different body movement when the muscle contracts.

Tenesmus

A feeling of incomplete emptying of the bowel in which the urge to pass feces is accompanied by ineffective straining. Tenesmus may be a symptom of a disorder of the *rectum*, such as polyps or cancer, or of severe inflammation caused by *ulcerative colitis* or *dysentery*.

Tennis elbow

A condition characterized by pain and tenderness on the outside of the *elbow* and in the back of the forearm. Its medical name is epicondylitis.

Tennis elbow is caused by inflammation of the *tendon* that attaches the extensor muscles (in this case the muscles that straighten the fingers and wrist) to the *humerus*. The condition results from overuse of these muscles, causing constant tugging of the tendon at its point of attachment to the humerus. Tennis elbow may be caused by playing tennis (or other racket sports) with a faulty grip, but more commonly it is due to other activities, such as gardening.

TREATMENT
Treatment consists of resting the arm, applying *ice packs*, and taking *analgesic drugs* (painkillers) and/or *nonsteroidal anti-inflammatory drugs* (NSAIDs). *Ultrasound treatment* may help reduce the inflammation. If the pain is severe or persistent, injection of a *corticosteroid drug* may be required. Surgery to release the tendon is occasionally required (see *Tendolysis*).

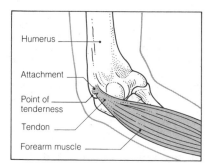

Site of tennis elbow
Pulling of the forearm muscles where they attach to the humerus causes tenderness on the outer side of the elbow.

Humerus

Attachment

Point of tenderness

Tendon

Forearm muscle

If the pain has occurred after playing a racket sport, it is wise to take a break from the sport for a week or two and to consult a professional about playing technique and equipment.

Tenosynovitis

Inflammation of the thin inner lining of the sheath that surrounds a *tendon*. Tenosynovitis is usually caused by excessive friction due to overuse; it is often brought on by working in an awkward position to do a job that involves repetitive movements. A rare cause is bacterial infection. Tendons in the hand and wrist are most commonly affected.

Symptoms include pain, tenderness, and swelling over the tendon. There is also occasionally *crepitus* (a grating noise or sensation) when the tendon is moved. Persistent or recurrent tenosynovitis may lead to restricted movement as a result of the formation of *adhesions* (fibrous bands) between the tendon and its sheath.

TREATMENT
If infection is the cause, *antibiotic drugs* are prescribed. Otherwise, treatment usually consists of *nonsteroidal anti-inflammatory drugs* (NSAIDs) or an injection of a *corticosteroid drug* around the tendon. The hand and wrist may need to be immobilized in a *splint* for a few weeks. If the condition does not improve, surgery may be required to release adhesions (see *Tendolysis*).

Tenovaginitis

Inflammation or thickening of the fibrous wall of the sheath that surrounds a *tendon*. The cause is unknown. Tenovaginitis affecting the sheath of one of the tendons that bends a finger results in *trigger finger*.

TENS

The abbreviation for transcutaneous electrical nerve stimulation. TENS is a method of pain relief achieved by the application of minute electrical impulses to nerve endings that lie beneath the skin. The procedure seems to work by blocking pain messages to the brain by providing an alternative stimulus. TENS is carried out to relieve severe or persistent pain that has not been satisfactorily controlled by *analgesic drugs*. TENS is sometimes used during childbirth.

HOW IT IS DONE
A TENS unit provides electrical impulses to electrodes that are placed on the skin or sometimes surgically implanted. Adjustments can be made by the patient to achieve best relief.

RISKS
TENS must not be used by anyone with a cardiac *pacemaker*; the electrical impulses from the transmitter may interfere with the pacemaker's action.

OUTLOOK
TENS may produce pain relief only during stimulation; sometimes, pain relief persists after treatment.

Tension

A feeling of mental and physical strain associated with *anxiety*. Sufferers feel unpleasantly keyed up, cannot relax, and may have feelings of bottled-up anger. Muscle tension accompanies the mental symptoms and may result in headaches and muscular stiffness and pain, particularly in the back and shoulders. Persistent tension is related to *generalized anxiety disorder*. (See also *Stress*.)

Teratogen

An agent that causes physical abnormalities in a developing *embryo* or *fetus*. Examples of teratogens include the *rubella* virus and the drug *thalidomide*. For a drug to be categorized as teratogenic, there must be substantive evidence that taking the drug during pregnancy causes an increased incidence of *congenital* abnormalities and that these cannot be explained by other factors.

Many chemicals that are known to be teratogenic in some species (such as rats) have not been proved to be teratogenic in humans. Drug regulatory organizations usually refuse to license drugs for use during pregnancy if they have been found to be teratogenic for any species.

Teratoma

A primary *tumor* consisting of cells that bear no resemblance to those normally found in that part of the body. For example, teratomas that develop in the ovary—one of the most common sites for this type of tumor—often form cysts (called *dermoid cysts*) that may contain skin, hair, teeth, or bone. Other sites in which teratomas may occur include the testes, the pineal gland in the brain, and the mediastinum (the space between the lungs).

Terbutaline

A *bronchodilator drug* used in the treatment of *asthma*, chronic *bronchitis*, and *emphysema*. Terbutaline also relaxes the muscles of the uterus, making it useful for the prevention of premature labor (see *Prematurity*).

T

Possible adverse effects are tremor, nervousness, restlessness, nausea, and, in rare cases, palpitations.

Terfenadine

An *antihistamine drug* used to treat allergic *rhinitis* (hay fever) and allergic skin conditions, such as *urticaria* (hives). Terfenadine has less sedative effect than some other antihistamines and is therefore useful for people who need to avoid drowsiness. Possible adverse effects include nausea, headache, loss of appetite, and rash.

Terminal care

Terminal care is broadly defined as any care given to a patient within 12 months of the anticipated time of death. Three types of care may be administered to terminal patients: basic nutrition, standard medical care, and extraordinary care. In earlier years, the physician made care decisions without consulting the patient or the patient's relatives. Today, the paternalistic philosophy has given way to the patient autonomy model in which an informed patient makes decisions about the type and amount of treatment he or she shall receive.

Competent terminal patients are increasingly considering "the right to die," and refusing, either beforehand or at the time it is offered, certain forms of, or all treatment. The law in this area is evolving rapidly, but there are conditions under which a patient (or relatives acting on the patient's behalf) can make decisions that affect the performance of all three of the types of care mentioned above. (See also *Dying, care of the*.)

Termination of pregnancy

See *Abortion, induced*.

Testicle

See *Testis*.

Testicular feminization syndrome

A rare inherited condition in which, despite having the external appearance of a female, the affected individual is genetically a male with internal testes. Testicular feminization syndrome is a form of *intersex* and is the most common form of male *pseudohermaphroditism*. It is sometimes alternatively known as androgen resistance syndrome.

CAUSE

Testicular feminization syndrome is caused by a defective response of the body's tissues to *testosterone* (male sex hormone), even though a normal male level of the hormone is produced. The genes that cause testicular feminization syndrome are transmitted on the X chromosome (see *Genetic disorders*). Females can therefore carry the causative genes and transmit them to their sons.

SYMPTOMS AND SIGNS

Affected individuals appear to be girls throughout childhood. Most develop normal female secondary *sexual characteristics* at *puberty*, but menstruation does not occur because there is no uterus and the vagina is short and blind-ending. People with testicular feminization syndrome tend to be tall and are of normal intelligence.

DIAGNOSIS

The condition may be diagnosed before puberty if a girl is found to have an inguinal *hernia* or a swelling in the labia that turns out to be a testis. Otherwise, the diagnosis is usually made at puberty during investigations to find the cause of *amenorrhea* (failure to menstruate).

The diagnosis is made by *chromosome analysis*, which shows the normal male chromosomal status, and by blood tests, which indicate male levels of testosterone.

TREATMENT AND OUTLOOK

Treatment involves surgical removal of the testes at puberty (because of an increased risk of testicular cancer) and hormonal therapy with *estrogen drugs*. An affected individual can never be fertile, but can lead an otherwise normal life as a woman.

Testis

One of two male sex organs, also called testicles, that produce *sperm* and the male sex hormone *testosterone*.

The testes are formed within the abdomen near the kidneys early in the development of the male fetus. In response to hormones produced by the mother and to hormones produced in the testes themselves, the testes gradually descend through the inguinal canal in the groin. At birth, they have usually reached the surface of the body, where they hang suspended in a pouch of skin called the *scrotum*.

STRUCTURE

Within each testis are the seminiferous tubules, delicate coiled tubes that produce sperm. The seminiferous tubules lead via the vasa efferentia (small ducts) to the *epididymis*, a structure lying behind the testis in which the newly formed sperm mature. Interstitial cells between the seminif-

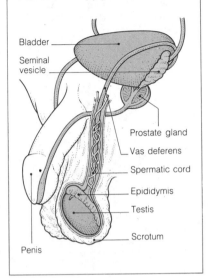

LOCATION OF THE TESTIS
Each testis is suspended in the scrotum by a spermatic cord, which contains the vas deferens, and the arteries, veins, and nerves that supply the testis.

Bladder

Seminal vesicle

Prostate gland

Vas deferens

Spermatic cord

Epididymis

Testis

Scrotum

Penis

crous tubules produce the male sex hormone testosterone, which passes into small blood vessels in the testis and then into the circulation.

Each testis is protected by a tough, fibrous capsule, the tunica albuginea, and is attached by the spermatic cord, composed of the *vas deferens* (the tube that transports sperm from the epididymis to the urethra) and a number of blood vessels and nerves.

DISORDERS

A direct blow sometimes tears the wall of the testis, resulting in severe pain and bleeding into the scrotal tissue. An operation may be required to drain the blood and repair the testis.

Occasionally, a testis fails to develop completely, does not descend fully into the scrotum (see *Testis, undescended*), or descends into an abnormal position (see *Testis, ectopic*).

Inflammation of the testis, known as *orchitis*, usually results from infection with the mumps virus. Inflammation of the testis and the epididymis occurs in *epididymo-orchitis*, which is usually caused by a bacterial infection.

Painless swelling of the tissues surrounding the testis usually results from a *hydrocele* (collection of fluid in the scrotum). Other causes of testicular swelling include a *varicocele* (swollen veins within the scrotum), an *epididymal cyst* (fluid-filled swell-

T

SELF-EXAMINATION OF THE TESTIS

A lump that can be felt in the testis must be considered potentially malignant until surgical exploration proves otherwise. Cancers are usually firm to the touch and not tender or painful when pressed.

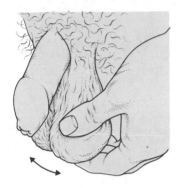

Procedure
Only regular self-examination can detect a tumor early enough to provide assurance of a cure. The entire surface of both testes should be felt. The skin over the testes moves freely, making palpation easy.

ing of the epididymis), and a *spermato-cele* (a sperm-filled swelling of the epididymis).

Torsion of the testis, in which the spermatic cord becomes twisted, cutting off the blood supply to the testis, is most common at the time of *puberty* (see *Testis, torsion of*).

In rare cases, the testis is affected by cancer (see *Testis, cancer of*).

Various conditions affecting the testis may cause a reduction or absence of sperm production; if both testes are affected, *infertility* may result.

Testis, cancer of

A malignant tumor of the *testis*. Cancer of the testis is rare. It occurs most commonly in young to middle-aged men, and is very rare before *puberty* or in old age. The risk of testicular cancer is higher in men who have a history of undescended testis (see *Testis, undescended*).

TYPES

The most common types of testicular cancer are seminomas and *teratomas*. Seminomas are made up of a single type of cell (probably developing from the cells that produce sperm). Teratomas consist of several different types of cell. Other cancers affecting the tes-

tis are extremely rare and develop from testicular tissue or from lymphatic tissue within the testis (see *Lymphoma*). Testicular cancer most commonly appears as a firm, painless swelling of one testis. Men are recommended to examine their testes regularly to check for lumps (see illustrated box). In some cases, there may be pain and inflammation.

The physician first examines the testis and may perform tests to exclude other causes of testicular swelling (see *Testis, swollen*).

The diagnosis of testicular cancer can be confirmed only by *orchiectomy* (surgical removal of the testis) and microscopic examination of the testicular tissue. This confirms the presence of cancer and also shows the type of cancer that is present. Other tests, including *CT scanning, ultrasound scanning*, and *blood tests*, are performed to look for any signs that indicate that the cancer has spread to other parts of the body.

TREATMENT

Orchiectomy may be sufficient to cure testicular cancer in its early stages. However, in patients in whom there is a high risk of spread, preventive treatment, consisting of *anticancer drugs* or *radiation therapy* to lymph nodes in the abdomen, may be carried out even if there are no signs that the disease has spread. Cancer that has spread beyond the testis is usually treated with both orchiectomy and anticancer drugs. Surgery to remove cancerous tissue from the abdomen is occasionally needed.

OUTLOOK

The outlook, which varies according to the type of cancer and how advanced it was when first discovered, is generally good. The cure rate for early testicular cancer is 95 to 100 percent; the cure rate for advanced disease is 80 to 90 percent. Provided the other testis is healthy, treatment with radiation therapy and/or anticancer drugs generally does not cause infertility in the remaining testis.

Testis, ectopic

A *testis* that is absent from the *scrotum* because it has descended into an abnormal position, usually in the groin or at the base of the penis. An ectopic testis is most often discovered soon after birth during a routine physical examination. Treatment involves an *orchiopexy*, a surgical operation to place the testis in the scrotum. (See also *Testis, undescended*.)

Testis, pain in the

Even mild injury to the *testis* may result in pain. Usually, no damage is caused, but a direct blow such as a kick may tear the wall of the testis. In this case, the pain is particularly severe, and an operation may be required to drain any accumulated blood and repair the testis.

Severe pain and swelling are a feature of *orchitis* (inflammation of the testis), *epididymo-orchitis* (inflammation of the testis and epididymis), and torsion of the testis (see *Testis, torsion of*). Cancer of the testis (see *Testis, cancer of*) does not usually cause pain.

Pain that seems to come from the testis is occasionally caused by a small kidney stone lodged in the ureter (see *Calculus, urinary tract*).

A physician can sometimes find no cause for testicular pain; in most of such cases the problem disappears without treatment.

Testis, retractile

A *testis* that is drawn up high into the groin by a pronounced muscle reflex in response to cold or touch. Retractile testis is normal in young children but usually disappears by *puberty*. Failure to feel the testis in the scrotum sometimes causes the condition to be confused with undescended testis (see *Testis, undescended*).

Testis, swollen

Swelling of the *testis* or its surrounding tissues in the *scrotum*, which may or may not be accompanied by pain. Most scrotal swellings are harmless and the testis itself is usually not affected. However, swelling of a testis should always be reported to a physician to rule out the possibility of a serious underlying disorder.

PAINLESS SWELLINGS

There are several types of harmless, painless swelling, the most common of which is a *hydrocele* (a collection of fluid in the scrotum). Other usually painless swellings include an *epididymal cyst* (fluid-filled swelling of the epididymis), a *spermatocele* (sperm-filled swelling of the epididymis), a *varicocele* (varicose veins in the scrotum), and a hematocele (a swelling that contains blood and that results from injury).

Cancer of the testis (see *Testis, cancer of*) may also cause a painless swelling in the scrotum, which requires prompt treatment.

PAINFUL SWELLING

Painful swelling of the scrotum may be caused by a sudden event, such as twisting of the spermatic cord (see *Testis, torsion of*) or a direct blow. When associated with fever, the swelling is usually due to infection of the testis (see *Orchitis*) or of the testis and epididymis (see *Epididymo-orchitis*). In very rare cases, a painful swelling is due to cancer of the testis.

Testis, torsion of

Twisting of the spermatic cord, causing acute, severe pain and swelling of the *testis*. Unless the condition is treated within a few hours, the testis is damaged permanently and sperm production ceases.

Torsion of the testis is most common around *puberty*, but may also occur in infants or in young adults. The condition is more likely to occur if the testis is unusually mobile within its covering in the *scrotum*.

Pain develops rapidly and is occasionally accompanied by abdominal pain and nausea. The testis becomes swollen and very tender, and the scrotal skin becomes discolored.

TORSION OF THE TESTIS
If a testis rotates, veins in the spermatic cord become obstructed and there is severe swelling and pain. Torsion of the testis most commonly occurs around puberty.

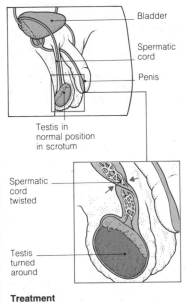

Bladder

Spermatic cord

Penis

Testis in normal position in scrotum

Spermatic cord twisted

Testis turned around

Treatment
Spontaneous untwisting sometimes occurs but unrelieved torsion is dangerous. Torsion must be treated urgently by surgery.

A diagnosis is made from a physical examination.

Treatment is by surgery. An incision is made in the skin of the scrotum and, if the diagnosis is confirmed, the testis can be immediately untwisted. If blood flow resumes, the testis is anchored in the scrotum with small stitches to prevent a recurrence of the problem. If irreversible damage exists, *orchiectomy* (removal of the testis) is performed. In all cases, the other testis is also anchored to the scrotum to prevent torsion on that side.

OUTLOOK
Recovery from the operation is rapid. If treatment was prompt, the testis recovers completely. Even if one testis is removed, the other is usually capable of maintaining fertility.

Testis, undescended

A *testis* that has failed to complete its normal passage from within the abdomen to the *scrotum*. Not all testes that are absent from the scrotum are undescended (see *Testis, ectopic*; *Testis, retractile*). Undescended testis is found in about 1 percent of full-term and in up to 10 percent of premature male babies. Usually, only one testis fails to descend. In many cases, an undescended testis descends of its own accord within several months of birth; an undescended testis rarely, if ever, descends of its own accord after this time.

CAUSES AND SYMPTOMS
The final descent of the testis through the inguinal canal to the scrotum is controlled by hormones from the mother and from the testis itself. If these stimuli do not have an effect, the spermatic cord (which carries the vas deferens and the blood vessels to the testis) fails to lengthen sufficiently to allow full descent. Alternatively, a normal testis may be prevented from reaching the scrotum by the presence of fibers that interrupt its route and cause it to remain in the groin.

An undescended testis does not develop normally and is not capable of normal sperm production. If both testes are undescended, *infertility* results. A testis that fails to descend normally is at increased risk of testicular cancer (see *Testis, cancer of*).

DIAGNOSIS AND TREATMENT
The diagnosis is made during examination of the newborn or later in infancy. It is rare for the condition to remain unnoticed into adult life.

Treatment is by *orchiopexy*, an operation in which the undescended testis

is lowered into the scrotum. Surgery within the first few years of life gives the testis the best chance of developing normally. If the undescended testis is very poorly developed and the other testis is normal, the undescended testis is removed.

Test meal

A procedure used to measure the output of acid by the *stomach*. The name test "meal" derives from the fact that gruel used to be given to stimulate the stomach to secrete fluid. Today, an injection of *histamine* or more commonly of pentagastrin (a synthetic preparation of the hormone gastrin) is given instead.

In some instances, an *insulin* test (in which an injection of insulin is given) is performed to confirm the completeness of a *vagotomy* (an operation in which the vagus nerve is cut).

HOW IT IS DONE
A *nasogastric tube* is passed via the nose into the stomach after an overnight fast, and an initial sample of gastric fluid is sucked up through the tube. The injection is then given and further samples of stomach fluid are taken at intervals for a period of up to two hours. The samples are analyzed for the amount of hydrochloric acid they contain.

RESULTS
High levels of acid are found in people with a duodenal ulcer (see *Peptic ulcer*) or *Zollinger-Ellison syndrome*. Absence of acid is characteristic of pernicious anemia (see *Anemia, megaloblastic*).

An insulin test done following a complete vagotomy will not result in the normal secretion of gastric acid that would occur if the vagus nerve were intact.

Testosterone

The most important of the *androgen hormones* (male sex hormones). Testosterone stimulates bone and muscle growth and sexual development. It is produced by the *testes* and in very small amounts by the *ovaries*.

DRUG THERAPY
Synthetic or animal testosterone is used to stimulate *puberty* or to treat *infertility* in males suffering from deficiency caused by disorders of the testes or *pituitary gland*. Testosterone was formerly used in the treatment of *breast cancer* but is now rarely used for this purpose.

Excess testosterone given to stimulate puberty may interfere with normal growth or cause over-rapid sexual development. In males, testosterone

T

may cause *priapism* (painful, persistent erection). In females, high doses of testosterone may cause deepening of the voice, excessive hair growth, or hair loss. Treatment with some orally administered forms of testosterone may cause liver damage.

Tests, medical

Medical tests may be performed to investigate the cause of a person's symptoms and thus establish a *diagno-sis*, to monitor the course of a disease, or to assess a patient's response to treatment. Tests are also sometimes performed on apparently healthy people to find disease at an early stage; this is known as *screening*.

To be of value, a medical test must be reasonably accurate in identifying or excluding the presence of a particular disease. The degree of accuracy is based on three factors: sensitivity, specificity, and predictive value.

Sensitivity is the ability of a test to show a positive (abnormal) value when the disease being tested for is actually present. A test that always detects a specific disease is said to have 100 percent sensitivity. One that shows positive results in only 80 people out of a hundred who have the disease is said to have 80 percent sensitivity; the 20 percent of the cases missed on the test reflect the false-negative test results.

Specificity is the extent to which a test shows false-positive results in healthy people. For example, a test that shows false results in 20 percent of the people tested is said to have 80 percent specificity.

Sensitivity and specificity may vary with the controls used in different laboratories and with the criteria for normal values.

The third measure of a test's accuracy is its predictive value. This is determined by a mathematical formula that includes the number of times the test is accurate (the true-negative test results plus the true-positive test results) and the total number of tests performed. The predictive value thus determines the probability that a patient who has a positive test result actually has the disease or, conversely, that a patient who has a negative test result does not have the disease.

Of course the test's predictive value is dependent on the *prevalence* of the disease in the group being tested; in situations where a disease is rare, a positive result is much more likely to be significant.

There is tremendous variation in accuracy among tests. For example, the fecal occult blood test (see *Occult blood, fecal*) used to detect cancer of the stomach or intestine is very sensitive; a person whose test results are negative (normal) is unlikely to have the disease. However, the test is not highly specific and many people whose test results are positive (abnormal) do not have the disease. More tests are required to confirm the diagnosis before any remedial treatment is performed.

An *ECG* to diagnose acute *myocardial infarction* (heart attack) is reasonably specific. A person whose test results are positive is almost definitely affected and is admitted to an intensive-care unit for treatment. However, the test is not sensitive; about half the people with severe chest pain who have negative test results may also need treatment.

TYPES OF MEDICAL TESTS

Brain and nervous system	EEG
	Evoked responses
	Hearing tests
	Vision tests
	Lumbar puncture
	Intelligence tests
		Myelography
		Brain imaging
		  CT scanning
		  MRI
		  PET scanning

Skin, bones, and muscles	EMG Biopsy	Bone imaging X rays
Endocrine system and metabolism	Thyroid function tests Thyroid scanning	Blood tests Urinalysis
Blood and immune system	Blood tests Lymphangiography	Skin tests Bone marrow biopsy

Heart and circulation	Heart imaging
	  Chest X ray
	  Angiography
	  Echocardiography
	  Venography
		ECG
		Catheterization, cardiac
		Cardiac stress test

Lungs	Pulmonary function tests
	  Blood gases
	  Peak flow meter
	  Spirometry
		Chest X ray
		Bronchoscopy

Biliary system	Liver function tests Liver imaging Ultrasound scanning Cholangiography	Cholecystography ERCP Liver biopsy

Gastrointestinal tract	Endoscopy
	  Colonoscopy
	  Gastroscopy
		Barium X ray examinations
		Jejunal biopsy
		Occult blood, fecal

Urinary tract	Kidney imaging
	  Urography
	  Ultrasound scanning
		Urinalysis
		Kidney function tests
		Cystoscopy

Reproductive system	Pregnancy tests Hysterosalpingography Mammography Ultrasound scanning Laparoscopy	Amniocentesis Cervical smear test Chorionic villus sampling Chromosome analysis Semen analysis

The table above lists some commonly performed medical tests, classified according to the body system they are used to study. Each test listed in the table has its own entry. Only some of the most important imaging techniques for each body organ have been included; a complete list appears in the appropriate imaging article.

T

The best tests have both high specificity and high sensitivity, and therefore high predictive value. Today's tests for *syphilis*, for example, have almost 100 percent predictive value; they almost always show a positive result in someone who has the disease and a negative result in someone who does not have the disease.

Tetanus

A serious, sometimes fatal, disease of the *central nervous system* (brain and spinal cord) caused by infection of a wound with spores of the bacterium *CLOSTRIDIUM TETANI*.

CAUSES AND INCIDENCE

The spores live mainly in soil and manure, but are also found in the human intestine and elsewhere. If spores that have entered the body through a wound infect tissues that are poorly supplied with oxygenated blood, they multiply and produce a *toxin* that acts on the nerves controlling muscle activity.

About half a million cases of tetanus occur worldwide each year; in Canada, fewer than five cases are reported annually. All occur in nonimmunized people, mostly in those aged over 50. In developing countries, tetanus often causes death in newborn infants as a result of contamination of the umbilical stump by spores.

PREVENTION

DPT vaccination (combined immunization against diphtheria, pertussis, and tetanus) is given routinely in Canada during childhood. Thereafter, tetanus immunization booster shots are recommended every 10 years. Any wound, particularly a deep or dirty one, should be cleaned and treated with an *antiseptic*.

SYMPTOMS AND SIGNS

The most common symptom is *trismus* (stiffness of the jaw, commonly known as lockjaw), which makes it difficult to open the mouth. Other symptoms include stiffness of abdominal and back muscles, and contraction of facial muscles, producing a fixed, mirthless smile. There may also be a fast pulse, slight fever, and profuse sweating. Eventually, painful muscle spasms develop. If these affect the larynx or chest wall, *asphyxia* may result. The spasms usually subside after 10 to 14 days.

DIAGNOSIS AND TREATMENT

The diagnosis is made from the patient's symptoms and signs, and a course of tetanus *antitoxin* injections is started. Severe cases may require a *tracheostomy* (insertion of a breathing tube into the windpipe) and maintenance of respiration using a *ventilator*. Given prompt treatment, most people recover completely.

Tetany

Spasms and twitching of the *muscles*, most commonly those in the hands and feet, although the face, larynx (voice box), or spinal muscles may also be affected. Initially, the spasms are painless; if the condition persists, they tend to become increasingly painful. In some cases, muscle damage eventually results if the underlying cause is not treated. Tetany is a symptom of a biochemical disturbance in the body, and should not be confused with *tetanus*, an infection.

The most common cause of tetany is *hypocalcemia* (a low level of calcium in the blood), which may be due to a diet lacking in *vitamin D*. Other causes include hypokalemia (a low blood level of *potassium*), which is commonly a result of prolonged diarrhea or vomiting; *hyperventilation* (abnormally deep or rapid breathing), which is most often a result of anxiety; or, more rarely, *hypoparathyroidism* (underactivity of the parathyroid glands).

Tetracaine

A powerful local *anesthetic*, given by injection or in the form of eye drops only under medical supervision. It has a rapid onset and a short duration of action.

Tetracycline drugs

COMMON DRUGS

Minocycline Oxytetracycline Tetracycline

A group of *antibiotic drugs* commonly used in the treatment of *acne*, *bronchitis*, *syphilis*, *gonorrhea*, *nonspecific urethritis*, and certain types of *pneumonia*. Tetracyclines are also prescribed for various other infections, such as *cholera*, *brucellosis*, and *Rocky Mountain spotted fever*.

Possible adverse effects include nausea, vomiting, diarrhea, and, less commonly, rash and itching. Tetracyclines may discolor developing teeth and are therefore not usually prescribed for children under the age of 12 or for pregnant women. Tetracyclines may worsen kidney function in people with a kidney disorder.

Tetrahydroaminoacridine

A drug that has been investigated for use in the treatment of *Alzheimer's disease*. In Alzheimer's disease, the level of the brain chemical *acetylcholine* is abnormally low. It is thought that tetrahydroaminoacridine increases the production of this chemical. The drug does not, however, halt degeneration of brain tissue and cannot provide a cure for Alzheimer's disease.

In a small clinical trial with the drug, memory loss improved in people with Alzheimer's disease. A large clinical trial intended to establish the effectiveness of tetrahydroaminoacridine was, however, discontinued because the drug caused an unacceptable incidence of impaired liver function. The risk of permanent liver damage from long-term treatment is unknown.

Tetralogy of Fallot

A form of congenital *heart disease* in which there are four heart anomalies: displacement of the aorta, narrowing of the pulmonary valve, a hole in the ventricular septum, and thickening of the wall of the right ventricle (see diagram). As a result of these defects, blood pumped to the body from the

NORMAL HEART

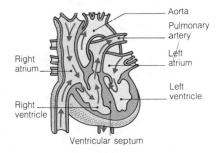

Aorta
Pulmonary artery
Left atrium
Left ventricle
Right atrium
Right ventricle
Ventricular septum

TETRALOGY OF FALLOT

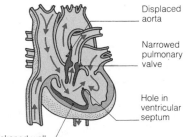

Displaced aorta
Narrowed pulmonary valve
Hole in ventricular septum
Thickened wall of right ventricle

Defects in tetralogy of Fallot
The four defects are shown above. Insufficient blood passes to the pulmonary artery and lungs to be oxygenated, and the large volume of blood pumped to the body via the aorta is therefore lacking in oxygen.

T

heart is insufficiently oxygenated, which typically leads to *cyanosis* (bluish-purple coloration) and breathlessness. Tetralogy of Fallot occurs in about 1 in 1,000 babies.

SYMPTOMS AND SIGNS

Affected infants appear normal at birth, although disturbance of blood flow in the heart can be detected as *murmurs* by a physician using a stethoscope. Severely affected babies may become cyanosed and breathless early in life. Less severely affected children may show a gradual increase in the degree of cyanosis and breathlessness. In such children, spells of cyanosis may be brought on by feeding, exertion, or infections. Other symptoms include failure to gain weight and poor development.

In older children who remain untreated, *clubbing* of the fingers and toes is usually evident. Another feature in older children is the adoption, after exertion, of a squatting position, knees up to the chest, to help them recover from breathlessness.

DIAGNOSIS

The condition is suspected from the child's symptoms and from a physical examination. A chest *X ray* shows a characteristic shape of the heart. An *ECG*, echocardiogram (see *Echocardiography*), and in some cases cardiac *catheterization* are performed in order to determine the severity of the abnormality.

TREATMENT AND OUTLOOK

Surgery is necessary for permanent correction of the disorder. The optimal time for surgical repair is before the child starts school.

A temporary procedure is usually performed first. A duct is created between the aorta and pulmonary artery. In this way some of the blood pumped into the aorta is diverted to the lungs instead.

Subsequently, corrective *open heart surgery* is performed. The narrowed pulmonary artery is widened and the hole in the heart is closed. If this corrective operation is successful, no further surgery should be necessary.

Tetraplegia

An alternative name for *quadriplegia* (*paralysis* in all four limbs).

Thalamus

A structure within the *brain* consisting of an egg-shaped mass of nerve tissue, about the size of a walnut. The two thalami sit at the top of the *brain stem* and are connected by many tracts to all parts of the brain.

LOCATION OF THE THALAMUS

The two thalami are situated deep within the brain, just above the brain stem.

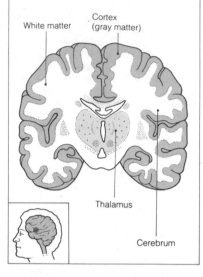

White matter · Cortex (gray matter)

Thalamus

Cerebrum

FUNCTION

The thalamus is an important relay center for sensory information flowing into the brain. Different clusters of nerve cells within the thalamus receive information from the sense organs, such as the eyes and ears, and, via the spinal cord, from touch and pressure receptors in the skin. Some basic sensations, such as *pain*, may actually reach consciousness within the thalamus. Other types of sensory information are processed and relayed to parts of the cerebral cortex (outer layer of the brain), where the sensations are perceived.

The thalamus seems to act as a filter, selecting only information of particular importance from the mass of sensory signals entering the brain. This is important for the ability to concentrate on a particular task. Certain centers within the thalamus may also play a part in long-term memory.

DISORDERS

Damage to the thalamus due to a *stroke* or *brain tumor* usually causes loss of sensation, but in some cases causes heightened sensitivity to pain, temperature, and other sensory stimuli.

Thalassemia

A group of inherited *blood* disorders in which there is a fault in the production of *hemoglobin*, the oxygen-carrying substance that is synthesized in the *bone marrow* for incorporation into red blood cells. Many of the red cells pro-

duced are fragile and rapidly hemolyzed (broken up), leading to anemia (see *Anemia, hemolytic*).

Thalassemia is prevalent in the Mediterranean region, the Middle East, and Southeast Asia. In Canada, it is most prevalent in people of Chinese, Greek and Italian origin. Major centers offer screening programs.

CAUSES, TYPES, AND INCIDENCE

The hemoglobin of healthy people contains two pairs of globins (protein chains), known as alpha chains and beta chains. In thalassemia, synthesis of either the alpha or the beta chains is reduced, causing an imbalance between the alpha and beta chains in much of the hemoglobin that is produced.

Abnormal hemoglobin production in thalassemia is caused by inheritance of a defective *gene*. Most commonly, it is the production of beta chains that is disturbed, leading to beta-thalassemia.

This condition is inherited in an autosomal recessive pattern (see *Genetic disorders*). If a person inherits one defective gene for the disease, he or she is said to have beta-thalassemia minor or thalassemia trait, which is never severe. If two defective genes are inherited—one from each parent—the result is a much more severe condition called beta-thalassemia major, or Cooley's anemia. In situations where two people with the minor trait have offspring, each child has a one in four chance of suffering from beta-thalassemia major.

Alpha-thalassemia is much less common than the beta type. If there is a severely reduced production of alpha chains, the lack of normal hemoglobin is incompatible with life and an affected infant dies within a few hours of birth. Lesser degrees of alpha-thalassemia also occur.

SYMPTOMS

Beta-thalassemia major produces the symptoms of hemolytic anemia, including fatigue and shortness of breath with *jaundice* and enlargement of the *spleen* due to the rapid breakup of red blood cells. These symptoms first appear three to six months after birth. In untreated cases, to compensate for the reduced life span of red cells, the bone marrow expands greatly and may cause bones to grow abnormally. This leads to a characteristic enlargement of the skull in untreated patients. Normal body growth is arrested and, without treatment, death occurs during early childhood.

T

In the forms of alpha-thalassemia compatible with life, there are also symptoms of anemia but these are generally less severe.

DIAGNOSIS AND TREATMENT

The diagnosis of beta-thalassemia major is made from microscopic examination of the blood, which shows many small, pale red blood cells, and from other blood tests that show reduced levels of adult hemoglobin in the blood.

Treatment is with blood transfusions, which should allow an affected child to grow normally. In addition, the spleen may be removed when the child is older (see *Splenectomy*). However, as each blood transfusion is administered, some iron is absorbed and eventually the internal organs become overloaded with iron, a condition known as *hemosiderosis*. This can lead to liver *cirrhosis*, to gland disorders such as *diabetes mellitus*, and to *heart failure*, which is a frequent cause of death in young adults with the disease. Compounds called *chelating agents* can help to reduce the iron overload. *Bone marrow transplants* are under investigation as a possible cure for the disease.

OUTLOOK

Parents or other close relatives of a child with thalassemia, and any person known to have beta-thalassemia minor (thalassemia trait), may derive benefit from *genetic counseling*. Beta-thalassemia major can now be diagnosed by *prenatal screening*.

Thalidomide

A *sleeping drug* that was withdrawn in Canada in 1962, after it was found to cause limb deformities in many of the babies born to women given this drug during pregnancy. Of some 8,000 thalidomide children born worldwide, about 125 were born in Canada. Of these, 75 to 100 are still alive.

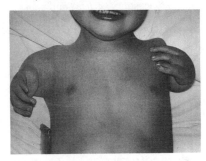

Thalidomide child
Phocomelia (stunted limbs) was a common result of the action of thalidomide on the fetus at an early stage of development.

Although it is no longer marketed in Canada, thalidomide is still available here under the emergency release program. It is used to combat *graft-versus-host* disease in persons receiving bone marrow transplants and in treating *Hansen's disease* (leprosy) and *Behçet's syndrome*.

Thallium

A rare metallic element that does not occur naturally in its pure form but is present (in minute amounts) as various compounds in certain ores of zinc and lead. Accidental poisoning may occur from swallowing rat poison and is characterized by loss of hair, disorders of the nerves in the limbs, and disturbance of the stomach and intestines.

Thallium 201 (an artificial radioactive isotope of the element) is sometimes used in *radionuclide scanning* of the heart. In this role, it reveals areas of heart muscle that have a poor blood supply or that have been damaged by a *myocardial infarction* (heart attack).

THC

The abbreviation for tetrahydrocannabinol (dronabinol), the active ingredient in *marijuana*. This drug is used to treat nausea and vomiting in cancer patients undergoing radiation therapy or anticancer drug treatment.

Theophylline

A *bronchodilator drug* used primarily in the treatment of *asthma* and to prevent attacks of *apnea* (cessation of breathing) in premature infants. Theophylline may also be used to treat *heart failure* because it stimulates the heart rate and increases excretion of urine.

Possible adverse effects include dizziness, nausea, vomiting, diarrhea, palpitations, and seizures.

Therapeutic

A term meaning related to treatment. The therapeutic dose of a drug is the amount required to have the most beneficial effect.

Therapeutic community

A method of treating antisocial behavior that entails patients living together as a group in a nonhospital environment usually under the supervision of medical and nursing staff. Therapeutic communities are used for treating *drug dependence*, *alcohol dependence*, and certain *personality disorders*.

Staff and patients share all decisions at regular group meetings, and unacceptable behavior and its effects are confronted and discussed openly. All aspects of day-to-day activity thus provide a focus for learning appropriate social and interpersonal skills. (See also *Social skills training*.)

Therapy

The treatment of any disease or abnormal physical or mental condition. Examples of therapy include *radiation therapy* for cancer and *psychotherapy* for certain psychiatric disorders.

Thermography

A technique in which temperature patterns on the surface of the skin are recorded in the form of an image.

WHY IT IS DONE

Thermography provides clues to the presence of diseases and abnormalities that alter the temperature of the skin, such as circulatory problems, inflammation, and tumors. However, because so many conditions affect skin temperature, further examination and tests are necessary to confirm the underlying cause.

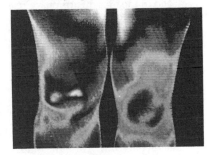

Thermographic image of the knees
Areas with different surface temperatures show up as different shades in thermographic images. Excess heat indicates either inflammation or rich blood flow.

HOW IT IS DONE

Two techniques are used in thermography to detect skin temperature. In one, a special camera or scanner picks up infrared radiation naturally emitted from the skin. In the other, sheets of special temperature-sensitive liquid crystals are applied to the skin and change color in response to changes in temperature.

Thermography is a safe technique. Results have not proved sufficiently reliable for thermography to fulfill hopes that it might prove useful as an early screening test for breast cancer.

Thermometer

An instrument used to measure *temperature*. A traditional clinical thermometer consists of a glass capillary

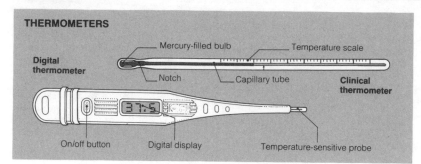

THERMOMETERS

Digital thermometer

Mercury-filled bulb

Temperature scale

Notch

Capillary tube

Clinical thermometer

On/off button

Digital display

Temperature-sensitive probe

tube (a tube with a very fine bore) that is sealed at one end and has a mercury-filled bulb at the other. Different styles of thermometer may be used to measure the temperature in the mouth, armpit, and rectum.

Clinical thermometers may be calibrated in *Celsius* (centigrade), *Fahrenheit*, or sometimes both. The wall of the thermometer is thickened on one side to form a cylindrical lens that makes the mercury easier to see.

When the bulb of the thermometer is placed in the mouth, armpit, or rectum, the mercury expands up the capillary tube. The thermometer is removed and the body temperature—indicated by the level of the mercury—is then read against a scale on the glass. There is a small kink in the capillary tube just above the bulb to prevent the mercury from moving down the tube when the thermometer is removed. Before the thermometer can be used again, the mercury must be shaken back down into the bulb.

A modern version of the traditional clinical thermometer uses an electronic probe connected to a digital readout display. In recent years, there has been a trend toward using disposable skin thermometers that employ heat-sensitive chemicals that change color at specific temperatures. Disposable skin thermometers are generally less accurate than the mercury or digital types because they are more likely to be affected by external factors, such as the temperature of the environment.

Thiabendazole

An *anthelmintic drug* used to treat *worm infestations*, including *strongyloidiasis*, *trichinosis*, and *toxocariasis*.

Thiabendazole may cause dizziness, loss of appetite, nausea, vomiting, headache, drowsiness, and diarrhea. Rarely, an allergic reaction to the drug occurs, leading to fever, rash, facial swelling, and, in severe cases, causing collapse.

Thiamine

See *Vitamin B complex*.

Thiopental

A *barbiturate drug* that is widely used as a general anesthetic (see *Anesthesia, general*). Thiopental is given by intravenous injection and quickly produces unconsciousness. The effects are relatively short-lived, and a different anesthetic agent is therefore used to maintain anesthesia.

Thioridazine

An *antipsychotic drug* used to treat *schizophrenia* and *mania*. Although thioridazine does not cure the underlying disorder, its tranquilizing effect reduces the abnormal experiences of patients who suffer from these conditions, and helps relieve their *anxiety* and *depression*.

Thioridazine may cause *dyskinesia* (abnormal movements) but is less likely to do so than some other antipsychotic drugs. Drowsiness, dry mouth, muscle stiffness, and dizziness may occur. High doses of thioridazine taken over long periods may damage the retina.

Thiothixene

An *antipsychotic* drug used primarily in the treatment of schizophrenia.

Thirst

The desire to drink. Thirst is one means by which the amount of water in the body is controlled (the other is the volume of urine excreted).

Thirst is stimulated by an increase in the concentration of salt, sugar, or certain other substances in the blood. Concentration of these substances in the serum (the liquid portion of blood) rises if fluid intake falls or if dietary intake of the substances (most commonly salt) increases. As the concentrated blood passes through the *hypothalamus* in the brain, special nerve receptors are stimulated, inducing the sensation of thirst.

Thirst is also stimulated if the volume of blood decreases as a result of sweating, vomiting, diarrhea, severe bleeding, or extensive burns. Thirst may also be caused by a dry mouth, even when a person is adequately hydrated; this can usually be relieved by moistening the mouth.

Damage to the hypothalamus (as a result of a head injury, for example) may cause loss of the desire to drink and consequent *dehydration*.

Thirst, excessive

A strong and persistent need to drink, most commonly due to *dehydration*. Excessive thirst is a symptom of untreated *diabetes mellitus* and *diabetes insipidus*. Other causes of excessive thirst include *kidney failure*, treatment with certain drugs (such as *phenothiazine drugs*), and severe blood loss. Abnormal thirst may also be psychological in origin, a condition known as psychogenic polydipsia.

Thoracic outlet syndrome

A condition in which pressure on the *brachial plexus* (the nerve roots that pass into either arm from the neck) causes pain in the arms and shoulders, a pins and needles sensation in the fingers, and weakness of grip and other hand movements.

Severe symptoms are usually caused by a *cervical rib*, which is an extra rib above the first rib that is linked to the first rib by a fibrous band of tissue which presses on the brachial plexus. Thoracic outlet syndrome may also result from pressure on the brachial plexus due to drooping shoulders, an enlarged scalenus muscle in the neck, or a tumor. The condition is made worse by lifting and carrying heavy loads or by an increase in body weight.

Treatment usually involves exercises to improve posture. *Nonsteroidal anti-inflammatory drugs* and *muscle-relaxant drugs* are sometimes helpful. Severe cases may be treated by surgical removal of the first rib.

Thoracic surgery

A surgical specialty concerned with operations on organs within the chest cavity, excluding the heart. Thoracic surgery is concerned particularly with disorders of the *lungs*, *esophagus*, and *trachea* (windpipe).

Thoracotomy

An operation in which the chest is opened to provide access to organs in the chest cavity.

T

A thoracotomy is usually performed to allow a surgeon to operate on a diseased *heart, lung,* or other organ in the chest cavity, such as the *esophagus.* It may also be carried out as an emergency procedure following a severe chest injury.

HOW IT IS DONE

There are two types of thoracotomy: lateral and anterior. Both are performed under general anesthesia.

A lateral thoracotomy provides access to the lungs, major blood vessels, and esophagus. A curved incision is made from between the shoulder blades, around the side of the trunk beneath the armpit, to just below the nipple. The necessary operation is then performed. Afterward, a drainage tube is inserted into the pleural cavity (the space between the membrane covering the lung and the membrane lining the chest wall) to allow fluid to drain and to prevent the lung from collapsing. The incision is then closed with stitches.

An anterior thoracotomy provides access to the heart and coronary arteries. A vertical incision is made from between the clavicles (collarbones) at the base of the neck to the lower end of the sternum (breastbone). The sternum is divided with a saw and prised apart. The heart is then exposed and the necessary surgery performed. Following insertion of a drainage tube into the pleural cavity, the sternum is closed with strong stitches (sometimes wire) and the overlying skin is sewn up.

RECOVERY PERIOD

Despite drainage, secretions in the air passages often cause breathing problems after surgery. To clear the passages, the patient is encouraged to breathe deeply and cough and is given *physiotherapy.* The drainage tube is usually removed within 48 hours after surgery.

Thorax

The medical name for the chest. The thorax extends from the base of the neck to the *diaphragm muscle* and is supported and protected by the *ribs, sternum* (breastbone), and *vertebrae* (spinal bones). The main structures in the thorax are the *heart, lungs, esophagus,* and large blood vessels such as the *aorta* and pulmonary arteries.

Thought

A mental activity that enables humans to reason, form judgments, and solve problems. The essential features of thought are the substitution of symbols (in the form of words, numbers, or images) for objects, the formation of these symbols into ideas, and the arrangement of ideas into a certain order in the mind. A person's thoughts are represented to others by speech, writing, and behavior.

Aspects of thought that can be examined or tested include speed and efficiency, content of ideas, and the logical relationship between ideas.

Thought disorders

Abnormalities in the structure or content of *thought* as reflected in a person's speech, writing, or behavior.

In the thought disorder characteristic of *schizophrenia,* sometimes referred to as formal thought disorder, associations lose their logical connection. The individual may jump from one subject to another that is apparently unrelated, or may make indirect associations or "clang" associations (the relating of words that sound the same rather than connect logically).

Other thought disorders that occur in schizophrenia include the invention of new words (see *Neologisms*), thought blocking (sudden interruption in the train of thought), experiencing thoughts as being inserted into or withdrawn from the mind by some outside force, and auditory *hallucinations,* in which a voice is heard dictating or repeating the subject's thoughts.

An inability to think clearly and coherently occurs in all types of *confusion,* including *dementia* and delirium. Rapidly jumping from one idea to another ("flight of ideas") as a result of a loosening of associations is characteristic of *hypomania* and *mania.* In someone suffering from *depression,* the opposite occurs: thinking becomes slow, there is a lack of ideas and associations, and the person tends to dwell in great detail on trivial subjects. Recurrent ideas that seem to come into a person's mind involuntarily are characteristic of *obsessive-compulsive behavior.*

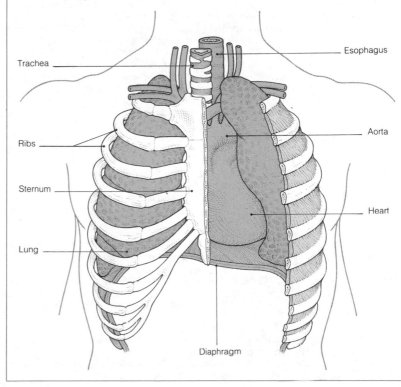

ANATOMY OF THE THORAX

The heart, lungs, and large blood vessels (such as the aorta) occupy almost all of the thoracic cavity; part of the esophagus and trachea are also in the thorax. The thoracic contents are protected and supported by the ribs, sternum (breastbone), and vertebrae.

Trachea

Esophagus

Ribs

Aorta

Sternum

Heart

Lung

Diaphragm

T

Delusions (false beliefs that do not respond to reasoned argument), which occur in schizophrenia and other psychotic illnesses, may be an expression of distorted thinking.

Threadworm infestation
See *Strongyloides.*

Thrill
A vibrating sensation felt when the flat of the hand is held against the front of the chest. A thrill is caused by abnormal blood flow in the *heart* due to a diseased heart valve or to some form of congenital *heart disease*. A thrill is always accompanied by an audible heart *murmur.*

Throat
A popular term for the *pharynx*, the passage running down from the back of the mouth and nose to the upper part of the *esophagus* and the opening into the *larynx* (voice box). The term throat is also used to refer to the front of the neck. (See also *Sore throat.*)

Throat cancer
See *Pharynx, cancer of.*

Thrombectomy
The removal of a *thrombus* (blood clot) that is partly or completely blocking a blood vessel.

Thrombectomy may be performed as an emergency procedure if a thrombus is blocking a major artery (such as one supplying blood to the brain, lungs, or intestines). It may also be performed as a precautionary measure if there is a risk of an *embolus* (fragment) breaking off from a thrombus and being carried into the bloodstream to block an artery.

Before surgery, the site of the thrombus is established by *angiography* and the patient is given *anticoagulant drugs* (drugs that prevent the blood from clotting). With the patient under general anesthesia, incisions are made to uncover the affected blood vessel. The blood vessel is then opened and the thrombus aspirated (sucked out). The incision is closed with delicate stitches.

Thromboangiitis obliterans
Another name for *Buerger's disease.*

Thrombocytopenia
A reduction in the number of *platelet* cells in the blood. Because platelets play a vital role in the arrest of bleeding (by plugging any small breaks that develop in the walls of blood vessels), thrombocytopenia causes a tendency to bleed, especially from the smaller blood vessels. The result may be thrombocytopenic purpura (abnormal bleeding into the skin and from other parts of the body).

CAUSES AND SYMPTOMS
Thrombocytopenia may be caused by a reduced rate of production of platelets by the *bone marrow* or by a fast rate of destruction of the platelets.

In a form of thrombocytopenia known as idiopathic thrombocytopenic purpura (ITP), the underlying cause is not apparent. However, this type of thrombocytopenia commonly follows a viral infection and may be an *autoimmune disorder* in which the infection triggers destruction of the platelets by the immune system. ITP occurs mainly in children and young adults. The symptoms may include purple bruises or bleeding points in the skin, nosebleeds, *hematuria* (blood in the urine), bleeding in the mouth, and *menorrhagia* (heavy menstrual bleeding). There is a small risk of *brain hemorrhage*, the warning signs for which are headache and dizziness.

Thrombocytopenia can be a feature of *leukemia, lymphoma*, other malignant diseases, megaloblastic *anemia*, systemic *lupus erythematosus*, or *hypersplenism* (overactivity of the spleen). Another possible cause is the rare disorder thrombotic thrombocytopenic purpura (TTP), which also causes damage to the kidneys and the brain and spinal cord.

Thrombocytopenia may also occur after exposure to X rays or radiation, in severe fevers, and as a reaction to certain drugs.

DIAGNOSIS
Thrombocytopenia is diagnosed from the patient's symptoms and from the presence of low numbers of platelets when a *blood count* is performed. A diagnosis of ITP is made by excluding other possible causes.

TREATMENT AND OUTLOOK
Any underlying disease will be treated if possible, and any causative drug withdrawn.

Children with ITP may not require treatment, but most adults are given *corticosteroid drugs*. In most cases, ITP lasts a few days to a few weeks before clearing up, although sometimes, particularly in adults, the bleeding tendency may recur from time to time. If ITP persists for many weeks or becomes recurrent, *splenectomy* (removal of the spleen) may be performed, giving a lasting cure in about three quarters of cases.

Thromboembolism
The blockage of a blood vessel by a fragment that has broken off from a thrombus (blood clot) and been carried elsewhere in the circulation. (See also *Embolism; Thrombosis.*)

Thrombolytic drugs

COMMON DRUGS

Streptokinase
Tissue-plasminogen activator

A group of drugs, also sometimes known as fibrinolytic drugs, used to dissolve blood clots occurring in *thrombosis, embolism*, and *myocardial infarction* (heart attack).

Thrombolytic drugs work by increasing the blood level of plasmin (an enzyme that dissolves fibrin, the main constituent of blood clots).

Treatment with thrombolytic drugs is carefully monitored because of the risk of abnormal bleeding. An allergic reaction, causing rash and breathing difficulty, may also occur.

Thrombophlebitis
Inflammation of part of a vein, usually near the surface of the body, along with clot formation in the affected segment. The condition can occur after minor injury to a vein (such as after an injection or intravenous infusion) and is particularly common in intravenous drug abusers. Thrombophlebitis can develop as a complication of *varicose veins* and also in blood vessel disorders such as *Buerger's disease.*

There is obvious swelling and redness along the affected segment of vein, which is extremely tender when touched. Fever and malaise often occur. Serious complications are uncommon, although sometimes far more dangerous clot formation develops in deeper veins (see *Thrombosis, deep vein*).

Treatment includes use of an elastic bandage to give gentle support, *nonsteroidal anti-inflammatory drugs*, and, if infection of the vein is suspected, *antibiotic drugs.*

Thrombosis
The formation of a thrombus (blood clot) within an intact blood vessel. Clotting is a normal response that prevents bleeding when a blood vessel wall is injured. Thrombus formation is abnormal if it occurs when a vessel wall has not been cut or punctured.

A thrombus within an artery may eventually grow to block the artery, preventing blood and oxygen from

T

reaching the organ or tissue supplied by the artery. Thrombi of this type are an important cause of death and disability in developed countries. A thrombus that forms within one of the arteries supplying the heart muscle, a condition known as coronary thrombosis, is the usual cause of *myocardial infarction* (heart attack). A thrombus within one of the arteries supplying the brain, a condition known as cerebral thrombosis, is a common cause of *stroke*.

Thrombi may also block arteries supplying blood to the legs, kidneys, retinas, intestines, and other organs, sometimes causing severe damage and symptoms such as pain and loss of function. Another danger is that an embolus (fragment of thrombus) may break off and be carried in the bloodstream to block an important blood vessel perhaps at some distance from its site of origin.

Thrombi sometimes form in veins—either in inflamed veins near the surface, a condition known as *thrombophlebitis*, or in deeper veins (see *Thrombosis, deep vein*). In deep vein thrombosis, the risk of large emboli breaking off and being carried to the heart and lungs is particularly serious, the result potentially fatal.

CAUSES

In the blood there is a fine balance between the mechanisms that encourage and discourage clotting, so there is neither a tendency to bleed nor to form clots (see *Blood clotting*). Thrombosis can occur if there is an upset in favor of clotting.

In arteries, the clotting process may be encouraged by a build-up of atheroma (fatty deposits) on blood vessel walls. Any of the factors that encourage *atherosclerosis*—such as smoking, obesity, *diabetes mellitus*, or *hypertension* (high blood pressure)—is similarly associated with an increased tendency to form clots. Clot formation may also be encouraged by damage to blood vessel walls from inflammation, which occurs in *arteritis* and phlebitis. Abnormal clotting may also be due to spread of infection in the blood, either to local blood vessels or throughout the circulation in *septicemia* (spread and multiplication of bacteria through the blood).

A clotting tendency may result from an increase in the level of coagulation factors in the blood, which may occur in pregnancy or when using *oral contraceptives*. A clotting tendency may also result from a liver disease that leads to deficient production of anti-

thrombin, an anticlotting factor. Any circumstance that causes a slowing down of blood flow to a particular area (such as inactivity during a long air flight, or general anesthesia induced for a surgical operation) may also result in a clotting tendency.

SYMPTOMS AND DIAGNOSIS

An arterial thrombus may cause no symptoms until it impairs the flow of blood through a blood vessel. At this point it may cause reduced function of the organ or tissue supplied by the blood vessel and, in some cases, severe pain. Venous thrombosis may also cause pain and swelling.

When thrombosis is a suspected cause of symptoms, it is investigated by *angiography* or by *venography* (X rays of blood vessels taken after the injection of a radiopaque substance).

TREATMENT

Treatment may include the use of *anticoagulant drugs*, which discourage clotting, or *thrombolytic drugs*, which help break down clots that have already formed. *Nonsteroidal anti-inflammatory drugs* are often given to relieve the inflammation of thrombophlebitis. Other treatment, such as *antibiotic drugs* if infection is the cause of thrombosis, may be necessary. In cases where a clot is life-threatening, surgical removal may be required (see *Thrombectomy*).

Thrombosis, deep vein

The formation of a thrombus (blood clot) within deep-lying veins, usually in the legs.

CAUSES AND INCIDENCE

Deep vein thrombosis is generally caused by a combination of sluggish blood flow through one part of the body and some condition that increases the natural tendency of the blood to clot.

Sluggish blood flow occurs when a person lies or sits still for long periods. An increase in the level of coagulation factors in the blood, which occurs after an operation or injury, during pregnancy, and in women taking *oral contraceptives*, causes an increased tendency for the blood to clot.

An increased tendency to form clots can also occur as a result of *polycythemia* (increased numbers of red cells in the blood), severe infection, liver disease, and certain types of cancer. Deep vein thrombosis is common in people with *heart failure* and in those who have had a *stroke* or who are immobilized for long periods. Other causes include injury to the veins or the spread of *thrombophlebitis*

(inflammation and clot formation in superficial veins) to deeper veins. Age and obesity both predispose to thrombosis.

SYMPTOMS AND COMPLICATIONS

If a deep vein thrombosis occurs somewhere other than in a leg, there are often no symptoms. Clots in the leg veins may cause symptoms such as pain, tenderness, swelling, discoloration, and ulceration of the skin (see illustrated box, p. 986).

Deep vein thrombosis is not always of serious significance. However, if clots are extensive, part of a clot may break free and be carried up to the heart and from there to the lungs, where it may block an artery. This is called a *pulmonary embolism*.

DIAGNOSIS

The presence and extent of deep vein thrombosis is diagnosed by *venography* (introduction of a radiopaque substance into the veins followed by X rays) and by a type of *radionuclide scanning* called the radioactive fibrinogen test. Doppler *ultrasound scanning* may also be used to detect thrombi.

TREATMENT

Treatment depends on the site and extent of the blood clots. If they are small, confined to the calf, and the patient is mobile, treatment may be unnecessary, as the clots often break up spontaneously. In some cases, *anticoagulant drugs* may be given to prevent extension of the clots. In other cases, *thrombolytic drugs*, which actively dissolve the clots, may be given. If there is a high risk of a clot breaking off and causing a pulmonary embolism, *thrombectomy* may be performed to remove the clot surgically.

PREVENTION

The incidence of deep vein thrombosis has been reduced by encouraging people to get up as soon as possible after an operation or childbirth. If a person is immobilized for a long period, he or she should wiggle the toes and flex the ankles and knees to keep the blood moving. Blood flow in the legs of an immobilized person may also be stimulated by the pumping up and down of inflatable bags around the legs.

When an operation is performed on someone thought to be particularly susceptible to deep vein thrombosis, anticoagulant drugs may be given.

Thrombus

A blood clot that has formed inside an intact blood vessel—as distinct from one that has formed to seal the wall of a blood vessel after injury.

T

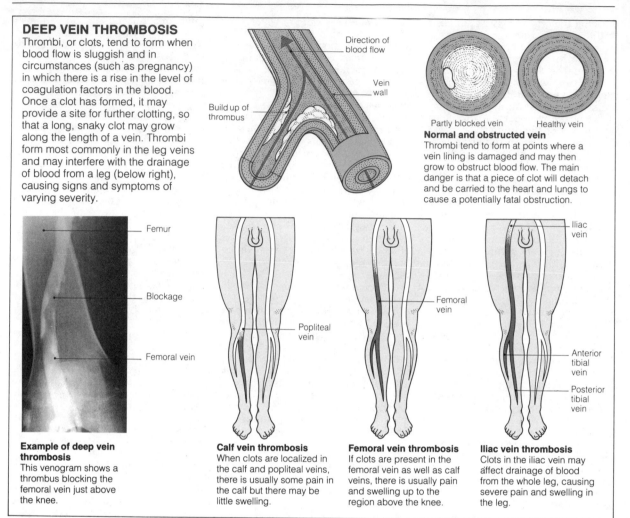

DEEP VEIN THROMBOSIS

Thrombi, or clots, tend to form when blood flow is sluggish and in circumstances (such as pregnancy) in which there is a rise in the level of coagulation factors in the blood. Once a clot has formed, it may provide a site for further clotting, so that a long, snaky clot may grow along the length of a vein. Thrombi form most commonly in the leg veins and may interfere with the drainage of blood from a leg (below right), causing signs and symptoms of varying severity.

Direction of blood flow

Vein wall

Build up of thrombus

Partly blocked vein   Healthy vein

Normal and obstructed vein
Thrombi tend to form at points where a vein lining is damaged and may then grow to obstruct blood flow. The main danger is that a piece of clot will detach and be carried to the heart and lungs to cause a potentially fatal obstruction.

Femur

Blockage

Femoral vein

Example of deep vein thrombosis
This venogram shows a thrombus blocking the femoral vein just above the knee.

Popliteal vein

Calf vein thrombosis
When clots are localized in the calf and popliteal veins, there is usually some pain in the calf but there may be little swelling.

Femoral vein

Femoral vein thrombosis
If clots are present in the femoral vein as well as calf veins, there is usually pain and swelling up to the region above the knee.

Iliac vein

Anterior tibial vein

Posterior tibial vein

Iliac vein thrombosis
Clots in the iliac vein may affect drainage of blood from the whole leg, causing severe pain and swelling in the leg.

A thrombus is life-threatening if it grows to obstruct the blood supply to an organ such as the heart or brain. Even a thrombus in a less vital blood vessel can be dangerous because it may produce *gangrene* in part of an organ or extremity served by the blood vessel, or lead to *embolism*, in which a fragment of the thrombus breaks off and is carried to obstruct the blood circulation elsewhere. (See also *Blood clotting; Thrombosis*.)

Thrush
A common name for the fungal infection *candidiasis*.

Thumb-sucking
A common habit in young children. For the young child, thumb-sucking provides comfort (especially before falling asleep), oral gratification, amusement if the child is bored, and reassurance, especially in periods of stress, such as the birth of a new baby in the family.

Thumb-sucking tends to decrease after the age of about 3. Only a few children do not grow out of the habit by 6 or 7. In general, it is best for parents to ignore a child's thumb-sucking; constant reprimands may make the habit worse.

COMPLICATIONS
In most cases, there is no evidence that thumb-sucking is harmful. However, *malocclusion* (incorrect bite) of the second teeth may develop if the habit continues after about the age of 7. The effect on the teeth is usually only temporary; their position improves considerably or even returns completely to normal after thumb-sucking stops. In severe cases, treatment with an *orthodontic appliance* may be recommended.

Thymoma
A tumor of the *thymus* gland. Thymomas are rare and are classified according to the type of thymus tissue from which they arise. An epithelial thymoma, arising from *epithelium*, is a slow-growing tumor that rarely spreads to other parts of the body. A lymphoid thymoma arises from lymphoid tissue, eventually resulting in generalized non-Hodgkin's *lymphoma*. A granulomatous thymoma consists of a mixture of epithelial and lymphoid tissue, and closely resembles *Hodgkin's disease*. The other main type of thymoma is a thymic *teratoma* (a tumor consisting of tissue that is not normally found in the thymus), which is usually benign in women but malignant in men.

Thymomas may affect function of the *immune system*, causing increased susceptibility to infection. They are

T

commonly associated with *myasthenia gravis* (an autoimmune disease), which can sometimes be cured by removal of the thymoma.

Thymoxamine

A *vasodilator drug* occasionally used in the treatment of *Raynaud's disease*. Thymoxamine is not sold in Canada, but it is available under the Emergency Drugs Release Program.

Thymus

A gland that forms part of the *immune system*. The thymus is situated in the upper part of the chest, behind the sternum (breastbone), and consists of two lobes that join in front of the trachea (windpipe). Each lobe is made up of tissue consisting of tightly packed *lymphocytes, epithelium,* and fat.

The thymus plays a part in the body's immune response from about the 12th week of gestation until puberty. The gland gradually enlarges until puberty, when it begins to shrink. Lymphoid and epithelial tissues are gradually replaced by fat, although some glandular tissue remains until after middle age.

The function of the thymus is to condition lymphocytes to become *T cells*, part of the body's defense against viruses and other infections.

DISORDERS

Abnormal enlargement of the thymus may occur in several conditions, including *myasthenia gravis, acromeg-* aly, *thyrotoxicosis,* and *Addison's disease*. Myasthenia gravis is also sometimes associated with *thymomas* (tumors of the thymus). In children, *immunodeficiency disorders* may arise as a result of abnormal development of the thymus.

Thyroglossal disorders

Congenital defects arising from failure of the thyroglossal duct to disappear during embryonic development. In the *embryo*, this duct runs from the base of the tongue to the thyroid gland in the neck. Abnormal development may cause the duct to persist in its entirety or partly as a cyst.

A thyroglossal cyst almost always becomes infected and swollen, a condition that may be mistaken for an abscess. Infection may lead to formation of a thyroglossal fistula (abnormal passage between the cyst and the surface of the neck).

Because of the danger of repeated infection, a thyroglossal cyst or fistula should be completely removed surgically, along with any remaining parts of the thyroglossal duct.

Thyroid cancer

Cancer of the *thyroid gland* is relatively rare, accounting for only about 1 percent of all cases of cancer. In most cases, the cause of the condition is unknown, although it is one of the cancers associated with exposure to radioactive fallout. Thyroid cancer has one of the highest cure rates of all types of cancer.

SYMPTOMS AND SIGNS

A thyroid cancer is usually first noticed as a single, firm nodule in the neck. The tumor may grow slowly or rapidly, depending partly on the particular type of cancer and partly on the age of the patient (growth tends to be slower in younger people). Thyroid cancers are painless in many cases; symptoms arise when tumors press on other structures in the neck. Such symptoms may include severe hoarseness or loss of voice, caused by pressure on the nerves to the larynx (voice box), or difficulty in swallowing, caused by pressure on the pharynx (throat). Spread of the cancer to the lymph nodes, which often occurs at an early stage, causes enlargement of the nodes. Advanced cancers are usually hard and irregularly shaped and are often firmly attached to adjacent structures in the neck.

DIAGNOSIS

A physician's initial physical examination cannot differentiate between a

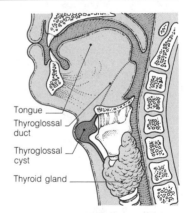

Tongue
Thyroglossal duct
Thyroglossal cyst
Thyroid gland

Thyroglossal duct and cyst
The thyroglossal duct, lying between the tongue and the thyroid, sometimes persists after fetal life, and a cyst may form.

cancerous and a noncancerous nodule. For this reason, single thyroid nodules are always imaged (see *Thyroid scanning*). In some cases, tissue is removed for microscopic analysis. This may be done either by a needle *biopsy* or surgically. If there are several nodules, they are likely to be benign rather than cancerous.

TREATMENT

Treatment is usually by total *thyroidectomy* (surgical removal of the entire gland); occasionally, it is also necessary to remove surrounding tissues. The loss of thyroid tissue results in a lack of natural *thyroid hormones*, and patients usually need to take thyroxine for the rest of their lives. Such supplements may also help to control *metastases* (secondary growths).

In virtually all cases, treatment with radioactive *iodine* is used after surgery. Because it is selectively taken up and concentrated in the thyroid, radioactive iodine has the advantage of destroying any residual cancer while leaving normal body tissue undamaged. This treatment may be repeated at one- to five-year intervals if any residual tissue is detected.

OUTLOOK

If thyroid cancer is diagnosed and treated at an early stage (even if local spread has occurred), the outlook is generally good.

Thyroidectomy

Surgical removal of all or part of the *thyroid gland*.

WHY IT IS DONE

Thyroidectomy is performed to treat *thyroid cancer*, some cases of *hyperthyroidism* that cannot be controlled by drugs, *goiter* (enlargement of the thy-

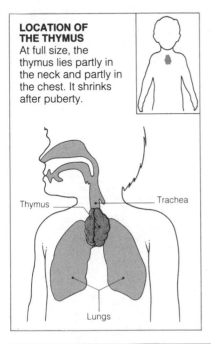

LOCATION OF THE THYMUS
At full size, the thymus lies partly in the neck and partly in the chest. It shrinks after puberty.

Thymus
Trachea
Lungs

T

SUBTOTAL THYROIDECTOMY

This operation entails removal of only part of the thyroid. The parathyroids (at the rear of the gland) are left intact.

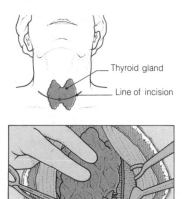

Thyroid gland

Line of incision

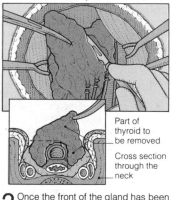

1 After administration of a general anesthetic, an incision is made in the neck. Layers of skin and muscle are then drawn aside to expose the thyroid gland underneath.

Part of thyroid to be removed

Cross section through the neck

2 Once the front of the gland has been detached from its blood supply, much of it is cut away (with care taken not to damage nearby nerves), and bleeding vessels are sealed.

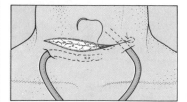

3 Tubes are sometimes placed in the site of the removed gland to drain blood that accumulates. The muscle and skin layers are replaced and the incision is closed with sutures or clips.

---

roid gland) that is causing breathing or swallowing difficulties or unsightly swelling, or a benign tumor of the thyroid gland.

HOW IT IS DONE

With the patient under general anesthesia, an incision is made in the neck and all or part of the thyroid gland is removed. A common form of operation to remove part of the thyroid (subtotal thyroidectomy) is shown in the illustrated box at left.

RECOVERY PERIOD

The wound usually heals quickly. The stitches and drainage tube can usually be removed within a few days of the operation, after which the patient leaves hospital.

Removal of all—or a large part—of the thyroid gland necessitates lifelong hormone replacement therapy with *thyroid hormones*.

COMPLICATIONS

There is a very small risk of damage to structures close to the thyroid gland. Injury to the nerve supplying the vocal cords can lead to hoarseness; damage to the *parathyroid glands* can result in a low calcium level in the blood and *tetany* (painful muscle spasms in the hands, feet, and face). After the operation, careful monitoring is required to ensure that hormone levels are in the normal range.

Thyroid function tests

A group of procedures used to evaluate the function of the *thyroid gland* and to detect or confirm any disorder of the gland.

Thyroid function can be measured by carrying out *blood tests* to determine the level of thyroxine (T_4) and triiodothyronine (T_3) in the blood. A sample of blood is taken from the patient's vein and the serum (liquid part of the blood) is tested.

The main function of the thyroid gland is to convert tyrosine (an amino acid) and *iodine* into T_4 and T_3. One way of measuring thyroid function is therefore to measure the rate at which iodine is accumulated by the gland. This can be done by introducing into the body a radioactive isotope of iodine (or *technetium*, which behaves in a similar way to iodine) and then measuring the level of radioactivity in the gland (see *Thyroid scanning*).

The thyroid secretes T_4 and T_3 into the bloodstream under the direct control of thyroid-stimulating hormone (TSH) from the *pituitary gland*. Measurement of the amount of TSH in the blood provides a sensitive means of diagnosing thyroid malfunction.

Various indices created by ratios of T_3 and T_4 enable the specialist to give a more accurate diagnosis of the patient's condition.

Thyroid gland

One of the main *endocrine glands*, which helps regulate the body's energy level. The thyroid gland is situated in the front of the neck, just below the larynx (voice box). It consists of two lobes, one on each side of the trachea (windpipe), joined by a narrower portion of tissue called the isthmus.

STRUCTURE

Thyroid tissue is composed of two types of secretory cells: follicular cells and parafollicular cells (or C cells). Follicular cells, which make up most of the gland, are arranged in the form of hollow, spherical follicles. These cells secrete the iodine-containing hormones thyroxine (T_4) and triiodothyronine (T_3). The space inside the follicles is filled with a yellow, semifluid, colloid material that is essential for the production of T_4 and T_3.

Parafollicular cells occur singly or in small groups between the follicles. These cells secrete the hormone *calcitonin*. Also between the follicles are blood capillaries, small lymphatic vessels, and connective tissue.

FUNCTION

T_4 and T_3 play an important role in controlling body *metabolism*. Calcito-

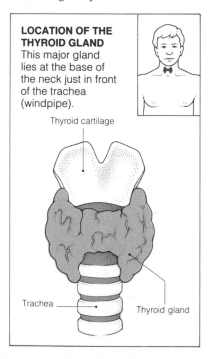

LOCATION OF THE THYROID GLAND

This major gland lies at the base of the neck just in front of the trachea (windpipe).

Thyroid cartilage

Trachea

Thyroid gland

T

nin acts in conjunction with parathyroid hormone to regulate the balance of calcium in the body. (See also *Thyroid gland* disorders box; *Thyroid hormones*.)

Thyroid hormones

The hormones thyroxine (T_4), triiodothyronine (T_3), and *calcitonin*, produced by the *thyroid gland*.

FUNCTION

T_4 (the hormone produced in greatest amounts by the thyroid gland) and T_3 regulate *metabolism* (the chemical activity in cells that releases energy from nutrients or uses energy to create other substances, such as proteins). In children, these hormones are also essential for normal physical growth and mental development.

Calcitonin acts in conjunction with parathyroid hormone to regulate the level of calcium in the body.

REGULATION

T_4 AND T_3 The secretion of T_4 and T_3 by the thyroid gland is controlled by a complex hormonal feedback system involving the *pituitary gland* and *hypothalamus*.

CALCITONIN The secretion of calcitonin by the thyroid is regulated directly by the level of calcium in the blood. Raised blood calcium stimulates calcitonin secretion, stimulating deposition of calcium in bone and thereby reducing the calcium level; decreased blood calcium inhibits calcitonin output to help increase the calcium level. This feedback regulation occurs independently of the pituitary gland or hypothalamus.

DEFICIENCY AND EXCESS

Insufficient thyroid hormone production is known as *hypothyroidism*. The symptoms include tiredness, dry skin, hair loss, weight gain, constipa-

tion, and sensitivity to cold. In childhood, deficiency of thyroid hormone may cause *cretinism* (a condition characterized by severe growth retardation, coarseness of the facial features and mental impairment).

Overproduction of thyroid hormones is known as *hyperthyroidism*. Symptoms of hyperthyroidism include fatigue, anxiety, palpitations, sweating, weight loss, diarrhea, and intolerance of heat.

DRUG THERAPY

The most commonly used thyroid hormone drugs are the synthetic thyroid hormone preparations levothyroxine and liothyronine. These drugs are used to treat hypothyroidism, to prevent hypothyroidism, to reduce thyroid enlargement in certain types of *goiter*, and to treat *thyroid cancer*.

Because a sudden increase in the body's thyroid hormone level may strain the heart, levothyroxine and liothyronine are usually prescribed in low doses that are gradually increased. Since too high a dose may cause symptoms of hyperthyroidism, regular visits to the physician are essential; when necessary, blood tests are carried out to monitor the level of thyroid hormones.

Calcitonin is used to treat *Paget's disease*, *osteoporosis*, and *hypercalcemia*.

Thyroiditis

The medical term for inflammation of the *thyroid gland*. Thyroiditis can be caused by a variety of factors, and occurs in several different forms.

The most common form is *Hashimoto's thyroiditis*, an autoimmune disorder causing *hypothyroidism* (underactivity of the thyroid gland).

Subacute thyroiditis, also known as de Quervain's thyroiditis, is a less common form in which the thyroid becomes tender and painful. Pain, which may be referred (see *Referred pain*) to the jaw, ears, or back of the head, may be accompanied by fever, weight loss, and a general feeling of illness. The precise cause of subacute thyroiditis is unknown. The condition may persist for several months, but in most cases eventually subsides on its own. In severe cases, treatment with *corticosteroid drugs* may be given to reduce the inflammation.

Thyroiditis due to infection is rare; when it does occur, it is usually as a result of an infection that has spread from elsewhere in the body. In some cases, an abscess forms in the gland, which may require surgical drainage.

CONTROL OF THYROID HORMONE PRODUCTION

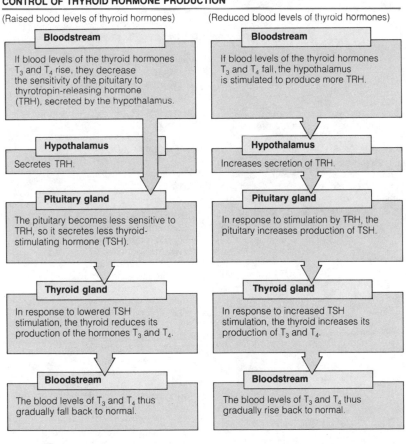

(Raised blood levels of thyroid hormones)

Bloodstream
If blood levels of the thyroid hormones T_3 and T_4 rise, they decrease the sensitivity of the pituitary to thyrotropin-releasing hormone (TRH), secreted by the hypothalamus.

Hypothalamus
Secretes TRH.

Pituitary gland
The pituitary becomes less sensitive to TRH, so it secretes less thyroid-stimulating hormone (TSH).

Thyroid gland
In response to lowered TSH stimulation, the thyroid reduces its production of the hormones T_3 and T_4.

Bloodstream
The blood levels of T_3 and T_4 thus gradually fall back to normal.

(Reduced blood levels of thyroid hormones)

Bloodstream
If blood levels of the thyroid hormones T_3 and T_4 fall, the hypothalamus is stimulated to produce more TRH.

Hypothalamus
Increases secretion of TRH.

Pituitary gland
In response to stimulation by TRH, the pituitary increases production of TSH.

Thyroid gland
In response to increased TSH stimulation, the thyroid increases its production of T_3 and T_4.

Bloodstream
The blood levels of T_3 and T_4 thus gradually rise back to normal.

Why control is necessary
The blood levels of the hormones T_3 (triiodothyronine) and T_4 (thyroxine) produced by the thyroid must be kept within narrow limits, otherwise

hyperthyroidism or hypothyroidism may result. The control systems above exist to achieve this balance but certain disorders may interfere with the system.

T

DISORDERS OF THE THYROID GLAND

The function of the thyroid gland is controlled by both the pituitary gland and the hypothalamus, so thyroid disorders may be due not only to defects in the gland itself, but also to disruption of the hypothalamic-pituitary hormonal control system. Thyroid disorders may cause symptoms due to overproduction of thyroid hormones (*hyperthyroidism*), underproduction of these hormones (*hypothyroidism*), or enlargement or distortion of the gland. *Myxedema*, *Graves' disease*, and *Hashimoto's thyroiditis* are the common disorders of thyroid function. *Goiter* (enlargement of the thyroid gland) may sometimes occur without any accompanying abnormality of thyroid function.

CONGENITAL DEFECTS

In rare cases, the thyroid gland is missing completely at birth, producing severe *cretinism*. However, congenital thyroid deficiency more often takes the form of underdevelopment or maldevelopment, in which there is sufficient hormone-producing thyroid tissue to avoid cretinism but insufficient tissue to produce normal amounts of hormones. If untreated, this may lead to juvenile myxedema.

Sometimes the thyroid develops in an abnormal position in the neck; in rare cases, this causes difficulty in swallowing or breathing.

GENETIC DISORDERS

A genetic disorder may impair the thyroid's ability to secrete hormones. The low blood level of thyroid hormones results in greatly increased secretion by the pituitary gland of thyroid-stimulating hormone (TSH), which, in turn, causes the thyroid to enlarge. This is one way in which a goiter may develop.

INFECTION

Thyroid infection is uncommon, but sometimes occurs as a complication of infection elsewhere in the body. The resulting *thyroiditis* may require treatment with antibiotics. If an abscess forms, a minor operation may be necessary to open and drain it. Viral infection of the thyroid can cause temporary hyperthyroidism as well as an extremely painful gland.

Tumors
Most lumps in the thyroid are benign, and some thyroid cancers are not highly malignant. A stone-hard, rapidly growing lump is an indication of thyroid cancer.

Autoimmune diseases
These are common causes of thyroid disorders. In Hashimoto's thyroiditis, much of the thyroid's glandular tissue is replaced by masses of lymphocytes.

Goiter
Enlargement of the thyroid (goiter) may result from hormonal imbalances at puberty or during pregnancy. Goiter may also be due to autoimmune disease, or, rarely, to iodine deficiency.

TUMORS

Thyroid tumors may be benign or malignant. Thyroid *adenomas* are benign tumors that may secrete thyroid hormone, sometimes in sufficient amounts to cause hyperthyroidism. *Thyroid cancers* vary greatly in their malignancy and rate of growth. They are relatively rare but may be suspected if a single firm or hard lump can be felt in the gland. One particular type of thyroid tumor secretes the hormone calcitonin.

AUTOIMMUNE DISORDERS

Graves' disease is a form of thyroid overactivity whose chief feature is hyperthyroidism. The disease is thought to be due to the body producing an "autoantibody" that stimulates the thyroid to secrete excessive amounts of hormones. Autoantibodies are also believed to be associated with certain other thyroid disorders, notably Hashimoto's thyroiditis, in which the antibodies damage glandular cells.

MYXEDEMA

Deficiency of thyroid hormone (hypothyroidism) may be associated with Hashimoto's thyroiditis or atrophy of the thyroid, or may be a consequence of treatment for hyperthyroidism. The result is myxedema, a condition in which the skin becomes dry and thickened, and facial features become coarse. Constipation, cold intolerance, and fatigue are other common symptoms. In many cases, the cause of myxedema is not known.

HORMONAL DISORDERS

Hormonal changes during puberty or pregnancy are a relatively common cause of a minor degree of goiter, which usually subsides when hormone levels return to normal. Hyperthyroidism due to excessive production of TSH by the pituitary gland is rare but can occur as a result of a pituitary tumor.

NUTRITIONAL DISORDERS

Because iodine is necessary for the production of thyroid hormone, deficiency of this mineral may lead to goiter. Severe iodine deficiency in children may cause myxedema. These problems can be avoided by using table salt that contains iodine.

RADIATION

Irradiation of the head or neck increases the likelihood of thyroid tumors, although it may be 25 years or more until such tumors develop.

INVESTIGATION

Suspected disturbances of thyroid function are investigated initially by taking a medical history and performing a physical examination. Blood samples may also be taken for *thyroid function tests*, in which the levels of thyroid or pituitary hormones are measured, and the gland itself may be imaged by various *thyroid scanning* techniques. In some cases, such as a suspected thyroid tumor, a fine-needle *biopsy* may be carried out to obtain a sample of thyroid tissue for examination under the microscope.

T

Rarer still is a condition known as Riedel's thyroiditis or Riedel's struma, in which deposits of dense, fibrous tissue form in the gland and surrounding tissues, resulting in a hardening of the entire area.

Thyroid scanning

Techniques used to provide information about the location, anatomy, and function of the *thyroid gland*. The technique of *radionuclide scanning* is commonly used to investigate disorders of the gland, but *ultrasound scanning* can be useful in some cases.

HOW IT IS DONE

For radionuclide scanning, an injection or an oral preparation containing a radioisotope (radioactive substance) is given, followed after an interval by the recording of images on a gamma camera. The radioisotope preparation usually contains a tiny dose of specially prepared *technetium* or *iodine*, both of which are taken up avidly by thyroid tissue, but hardly at all by other body tissues.

For ultrasound scanning, a transducer producing high-frequency sound waves that penetrate tissue is moved back and forth across the skin over the thyroid gland. Echoes of the sound waves are transformed electronically into an image.

WHY IT IS DONE

Radionuclide scanning reveals the position of any functioning thyroid tissue and is therefore useful in showing whether the gland is abnormally located or absent. The scan also shows the amount of radioisotope taken up by the gland, thus indicating *hyperthyroidism* (overactivity of the thyroid gland) or *hypothyroidism* (underactivity of the thyroid gland).

A radionuclide scan may suggest whether a thyroid nodule or tumor is cancerous or noncancerous and can

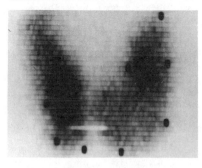

Radionuclide thyroid scanning
In this scan the diffuse darker areas indicate regions of overactive thyroid tissue (the small black ovals are markers).

show whether it is active or inactive. This technique can also detect malignant thyroid tissue that has spread to other parts of the body, therefore playing an important part in planning the treatment of *thyroid cancer*.

Ultrasound scanning is of more limited use because it can show only the structure of thyroid tissue. This technique can be useful in showing whether a *goiter* is solid, cystic (fluid-filled), or a mixture of the two.

Thyrotoxicosis

A term for any toxic condition that results from *hyperthyroidism* (overactivity of the thyroid gland). The term thyrotoxicosis is often used as a synonym for *Graves' disease*.

Thyroxine

See *Levothyroxine*.

Tiaprofenic acid

A *nonsteroidal anti-inflammatory drug* that reduces the pain of arthritic disorders. Like other drugs in this group, tiaprofenic acid is likely to cause gastrointestinal distress.

Tibia

The inner and thicker of the two long bones in the lower leg, also called the shin. The tibia is the supporting bone of the lower leg. It runs parallel to the narrower lower leg bone, the *fibula*, to which it is attached by *ligaments*.

The front surface of the tibia lies just beneath the skin and is easily felt. The upper end articulates with the *femur* (thigh bone) to form the *knee* joint and the lower end forms part of the *ankle joint*. On the inside of the ankle, the tibia is widened and protrudes to form a large bony prominence called the medial malleolus.

FRACTURE

The tibia is one of the most commonly fractured bones. It may break across the shaft as a result of a direct blow to the front of the leg, or at the upper end from a blow to the outside of the leg below the knee. Fracture of the lower end of the tibia may accompany dislocation of the ankle and fracture of the fibula in a *Pott's fracture*, caused by violent twisting of the ankle. Prolonged running or walking on hard ground may cause a *stress fracture* of the tibia. Some fractures of the shaft heal satisfactorily if the leg is immobilized in a plaster *cast*, usually for about six to eight weeks. If the bone ends are displaced or unstable, an operation may be needed to fasten them together with a nail or screw.

Tic

A repeated, uncontrolled, purposeless contraction of a *muscle* or group of muscles, most commonly in the face, shoulders, or arms. Typical tics include pointless blinking, mouth twitching, and shrugging.

Tics are often a sign of a usually minor psychological disturbance. Most develop in childhood, occurring in as many as a quarter of children and affecting three times more boys than girls. Tics are made worse by stress or by drawing attention to them, but often disappear when the child is deeply absorbed or asleep.

Tics usually stop within a year of onset but in some cases persist into adult life. Most can be controlled for short periods of time by will. However, such control is of questionable value because tics appear to release emotional tension.

In rare cases, tics become so severe that they require treatment with *benzodiazepine drugs* or *antipsychotic drugs*. Examples include involuntary contractions of the diaphragm (the muscle that separates the chest from the abdomen), resulting in grunting noises, and *Gilles de la Tourette's syndrome*, a disorder that is characterized by widespread tics and involuntary noises and words.

Tic douloureux

Another name for *trigeminal neuralgia*.

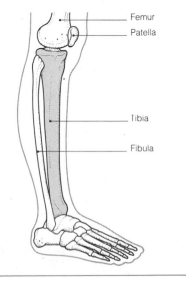

LOCATION OF THE TIBIA
Also called the shin, the tibia can easily be felt beneath the skin of the lower leg.

Femur
Patella
Tibia
Fibula

T

Ticks and disease

Ticks are small, eight-legged animals that feed on blood and sometimes transmit diseases to humans via their bites. Ticks are about 3 mm long before feeding; when bloated with blood, they become much larger. A person may pick up ticks when in various rural habitats, such as long grass, scrub, woodland, or caves. The ticks attach themselves by their mouthparts to the skin of animal or human hosts.

Ticks can spread infectious organisms from animals to humans via their bites. Diseases transmitted by ticks in various parts of North America include *Lyme disease*, *relapsing fever*, *Rocky Mountain spotted fever*, *Q fever*, *tularemia*, and certain types of viral *encephalitis*. The prolonged bite of certain female ticks can cause a condition called tick paralysis, in which a toxin in the tick saliva affects the nerves that control movement. In extreme cases, this can lead to paralysis of the respiratory muscles and can be fatal.

Tietze's syndrome

Chest pain localized to an area on the front of the chest wall, usually made worse by movement of the arms or trunk or by pressure from the fingers. Tietze's syndrome is caused by inflammation of one or several *rib* cartilages. Symptoms may persist for several months. Treatment is with *analgesic drugs* (painkillers) and *nonsteroidal anti-inflammatory drugs*.

Timolol

A *beta-blocker drug* used in tablet form to treat *hypertension* (high blood pressure) and *angina pectoris* (chest pain due to inadequate blood supply to the heart muscle). Timolol is also given after a *myocardial infarction* (heart attack) to prevent further damage to the heart muscle. In eye drop form, timolol is used to treat *glaucoma*.

Possible adverse effects are typical of other beta-blocker drugs. Eye drops may cause irritation, blurred vision, and headache.

Tinea

Any of a group of common *fungal infections* of the skin, hair, or nails. Most infections are caused by a group of fungi called the dermatophytes and are often called ringworm.

Tineal infections may be acquired from another person, from an animal, from soil, from the floors of showers, or from chairs or carpets.

The word tinea is sometimes followed by the Latin term for the affected part of the body. For example, tinea pedis affects the feet and tinea cruris affects the groin.

TYPES AND SYMPTOMS

The appearance and symptoms of tinea vary according to the site. The most common type is tinea pedis, also called *athlete's foot*, which causes cracking and itching between the toes.

Tinea corporis (ringworm of the body) is characterized by itchy patches on the body that are usually circular with a prominent edge. Tinea cruris (also commonly called jock itch) produces a reddened, itchy area spreading from the genitals outward over the inside of the thigh. This form of tinea is more common in males.

Tinea capitis (ringworm of the scalp) causes one or several round, itchy patches of hair loss on the scalp; it occurs mainly in children and is more common in large cities and overcrowded conditions. Ringworm of the nails, also called tinea unguium or onychomycosis, is often accompanied by scaling of the soles or palms. The nails become thick and turn white or yellow.

DIAGNOSIS AND TREATMENT

Most types of tinea are diagnosed by a physician from their appearances. However, the diagnosis should be confirmed, and the type of fungus identified, by culturing the organisms in a laboratory. Some scalp infections exhibit fluorescence under a filtered *ultraviolet light* (Wood's light), but most do not.

For most types of tinea, treatment is with *antifungal drugs* in the form of skin creams, lotions, or ointments. However, for widespread infections or those affecting the hair or nails, an antifungal drug in tablet form (usually griseofulvin) may be necessary.

Treatment may be continued for some time after symptoms have subsided to eradicate the fungi and prevent recurrence. For mild infections on the skin surface, there may need to be four to six weeks of treatment; for toenail infections, treatment may be necessary for up to one or two years.

Tinea versicolor

A common skin condition that produces patches of white, brown, or salmon-colored finely flaking skin over the trunk and neck. Also known as pityriasis versicolor, it is caused by colonization of the dead outer layer of skin by a fungus that exists unnoticed on most people's skin. The condition

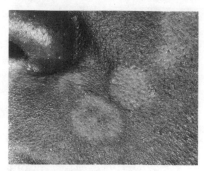

Appearance of tinea versicolor
This fungal infection causes patches of color change in the skin and is particularly common in tropical and subtropical areas.

primarily affects young and middle-aged adults and is more common in men. It is not contagious.

The condition is usually noticed because of the contrast in color between the affected and surrounding skin. Exposure to sunlight can make it more noticeable.

Treatment consists of applying an antifungal cream or lotion at night and washing underclothes and nightclothes thoroughly. It is important to treat the entire trunk, neck, arms, and upper legs each time the preparation is applied. Otherwise, a spot may be missed and the fungus will recur. This treatment usually clears the condition, but the spots may take months to return to normal skin color.

Tingling

See *Pins and needles*.

Tinnitus

A ringing, buzzing, whistling, hissing, or other noise heard in the *ear* or ears in the absence of a noise in the environment.

CAUSES

In tinnitus, the *acoustic nerve* transmits impulses to the *brain* not as the result of vibrations produced by external sound waves but, for reasons not fully understood, as the result of stimuli that originate inside the head or within the ear itself. The condition is almost always associated with hearing loss, particularly with deafness due to *presbycusis* and continuous exposure to loud noise.

Tinnitus can occur as a symptom of many ear disorders, including *labyrinthitis*, *Meniere's disease*, *otitis media*, *otosclerosis*, *ototoxicity*, and blockage of the outer ear canal with *earwax*. In rare cases, tinnitus is a symptom of an *aneurysm* or a tumor pressing on a blood vessel in the head. Tinnitus may

T

also be caused by certain drugs, such as *ASA* or *quinine*, or may follow a *head injury*.

SYMPTOMS

The noise in the ear may sometimes change in nature or intensity. In most cases it is present continuously but the sufferer's awareness of it is usually intermittent. Tolerance of tinnitus varies considerably from one person to another and is largely determined by the sufferer's personality. Many people learn to accept the condition without distress, but some find it almost intolerable.

Any underlying disorder is treated if possible. Many sufferers make use of a radio, television, cassette player, or headphones to block out the noise in their ears. Some find a tinnitus masker—headphones that play white noise (a random mixture of sounds of a wide range of frequencies)—particularly effective.

Tiredness

A common complaint that is usually the result of overwork or lack of sleep. In some people, persistent tiredness is caused by *depression* or *anxiety*. Tiredness may be due to a more serious condition, such as *anemia* or *cancer*, but in such cases there are usually also other symptoms.

Tissue

A collection of *cells* specialized to perform a particular function. Examples of tissues include muscle tissue, which consists of cells that are specialized to contract; epithelial tissue, which forms the *skin* and *mucous membranes* that line the respiratory and other internal tracts; nerve tissue, comprising cells specialized to conduct electrochemical nerve impulses; and *connective tissue*, which includes *adipose tissue* (fat), and the various fibrous and elastic tissues (such as tendons and cartilage) that hold the body together.

Tissue fluid

The watery liquid present in the tiny gaps between body cells, also known as interstitial fluid. Tissue fluid is one component of extracellular fluid (any body fluid outside the cells, including blood and lymph).

To reach cells, oxygen and nutrients must pass from the blood vessels and into the tissue fluid. Similarly, there is a reverse movement of carbon dioxide and other waste products from the cells into the tissue fluid, and then into the bloodstream.

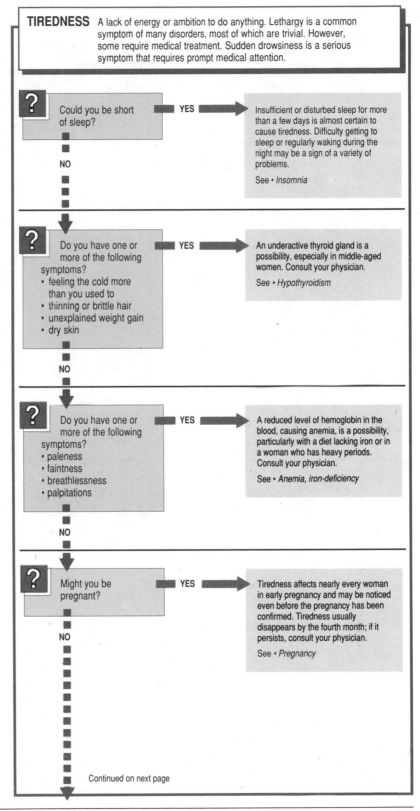

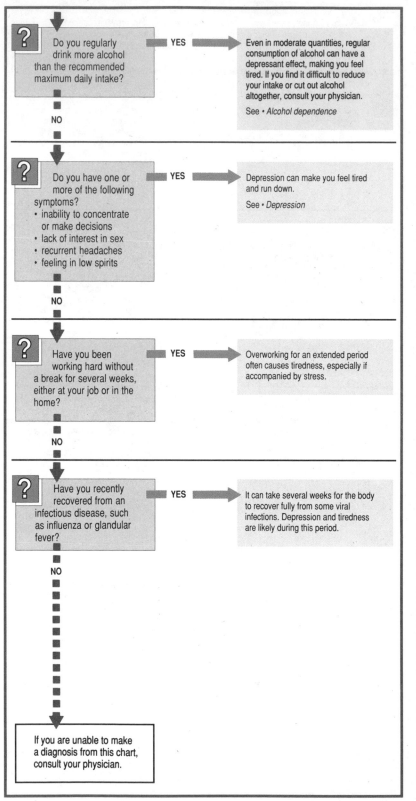

In addition to nutrients and wastes, tissue fluid also contains *ions*. This fluid contains a much higher level of sodium ions, and a much lower level of potassium ions, than intracellular fluid. It is this difference in ion levels that helps control the movement of water into and out of cells by *osmosis*; ion levels also play a role in the transmission of electrical impulses through nerves and muscles.

Tissue fluid is formed by the filtration of liquid out through the walls of the first part of blood capillaries (that is, the part nearest an arteriole), where it is forced out by the high blood pressure. In the last part of capillaries (nearest to a venule), blood pressure is much lower, and tissue fluid passes back into the capillaries; some tissue fluid is also drained away into the lymphatic vessels. Thus, there is a continual flow that keeps the amount of tissue fluid constant. Various disorders—such as *hypertension* (high blood pressure)—may disrupt the balance between formation and drainage of tissue fluid, leading to the accumulation of excess fluid in the tissues, a condition called *edema*.

Tissue-plasminogen activator

A substance produced by body tissues that prevents abnormal *blood clotting*. Also called TPA, it is produced in small amounts by the inner lining of blood vessels and by the muscular wall of the uterus.

DRUG THERAPY

TPA can be prepared artificially by *genetic engineering* techniques for use as a *thrombolytic drug* (a drug that dissolves blood clots). It is used in the treatment of *myocardial infarction* (heart attack), severe *angina pectoris* (chest pain caused by inadequate blood supply to the heart muscle), and arterial *embolism* (blockage of an artery), including *pulmonary embolism*.

HOW IT WORKS

Given by *intravenous infusion*, TPA dissolves blood clots by converting plasminogen (a chemical in the blood) to the enzyme plasmin. Plasmin in turn breaks down fibrin, the main constituent of blood clots.

POSSIBLE ADVERSE EFFECTS

Bleeding or the formation of a *hematoma* (collection of blood) may occur at the site of injection. TPA may also cause bleeding elsewhere but this can usually be controlled because TPA has a short-lived action. An allergic reaction to TPA may occur, but this is less likely than with other thrombolytic drugs. (See also *Fibrinolysis*.)

T

Tissue-typing

The classification of certain characteristics of the tissues of prospective organ donors and recipients.

WHY IT IS DONE

Tissue-typing is necessary to help match recipient and donor tissues for *transplant surgery*, thus minimizing the risk of rejection of a donor organ by the recipient's *immune system*.

The main features by which a person's immune system distinguishes his or her own tissues from those of other people are called *histocompatibility antigens*. Most important of these are the human leukocyte antigens (HLAs), which are present on the surface of human cells. A person's set of HLAs is inherited and unique to that person (except for identical twins, who have the same set). Hence, perfect tissue matching is achieved only between identical twins. Nevertheless, close relatives often have closely matching HLA types.

HOW IT IS DONE

A person's tissue-type, or HLA "fingerprint," is established by tests in the laboratory on cells from a sample of the person's blood. There are many different possible HLAs and the presence or absence of each must be tested individually. In one of the simpler methods, an *antiserum* containing *antibodies* (substances that react with a particular antigen—in this case, a particular HLA) is added to the test specimen. If the antigen is present, it is detected by an observable color or other change.

For organ transplantation, once a recipient has been tissue-typed, a selection is made of a donor whose HLA grouping best matches that of the recipient. This helps reduce the chances of *rejection*. It is easiest to find such donors among close relatives.

Titanium dental implants

See *Implants, dental*.

TMJ syndrome

See *Temporomandibular joint syndrome*.

Toadstool poisoning

See *Mushroom poisoning*.

Tobacco

 The dried leaf of the plant *NICOTIANA TABACUM*. Indigenous to America, the tobacco plant is now cultivated in many parts of the world. Tobacco is used for *tobacco smoking*, tobacco chewing, or as *snuff* by billions of people all over the world.

Tobacco contains a variable percentage of *nicotine*, which is a toxic chemical, and several carcinogenic (cancer-inducing) substances. There is a direct proportion between the amount of tobacco used, the period over which it is used, and the likelihood of cancer. Increased exposure to heavy concentrates of carcinogens in tobacco has been shown to result in an increased risk of tumor development in exposed tissues.

Tobacco smokers have an increased risk of *lung cancer, bladder cancer, kidney cancer*, and pancreatic cancer (see *Pancreas, cancer of*). All tobacco users have an increased risk of cancers of the oral cavity (see *Mouth cancer*), pharynx (see *Pharynx, cancer of*), larynx (see *Larynx, cancer of*) and esophagus (see *Esophagus, cancer of*). The majority of people with head and neck cancers have a history of heavy alcohol and tobacco use.

Tobacco smoking

Despite its practice in Western countries for more than 400 years—and for much longer in some other parts of the world—tobacco smoking has only relatively recently been accepted as a major health hazard. It is estimated that 20 percent of all deaths in developed countries are due to tobacco smoking.

CANCER DEATHS

Tobacco smoke contains 3,800 compounds; many are toxic and some are *carcinogenic*. About 30 percent of all cancer deaths can be attributed to smoking. In Canada, *lung cancer* kills about 12,250 men and 8,800 women each year, and the incidence of this cancer is still rising. Probably 90 percent of lung cancer is due to smoking. Because pipe and cigar smokers tend not to inhale tobacco smoke, they have a slightly lower risk of lung cancer, although the risk is still significantly greater than for nonsmokers. The risk of developing lung cancer begins to diminish as soon as smoking is stopped.

All forms of tobacco smoking increase the risk of cancer in other parts of the body—the bladder, the mouth, the lip, and the throat (see *Pharynx, cancer of*).

DISEASES OF THE HEART AND ARTERIES

The risk of *coronary artery disease* in a young man who smokes 20 cigarettes a day is about three times that of a nonsmoker, and the risk increases proportionally with the number of cigarettes smoked. *Coronary artery disease* causes 57,000 deaths in men and 32,000 deaths in women, and 30 percent of these are attributed to smoking. *Stroke* and *peripheral vascular disease* are also much more likely in smokers. (See also *Buerger's disease*.)

CHRONIC LUNG DISEASE

Most of the 100,000 Canadians who are disabled from chronic lung disease (see *Lung disease, chronic obstructive*) have been heavy smokers, and 85 percent of deaths from this cause are attributable to smoking.

SMOKING DURING PREGNANCY

Smoking is extremely harmful during pregnancy. Babies born to mothers who smoke are more likely to be premature, which means they have a lower survival rate than babies of nonsmoking mothers. Some studies have also shown that such babies are more likely to die in infancy than babies of mothers who do not smoke. The fetus is apparently very sensitive to the products of tobacco smoke in the mother's blood: even smoking 10 cigarettes a day may produce harmful effects on the fetus.

PASSIVE SMOKING

Nonsmokers often experience eye and nose irritation when exposed to tobacco smoke. Exhaled or environmental tobacco smoke contains not only smoke that the smoker has exhaled, but even more toxic "sidestream" smoke that escapes into the air without being inhaled. Legislation and public pressure have been directed against smoking in public places, but there is no convincing evidence that the levels or durations of exposure in public buildings are harmful to the occasional visitor.

The situation is very different in the home (where there is no legislation to protect the victims). Involuntary inhalation of tobacco smoke has been shown to cause or aggravate severe respiratory infections and chronic respiratory conditions such as asthma in children. There is some evidence that nonsmoking spouses of heavy smokers are at increased risk of lung cancer. Recent studies also have suggested that passive smokers have an increased risk of *coronary heart disease*.

HOW SMOKING CAUSES HARM

Tobacco contains a variety of noxious substances, but the dangers of three are particularly important.

Nicotine is the substance that causes addiction to tobacco. It acts as a tranquilizer, but also stimulates the release of *epinephrine* into the smoker's bloodstream, which may explain why some smokers are found to have raised blood pressure.

TOBACCO SMOKING

Some 50,000 deaths per year in Canada are attributed to smoking. The main harmful effects of smoking are respiratory diseases (lung cancer, bronchitis, and emphysema) and cardiovascular diseases (coronary artery disease and peripheral vascular disease).

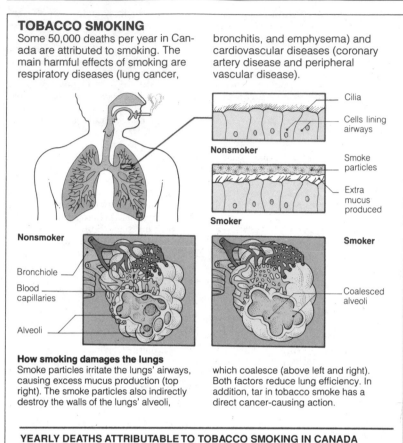

How smoking damages the lungs
Smoke particles irritate the lungs' airways, causing excess mucus production (top right). The smoke particles also indirectly destroy the walls of the lungs' alveoli, which coalesce (above left and right). Both factors reduce lung efficiency. In addition, tar in tobacco smoke has a direct cancer-causing action.

YEARLY DEATHS ATTRIBUTABLE TO TOBACCO SMOKING IN CANADA

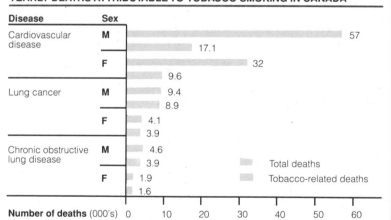

Disease	Sex	Value
Cardiovascular disease	M	57
		17.1
	F	32
		9.6
Lung cancer	M	9.4
		8.9
	F	4.1
		3.9
Chronic obstructive lung disease	M	4.6
		3.9
	F	1.9
		1.6

Total deaths
Tobacco-related deaths

Number of deaths (000's) 0 10 20 30 40 50 60

Major health hazards of smoking
This chart of the annual number of smoking-related deaths in Canada does not include other tobacco-related cancers —of the lips, tongue, pharynx, larynx, and bladder. Such cancers may account for several thousand additional tobacco-related deaths each year, most of them in men. Even though the proportion of smoking-related deaths from cardiovascular disease is much lower than that due to cancer and chronic lung disease, because cardiovascular disease is the commonest cause of death, smoking causes more unnecessary deaths from cardiovascular disease than all other causes combined. Of those at risk through exposure to others' smoke, young children are especially vulnerable: they may suffer chronic respiratory infections.

Tar in tobacco produces chronic irritation of the respiratory system and is thought to be a major cause of lung cancer.

Carbon monoxide passes from the lungs into the bloodstream, where, in competition with oxygen, it easily combines with *hemoglobin* and thus interferes with oxygenation of tissues. This reduces the activity of the muscles, causing fatigue and poor exercise tolerance.

STOPPING SMOKING

The most important prerequisite for stopping smoking is an absolute commitment to giving up the habit. Most successful "quitters" do so on their own, after one or several attempts. Almost always, stopping suddenly is the only way. A number of programs, both commercial and sponsored by health professionals, are offered. Success rates vary from 5 percent to 25 percent at the end of a year. Physicians have employed a number of methods such as acupuncture, hypnosis, self-reinforcement techniques, and chewing nicotine-containing gum with varying success.

Many smokers are concerned about weight gain after stopping smoking. Smoking inhibits the sense of smell and taste, and reduces appetite; the amount of weight a smoker will gain after quitting is much less harmful to health than the smoking habit. Many smokers will find a moderate exercise program will help them quit smoking and curb weight gain at the same time.

PREVENTION

In the 1960s, 53 percent of men and 32 percent of women smoked 66 billion cigarettes in Canada each year. Now, the figures are 30 percent, 25 percent, and 40 billion. Nevertheless, as domestic sales dwindle, tobacco companies are more than making up the deficit by promoting their toxic product to minorities and developing countries. Tobacco smoking threatens to become the world's most serious preventable health problem.

The best hope for reducing the health toll of smoking in the future lies in raising a "smoke-free generation" by increasing the social disapproval of smoking, making accurate and meaningful health information available to all, and restricting and eventually outlawing the promotion and sale of tobacco.

Tobramycin

An *antibiotic drug* used to treat *peritonitis, meningitis,* and severe infections of the lungs, skin, bones, and joints.

Tobramycin is given by injection, usually in combination with a *penicillin drug*. Eye drops containing tobramycin are sometimes used to treat *conjunctivitis* and *blepharitis* (inflammation of the eyelids).

High doses of tobramycin given by injection may cause kidney damage, deafness due to inner ear damage, nausea, vomiting, and headache. Any preparation that contains tobramycin may cause rash and itching.

Tocainide

An *antiarrhythmic drug* that is used to prevent and treat certain irregularities in the pattern of the heartbeat (see *Arrhythmia, cardiac*).

There is a high risk of adverse effects, including nausea, dizziness, tremor, loss of appetite, diarrhea, confusion, and hallucinations. Prolonged treatment may cause blood disorders such as *thrombocytopenia*.

Tocography

An obstetric procedure for recording muscular contractions of the uterus during *childbirth*. The procedure known as cardiotocography combines tocography with *fetal heart monitoring*.

Tocopherol

A constituent of *vitamin E*. Four tocopherols (alpha, beta, gamma, and delta) and several tocopherol derivatives together make up the substance known as vitamin E. Tocopherols are fat-soluble and occur in many foods. Dietary deficiency of tocopherols is extremely rare.

Todd's paralysis

Weakness in part of the body following some types of epileptic seizure (see *Epilepsy*). The weakness may last for minutes, hours, or occasionally days, but there is no lasting effect. The affected part of the body is usually a part that twitched during the seizure. Todd's paralysis is thought to be caused by damage to, or a tumor in, the motor cortex (the part of the *brain* that controls movement).

Toe

One of the digits of the foot. Each toe has three phalanges (bones), except for the hallux (big toe), which has two. The phalanges join at hinge joints, which are moved by muscle tendons that flex (bend) or extend (straighten) the toe. A small artery, vein, and nerve run down each side of the toe. The entire structure is enclosed in skin with a nail at the top.

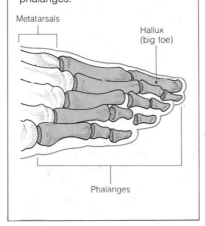

ANATOMY OF THE TOES
Each hallux, or big toe, has two bones called phalanges, which are connected by hinge joints. All the other toes have three phalanges.

Metatarsals

Hallux (big toe)

Phalanges

The main function of the toes is to maintain balance during walking. People without hands often learn to use their toes to perform tasks, typing and painting for example, which are usually performed with the fingers.

DISORDERS
Congenital disorders include *polydactyly* (extra toes), missing toes, *syndactyly* (fused toes), or *webbing* (skin flaps between the toes).

Injuries to the toes are fairly common, particularly bruises or fractures. Inflammation of one or several toe joints, causing stiffness, pain, swelling, and deformity, may be caused by *osteoarthritis*, *rheumatoid arthritis* or *gout*.

Infections may occur under the nail as a complication of an ingrowing toenail (see *Toenail, ingrown*; see also illustration on preventing ingrowth).

Impaired blood supply, usually due to *peripheral vascular disease* (narrowing of arteries in the legs), causes pain and blueness of the toes and can eventually lead to *gangrene*. Numbness and a pins and needles sensation in the toes may be caused by damage to peripheral nerves, which is common in *diabetes mellitus*.

A common deformity of the big toe is *hallux valgus*, in which the joint at the base projects outward while the top of the toe turns inward. Hallux valgus often results in a *bunion* (a firm, fluid-filled swelling over the joint). Abnormality of a tendon in one of the toes may cause the main joint to remain bent (see *Hammer toe*).

Toenail, ingrown

A painful condition of a toe (usually the big toe) in which one or both edges of the *nail* press into the adjacent skin, leading to infection and inflammation. The condition usually results from cutting the nail incorrectly, from wearing tight-fitting shoes, and from poor personal hygiene.

TREATMENT AND PREVENTION
Temporary relief from pain can be obtained by bathing the foot once or twice daily in a strong, warm, salt solution; after bathing, the nail should be covered with a dry gauze dressing. *Antibiotic drugs* may be given to control infection. In some cases, the edge of the affected nail is removed under local anesthesia.

Unless preventive measures are taken, the problem is likely to recur. The nail should be cut straight across to avoid exposing tender skin that easily becomes infected if a splinter of nail from the cut edge grows into it.

Toilet training

The process of teaching a young child to acquire complete bowel and bladder control and to make appropriate use of toilet facilities.

WHEN TO START
There is no reason to start toilet training until the child's nervous system is sufficiently mature. Up to the age of about 18 months, emptying of the bladder and bowel is a totally automatic reaction. The child is not yet able to connect the actions of defecation and urination with their results, and does not have the ability to control these actions at will.

At around 18 months, a child is able to indicate that he or she has passed urine or a bowel movement, but is not yet aware when he or she is about to do so. At this stage, the child is not quite ready to use the potty, but should become familiar with it, be told

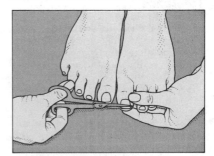

Preventing ingrown toenails
Cutting the toenails straight across does not damage the skin at the corners of the nails and helps to prevent ingrowing of the nails.

997

what it is for, and practice sitting on it. At around 24 months, the child becomes aware when he or she is about to pass urine or a bowel movement, and says so. At this stage, the child is ready to start using the potty.

USING THE POTTY AND TOILET
Toilet training should be approached in a relaxed, unhurried manner. The child may rebel if the potty is introduced too early or if he or she is forced to sit on it. If possible, wait until your child shows an interest in using the potty. Boys initially urinate sitting on the potty but soon learn to urinate standing up.

When the child has gained proficiency in using the potty, he or she should be introduced to the toilet. A useful intermediate step is to place the potty near the toilet. The child continues to use the potty for a while, but is taught to use toilet paper and to flush the toilet. When reasonable control has been achieved, the child can be taken out of diapers during the day. Diapers should be worn at night until the child is usually dry on waking.

Children differ in the age at which they become toilet trained and more so in the age at which they are dry both during the day and at night. A child is unlikely to be completely toilet trained or to be able to empty the bladder on demand before his or her third birthday. Toilet accidents, particularly wetting, are common up to the age of 5 because a young child can delay urination for only a few minutes after the initial urge to urinate. Some toilet trained children may revert to soiling or wetting when anxious or under stress. (See also *Encopresis; Enuresis; Soiling*.)

Tolbutamide
An oral hypoglycemic drug (see *Hypoglycemics, oral*).

Tolerance
The need to take increasingly higher doses of a *drug* to attain the same physical or mental effect. Tolerance develops after taking a drug over a period of time and usually results either from the liver becoming more efficient at breaking down the drug or from the body tissues becoming less sensitive to it.

The most familiar example of tolerance occurs in heavy drinkers who become so tolerant of *alcohol* that they are capable of drinking amounts that would render occasional drinkers unconscious. (See also *Alcohol dependence; Drug dependence*.)

Tolmetin
A *nonsteroidal anti-inflammatory drug* (NSAID) used to relieve pain, stiffness, and inflammation in *osteoarthritis, rheumatoid arthritis*, and *ankylosing spondylitis*. Tolmetin is also given to treat pain caused by minor injuries.

Tolnaftate
An *antifungal drug* used to treat and sometimes to prevent the recurrence of types of *tinea*, including *athlete's foot*. Tolnaftate, which is available over-the-counter as a cream, may in rare cases cause skin irritation or rash.

Tomography
An *imaging technique* that produces a cross-sectional image ("slice") of an organ or part of the body.

In *X-ray* tomography, the X-ray machine and film are positioned so that tissue is in focus at one depth only. All background and foreground structures appear blurred. By taking a series of tomograms it is possible to build an outline image of a part of the body which, on an ordinary X-ray film, would be hidden by other structures. Tomography is often used to obtain a clear outline of the kidneys during intravenous *urography*, when the kidneys would otherwise be obscured by gas or fecal matter.

Most tomography today is performed using computed techniques (see *CT scanning*), which produce images that are extremely accurate and highly detailed.

-tomy
A suffix denoting the operation of cutting or making an incision, as in thoracotomy, a surgical operation in which the thorax (chest) is opened.

Tone, muscle
The natural tension in the fibers of a *muscle*. At rest, all muscle fibers are maintained in a state of partial contraction by nerve impulses from the spinal cord. This resting muscle tone helps control posture, keeps the eyes open, and allows muscles to contract more efficiently.

Abnormally high muscle tone causes *spasticity*, rigidity, and an increased resistance to movement. Abnormally low muscle tone causes floppiness of the body part (see *Hypotonia; Hypotonia in infants*).

Tongue
A muscular, flexible organ occupying the floor of the *mouth* and important for taste, speaking, and eating.

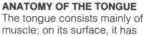

ANATOMY OF THE TONGUE
The tongue consists mainly of muscle; on its surface, it has various types of papillae that contain the taste buds.

Vallate papillae   Epiglottis

Fungiform papillae

Filiform papillae

STRUCTURE AND FUNCTION
The tongue is composed of a mass of muscles covered by *mucous membrane*. These muscles are attached to the mandible (lower jaw) and to the hyoid bone above the larynx. Minute nodules called papillae project from the upper surface of the tongue, giving it a rough texture. Situated between the papillae at the sides and base of the tongue are minute sensory organs called taste buds, which are responsible for the sense of *taste*.

As well as being the organ of taste, the tongue is essential for *mastication* (chewing), *swallowing*, and *speech*.

DISORDERS
A large tongue is a feature of *Down's syndrome, cretinism*, and *acromegaly*. Temporary enlargement of the tongue as a result of swelling and inflammation occurs in *glossitis*.

Fissures on the tongue are common and usually cause no trouble, but in some cases they are so deep that food particles collect in them, causing discomfort. Unnatural smoothness of the tongue, accompanied by redness and soreness, is a feature of pernicious anemia (See *Anemia, megaloblastic*), iron-deficiency anemia (see *Anemia, iron-deficiency*), *syphilis*, and *glossitis*.

In rare cases, the papillae on the tongue become elongated and turn black or brown, a condition known as

T

black tongue. This disorder, of which the cause is unknown, is harmless but persistent. The unsightly discoloration can be removed by cleaning the tongue twice a day with a soft toothbrush dipped in an antiseptic mouthwash.

The tongue can be a site for *mouth ulcers* and *leukoplakia* (thickened white or gray patches), a condition that occasionally becomes cancerous (see *Tongue cancer*). Any ulcer or lump on the tongue that does not disappear within about three weeks should be reported to a physician because of the risk of cancer.

Tongue cancer

The most serious type of *mouth cancer* because of its rapid spread. Tongue cancer is one of the two most common types of mouth cancer (the other being *lip cancer*). Cancer of the tongue mainly affects people over 40. This form of cancer is usually associated with tobacco smoking and heavy consumption of alcohol, particularly liquor; poor oral hygiene is commonly also a contributing factor.

SYMPTOMS AND SIGNS
The edge of the tongue is most commonly affected. The first sign may be a small ulcer with a raised margin, a white patch of thickened tissue known as *leukoplakia*, a deep fissure with hard edges, or a raised, hardened mass. Pain is rare until the cancer is advanced, when there is also excessive salivation, stiffness of the tongue, difficulty in swallowing, and, in some cases, offensive breath.

The tumor may become very large, obstructing the throat and occasionally causing asphyxia. Tongue cancer spreads rapidly to any or all of the following: the gums, the lower jaw, and the lymph nodes in the floor of the mouth and the neck.

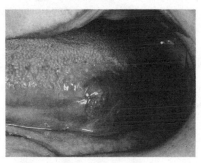

Appearance of tongue cancer
The cancer often starts at the edge of the tongue. It may appear (as here) as a raised mass, as a fissure, or as an ulcer.

DIAGNOSIS AND TREATMENT
Any physical change in the tongue that does not clear up within about three weeks should be reported to a physician. Cancer is diagnosed by means of a tongue *biopsy* (the removal of a small sample of tissue for microscopic examination).

Small tumors, especially those at the tip of the tongue, are usually removed surgically. Larger tumors or tumors that have spread often require *radiation therapy*. If a tumor is very large and has spread to affect the lymph nodes, the surgeon may remove the whole tongue, the lymph nodes, and sometimes the lower jaw, although *anticancer drugs* and occasional radiation therapy may reduce the need for such drastic surgery.

Unless the cancer is detected very early, its spread makes the outlook poor. In about half of all sufferers, the lymph nodes are involved by the time of diagnosis. About half of affected women but only a quarter of men survive for five years or more.

Tongue depressor

A flat wooden or metal instrument for holding down the tongue against the floor of the mouth to allow examination of the back of the throat.

Tongue-tie

A minor defect of the *mouth*, also called ankyloglossia, in which the frenulum (the band of tissue attaching the underside of the *tongue* to the floor of the mouth) is too short and extends forward to the tip of the tongue. There are usually no symptoms other than limited movement of the tongue. In rare cases, the condition causes a speech defect, in which case a minor operation is required to divide the frenulum.

Tonic

One of a diverse group of remedies intended to relieve symptoms such as malaise, lethargy, and loss of appetite. Most tonics contain herbal extracts, vitamins, and minerals. Medical evidence suggests that tonics mainly have a *placebo* effect.

The term tonic is also used adjectivally to relate to muscle tone (see *Tone, muscle*), as in the tonic neck reflex, one of the primitive *reflexes* occurring in newborn babies.

Tonometry

The procedure for measuring the pressure of the fluid within the *eye*. A rise in intraocular pressure is one of the signs of *glaucoma*. Tonometry is usually performed by an ophthalmologist during an eye examination (see *Eye, examination of*).

HOW IT IS DONE
The standard method of measuring pressure in the eye is called applanation tonometry. The ophthalmologist applies a drop of quick-acting anesthetic and a trace of *fluorescein* to each cornea; he or she then measures the pressure within the eye by means of a tonometer (measuring device) mounted on a *slit lamp* (light source with a magnifying viewer). The head of the tonometer is illuminated and touched gently against the anesthetized cornea. A visible circle of fluorescein-stained tear film is formed, which the ophthalmologist views through the slit lamp microscope. The force with which the tonometer head is pressed against the cornea is gradually increased until the area of the circle reaches a fixed standard. The force needed to achieve this degree of corneal flattening is a measure of the pressure within the eye.

Tonsil

A pair of oval tissue masses at the back of the throat. The tonsils are made up of lymphoid tissue and form part of the *lymphatic system*, which is an important part of the body's defense against infection. Along with the *adenoids* at the base of the tongue, the

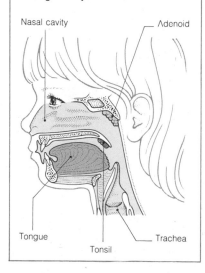

LOCATION OF THE TONSILS
The tonsils can be easily seen on either side of the back of the throat. They reach maximum size at about the age of 7 years and then shrink.

Nasal cavity

Adenoid

Tongue

Tonsil

Trachea

T

tonsils protect against upper *respiratory tract infections*. The tonsils gradually enlarge from birth, reach their maximum size at about 7 years of age, and then shrink substantially.

Tonsillitis (inflammation of the tonsils) is a common childhood infection. Rarely, *quinsy* may develop.

Tonsillectomy

Surgical removal of the *tonsils*.

WHY IT IS DONE

Tonsillectomy was once a common childhood operation; it is now performed only if a child suffers frequent recurrent attacks of severe *tonsillitis*. Less common problems that may necessitate the operation are *quinsy* (an abscess around the tonsil) or a single tonsil growing larger or becoming deeply ulcerated and therefore coming under suspicion of being malignant. In rare cases, removal of the tonsils may be advised for adolescents or young adults suffering from recurrent bouts of tonsillitis.

HOW IT IS DONE

The operative technique is shown in the illustrated box.

RECOVERY PERIOD

In the first 24 hours after the operation there may be bleeding from the throat; the patient must lie on his or her side to avoid choking and to allow bleeding to be detected. Postoperative pain

---

PROCEDURE FOR TONSILLECTOMY

Tonsillectomy is most commonly carried out around the age of 6 or 7. The adenoids may be removed at the same time.

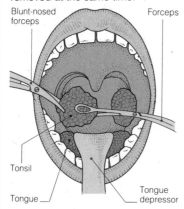

Blunt-nosed forceps

Forceps

Tonsil

Tongue

Tongue depressor

Standard technique

With the patient under a general anesthetic, the tongue is depressed and the tonsils prised from the back of the throat and then cut away.

---

in the throat and sometimes the ears is common and may require an *analgesic drug* (painkiller). Fluids and soft, easily swallowed foods such as ice cream are usually given for a day or two until the patient can eat normally.

Sore throat, particularly at mealtimes, may persist for up to two weeks after the operation. Full recovery usually takes place within three weeks. In some people, bleeding occurs a week or so after the operation, requiring medical attention and possible readmission to hospital.

Tonsillitis

Inflammation of the *tonsils* due to infection. Tonsillitis mainly occurs in childhood, most children suffering at least one attack.

CAUSES AND INCIDENCE

The function of the tonsils is to help protect against upper *respiratory tract infection*. Sometimes, however, the tonsils themselves become repeatedly infected by the microorganisms they fight. Tonsillitis is most common in children under the age of 9; it also occurs infrequently in adolescents and young adults.

SYMPTOMS AND SIGNS

The main symptoms are a sore throat and difficulty in swallowing (very young children may refuse to eat). The throat is visibly inflamed. Other common symptoms are fever, headache, earache, enlarged and tender lymph nodes in the neck, and unpleasant-smelling breath. Occasionally, the illness causes temporary deafness or *quinsy* (an abscess around the tonsil). If symptoms persist for more than 24 hours or if pus can be seen on the tonsils, a physician should be consulted.

TREATMENT

Tonsillitis is treated with bed rest, plenty of fluids, and an *analgesic drug* (painkiller), such as *acetaminophen*. In some cases, *antibiotic drugs* may also be prescribed.

Tooth abscess

See *Abscess, dental*.

Toothache

Pain coming from one or more *teeth* and sometimes also from the *gums*, felt as a dull throb or a sharp twinge.

CAUSES

Early dental *caries* (decay) may cause mild toothache when eating sweet or very hot or cold food. More advanced decay or, less commonly, a fracture in a tooth (see *Fracture, dental*) or a deep, unlined filling (see *Filling, dental*) may

result in inflammation of the pulp. This usually causes sharp, stabbing pain, which is often worse when the sufferer is lying down.

If the inflammation spreads, periapical *periodontitis* (inflammation of supporting tissues around the root tip) may develop, causing localized pain that is brought on mainly by biting and chewing. A dental abscess (see *Abscess, dental*) may also occur. In this case, pain is severe and often continuous, the gum surrounding the affected tooth is tender and swollen, and there may be swelling of the face and neck accompanied by fever.

Chronic periodontitis, which affects all the supporting tissues around the tooth and which causes the gums to recede, results in aching around exposed tooth roots when hot, cold, or sweet food is eaten. Gums around the affected teeth are tender and swollen.

A filling that is not quite level or a blow to a tooth may also result in inflammation of supporting tissues, causing pain when biting.

Sometimes toothache is not caused by a disorder of the teeth or gums. For example, in *sinusitis* (inflammation of the mucous membrane lining the facial air cavities) pain may be referred to the upper molar and premolar teeth (see *Referred pain*).

TREATMENT

Analgesic drugs (painkillers) may provide temporary relief until a visit to the dentist can be arranged. An emergency appointment should be made if the symptoms suggest there is an abscess. The treatment carried out by the dentist depends on the underlying cause of the toothache.

Toothbrushing

Cleaning of the *teeth* with a brush to remove plaque and food particles from tooth surfaces, and to stimulate the *gums*.

Toothbrushing should be carried out at least once a day using a fluoride *dentifrice* (usually toothpaste); children should brush their teeth after every meal and at bedtime. For complete *oral hygiene*, flossing (see *Floss, dental*) should be performed daily.

A safe and effective toothbrush for general use has an easily gripped handle and soft, round-ended or polished bristles. The size and shape of the head of the brush must allow every tooth to be reached; children need a smaller toothbrush than adults. Toothbrushes should be rinsed after each use and replaced as soon as the

T

BASIC TOOTHBRUSHING

Efficient toothbrushing is essential for the preservation of the teeth and the health of the gums. The enemy is plaque, a mixture of food debris, dried saliva, and bacteria, which develops at the gum margins and leads to caries (tooth decay) and gum disease.

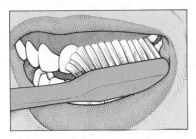

1 With the bristle tips set at 45 degrees to the plane of the teeth, scrub gently along the gum line using short strokes. The bristle tips should do the work.

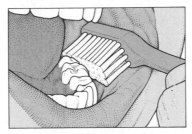

2 Keep the bristles angled against the line of the gums and work over the outer and inner surfaces of the upper and lower teeth. Keep the strokes short.

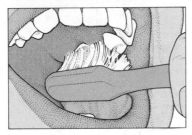

3 Don't forget to scrub over the chewing surfaces of all four sets of premolar and molar teeth. Move slowly over the surfaces, cleaning each tooth in turn.

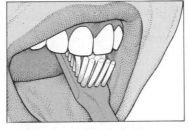

4 Remember to brush the inside surfaces of the front teeth. Hold the brush almost vertical and scrub with an up-and-down movement.

bristles become frayed or bent. Interspace brushes, which have small, round heads, are useful for cleaning around *bridges* and fixed *orthodontic appliances*.

Electric toothbrushes are also available and may make brushing easier for people suffering from certain physical disabilities.

Tooth decay
See *Caries, dental.*

Tooth extraction
See *Extraction, dental.*

Toothpaste
See *Dentifrice.*

Tophus
A collection of *uric acid* crystals deposited in the tissues, especially around joints (such as the elbow) but occasionally in other places (such as the ear). A tophus is a sign of *hyperuricemia*, which accompanies *gout*. Tophi may occasionally ulcerate and discharge chalky white material.

Topical
A term describing a *drug* that is applied to the surface of the body, as opposed to being swallowed or injected. Topical refers not only to drugs applied to the skin, but also to those administered into the ear canal, onto the surface of the eye, or as suppositories into the vagina or rectum.

Torsion
A term that means twisting. Almost any structure that is relatively free to move in the body may become twisted, such as the intestine (see *Volvulus*), the spermatic cord from the testis (see *Testis, torsion of*), or a *cyst* on a stalk. One of the principal dangers of torsion is obstruction of the blood supply to the affected part; if this occurs, pain is usually the first symptom. If the torsion is not corrected, tissue death may develop.

Torticollis
Twisting of the neck, causing the head to be rotated and tilted into an abnormal position, in which it remains.

Also known as wry neck, torticollis is often accompanied by pain and stiffness in the neck.

CAUSES
The condition usually results from a minor neck injury that causes irritation of cervical nerves and consequent spasm of neck muscles. Torticollis may also result from muscle spasm caused by sleeping in an awkward position or by anxiety. Injury to a neck muscle at birth can also cause torticollis, as can a burn or other injury that has resulted in heavy scarring and contracture (shrinkage) of the skin.

TREATMENT
Treatment for torticollis due to muscle spasm may include wearing an orthopedic collar (see *Collar, orthopedic*), heat treatment, ultrasound treatment, or *physiotherapy*. When the cause is an injury arising from birth, the muscle is gently stretched several times each day; occasionally, an operation is required to cut the lower end of the muscle. Skin contracture may be treated by *Z-plasty*, which relieves tension in the scar tissue.

Touch
The sense by which certain characteristics of objects, such as their size, shape, temperature, and surface texture, can be ascertained through physical contact. Many types of touch *receptors* are present in the skin. In hairy skin areas, some of the receptors consist of webs of sensory nerve cell endings wrapped around the hair bulbs. These are triggered if the hairs are moved. Other receptors are more common in nonhairy areas of the body, such as the lips and fingertips; these receptors consist of nerve cell endings that may be free or surrounded by bulblike structures.

Signals from touch receptors pass, via sensory nerves, to the spinal cord, from there to the thalamus in the

T

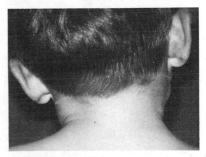

Child with torticollis
The muscles on one side of the neck have gone into spasm, pulling the head over to that side and causing pain.

THE SENSE OF TOUCH

The skin contains many thousands of specialized cells that respond to external stimuli, such as touch, heat, cold, and pressure. These cells (receptors) are divided into two types. One type of receptor consists only of a thin nerve fiber, which may wrap around an individual hair and respond to its movement. The other type has a specialized structure, known as an end organ, surrounding the nerve ending. Some skin receptors consist of several layers of cells attached to one nerve fiber. Others contain several nerve fibers arranged in a loop or coil. Probably several varieties of receptors play a part in each touch modality.

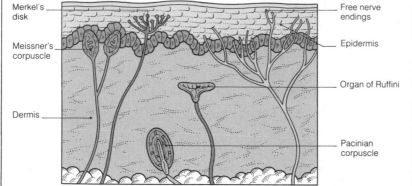

Merkel's disk

Meissner's corpuscle

Dermis

Free nerve endings

Epidermis

Organ of Ruffini

Pacinian corpuscle

Skin receptors

These receptors vary from free nerve endings to corpuscular or bulblike structures. Individual receptors do not seem to be associated exclusively with any one touch sensation (e.g., cold or pain).

Delicate touch
The ability to detect light contact between an object and the skin. Areas with more receptors are more sensitive.

Pain
Pain warns the brain about possible injury from an external stimulus and can trigger a reflex withdrawal.

Heat
Some free nerve endings respond specifically to heat. The skin of the wrist is good for testing temperature.

Cold
Cold on the skin is detected by specialized end organs. Extreme cold also stimulates pain receptors.

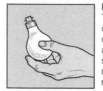

Pressure
A change in pressure on the skin is detected by specialized end organs called pacinian corpuscles.

TOUCH PERCEPTION

General sensations from various parts of the body are perceived at specific points within the brain's cerebral cortex. Highly sensitive body parts, such as the lips and hands, are represented by correspondingly large regions within the cortex.

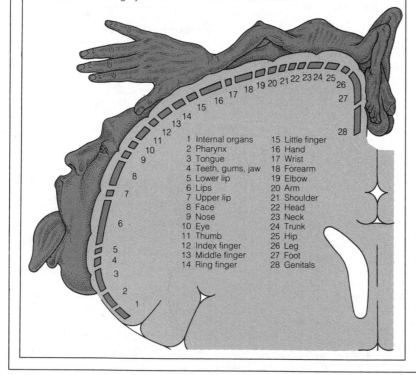

1 Internal organs
2 Pharynx
3 Tongue
4 Teeth, gums, jaw
5 Lower lip
6 Lips
7 Upper lip
8 Face
9 Nose
10 Eye
11 Thumb
12 Index finger
13 Middle finger
14 Ring finger
15 Little finger
16 Hand
17 Wrist
18 Forearm
19 Elbow
20 Arm
21 Shoulder
22 Head
23 Neck
24 Trunk
25 Hip
26 Leg
27 Foot
28 Genitals

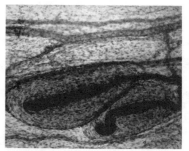

Pacinian corpuscle
These receptors are 1 mm to 4 mm long and occur in hairless areas of skin, especially the fingers.

T

brain, and on to the *sensory cortex*, where touch sensations are perceived and interpreted.

According to the number and distribution of receptors, the various parts of the body differ in their sensitivity to painful stimuli and in touch discrimination (the ability to distinguish between a single pinprick and two pinpricks placed slightly apart). For example, the cornea is several hundred times more sensitive to painful stimuli than are the soles of the feet. The fingertips are remarkably good at touch discrimination but in comparison relatively insensitive to painful stimuli.

Touch sense becomes much more developed in people deprived of other senses, particularly blind people; it is this capacity for touch development that is used by systems such as *braille*. (See also *Sensation*.)

Tourette's syndrome

See *Gilles de la Tourette's syndrome*.

Tourniquet

A device placed around a limb to compress blood vessels. A tourniquet may be used to help locate a vein for an intravenous injection or for the withdrawal of blood. By preventing blood from flowing back to the heart, a tourniquet causes veins in the limb below it to swell and become prominent.

An inflatable tourniquet, called an *Esmarch's bandage*, is used to control blood flow in some limb operations. An inflatable tourniquet also forms part of a *sphygmomanometer*, an instrument for measuring *blood pressure*.

Tourniquets have caused more problems than they have solved. In the past, they were used as a first aid measure to stop severe bleeding. This use is now discouraged because leaving a tourniquet in place for too long can cause *gangrene* (tissue death). First aid courses now teach the control of bleeding by pressure over the bleeding site (see *Pressure points*).

Toxemia

The presence in the bloodstream of *toxins* (poisons) produced by *bacteria*. Toxemia may be a feature of *septicemia* (the spread and multiplication of bacteria within the bloodstream from a localized site of infection), but it can also occur without any evidence of bacteria in the blood. Toxemia with or without septicemia is sometimes called blood poisoning.

Toxemia may cause symptoms such as a fever and headache and other symptoms specific to the particular toxin (e.g., muscle spasms caused by the toxin released by *tetanus* bacteria). Toxemia can lead to the very dangerous condition of *septic shock*, in which there is widespread tissue damage and a drop in blood pressure.

Treatment of toxemia is as for septicemia and septic shock—*antibiotic drugs*, removal of a localized site of infection if one can be found, and measures to treat shock, including *intravenous infusions*. For some types of toxemia, an *antitoxin* may be given. (See also *Toxemia of pregnancy; Toxic shock syndrome*.)

Toxemia of pregnancy

A disorder of pregnant women characterized by raised blood pressure, tissue swelling, and leakage of protein from the kidneys into the urine (see *Preeclampsia*). If severe, toxemia of pregnancy may progress to seizures and coma (see *Eclampsia*). Toxemia of pregnancy has some features common to other forms of *toxemia*, but no toxin has ever been identified.

Toxicity

The property of being poisonous. The term is also used to refer to the severity of adverse effects or illness produced by a *toxin* (a poisonous protein produced by certain bacteria, animals, or plants), by a *poison*, or by a drug overdose (see *Drug poisoning*).

Toxicology

The study of *poisons*, including their chemical composition, preparation, identification, effects on the body, and, where appropriate, their antidotes. (See also *Poisoning*.)

Toxic shock syndrome

An uncommon severe illness caused by a *toxin* produced by the bacterium *STAPHYLOCOCCUS AUREUS*. Toxic shock syndrome was first recognized in the late 1970s and many cases were diagnosed in young women in the early 1980s, particularly in the US. About 70 percent of cases occur in women who are using vaginal tampons at the time of onset.

Overgrowth of *STAPHYLOCOCCUS AUREUS* bacteria in the vagina and increased production of the toxin they produce have been associated with prolonged use of certain brands of tampons. These brands of highly absorbent tampons have now been taken off the market.

Of the cases that do not occur in association with menstruation, some have been linked to use of a contraceptive cap, diaphragm, or sponge. Other cases arise from skin wounds or infections caused by *STAPHYLOCOCCUS AUREUS* elsewhere in the body.

SYMPTOMS

The onset of toxic shock syndrome is sudden, with high fever, vomiting, diarrhea, headache, muscular aches and pains, dizziness, and disorientation. A skin rash resembling sunburn develops on the palms and soles, and peels within one or two weeks. The blood pressure may fall dangerously low, and *shock* may develop.

Other serious complications of this condition include *kidney failure* and *liver failure*. The mortality rate for toxic shock syndrome is about 3 percent. Death usually occurs as a result of a prolonged fall in blood pressure or because of lung complications.

TREATMENT

Treatment is with *antibiotic drugs*. *Intravenous infusion* may be necessary to treat shock, and more treatment may be needed for complications.

Recurrence is common; women who have had toxic shock syndrome are advised not to use tampons, caps, diaphragms, or sponges.

Toxin

A poisonous protein produced by pathogenic (disease-causing) bacteria, such as *CLOSTRIDIUM TETANI*, which causes *tetanus*; various animals, notably venomous snakes (see *Snakebites*); or certain plants, such as the death cap mushroom *AMANITA PHALLOIDES* (see *Mushroom poisoning*).

Bacterial toxins are sometimes subdivided into three categories: *endotoxins*, which are released only from the inside of dead bacteria; *exotoxins*, which are released from the surface of live bacteria; and *enterotoxins*, which inflame the intestine. (See also *Poison; Poisoning; Toxemia*.)

Toxocariasis

 An infestation of humans, usually children, with the larvae of *TOXOCARA CANIS*, a small, threadlike worm that lives in the intestines of dogs. The disease is also sometimes known as visceral larva migrans.

CAUSES AND INCIDENCE

The causes and course of an infestation are shown in the illustrated box on the next page.

PREVENTION

Dogs that live with children should be dewormed monthly until the dog is 6 months old, and then annually.

ORIGINS OF TOXOCARIASIS

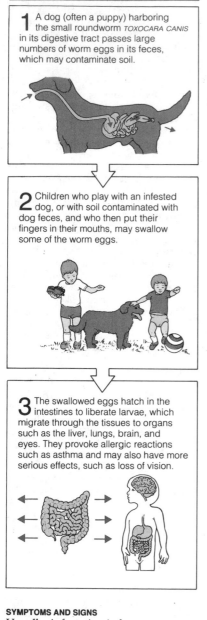

1 A dog (often a puppy) harboring the small roundworm *TOXOCARA CANIS* in its digestive tract passes large numbers of worm eggs in its feces, which may contaminate soil.

2 Children who play with an infested dog, or with soil contaminated with dog feces, and who then put their fingers in their mouths, may swallow some of the worm eggs.

3 The swallowed eggs hatch in the intestines to liberate larvae, which migrate through the tissues to organs such as the liver, lungs, brain, and eyes. They provoke allergic reactions such as asthma and may also have more serious effects, such as loss of vision.

SYMPTOMS AND SIGNS
Usually, infestation in humans causes only mild fever and malaise, which soon clears up. However, following some cases of heavy infestation, *pneumonia* and *seizures* may develop. Another possible complication is loss of vision, which may occur if a larva enters the eye and dies there.

DIAGNOSIS AND TREATMENT
Toxocariasis is diagnosed from sputum (phlegm) analysis, and by a *liver biopsy* (removal of a small sample of the organ for analysis).

Severe cases of toxocariasis require treatment in hospital, where the patient may be given *thiabendazole* (an *anthelmintic drug*) to control the infestation, and an *anticonvulsant drug* to control seizures.

Toxoid
An inactivated bacterial *toxin* (poisonous protein). Inactivation, usually by heat or chemicals, removes the toxicity of the toxin but preserves its property of stimulating antibody production by the *immune system*. Certain toxoids are used to immunize against specific diseases, *diphtheria* or *tetanus* for example.

Toxoplasmosis
An infection of mammals, birds, and reptiles that is also common in humans. Toxoplasmosis usually produces no ill effects except when it is transmitted by a pregnant woman to her unborn child or in people who have an *immunodeficiency disorder*, such as *AIDS*.

CAUSES AND INCIDENCE
The infection is caused by the protozoan (single-celled microorganism) *TOXOPLASMA GONDII*. Humans are most commonly infected by eating undercooked meat from infected animals. An estimated 25 percent of pork and 10 percent of lamb eaten by humans contains toxoplasma organisms. The protozoa also multiply in the intestines of cats, and about 1 percent of cats excrete cysts containing toxoplasma eggs in their feces. Infection in humans can occur through failure to wash the hands after handling the cat or its feces.

Toxoplasmosis contracted by a woman during pregnancy is transmitted to the child in about one third of cases, often with severe effects. Infection is extremely common worldwide. However, recognized illness or effects on the fetus are rare in Canada.

SYMPTOMS AND SIGNS
In most cases, the body's *immune system* provides adequate protection against the protozoa, so that the infection produces no symptoms. In some people with a normal immune system, however, the infection causes a feverish illness resembling infectious *mononucleosis*. It may also cause retinitis (inflammation of the retina) and *choroiditis* (inflammation of the blood vessels behind the retina).

Infection of an unborn child during early pregnancy may result in miscarriage or stillbirth. Infants may have enlargement of the liver and spleen, *hydrocephalus*, blindness, mental retardation, and may die during infancy. Infection in late pregnancy usually has no ill effects. Toxoplasmosis may also take a severe course in people with an immunodeficiency disorder, causing lung and heart damage and severe *encephalitis*.

DIAGNOSIS AND TREATMENT
The diagnosis is made from *blood tests*. Treatment is necessary only in pregnant women, in children born with severe symptoms, in people with an immune system deficiency, and in cases of retinitis or choroiditis. Treatment is usually with the antimalarial drug *pyrimethamine* combined with a *sulfonamide drug*.

TPA
The abbreviation for *tissue-plasminogen activator*.

Trabeculectomy
A surgical procedure performed to reduce pressure in the *eye*. Trabeculectomy is used to control *glaucoma* when medication cannot keep the intraocular pressure within safe limits or when, despite medical treatment, loss of *visual field* due to damage to the *optic nerve* is progressing.

Trabeculectomy creates an alternative outlet from the eye for aqueous humor (fluid in the front chamber of the eye) so that a better balance is achieved between the rate of secretion of aqueous humor and its rate of outflow. In this way, the pressure can be kept within normal limits and further damage to the optic nerve fibers is reduced.

HOW IT IS DONE
The *conjunctiva* (mucous membrane covering the front of the eyeball) above the upper edge of the *cornea* is opened and a half-thickness flap of *sclera* (white of the eye) is cut and folded forward. A small rectangle is removed from the inner layer at the scleral-corneal junction, so that a connection is made into the front chamber of the eye. The outer flap is replaced and secured with delicate stitches and the conjunctiva closed over it.

Trace elements
A group of *minerals* that are required in the diet only in minute amounts to maintain health. The principal trace elements include *chromium, copper, selenium,* and *zinc*. Although only tiny amounts are needed, they are vital to numerous chemical processes in the body. (See also *Nutrition*.)

Tracer

A radioactive substance introduced into the body so that its distribution, processing, and elimination from the body can be monitored (by using a radiation detector). For example, radioactive iodine may be used as a tracer to study the functioning of the thyroid gland.

Trachea

The anatomical name for the windpipe. The trachea begins immediately below the *larynx* (voice box) and runs down the center of the front of the neck to end behind the upper part of the sternum (breastbone), where it divides to form the two main *bronchi*.

The trachea consists of fibrous and elastic tissue and smooth muscle. It also contains about 20 rings of cartilage, which help keep the trachea open even during extremes of neck movement. The lining of the trachea includes cells that secrete mucus (called goblet cells) and other cells that bear minute, hairlike cilia. The mucus helps trap tiny particles in inhaled air; the beating of the cilia moves the mucus upward and out of the respiratory tract, thereby helping to keep the *lungs* and airways free.

DISORDERS

One of the most common disorders is *tracheitis* (inflammation of the lining of the trachea), which is usually caused by an infection (often by a virus) and is frequently associated with *bronchitis* or *laryngitis*. The principal symptoms are difficult, painful breathing and a harsh cough.

Obstruction of the trachea by an inhaled foreign object is rare because the narrowest part of the upper respiratory tract is the larynx, and any objects that pass through it usually continue through the trachea into a bronchus. However, the trachea may become obstructed by a tumor or narrowed as a result of scarring caused by the prolonged presence of a *tracheostomy* tube inserted to create an artificial airway through the front of the neck. Tracheal obstruction results in breathlessness and the condition produces a loud, harsh, vibrating sound during breathing.

Rarely, a congenital malformation occurs in which a channel forms between the trachea and the esophagus, situated immediately behind it (a condition called a *tracheoesophageal fistula*).

The trachea is sometimes injured by a direct blow or by strangulation. The seriousness of such an injury depends on the extent to which the airway is obstructed. In extreme cases, the trachea may collapse completely, which may be rapidly fatal unless an emergency tracheostomy is performed to reestablish an airway.

Tracheitis

Inflammation of the *trachea* (the windpipe). Tracheitis is usually caused by a viral infection and aggravated by inhaled fumes, especially tobacco smoke. It often occurs with *laryngitis* and *bronchitis*, a condition known as laryngotracheobronchitis, which is the most common cause of *croup* in young children.

Typical symptoms of tracheitis include a dry cough and hoarseness. In most cases, the condition is of short duration and requires no treatment.

Tracheoesophageal fistula

A rare *birth defect* in which an abnormal passage connects the *trachea* (windpipe) with the *esophagus*. About three babies per 10,000 are born with a tracheoesophageal fistula. In the most common form, the lower end of the esophagus connects with the trachea, and the upper end of the esophagus is underdeveloped, forming a blind-ending pouch.

SYMPTOMS AND SIGNS

The affected baby cannot swallow saliva and as a result drools constantly. During feeding, food is regurgitated and enters the lungs, causing the baby to choke, cough, and sometimes turn blue because of lack of oxygen. The abdomen becomes swollen because inhaled air passes into the stomach through the fistula. The acidic fluid in the stomach passes up into the lungs through the fistula, leading to *pneumonia* and *atelectasis* (lung collapse).

DIAGNOSIS AND TREATMENT

In most cases the condition is discovered soon after birth. Milder forms of tracheoesophageal fistula may not be detected until childhood or even adult life, usually after recurrent attacks of pneumonia. The diagnosis may be confirmed by *chest X ray* and other radiological studies.

Treatment consists of an operation to close the fistula and to connect the trachea and esophagus correctly. Before the 1940s, the condition was untreatable; today the survival rate is about 90 percent.

Tracheostomy

A surgical opening in the *trachea* and insertion of a tube to maintain an effective airway.

WHY IT IS DONE

Tracheostomy may be performed to treat an emergency or as a planned procedure. Today, acute airway problems are usually handled by an *endotracheal tube* passed via the mouth or nose. A tracheostomy is preferable, however, for the emergency treatment of airway problems (such as a foreign body) involving the larynx.

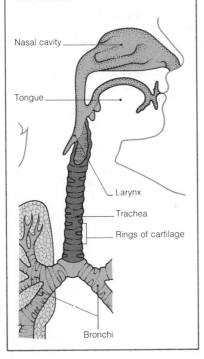

LOCATION OF THE TRACHEA
The trachea extends down from the larynx for about 10 cm to the point where it divides into the two bronchi.

Nasal cavity

Tongue

Larynx

Trachea

Rings of cartilage

Bronchi

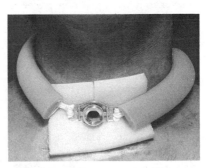

Tracheostomy tube
The tube readily becomes blocked by secretions; it has a metal inner lining that can be removed for cleaning.

A planned tracheostomy is most commonly performed on a person who has lost the ability to breathe naturally and is undergoing long-term *ventilation* (the pumping of air into the lungs by a machine) or who has lost the ability to keep saliva and other secretions out of the trachea because of coma or a specific airway or swallowing problem. In such cases, tracheostomy is performed after passing an endotracheal tube through the nose or mouth and into the trachea. Permanent tracheostomy is necessary after *laryngectomy* (surgical removal of the larynx).

HOW IT IS DONE
The operation is carried out under local or general anesthetic.

An incision is made in the skin overlying the trachea, between the Adam's apple and the clavicles (collarbones). The neck muscles are pulled apart, and the thyroid gland, which surrounds the trachea, is usually severed. A small vertical incision (called a "window") is made in the trachea so that a metal or plastic tube can be inserted. If the patient cannot breathe unaided, the tube is connected to a *ventilator*.

If a laryngectomy is being performed, the cut edges of the trachea are brought forward and stitched to the edges of the skin wound before the tube is inserted.

RECOVERY PERIOD
For patients who are able to breathe unaided, the air in the room is humidified to reduce the drying of mucus in the airway. Air from a ventilator is humidified before it passes into the tube. Any excessive mucus that accumulates in the airway is sucked away through a catheter.

While the tube is in place, the patient is usually unable to speak and is therefore provided with a bell or buzzer and with pen and paper for communication. After laryngectomy, the tube is removed after several days, and a permanent opening remains. In other cases, the tube is removed when the patient has recovered from the condition that necessitated the operation, and the opening soon closes and heals.

Tracheotomy
Cutting of the trachea (windpipe). (See also *Tracheostomy*.)

Trachoma
A persistent infectious disease of the *conjunctiva* and *cornea*. Trachoma is caused by an organism, CHLAMYDIA TRACHOMATIS, that is spread by direct contact and possibly by flies (see *Chlamydial infections*). Untreated trachoma leads to complications that may cause blindness. Trachoma is uncommon where standards of personal hygiene are high.

SYMPTOMS AND SIGNS
Infection by CHLAMYDIA TRACHOMATIS causes acute *conjunctivitis*, with pain, *photophobia*, and watering of the eyes. The eyes become red and inflamed, and the conjunctiva that lines the lids becomes thickened and roughened with scar tissue and studded with small lumps called follicles. Damage to the mucus-secreting cells of the conjunctiva and to the lacrimal (tear-producing) glands may lead to *keratoconjunctivitis sicca* (inflammation and dry eye).

An abnormal growth of blood vessels can extend down from the conjunctiva into the upper part of the cornea, leading to opacity (loss of transparency) and loss of vision. More severe damage to the cornea occurs later when fibrous scarring of the inside of the upper lid causes it to be rolled inward so that the lashes rub against the cornea, causing ulceration and encouraging secondary bacterial infection. Secondary infection may lead to extensive ulceration, scarring, and even *perforation*, with spread of infection into the eye and permanent loss of vision.

Antibiotic drugs may be applied to the eye or taken by mouth in an attempt to eradicate the causative organism. No further treatment may be necessary in the early stages of the disease. In established trachoma, however, after scarring has occurred, surgery to correct lid deformities or corneal grafting to restore transparency and vision may be needed.

Tract
A group of organs that form a common pathway to perform a particular function. For example, the urinary tract comprises the kidneys, ureters, bladder, and urethra, which together form a series of connected structures for the removal of waste products from the body. The *alimentary tract* extends from the mouth, through the pharynx, esophagus, stomach, and intestines, to the anus.

The term tract also refers to a bundle of nerve fibers that have a common function, as in the pyramidal tract, a bundle of nerve fibers in the spinal cord that carry nerve impulses from the brain to the muscles.

Traction
A procedure in which part of the body is placed under tension to correct the alignment of two adjoining structures or to hold them in position.

WHY IT IS DONE
The most common use of traction is in the treatment of a *fracture* in which muscles around the bone ends are pulling the bones out of alignment. Fractures of the shaft of the *femur* (thighbone) are most likely to be treated in this way. Traction is also used to align and immobilize unstable fractures of the cervical spine (neck) when any movement of the vertebrae might damage the spinal cord (see *Spinal injury*).

HOW IT IS DONE
To apply traction to a lower limb fracture, the person lies on a bed with the injured limb supported by attachments from an overhead frame. The upper end of the fractured bone is held immobilized while the lower end is pulled in a straight line away from it by a system of weights and pulleys. The traction grip is obtained by a pin inserted through the tibia (shin) or through a plaster cast applied to the fractured limb.

For spinal fractures, the patient lies flat on a firm surface and weights are attached to tongs inserted into holes drilled on either side of the skull. Both limb and spinal fractures are maintained in continuous traction until healing has occurred.

Training
A program of *exercises* undertaken to prepare for a particular sport. Training may be concentrated on improving particular skills or on improving physical *fitness*.

Fitness training should include both *aerobic* and anaerobic exercises, which together build up strength, flexibility, and endurance (the capacity to exercise for long periods).

Interval training is a type of fitness program in which a particular exercise, such as running a set distance at a timed pace, is repeated several times with a rest period between. Circuit training consists of performing a set number of different exercises, such as push-ups, sit-ups, and step-ups, one after the other.

The selection of an appropriate training program requires specialized assessment and advice. Self-imposed training schedules may be damaging to health; for example, bone and muscle disorders may develop in runners if their training is unsupervised.

T

TRACTION FOR FEMORAL FRACTURE

Because of the power of the thigh muscles and their tendency to go into spasm, fractures of the femur (thighbone) tend to override.

Without traction to prevent this, the bone would heal with overlapping ends and the leg would be permanently shortened.

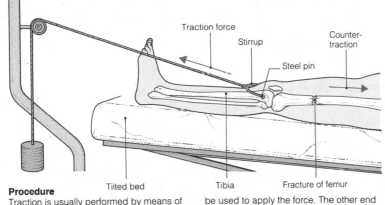

Traction force

Stirrup

Counter-traction

Steel pin

Tilted bed

Tibia

Fracture of femur

Procedure
Traction is usually performed by means of a narrow steel pin through the upper end of the tibia (shin), to which a steel stirrup is attached so that a cord and weight can be used to apply the force. The other end of the femur must be immobilized (or countertraction applied) to keep the fractured bone ends aligned.

Trait

Any characteristic or condition that is inherited (determined by a *gene* or genes). Blue or brown eye color, dark or light skin, body proportions, and nose shape are all genetic traits.

The majority of common traits (such as eye color) have no obvious effect on health. Others may have marginally advantageous effects in particular environments (such as dark skin in a sunny climate) or mildly disabling effects (such as *color vision deficiency*). Severely handicapping traits, such as *cystic fibrosis* or *osteogenesis imperfecta*, are individually rare, but the fact that there are many different types means that they are collectively quite common (see *Genetic disorders*).

The term trait is also used in a more restricted sense to describe a mild form of a recessive genetic disorder. For example, a person who inherits the sickle cell gene in a single dose is said to have sickle cell trait. A double dose of the same gene causes serious *sickle cell anemia*.

Trance

A sleeplike state in which consciousness is reduced, voluntary actions are lessened or absent, and bodily functions are diminished. A trance usually results from separation of a group of mental processes from the rest of the mind rather than from any physical brain disturbance.

Trances are claimed to be induced by *hypnosis* and have been reported as part of a group experience, particularly in a religious context. Trances are sometimes a feature of *catalepsy*, *automatism*, and petit-mal *epilepsy*.

Tranquilizer drugs

Drugs with a sedative effect, subdivided into major tranquilizers (see *Antipsychotic drugs*) and minor tranquilizers (see *Antianxiety drugs*).

Transcutaneous electrical nerve stimulation

A method of pain relief achieved by the application of minute electrical impulses to nerve endings under the skin. (See *TENS*.)

Transdermal patch

A type of dressing that releases a drug when in contact with the skin.

Transference

The unconscious displacement of emotions from people who were important during one's childhood, such as parents, to other people when one is an adult. Transference is important in *psychoanalysis*.

Transfusion

See *Blood transfusion*.

Transfusion, autologous

See *Blood transfusion, autologous*.

Transient ischemic attack

A brief interruption of the blood supply to part of the *brain* that results in temporary impairment of vision, speech, sensation, or movement. Typically, the episode lasts for several minutes or, at the most, for a few hours. Any attack with effects that last for more than 24 hours is called a *stroke*. Transient ischemic attacks (TIAs) can be the prelude to a full-scale stroke.

CAUSES
Some TIAs occur when an artery supplying the brain becomes temporarily blocked by a flake of clotted blood carried from elsewhere in the bloodstream (see *Embolism*). Other attacks are caused by narrowing of an artery due to *atherosclerosis*.

SYMPTOMS AND SIGNS
Symptoms occur suddenly, and vary widely, according to the site and duration of the interruption to the flow of blood to the brain. Common symptoms include weakness or numbness in an arm or leg, *aphasia* (disturbance of language functions), dizziness, or partial blindness. An attack is always followed by full recovery.

DIAGNOSIS
Diagnostic testing may include *CT scanning* to rule out the possibility of a *brain tumor* or a subdural *hematoma* (a swelling containing blood), which sometimes produce TIA-like symptoms. Blood tests to look for blood-clotting abnormalities may also be done. Other tests, including *ultrasound scanning*, digital subtraction *angiography*, or conventional angiography, may be used to look at the vessels for evidence of atherosclerosis. In some cases, the heart is studied as a possible source of blood clots.

TREATMENT
Treatment is aimed at preventing a major stroke, which occurs within five years in from one quarter to one third of the patients with TIA. Possible treatments include *endarterectomy*, anticoagulant drugs, or *ASA* (which reduces the stickiness of platelets in the blood). Thus far, only ASA has proved to be effective.

Transillumination

A procedure sometimes carried out during physical examination of a lump or swelling. Light from a small torch is shone against one side of the lump; if light can be seen on the other side, the physician knows that the lump contains clear fluid because fat or other tissue would block the light. For example, a *hydrocele* (a fluid-con-

T

taining swelling in the scrotum) allows light to pass, whereas a *varicocele* (a mass of enlarged veins) in the scrotum does not.

Translocation

A rearrangement of the *chromosomes* inside a person's cells. Translocation is a type of *mutation* (change in the genetic material). Sections of chromosomes may be exchanged, or the main parts of two chromosomes may be joined. A translocation may be inherited or acquired as the result of a new mutation.

Often, because there has been no net loss or gain of chromosomal material within the person's cells, a translocation has no outward effect, and causes no abnormality. However, the translocation can mean that some of the person's egg or sperm cells carry too much or too little chromosomal material, which leads to a risk of a *chromosomal abnormality*, such as *Down's syndrome*, in the person's children (see illustrated box).

When a chromosomal abnormality occurs, the child's and the parents' chromosomes are checked to discover whether a translocation is the cause (see *Chromosome analysis*). *Genetic counseling* can help determine the risk of another child's being affected and can provide advice about prenatal diagnosis.

Transmissible

A term meaning capable of being passed from one person to another, or from one organism to another of the same or a different species. The term may be applied to an *infectious disease* or to an inherited *genetic disorder*.

Transplant surgery

The replacement of a diseased organ or tissue with a healthy, living substitute. The organ is usually taken from a person who has just died. Some transplanted kidneys (about 13 percent in Canada) are taken from living relatives of the patient (see *Organ donation*).

The earliest successful transplant operation was *corneal grafting*, carried out early this century. The cornea is not affected by the *rejection* process (the automatic attempt by the body's *immune system* to reject foreign cells and destroy them) because it has no blood supply, and therefore no white blood cells and antibodies to bring about rejection.

Kidney transplantation was shown to be technically possible in the 1950s,

T

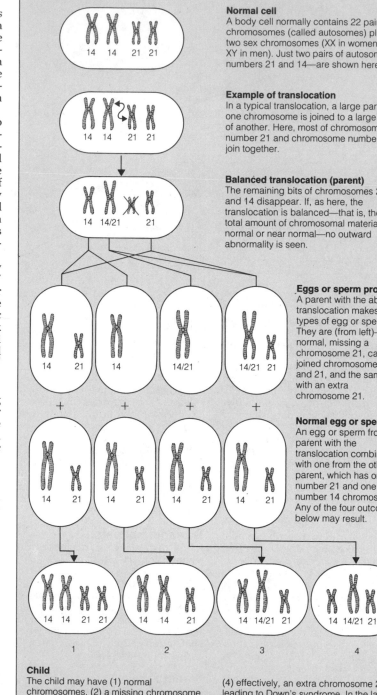

EFFECT OF CHROMOSOMAL TRANSLOCATION

A translocation is a rearrangement of the chromosomes in body cells. A person carrying a translocation may show no abnormality but there is a risk of his or her child having a chromosomal abnormality.

Normal cell
A body cell normally contains 22 paired chromosomes (called autosomes) plus two sex chromosomes (XX in women and XY in men). Just two pairs of autosomes—numbers 21 and 14—are shown here.

Example of translocation
In a typical translocation, a large part of one chromosome is joined to a large part of another. Here, most of chromosome number 21 and chromosome number 14 join together.

Balanced translocation (parent)
The remaining bits of chromosomes 21 and 14 disappear. If, as here, the translocation is balanced—that is, the total amount of chromosomal material is normal or near normal—no outward abnormality is seen.

Eggs or sperm produced
A parent with the above translocation makes four types of egg or sperm. They are (from left)—normal, missing a chromosome 21, carrying joined chromosomes 14 and 21, and the same with an extra chromosome 21.

Normal egg or sperm
An egg or sperm from the parent with the translocation combines with one from the other parent, which has one number 21 and one number 14 chromosome. Any of the four outcomes below may result.

Child
The child may have (1) normal chromosomes, (2) a missing chromosome 21 (incompatible with life), (3) a balanced translocation (like the parent), and (4) effectively, an extra chromosome 21, leading to Down's syndrome. In the last case, the parents may benefit from genetic counseling.

TRANSPLANTS PERFORMED IN CANADA IN 1988

Kidney	902
Heart and heart/lung	185
Liver	125
Lung (single and double)	14
Pancreas and kidney/pancreas	8

Factors affecting transplantation
In Canada, as elsewhere, there is a shortage of suitable donor organs at almost all times. The number of transplant operations performed is limited by this shortage and, to a lesser extent, by access to specialist centers that can perform the operation and provide suitable postoperative care.

but early transplant operations ended in failure because of rejection. In the 1960s, however, *corticosteroid drugs* and cytotoxic agents (see *Anticancer drugs*) were found to suppress the rejection response, making transplantation practicable. The discovery in the 1970s and introduction in the early 1980s of *cyclosporine*, a more effective *immunosuppressant drug*, substantially improved success rates.

A second important factor in improving the results of transplant surgery has been the steady improvement in techniques for matching donors and recipients. Organ transplantation proceeds most smoothly when the donor and recipient share most of the same tissue types (see *Histocompatibility antigens; Tissue-typing*). Matching of tissue types has become less important, however, since the introduction of cyclosporine.

A third factor that has contributed to higher success rates is the development of techniques for organ preservation. After removal from the donor, the organ is washed with an oxygenated fluid and cooled; this reduces the risk of damage due to lack of blood. Nevertheless, it is still important to keep to a minimum the time the organ is deprived of a normal blood supply. In most cases of heart or liver transplantation, the organs are removed from the donor while the heart is still functioning, but after *brain death* has been certified.

Every patient who undergoes an organ transplant operation must take immunosuppressant drugs indefinitely; this damping down of the body's natural defenses exposes him or her to a greater risk of infection,

especially with fungi (see *Fungal infections*) and protozoal *parasites*. Patients undergoing long-term immunosuppressant treatment are also at increased risk of certain types of cancer, especially *lymphomas*. (See also *Heart-lung transplant; Heart transplant; Liver transplant; Kidney transplant.*)

Transposition of the great vessels
A form of congenital *heart disease* in which the two major vessels that carry blood away from the heart—the aorta and the pulmonary artery—are in each other's normal position. This means that, unless the baby also has a septal defect (hole in the heart) through which blood can flow, insufficient oxygenated blood is supplied to the body's tissues. Transposition of the great vessels occurs in about 40 babies per 100,000 born.

SYMPTOMS
Cyanosis (blueness of the skin) usually develops and the baby becomes increasingly short of breath; the baby also feeds poorly. Symptoms vary in severity according to the amount of oxygenated blood passing through the septal opening.

A firm diagnosis can be made only after a *chest X ray, ECG, echocardiography*, and cardiac *catheterization* (in which a catheter is introduced into the heart via a blood vessel).

The cardiac catheter may be used to make a hole in the septum. Alternatively, emergency surgery may be performed to create or enlarge an existing septal hole. These techniques allow enough oxygenated blood to reach the body tissues and keep the child alive. Later, reconstructive *open heart surgery* is performed to create a nearly normal circulation.

Transsexualism
A rare disorder in which a person feels persistently uncomfortable about his or her anatomical sex, and wishes to live as a member of the opposite sex. Usually developing in early adulthood, transsexualism is much more common in men than in women. The condition may be associated with a disturbed child-parent relationship and may follow a period of cross-dressing (see *Transvestism*).

Features associated with transsexualism include *personality disorder, alcohol dependence, drug dependence, anxiety, depression*, and work problems. In many transsexuals, sexual drive is quite low. Some transsexuals are actively homosexual.

Transsexualism should be distinguished from the delusion (false belief not responding to reasoned argument) of belonging to the other sex, which sometimes occurs in *schizophrenia*, and from physical *intersex* (in which there are congenital abnormalities of the sexual structures).

Transsexuals commonly seek hormonal or surgical treatment to bring about a physical *sex change*. A careful psychiatric evaluation and physical examination are necessary before such treatment is undertaken.

Transvestism
A persistent desire by a man to dress in women's clothing, also called cross-dressing. Transvestism commonly starts in childhood with secret masturbation while dressed in the underwear of a female relative. Transvestism should be differentiated from female impersonation, which does not involve the component of sexual arousal.

Transvestism ranges from the occasional wearing of female underclothes to constant, public dressing in women's clothes and extensive involvement in transvestite subculture. For some individuals, cross-dressing serves to relieve anxiety; for others it provides sexual excitement. Occasionally, transvestism develops into *transsexualism*.

Transvestites rarely seek medical or psychiatric treatment. Most transvestites are heterosexual and have a sexual relationship with a female partner who knows and can accept the cross-dressing as a special need. A crisis may occur, however, if transvestism is accidentally revealed to a partner or family member. Psychiatric intervention in such cases consists of helping the partner and family to understand that transvestites are not dangerous and that their behavior does not break the law.

Tranylcypromine
A monoamine-oxidase inhibitor *antidepressant drug* used mainly in patients with severe depression.

Trapezius muscle
A large, diamond-shaped *muscle* that extends from the back of the skull to the lower part of the thoracic spine (the part of the spine in the chest) and, at its broadest point, across the width of the shoulders.

At the shoulders, the trapezius is attached to the top and back of the scapula (shoulder blade) and to the

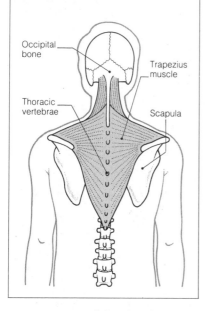

LOCATION OF THE TRAPEZIUS MUSCLE
The trapezius is a large, diamond-shaped muscle in the upper part of the back. It helps to support the neck and head, and is also involved in raising the arms.

Occipital bone

Trapezius muscle

Thoracic vertebrae

Scapula

outermost part of the clavicle (collarbone). Along its midline, the trapezius is also attached by ligaments to the vertebrae (spinal bones).

The trapezius muscle helps support the neck and spine. It is also involved in movements of the arm. When an arm is raised, the trapezius on that side contracts, thereby causing the scapula to rotate.

Trapped nerve
A compressed or stretched nerve. See *Nerve, trapped*.

Trauma
A physical injury or a severe emotional shock. The psychological condition that can result from physical or emotional trauma is known as *post-traumatic stress disorder*.

Trauma surgery
See *Traumatology*.

Traumatology
Emergency treatment of patients suffering from acute trauma (physical injury), commonly as a result of road traffic accidents, industrial accidents, domestic accidents, shootings, or stabbings.

In cases of life-threatening trauma, the priorities are to prevent *asphyxia* by maintaining a clear airway, to arrest *bleeding*, to treat *shock*, and to deal with major chest wounds affecting the heart or lungs. If there are abdominal injuries, an exploratory operation called a *laparotomy* or, in the case of head injuries, a *craniotomy*, may be required. Multiple injuries require coordinated treatment by different specialists.

Once the patient's condition is stable, other injuries are treated. (See also *Accidental death*.)

Traveler's diarrhea
A form of *gastroenteritis* that afflicts people visiting foreign countries. Episodes of diarrhea range in severity from inconvenient to debilitating.

Travel immunization
Any person planning to travel outside Canada, Europe, the US, Australia, and New Zealand may need immunizations before departure. Few immunizations are now compulsory for international travel. Nevertheless, some immunizations are advisable for the traveler's own protection.

Travel agents and tour operators often include information about which immunizations may be required. More detailed information is available at travel clinics of major urban hospitals, from the *Medical officer of health*, or from a physician, who will be able to take into account the individual's previous vaccinations and medical history.

All travelers should be up-to-date on their childhood vaccinations (see *Immunization*); in some instances, booster doses may be advisable. Some vaccines must be given in two or three doses several weeks apart, so any one planning a foreign trip should consult the physician at least two to three months before departure. Antimalarial drugs (see *Malaria*) may be advisable for those visiting certain destinations.

Because of the danger of *AIDS* transmitted by unsterile needles in many developing countries, especially in Africa, travelers who require injections or who will be exposed to dangerous situations that may create injuries requiring medical treatment should carry a kit of syringes and needles. These are available in many pharmacies. The needles will not, of course, reduce the risk of acquiring AIDS in a contaminated blood transfusion.

Travel sickness
See *Motion sickness*.

Trazodone
An *antidepressant drug*. Trazodone has a strong sedative effect and is particularly useful in the treatment of *depression* that is accompanied by *anxiety* or *insomnia*. Possible adverse effects include drowsiness, constipation, dry mouth, dizziness, and, rarely, *priapism* (painful, persistent erection).

Treatment
Any measure taken to prevent or cure a disease or disorder or to relieve symptoms. Examples include *drug treatment*, *radiation therapy*, *surgery*, bed rest and *physiotherapy*.

Trematode
The scientific name for any *fluke* or *schistosome* (flattened worm that may parasitize humans).

Trembling
See *Tremor*.

Tremor
An involuntary, rhythmic, oscillating movement in the *muscles* of part of the body, most commonly the hands, feet, jaw, tongue, or head. Tremor is caused by rapidly alternating contraction and relaxation of the muscles.

Occasional temporary tremors are experienced by almost everyone, usually at times of heightened emotion, and are due to increased production of the hormone *epinephrine*.

A slight persistent tremor unrelated to any disease is common in elderly people. Another type of persistent tremor not associated with disease is known as essential tremor.

This is a fine-to-moderate tremor (six to 10 movements per second) that runs in families and may be temporarily relieved by a small amount of alcohol or by taking *beta-blocker drugs*. Both these types of tremor increase when the affected part of the body is moved.

Some types of persistent tremor indicate an underlying disorder. Coarse tremor (four to five muscle movements per second) present at rest but reduced during movement is often a sign of *Parkinson's disease*. An intention tremor (tremor that is worse on movement of the affected part) may be a sign of *cerebellar ataxia*. Other disorders marked by tremor include *multiple sclerosis*, *Wilson's disease*, *mercury poisoning*, *thyrotoxicosis*, and hepatic *encephalopathy*.

T

GUIDELINES FOR TRAVEL IMMUNIZATION

Immunization	Reason for immunization	Effectiveness
Yellow fever	Compulsory for entry to some countries and advisable for visits to others within yellow fever zones in Africa and South America. May also be needed when traveling from yellow fever zones to some Asian countries.	Almost 100 percent protection for at least 10 years. Certificate provided.
Cholera	Occasionally compulsory for entry to some countries in Asia and Africa. Also advisable when traveling to many other Asian and African countries.	Gives moderate protection for six months. Other precautions against cholera needed in epidemic areas.
Typhoid fever	Recommended when traveling anywhere outside Canada, Europe, the US, Australia, and New Zealand for anyone who has not received immunization or a booster within the past three years.	Gives moderate protection for about three years, after which a booster is needed.
Tetanus	Advisable for anyone who has not received childhood immunization or a booster within the past 10 years.	Highly effective, with booster needed every 10 years.
Polio-myelitis	Advisable for anyone who has not received childhood immunization or a booster within the past 10 years.	Highly effective, with booster needed every 10 years.
Immuno-globulin	Recommended for protection against viral hepatitis type A when traveling to any country where hygiene and sanitary standards are low.	Moderate protection for up to six months.
Measles	Advisable for anyone who has not received childhood immunization and who has not had measles.	Highly effective; gives lifelong protection.
Diphtheria	Advisable for anyone who has not received childhood immunization and who is shown by a test to be nonimmune.	Highly effective.
Hepatitis B Rabies Meningitis	Recommended only for people who are at special risk because of their occupation or the nature of their visit abroad.	All highly effective.
Smallpox	No longer necessary as the disease has been eradicated.	

Tremor may also be caused by drugs, among them *amphetamine drugs*, *antidepressant drugs*, *antipsychotic drugs*, *lithium*, and *caffeine*. Withdrawal may also result in tremor. The so-called morning shakes may be an indication of *alcohol dependence*.

Trench fever
An infectious disease that was common among troops in the trenches of World War I and World War II, but is now rare or unknown in most parts of the world. Like epidemic *typhus*, which it resembles, the disease is caused by *rickettsiae* (microorganisms similar to bacteria) spread by body *lice*. The symptoms include headache and muscle pains as well as fever, which may occur in bouts. Trench fever is treated with *antibiotic drugs*.

Trench foot
See *Immersion foot*.

Trench mouth
See *Gingivitis, acute ulcerative*.

Trephine
A hollow, cylindrical instrument with a saw-toothed edge used for cutting a circular hole, usually in bone. Trephines are most often used to bore holes in the skull to form a removable flap before operations on the brain.

Perforation of the skull to relieve excess pressure is a recent innovation and is part of conventional surgery. Ancient peoples used trephines on the skull (as evidenced by the skulls found by paleontologists) but the reason they did so is unknown; most likely it was done by witch doctors to encourage the release of evil spirits.

Tretinoin
A drug chemically related to *vitamin A*, which is applied to the skin to treat *acne* and certain skin disorders characterized by scaling and thickening, such as *ichthyosis*. Tretinoin is also being evaluated as a treatment for the wrinkling of the skin with age, especially in people who have been exposed to strong sunlight.

Tretinoin may aggravate acne in the first few weeks of treatment but usually improves the condition within three to four months. In some people, tretinoin causes skin irritation and peeling. Excessive exposure to sunlight while using tretinoin may aggravate any irritation and lead to *sunburn*. In rare cases, tretinoin may bleach or darken the skin.

Trial, clinical
A test on human volunteers of the effectiveness and safety of a drug, or a systematic comparison of alternative forms of medical or surgical treatment for a particular disorder. Clinical trials are also used to test the usefulness of new medical or surgical appliances, dressings, or equipment.

In the development of new drugs, clinical trials follow animal tests that mainly evaluate toxic effects (see *Animal experimentation*); clinical trials are usually undertaken at a late stage before the manufacturer proceeds to commercial production. The purpose of clinical trials is to demonstrate that the new drug is effective, safe, and superior to, or at least as good as, existing drugs. Such trials are also useful in revealing effects that may not have been suspected from results of the animal tests.

Careful precautions are necessary to ensure that the results of clinical

T

trials are not misleading. Trials that fail to eliminate the effects of personal bias or the *placebo* effect may be of little value. For these reasons, most clinical trials are carried out in the form of randomized, *controlled trials*.

Triamcinolone
A *corticosteroid drug* used to treat inflammation of the mouth, gums, skin, and joints. Triamcinolone is also used to treat *asthma* and certain blood disorders, such as *thrombocytopenia* and *leukemia*.

Triamterene
A potassium-sparing *diuretic drug*. Triamterene is used with thiazide or loop diuretics to treat *hypertension* (high blood pressure) and *edema* (accumulation of fluid in tissues). Possible adverse effects include nausea, vomiting, weakness, and rash.

Triazolam
A *benzodiazepine drug* used in the short-term treatment of *insomnia*.

Triceps muscle
The name (meaning "three heads") of the *muscle* at the back of the upper arm. At the upper end of the triceps, one of the three heads is attached to the outer edge of the scapula (shoul-

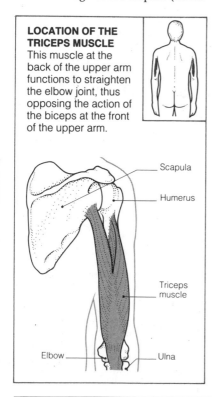

LOCATION OF THE TRICEPS MUSCLE
This muscle at the back of the upper arm functions to straighten the elbow joint, thus opposing the action of the biceps at the front of the upper arm.

Scapula

Humerus

Triceps muscle

Elbow

Ulna

der blade); the other two heads are attached to either side of the upper part of the humerus (upper arm bone). The lower part of the triceps is attached by a large *tendon* to the olecranon process of the ulna (the bony prominence at the back of the elbow). Contraction of the muscle straightens the arm. (See also *Biceps muscle*.)

Trichiasis
An alteration in the direction of growth of the eyelashes in which the lashes grow inward toward the eyeball. The abnormally directed lashes can rub against the eye, causing severe discomfort and sometimes damage to the *cornea*. Trichiasis can result from the inflammation and scarring that occurs in *trachoma*. Severe scarring may lead to *entropion* (turning in of the lid margin).

Temporary treatment involves removal of the offending lashes, but the lashes regrow and may again cause pain and damage. Permanent treatment may be by *electrolysis* to destroy the growth follicles of the eyelashes involved, or by minor surgical adjustment of the lid margin.

Trichinosis
 An infestation with the larvae of a tiny worm, *TRICHINELLA SPIRALIS*, usually acquired by eating undercooked pork or pork products, such as ham or sausages.

CAUSES AND INCIDENCE
Worm larvae are present as cysts in the muscles of infested animals, such as pigs, dogs, and rats. Humans can become infected by eating undercooked or raw pork, beef, bear or walrus meat. Serious outbreaks of trichinosis have occurred in arctic communities.

If a person eats the raw or undercooked meat of an infested animal, the larvae are released from the cysts and develop into adults in the person's intestines. The adult worms discharge fresh larvae, which travel around the body in the bloodstream to various tissues and organs, including the heart and brain, and to the muscles, where they form cysts.

The principal preventive measure is thorough cooking of pork and pork products. Freezing to a temperature below −18°C for 24 hours also kills the larvae.

SYMPTOMS AND COMPLICATIONS
Infestation with only a few worms usually causes no symptoms. A heavy infestation may cause diarrhea and

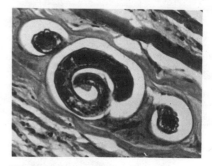

Biopsy specimen showing trichinosis
This photomicrograph of a section of a patient's muscle shows a cyst formed by a *TRICHINELLA SPIRALIS* larva.

vomiting within a day or two of eating infested meat, followed, a week or so later, by more symptoms as new larvae circulate through the body. Symptoms may include fever, swelling around the eyelids, and severe muscle pains, which may last for several weeks. In most people, the symptoms subside and gradually disappear. Very rarely, an infected person becomes seriously ill and may die.

DIAGNOSIS AND TREATMENT
Trichinosis may be suspected by a physician from the symptoms. The diagnosis is confirmed by *blood tests*, which detect antibodies to the larvae, or by a muscle *biopsy*, which shows the larvae themselves.

The disease is treated with an *anthelmintic drug* (usually *thiabendazole*) that kills adult worms in the intestines and attacks larvae in the tissues. *Corticosteroid drugs* are given to reduce inflammation. This treatment generally leads to recovery within a period of a few days to weeks.

Trichomoniasis
 An infection caused by the protozoan (single-celled microorganism) *TRICHOMONAS VAGINALIS*. Trichomoniasis is a common cause of *vaginitis* in women. In most cases, the infection is sexually transmitted, but it is occasionally contracted indirectly, such as from an infected towel. Trichomoniasis is less commonly reported in men, in whom the infection affects the urethra but usually does not cause symptoms. Occasionally, trichomoniasis is transmitted by a woman to her baby during the process of childbirth.

Trichomoniasis, which itself is not a serious condition, may occur in conjunction with other sexually transmitted diseases.

T

SYMPTOMS AND SIGNS

In women, the causative organism may inhabit the vagina for years without causing symptoms. If symptoms do occur, they include painful inflammation of the vagina and vulva, and a profuse, yellow, frothy, offensive discharge. Sexual intercourse may be painful. Men usually have no symptoms but some suffer from urethral discomfort and signs of *nonspecific urethritis*.

DIAGNOSIS AND TREATMENT

The diagnosis is made from a laboratory examination of a sample of the vaginal discharge or of swabs taken from the urethra. Diagnosis is usually difficult in men. Treatment is with *metronidazole*, which usually clears up the condition. An infected person's sexual partner or partners should be traced, examined, and treated at the same time to prevent reinfection.

Trichotillomania

The habit of constantly pulling out one's own hair. Trichotillomania can be associated with severe *mental retardation* or with a psychotic illness, such as *schizophrenia*. It may also occur in psychologically disturbed children as an outward expression of anxiety and frustration.

The sufferer typically pulls, twists, and breaks off chunks of hair from the scalp, leaving bald patches; occasionally, pubic hair is pulled out. Children sometimes eat the removed hair, which may form a hairball in the stomach, known medically as a trichobezoar (see *Bezoar*).

Treatment depends on the cause and may consist of *psychotherapy* or *antipsychotic drugs*.

Tricuspid insufficiency

Failure of the tricuspid valve of the *heart* to close properly, allowing blood to leak back into the right atrium (upper chamber) during contractions of the right ventricle (lower chamber). This lowers the pumping efficiency of the heart. The condition is also known as tricuspid insufficiency.

CAUSES AND INCIDENCE

Tricuspid incompetence is usually due to an increased work load on the right side of the heart as a result of *pulmonary hypertension* (high pressure in the blood supply to the lungs). This causes the right ventricle to distend and leads to widening of the opening in which the tricuspid valve is situated.

In rare cases, tricuspid insufficiency occurs in people who have had

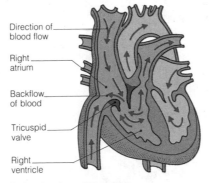

Direction of blood flow

Right atrium

Backflow of blood

Tricuspid valve

Right ventricle

Defect in tricuspid insufficiency
The tricuspid valve lies between the atrium and ventricle in the right side of the heart. Insufficiency means that when the right ventricle contracts, some blood escapes back into the right atrium.

rheumatic fever. It may also result from bacterial infection of the heart in intravenous drug abusers. In both these groups of people, tricuspid insufficiency may be accompanied by other heart valve disorders.

SYMPTOMS

The tricuspid insufficiency causes symptoms of right-sided *heart failure*, notably *edema* (fluid collection and swelling) affecting the ankles and abdomen. The liver is congested with blood and is swollen and tender. Veins in the neck are distended.

DIAGNOSIS

The condition is diagnosed from the patient's symptoms, from a characteristic *murmur* heard through a stethoscope, and by tests that may include an *ECG*, *chest X rays*, *echocardiography*, and cardiac *catheterization*.

TREATMENT

Treatment for heart failure, with *diuretic drugs* and *ACE inhibitor drugs*, often clears up the symptoms. If symptoms persist, *heart valve surgery* may be performed to repair or replace the malfunctioning valve.

Tricuspid stenosis

Narrowing of the opening of the tricuspid valve in the *heart* between the right atrium (upper chamber) and right ventricle (lower chamber). Tricuspid stenosis is an uncommon type of heart valve disorder. When it does occur, it is usually in a person who has previously had *rheumatic fever*. Tricuspid stenosis may also occur in intravenous drug abusers as a result of bacterial infection of the heart.

Tricuspid stenosis is usually accompanied by other types of heart valve disorder, such as *mitral stenosis*.

The right atrium must work harder to pump blood through the narrowed valve, causing it to enlarge. The symptoms are very similar to those of *tricuspid insufficiency*; the condition is diagnosed by the same procedures.

Drug treatment is given with *diuretic drugs* to reduce *edema* (accumulation of fluid in tissues) and sometimes a *digitalis drug* to increase the force of the heart's contractions. If symptoms persist, *heart valve surgery* may be carried out to repair or replace the defective valve.

Trifluoperazine

An *antipsychotic drug* used principally in the treatment of *schizophrenia*.

Trifluridine

An *antiviral drug* effective in the form of eye drops against *herpes* infections.

Trigeminal nerve

The fifth *cranial nerve*. The trigeminal nerves, one on each side, arise from the pons (part of the *brain stem*). Each nerve divides into three main branches, which then subdivide into a complex network of nerves.

The trigeminal nerves and their branches supply sensation to the face, scalp, nose, teeth, lining of the mouth, upper eyelid, sinuses, and front two thirds of the tongue. They also stimulate contraction of the jaw muscles responsible for chewing, and control the production of saliva by the salivary glands and of tears by the lacrimal glands.

Damage to, or disease in, one area supplied by a branch of the trigeminal nerve may cause *referred pain* in another area supplied by a different branch of the nerve. For example, sinusitis (infection of the sinuses) may cause toothache.

Trigeminal neuralgia

A disorder of the trigeminal nerve (fifth *cranial nerve*) in which episodes of severe, stabbing pain affect the cheek, lips, gums, or chin on one side of the face. The pain is very brief (lasting only a few seconds to minutes) but is often so intense that the sufferer is unable to do anything for the duration of the attack. The pain often causes wincing and for this reason is commonly called tic douloureux (literally, "painful twitch").

Trigeminal neuralgia is unusual under the age of 50. When the condition occurs in younger people, it may be associated with *multiple sclerosis*. Attacks occur in bouts that may last

T

LOCATION OF THE TRIGEMINAL NERVE

The trigeminal nerve splits into three main branches. The ophthalmic nerve supplies most of the scalp, the upper eyelid, tear gland, and cornea; the maxillary nerve supplies the upper jaw; and the mandibular nerve supplies the tongue, lower jaw, and jaw muscles.

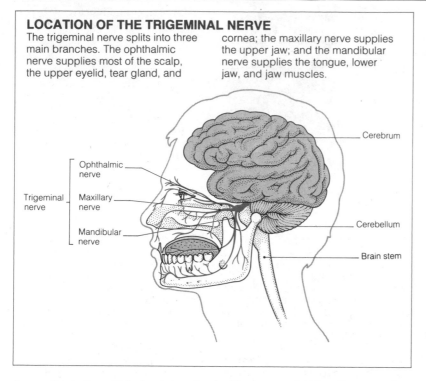

- Cerebrum
- Ophthalmic nerve
- Trigeminal nerve
- Maxillary nerve
- Mandibular nerve
- Cerebellum
- Brain stem

for weeks at a time. Pain-free intervals between attacks tend to become shorter with time.

The cause of trigeminal neuralgia is uncertain. The pain nearly always starts from one trigger point on the face and can be brought on by touching the face, washing, shaving, eating, drinking, or even talking.

Treatment is difficult. *Carbamazepine* suppresses the pain in most sufferers, but a few people develop resistance to the drug or are unable to tolerate a high enough dosage to relieve the pain. If the disorder is not helped by drug treatment, several surgical options are available.

Trigger finger

Locking of one or several fingers in a bent position. Forcible straightening of an affected finger usually causes an audible click.

Trigger finger is caused by inflammation of the fibrous sheath that encloses the *tendon* of the affected finger and is accompanied by localized swelling of the tendon. When the finger is bent, the enlarged tendon is forced out of the narrowed mouth of the sheath and is then unable to re-enter it. There is usually tenderness at the base of the affected finger. In addition, a small swelling may be felt over the tendon.

Treatment of trigger finger involves either the injection of a *corticosteroid drug* into the sheath to reduce inflammation, or a surgical procedure to widen the opening of the sheath.

Trihexyphenidyl

A drug used in the treatment of *Parkinson's disease* since the 1940's. Trihexyphenidyl is useful in relieving rigidity and tremor in the early stages of the disease. It has side effects typical of the *anticholinergic* drugs.

Trimeprazine

An *antihistamine drug* used mainly to relieve itching in allergic conditions, such as *urticaria* (hives) and atopic

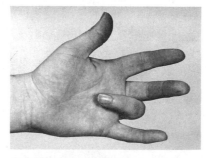

Appearance of trigger finger
The disorder is caused by inflammation of the sheath of one of the tendons involved in controlling the finger's movements.

eczema. Because trimeprazine has a sedative effect, it is useful in the relief of itching that interferes with sleep. Trimeprazine is also used as a surgery *premedication* for children.

The adverse effects of trimeprazine are typical of other antihistamines, although trimeprazine is more likely to cause drowsiness.

Trimethoprim

An *antibacterial drug* prescribed for a wide variety of infections. Trimethoprim is used on its own to treat *urinary tract infection, prostatitis*, and *bronchitis*. The drug *co-trimoxazole* is a combination of trimethoprim and another antibacterial drug, *sulfamethoxazole*.

Possible adverse effects of trimethoprim include rash, itching, nausea, vomiting, diarrhea, and sore tongue.

Trimipramine

A tricyclic *antidepressant drug*. Trimipramine has a strong sedative effect and is used to treat *depression* accompanied by *anxiety* or *insomnia*. It elevates mood, increases physical activity, improves appetite, and restores interest in everyday activities. Possible adverse effects include dry mouth, blurred vision, dizziness, constipation, and nausea.

Triple vaccine

See *DPT vaccination*.

Triprolidine

An *antihistamine drug* used to treat allergies, such as allergic *rhinitis* (hay fever) and *urticaria* (hives). Triprolidine is also a common ingredient of *cough remedies* and *cold remedies*. It is occasionally given to treat or prevent allergic reactions to *blood transfusions* or certain foods.

Possible adverse effects include dry mouth, dizziness, difficulty in passing urine, and, in children, *hyperactivity*.

Trismus

Involuntary contraction of the *jaw* muscles, resulting in the mouth's becoming tightly closed, a condition commonly known as lockjaw.

Trismus may occur as a symptom of *tetanus, tonsillitis, quinsy, mumps*, acute ulcerative *gingivitis*, an abscess around a back tooth (see *Abscess, dental*), nasopharyngeal cancer (see *Nasopharynx, cancer of*), or *Parkinson's disease*. Occasionally, trismus is psychological in origin; for example, it sometimes occurs in *anorexia nervosa*.

Treatment of trismus is of the underlying cause.

T

Trisomy

The presence, within a person's cells, of an extra chromosome so that there are three *chromosomes* of a particular number, instead of the usual two. The result can range from the death and miscarriage of an affected embryo to a range of physical abnormalities in a live-born child.

CAUSES AND INCIDENCE

A trisomy may result from a fault by which an extra chromosome gets into an egg or sperm cell during the cell's formation. If an affected egg or sperm takes part in fertilization, the resulting embryo also has an extra chromosome, causing trisomy. Most types of trisomy are more common with advanced maternal age.

By far the most common trisomy in live-born infants is trisomy 21, also called *Down's syndrome* (formerly called mongolism), in which there are three number 21 chromosomes. Much less common are trisomy 18 (Edwards' syndrome) and trisomy 13 (Patau's syndrome). Trisomy 8 and trisomy 22 are extremely rare. Partial trisomies, in which only part of a chromosome is in triplicate, have also been found.

All full trisomies cause multiple abnormalities, such as skeletal and heart defects, facial anomalies, and mental deficiency. Babies with full trisomies other than Down's syndrome usually die early in infancy. The effect of a partial trisomy is variable, depending on how much extra chromosomal material is present.

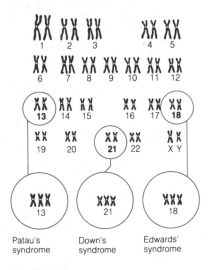

Types of trisomy
In all trisomies a child has three, instead of the usual two, chromosomes of a particular number. Down's syndrome is by far the most common trisomy.

DIAGNOSIS AND TREATMENT

Trisomies are diagnosed by *chromosome analysis* of cells. There is no specific treatment for these disorders. Parents of an affected baby should obtain *genetic counseling* to assess the risk of a future child being affected. Prenatal diagnosis, particularly by means of *amniocentesis* and chromosome analysis of the cells obtained, can be performed if a pregnancy is considered to be at risk.

Trisomy 21 syndrome

A set of abnormalities caused when a child has three, instead of the usual two, number 21 chromosomes in each of his or her cells. It is better known as *Down's syndrome.*

Trochlear nerve

The fourth *cranial nerve.* The trochlear nerves, one on each side of the brain, arise from the midbrain (part of the *brain stem*) and pass through the skull to enter the eye sockets through gaps in the skull bones. Each trochlear nerve supplies only one eye muscle: the superior oblique muscle. Contraction of this muscle rotates the eye downward and outward.

Damage to the trochlear nerve (as a result of a skull fracture, for example) may lead to *double vision.*

Trophoblastic tumor

A growth arising from the tissues that develop into the *placenta.* The most common type of trophoblastic tumor is a benign growth called a *hydatidiform mole.* A malignant trophoblastic tumor that spreads outside the uterus is called a *choriocarcinoma.*

Tropical diseases

Many diseases are virtually confined to tropical areas. In most cases, this is not due primarily to tropical geographical factors (such as temperature, humidity, or disease-carrying insects), but to the fact that large populations in many tropical countries live in poverty and squalor.

DISEASES OF POVERTY

Malnutrition is one of the major causes of illness in the tropics. Apart from causing nutritional deficiency disorders, a poor diet weakens the body's ability to fight infectious diseases such as *measles* and *diphtheria.* Overcrowded living conditions are a cause of such diseases as *tuberculosis.*

Low standards of public health administration, food inspection and handling, and a lack of sanitary facilities, which encourage water and soil

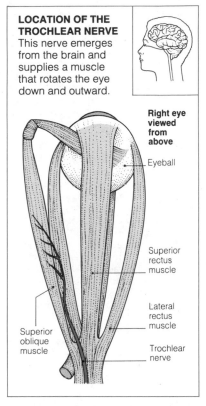

LOCATION OF THE TROCHLEAR NERVE
This nerve emerges from the brain and supplies a muscle that rotates the eye down and outward.

Right eye viewed from above

Eyeball

Superior rectus muscle

Lateral rectus muscle

Trochlear nerve

Superior oblique muscle

contamination with human excrement, are the cause of a vast number of diseases, including *typhoid fever, shigellosis, cholera, amebiasis,* and *tapeworm infestation.* Most of these diseases were common in temperate zones before improvements in public health and sanitation brought them under control in such regions. Only some diseases, such as *hookworm infestation* and *schistosomiasis,* appear to be related to temperature or soil conditions found only in the tropics in addition to the lack of community sanitation and walking barefoot.

DISEASES SPREAD BY INSECTS

Some tropical diseases depend on the coincidence of a parasite and a specific insect *vector* (agent responsible for spread) such as a mosquito. These diseases include *malaria, yellow fever, sleeping sickness,* and *leishmaniasis.* It is worth noting, however, that at least some of the relevant insect vectors can survive in temperate zones; malaria was once common in parts of Canada.

LIGHT AND HEAT

Certain conditions arise as a result of exposure to tropical sunlight. The most common is skin damage from *ultraviolet light,* leading to wrinkling, loss of elasticity, and an increased ten-

T

dency to *skin cancer*, especially in white people with fair coloring. Ultraviolet light also damages the outer tissues of the eye (the conjunctiva and the cornea) and may lead to the development of *pinguecula* and *pterygium*. Undue exertion in the tropics, with inadequate water intake and salt replacement, may lead to *heat exhaustion*; prolonged exposure to high temperatures may lead to *heatstroke*.

Tropical ulcer

An area of persistent skin and tissue loss caused by infection, a condition that occurs mainly in tropical regions. The ulcers are most common in people who are malnourished.

The classic form of tropical ulcer results from contamination of a cut or abrasion (usually on a foot or leg) by a mixture of various types of bacteria. Infections spread beneath the skin, and the affected tissue dies and is shed, leaving the ulcer in place.

Treatment consists of thorough cleaning of the ulcer, which is then dressed; the patient also needs *antibiotic drugs* and a nourishing, protein-rich diet. With this treatment, the ulcer usually heals, although it may leave some scarring and deformity.

Similar types of ulcer can occur as a result of more specific infections, such as *diphtheria* of the skin, cutaneous *leishmaniasis*, and *yaws*. Treatment is as described above, except that drug therapy may vary according to the causative organisms.

To avoid tropical ulcers, it is particularly important to wash any cuts, sores, or abrasions thoroughly and cover them with a sterile dressing.

Tropicamide

A drug used to dilate the *pupil* before an eye examination and, occasionally, before eye surgery. Rare adverse effects include blurred vision, increased sensitivity to light, stinging, dry mouth, flushing, and *glaucoma* (increased pressure in the eye).

Trunk

The central part of the body, comprising the thorax (chest) and abdomen, to which the head and limbs are attached. The term trunk also refers to any large blood vessel or nerve from which smaller vessels or nerves branch off.

Truss

An elastic, canvas, or padded metal appliance used to hold an abdominal *hernia* (protrusion of part of the intes-

tine through a weakened area in the abdominal wall) in place. The hernia is pushed back through the abdominal wall before the truss is put on, usually while the person lies down. A truss may be used to treat a hernia that is causing discomfort or is unsightly in people who are waiting for an operation to repair the hernia or who are unfit for surgery.

Trypanosomiasis

A tropical disease caused by protozoan (single-celled) parasites known as trypanosomes. In Africa, trypanosomes spread by tsetse flies are the cause of *sleeping sickness*. In South America, other trypanosomes, spread by beetlelike insects, are the cause of *Chagas' disease*.

Tryptophan

An *antidepressant drug*. Tryptophan may take at least two weeks to have an effect. Elderly people and women taking oral contraceptives may have to take *pyridoxine* (vitamin B_6) during treatment to prevent an adverse reaction. Possible side effects include nausea, drowsiness, and headache.

Tsetse fly bites

Tsetse flies are found in Africa, where they spread the parasitic disease *sleeping sickness*. They are brown, about the size of houseflies, and have a projecting proboscis (feeding apparatus). The bites of tsetse flies can be painful. Measures to minimize the risk of bites include use of insecticide sprays and protective clothing.

T-tube cholangiography

An *imaging technique*, also called operative or postoperative choledochography, performed to check that there are no residual *gallstones* in the common bile duct after *cholecystectomy* (surgical removal of the *gallbladder*).

The T-shaped rubber tube used in this type of cholangiography is inserted when the gallbladder is removed. The short arms of the T are inserted into the common bile duct, and the main body of the tube is brought out through a small incision in the abdomen.

T-tube cholangiography is carried out eight to 10 days after surgery on the gallbladder. Contrast medium is injected into the T-tube and *X rays* are taken. If no residual gallstones are found, the T-tube is removed. Otherwise, the tube is left until a decision is made concerning treatment.

Tubal ligation

See *Sterilization, female*.

Tubal pregnancy

See *Ectopic pregnancy*.

Tubercle

Any of several small, nodular masses apparent in tissues that have been infected by the bacterium that causes *tuberculosis*. Such tubercles are gray and semitransparent.

The term tubercle (or tuberculum or tuberosity) also refers to any small, rounded protrusion on the surface of a bone. For example, the tibial tubercle is a bump at the top of the *tibia* (main bone of the lower leg), immediately below the knee.

Tuberculin tests

Skin tests used to determine whether or not a person has been previously infected with *tuberculosis*. Tuberculin tests are performed in the diagnosis of suspected tuberculosis and are also carried out before *BCG vaccination*.

HOW THEY ARE DONE

The skin of the forearm is first cleaned with alcohol. A small dose of tuberculin (a purified protein extracted from the bacteria that cause tuberculosis) is then introduced into the skin by one of various techniques. In the Mantoux test, tuberculin is injected into the skin with a needle. In the Heaf test, a drop of tuberculin is put on the forearm and a spring-loaded device with a circle of sharp prongs is used to force the tuberculin through multiple tiny punctures in the skin. The tests are nearly painless.

RESULTS

The forearm is examined after a few days and the skin reaction at the test site noted. If there is no change in the skin, the reaction is said to be negative. This indicates that the person has never been exposed to and has no immunity against tuberculosis. If the test area of skin becomes red, hard, and raised, the reaction is positive. A positive reaction indicates previous exposure to tuberculosis, either through BCG vaccination or through actual infection.

Tuberculosis

An infectious disease, commonly called TB, caused in humans by the bacterium MYCOBACTERIUM TUBERCULOSIS. Tuberculosis was once common worldwide and was a major killer in childhood and early adult life. In Europe, it was responsible for about a quarter of all deaths in the mid-19th

T

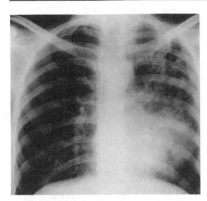

Chest X ray showing tuberculosis
The right lung appears normal, but the left lung shows dense opacities (white areas) adjoining the heart shadow.

century. Its incidence has fallen and continues to fall in developed countries, but tuberculosis remains a major problem in poorer countries.

CAUSES
Infection is passed from person to person in airborne droplets (produced by coughing or sneezing). The bacteria breathed into the *lungs* then multiply to form an infected "focus." In a high proportion of cases, the body's *immune system* then halts the infection and healing occurs, leaving a scar.

In about 5 percent of cases, however, the primary infection does not resolve. Spread occurs via the vessels of the *lymphatic system* to the lymph nodes. Sometimes at this stage bacteria enter the bloodstream and spread to other parts of the body; this is called miliary tuberculosis and may occasionally be fatal. In some people, the bacteria go into a dormant state in the lungs and other organs, only to become reactivated many years later. Progressive damage may then occur, such as the formation of cavities in the lungs.

In some cases, the primary infection is not in the lungs but in the lymph nodes (particularly of the neck), intestines, bones, kidneys, or other organs.

INCIDENCE
Worldwide, there are 30 million people with active tuberculosis; about 3 million die from the disease annually. Tuberculosis is most prevalent where resistance has been lowered by disease or malnutrition.

The incidence of tuberculosis in Canada is about 2,000 cases annually. The incidence is up to 10 times higher in native peoples, and five times higher in immigrants, than it is in the

Canadian population as a whole. The poor and those suffering from *immunodeficiency diseases*, *diabetes mellitus*, or *alcohol dependence* are also at higher risk of tuberculosis. Most cases of tuberculosis can be traced to close contact with another person who has the disease.

PREVENTION
In Canada, *BCG vaccination* is used in high-risk groups such as native peoples. Another preventive measure is *contact tracing* so that relatives and close friends of a tuberculosis victim can be examined, x-rayed, and given a *tuberculin test*. Contact tracing thus makes it possible to detect tuberculosis at an early stage and to reduce the risk of spread to other people.

SYMPTOMS AND COMPLICATIONS
Because tuberculosis usually affects the lungs, the main symptoms include coughing (sometimes bringing up blood), chest pain, shortness of breath, fever and sweating (especially at night), poor appetite, and weight loss. The main complications of tuberculosis of the lungs are *pleural effusion* (collection of fluid between the lung and the chest wall), *pneumothorax* (air between the lung and chest wall), and, in some cases, progression of the disease to death.

DIAGNOSIS
The diagnosis is made from the patient's symptoms and signs, and from a *chest X ray* and tests on the sputum (phlegm) and skin. The chest X ray is almost always abnormal. The upper parts of the lung are most commonly affected and may show cavities. Old healed areas of tuberculosis often remain as persistent shadows.

The sputum is examined for tuberculosis organisms. Attempts are also made to grow the bacteria from the sputum or other body fluids, although this procedure can take as long as six weeks. A tuberculin test may be carried out. A positive test result indicates that the person has either been immunized against tuberculosis or has been infected. Occasionally, *bronchoscopy* or the removal and examination of a piece of tissue (e.g., from a lymph node) may be necessary to make a firm diagnosis.

TREATMENT AND OUTLOOK
Modern drugs are very effective against tuberculosis, although at least two different *antibiotic drugs* must be taken to avoid bacterial *resistance* to the drugs. In Canada, new cases are usually treated with three or four drugs daily for two months, followed by two drugs, usually *isoniazid* and

rifampin, either daily or twice a week under direct observation by a health care worker. An adverse drug reaction (usually a rash or fever) develops in about 5 percent of patients, who then require a modification of treatment. Blood tests are often performed to ensure that the drugs are not causing toxic effects on the liver.

Provided the full course of treatment is taken, the majority of patients are fully restored to health and suffer no recurrences.

Tuberosity

A prominent area on a *bone* to which *tendons* are attached. For example, the gluteal tuberosity is a ridge on the upper back part of the shaft of the femur (thigh bone) to which tendons of part of the gluteus maximus muscle are attached. Other bones with tuberosities include the ischium (one of the three fused bones that form the pelvis), the humerus (upper arm bone), and the radius and the ulna (lower arm bones).

Tuberous sclerosis

An inherited disorder affecting the *skin* and *nervous system*. The most typical skin feature of tuberous sclerosis is adenoma sebaceum (an acnelike condition of the face) but a variety of other skin conditions may also occur. Affected people characteristically suffer from *epilepsy* and *mental retardation*, although intelligence may be normal in mild cases.

Other associated problems include the development of noncancerous tumors, especially of the brain, kidney, retina, and heart.

There is no cure for tuberous sclerosis. Treatment, including *anticonvulsant drugs* and the removal of tumors, is aimed at relieving troublesome symptoms. Seriously affected people may not live beyond the age of 30. *Genetic counseling* is recommended for affected families who are considering having children. In some cases, the gene for tuberous sclerosis can be detected in the fetus at an early stage in the pregnancy.

Tuboplasty

An operation in which a damaged fallopian tube is repaired to treat *infertility*. Tuboplasty is performed if a tube has become scarred and blocked, usually following *salpingitis* (infection of the fallopian tubes) or *pelvic inflammatory disease*. The procedure is sometimes performed using *microsurgery* techniques.

T

The fertility rate following tuboplasty varies from less than 5 to about 50 percent, depending on the severity of the problem and on whether there are other reasons for the infertility. *Ectopic pregnancy* is more common in women who have had diseased tubes or tuboplasty than in those with healthy fallopian tubes.

Tularemia

An infectious disease of wild animals, such as rabbits and squirrels, that is occasionally transmitted to humans.

CAUSES AND INCIDENCE

Humans may be infected through direct contact with an infected animal or its carcass, in which cases the causative bacteria enter the body via a cut or abrasion in the skin. Tularemia can also be acquired through a bite from an infected tick, flea, fly, or louse or, in rare cases, by eating infected meat.

Tularemia is diagnosed by a blood test that detects *antibodies* formed against the bacteria. Treatment is with *antibiotic drugs*. Without treatment, tularemia is fatal in about 5 percent of cases; with treatment, the fatality rate is less than 1 percent.

Tumor

By strict definition, any swelling. In its more usual meaning, tumor is synonymous with neoplasm and refers to an abnormal mass of tissue that forms when cells in a specific area reproduce at an increased rate. Tumors may be *malignant* (cancerous) or *benign* (noncancerous).

Malignant tumors invade surrounding tissues and may also spread via the bloodstream or lymphatic system to form a secondary growth (called a *metastasis*) elsewhere in the body. *Cancer* is the general term used to refer to all types of malignant tumors. A malignant tumor that arises from epithelial tissues (such as skin) is termed a *carcinoma*; one that arises from connective tissue (such as muscle, bone, or fibrous tissue) is called a *sarcoma*.

Benign tumors usually grow slowly and do not metastasize, although they may sometimes be multiple. They tend to remain confined within a fibrous capsule, making surgical removal relatively straightforward. However, benign tumors may grow large enough to cause damage by pressing on nearby structures, which can be particularly dangerous in confined spaces, such as when they form inside the skull.

At the microscopic level, one essential difference between benign and malignant tumors is that benign tumors retain many of the features of the tissue from which they arise. In contrast, malignant tumors tend to comprise small, rapidly growing cells that form masses of tissue with fewer recognizable features of the tissue from which they originate.

Tumor-specific antigen

A substance secreted by a specific type of *tumor* (or class of tumors) that is detectable in the blood. Tumor-specific antigens, also known as tumor-associated antigens, do not provide conclusive results when screening for malignant tumors because most of the substances can also be produced in nonmalignant conditions. Repeated measurements of the levels of tumor-specific antigens are, however, helpful in monitoring a patient's response to therapy.

Examples of tumor-specific antigens include carcinoembryonic antigen and *alpha-fetoprotein*, which are both produced by immature fetal tissue and known as onco-fetal antigens. Carcinoembryonic antigen is produced in abnormal amounts by about half of all tumors of the colon, stomach, breast, lungs, and pancreas. Alpha-fetoprotein levels in blood serum are raised in 70 percent of cases of hepatoma (a primary *liver cancer*) and in most cases of *teratoma* of the testis (see *Testis, cancer of*).

Tunnel vision

Constriction of the *visual field* so that only objects straight ahead can be clearly seen.

CAUSES

The most common cause of tunnel vision is chronic simple *glaucoma*, in which raised pressure within the eye results in the destruction of *optic nerve* fibers. As a result of this destruction, peripheral vision is gradually lost until the visual field is reduced to only a few degrees across.

Tunnel vision may also be caused by a tumor or other brain disorder that interferes with the fibres that connect the *optic nerve* to the brain. *Pituitary tumors*, for example, can press on the point where the optic nerves come together, causing loss of the right half of the right eye's visual field and the left half of the left eye's visual field. *Retinitis pigmentosa* (retinal degeneration) may cause the loss of peripheral vision and lead to the development of tunnel vision.

Turner's syndrome

A disorder caused by a *chromosomal abnormality* that affects only females.

INCIDENCE AND CAUSES

Approximately one in 3,000 live-born girls is born with Turner's syndrome. The chromosomal abnormality may arise in one of three ways. Most affected females have only 45 chromosomes compared with the normal complement of 46, the missing chromosome being one of the X chromosomes. Sometimes, however, both X chromosomes are present but one is defective. Occasionally, the condition arises as a type of *mosaicism*, in which some cells are missing one X chromosome, some have extra chromosomes, and others have their normal number of chromosomes.

SIGNS

The main features of the syndrome are shortness of stature, webbing of the skin of the neck, absence or very retarded development of secondary sexual characteristics (see *Sexual characteristics, secondary*), *amenorrhea* (absence of menstruation), *coarctation of the aorta*, abnormalities of the eyes and bones, and a degree of *mental retardation*. Without treatment, the average adult height is 1.35 metres.

TREATMENT

Coarctation of the aorta is treated by surgery at an early age. Menstruation may be induced by *estrogen drugs* but sufferers continue to be infertile. To increase the girl's final height, growth hormone may be given.

Twins

Two offspring resulting from one pregnancy. Twins may develop from a single ovum (egg) or from two ova.

Monozygotic or monovular (identical) twins develop when a single, fertilized ovum divides completely and equally at an early stage of development; if this division is incomplete it results in *Siamese twins* (also known as conjoined twins). Monozygotic twins share the same placenta. Although one is often much bigger than the other at birth, they are always of the same sex and look remarkably alike.

Twins from two ova are called dizygotic or binovular (fraternal) twins. The ova from which they develop may be released by the same or different ovaries; fertilization of the two ova occurs simultaneously. Each dizygotic twin has its own placenta. The twins may be of the same or of different sexes, and may look quite different.

Twins occur in about one in 80 pregnancies. Dizygotic twins are more

T

TWO TYPES OF TWINS

During each menstrual cycle, either one ovum or a small number of ova may be released. If one ovum is fertilized and the two cells formed from its first division develop independently, the result is identical twins. If two ova are fertilized and mature normally, nonidentical twins result.

IDENTICAL TWINS

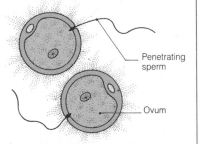

Penetrating sperm

Ovum

Identical twins come from a single fertilized ovum. When the ovum splits, the two cells formed develop independently.

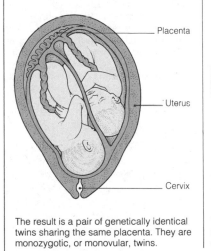

Placenta

Uterus

Cervix

The result is a pair of genetically identical twins sharing the same placenta. They are monozygotic, or monovular, twins.

NONIDENTICAL TWINS

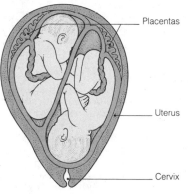

Penetrating sperm

Ovum

Nonidentical twins come from two separate ova that have been fertilized by two separate sperm.

Placentas

Uterus

Cervix

The resulting individuals are genetically distinct and have separate placentas. They are dizygotic, or binovular, twins.

likely to occur in older women, in women who have had many previous pregnancies, and in women who have a history of twins in the family; a woman whose mother had fraternal twins is almost twice as likely to have twins as a woman who has never had any twins in her family. Dizygotic twins are also more common in Africa and Asia. These factors do not have any bearing on the incidence of monozygotic twins.

Twins face greater difficulties from the start. Deaths are more frequent before, during, or just after birth. When rearing twins, especially monozygotic twins, it is important to emphasize that they are two individuals, not half of a pair. (See also *Pregnancy, multiple.*)

Twins, conjoined
Another name for *Siamese twins*.

Twitch
See *Fasciculation; Tic*.

Tylectomy
A term sometimes used for lumpectomy (removal of a lump), especially in *breast cancer*. (See *Mastectomy*.)

Tympanometry
A type of *hearing test*, also called impedance audiometry.

Tympanoplasty
An operation on the *ear* to repair a hole in the eardrum (see *Myringoplasty*) or to reposition or reconstruct diseased ossicles.

WHY IT IS DONE
In a healthy ear, sound waves are conducted from the eardrum to the oval window of the inner ear by a chain of three bones called ossicles. Chronic *otitis media* (middle ear infection) can fuse these bones in position or erode them, interfering with sound conduction. In such cases, a procedure such as tympanoplasty offers the only chance of restoring some of the lost hearing.

HOW IT IS DONE
Under general anesthesia, an incision is made to provide access to the middle ear. Viewing the ear through an operating microscope, the surgeon then repositions or repairs the chain of ossicles. This may involve one or more of a number of procedures such as reshaping and transposing one of the bones, replacing an ossicle with a plastic substitute, grafting an ossicle taken from a donor, or fashioning an ossicle from cartilage. The bones are then reset in position and the eardrum repaired.

RESULTS
Tympanoplasty results in a considerable improvement in hearing in the majority of patients, but a successful outcome of the operation cannot be guaranteed in some instances. (See also *Stapedectomy*.)

Tympanum
Part of the *ear*, comprising the middle ear cavity (tympanic cavity) and eardrum (tympanic membrane). (See also illustration below.)

Typhoid fever
An infectious disease contracted by eating food or drinking water contaminated with the bacterium SAL-MONELLA TYPHI. An almost identical disease, *paratyphoid fever*, is caused by related bacteria.

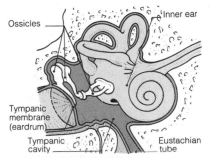

Inner ear

Ossicles

Tympanic membrane (eardrum)

Tympanic cavity

Eustachian tube

Anatomy of the tympanum
The tympanic cavity contains three movable bones (malleus, incus, and stapes), which transmit sound from the tympanic membrane (eardrum) to the inner ear.

CAUSES AND INCIDENCE

The infection is contracted from the feces of a person who has the disease or who is a symptomless carrier of the causative bacteria. In areas of poor sanitation, typhoid is commonly spread by the contamination of drinking water with sewage, or by flies carrying the bacteria from infected feces to food. Elsewhere, infection is usually due to the handling of food by typhoid carriers. Shellfish that have been contaminated by sewage are an occasional source of typhoid.

During the development of the disease, the bacteria pass from the intestines into the blood, and then to the spleen and liver, where they multiply. The organisms are excreted from the liver, accumulate in the gallbladder, and are released in enormous numbers into the intestine. Carriers, after recovering from typhoid fever, may continue to harbor typhoid bacteria in the gallbladder and shed them in the feces for many years.

Typhoid is uncommon in developed countries but epidemics occur regularly in developing countries. There are about 50 cases a year in Canada, most of which are acquired abroad.

PREVENTION

Typhoid is a *notifiable disease*, and people with the disease should be medically isolated.

Immunization against typhoid is generally advisable before traveling anywhere outside North America, northern Europe, Australia, and New Zealand. The vaccine is given in two doses, followed every three years by a booster dose. Typhoid immunization often causes swelling and pain at the site of injection, lasting for one to two days.

The vaccine does not provide complete protection; travelers at risk should drink only boiled water or bottled drinks and take care over what they eat (see *Food-borne infection*).

SYMPTOMS AND SIGNS

Typhoid has an incubation period of seven to 14 days. The course of the infection varies from a mild upset to a major life-threatening illness. The first symptom is usually severe headache, followed by fever, loss of appetite, malaise, abdominal tenderness, constipation, and often delirium. Constipation soon gives way to diarrhea. During the second week of the illness, small, raised pink spots can be seen on the chest and abdomen for several days, and there is enlargement of the liver and spleen.

The illness usually clears up within four weeks. However, if treatment is delayed, severe, and sometimes fatal, complications may develop. Possible gastrointestinal complications include intestinal bleeding, and *perforation* of the intestine leading to *peritonitis*. Among other possible complications are *urinary tract infection* and *kidney failure*.

DIAGNOSIS AND TREATMENT

The diagnosis is confirmed by obtaining a *culture* of typhoid bacteria from a sample of blood, feces, or urine, or by a *blood test* that reveals the presence of *antibodies* against typhoid bacteria.

Either *chloramphenicol* or *amoxycillin* usually brings the disease under control within a few days and prevents complications; severely ill patients may require supplementary treatment with *corticosteroid drugs*. An operation may be needed if widespread peritonitis or severe bleeding develops.

OUTLOOK

Given early diagnosis and proper treatment, the outlook is usually excellent, although relapses are common within a few weeks of treatment.

Typhus

 Any of a group of infectious diseases, with similar symptoms, caused by *rickettsiae* (microorganisms similar to bacteria) and spread by insects or similar animals.

TYPES

Of the various types of typhus, epidemic typhus is historically the most important. This disease formerly occurred in epidemics that killed hundreds of thousands of people in times of war, famine, or other natural disasters. Today, epidemic typhus is rare except in some highland areas of tropical Africa and South America.

CAUSES

Epidemic typhus is spread between humans by body lice, which ingest the causative organism, RICKETTSIA PROWAZEKI, from the blood of infected people, and deposit infected feces onto the skin of other people. The rickettsiae are introduced into the bloodstream by scratching.

Endemic typhus, also called murine typhus, is a disease of rats that is occasionally spread to humans by fleas; sporadic cases occur in North and Central America. Scrub typhus is spread by mites and occurs in India and Southeast Asia.

PREVENTION

Epidemic typhus can be prevented through control of human louse infestation with insecticides. A vaccine also exists against the disease. Preventive measures are especially important in crowded conditions following natural disasters.

Other types of typhus can be prevented by taking measures, such as the use of protective clothing, to discourage bites by fleas, mites, or ticks.

SYMPTOMS AND SIGNS

In epidemic typhus, severe headache, back and limb pain, coughing, and constipation develop suddenly and are followed by high fever, confusion, a rash similar to that of measles, prostration, a weak heartbeat, and, in many cases, delirium. Without treatment, death may occur from *septicemia, heart failure, kidney failure*, or *pneumonia*.

Other types of typhus have similar symptoms and signs, and similar complications.

DIAGNOSIS AND TREATMENT

Particular types of typhus fever are diagnosed by tests that can detect blood products formed in reaction to the rickettsial organisms. Typhus fevers are treated with *antibiotic drugs*. Other measures may be required to relieve severe symptoms and to treat complications. Convalescence is often slow, particularly in the elderly.

Typing

A general term for procedures by which blood or tissues are classified. (See *Blood groups*; *Tissue-typing*.)

U

Ulcer

An open sore on the *skin* or on a *mucous membrane* that results from the destruction of surface tissue. Ulcers may be shallow, or deep and crater-shaped, and are usually inflamed and painful.

Skin ulcers most commonly occur on the leg (see *Leg ulcer*), usually as the result of inadequate blood supply to, or drainage from, the limb. Among the rarer forms of skin ulcers are *basal cell carcinomas*, which are a form of skin cancer.

Ulcers on mucous membranes most commonly develop within the digestive tract, occurring in the mouth (see *Mouth ulcer*), the stomach or the duodenum (see *Peptic ulcer*), or in any part of the small or large intestines (see *Ulcerative colitis*).

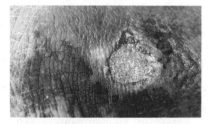

Ulcer on the forehead
An ulcer on this area of the skin is often due to a basal cell carcinoma—a type of skin cancer that is easily treated.

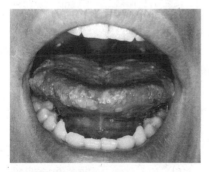

Ulcers in the mouth
Aphthous ulcers are common, painful, and typically last for one to two weeks. Most heal well, without leaving scars.

The skin or mucous membranes of the genitalia may also be affected by ulcers (see *Genital ulceration*). Most genital ulcers are caused by sexually transmitted disease. Examples of this type of ulcer are hard chancres, which develop during the first stage of *syphilis*, and soft chancres (see *Chancroid*).

Ulcers may also develop on the cornea, the transparent covering at the front of the eyeball (see *Corneal ulcer*).

Ulcer, aphthous

A small, painful *ulcer* that occurs alone or in a group on the inside of the cheek or lip or underneath the tongue.

INCIDENCE
Minor aphthous ulcers affect about 20 percent of the population at any given time. They are most common between the ages of 10 and 40 and affect women more than men. The most severely affected people have continuously recurring ulcers; others have just one or two ulcers per year.

SYMPTOMS
Each ulcer is usually small and oval with a gray center and a surrounding red, inflamed halo. The ulcer usually lasts for one to two weeks.

CAUSES
The ulcer may be a hypersensitive reaction to hemolytic streptococcus bacteria, which have often been isolated from aphthous ulcers. Other factors commonly associated with the occurrence of these ulcers are minor injuries (such as at an injection site or from a toothbrush), acute stress, and allergies (such as allergic *rhinitis*). In women, ulcers are most common during the premenstrual period. Ulcers may also be more likely to occur if other members of the family suffer from recurrent ulceration.

TREATMENT
Analgesic mouth gels or mouthwashes may ease the pain of an aphthous ulcer. Some ointments form a waterproof covering that protects the ulcer while it heals. Ulcers will heal by themselves if left alone, but a physician may prescribe an ointment containing a *corticosteroid drug* or a mouthwash containing a *tetracycline drug* to speed up the healing process.

Ulceration

The formation or presence of one or more *ulcers*.

Ulcerative colitis

Chronic inflammation and ulceration of the lining of the *colon* and *rectum*. The disease sometimes begins by affecting only the rectum.

CAUSES AND INCIDENCE
The cause of ulcerative colitis is unknown. In Canada, the disease affects between 40 and 50 people per 100,000. It is most common in young and middle-aged adults.

SYMPTOMS AND SIGNS
The main symptom is bloody diarrhea; the feces may also contain pus and mucus. In severe cases, diarrhea and bleeding are extensive and there may be abdominal pain and tenderness, fever, and general malaise. The incidence of attacks varies considerably from person to person. Most commonly, attacks occur at intervals of a few months; however, in some cases, symptoms are either continuous or occur infrequently.

One of the principal dangers of severe ulcerative colitis is *anemia*, caused by loss of blood. Other complications include a toxic form of *megacolon* (an abnormally enlarged colon), which may become life-threatening; rashes; mouth ulcers; *arthritis*; and inflammation of the eye in the form of *conjunctivitis* or *uveitis*. In addition, people whose entire colon has been inflamed for more than 10 years are at increased risk of developing cancer of the colon (see *Colon, cancer of*).

DIAGNOSIS
The diagnosis is based on examination of the rectum and lower colon (see *Sigmoidoscopy*) or of the entire colon (see *Colonoscopy*) with a viewing instrument, or by a barium enema (see *Barium X-ray examinations*). During sigmoidoscopy or colonoscopy, a *biopsy* (removal of a small sample of tissue for microscopic analysis) may be performed. Samples of feces may also be taken for analysis to exclude the possibility of infection (by bacteria or parasites) as a cause of the symptoms. *Blood tests* may be required.

People who have had ulcerative colitis for many years require periodic colonoscopy and biopsy to check for the development of cancer.

TREATMENT
In most cases, medical treatment effectively controls the disease. Treatment usually consists of *corticosteroid drugs* (to control symptoms by reducing inflammation) and *sulfasalazine* (to maintain long-term freedom from symptoms). Newer drug treatments using salicylate derivatives of sulfasalazine are also being investigated.

Colectomy (surgical removal of the colon) may be required if inflammation is extensive, severe, and uncontrollable; colectomy is required for most patients with toxic megacolon.

U

This operation usually produces a dramatic improvement in the patient's health, although he or she is usually left with an *ileostomy* (an opening in the surface of the abdomen through which the feces are passed).

Ulcer-healing drugs

COMMON DRUGS

H₂-receptor antagonists
Cimetidine Famotidine Nizatidine Ranitidine

Others
Antacids Bismuth salts Carbenoxolone Pirenzepine Sucralfate

A group of drugs used to treat and prevent stomach and duodenal ulcers (see *Peptic ulcer*).

HOW THEY WORK
Ulcer-healing drugs work in one of two ways.

H₂-receptor antagonists work by blocking the effects of histamine, an action that reduces the secretion of acid in the stomach and thus promotes the healing of ulcers. *Antacid drugs* taken regularly may be effective in healing duodenal ulcers, because they neutralize the excess acid.

Other ulcer-healing drugs, such as *sucralfate*, are believed to form a protective barrier over the ulcer, thereby allowing the tissues time to heal.

Ulcer-healing drugs usually relieve symptoms within one to two weeks and, in most cases, the ulcer heals within eight weeks. Once the ulcer has healed, a maintenance dose may be prescribed. Without continuing treatment, the chance of an ulcer's recurring is somewhere between 60 and 70 percent.

POSSIBLE ADVERSE EFFECTS
Adverse effects may include confusion, headaches, and dizziness. Ulcer-healing drugs may mask the symptoms of *stomach cancer*. These drugs are therefore not usually prescribed for periods longer than two months unless the possibility of cancer has been ruled out.

Ulna

The longer of the two bones of the forearm; the other is the *radius*. With the palm forward, the ulna is the inner bone (i.e., the bone nearer the trunk) running down the forearm on the side of the little finger.

The upper end of the ulna articulates with the radius and extends into a rounded projection (called the *olecranon* process) that fits around the lower end of the *humerus* (upper-arm bone)

to form part of the *elbow* joint. The lower end of the ulna is rounded and articulates with the carpals (*wrist* bones) and lower part of the radius.

Ulna, fracture of

Fractures of the *ulna* typically occur across the shaft or at the *olecranon* process (the rounded projection at the tip of the elbow).

A shaft fracture is usually caused by a blow to the forearm or a fall onto the hand. In some cases, the radius is fractured at the same time (see *Radius, fracture of*). An operation is usually needed to reposition the broken bone ends and fix them together, using either a plate and screws or a long nail down the center of the bone. The arm is then immobilized in a plaster *cast*, with the elbow at a right angle, until the fracture heals.

A fracture of the olecranon process is usually caused by a fall onto the elbow. If the bone ends are not displaced, the arm is immobilized in a plaster cast that holds the elbow at a right angle. If the bone ends are displaced, they are fitted together during a surgical operation and fixed with a metal screw; if the bone is broken into several pieces, the smallest bone fragments are removed and the *triceps muscle* is reattached to the broken end of the ulna.

Ulnar nerve

One of the principal *nerves* of the arm, running down its full length into the hand. A branch of the *brachial plexus*,

---

LOCATION OF THE ULNA
The ulna hinges at the elbow on the inner side of the lower end of the humerus (upper-arm bone). It is less mobile than the radius.

Right arm

Humerus

Radius
Ulna

Carpals
Thumb

---

the ulnar nerve controls muscles that move the thumb and fingers. It also conveys sensation from the fifth and part of the fourth fingers, and from the palm at the base of these digits.

DISORDERS
A blow to the *olecranon* process (the rounded projection at the tip of the elbow), over which the ulnar nerve passes, causes a pins and needles sensation and pain in the forearm and in the fourth and fifth fingers.

Persistent numbness and muscle weakness in the areas controlled by the nerve may be caused by pressure from an abnormal bony outgrowth from the *humerus* (upper-arm bone). Such a growth may be due to *osteoarthritis* or to a fracture of the humerus. If an operation is not performed to relieve the pressure on the nerve, the hand muscles controlled by the nerve may become permanently damaged, resulting in a *clawhand*.

Ultrasound

Sound with a frequency greater than the human ear's upper limit of perception—that is, with a frequency higher than 20,000 hertz (cycles per second). Ultrasound used in medicine for diagnosis or treatment is typically in the frequency range of one million to 15 million hertz (see *Ultrasound scanning; Ultrasound treatment*).

Ultrasound scanning

A diagnostic technique in which very high frequency sound waves (inaudible to the human ear) are passed into the body, and the reflected echoes are detected and analyzed to build a picture of the internal organs or of a fetus in the uterus. The procedure is painless and considered safe.

Also called sonography, ultrasound scanning was originally a spin-off from naval sonar (used to detect submarines in World War II) and was first used medically in the 1950s. The original ultrasound scanners produced still images; most modern scanners produce moving pictures, which are easier to interpret.

HOW IT WORKS
The illustrated box (facing page) explains how ultrasound scanners work and how they are operated.

WHY IT IS DONE
Ultrasound waves pass readily through soft tissues and fluids, making this procedure particularly useful for examining fluid-filled organs (such as the uterus in pregnancy, and the gallbladder) and soft organs (such as the liver). Ultrasound

U

waves cannot, however, pass through bone or gas. They are thus of limited use for examining regions that are surrounded by bone (such as the adult brain) or that contain gas (such as the lungs or intestines).

OBSTETRIC USES One of the most common uses of ultrasound is to view the uterus and fetus in pregnancy.

Ultrasound scanning is often performed about 16 to 18 weeks into the pregnancy, but may be performed at

HOW ULTRASOUND SCANNING WORKS

Ultrasound waves are emitted by a device called a transducer, which is placed on the skin over the part of the body to be viewed. The transducer contains a crystal that converts an electric current into sound waves. The waves used have frequencies in the range of 1 to 15 million hertz. At these high frequencies, the waves can be focused into a fine parallel beam, which passes through a "slice" of the body if the transducer crystal is

made to oscillate back and forth. Some of the waves are reflected at tissue boundaries, so a series of echoes is returned. The transducer also acts as a receiver, converting these echoes into electrical signals, which are processed and displayed on a screen to give a two-dimensional image of the scanned body slice. By moving the transducer, different slices through the body can be seen.

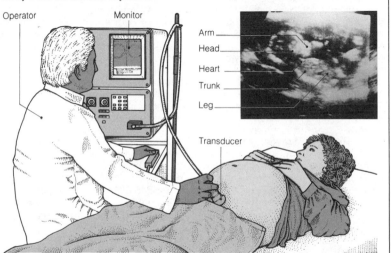

Operator — Monitor

Arm — Head — Heart — Trunk — Leg

Transducer

Ultrasound has wide applications in medicine and is especially useful in obstetrics. It offers no known risk to the baby. By moving the transducer across

the outer wall of the abdomen, views of the growing fetus are obtained from various angles, so it is possible to screen for abnormalities.

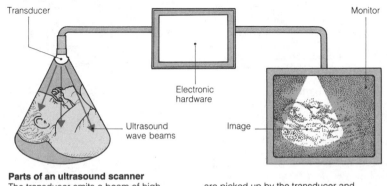

Transducer

Electronic hardware

Ultrasound wave beams

Monitor

Image

Parts of an ultrasound scanner
The transducer emits a beam of high frequency waves, which are passed through a slice of the body; the echoes

are picked up by the transducer and converted by the electronic hardware into an image displayed on the monitor.

any stage. If the date of conception is known, the scan shows whether the fetus is of the expected size; conversely, fetal size can help establish the accurate date of conception and therefore predict the expected date of delivery. The scan also reveals whether there is a multiple pregnancy (see *Pregnancy, multiple*). It is also possible to identify certain gross abnormalities, such as *anencephaly* or *spina bifida*. Congenital *heart disease* can sometimes be detected, enabling the baby to be delivered in a hospital that specializes in correcting such defects soon after birth. The scan also shows the position of the placenta. If the placenta is in a position that could obstruct normal childbirth (a condition known as *placenta previa*), delivery by *cesarean section* may be necessary.

Scans earlier in pregnancy may be performed if the physician suspects an *ectopic pregnancy* (presence of an embryo outside the uterus), *hydatidiform mole* (abnormal tumor in the uterus), impending *miscarriage*, or early death of the fetus.

Ultrasound is also vital for the procedure of *amniocentesis* (removal of amniotic fluid via a needle for analysis) and is used during *chorionic villus sampling* (removal of tissue from the placenta for analysis). A scan shows the position of the fetus and placenta before either of these procedures and also helps in guiding the needle into the uterus.

Later in pregnancy, a scan may be carried out if the growth rate of the fetus seems slow, if fetal movements cease or are excessive, or if the mother experiences vaginal bleeding. For high-risk or overdue pregnancies, a scan may be carried out before delivery to check on fetal size, development, and position in the uterus, the amount of amniotic fluid, and to recheck the position of the placenta.

NONOBSTETRIC USES In the newborn child, ultrasound can be used to scan the brain, via a gap (the anterior fontanelle) in the skull, to investigate *hydrocephalus* or to diagnose a *brain tumor* or brain hemorrhage.

Echocardiography is a type of ultrasound technique used to look at the heart. This technique is particularly useful for investigating congenital heart disease and disorders of the heart valves.

The liver can be clearly viewed by ultrasound, which can be used to diagnose liver disorders such as *cirrhosis*, cysts, abscesses, or tumors. Ultrasound shows the presence of

U

gallstones in the gallbladder or bile ducts. In a patient with *jaundice*, a scan can help establish whether the jaundice is due to obstruction of the bile ducts or to liver disease. The pancreas can be scanned for cysts, tumors, or *pancreatitis*, and the kidneys for congenital defects, cysts, tumors, and *hydronephrosis* (swelling due to obstruction to the outflow of urine). Other organs that may be scanned by ultrasound for diagnostic purposes (primarily to look for cysts, solid tumors, or foreign bodies) include the thyroid gland, breasts, bladder, testes, ovaries, spleen, and eyes.

Ultrasound scanning is also used during needle *biopsy* (insertion of a very thin hollow needle into an organ to remove cells, tissue, or fluid for examination) to help guide the needle accurately to a specific spot.

ELECTROMAGNETIC SPECTRUM

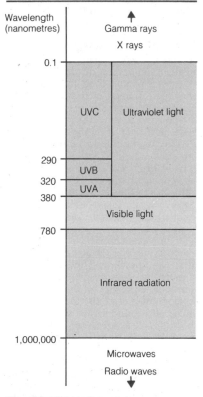

Ultraviolet light in the spectrum
Different types of electromagnetic radiation are defined according to their wavelengths. The diagram shows the different types—which together make up the electromagnetic spectrum—and their wavelength limits in nanometres (one nanometre equals one thousand-millionth of a metre). Ultraviolet light is the part of the electromagnetic spectrum between visible light and X rays.

Doppler ultrasound is a modified form of ultrasound that exploits the *Doppler effect* (the change in pitch that occurs when a sound source is moving relative to the detector) to investigate moving objects. One important use of Doppler ultrasound is to examine the fetal heartbeat.

Doppler ultrasound is frequently used in the technique, by which information can be obtained about the rate of blood flow through blood vessels. This procedure enables the physician to detect narrowing of vessels or turbulence in the flow of blood.

HOW IT IS DONE
For a scan in early pregnancy, the woman is usually asked not to pass urine for a few hours beforehand; a full bladder helps improve the view of the uterus by displacing nearby loops of intestine. For a liver or gallbladder scan, the patient is usually asked to fast for several hours beforehand.

Clothing over the region to be scanned is removed, and oil or jelly is smeared over the skin to achieve good contact when the transducer is passed back and forth over the skin. During the scan, which takes about 15 minutes (or sometimes less), the patient can usually lie back and watch the images appearing on the screen.

The ultrasonic waves produce no detectable sensation. When a scan is performed in conjunction with a technique involving insertion of a needle, a local anesthetic is used and there is usually little or no discomfort.

Ultrasound treatment
The use of high-frequency sound waves to treat *soft-tissue injuries* (such as injuries to ligaments, muscles, and tendons). The treatment reduces inflammation and speeds up healing. It is thought to work by improving blood flow in tissues under the skin.

During treatment, there may be a feeling of warmth and a slight tingling sensation. Occasionally, severe pain occurs if the sound waves are pointed at a bone surface just under the skin.

Ultraviolet light
Invisible light from the part of the electromagnetic spectrum immediately beyond the violet end of the visible light spectrum (i.e., between visible light and *X rays*). Long wavelength ultraviolet light (i.e., that nearest visible light) is often termed UVA; intermediate wavelength ultraviolet light is designated UVB; and short wavelength ultraviolet light (i.e., that nearest X rays) is called UVC.

Ultraviolet light occurs naturally in sunlight, but much of it—including all UVC and much UVB (both of which are potentially harmful)—is absorbed by the *ozone* layer of the atmosphere. The ultraviolet light that reaches the earth's surface, mainly UVA with some UVB, is responsible for the tanning and burning effects of sunlight and for the production of *vitamin D* in the skin. However, it is repeated overexposure to the ultraviolet component of sunlight that can have harmful effects (see *Sunlight, adverse effects of*), such as *skin cancer*, especially in fair-skinned people.

Suntan lamps, which produce ultraviolet light artificially, are designed to emit only UVA rays. In practice, however, they also give off a small amount of UVB light and may pose a significant health risk. Ultraviolet light is also produced by certain other types of equipment, such as welding torches, carbon arcs, and lasers. Special precautions, such as the use of goggles, should always be taken when using such equipment.

MEDICAL USES
Ultraviolet light is sometimes used in *phototherapy* to treat certain skin conditions, such as *psoriasis* and *vitiligo*, and also jaundice of the newborn (see *Jaundice, neonatal*).

A mercury-vapor lamp (Wood's light) can also be used to produce ultraviolet light artificially. This light is used to diagnose certain skin conditions, such as *tinea*, because it causes the infected area to fluoresce.

Umbilical cord
The ropelike structure connecting the fetus to the *placenta* that supplies oxygen and nutrients from the mother's

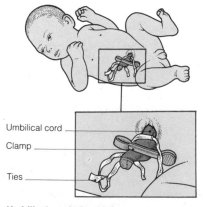

Umbilical cord after birth
The cord ceases to function after birth and is clamped and cut; the baby now obtains oxygen through his or her own lungs.

circulation. The umbilical cord is usually 40 to 60 cm long and consists of a jellylike substance in which two arteries and a vein are embedded.

Several minutes after delivery, the umbilical cord is clamped and then cut about 2.5 cm from the baby's abdominal wall. The stump falls off within a couple of weeks, leaving a scar called the *umbilicus* (navel).

DISORDERS

In rare cases, the umbilical cord protrudes down through the mother's cervix during labor. This is dangerous because the baby's oxygen supply can be cut off. Prompt delivery, by *cesarean section* or a *forceps delivery*, is necessary. Sometimes the cord pulls tightly around the baby's neck during delivery, but can usually be freed by slipping it over the baby's head.

Rarely, there is only one artery in the umbilical cord. This condition may be associated with birth defects.

The newborn baby's umbilical stump sometimes becomes infected and may ooze pus. This condition, called omphalitis, generally begins during the first week of life. Treatment involves gently wiping the umbilicus with sterile cotton wool and water. Treatment with *antibiotic drugs* may also be necessary.

Quite commonly, a fleshy protuberance called a *granuloma* grows on the umbilical stump, sometimes as a result of chronic infection. Umbilical granulomas may be destroyed by local application of *silver nitrate*. Umbilical polyps (also called umbilical adenomas) are shiny, bright red, raspberrylike growths which may also appear in the newborn period. Such polyps may require surgical removal.

Umbilicus

The scar on the abdomen that marks the site of attachment of the *umbilical cord* to the fetus. The umbilicus is commonly called the navel.

DISORDERS

An umbilical *hernia* is a soft swelling at the umbilicus caused by protrusion of the abdominal contents through a weak area of the abdominal wall.

Umbilical hernias are quite common in newborn infants, occurring twice as commonly in boys as in girls. When the baby cries, the swelling increases in size and may cause discomfort. Umbilical hernias usually disappear without treatment by the time a child is about 2 years old. If an umbilical hernia has not disappeared spontaneously by the age of about 4, surgery may be necessary.

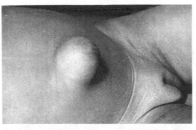

Umbilical hernia
This condition, present from birth, is due to a localized weakness in the abdominal wall. It usually disappears without treatment.

Occasionally, umbilical hernias develop in adults, especially in women following childbirth. Surgery may be necessary if such hernias are large, persistent, or disfiguring.

In rare cases, a discharge from the umbilicus develops due either to an infection or to an abnormal connection between the umbilicus and the urinary, biliary, or intestinal tract. Possible causes of the abnormal connection, which can be corrected surgically, include a birth defect, cancer, or tuberculosis.

Occasionally, benign or malignant tumors develop in the umbilicus. Such tumors may be secondary to cancers in the breast, colon, ovary, or stomach.

In rare cases, women develop *endometriosis* in the umbilicus, causing it to bleed periodically. Surgery may be necessary in such cases.

Unconscious

A specific part of the mind in which ideas, memories, perceptions, or feelings that a person is not currently aware of are stored and actively processed. The contents of the unconscious mind are not easily retrievable,

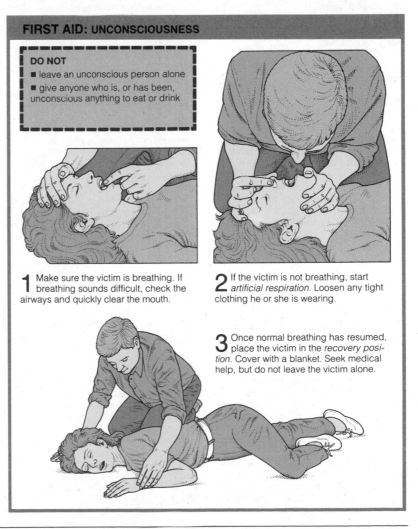

FIRST AID: UNCONSCIOUSNESS

DO NOT
- leave an unconscious person alone
- give anyone who is, or has been, unconscious anything to eat or drink

1 Make sure the victim is breathing. If breathing sounds difficult, check the airways and quickly clear the mouth.

2 If the victim is not breathing, start *artificial respiration*. Loosen any tight clothing he or she is wearing.

3 Once normal breathing has resumed, place the victim in the *recovery position*. Cover with a blanket. Seek medical help, but do not leave the victim alone.

U

in contrast to those of the *subconscious*. *Freudian theory* stresses the importance of the unconscious in determining behavior and causing neurotic symptoms. *Jungian theory* describes a collective unconscious, inherited by every person and derived from experiences in our distant past.

Unconsciousness

Abnormal loss of awareness of the self and of one's surroundings, resulting from a reduced level of activity in the reticular formation of the *brain stem*. *Sleep* is a normal state of altered consciousness from which a person can be roused easily; an unconscious person can be roused only with difficulty or not at all. Unconsciousness may be brief and light, as in *fainting*, or deeper and more prolonged (see *Coma*). The term *concussion* refers to a brief transient state of unconsciousness following a head injury.

Underbite

See *Prognathism*.

Unsaturated fats

See *Fats and oils*.

Uranium

A radioactive metallic element which does not occur naturally in its pure form but is widely distributed in various compounds in ores such as pitchblende, carnotite, and uraninite.

Natural radioactive decay of uranium yields a series of radioactive products, including *radium* and *radon*, and progresses ultimately to lead. During the various decay stages, *radiation* is emitted as alpha and beta particles and gamma rays. In addition to its *radiation hazards*, uranium is chemically poisonous, causing damage to the urinary system.

Urea

A waste product of the breakdown of proteins and the main nitrogenous (nitrogen-containing) constituent of *urine*. Proteins in food are digested in the intestine to form *amino acids*, which are absorbed into the bloodstream and transported to the *liver*. In the liver, amino acids in excess of the body's requirements are converted into urea, which is transported by the bloodstream to the *kidneys* and excreted in the urine.

The kidneys are usually highly efficient at eliminating urea from the body. A high-protein diet increases the amount of urea produced. Healthy kidneys are able to cope with increased urea production, but *kidney failure* impairs the kidneys' ability to eliminate urea and leads to *uremia* (abnormally high blood levels of urea). For this reason, measurement of urea levels in the blood is one of the routine *kidney function tests*.

Urea is also formed in the body from the breakdown of cell proteins. If there is a large increase in urea from this source (due, for example, to severe tissue damage resulting from injury or surgery), the kidneys are sometimes unable to cope and uremia results.

Certain conditions (such as liver damage) may lead to a decrease in the blood level of urea. Blood levels of urea also fall during pregnancy, when the blood is more dilute than usual.

MEDICAL USES

Urea is used in various creams and ointments to moisturize and soften the skin in the treatment of disorders such as *psoriasis*, atopic *dermatitis*, *ichthyosis*, and other conditions in which the skin is dry and scaly. Occasionally, urea is used as an osmotic *diuretic drug*, primarily to reduce pressure in the skull due to cerebral *edema* or to reduce pressure in the eye caused by *glaucoma*.

Uremia

The presence of excess *urea* and other chemical waste products in the *blood*. Uremia results from *kidney failure*.

Ureter

One of the two tubes that carry *urine* from the *kidneys* to the *bladder*. Each ureter is about 25 to 30 cm long. The walls of the ureters have three layers: a fibrous outer layer; a muscular middle layer; and an inner watertight layer (known as transitional epithelium). Each ureter is supplied by blood vessels and nerves.

Urine flows down the ureters partly due to gravity but mainly as a result of the pumping action known as peristalsis in which wavelike contractions pass several times a minute through the muscular ureter walls. Each ureter enters the bladder via a tunnel in the bladder wall, which is angled to prevent reflux (backflow) of urine into the ureter when the bladder muscle contracts.

DISORDERS

Some people are born with double ureters, on one or both sides of the body, usually in association with partial duplication of the kidney on an affected side. Double ureters may be completely distinct along their entire

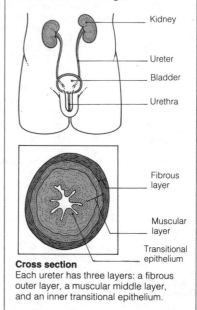

ANATOMY OF THE URETER
The ureters are tubes that carry urine from the kidneys to the bladder. They enter the back of the bladder at an angle.

Kidney

Ureter

Bladder

Urethra

Fibrous layer

Muscular layer

Transitional epithelium

Cross section
Each ureter has three layers: a fibrous outer layer, a muscular middle layer, and an inner transitional epithelium.

length or may join to form a Y shape. In many cases, ureteric duplication causes no problems, but there may be a tendency for urine to reflux up one of the tubes if the duplicated ureters enter the bladder separately. There may also be problems, such as *incontinence* or infection, if a ureter enters the urethra or the vagina instead of the bladder. Corrective surgery can be performed if necessary.

Spasms of the ureter may result if a stone (see *Calculus, urinary tract*) passes down or becomes stuck in a ureter. This extremely painful condition is commonly known as *renal colic*.

Ureteritis is an inflammatory condition of the ureter, which may be caused by blockage of the ureter by a stone, or by the spread of infection from the bladder.

Ureteral colic

See *Renal colic*.

Ureterolithotomy

The surgical removal of a stone (see *Calculus, urinary tract*) that is stuck in a *ureter* (tube that carries urine from a kidney to the bladder). In some cases, calculi are removed by means of *cystoscopy* or *lithotripsy* rather than by ureterolithotomy.

U

HOW IT IS DONE

Ureterolithotomy is preceded by intravenous *urography* to locate the calculus. With the patient under general anesthesia, the surgeon makes an abdominal incision and feels the ureter to locate the calculus. The ureter is then opened with a longitudinal cut, the calculus is removed with forceps, and a check is made for more calculi. The ureter and abdomen are then sewn up, leaving a tube inserted into the abdomen to drain any urine that leaks from the ureter. This tube is removed four or five days later and the patient can then leave hospital.

Urethra

The tube by which *urine* is excreted from the *bladder*. In females, the urethra is short and opens to the outside just in front of the vagina between the labia minora. In males, the urethra is much longer. It is surrounded by the prostate gland at its upper end and then forms a channel through the length of the penis. The location and relative length of the male and female urethras are shown in the illustrated box.

DISORDERS

Although urethral infections, scarring, and congenital abnormalities occur in both sexes, these disorders are much more common and serious in males than in females.

In male infants, a urethral valve is sometimes present. This is a flap that arises from the lining of the urethra and impedes the flow of urine. The resulting bottleneck causes back pressure on the *kidneys* as urine overfills the bladder, ureters, and collecting ducts of the kidneys. Permanent and severe damage to the kidneys can occur if the urethral valve is not removed surgically.

Urethritis (inflammation of the urethra) may be due to infection, irritation, or minor injury. Inflammation may be followed by scarring and formation of a *urethral stricture* (a narrowed section of the urethra).

The male urethra is easily damaged in accidents involving pelvic injury and may require surgical repair. Injury to, or surgery on, the urethra may lead to urethral stricture.

Urethral dilatation

A procedure in which a *urethral stricture* (narrowed urethra) in a male is widened by means of a slim, round-tipped instrument inserted through the opening of the urethra at the tip of the penis. Urethral dilatation is performed under either local or general anesthesia. The procedure may need to be repeated.

Urethral discharge

A fluid that flows from the *urethra* in some cases of *urethritis* caused by infection. In *gonorrhea*, the discharge is yellow and purulent (pus-containing); in other types of infection the discharged fluid is clear.

Urethral stricture

An uncommon condition in which the male *urethra* becomes narrowed and sometimes shortened along part of its length as a result of shrinkage of scar tissue within its walls.

CAUSES AND SYMPTOMS

Scar tissue may form after injury to the urethra or after persistent *urethritis* (inflammation of the urethra). In the past, urethritis was most commonly due to *gonorrhea*, but modern antibiotic treatment has made strictures from this cause uncommon.

A urethral stricture may make it difficult or painful to pass urine or to ejaculate, and may cause some deformation of the penis when erect.

In some cases, a urethral stricture may lead to kidney damage due to back pressure from the build-up of urine. A urethral stricture may also encourage the development of *urinary tract infection*.

TREATMENT

A urethral stricture is usually treated by *urethral dilatation* (widening of the urethra by inserting a slim, round-tipped instrument through the urethral opening at the tip of the penis). If dilatation fails, an instrument called a urethrotome may be inserted to cut through the scar tissue. In some cases, a urethral stricture may be completely removed and the urethra reconstructed by plastic surgery.

Urethral syndrome, acute

A set of symptoms of uncertain cause experienced by some women and, very rarely, by some men. The symptoms consist of pain and discomfort in the lower abdomen, a frequent urge to pass *urine*, and, in women, pain around the vulval region. Middle-aged women are the most commonly affected by this syndrome.

In most cases, the physician cannot discover any causative infection, and the patient's *kidney* function and *urinary tract* anatomy are normal. Emotional and psychological factors may contribute. In women who have gone through the menopause, the symptoms may be due to inflammation of the vulva associated with thinning of tissues (see *Vulvitis*).

Treatment may be difficult. Cases due to vulvitis may be relieved by use of *estrogen drugs* or *corticosteroid drugs* in cream form. Antiseptic creams and strong soaps should be avoided because they may cause irritation or an allergic reaction that worsens the symptoms. Scrupulous personal hygiene and a high fluid intake are usually recommended.

Urethritis

Inflammation of the *urethra*, usually due to an infection but sometimes having other causes.

LOCATION OF THE URETHRA

The urethra is the tube through which urine is passed from the bladder. There is no voluntary muscle in the urethra. The flow of urine is controlled by muscles in the wall and outlet of the bladder.

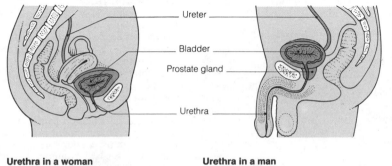

Ureter

Bladder

Prostate gland

Urethra

Urethra in a woman
The female urethra is short—about 4 cm long—and runs down to open to the exterior just in front of the vagina.

Urethra in a man
The male urethra is about 18–20 cm long. It passes through the prostate gland and along the full length of the penis.

U

CAUSES

Urethritis may be caused by various infectious organisms, including the bacterium that causes *gonorrhea*. *Nonspecific urethritis* may be caused by any of a large number of different types of microorganisms, including bacteria, yeasts, and *chlamydial infection*. Bacteria from the skin or rectum sometimes spread to infect the urethra.

Urethritis may also be caused by damage from an accident or from a surgically introduced catheter or cystoscope (viewing instrument for examining the bladder). Other possible causes include exposure to irritant chemicals, such as antiseptics and some spermicidal preparations.

SYMPTOMS AND COMPLICATIONS

Urethritis causes a burning sensation and pain when passing urine. The pain can be severe and is sometimes likened to passing small fragments of broken glass. The urine may be blood-stained and, particularly when gonorrhea is the cause, there is often a yellow, pus-filled, discharge.

Urethritis may be followed by scarring and the formation of a *urethral stricture* (narrowing of a section of the urethra), which can make the passing of urine difficult.

TREATMENT

Infections are treated with an appropriate *antibiotic drug*. Antibiotic treatment may also be needed if bacterial infection follows urethritis due to a noninfective cause. Urethral strictures are usually treated by the technique of *urethral dilatation*.

Urethrocele

An anatomical abnormality caused by a weakness in the tissues in the front wall of the *vagina*. This weakness allows the overlying *urethra* to bulge backward and downward into the vagina. A urethrocele may be congenital (present from birth), may develop after *childbirth*, or may be associated with *obesity*.

A urethrocele may cause difficulty in emptying the bladder and pain during sexual intercourse (see *Intercourse, painful*). It also increases susceptibility to *urinary tract infection*.

The usual treatment for a urethrocele is a surgical operation to tighten the tissues at the front of the vagina, thus giving the urethra better support (see *Vaginal repair*).

-uria

A suffix relating to *urine*, as in *proteinuria*, the term for presence of protein in the urine.

Uric acid

A waste product of the breakdown of *nucleic acids* in body cells. A small amount of uric acid is also produced by the digestion of foods rich in nucleic acids, such as liver, kidneys, and other offal.

Most uric acid produced in the body passes, via the bloodstream, to the *kidneys*, which remove the acid from the blood and excrete it in the urine. However, some uric acid passes into the intestine, where it is broken down by bacteria into chemicals which are excreted in the feces.

The kidneys of a healthy person maintain blood levels of uric acid within acceptable limits. When uric acid excretion is disrupted, it may result in *hyperuricemia* (abnormally high levels of uric acid in the blood), which, in turn, may lead to *gout* or kidney stones (see *Calculus, urinary tract*). Causes of hyperuricemia include kidney disease, *leukemia*, *hemolytic anemia*, genetic disorders in which an enzyme involved in uric acid excretion is lacking, and certain drugs, including some *diuretic drugs* and *anticancer drugs*.

Urinal

A container for *urine*, useful for bedridden men (women use a *bedpan*). Also known as a urinal is an appliance for men suffering from urinary *incontinence*, which consists of a thick rubber tube connected by a plastic tube to a drainage bag strapped on the leg.

Urinalysis

A battery of tests on a patient's *urine*, including measurements of the urine's physical characteristics (such as color, concentration, and cloudiness), microscopic examination, and chemical testing. Urinalysis can be used to check kidney function and to detect and diagnose *urinary tract* and other disorders.

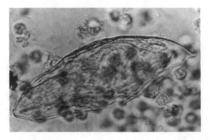

Schistosome egg in urine
The tropical disease schistosomiasis may be diagnosed by the finding of schistosome (worm) eggs on urinalysis.

TYPES OF TESTS

MICROSCOPIC EXAMINATION Microscopy of urine may reveal *hematuria* (red blood cells in the urine), indicating damage to the glomeruli (filtering units of the kidneys) or some other disorder of the kidneys or urinary tract. Fragments of protein and kidney cells, called casts, in the urine may indicate various types of kidney disease. *Urinary tract infection* results in the presence of pus or bacteria in the urine. Crystals in the urine indicate the possibility of an inborn error of metabolism (see *Metabolism, inborn errors of*) or susceptibility to stones (see *Calculus, urinary tract*). The parasitic disease *schistosomiasis* may be diagnosed from the presence of worm eggs in the urine.

CULTURE If a single drop of fresh urine is spread thinly on the surface of a nutrient gel and incubated, any bacteria present will multiply and produce colonies. The appearance of these colonies under microscopic examination allows the microbiologist to identify the organism causing a urinary tract infection.

CHEMICAL TESTS A range of simple stick or strip tests is available to show the presence of various substances in the urine, and to measure properties of the urine, such as its acidity and concentration (ratio of dissolved substances to water). These tests rely on a simple color change when the stick or strip is dipped into the urine. Substances tested for include glucose (a high level usually means that the patient has *diabetes mellitus*), blood, protein, and bile. Detection of human chorionic gonadotropin in the urine is the basis of many *pregnancy tests*. Urine tests are also useful in determining whether a person has been taking a particular drug. (See also *Kidney function tests*.)

Urinary diversion

Any surgical procedure performed to allow passage of urine when the normal outlet channel of the *urinary tract*, via the bladder and urethra, is obstructed or cannot be used, or when the bladder has been surgically removed.

TEMPORARY DIVERSION

Temporary urinary diversion is sometimes required when passage of urine is blocked by enlargement of the *prostate gland* or by *urethral stricture*. In such cases, a small opening is made through the abdominal wall just above the pubic bone, and a tube is passed directly into the bladder (see *Catheterization, urinary*). Temporary

URINARY DIVERSION USING ILEAL CONDUIT

This is a standard operation performed when the bladder has been removed or is seriously malfunctioning and beyond hope of repair. A midline incision in the abdomen is used; before making it, the surgeon creates an opening through the abdominal wall in a good position for later attachment of the collecting bag.

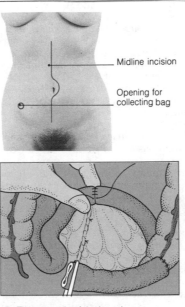

Midline incision

Opening for collecting bag

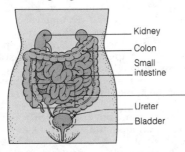

Kidney

Colon

Small intestine

Ureter

Bladder

1 A short length is cut out of the ileum (the lower part of the small intestine), retaining the mesentery (supporting folds of tissue) and the essential blood vessels that supply the freed section.

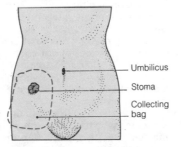

2 The cut ends of the intestine are stitched together to reestablish continuity. One end of the freed length of intestine is closed and the other end is temporarily clamped.

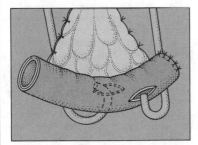

3 The ureters are now implanted into the isolated length of ileum. The open end of this segment is brought through the abdominal wall and stitched in place.

Umbilicus

Stoma

Collecting bag

4 A collecting bag for receiving the patient's urine is fixed with adhesive around the new stoma (opening) in the wall of the abdomen.

diversion is also required after some operations on the urinary tract; a small tube is introduced into the kidney and brought to the abdominal surface, bypassing the ureters and allowing healing to take place.

PERMANENT DIVERSION
Permanent urinary diversion is needed when the bladder has been removed, usually to treat advanced bladder cancer, or when neurological control of the bladder is severely disturbed, such as after severe spinal injury. Permanent diversion may also be required if there is an irreparable *fistula* (abnormal opening) between a female patient's bladder or urethra and the vagina.

Permanent diversion is usually achieved by creating what is known as an ileal conduit (see illustrated box). A section of the ileum is removed to create a substitute bladder, into one end of which the surgeon implants the ureters. The other end of the substitute bladder is then brought out through an incision in the abdominal wall, as in an *ileostomy*. The patient wears a bag attached to the skin to collect urine.

In recent years, the use of so-called continent urinary diversions has been investigated. These permit the patient to control the drainage of urine by periodically emptying an internal ileal conduit pouch with a catheter, there-

by permitting a degree of continence. Initial results have been encouraging, although this treatment is still considered experimental.

Urinary retention

Inability to empty the *bladder* or difficulty in doing so. Urinary retention may be complete, in which case urine cannot voluntarily be passed at all (although some may leak out), or incomplete, in which case some urine may be passed but the bladder fails to empty completely.

CAUSES
Retention may be due to an obstruction to the flow of urine. This problem predominantly affects males. Causes include *phimosis* (tight foreskin), *urethral stricture*, a stone in the bladder (see *Calculus, urinary tract*), *prostatitis* (inflammation of the prostate), enlargement of the prostate (see *Prostate, enlarged*), or a tumor of the prostate (see *Prostate, cancer of*). In women, urinary retention may result from pressure on the urethra from uterine *fibroids* or from a fetus in the uterus. In either sex it may be due to a *bladder tumor*.

Alternatively, retention may be due to defective functioning of the nerve pathways concerned with the sensing of bladder enlargement and with the triggering of bladder emptying. This may be induced by a general or spinal anesthetic, by drugs that act on the bladder, or by surgery. Defective nerve functioning may also be due to injury to the nerve pathways or to disease of the spinal cord.

SYMPTOMS AND COMPLICATIONS
Except when nerve pathways are defective, complete urinary retention causes discomfort and pain in the lower abdomen, which may be severe. The filled bladder can be felt on examination as a swelling above the pubic bone. Chronic or partial retention, by contrast, may not cause any serious symptoms and the sufferer may be unaware of it.

There is a risk that retention will lead to kidney damage from back pressure up the urinary tract. Incomplete emptying often leads to a *urinary tract infection*.

TREATMENT
Urinary retention is treated by inserting a drainage tube into the bladder, usually via the urethra (see *Catheterization, urinary*). The cause of the retention is then investigated if it is not already known. When obstruction is the cause, it can usually be treated; if nerve damage is the cause, the pros-

U

pects are less hopeful; permanent or intermittent catheterization is sometimes necessary in such cases.

Urinary system
See *Urinary tract*.

Urinary tract
The part of the body concerned with the formation and excretion of *urine*. The urinary tract consists of the *kidneys* (with their blood and nerve supplies), renal pelvises (funnel-shaped ducts that channel urine from the kidneys), *ureters, bladder,* and *urethra.*

The kidneys make urine by filtering blood. The urine collects in the renal pelvises and then passes down the ureters into the bladder by the actions of gravity and peristalsis (wavelike contractions of the walls of the ureters). Urine is then stored in the bladder until a sufficient amount is present to stimulate micturition (passage of urine). When the bladder contracts, the urine is expelled from the body through the urethra.

Urinary tract infection
An infection anywhere in the *urinary tract*. *Urethritis* (inflammation of the urethra) may be caused by mechanisms other than infection, but *cystitis* (inflammation of the bladder) and *pyelonephritis* (inflammation of the kidneys) are nearly always caused by a bacterial infection.

Urethral infections are more common in men than in women. However, infections further up the urinary tract are more common in women because of the shorter female urethra.

CAUSES
Urethritis is often due to a *sexually transmitted disease,* such as *gonorrhea* or *nonspecific urethritis.* Other urinary tract infections are usually caused by organisms that have spread from the rectum, via the urethra, to the bladder or kidneys. Infections can also be carried to the urinary tract in the blood.

In men, there is often an identifiable predisposing factor, usually some condition that impairs the drainage of urine, such as an enlarged prostate gland (see *Prostate, enlarged*) or a *urethral stricture*. In women, urinary tract infections often occur without any identifiable underlying cause. Such infections are, however, more common during pregnancy.

In both sexes, urinary tract infection may be caused by a stone (see *Calculus, urinary tract*), a *bladder tumor*, or a congenital abnormality of the urinary tract, such as a double kidney on one side. Defective bladder emptying as a result of *spina bifida* or of damage to the spinal cord in a *spinal injury* leads almost inevitably to urinary tract infection.

The risks of a urinary tract infection can be reduced by careful personal hygiene, by drinking plenty of fluids, and by regular emptying of the bladder.

SYMPTOMS
Urethritis causes a burning sensation when passing urine. Cystitis causes a frequent urge to pass urine, lower abdominal pain, *hematuria* (blood in the urine), and, in many cases, general malaise with a mild fever. Pyelonephritis causes pain in the loins and high fever.

COMPLICATIONS
Urethritis can lead to scarring of the urethra and formation of a *urethral stricture*. Cystitis does not usually produce complications unless infection spreads up to the kidneys. Without proper treatment, pyelonephritis can lead to permanent kidney damage, *septicemia* (spread of infective organisms to the blood), and *septic shock*. If a calculus in a kidney is the underlying cause of infection, it may grow rapidly during the course of the infection.

DIAGNOSIS
Infection is diagnosed by examination of a *culture* of a few drops of urine. The urine specimen is taken midstream to avoid contamination of the specimen by organisms that normally live in the last part of the urethra.

Further investigation is usually needed for men who have any urinary tract infection or for women suffering from recurrent cystitis or pyelonephritis. Such investigation is performed by *urography* (an X-ray procedure for examining the urinary tract after injection of a radiopaque contrast medium) or by *ultrasound scanning*.

TREATMENT
Most urinary tract infections are treated with *antibiotic drugs*; the specific drug used depends on the type of infection.

Urination, excessive
The production of more than about 2.5 litres of *urine* per day. Excessive urination is known as polyuria.

CAUSES
Excessive urination is sometimes due to psychiatric problems, which may cause a person to drink compulsively. The high intake of fluid leads inevitably to a high urine output.

Various diseases may cause abnormal amounts of certain substances to be excreted in the urine; these substances draw water with them, increasing the urine volume. The most important disease in this group is *diabetes mellitus*, in which excess glucose in the blood spills into the urine. Certain kidney diseases lead to excessive salt loss in the urine, with an accompanying increase in volume.

In the disorder known as central *diabetes insipidus*, excessive urination results from reduced production of *ADH* (antidiuretic hormone) by the pituitary gland. This leads to a marked increase in urine volume because ADH normally acts on the kidneys to concentrate the urine. In nephrogenic diabetes insipidus, which may result from various kidney disorders, normal amounts of ADH are produced but the kidneys fail to respond to it.

DIAGNOSIS
Any person who passes large quantities of urine should discuss the matter with a physician.

In a compulsive drinker, urine volume soon drops if water intake is restricted, but no such drop occurs in a patient with diabetes insipidus. Central diabetes insipidus improves after administration of synthetic ADH, but nephrogenic diabetes insipidus does not.

In patients with diabetes mellitus, the glucose level in the blood and urine is high; in salt-losing patients, an excessive amount of sodium is detectable in the urine.

TREATMENT
Treatment of excessive urination depends on the underlying cause. (See also *Urination, frequent*.)

Urination, frequent
The passing of urine more frequently than usual, also called simply "frequency." Most people pass urine an average of four to six times daily and only occasionally need to urinate at night. A marked increase in this rate constitutes frequency.

In some cases, frequency is the inevitable result of excessive production of urine (see *Urination, excessive*). In other cases, the total volume of urine produced is not high or may even be lower than usual.

Frequency is commonly due to *cystitis* (inflammation of the bladder) caused by infection. Reducing fluid intake in such cases has the effect of making the urine more concentrated (and thus more irritant), which increases urinary frequency. Sufferers from cystitis should drink more than usual, not less.

U

THE URINARY TRACT

Also known as the urinary system, the urinary tract consists of the kidneys, in which urine is formed to carry away waste materials from the blood; the ureters, which transport the urine from the kidneys; the bladder, where the urine is stored until it can be conveniently disposed of; and the urethra, through which the bladder is emptied to the outside. The kidneys require a large blood supply and are connected close to the body's main artery, the aorta. More than a litre of blood passes through the kidneys every minute.

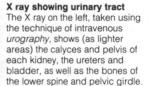

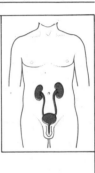

X ray showing urinary tract
The X ray on the left, taken using the technique of intravenous *urography*, shows (as lighter areas) the calyces and pelvis of each kidney, the ureters and bladder, as well as the bones of the lower spine and pelvic girdle.

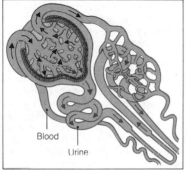

The filtering units
Each kidney has about one million of these units, which form dilute urine by filtering the blood.

Blood

Urine

Pelvis

Calyces

Medulla

Cortex

Aorta

Vena cava

Renal vein

Renal artery

Kidneys
The two kidneys lie within large pads of fat on the inside of the back wall of the abdomen, close to, and on either side of, the spine. Each kidney consists of an outer cortex, an inner medulla, and a urine-collecting system that includes the calyces and the pelvis of the kidney.

COMPOSITION OF URINE

Urine consists almost entirely of water, with only small amounts of urea (the main waste product), other waste products (e.g., creatinine and uric acid), and sodium chloride (salt).

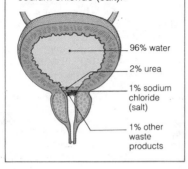

96% water

2% urea

1% sodium chloride (salt)

1% other waste products

Interior of bladder
The two ureteral openings and the urethral orifice form a triangle at the base of the bladder. In males, the urethra runs through the body of the prostate gland situated below the bladder.

Collecting system
From the tubules that lead from the filtering units, much of the water and some other substances are reabsorbed into the blood. The remaining, more concentrated, urine runs into collecting ducts and then into the pyramid-shaped calyces of the kidney and the kidney pelvis. From there, the urine passes into the ureter.

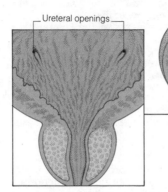

Ureteral openings

Ureters

Bladder
The muscular bladder wall can stretch to accommodate about half a litre of urine, but at this volume the desire to pass urine is very strong.

Urethra

Prostate (male only)

U

Anxiety is a common cause of increased frequency. Other causes include stones in the bladder (see *Calculus, urinary tract*), an enlarged prostate gland (see *Prostate, enlarged*) in men, and, in rare cases, a *bladder tumor*. Some people who are suffering from *kidney failure* also notice that they pass urine more frequently, particularly during the night.

Treatment of urinary frequency is always of the underlying cause once it has been diagnosed.

Urination, painful

Pain or discomfort when passing urine, also known medically as *dysuria*. The pain is often described as having a burning or scalding quality. Sometimes it is preceded by difficulty in starting the flow. Pain after the flow has ceased, with a strong desire to continue, is called *strangury*.

The most common cause of dysuria is *cystitis* (inflammation of the bladder), especially in women. Dysuria may also be caused by a *bladder tumor* or stone (see *Calculus, urinary tract*), especially if blood clots or small stones or crystals are passed in the urine. Strangury is usually due to spasm of an inflamed bladder wall, but may also be caused by bladder stones.

Other possible causes of dysuria include *urethritis* (inflammation of the urethra), often due to *gonorrhea*; in men, *prostatitis* (inflammation of the prostate gland) or *balanitis* (inflammation of the glans of the penis); and in women, vaginal *candidiasis* (thrush) or an allergy to vaginal deodorants.

Mild discomfort when passing urine may be caused by highly concentrated urine, which may result from fever or excessive sweating.

Dysuria may be investigated by physical examination, *urinalysis*, *urography*, or *cystoscopy*. (See also *Urethral syndrome, acute*.)

Urine

The pale yellow fluid produced by the *kidneys* and excreted from the body via the *ureters*, *bladder*, and *urethra*. Waste products and excess water or chemical substances are eliminated from the body in the urine.

URINE PRODUCTION

Urine is produced by the filtration of blood through the kidneys. The filtering units of the kidneys remove about 110 litres of watery fluid from the blood every day. Nearly all of this fluid is then reabsorbed into the blood; the remainder is passed from the body as urine.

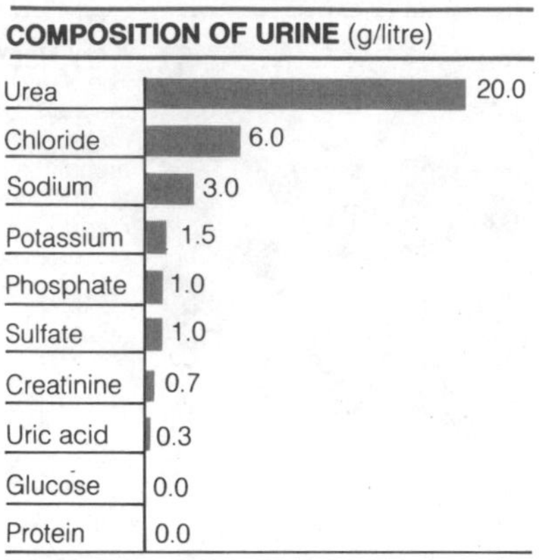

COMPOSITION OF URINE (g/litre)

Urea	20.0
Chloride	6.0
Sodium	3.0
Potassium	1.5
Phosphate	1.0
Sulfate	1.0
Creatinine	0.7
Uric acid	0.3
Glucose	0.0
Protein	0.0

Composition of urine
The chart shows the normal average contents of urine, other than water. The main waste products excreted are urea, creatinine, and uric acid. Variable amounts of sodium, chloride, hydrogen, and other ions are excreted to adjust the body's water, salt and acid-base balance.

A healthy adult may produce between about 0.5 and 2 litres of urine per day. The minimum volume of urine needed to remove all waste products is about 0.5 litre; any volume produced above this level consists of excess water. A high fluid intake increases the amount of urine produced; a high fluid loss from sweating, vomiting, or diarrhea leads to reduced production.

COMPOSITION

The average composition of urine excreted by a healthy person is shown in the diagram.

The volume, acidity, and salt concentration of the urine are carefully regulated by hormones such as *ADH* (antidiuretic hormone), *atrial natriuretic peptide*, and *aldosterone*. These hormones act on the kidneys to ensure that the body's water, salt, and *acid-base balance* (acidity or alkalinity of the blood and tissue fluids) is kept within narrow limits.

Measurements of the composition of urine are useful in the diagnosis of a wide variety of conditions, from kidney disease and diabetes to pregnancy (see *Urinalysis*).

Urine is normally sterile when passed and has only a faint odor. The unpleasant smell of stale urine is due to the action of bacteria, which causes the release of ammonia.

Urine, abnormal

Urine may be produced in abnormal amounts or may have an abnormal appearance or composition.

ABNORMAL VOLUME

Production by an adult of more than about 2.5 litres of urine per day is unusual unless he or she is drinking excessively or has a disease (see *Urination, excessive*).

Abnormally low urine production (*oliguria*) of less than about 0.4 litre per day may occur in severe *dehydration* and in cases of acute *kidney failure*. It also occurs when the kidneys are not receiving their normal blood supply due, for example, to *heart failure, shock*, or advanced liver disease.

No production of urine by the kidneys (*anuria*) may occur in extreme cases of kidney damage. However, lack of the passage of urine from the bladder is more commonly caused by obstruction in the lower part of the urinary tract as a result of a *bladder tumor*, stone (see *Calculus, urinary tract*), or an enlarged prostate gland (see *Prostate, enlarged*).

ABNORMAL APPEARANCE

Cloudy urine may be due to a *urinary tract infection*, in which case it may have an offensive smell. Urinary tract calculi can also produce cloudy urine, which is not necessarily infected. Cloudy urine may be caused by the presence of certain salts, such as phosphates. In rare instances, *lymph* enters the urine and gives it a milky appearance.

Slight *hematuria* (blood in the urine) produces a smoky appearance. Larger amounts of blood produce easily recognizable red urine, which may contain clots. Red urine is not always due to blood, however. Some dyes used in confectionery may be excreted in the urine, and a wide variety of drugs can discolor it (for example, rifampicin turns urine orange). People who eat beets may pass red urine. In some patients with *porphyria*, the urine turns red if it is left to stand; in some patients with *jaundice*, the urine is orange or brown. Frothy urine, particularly if the froth persists after shaking, may contain an excess of protein.

ABNORMAL COMPOSITION

In *diabetes mellitus*, the excess glucose present in the blood spills into the urine, causing *glycosuria*. In *glomerulonephritis* (inflammation of the filtering units of the kidneys) and in *nephrotic syndrome*, there may be excess protein present in the urine (*proteinuria*). In *kidney failure*, the total amount of waste products in the urine (such as urea) is reduced.

Other kidney disorders, such as *Fanconi's syndrome* and *renal tubular acidosis*, may make the urine too acid

U

or too alkaline, or may cause it to contain excess amino acids, phosphates, salt, or water.

Urine tests
See *Urinalysis*.

Urography
A procedure for obtaining *X-ray* pictures of the *urinary tract* (kidneys, ureters, and bladder), also known as pyelography. The technique involves the introduction into the bloodstream of a radiopaque medium that shows up on X rays when it is excreted by the kidneys, ureters, and bladder.

WHY IT IS DONE
Urography is performed, for example, to investigate recurrent *urinary tract infections*, *hematuria* (blood in the urine), and suspected stones (see *Calculus, urinary tract*).

Urography is also performed to discover whether kidney disease is the cause of *hypertension* (high blood pressure) in a young person.

HOW IT IS DONE
INTRAVENOUS UROGRAPHY (IVU) The patient is told not to drink for four hours before the IVU, and is given a laxative to empty the bowel (to improve the quality of the X-ray films).

With the patient lying down, X rays of the abdomen are taken. An *iodine*-based contrast medium is then injected into the bloodstream via a vein in the arm, from where it travels to the kidneys and urinary tract. Further X rays are taken immediately after the injection, and then five, 10, and 30 minutes later. Between the 5- and 10-minute X rays, pressure may be applied to the abdomen to improve the definition of the central cavities of the kidneys. After the bladder has filled with contrast medium, the patient is asked to urinate while another X ray is taken.

RETROGRADE PYELOGRAPHY Under anesthesia, a cystoscope (a type of viewing instrument) is passed into the bladder (see *Cystoscopy*). A fine tube is then threaded through the cystoscope and up the ureter to the kidney. A small quantity of contrast medium is injected and X rays are taken.

RESULTS
The X rays obtained by IVU allow the radiologist to see the size, shape, and position of the kidneys, the course of the ureters, the size and position of the bladder, and whether there are any obvious obstructions in the ureters. The X ray taken after urination shows whether or not the bladder has emptied completely.

COMPLICATIONS
Urography is generally very safe, but must not be used in people who are sensitive to iodine. With retrograde pyelography, there is a risk of aggravating any infection that may be present in the urinary tract.

Urokinase
A *thrombolytic drug* prepared from human urine or from a *culture* of human kidney tissue. Urokinase is given to dissolve blood clots in people who have had a recent *myocardial infarction* (heart attack) or *pulmonary embolism*. Given by injection in the early stages of a myocardial infarction, urokinase may limit the extent of damage that is caused to the heart muscle.

Treatment with urokinase is strictly supervised due to a risk of excessive bleeding. Urokinase sometimes produces a mild allergic reaction that causes rash or fever.

Urology
A branch of medicine concerned with the structure, functioning, and disorders of the *urinary tract* in males and females, and of the *reproductive system* in males.

Problems that are investigated and treated by urologists include congenital abnormalities of the urinary tract, *incontinence, urinary retention, urinary tract infection, bladder tumors*, and stones (see *Calculus, urinary tract*). Many urological problems are treated by surgery.

Investigative techniques commonly used in urology include *urography, cystoscopy, ultrasound scanning, cystometry*, and *urinalysis*.

Uropathy, obstructive
A general term for damage to the urinary system caused by partial or complete obstruction to the flow of urine. The commonest points for obstruction are in the collecting system of the kidney (*calyces*), in one or both of the *ureters*, and in the bladder, usually at the opening of the urethra. Common symptoms are infrequent urination, pain on urination, and *uremia*, the accumulation of nitrogenous waste products in the blood. The most serious consequence is kidney damage; in extreme cases, kidney function may be impaired or cease altogether, although considerable improvement may result when the obstruction is relieved. The commonest causes of obstructive uropathy are stones and tumors.

Urticaria
A *skin* condition, also known as hives or nettle rash, characterized by the development of itchy wheals (raised white or yellow lumps surrounded by an area of red inflammation). Wheals vary considerably in size, and large ones may merge to form irregular, raised patches. The rash is most common on the limbs and trunk but may appear anywhere on the body.

Urticaria usually lasts for no more than a few hours, but some people develop a persistent or recurrent form of the disorder. Urticaria sometimes occurs with *angioedema* (an allergic condition in which swelling occurs in various parts of the body). *Dermographism* is a less common form of urticaria in which wheals form after the skin is stroked.

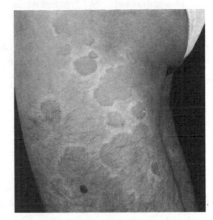

Appearance of urticaria
This skin condition is characterized by itchy wheals with a white or yellow center and an outer area of inflammation.

The cause of urticaria is often not known. Of known mechanisms, the most common is an allergic reaction (see *Allergy*) in which the chemical *histamine* is released from skin cells, causing fluid to leak from tiny blood vessels into the skin tissues. Urticaria often results from an allergic reaction to a particular kind of food (such as milk, eggs, shellfish, strawberries, or nuts), *food additive* (such as tartrazine, a food colorant), or *drug* (such as penicillin or ASA).

Urticaria may also be caused by exposure to heat, cold, or sunlight. Less commonly, urticaria may be associated with another disorder, such as *vasculitis*, systemic *lupus erythematosus*, or *cancer*.

TREATMENT AND PREVENTION
Itching can be relieved by applying *calamine* lotion or by taking *antihista-*

U

mine drugs. More severe cases may require *corticosteroid drugs*. Identifying and avoiding known trigger factors can help prevent future allergic reactions. Even if the cause cannot be identified, however, a tendency to urticaria often disappears in time without any treatment.

Urticaria, neonatal

A very common skin condition, also known as erythema neonatorum or toxic erythema, that affects newborn infants. Neonatal urticaria consists of a blotchy rash in which raised white or yellow lumps are surrounded by ill-defined red areas of inflammation. The rash usually appears on the second day after birth, occurring predominantly over the face, chest, arms, and thighs. The cause of neonatal urticaria is unknown. No treatment is necessary and the rash usually clears up within a few days.

Uterus

The hollow, muscular organ of the female *reproductive system* in which the fertilized *ovum* (egg) normally becomes embedded and in which the *embryo* and *fetus* develop. It is also commonly known as the womb.

The uterus is situated in the pelvic cavity, behind the bladder and in front of the intestines.

STRUCTURE

The uterus of a nonpregnant woman measures 7.5 to 10 cm in length and weighs about 60 to 90 g. In shape, it resembles an upside-down pear. The lower, narrow part of the uterus opens into the *vagina* at the *cervix* (neck of the uterus); the upper part opens into the *fallopian tubes*.

In most women, the uterus is anteverted (tilts forward) at an angle of 90 degrees to the vagina. In about 20 percent of women, the uterus is retroverted (tilts backward; see *Uterus, retroverted*).

The uterus is lined with *endometrium*, which is a specialized type of tissue that undergoes changes during the menstrual cycle. The endometrium builds up under the influence of hormones from the *ovary*. When hormonal support is withdrawn at the end of each menstrual cycle, the blood supply to the endometrium is cut off and the layer of tissue is shed (see *Menstruation*).

During *pregnancy*, the uterus expands in size to accommodate the growing baby. Muscle bulk also increases dramatically. At full term, the uterus weighs about 1 kg, and the powerful uterine muscles expel the baby through the birth canal (see *Childbirth*).

After the *menopause*, the endometrium atrophies (becomes thinner), and the uterine muscle and connective tissue are reduced.

Uterus, cancer of

A malignant growth in the tissues of the *uterus*. Cancer of the uterus affects two main sites—the cervix (see *Cervix, cancer of*) and the *endometrium* (lining of the uterus). In rare cases, the uterine muscle is affected by a type of cancer known as a leiomyosarcoma. The term uterine cancer is more usually taken to refer only to cancer of the endometrium.

INCIDENCE AND CAUSES

In Canada, endometrial cancer is the commonest cancer of the female reproductive tract. About 3,000 new cases are diagnosed each year, compared with 2,000 new cases of ovarian cancer and 1,500 of cervical cancer.

Endometrial cancer occurs more commonly in women who have had an excess of *estrogen hormone* in their systems, particularly if *progesterone hormone* levels are low. Factors that may raise the estrogen level include

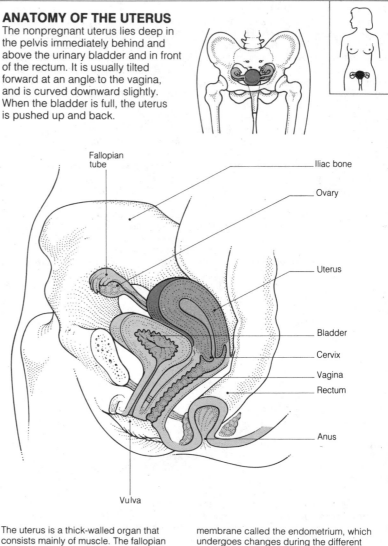

ANATOMY OF THE UTERUS

The nonpregnant uterus lies deep in the pelvis immediately behind and above the urinary bladder and in front of the rectum. It is usually tilted forward at an angle to the vagina, and is curved downward slightly. When the bladder is full, the uterus is pushed up and back.

Fallopian tube

Iliac bone

Ovary

Uterus

Bladder

Cervix

Vagina

Rectum

Anus

Vulva

The uterus is a thick-walled organ that consists mainly of muscle. The fallopian tubes enter on both sides of the uterus just below its uppermost point. The small uterine cavity is lined with a mucous membrane called the endometrium, which undergoes changes during the different phases of the menstrual cycle. The cervix is lined with a flatter mucous membrane identical to that of the vagina.

U

DISORDERS OF THE UTERUS

Conditions that affect the uterus include congenital disorders, infection, benign or malignant growths, and hormonal imbalances that may affect menstrual flow.

CONGENITAL DISORDERS

In embryonic life, the uterus develops in two halves, which fuse along the midline. One percent of women have a congenital malformation of the uterus, usually resulting from a fusion error. Malformation is not usually serious, but may predispose a woman to premature labor, *breech* presentation, or retention of the placenta after childbirth. Less commonly, the uterus may be absent, or there may be separate right and left halves, each with its own cervix and vagina. If a congenital malformation makes it difficult or impossible for a woman to conceive or to carry a pregnancy to term, surgical correction may be necessary.

INFECTION AND INFLAMMATION

Endometritis (infection and inflammation of the lining of the uterus) may originate in the uterus or be caused by infection spreading from elsewhere in the reproductive tract, such as the cervix or fallopian tubes. Endometritis may also develop if placental fragments are retained after childbirth or a *miscarriage*.

TUMORS

Benign tumors of the uterus include *polyps* and *fibroids*. Malignant tumors include cancer of the endometrium (see *Uterus, cancer of*).

Endometriosis
The lining of the uterus may grow in abnormal places.

Polyps
These may arise from the cervix or endometrium. If polyps bleed, they require investigation.

Cancer of the endometrium
This is a relatively common cancer in women; it causes abnormal bleeding.

Fibroids
These may cause excessive menstrual bleeding.

Endometritis
This infection of the uterus may be part of a more extensive infection of the reproductive tract.

Tumors may also affect placental tissue. Such tumors include *hydatidiform mole*, which is usually benign, and *choriocarcinoma*, which is malignant.

HORMONAL DISORDERS

Excessive production of *prostaglandins* by the uterus may lead to *dysmenorrhea* (painful periods) or *menorrhagia* (heavy periods).

Hormonal disorders affecting the *ovary* or other organs may disrupt the normal build-up of endometrium during the menstrual cycle, causing menstrual disorders (see *Menstruation, disorders of*), especially *amenorrhea* (absence of periods), or irregular, heavy bleeding.

INJURY

Injury to the uterus is rare, except following surgery, particularly an *abortion*. In rare cases, the uterus may be perforated by an *IUD*.

OTHER DISORDERS

The uterus may move from its normal position (see *Uterus, prolapse of*).

Adenomyosis (invasion of the uterine muscle by endometrium) may lead to dysmenorrhea, menorrhagia, and pain during intercourse.

Endometriosis (the presence of endometrium outside the uterus) may be symptomless or may be associated with dysmenorrhea, menorrhagia, painful intercourse, and *infertility*.

INVESTIGATION

A physical examination may be followed by *blood tests*, a *biopsy* (removal of a sample of tissue for microscopic analysis), imaging of the uterus by *hysterosalpingography* or *ultrasound scanning*, or *laparoscopy* (examination of the abdominal cavity through a viewing tube).

---

obesity, a history of failure to ovulate, or long-term taking of estrogen hormones if these are not balanced by taking *progestogen drugs*.

Unlike cervical cancer, which is rare among women who have not had sexual intercourse, endometrial cancer may occur in virgins; it is more common in women who have had few or no children.

The first symptom of endometrial cancer in a postmenopausal woman is usually a bloodstained vaginal discharge. In a younger woman, the first symptom may be *menorrhagia* (heavy periods), bleeding between periods, or bleeding after sexual intercourse. A variety of other conditions can also cause such bleeding.

DIAGNOSIS

Diagnosis must be made from a sample of uterine lining obtained either by *biopsy* or by *D and C* (dilatation and curettage). A *cervical smear test* is not an effective screening test for cancer of the uterus.

TREATMENT

Very early endometrial cancer is usually treated by simple *hysterectomy* and removal of the fallopian tubes and ovaries. Some surgeons recommend removal also of lymph nodes in the pelvis and abdomen. If the cancer has spread, *radiation therapy* may be recommended. Treatment with *anticancer drugs* may also be used.

With early treatment, the five-year survival rate is over 80 percent.

Uterus, prolapse of

A condition in which the *uterus* descends from its normal position down into the *vagina*. The degree of prolapse varies from first-degree prolapse, in which there is only slight displacement of the uterus, to third-degree prolapse, in which the uterus can be seen outside the vulva. Third degree prolapse is also known as procidentia.

Related conditions include *cystocele* (in which the bladder bulges into the front wall of the vagina); *urethrocele* (in which the urethra bulges into the front wall of the vagina; and *rectocele* (in which the rectal wall bulges into the back wall of the vagina). A general term for these conditions is pelvic relaxation. Prolapse of the uterus

U

PROLAPSE OF THE UTERUS

This condition is caused by weakening and slackness of the various ligaments, muscles, and connective tissues that help to keep the uterus in position in the pelvis. Prolapse of the uterus, which is more common in women who have had children, may occur in conjunction with a rectocele or cystocele. There are three degrees of uterine prolapse, as shown below.

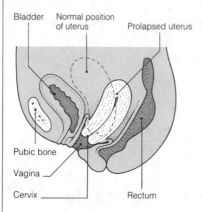

Bladder Normal position of uterus Prolapsed uterus

Pubic bone
Vagina
Cervix
Rectum

First-degree prolapse
In this, the least severe degree of prolapse, strain causes the cervix (neck) of the uterus to move farther down in the vagina; however, it remains well within the vagina.

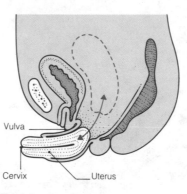

Vulva
Cervix
Uterus

Third-degree prolapse
The whole uterus projects outside the vulva. The surface of the cervix and the everted vaginal wall eventually dry out and are replaced by thick white tissue.

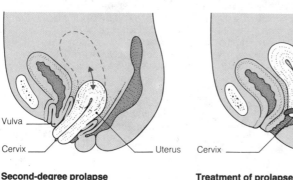

Vulva
Cervix
Uterus

Second-degree prolapse
The cervix protrudes beyond the vulva during straining, but retracts on relaxation. The vagina is partly everted (turned inside out).

Cervix
Pessary

Treatment of prolapse
The uterus may be held in position by a plastic pessary inserted into the vagina; alternatively, a hysterectomy or vaginal repair may be performed.

always occurs with some degree of vaginal relaxation, but vaginal relaxation may occur without any prolapse of the uterus.

CAUSES AND INCIDENCE
Normally, the uterus is kept in position by supporting *ligaments*. Stretching of these ligaments (for example, during childbirth) is the most common cause of uterine prolapse. Retroversion of the uterus (see *Uterus, retroverted*) makes such a prolapse more likely.

Prolapse occurs most commonly in middle-aged women who have had children, although it can occur in childless women. The condition was more common in the past when women had more pregnancies and were in poorer general health. Prolapse is aggravated by obesity.

SYMPTOMS
There are often no symptoms, but sometimes there is a dragging feeling in the pelvis or a sensation that something is being displaced down-ward. In severe cases, the uterus is visible from the outside. Other symptoms, such as leakage of urine or difficulty in passing urine or feces, may result from an accompanying cystocele, urethrocele, or rectocele.

DIAGNOSIS
Prolapse of the uterus is diagnosed by physical examination. In some cases, it is discovered during a routine *pelvic examination*. Investigation of the urinary system may be necessary if the bladder is also prolapsed.

PREVENTION AND TREATMENT
Pelvic floor exercises strengthen the muscles of the vagina and thus reduce the risk of a prolapse, especially following childbirth.

If prolapse is severe, a vaginal *hysterectomy* (removal of the uterus through the vagina), along with tightening of the support ligaments and, in some cases, *vaginal repair* may be recommended. For women who do not want surgery, or who are not fit enough to undergo general anesthesia, a plastic ring-shaped *pessary* may be inserted into the vagina to hold the uterus in position. Such pessaries need to be replaced under medical supervision at regular intervals.

Uterus, retroverted

A condition in which the *uterus* inclines backward rather than forward. A retroverted uterus was formerly believed to be the cause of various gynecological symptoms. It is now generally considered to be a harmless variation of the normal.

CAUSES AND INCIDENCE
About 20 percent of women have a uterus that is retroverted. Retroversion occurs in some women because the uterus has stayed in the retroverted position usual in infancy rather than becoming anteverted (tilting forward) as it matures. In others, the position of the uterus changes after childbirth—either becoming retroverted when it was previously anteverted, or vice versa. Less commonly, retroversion of the uterus is caused by a disease, such as a tumor, scarring as a result of *endometriosis*, or *pelvic inflammatory disease*.

SYMPTOMS
Retroversion usually causes no symptoms, but an underlying disease may produce symptoms such as *dysmenorrhea* (painful periods), painful intercourse, and *infertility*.

DIAGNOSIS AND TREATMENT
A retroverted uterus is diagnosed by physical examination of the pelvis (see *Pelvic examination*).

U

RETROVERTED UTERUS

In about 80 percent of women, the uterus is anteverted (tilted forward). In addition, the body of the organ is anteflexed (bent forward). In simple retroversion, the organ is tilted back, but not bent back. A retroverted uterus may also be retroflexed (bent back). Retroversion may or may not cause symptoms.

ANTEFLEXION

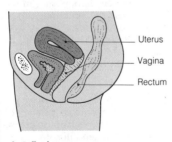

Anteflexion
The illustration shows the usual position of the uterus, lying bent and tilted forward, at right angles to the vagina.

RETROVERSION

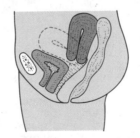

Retroversion
A retroverted uterus that can easily be anteverted by manipulation seldom causes any symptoms.

RETROFLEXION

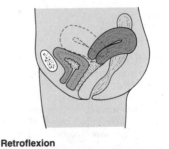

Retroflexion
If the retroversion and retroflexion are the result of disease, there are usually symptoms. Intercourse may be painful.

Treatment is unnecessary if there are no symptoms. In the rare cases in which a retroverted uterus does cause symptoms, the gynecologist may manipulate the uterus into a forward position and then insert a plastic vaginal pessary to hold the uterus in place. If this procedure relieves the symptoms, surgery may be performed to change the position of the uterus permanently.

If an underlying gynecological disease is suspected of being the cause of the retroversion, *laparoscopy* (examination of the abdominal cavity through a viewing instrument) may be suggested.

Uvea

Part of the *eye*, comprising the *iris* (the pigmented area around the pupil), the ciliary body and its muscle that focuses the lens, and the *choroid* (the blood-vessel-containing layer just under the retina).

The uvea contains many blood vessels. In the iris, these supply the active muscles that control the dilation (widening) and constriction (narrowing) of the pupil. The blood vessels in the choroid supply oxygen and nutrients to the retina.

Pigment cells give the eye its color and improve optical efficiency. In the uvea, pigment cells are concentrated in the back layer of the iris and scattered throughout the choroid. (See also *Uveitis*.)

Uveitis

Inflammation of the *uvea*, which may seriously affect vision. Uveitis may affect any part of the uvea, including the iris (when it is called iritis), the ciliary body (when it is known as cyclitis), or the choroid (when it is called choroiditis).

CAUSES
Uveitis is most commonly caused by an *autoimmune disorder*. Infections that sometimes cause uveitis include *tuberculosis* and *syphilis*.

TREATMENT
Treatment involves monitoring the inflammation with a *slit lamp*. Corticosteroid drugs, usually in the form of eye drops, are given to relieve inflammation. Eye drops containing a substance related to *atropine* are given to block nerve impulses to the muscles of the iris and ciliary body. Other drugs may be given to treat uveitis that is due to infection.

Uvula

The small, conical, fleshy protuberance that hangs from the middle of the lower edge of the soft palate. The uvula is composed of muscle and connective tissue, with a covering of mucous membrane. Some people are born with a bifid (forked) uvula. This is of little significance, but may be associated with cleft palate (see *Cleft lip and palate*).

LOCATION OF THE UVEA
The uvea consists of the iris, ciliary body, and choroid.

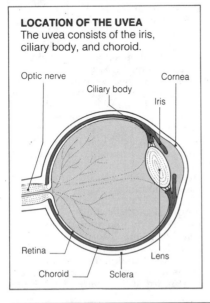

LOCATION OF THE UVULA
This conical fold of loose, wet tissue hangs down from the middle of the soft palate.

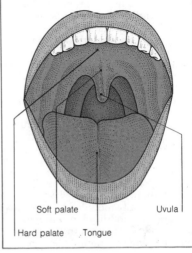

U

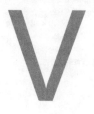

Vaccination

One of the main types of *immunization* (a procedure to stimulate or bolster the body's *immune system*). Vaccination is another term for active immunization, in which killed or weakened microorganisms are introduced into the body, usually by injection. These microorganisms sensitize the immune system so that if disease-causing organisms of the same type later enter the body, they are quickly destroyed through the action of *antibodies* or by other immune mechanisms.

Vaccination does not encompass the other main type of immunization procedure—passive immunization—in which ready-made antibodies are given by injection to provide short-term immunity.

Vaccine

A preparation given to induce *immunity* against an infectious disease. A vaccine works by sensitizing the body's *immune system* to a particular disease-causing bacterium, bacterial toxin, or virus. If the particular infectious agent invades the body at a later time, the sensitized immune system quickly produces *antibodies*, which help destroy either the agent itself or the toxin it produces.

Most vaccines are preparations containing the organisms (or parts of the organisms) against which protection is sought. So that these organisms themselves do not cause disease, they are killed or weakened. The term "live attenuated organisms" describes strains of organisms that have been rendered harmless. Attenuation is achieved either by artificially altering their genes or by successively infecting laboratory animals, thus producing small changes in the organisms which considerably reduce the ability of the organisms to cause disease without reducing their ability to induce immunity. Other vaccines contain chemically modified bacterial *toxins*. Again, modification removes the dangerous qualities of the toxin without affecting the immune features.

Vaccines are now available to protect against a wide variety of infectious diseases. Examples of live attenuated vaccines are those given to protect against *measles, mumps*, and *rubella* (see *MMR vaccination*), *yellow fever*, and *poliomyelitis. Diphtheria* and *tetanus* vaccines contain inactivated bacterial toxins. *Cholera, typhoid fever, pertussis, rabies*, and *influenza* vaccines contain killed organisms. *Hepatitis B* vaccine is now produced by *genetic engineering*.

Vaccines are usually given by injection into the upper arm. Oral polio vaccine is given on a sugar lump or by drops on the tongue. Some vaccines require several doses, spaced some weeks apart; others require only one dose. The effectiveness of vaccines varies from near total protection in most cases to only partial or weak protection (for example, against typhoid fever or cholera). The duration of effectiveness also varies from a few months to lifelong. (See also *Immunization*.)

Vacuum extraction

An obstetric procedure to facilitate delivery of a baby. Vacuum extraction was introduced in the 1950s as an alternative to *forceps delivery*. It may be used if the second stage of labor (see *Childbirth*) is prolonged, if the mother becomes exhausted, or if the baby shows signs of *fetal distress*.

HOW IT IS DONE

Vacuum extraction is performed using an instrument called a ventouse, or vacuum extractor, consisting of a suction cup connected to a vacuum bottle. The cup is placed on the baby's head in the birth canal and the

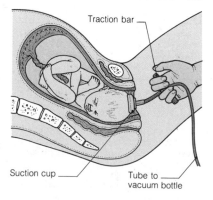

Traction bar

Suction cup

Tube to vacuum bottle

Technique of vacuum extraction
Once the suction cup is attached to the baby's head, the obstetrician pulls on the traction bar during each contraction, and the baby is drawn out through the vagina.

vacuum machine is turned on; this sucks the baby's scalp firmly into the cup. The obstetrician draws the baby out of the mother's vagina by gently pulling on the cup with each uterine contraction.

Delivery by vacuum extraction is generally slower than with forceps, but there is less risk of damage to the mother's genital tract. The baby is born with a swelling on the scalp, but this disappears after a few days, usually without treatment.

Vagina

The muscular passage, forming part of the female *reproductive system*, that connects the *cervix* (neck of the uterus) with the external genitalia.

STRUCTURE

The vagina is 7 to 10 cm in length, the back wall being slightly longer than the front. The vagina is H-shaped in cross section. The muscular walls have a ridged inner surface and are richly supplied with blood vessels. The walls are usually in contact with each other, except during sexual arousal and intercourse when they become engorged with blood.

FUNCTION

The vagina has three functions. It is a receptacle for the penis during *sexual intercourse*, bringing sperm closer to an ovum for fertilization; it provides an outlet for blood shed at *menstruation*; and, during *childbirth*, it stretches considerably to allow the baby to pass through.

DISORDERS

Vaginal discharge is a common symptom, which may indicate a disorder in the vagina or cervix.

Congenital abnormalities include vaginal atresia (partial or complete absence of the vagina) and blocking of the external opening of the vagina by an imperforate *hymen*.

Infections (see *Vaginitis*) and prolapse of the vagina (see *Cystocele; Rectocele; Urethrocele*) are the most common disorders. Cancer of the vagina occurs very rarely.

In *vaginismus*, sexual intercourse and pelvic examination are rendered impossible by abnormal (and painful) spasm of the muscles around the vaginal entrance.

Vaginal bleeding

Bleeding, via the *vagina*, that may come from the *uterus*, the *cervix*, or from the vagina itself.

The most common source of bleeding is the uterus and the most likely reason for it is *menstruation*. From

STRUCTURE OF THE VAGINA

The vagina has muscular walls, which are highly elastic to allow intercourse and childbirth; it has a ribbed inner lining that secretes a lubricating fluid during sexual arousal and intercourse.

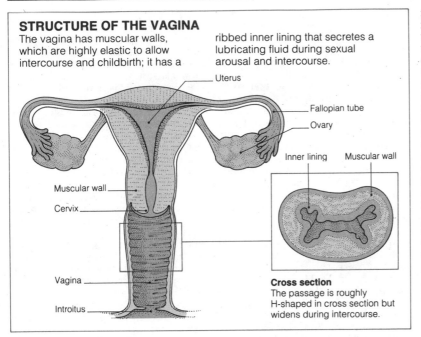

Uterus
Fallopian tube
Ovary
Inner lining
Muscular wall
Muscular wall
Cervix
Vagina
Introitus

Cross section
The passage is roughly H-shaped in cross section but widens during intercourse.

puberty to the menopause, menstrual bleeding usually occurs at regular intervals. However, problems may occur with either the character or the timing of the bleeding (see *Menstruation, disorders of*).

Nonmenstrual bleeding from the uterus may be due to a variety of causes. Hormonal drugs, such as *oral contraceptives*, can cause spotting (see *Breakthrough bleeding*). Other possible causes include *endometritis* (infection of the uterine lining), endometrial cancer (see *Uterus, cancer of*), and *fibroids*. Bleeding from the uterus may also occur during pregnancy. In the early months, bleeding may be a sign of threatened *miscarriage*. Later in pregnancy, it may indicate serious problems with the placenta, such as *placenta previa* or placental abruption (see *Antepartum hemorrhage*).

Bleeding from the cervix may be due to *cervical erosion*, in which case it may occur after sexual intercourse. *Cervicitis* (infection of the cervix) and *polyps* may also cause bleeding. More seriously, bleeding from the cervix may be a sign of cervical cancer (see *Cervix, cancer of*).

Vaginal bleeding originating from the walls of the vagina is less common than bleeding from the uterus or the cervix. The most likely cause is injury during intercourse, especially after the menopause, when the walls of the vagina become thinner and more fragile. In extreme cases, the vaginal wall in women after the menopause may be so fragile that bleeding occurs without any apparent precipitating cause. Occasionally, severe *vaginitis* causes vaginal bleeding. In rare cases, vaginal bleeding is caused by cancer of the vagina.

Any bleeding not caused by menstruation should be investigated by a physician. Infections can be treated with *antibiotic drugs*. Breakthrough bleeding can be prevented by the adjustment of hormone dosages. Fragile vaginal walls can be helped by use of a cream containing *estrogen drugs*. Growths, such as polyps, fibroids, or cancer of the uterus or cervix, may require surgical treatment.

Vaginal discharge

The normal or abnormal emission of secretions from the *vagina*.

Some mucous secretion from the walls of the vagina and from the cervix is normal in the reproductive years. The amount and nature of the discharge varies considerably from woman to woman and at different times in the menstrual cycle (see *Menstruation*). *Oral contraceptives* can increase or decrease the discharge, and secretions are usually greater during pregnancy. Sexual stimulation, with or without intercourse, also produces increased vaginal discharge.

Discharge may be abnormal if it is excessive, offensive-smelling, yellow or green, or if it causes itching. Abnor-mal vaginal discharge often occurs in *vaginitis*, and may be caused by various microorganisms. Infection with the fungus CANDIDA ALBICANS causes a thick, white discharge (see *Candidiasis*). Infection with the protozoan parasite TRICHOMONAS VAGINALIS causes a profuse green-yellow discharge (see *Trichomoniasis*). A forgotten tampon or a retained pessary may cause a profuse and highly offensive discharge. Very rarely, a vaginal discharge may occur in childhood; this is usually the result of infection or a foreign body. Abnormal vaginal discharge is often accompanied by vaginal and vulval itching.

Treatment depends on the cause. Infections are treated with an *antibiotic drug* or *antifungal drug*. Foreign bodies are removed.

Vaginal itching

Irritation in the *vagina*, which commonly occurs with *vulval itching*.

In many cases, vaginal itching is a symptom of *vaginitis*, which may result from infection or from an allergic reaction to chemicals in deodorants, spermicides, creams, and douches. Vaginal itching is very common after the *menopause*, when it is caused by low estrogen levels.

Depending on the cause, treatment for vaginal itching may be with *antibiotic drugs* or hormones, sometimes taken orally and sometimes applied in the form of a cream.

Vaginal repair

An operation, also known as colporrhaphy, to correct prolapse (displacement) of the vaginal wall.

TYPES

There are two different types of vaginal repair operations: anterior colporrhaphy and posterior colpoperineorrhaphy. Either type may be accompanied by a vaginal *hysterectomy* if the uterus is also prolapsed (see *Uterus, prolapse of*).

ANTERIOR COLPORRHAPHY This operation is performed for prolapse affecting the front wall of the vagina.

The repair is performed through the vagina. A triangle of vaginal skin is removed, with its base toward the uterus. Supporting stitches are inserted through the skin at one side of the triangle, across the gap, and through the skin at the other side. The tissues are then drawn together, narrowing the vagina.

POSTERIOR COLPOPERINEORRHAPHY This procedure is performed for prolapse of the back wall of the vagina.

V

The repair is performed through the vagina. Triangles of skin are removed from the vagina and from the perineum (the area between the genitals and the anus), with the bases of the triangles at the vaginal opening. The perineal muscles are stitched tightly together and the skin on each side of the triangles is brought together and stitched, thereby narrowing the vagina.

Vaginismus

Painful, involuntary spasm of the muscles that surround the entrance to the *vagina*, interfering with *sexual intercourse*. When penetration is attempted, the woman's pelvic floor muscles tighten and virtually close the vaginal entrance, making penetration very painful; her legs may straighten and come together. This spasm also usually occurs when a physician attempts a vaginal examination, which may therefore have to be carried out under anesthesia.

CAUSES
Vaginismus usually occurs in women who fear that penetration will be painful. Often they have been previously unable to insert a tampon or a finger into the vagina. A traumatic experience with painful penetration, such as *rape* or a history of sexual abuse as a child (see *Child abuse*), may predispose a woman to vaginismus. Chronic *vaginitis* may result in painful intercourse and lead to vaginismus. Sufferers may also be particularly sensitive to the stretching sensation that occurs during penetration, which may trigger a spasm when intercourse is first attempted. A vicious circle of anxiety and spasm is then established.

In some women, a contributing factor may be underlying guilt or fear associated with the sexual act due to a restrictive upbringing or an inadequate sex education.

DIAGNOSIS
The physician first examines the woman to ensure that she does not have any anatomical abnormalities of the *vagina* that might be causing pain, leading to spasm. Common causes of vaginal pain are infections such as *candidiasis* and, in older women, atrophy (thinning of the vaginal lining) due to low hormone levels.

TREATMENT
Any medical problem that is contributing to vaginismus is given appropriate treatment.

Vaginismus is commonly treated by use of a series of graded dilators, which the woman introduces into her vagina. Starting with the smallest size, she practices inserting and removing the instrument. In the course of doing this, she also learns to relax and tighten her vaginal muscles with the dilator in place.

Over the course of several treatment sessions, the size of the dilator is gradually increased until the woman is comfortable with the largest size (about the size of the average erect penis). Sexual intercourse can then be attempted.

Results of treatment are usually excellent, with the woman experiencing no discomfort during penetration. (See also *Intercourse, painful; Psychosexual dysfunction*.)

Vaginitis

Inflammation of the *vagina*. Vaginitis may be caused by infection, allergic reaction, hormone deficiency associated with aging, or the presence of a foreign body, such as a forgotten tampon in the vagina.

Vaginal infection is commonly caused by the fungus CANDIDA ALBI-CANS (see *Candidiasis*) or the protozoan parasite TRICHOMONAS VAGINA-LIS (see *Trichomoniasis*), both of which cause irritation and *vaginal discharge*. Another common form of vaginitis, known as nonspecific vaginitis, is caused by bacteria that normally inhabit the vagina. In nonspecific vaginitis, these bacteria multiply for reasons that are not yet known but which may be linked to stress or a change of sexual partner. Unfortunately, this bacterial multiplication causes an offensive, fishy-smelling vaginal discharge.

Vaginitis may also be caused by a reaction to the spermicidal creams often used with barrier contraceptives, to chemicals in vaginal douches, or to the ingredients of soaps, bath oils, or bath salts.

After the *menopause*, the lining of the vagina becomes thin and dry and prone to inflammation. Such inflammation, known as atrophic vaginitis, is due to a reduction in the production of *estrogen hormones*.

TREATMENT
Infections are treated with *antibiotic drugs* or *antifungal drugs* as appropriate. In cases of allergy, irritant agents should be avoided. Any foreign body should be removed and any secondary infection treated with antibiotic drugs. Atrophic vaginitis is treated with *estrogen drugs* in cream or tablet form. (See also *Vulvitis; Vulvovaginitis*.)

Vagotomy

An operation in which the *vagus nerve*, which controls production of digestive acid by the stomach wall, is cut to treat some cases of *peptic ulcer*.

HOW IT IS DONE
The operation is performed under general anesthesia. An incision is made in the upper abdomen to expose the two branches of the vagus nerve, which lie in front of and behind the lower esophagus. In many cases, all the nerve fibers of the vagus nerve are then cut (a procedure known as a truncal vagotomy). Less commonly, only some of the nerve fibers are cut (procedures known as selective vagotomy and highly selective vagotomy).

A *pyloroplasty* (surgical widening of the lower outlet of the stomach) or a *gastrojejunostomy* (surgical creation of a connection between the stomach and jejunum) is usually performed with either a truncal or a selective vagotomy (but not with a highly selective vagotomy). These accompanying procedures are needed to allow free emptying of the stomach because a truncal or a selective vagotomy interferes with the normal emptying of the stomach.

RECOVERY PERIOD
After the operation the patient is given fluids by *intravenous infusion*

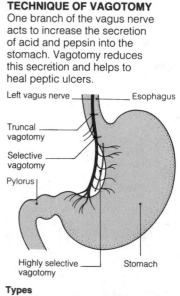

TECHNIQUE OF VAGOTOMY
One branch of the vagus nerve acts to increase the secretion of acid and pepsin into the stomach. Vagotomy reduces this secretion and helps to heal peptic ulcers.

Left vagus nerve — Esophagus
Truncal vagotomy
Selective vagotomy
Pylorus
Highly selective vagotomy — Stomach

Types
In a truncal vagotomy all the fibers of the vagus nerve are cut. In selective and highly selective vagotomies, only nerve fibers that supply the stomach are cut.

V

until the gastrointestinal tract can accept swallowed fluids (usually after two or three days).

OUTLOOK
The operation cures peptic ulcers in about 90 percent of cases, but occasionally there are troublesome side effects, including diarrhea and *dumping syndrome* (premature passing of food from the stomach into the intestine, causing a feeling of weakness and bloating after meals).

Vagus nerve
The 10th *cranial nerve* and the principal component of the parasympathetic division of the *autonomic nervous system*. The vagus nerve is the longest of the cranial nerves, and it branches most extensively. It emerges from the medulla oblongata (part of the *brain stem*), passes through the neck and chest to the abdomen, and has branches to most of the major organs in the body, including the larynx (voice box), pharynx (throat), trachea (windpipe), lungs, heart, and much of the digestive system.

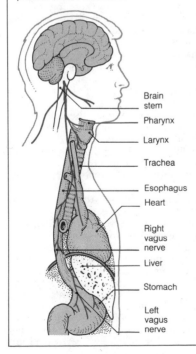

COURSE OF THE VAGUS NERVE
There are two vagus nerves, right and left. The right vagus nerve supplies the rear portion of the stomach; the left vagus nerve supplies the front portion of the stomach.

Brain stem
Pharynx
Larynx
Trachea
Esophagus
Heart
Right vagus nerve
Liver
Stomach
Left vagus nerve

The vagus nerve exerts its effects on target organs by releasing the chemical *acetylcholine*. This causes narrowing of the bronchi and slowing of the heart rate. Acetylcholine also stimulates the production of stomach acid and pancreatic juice; stimulates the activity of the gallbladder; and increases *peristalsis* (the rhythmic, muscular contractions that move food through the digestive tract).

Branches of the vagus nerve supply the muscles of the larynx and trachea and are thus involved in the actions of swallowing, coughing, sneezing, and speech quality.

Overactivity of the vagus nerve increases the production of stomach acid, which is a factor in the development of a *peptic ulcer*. Some cases of peptic ulcer may be successfully treated by a *vagotomy*.

The vagus nerve may be damaged by infection (such as *meningitis*), tumor, or *stroke*. In most such cases, the *glossopharyngeal nerve* (the ninth cranial nerve) and the *accessory nerve* (the 11th cranial nerve) are also affected. Possible effects of such damage include impairment or complete loss of the gag reflex, difficulty in swallowing, and hoarseness. In severe cases, death may result.

Valgus
The medical term for outward displacement of a part of the body.

Valproic acid
An *anticonvulsant drug* used to treat *epilepsy*. Although sodium valproic acid has less of a sedative effect than many other anticonvulsant drugs, it may occasionally cause drowsiness. Other possible side effects include abdominal discomfort, temporary hair loss, weight gain, and rash. Since prolonged treatment may in rare cases cause liver damage, regular blood tests are usually performed to monitor liver function.

Valsalva's maneuver
A forcible attempt to breathe out when the airway is closed. Valsalva's maneuver may be performed under certain circumstances without conscious effort or it may be carried out as a deliberate action.

Valsalva's maneuver occurs naturally when an attempt is made to breathe out while holding the *vocal cords* tightly together. This happens when lifting a heavy object, straining on the toilet, and at the beginning of a sneeze.

When performed deliberately by pinching the nose and holding the mouth closed, Valsalva's maneuver is useful in the prevention of pressure damage to the eardrums as it forces air through the ducts leading to the middle-ear cavities (see *Barotrauma*).

Valve
A structure that allows fluid or semifluid material to flow in one direction through a tube or passageway but closes to prevent reflux in the opposite direction. The most important valves in the body are at the exits from the *heart* chambers and in the *veins*. By ensuring that blood flows in one direction only, these valves are vital to the *circulatory system*; without them, the circulation of blood could not occur.

There are also small valves in the vessels of the *lymphatic system*. The muscular rings at the junction of the stomach and duodenum and between the small and large intestines are also sometimes called valves. In fact, these structures are flow-regulating devices and do not prevent backflow.

Defects of the *heart valves* include stenosis (narrowing) and/or insufficiency (inability to prevent reflex or backflow). Either defect can lead to *heart failure*. Insufficiency of the valves in the veins—most commonly in the legs—causes *varicose veins*.

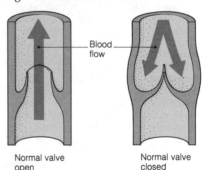

Blood flow

Normal valve open

Normal valve closed

Valves in the circulatory system
The valves are flaps that open to allow blood to flow in one direction but close to prevent blood flow in the opposite direction.

Valve replacement
A surgical operation to replace a defective or diseased heart valve. (See *Heart valve surgery*.)

Valvotomy
An operation performed to correct a stenosed (narrowed) *heart valve*. Cuts are made, or pressure is applied, to separate the flaps of the valve where they have joined and thus to reduce the degree of narrowing.

In the past, valvotomy operations were usually performed, with the heart still beating, by means of a dilating instrument or even a finger introduced into the heart via an incision. Today, valvotomy is usually performed with the heart opened up (see *Heart valve surgery*). Balloon *valvuloplasty* is a newer technique for treating a narrowed valve without the need to open the chest.

Valvular heart disease

A defect of one or more of the valves in the heart. (See *Heart valve*.)

Valvuloplasty

A reconstructive or repair operation on a defective heart valve (see *Heart valve surgery*).

Valvuloplasty can be performed as an open-heart operation (in which the patient is connected to a *heart-lung machine* and the heart opened up). However, the newer technique of balloon valvuloplasty makes it possible to treat a stenosed (narrowed) valve without opening the chest. A *balloon catheter* is passed through the skin into a blood vessel and from there to the heart. Inflation of the balloon via the catheter may then help separate the flaps of a narrowed valve.

Vancomycin

An antibiotic used primarily in the hospital to treat *endocarditis*, especially if it is due to *staphylococcal infection*.

Vaporizer

A device for converting a drug or water into an aerosol (fine spray) so that medication can be taken by inhalation or so that inhaled air can be moistened. A common example of a vaporizer is an *inhaler*, used to administer *bronchodilator drugs* and *corticosteroid drugs* in the treatment of asthma and other respiratory disorders. Vaporizers are also used to moisten air breathed by children suffering from croup.

Varicella

Another name for *chickenpox*.

Varices

Enlarged, tortuous, or twisted sections of vessels, usually veins. Varices is the plural of varix. A vein affected by varices is called a *varicose vein*. Although varicose veins can occur anywhere in the body, they most commonly occur in the legs. *Esophageal varices* are enlarged veins in the lower end of the esophagus.

Varicocele

Varicose veins surrounding the *testis*. Varicocele is a very common condition that affects about 10 to 15 percent of men. The condition almost exclusively affects the left testis.

Varicocele is caused by a failure of the venous valve system in the testicular vein at the point where the left testicular vein forms the renal vein. The condition is usually harmless, although there may be aching discomfort in the *scrotum* or an abnormally low sperm count.

Diagnosis is confirmed by examination of the scrotum while the patient is standing up. The aching may be relieved by wearing an athletic support or tight underpants. Further treatment is not usually required. However, an operation to divide and tie off the swollen veins is sometimes performed if the left testis is smaller than normal or if the sperm count is measured to be low.

Varicose veins

Enlarged, tortuous, or twisted superficial *veins* (veins just beneath the skin). Varicose veins in the legs are the best-known type. Examples of varicosities in other parts of the body include *hemorrhoids* (in the anus), *esophageal varices* (in the esophagus), and *varicoceles* (in the scrotum).

CAUSES

There are two principal systems of veins in the legs—the deep veins, which lie among the muscles and carry about 90 percent of the blood, and the superficial veins, which are often visible just under the skin and are less well supported by other surrounding tissues.

After oxygenating the tissues of the legs, the circulating blood is collected by the leg veins and pumped upward by contractions of the leg muscles. The blood then passes, via connecting veins, to veins in the abdomen, which return it to the heart.

Valves in the veins prevent blood from draining back down the leg under the force of gravity. However, these valves must support a high column of blood and, in many people, they become defective, causing pooling of blood in the superficial veins, which become swollen and distorted. Factors that may contribute to the development of varicose veins include *obesity*, hormonal changes and pressure on the pelvic veins during *pregnancy*, hormonal changes at the *menopause*, and standing for long periods of time.

Thrombophlebitis (inflammation and clotting of blood in veins) or deep vein *thrombosis* (clotting of blood in the deeper veins) may sometimes be associated with varicosities.

INCIDENCE

Varicose veins are extremely common, affecting about 15 percent of adults. Women are affected more often than men. The disorder tends to run in families.

SYMPTOMS AND SIGNS

The most common sites for varicose veins are the backs of the calves and the insides of the legs. The veins are blue, visibly enlarged, prominent, and tortuous.

Some people have no symptoms, but others experience a severe ache in the affected area (made worse by prolonged standing), swelling of the feet and ankles, and persistent itching of the skin. These symptoms become progressively worse during the day and can be relieved only by sitting with the legs raised. In women, symptoms are often most troublesome just before menstruation, potentially exacerbating premenstrual syndrome.

In severe cases, tissues in the leg become starved of oxygen and nourishment. This causes the skin to become thin, hard, dry, scaly, and discolored, and may lead to the formation of *leg ulcers*.

Injury to a large varicose vein may cause severe bleeding. (Such bleeding can be stopped by keeping the affected leg raised and by applying moderate pressure; a physician should then be consulted.)

DIAGNOSIS AND TREATMENT

Varicose veins in the legs are diagnosed from a physical examination performed while the patient remains standing.

For many people, the only treatment needed is the wearing of elastic support stockings, regular walking, as little standing still as possible, and sitting with the feet up.

In more severe cases, *sclerotherapy* may be carried out. The vein is first emptied of blood, then an irritant solution is injected into the varicose veins. After injection, firm pressure is applied so that the walls of the veins are pressed together. Compression is maintained by tight bandaging. The consequent scarring and blockage of the injected veins cause the venous blood to be diverted into other, healthy veins.

If varicose veins are very painful, ulcerated, or prone to bleed, they may require removal by an operation

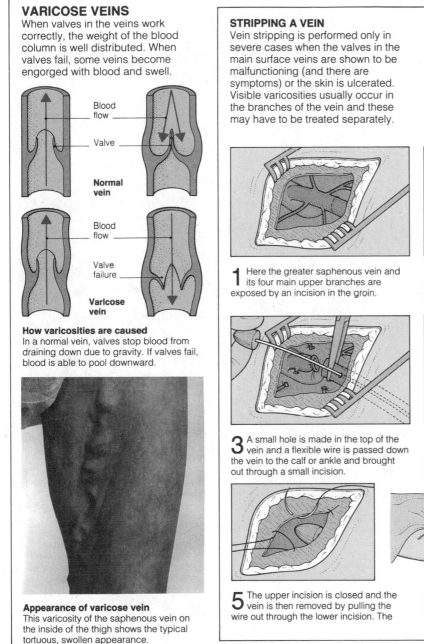

VARICOSE VEINS

When valves in the veins work correctly, the weight of the blood column is well distributed. When valves fail, some veins become engorged with blood and swell.

Blood flow

Valve

Normal vein

Blood flow

Valve failure

Varicose vein

How varicosities are caused
In a normal vein, valves stop blood from draining down due to gravity. If valves fail, blood is able to pool downward.

Appearance of varicose vein
This varicosity of the saphenous vein on the inside of the thigh shows the typical tortuous, swollen appearance.

STRIPPING A VEIN

Vein stripping is performed only in severe cases when the valves in the main surface veins are shown to be malfunctioning (and there are symptoms) or the skin is ulcerated. Visible varicosities usually occur in the branches of the vein and these may have to be treated separately.

Site of incision

1 Here the greater saphenous vein and its four main upper branches are exposed by an incision in the groin.

2 The vein is clamped and cut and both free ends tied off. The four branches are also securely tied off and cut. If branches remain, the operation may fail.

3 A small hole is made in the top of the vein and a flexible wire is passed down the vein to the calf or ankle and brought out through a small incision.

4 The upper end of the wire has a specially shaped metal head; the vein is tied firmly to the wire just below the head.

5 The upper incision is closed and the vein is then removed by pulling the wire out through the lower incision. The vein bunches up on the stripper and its branches tear off as it does so. Bleeding is not usually severe.

---

known as stripping (see illustrated box). The procedure itself takes very little time—usually no more than half an hour—and bleeding is seldom severe. However, the patient must keep the leg bandaged for several weeks after the operation.

Both sclerotherapy and surgery are usually successful, but varicose veins may later develop elsewhere.

Variola

Another name for *smallpox*, a highly infectious viral disease eradicated by vaccinations worldwide. The term variolation was once used to describe smallpox vaccination.

Varus

The medical term for an inward displacement of part of the body.

Vascular

Relating to the blood vessels (see *Circulatory system*).

Vasculitis

Inflammation of blood vessels. Vasculitis usually leads to damage to the lining of vessels, with narrowing or blockage, so that the blood flow is restricted or stopped. As a result, the

V

tissues supplied by the affected vessels are also damaged or destroyed by *ischemia* (lack of blood supply and, therefore, oxygen).

Vasculitis is thought to be caused in most cases by minute bodies in the circulating blood. These tiny bodies, known as immune complexes, consist of *antigens* (foreign materials, such as components of microorganisms) bound to *antibodies* that have been formed in response to the antigens. Normally, the immune complexes are destroyed by *phagocytes* (types of white blood cell), but sometimes they adhere to and settle in the walls of the blood vessels, where they cause severe inflammation. In some cases, the antigens are known to be *viruses*.

Vasculitis is the basic disease process in a number of conditions, including *polyarteritis nodosa, erythema nodosum, Schönlein-Henoch purpura, serum sickness, temporal arteritis,* and *Buerger's disease.*

Vas deferens
A narrow tube on each side of the body that carries and stores *sperm* released from one *testis* and *epididymis.* The plural form of the term is vasa deferentia. Each vas deferens is about 60 cm long and passes into the *prostate gland* at the base of the bladder to connect to a tube from the seminal vesicles to form the ejaculatory duct. Sperm and seminal fluid are passed through this duct into the urethra during *ejaculation.*

LOCATION OF THE VAS DEFERENS
The vas deferens passes from the epididymis, up and around the bladder, before entering the prostate, where it connects to a tube from the seminal vesicle to form the ejaculatory duct.

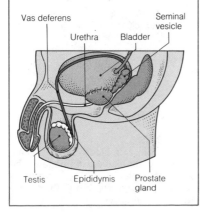

Vas deferens
Seminal vesicle
Urethra
Bladder
Testis
Epididymis
Prostate gland

HOW VASECTOMY IS PERFORMED
This operation blocks the passage of sperm from the testes but does not prevent the prostate and other glands from secreting the fluids that form most of the semen. Hence it has little effect on the volume of the ejaculate and no effect on orgasm.

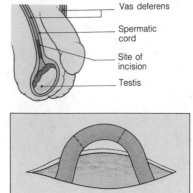

Vas deferens
Spermatic cord
Site of incision
Testis

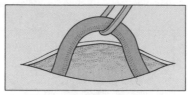

1 Incisions are made on both sides near the root of the penis; the vas deferens is cut free of the spermatic cord. Blood vessels are avoided.

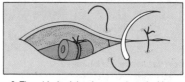

2 A loop of the vas deferens is freed and brought out through the incision. There are now several possibilities; usually, a length of the vas is cut out.

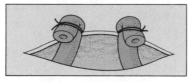

3 To prevent the cut ends from rejoining, they are often bent back and tightly closed with ligatures. They are then pushed back into the spermatic cord.

4 The skin incision is now closed with three or four sutures. When the local anesthetic wears off, there is usually a mild, dull, aching pain for a few days.

A *vasectomy* (male sterilization) involves blocking each vas deferens to prevent the passage of sperm.

Vasectomy
The operation of male sterilization. Vasectomy is a minor surgical procedure that consists of cutting the *vas deferens* (the duct that carries sperm from one testis to the seminal vesicle) on each side of the body. After the operation, the man continues to ejaculate as normal, but the *semen* no longer carries *sperm,* which are reabsorbed within the testes.

WHY IT IS DONE
Male sterilization provides a method of *contraception* that is safe and close to 100 percent effective; the risk of problems or complications is lower than for female sterilization. However, vasectomy is often irreversible, and the decision to have it performed should be carefully considered by the man and his partner.

HOW IT IS DONE
The operation is performed on an outpatient basis under a local anesthetic. The basic steps are shown in the illustrated box above. The procedure takes 15 to 20 minutes.

RECOVERY PERIOD
The patient should rest for 24 hours. There may be slight bruising of the *scrotum* and/or bleeding from the external wound for a few days. To relieve any pain, *acetaminophen* should be taken rather than *ASA,* which can prolong bleeding. Most men return to work within a few days, and sexual relations can be resumed as soon as the man is able, often within a week to 10 days. For two weeks, tight-fitting underpants or a jockstrap should be worn to support the scrotum.

After a vasectomy, a man remains fertile until the sperm already present in the vas deferens are ejaculated or die. Only after two consecutive specimens of semen are analyzed (about three months after the operation) and found to be sperm-free is a man considered sterile. Until that time, either he or his partner needs to use some other form of contraception.

In one in approximately 2,000 cases, sperm reappear (often long after the patient has been pronounced sterile) because the severed parts of a vas deferens reunite. If this occurs, the man can safely undergo another vasectomy operation.

V

Although most men who have a vasectomy experience no sexual problems as a result, the operation very rarely causes psychological problems that affect sexual performance. If *counseling* or *psychotherapy* fails to clear up these problems (or if a man strongly regrets that he has been sterilized) it may be possible to have the operation reversed. About 50 percent of all reversal operations are successful.

Vasoconstriction

Narrowing of blood vessels, causing reduced blood flow to a part of the body. Vasoconstriction under the skin occurs in response to cold and reduces heat loss from the body. It also occurs due to a fall in blood pressure in physiological *shock*. Vasoconstriction is also caused by *decongestant drugs*, which relieve *nasal congestion* by reducing blood flow to the lining of the nose.

Vasodilatation

Widening of blood vessels, causing increased blood flow to a part of the body. Vasodilatation under the skin occurs in response to hot weather and increases heat loss from the body. It also occurs as a response to *vasodilator drugs* and *alcohol*.

Vasodilator drugs

A group of drugs that widen blood vessels. Vasodilator drugs include *ACE inhibitor drugs, calcium channel blockers, nitrate drugs*, and *sympatholytic drugs*.

WHY THEY ARE USED

Vasodilator drugs are used to treat disorders in which abnormal narrowing of blood vessels reduces blood flow through tissues, impairing the supply of oxygen. Such disorders include *angina pectoris* (chest pain caused by inadequate blood supply to heart muscle) and *peripheral vascular disease* (poor blood flow in limbs).

Vasodilator drugs are also used to treat *hypertension* (high blood pressure) and *heart failure* (reduced pumping efficiency). Drugs of the vasodilator group are also occasionally prescribed in the treatment of senile *dementia*, although they rarely improve symptoms.

HOW THEY WORK

Vasodilator drugs widen blood vessels by relaxing surrounding muscles within the walls of the vessels; calcium channel blockers and nitrate drugs have a direct action on these muscles; sympatholytic drugs block the nerve signals that stimulate muscular contraction; and ACE inhibitors interfere with enzyme activity in the blood—an action that reduces the production of angiotensin II (a chemical that narrows blood vessels).

POSSIBLE ADVERSE EFFECTS

All vasodilator drugs may cause flushing, headaches, dizziness, fainting, and swollen ankles.

Vasopressin

An alternative name for *ADH* (antidiuretic hormone), a major factor in controlling the body's water balance.

Vasovagal attack

Temporary loss of consciousness due to sudden slowing of the heartbeat, usually brought on by severe pain, stress, shock, or fear. A vasovagal attack, which is a common cause of *fainting* in healthy people, is a result of overstimulation of the *vagus nerve*, which helps to control breathing and blood circulation.

VD

The abbreviation for venereal disease, another general term for *sexually transmitted disease*.

Vector

A term applied to any living carrier of an *infectious disease* but usually limited to insects and animals that transmit such diseases to human beings. A vector picks up disease organisms from a source of infection (such as an infected person's or animal's blood or feces), carries them within or on its body, and later deposits them where they infect a new host.

Mosquitoes, fleas, lice, ticks, and flies are the most important vectors of disease to humans. When an organism develops or completes part of its life cycle inside a vector, this vector is called a biological vector. For example, mosquitoes are biological vectors for malarial parasites, which develop and multiply inside the insect and are injected into the blood of a new host by the mosquito's bite.

When a vector is not essential to the life cycle of a disease organism, it is called a mechanical vector. For example, flies may act as mechanical vectors of *shigellosis* (bacterial dysentery) by carrying the bacteria on their legs from infected feces to food.

V

TYPES OF VASODILATOR DRUGS

The different types of vasodilator drugs work in various ways to prevent or reduce the contraction of muscle cells in blood vessel walls, thus helping to widen the blood vessels.

Constricted   Dilated

Action
A blood vessel is shown contracted and dilated (above). Vasodilators widen vessels, improving blood flow.

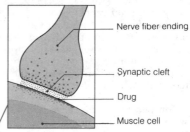

Nerve fiber ending

Synaptic cleft

Drug

Muscle cell

Sympatholytic drugs
Muscles in blood vessel walls are made to contract by the action of neurotransmitters. Sympatholytic drugs block the sites where neurotransmitters act.

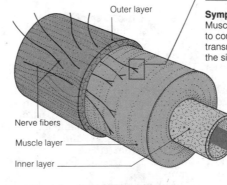

Outer layer

Nerve fibers

Muscle layer

Inner layer

Calcium channel blockers and nitrates
These drugs act directly on the contracted muscle cells in blood vessel walls, causing them to relax.

ACE inhibitors
These drugs work by blocking the activity of a particular enzyme in the blood—an action that reduces the production of angiotensin II, a chemical that acts to narrow blood vessels.

Vegetarianism

Eating a diet that excludes meat and fish, and sometimes all other animal products. Human beings do not need to eat meat or animal products to maintain health as long as the nutrients supplied by plant foods provide a balanced diet (see *Nutrition*).

TYPES

There are three main types of vegetarian diet. In a lacto-ovovegetarian diet all types of fish and meat are excluded, but milk, milk products and eggs are allowed. A lactovegetarian diet is basically the same, except that eggs are also excluded. A vegan diet excludes all foods of animal origin, including milk and milk products.

DIETARY RISKS

Although animal products are not essential to the human diet, any restriction on food choice calls for special care. Problems have arisen on vegan diets from a deficiency of *vitamin B_{12}*, giving rise to megaloblastic anemia (see *Anemia, megaloblastic*) because this vitamin is found virtually only in animal foods. Nowadays, vitamin B_{12} can be obtained from preparations made from extracts of some yeasts or from fermentation liquors.

Vegans, unlike lactovegetarians, cannot benefit from calcium-rich milk and milk products and must rely on less rich sources of calcium, such as grains, nuts, legumes, seeds, and dark-green leafy vegetables.

Although the iron in plant foods is poorly absorbed compared with that from meat, most vegetarians and vegans do not appear to suffer from *iron* deficiency, possibly because their diets are rich in *vitamin C*, which assists the absorption of iron.

A properly planned vegetarian diet contains sufficient protein.

BENEFITS

Vegetarian diets are relatively rich in fiber (see *Fiber, dietary*), which may help protect against *diverticular disease* and cancer of the intestine (see *Colon, cancer of*; *Rectum, cancer of*). Vegetarian diets are also unusually low in *fats*, especially saturated fats which are considered to be a contributory factor in *coronary artery disease*. Vegetarian diets are also likely to contain less *sodium* and more *potassium* than that of a meat-eater, and there is evidence that vegetarians have lower blood pressures than people who eat meat.

Vegetative state

A term sometimes used to describe a type of indefinite deep *coma*. Although the eyes may be open and occasional random movements of the head and limbs may occur, there are no other signs of consciousness and no responsiveness to stimuli. Only basic functions, such as breathing and heartbeat, are maintained.

Vein

A vessel that returns blood toward the *heart* from the various organs and tissues of the body.

The majority of veins carry deoxygenated (blue) blood. This blood collects in small vessels called venules in the tissues. The venules join to form veins, which deliver the blood to the two largest veins in the body, the venae cavae. The venae cavae then carry the deoxygenated blood to the right side of the heart to be pumped to the lungs.

The main exceptions to this design are the pulmonary veins in the chest, which carry oxygenated blood from the lungs to the left side of the heart. Another special vein is the portal vein, which carries nutrient-rich blood from the intestines to the liver.

The walls of veins, like those of arteries, consist of a smooth inner lining, a muscular middle layer, and a fibrous outer covering. However, blood pressure in veins is much lower than blood pressure in arteries. Correspondingly, the walls of veins are thinner, less elastic, less muscular, and weaker. Veins collapse when empty, whereas arteries do not.

The inner linings of many veins contain folds, which act as valves, ensuring that blood can flow only toward the heart. The blood is helped on its way through the veins by pressure on the vessel walls from the contraction of surrounding muscles. (See also *Circulatory system*.)

Veins, disorders of

The most common disorder affecting a *vein* is a *varicose vein*, in which the vein becomes enlarged, tortuous, or twisted. Varicose veins occur most commonly in the legs, where they are caused by failure of the valves farther up the vein. *Esophageal varices* are varicose veins in the lower part of the esophagus. These commonly result from back pressure through the circulation from *cirrhosis* of the liver. *Hemorrhoids* are varicose veins in the anus.

Inflammation of a vein is called phlebitis. This condition is almost always associated with a tendency to blood clotting in the affected vein, in which case it is called *thrombophlebitis*.

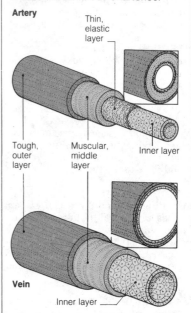

STRUCTURE OF A VEIN AND AN ARTERY

Like arteries, the walls of veins have a smooth inner layer, a muscular middle layer, and a fibrous outer layer. However, the walls are thinner and less muscular than those of arteries.

Artery

Thin, elastic layer

Tough, outer layer

Muscular, middle layer

Inner layer

Vein

Inner layer

Clot formation in the small veins near the surface is not significant, although clots may cause swelling and tenderness. However, clots that form in deeper, larger veins (see *Thrombosis, deep vein*) may become widespread, increasing the risk that part of a clot will break off and block an important artery elsewhere in the body.

The blood pressure in veins is much lower than that in arteries, causing an injured vein to bleed much more slowly than an artery of the same size. Bleeding from veins can usually be stopped by applying gentle pressure to the vein. It is also possible to stop bleeding from veins (but not from arteries) by raising an injured part of the body above the level of the heart.

Vena cava

Either of two very large *veins* into which all the circulating venous (deoxygenated) blood drains. The two venae cavae (the superior vena cava and the inferior vena cava) deliver venous blood to the right atrium (one of the upper chambers of the *heart*) for pumping to the lungs. Each vena cava measures nearly 2.5 cm in diameter.

V

The superior vena cava starts at the top of the chest, behind the lower edge of the right first rib and close to the sternum (breastbone). It travels some 7.5 cm downward, passing through the pericardium (outer lining of the heart) before connecting to the right atrium. The superior vena cava is formed from the right and left brachiocephalic veins, which themselves are formed from union of the subclavian veins (draining blood from the arms), the jugular veins (draining blood from the head), and several minor veins. The superior vena cava also receives blood from the azygos vein, which is responsible for draining much of the chest. The superior vena cava thus collects blood from the whole of a person's upper trunk, head, neck, and arms.

The inferior vena cava starts in the lower abdomen, in front of the fifth lumbar vertebra, and travels some 25 cm upward in front of the spine, behind the liver, and through the diaphragm before joining to the right atrium. It is formed from the union of the two common iliac veins, which receive blood from the legs and pelvic organs. The inferior vena cava also receives blood from the hepatic vein, which drains the liver, and the renal veins, which drain the kidneys.

Venereal diseases
See *Sexually transmitted diseases.*

Venereology
The medical discipline concerned with the study and treatment of *sexually transmitted diseases.*

Venesection
The process of withdrawing blood from a *vein*, also called phlebotomy, for *blood donation* or for therapeutic bloodletting. Regular bloodletting is used in the treatment of *polycythemia* (a disorder in which the blood is too thick); in *hemochromatosis* (a disorder of body iron chemistry) to reduce the amount of iron in the body; and very occasionally in some types of *heart failure* to reduce the blood volume and ease the heart's work load.

Venipuncture
A common procedure in which a *vein* is pierced with a needle to withdraw blood or to inject fluid. It is usually performed on a vein in the forearm.

HOW IT IS DONE
A *tourniquet* is applied to the upper arm, causing the veins to swell. A suitable vein, usually a large one that can be easily felt through the skin, is selected. The overlying skin is cleaned with alcohol, and a sterile needle is inserted into the vein. For taking blood or injecting medication, the needle has a syringe attached. For purposes of *intravenous infusion*, a cannula (narrow tube) is inserted into the vein via the needle; the needle is then withdrawn, and tubing for the fluid to flow through is attached to the cannula.

After the required amount of fluid has been injected or withdrawn, the needle or cannula is removed. The area is then covered with a piece of cotton wool and firm pressure applied for a minute or two until any bleeding has stopped.

Venipuncture is not usually painful but may cause some discomfort. Slight bruising may appear at the venipuncture site but usually fades in a few days.

Venography
A diagnostic procedure, also known as phlebography, that enables *veins* to be seen on an *X-ray* film after they have been injected with a substance opaque to X rays.

WHY IT IS DONE
Venography is used to detect anatomical abnormalities or diseases of the veins themselves—such as narrowing or blockage from *thrombosis* (abnormal clot formation) or a tumor—as well as disease or injury in organs that are supplied by the veins. This particular procedure is also used to evaluate the extent of disease before planning the patient's treatment.

The veins most frequently studied are those in the leg, usually because of suspected deep vein thrombosis (see *Thrombosis, deep vein*). Other commonly studied veins include the axillary veins in the arm, the superior and inferior venae cavae (the main veins leading to the heart), and the renal veins (leading from the kidney).

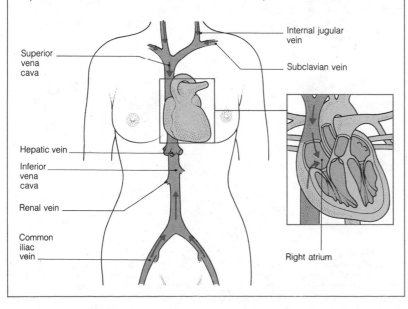

LOCATION OF THE VENAE CAVAE
All the circulating blood, after being pumped to the body, returns to the heart via the venae cavae. The superior vena cava collects blood from the whole of the upper trunk, head, neck, and arms. The inferior vena cava drains blood from all parts of the body below the chest.

Internal jugular vein

Superior vena cava

Subclavian vein

Hepatic vein

Inferior vena cava

Renal vein

Common iliac vein

Right atrium

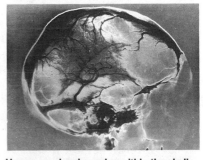

Venogram showing veins within the skull
This X-ray image of a skull shows both the veins and the venous sinuses (dark areas), which are wide blood drainage channels.

V

HOW IT IS DONE

Contrast medium is injected either through a needle directly into the veins to be examined or, if the veins are not readily accessible, through a catheter that has been guided, under X-ray control, along the venous system to the required vein. A sequence of X-ray pictures is taken so that blood flow along the veins can be studied. Leg venography takes about 20 minutes to perform; other types may take longer.

The newer technique of digital subtraction *angiography* adds to the information obtained through use of computer analysis to process images and remove unwanted shadowing.

Venomous bites and stings

The injection of venom (poison) by certain animals via their mouthparts (bites) or some other injecting apparatus (stings). Often, these venoms are carried for purely defensive purposes. Sometimes they are used to kill or immobilize prey. It is rare for a venomous animal to attack a person unless cornered, provoked, stepped on, or otherwise disturbed.

Specific antivenins are available to treat many, though not all, animal venoms. In cases of serious poisoning, administration of *antivenin* can sometimes be lifesaving.

TYPES OF VENOMOUS ANIMAL

For the better known types of venomous bites and stings, see *Insect stings; Jellyfish stings; Scorpion stings; Snakebites; Spider bites.* Other venomous animals include certain species of centipedes, millipedes, and fish.

CENTIPEDES AND MILLIPEDES Centipede bites can cause severe pain and local swelling but are not a danger to life. Certain millipedes secrete, and sometimes squirt out, an irritating liquid that may be dangerous if it enters the eyes. First aid is by thorough irrigation with water.

FISH STINGS Venomous fish inflict stings by means of certain fins or specialized spines on their bodies. Examples of venomous fish include weeverfish, scorpion fish, lionfish, and stonefish. Most of the venomous species of fish live in tropical waters, where they are a danger to swimmers, waders, snorkelers, and scuba divers.

Ventilation

The use of a machine called a *ventilator* to take over *breathing*, and thus maintain life, in a person who lacks or who has lost the ability to breathe in the natural way.

WHY IT IS DONE

Arrested or severe impairment of breathing may be caused by damage to the respiratory center in the *brain stem* due to *head injury*, brain disease, or an overdose of *narcotic drugs*. Breathing difficulties may also be due to damage to or malfunctioning of the breathing mechanism as a result of chest injury, respiratory disease, a nerve or muscle disorder, or major chest or abdominal surgery. Occasionally, difficulties arise as a result of problems during general *anesthesia*. Severely premature babies with *respiratory distress syndrome* may also need ventilation for a period until their lungs develop sufficiently to cope with breathing unaided.

HOW IT IS DONE

Artificial ventilation is usually carried out in an *intensive-care* unit or *operating room*. The patient is connected to the ventilator by means of an *endotracheal tube* passed through the nose or mouth into the trachea (windpipe); if prolonged ventilation is likely to be required, a tube is inserted into an opening made in the trachea, an operation called a *tracheostomy*. Conscious patients, and those nearing the end of anesthesia, are usually given muscle-relaxant and sedative drugs to prevent them from resisting the insertion and irritant presence of the tube.

During ventilation, the patient's *blood gases* (the amount of oxygen and other gases in the patient's blood) are checked by analyzing blood samples; *X rays* are taken to assess the state of the lungs; and the pulse, blood pressure, heart rhythm, and temperature are monitored.

The patient is unable to eat or drink when connected to the ventilator. Fluids are therefore given by *intravenous infusion*. Drugs may need to be given in the same way.

The patient's inability to cough may cause secretions to accumulate in the lungs. These are removed by suction apparatus, and intensive *physiotherapy* is given to prevent the secretions from building up again.

RECOVERY PERIOD

When the patient begins to recover, he or she is disconnected from the ventilator and allowed to breathe naturally for increasingly longer and more frequent periods. After the blood gases have returned to a normal level during spontaneous breathing, the patient is taken off the ventilator permanently.

TECHNIQUE OF ARTIFICIAL VENTILATION

Machine-assisted breathing may be needed when a person has lost the ability to breathe naturally—often following a severe head injury, narcotic drug overdose, or in various other medical emergencies. It may also be needed when a muscle relaxant has been given during an operation as part of a general anesthetic.

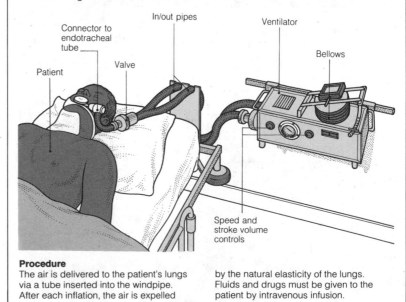

Connector to endotracheal tube

In/out pipes

Ventilator

Bellows

Patient

Valve

Speed and stroke volume controls

Procedure
The air is delivered to the patient's lungs via a tube inserted into the windpipe. After each inflation, the air is expelled by the natural elasticity of the lungs. Fluids and drugs must be given to the patient by intravenous infusion.

V

Ventilator

A device, also known as a respirator or a life-support machine, used for the artificial *ventilation* of a patient who is unable to breathe naturally.

A ventilator is an electrical pump connected to an air supply that works like bellows. The pump can be adjusted to vary the proportion of oxygen in the pumped air and to regulate the amount of air delivered according to the needs of the patient. The air is pumped through a humidifier, which adds sterile water vapor to prevent the lungs from drying out; the air is then directed through a tube that has been passed down the patient's trachea (windpipe). After the lungs have been inflated, the air is expelled by the natural elasticity of the lungs and rib cage. A valve on the ventilator prevents the expelled air from reentering the lungs.

Ventral

Relating to the front of the body, or describing the lowermost part of a body structure when a person is lying face down. In human anatomy, the term ventral means the same as anterior. The opposite of ventral is *dorsal* (or posterior).

Ventricle

A cavity or chamber. Both the *heart* and *brain* have anatomical parts known as ventricles.

The brain has four ventricles: one in each of the two cerebral hemispheres (which make up the cerebrum, or main mass of the brain); a third at the center of the brain, above the brain stem; and a fourth situated between the brain stem and the cerebellum. These cavities are filled with cerebrospinal fluid and are linked by ducts so that the fluid can circulate through them. The cavities are lined in part with tuftlike clusters of blood vessels called the choroid plexus, derived from vessels in the *meninges*, which secrete the *cerebrospinal fluid*.

The heart has two ventricles. These are the lower, pumping chambers of the heart, which receive blood from the atria (upper heart chambers) and pump it to the lungs.

Ventricular ectopic beat

A type of cardiac *arrhythmia* (abnormal heart rhythm) in which abnormal heartbeats are initiated from electrical impulses in the *ventricles* (lower chambers of the *heart*). In the normal heart, beats are initiated from electrical impulses in the sinoatrial node in the right atrium (upper heart chamber).

Many people, especially older people, have occasional ventricular ectopic beats that do not signify any disorder. Such beats may also be caused by *myocardial infarction* (heart attack), *heart failure*, disturbances of body chemistry, or *digitalis drugs*.

SYMPTOMS
Ventricular ectopic beats often do not cause any symptoms. Sometimes, a ventricular ectopic beat causes the sensation that the heart has stopped for a second and then restarts with a thump.

DIAGNOSIS
Ventricular ectopic beats may be detected on an *ECG* (measurement of electrical activity of the heart) as a broad, bizarre-looking wave (see illustrated box overleaf).

TREATMENT
If a person has frequent ventricular ectopic beats that cause symptoms, or has beats that arise from more than one site in the ventricles, treatment with an *antiarrhythmic drug* may be required.

Ventricular fibrillation

A life-threatening cardiac *arrhythmia* (abnormal heart rhythm) in which there are rapid, ineffective, uncoordinated contractions of the *heart*. Ventricular fibrillation is caused by abnormal *heartbeats* initiated by electrical activity in the ventricles (lower heart chambers). It is a common complication of *myocardial infarction* (heart attack) and may also be caused by electrocution or drowning. The heart ceases to pump blood effectively and the condition is fatal unless the normal heart rhythm is quickly restored.

The diagnosis of ventricular fibrillation is confirmed by *ECG* (measurement of electrical activity of the heart) which shows broad, irregular waves (see illustrated box overleaf).

Treatment is with *defibrillation* (administration of an electric shock to the heart) and *antiarrhythmic drugs*. *Cardiopulmonary resuscitation* may be an interim lifesaving measure.

Ventricular tachycardia

A serious cardiac *arrhythmia* (abnormal heart rhythm) in which each heartbeat is initiated from electrical activity in the ventricles (lower heart chambers) rather than the sinoatrial node in the right atrium (upper heart chamber). The result is an abnormally fast heart rate of between 140 and 220 beats per minute.

Ventricular tachycardia is caused by serious heart disease, such as *myocardial infarction* (heart attack) or *cardiomyopathy*. It may last for a few seconds or for several days. Diagnosis is confirmed by *ECG* (recording of the electrical activity of the heart), which shows broad, regular abnormal waves (see illustrated box overleaf).

LOCATION OF THE VENTRICLES

The location of the ventricles in the brain (seen from above) and in the heart is shown below. Of the heart ventricles, the right ventricle pumps blood to the lungs, the left pumps blood to the rest of the body.

VENTRICLES IN THE BRAIN
Together, these four irregularly shaped cavities contain about 25 ml of cerebrospinal fluid.

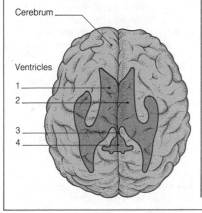

Cerebrum

Ventricles

1
2

3
4

VENTRICLES IN THE HEART
The ventricles of the heart are the large, lower chambers, separated by a muscular wall, the septum.

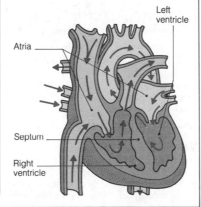

Left ventricle

Atria

Septum

Right ventricle

V

VENTRICULOGRAPHY

TYPES OF VENTRICULAR ARRHYTHMIA

The ventricles (lower chambers) of the heart usually beat regularly in response to excitatory waves spread from the upper chambers. If rhythm disturbances (which may be associated with heart disease) occur, they are visible on an electrocardiograph (ECG) recording.

Normal heartbeat

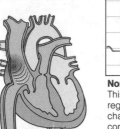

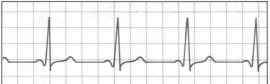

Normal heartbeat
This is the normal ECG appearance of the heartbeat. The regular spikes coincide with beats of the ventricles (lower heart chambers). The small rises before each spike coincide with contractions of the atria (upper chambers).

Ventricular ectopic beat

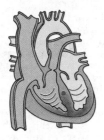

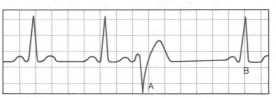

Ventricular ectopic beat
Here there is an abnormal beat, which has a broad, bizarre-looking wave form on the ECG; it occurs just before the expected normal beat. To the patient, the heart may seem to stop at time A and restart with a thump at time B.

Ventricular tachycardia

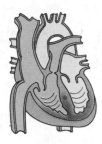

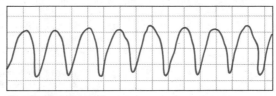

Ventricular tachycardia
Here there is a rapid succession of abnormal beats, caused by an abnormal focus of electrical activity in a ventricle. It usually indicates serious underlying heart disease. The rate of beating may be very high—up to 220 beats per minute.

Ventricular fibrillation

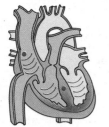

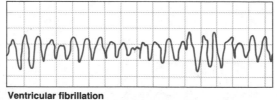

Ventricular fibrillation
This pattern is seen only when the heart is in a state of virtual arrest, usually after a heart attack, with the ventricles twitching in a rapid and totally irregular manner. Unless a normal rhythm can be restored, the condition is rapidly fatal.

Emergency treatment is with *defibrillation* (administration of an electric shock to the heart) or by injection of an *antiarrhythmic drug*, such as *lidocaine*. Use of the drug is usually continued by mouth for several months.

Ventriculography

An outdated procedure that enables the ventricles (cavities) within the *brain* to be seen on *X-ray* film after the introduction of air or a radiopaque contrast medium (a substance that is opaque to X rays). Ventriculography is performed very infrequently nowadays; *CT scanning* has largely taken its place.

Verapamil

A drug that acts as a *calcium channel blocker* used in the treatment of *hypertension* (high blood pressure), *angina pectoris*, and certain types of *arrhythmia* (abnormal heart rhythm).

Possible adverse effects include headache, facial flushing, dizziness, ankle swelling, and constipation.

Vernix

The white, greasy, cheeselike substance that covers the skin of a newborn baby. Vernix consists of fatty secretions and dead cells. It is thought to protect the baby's skin and insulate against heat loss before birth. Vernix lubricates the passage of the baby through the birth canal.

Verruca

The Latin name for a *wart*. The term is commonly applied to warts on the soles of the feet, known medically as plantar warts.

Version

A change in the direction in which a *fetus* lies so that a *malpresentation*, most often a breech (bottom-down) presentation, becomes the normal cephalic (head-down) presentation. Version is also the term for the obstetric procedure used to change the presentation of a fetus.

Many breech babies undergo version spontaneously, especially before the 34th week of pregnancy. If this does not occur, the obstetrician may be able to manipulate the fetus into the cephalic position by a procedure called external version. With one hand on the mother's abdomen over the baby's head and the other over the baby's buttocks, the obstetrician very gently attempts to rotate the baby, bringing its head down into the mother's pelvis. External version is performed between the 34th and 37th week of pregnancy and can be done with or without general anesthesia. Drugs may be used to relax the uterus.
POSSIBLE COMPLICATIONS
External version carries small risks of inducing premature labor (see *Prematurity*), rupture of the membranes, *antepartum hemorrhage*, or knotting of the umbilical cord. The risks of external version must be weighed against those of vaginal breech delivery and of *cesarean section*.

V

In internal version, the obstetrician turns the fetus by reaching inside the uterus. Internal version is rarely done: the most likely exception would be in the case of a second twin who is not in the normal position after delivery of the first twin.

Vertebra

Any of the 33 approximately cylindrical bones that form the *spine*. There are seven vertebrae in the cervical spine in the neck; 12 vertebrae in the thoracic spine in the chest; five vertebrae in the lumbar spine in the lower back; five fused vertebrae in the *sacrum*; and four fused vertebrae in the *coccyx* (see illustrated box). Between each pair of separate vertebrae is an intervertebral disk (see *Disk, intervertebral*).

Vertebrobasilar insufficiency

Intermittent episodes of dizziness, double vision, weakness, and difficulty in speaking caused by reduced blood flow to parts of the *brain*.

The obstruction to blood flow is usually caused by *atherosclerosis* (narrowing of arteries by fatty deposits) of the basilar and vertebral arteries and other arteries in the base of the brain. Vertebrobasilar insufficiency sometimes precedes a *stroke*.

Vertigo

An illusion that one or one's surroundings are spinning, either horizontally or vertically. Vertigo is a common complaint, but only rarely is it a sign of an underlying disorder. The term is sometimes used erroneously to describe the sensation of *dizziness* or faintness.

CAUSES

Vertigo results from a disturbance of the semicircular canals in the inner *ear* or the nerve tracts leading from them. It can occur in healthy people when sailing, on amusement park rides, or even when watching a film. Astronauts in zero gravity experience vertigo when moving their heads.

Severe vertigo, usually accompanied by other symptoms, may indicate a number of diseases. *Labyrinthitis* (inflammation of the semicircular canals) causes sudden vertigo accompanied by vomiting and unsteadiness. Labyrinthitis often occurs in conjunction with an infection, such as *influenza* or *otitis media* (infection of the middle ear), and usually clears up as the infection subsides. *Meniere's disease* is a more serious condition characterized by attacks of vertigo that are sometimes severe enough to cause the sufferer to fall to the ground. In victims of the disease, the attacks of vertigo may be accompanied by severe vomiting, *tinnitus* (noises in the ears), *nystagmus* (jerky eye movements), and unsteadiness.

Elderly people with *atherosclerosis* often suffer from vertigo as a result of suddenly moving the head. Vertigo is less commonly caused by a tumor of the *brain stem* or by *multiple sclerosis*. Vertigo may also be psychological in origin, in which case it is usually associated with *agoraphobia* (fear of open spaces).

V

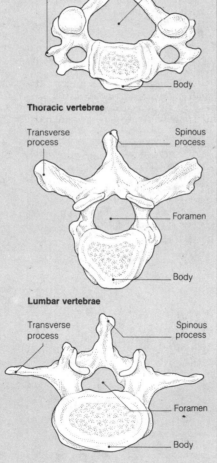

LOCATION AND STRUCTURE OF THE VERTEBRAE

The 33 vertebrae are arranged as shown. Apart from the top two, they all have a similar structure. The topmost cervical vertebra (the atlas) has no body. The second (the axis) forms a pivot on which the atlas can rotate, allowing the head to be turned in all directions.

The spine

Cervical vertebrae (7)

Thoracic vertebrae (12)

Lumbar vertebrae (5)

Sacral vertebrae (5)

Coccygeal vertebrae (4)

Cervical vertebrae

Transverse process — Spinous process — Foramen — Body

Thoracic vertebrae

Transverse process — Spinous process — Foramen — Body

Lumbar vertebrae

Transverse process — Spinous process — Foramen — Body

Arrangement

The vertebrae fall into five groups—cervical, thoracic, lumbar, sacral, and coccygeal. The top 24 are separated by disks of cartilage.

Structure

Three typical vertebrae are shown above. The foramen in each is the channel through which the spinal cord runs. The processes serve as muscle attachments.

INVESTIGATION

If disease is the suspected cause of vertigo, the physician performs an examination of the ears, eyes, and nervous system, sometimes including *CT scanning* of the brain.

TREATMENT

Vertigo that comes on suddenly is usually assumed to be due to laby-rinthitis and is treated with bed rest and with *antihistamine drugs* or *anticholinergic drugs*. If vertigo persists for more than a few days, the sufferer should walk as much as possible to allow the body to develop compensatory measures. In some cases, antihistamine drugs may be prescribed to prevent recurrent attacks.

Vesicle

A small skin blister, usually filled with clear fluid, that forms at the site of skin damage. The term vesicle is also used to refer to any small saclike structure in the body (e.g., the seminal vesicles, which store seminal fluid).

Vestibulitis

Inflammation of the nasal vestibule (the part of the nasal cavity just inside the nostril), usually as a result of bacterial infection.

Vestibulocochlear nerve

The eighth *cranial nerve* concerned with *balance* and *hearing*. Each vestibulocochlear nerve (one on each side) carries sensory impulses from the inner *ear* to the brain, which it enters between the pons and the medulla oblongata (parts of the *brain stem*). The vestibulocochlear nerve consists of two parts—the vestibular nerve and the cochlear nerve (the latter is also sometimes known as the acoustic nerve or auditory nerve).

The vestibular nerve carries sensory impulses from the semicircular canals in the inner ear to the *cerebellum* in the brain, which, in conjunction with information from the eyes and joints, controls balance. The cochlear nerve carries sensory impulses from the cochlea (the snail-shaped part of the inner ear responsible for detecting sound) to the hearing center in the brain, where the impulses are interpreted as sounds.

DISORDERS

A tumor of the cells that surround the vestibulocochlear nerve (see *Acoustic neuroma*) may cause loss of balance, *tinnitus* (ringing or other noises in the ear), and *deafness*. Deafness may also result from damage to the vestibulocochlear nerve, which is sometimes due to an infection, such as *meningitis* or *encephalitis*, or to an adverse reaction to a drug, such as *streptomycin*.

Viability

The capability of independent survival and development. A normal human fetus is widely accepted to be viable from 28 weeks' gestation onward. However, fetuses born as early as the 23rd to 24th week now commonly survive after care in a neonatal intensive-care unit.

Vibrator

A mechanical device applied to the body to tone or relax muscles and to massage the skin. Vibrators may also be used as an aid to sexual stimulation (possibly during *sex therapy*) or as an alternative to sexual intercourse for inducing orgasm.

Villus

A minute fingerlike projection from a membranous surface, particularly one of the countless millions of them that occur on the mucous lining of the small *intestine*. Although villi are present in all three sections of the small intestine, they are largest and most

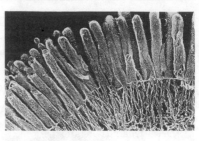

Microvilli in the intestine
This scanning electron micrograph shows numerous microvilli projecting from a single cell in the lining of the small intestine.

numerous in the duodenum and jejunum (the first and second parts), where most of the absorption of digested food occurs.

STRUCTURE

Each intestinal villus contains a small lymph vessel and a network of capillaries (tiny blood vessels). The outer surface of each villus is covered with hundreds of hairlike structures (called microvilli) which increase the surface area of the small intestine to an area approximately equal to that of a tennis court.

FUNCTION

The function of the intestinal villi is to provide a large surface area for the absorption of food molecules into the blood and lymphatic systems. Food particles that are broken down into small molecules by digestive enzymes reach the bloodstream via the capillaries of the villi.

Vincent's disease

A severe form of gingivitis in which bacterial infection causes painful ulceration of the gums (see *Gingivitis, acute ulcerative*). This condition is also sometimes called acute necrotizing ulcerative gingivitis, trench mouth, or Vincent's stomatitis.

Viremia

The presence of *virus* particles in the blood. Viremia can occur at certain stages in a variety of viral infections.

Some viruses, such as those responsible for viral *hepatitis*, *yellow fever*, and *poliomyelitis*, may simply be transported in the bloodstream. Symptoms arise when virus particles enter and start multiplying in target tissues rather than from the viremia.

Other viruses, such as the *rubella* virus and *HIV* (the virus that causes *AIDS*), exist within lymphocytes (types of white blood cell), which they use as a place to multiply as well as a means of spreading.

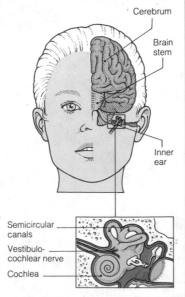

LOCATION OF THE VESTIBULOCOCHLEAR NERVE
This nerve conducts sensory impulses concerned with hearing and balance from different parts of the inner ear to the brain.

Cerebrum

Brain stem

Inner ear

Semicircular canals

Vestibulo-cochlear nerve

Cochlea

V

If viremia is a feature of a viral infection, there is a risk that the infection may be transmissible in blood or blood products, or by insects that feed on blood.

Virginity

The physical state of not having experienced *sexual intercourse*.

Virilism

Masculine characteristics that affect the physical appearance of a woman. Virilism is caused by excessive levels of *androgen hormones*. Androgens are male sex hormones which, in women, are normally secreted in small amounts by the adrenal glands and ovaries. Raised levels of these hormones induce various changes in women, including *hirsutism* (excessive hair growth); a male-pattern hairline with balding at the temples; disruption or cessation of menstruation; enlargement of the clitoris; loss of normal fat deposits around the hips; development of the arm and shoulder muscles; and deepening of the voice as a result of enlargement of the larynx. (See also *Virilization*.)

Virility

A term used to describe the quality of maleness, especially in sexual characteristics and performance.

Virilization

The process by which *virilism* occurs in women as a result of overproduction of *androgen hormones* (male sex hormones) by the adrenal glands and/or ovaries. This process, in turn, may be caused by various underlying conditions, such as certain *adrenal tumors*, polycystic ovary (see *Ovary, polycystic*) and some other *ovarian cysts*, or congenital *adrenal hyperplasia*.

Virion

A single, complete, virus particle. (See *Viruses*.)

Virology

The study of *viruses* and the *epidemiology* and treatment of diseases caused by viruses. In a more restricted sense, virology also means the isolation and identification of viruses to diagnose specific viral infections. To achieve this, a tissue or fluid sample must be obtained for analysis. Depending on the suspected virus, the type of sample studied may be a specimen of feces, sputum, blister fluid, blood, urine, cerebrospinal fluid, or even a brain biopsy specimen.

Unlike bacteria, viruses cannot be grown in a culture medium; they can multiply only within living cells. For this reason viruses must be grown in cultures of cells, which can be any of many types of animal or human cell that can easily be made to multiply in test tubes. The cell culture is exposed to the specimen or fluid sample that contains the virus, and the cells are then observed for distinctive changes that occur when they are infected.

Alternatively, virus particles or components of viruses can sometimes be detected directly in specimens by the use of *staining* techniques or an electron microscope. Sometimes, the virus particles must first be made to clump together by adding an *antiserum* (*antibodies* obtained from the blood of someone who has had the viral infection, and which will bind to the virus particles). *Immunoassay* techniques, in which "labeled" antibodies are added to the specimens and detected if they have bound to virus cell components, are another possible means of detecting infection.

Another method of diagnosing viral infections is to look for antibodies produced by the *immune system* to combat the viruses. A rapidly rising level of antibodies to a particular virus can provide good evidence of infection. Antibodies can be detected by immunoassay and by other laboratory techniques (see *Serology*).

Virulence

The ability of a microorganism to cause disease. Virulence can be assessed by measuring what proportion of the population exposed to the microorganism develops symptoms of disease, how rapidly the infection spreads through body tissues, or by the mortality from the infection.

Viruses

The smallest known types of infectious agent. Viruses are about one half to one hundredth the size of the smallest *bacteria*, from which they differ in having a much simpler structure and method of multiplication. Viral infections range from the trivial, such as *warts*, the common cold (see *Cold, common*), and other minor respiratory tract infections, to extremely serious diseases, such as *rabies* and *Lassa fever*. Viral infection also leads to the development of *AIDS*, and probably to various *cancers*.

NATURE OF VIRUSES

It is debatable whether viruses are truly living organisms or just collec-

tions of large molecules capable of self-replication under very specific favorable conditions. Their sole activity is to invade the cells of other organisms, which they then take over to make copies of themselves. Outside living cells, viruses are wholly inert. They are incapable of activities typical of life, such as metabolism (internal processing of nutrients).

The number of different kinds of virus probably exceeds the number of types of all other organisms. Viruses parasitize all recognized life-forms. Not all viruses cause disease, but many do.

STRUCTURE OF VIRUSES

A single virus particle (virion) consists simply of an inner core of *nucleic acid* surrounded by one or two protective shells (capsids) made of protein. These capsids are built from a number of identical protein subunits arranged in a highly symmetrical form, usually either as a 20-faced solid (an icosahedron) or as a spiral tube. Surrounding the outer capsid may be another layer called the viral envelope, which also consists mainly of protein. The viral envelope is often lost when the virus invades a cell.

The nucleic acid at the core is called the genome and consists of a string of *genes* that contain coded instructions for making copies of the virus. Depending on the type of virus, the nucleic acid may be either *DNA*, in which there are two complementary, intertwined strands of nucleic acid (the double helix), or *RNA*, consisting of a single strand.

REPLICATION OF VIRUSES

The basic process by which a virus replicates is shown in the illustrated box overleaf. Different viruses employ different strategies, some highly complex, to make copies of themselves once they have invaded a host cell. During replication of the viral nucleic acid, the viral genes may first have to code the manufacture of special *enzymes* called polymerases or transcriptases to assist in replication; alternatively, the virus may borrow these enzymes from the host cell. Sometimes the viral genome must invade the nucleus of the host cell and incorporate itself into the cell's *chromosomes* (genetic material) before it is able to replicate.

Sometimes, if the viral genome invades the nucleus of the host cell, it may not replicate immediately but may "hide" there, perhaps becoming reactivated months or years later. The viral genome may also interact with

V

VIRUSES AND DISEASE

All viruses have the same basic structure (right), but they come in various shapes and sizes. Examples from the main families are shown below (some in cross section). All are tiny—from about 15 to 300 nanometres in diameter (one nanometre equals one thousand-millionth of a metre); most are so small that they can be seen only with an electron microscope. All types of viruses can multiply only within cells of their host (far right).

Structure of a typical virus particle
Nucleic acid in the center is surrounded by one or more capsids made of protein subunits.

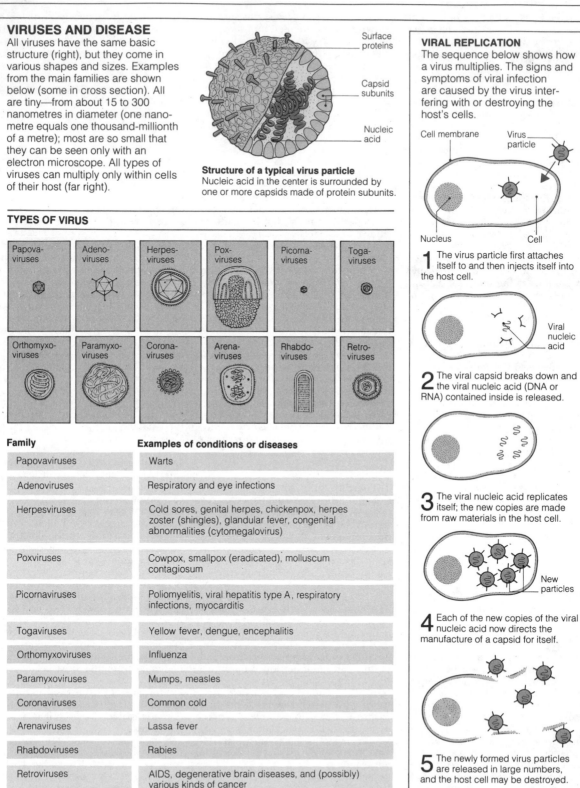

VIRAL REPLICATION

The sequence below shows how a virus multiplies. The signs and symptoms of viral infection are caused by the virus interfering with or destroying the host's cells.

1 The virus particle first attaches itself to and then injects itself into the host cell.

2 The viral capsid breaks down and the viral nucleic acid (DNA or RNA) contained inside is released.

3 The viral nucleic acid replicates itself; the new copies are made from raw materials in the host cell.

4 Each of the new copies of the viral nucleic acid now directs the manufacture of a capsid for itself.

5 The newly formed virus particles are released in large numbers, and the host cell may be destroyed.

TYPES OF VIRUS

Papovaviruses · Adenoviruses · Herpesviruses · Poxviruses · Picornaviruses · Togaviruses

Orthomyxoviruses · Paramyxoviruses · Coronaviruses · Arenaviruses · Rhabdoviruses · Retroviruses

Family	Examples of conditions or diseases
Papovaviruses	Warts
Adenoviruses	Respiratory and eye infections
Herpesviruses	Cold sores, genital herpes, chickenpox, herpes zoster (shingles), glandular fever, congenital abnormalities (cytomegalovirus)
Poxviruses	Cowpox, smallpox (eradicated), molluscum contagiosum
Picornaviruses	Poliomyelitis, viral hepatitis type A, respiratory infections, myocarditis
Togaviruses	Yellow fever, dengue, encephalitis
Orthomyxoviruses	Influenza
Paramyxoviruses	Mumps, measles
Coronaviruses	Common cold
Arenaviruses	Lassa fever
Rhabdoviruses	Rabies
Retroviruses	AIDS, degenerative brain diseases, and (possibly) various kinds of cancer

V

the cell's chromosomes—a process that may convert the host cell into a tumor cell.

TYPES

Viruses that cause human disease are grouped into more than 20 large families; the most important are shown in the table (facing page).

In recent years, special attention has been paid to the family of retroviruses, which include *HIV* (human immunodeficiency virus), the agent responsible for AIDS. HIV is an RNA virus and, after invading a cell, first manufactures an enzyme called reverse transcriptase, which it needs to make copies of itself. Research into this enzyme may reveal a means of attacking HIV.

HOW VIRUSES CAUSE DISEASE

Viruses gain access to the body by all possible entry routes. They are inhaled in droplets; swallowed in food and fluids; passed through the punctured skin in the saliva of feeding insects or rabid dogs or on infected needles; viruses are accepted directly by the mucous membranes of the genital tract during sexual intercourse and by the conjunctiva of the eye after accidental contamination.

Many viruses begin to invade cells and multiply near their site of entry. Some enter the lymphatic vessels and may spread to the lymph nodes, where many are engulfed by white blood cells. Some, such as HIV, invade and then multiply within *lymphocytes* (a type of white cell). Many pass from the lymphatics to the blood and within a few minutes are spread to every part of the body. They may then invade and start multiplying within specific target organs such as the skin, brain, liver, or lungs. Other viruses travel along nerve fibers to their target organs.

Viruses cause disease in a variety of ways. First, they may destroy or severely disrupt the activities of the cells they invade, possibly causing serious disease if vital organs are affected. Second, the response of the body's *immune system* to viral infection may lead to symptoms, such as fever and fatigue, or to a disease process. In particular, antibodies produced by the immune system may attach to viral particles and circulate as immune complexes in the bloodstream. The antibodies may then be deposited in various parts of the body and cause inflammation and severe tissue damage. Third, by interacting with the chromosomes of their host cells, viruses may cause cancer. Fourth, a virus may cause disease by weakening the cell-mediated arm of the immune system (i.e., the activity of T-lymphocytes). This is how HIV works, invading and disrupting one type of T-lymphocyte so that the body's normal defenses are lost.

VIRUSES AND CANCER

The chromosomes in all normal body cells contain 50 or more genes (known as *oncogenes*) that are necessary for the growth or *differentiation* of the cells. Certain retroviruses contain almost identical oncogenes. In the process of replication, these viruses may modify the chromosomes of the host cell. A small mutation in these can "switch on" the oncogenes inappropriately, thus prompting the cell to begin unrestrained division, leading to the formation of tumors.

To date, this process has been found to cause many cancers in animals but only one type of cancer in humans. The virus responsible is similar to the AIDS virus and can cause *leukemia* in the person it infects. However, other viruses are known to be at least potentially cancer-producing in humans, and this is a major area of research.

RESISTANCE TO VIRUSES

The immune system deals fairly rapidly with most viruses. Each mechanism of the immune system may be involved in resisting a viral attack—including white cells (macrophages) that engulf the viral particles, and lymphocytes that produce antibodies against the virus or attack virally infected cells. This leads to recovery from most viral infections within a few days to weeks. Furthermore, the immune system is often sufficiently sensitized by the infection to make a second illness from the same virus rare (as is the case with *measles*).

With some viruses, however, the speed of the attack is such that serious damage or even death may occur before the immune system can adequately respond (as is the case with rabies and some cases of *poliomyelitis*). In other cases, a virus is able to dodge or hide from the immune system, so that the infection becomes chronic or recurrent. This is common with many *herpes* virus infections (such as genital herpes and shingles) and with viral *hepatitis B*. Finally, the AIDS virus, by weakening the immune system, leaves the body open to many *opportunistic infections*.

FIGHTING VIRAL DISEASE

Viruses are more difficult than bacteria to combat with drugs because it is difficult to design drugs that will kill viruses without also killing the cells they parasitize. Nevertheless, there has been progress in the development of antiviral agents, especially against the herpes group of viruses (see *Antiviral drugs*). Such drugs may work by helping to prevent viruses from entering cells or by interfering with their replication in cells, and thus their spread to uninfected cells.

Interferon refers to a group of natural substances, produced by virus-infected cells, that protect uninfected cells. Some interferons can now be produced artificially (by means of *genetic engineering*) and have been tried in the treatment of various viral infections, including the common cold and viral hepatitis B.

Otherwise, treatment of viral infections depends largely on alleviating the patient's symptoms and trusting the body's immune defenses to bring about a cure.

A much more fruitful area in the fight against viruses is *immunization*. One viral disease, *smallpox*, has already been eradicated worldwide through a coordinated vaccination program. Highly effective vaccines are also now available to prevent many others, including poliomyelitis, measles, *mumps, rubella*, hepatitis B, *yellow fever*, and rabies.

Viscera

A collective term used to describe the internal organs.

Viscosity

The resistance to flow of a liquid or gas; the "stickiness" of a fluid. The viscosity of the blood affects its ability to flow through small blood vessels. An increase in the viscosity of the blood—caused by an increase in the proportion of red blood cells—increases the risk of *thrombosis* (abnormal clot formation).

Vision

The faculty of sight. Vision involves two main components—the *eye* and the *brain*.

When light-rays reach the eye, most of the focusing is done by the *cornea*. However, the eye also has an automatic fine-focusing facility, known as *accommodation*, that operates by altering the curvature of the crystalline *lens*. Together, these two systems provide sufficient optical power to form an image on the *retina*. The light-sensitive rods and cones in the retina convert the elements of this image into

V

THE SENSE OF VISION

Vision starts in the retina, the membrane at the back of the eye that contains the light-sensitive rod and cone cells. Much of the rest of the eye is concerned with focusing light, in the right quantities, onto the retina. Huge amounts of data are sent from the retina via the optic nerves to the brain for analysis.

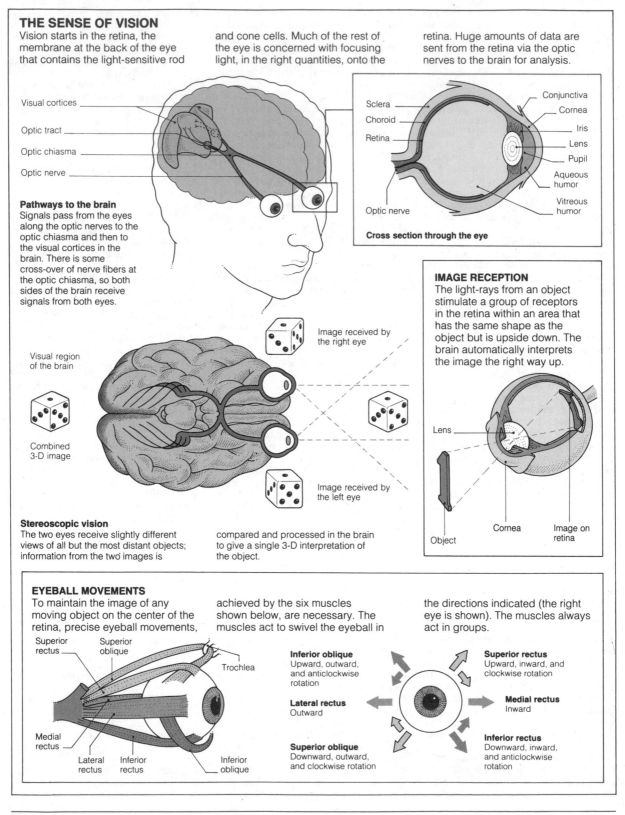

Visual cortices

Optic tract

Optic chiasma

Optic nerve

Sclera
Choroid
Retina
Optic nerve

Conjunctiva
Cornea
Iris
Lens
Pupil
Aqueous humor
Vitreous humor

Cross section through the eye

Pathways to the brain
Signals pass from the eyes along the optic nerves to the optic chiasma and then to the visual cortices in the brain. There is some cross-over of nerve fibers at the optic chiasma, so both sides of the brain receive signals from both eyes.

Visual region of the brain

Combined 3-D image

Image received by the right eye

Image received by the left eye

IMAGE RECEPTION
The light-rays from an object stimulate a group of receptors in the retina within an area that has the same shape as the object but is upside down. The brain automatically interprets the image the right way up.

Lens

Object
Cornea
Image on retina

Stereoscopic vision
The two eyes receive slightly different views of all but the most distant objects; information from the two images is compared and processed in the brain to give a single 3-D interpretation of the object.

EYEBALL MOVEMENTS

To maintain the image of any moving object on the center of the retina, precise eyeball movements, achieved by the six muscles shown below, are necessary. The muscles act to swivel the eyeball in the directions indicated (the right eye is shown). The muscles always act in groups.

Superior rectus
Superior oblique
Trochlea
Medial rectus
Lateral rectus
Inferior rectus
Inferior oblique

Inferior oblique
Upward, outward, and anticlockwise rotation

Lateral rectus
Outward

Superior oblique
Downward, outward, and clockwise rotation

Superior rectus
Upward, inward, and clockwise rotation

Medial rectus
Inward

Inferior rectus
Downward, inward, and anticlockwise rotation

V

nerve impulses that, after preliminary processing in the retina, pass into the visual cortex of the brain via the *optic nerves*. The rods, which are proportionately more concentrated at the periphery of the retina, are highly sensitive to light but not to color. The color-sensitive cones are concentrated more at the center of the retina (see *Color vision*).

Accurate alignment of the two eyes is achieved by coordination of the motor nerve impulses to the six tiny muscles that move each eye. This coordination is achieved in the brain, which correlates information from several sources, taking into account the brain's perception of the images, the position of the head, the position of the eyes relative to the head, and the position of the two eyes relative to each other.

Accurate alignment of the two eyes allows the brain to fuse the images from each eye, but because each eye has a slightly different view of a given object, the brain obtains information that is interpreted as solidity or depth. This stereoscopic vision is important in judging distance.

Vision, disorders of

The most common visual disorders are due to simple errors of *refraction*, such as *myopia*, *hyperopia*, and *astigmatism*. The blurring of vision from refractive errors can almost always be corrected by *glasses*. Defects of vision that cannot be eliminated in this way may have any of a wide variety of causes, including loss of binocular fusion (which can cause *double vision* or *amblyopia*), disorders of the *eye* or *optic nerve*, disorders of the nerve pathways that connect the optic nerves to the *brain*, and disorders of the brain itself.

VISUAL DEFECT FROM EYE AND OPTIC NERVE DISORDERS

Eye or optic nerve disease often affects vision in only one eye or in the two eyes to different degrees. Any interference with the transparency of the eye affects vision. Loss of transparency may result from corneal opacities (clouding of the cornea) following infection, ulceration, or injury; from *cataract* (opacification of the crystalline lens); or from *vitreous hemorrhage* (bleeding into the gel of the eye behind the lens).

Defects near the center of the retina cause loss of the corresponding parts of the *visual field* of the affected eye. This is especially serious if the central part of the retina, where sharp *visual*

acuity exists, is involved (see *Macular degeneration*). Peripheral retinal damage, which occurs in the early stages of chronic simple *glaucoma* or *retinitis pigmentosa*, may not cause noticeable visual disturbance if sharp central vision is unaffected.

Floaters (freely moving shadows perceived in the field of vision) are usually of no significance, but necessitate an eye examination. Floaters may signify a *retinal tear* or hemorrhage, or they may herald a *retinal detachment*, especially if accompanied by bright flashing lights at the periphery of the field of vision.

A defect in the optic nerve in front of the optic nerve crossing causes visual disturbance in one eye only, which often takes the form of a central *scotoma* (a blind spot in the center of the field of vision). This condition can be due to *optic neuritis*.

VISUAL DEFECT FROM NERVE PATHWAY DISORDERS

Disorders of one of the nerve pathways behind the optic nerve crossing always affect both eyes. This is because half of the fibers from each optic nerve—those from the inner half of each retina—cross over before they reach the back of the brain. Each pathway thus has contributions from both eyes, and any interruption thus causes loss of part of the visual field of each eye.

VISUAL DEFECT FROM BRAIN DISORDERS

Severe damage to one side of the visual area of the brain, such as from loss of blood supply in *stroke*, causes loss of the inner half of the field of vision of the eye on the same side and of the outer half of the field of the other eye. This condition, in which half of the field of vision is lost, is known as *hemianopia*.

Visual disturbance may also arise from involvement of the areas of the brain concerned with the psychological and associational aspects of vision. Disorders of these functions may cause visual *agnosia* (failure to recognize objects), visual perseveration (in which a scene continues to be perceived after the direction of gaze has shifted), or visual hallucinations.

Vision, loss of

An inability to see, which may develop slowly or suddenly, and may be temporary or permanent, depending on the cause. Vision loss may affect one or both eyes. It can cause complete blindness, or may affect only peripheral (side) vision or only central vision. A person suffering from loss of

central vision is usually aware of the fact, since it prevents reading and discernment of fine detail. However, loss of peripheral vision may pass unnoticed by the sufferer until it is well advanced and causes clumsiness.

SLOW VISION LOSS

A progressive loss of visual clarity is common with advancing age as a result of loss of transparency of the crystalline lenses of the eyes (see *Cataract*). Other common causes of gradual loss of vision are *macular degeneration* and chronic simple *glaucoma*, and complications of *diabetes mellitus*. Gradual visual loss may also be due to progressive opacity of the cornea from *keratopathy* (disease of the cornea) of any kind, or to progressive distortion from *keratoconus* (a conical deformity of the cornea). *Retinitis pigmentosa* causes a variable degree of visual loss in both eyes.

SUDDEN VISION LOSS

Sudden loss of vision may be caused by optical, vascular, or neurological disorders. *Hyphema* (bleeding into the aqueous humor) usually results from injury; the blood can block the normal passage of the light to the retina. Severe *uveitis* (inflammation of the uvea) may cause serious reduction in vision. *Vitreous hemorrhage* (bleeding into the gel of the eye) and retinal disorders, such as *retinal hemorrhage*, may also reduce vision suddenly.

Optic neuritis (inflammation of the optic nerve) can severely reduce vision in one eye. Any damage to the nerve connections between the eyes and the brain, or to the visual area of the brain itself, can cause loss of peripheral vision. Damage may sometimes be a result of *embolism*, *ischemia*, *tumor*, *inflammation*, or *injury*.

Vision tests

The part of an eye examination that determines if there is any reduction in the ability to see. Most vision tests are tests of *visual acuity* (sharpness of central vision). Tests of *visual field* (the total area of vision when looking ahead) may also be performed in order to assess disorders of the eye and the nervous system. Refraction tests are done to discover whether the patient has a refractive error (i.e., an error that can be corrected with glasses), such as *hyperopia*, *myopia*, or *astigmatism*. Refraction tests also show up *presbyopia* (a deficiency in the power of *accommodation*).

VISUAL ACUITY TESTS

Visual acuity is tested, one eye at a time, using a *Snellen's chart*. In the test,

V

the patient attempts to read letters of standard sizes from a standard distance of 6 m.

REFRACTION TESTS

Retinoscopy is one type of refraction test. A narrow beam of light is projected into the eye, from about 65 cm, and the tester observes the light reflected back through the pupil from the retina. Small movements of the light are made in various directions. Correction is determined from the power and type of lenses needed to neutralize the light's movement.

Refinement of the refraction is achieved by determining the person's subjective response to changes in his or her vision brought about by the use of different lenses.

ACCOMMODATION TESTS

The power of accommodation (ability to focus on near objects) may be measured by correcting any refractive error with *glasses*, and then determining the nearest distance at which very small print can be read.

VISUAL FIELD TESTS

Visual field tests can indicate disorders of the peripheral parts of the retinas, of the optic nerves, or of the optical pathways to the brain. Most visual field tests involve the use of large black screens or white hollow bowls. The patient's head is secured, one eye is covered, and the other is directed to a point at the center of the inside of the bowl. Small spots of light are projected onto the inner surface of the bowl; the spots appear for brief periods in various places or are moved inward from the periphery. The person being tested responds when he or she sees the spot. (See also *Eye, examination of*.)

Visual acuity

Sharpness of *vision*. Visual acuity is concerned with sharpness (discrimination) of central vision, not with the extent or clarity of the peripheral vision (see *Visual field*). Normal visual acuity is expressed as 20/20 (feet) or 6/6 (metres). A result of 20/30 means that the first line a patient sitting 20 feet away from the chart can read is the line that someone with normal visual acuity could read sitting 30 feet away.

Refractive errors (errors that can be corrected with glasses), such as *myopia*, *hyperopia*, and *astigmatism*, are the most common cause of poor visual acuity. Poor visual acuity for near objects occurs in *presbyopia*.

Visual field

The total area in which visual perception is possible while looking straight ahead. The visual fields normally extend outward over an angle of about 90 degrees on either side of the midline of the face, but are more restricted above and below, especially if the eyes are deep-set or the eyebrows are prominent. The visual fields of the two eyes overlap to a large extent so that a defect in the field of one eye may be concealed if both eyes are open.

The level of *visual acuity* (sharpness of vision) in the visual field is much lower in areas remote from the point

---

TYPES OF VISION TESTS

These tests are performed to measure a number of variables—the acuity of a patient's distance vision and the power of the lenses he or she may need (visual acuity and refraction tests), the extent of peripheral vision (visual field tests), and the ability to focus on near objects (accommodation tests).

VISUAL ACUITY TESTS

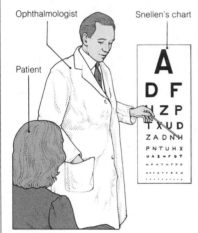

These tests use the familiar Snellen's chart. Visual acuity is measured according to how far down the chart the patient can read accurately.

REFRACTION TESTS

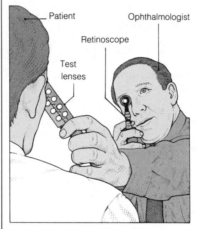

The effect of lenses on movements of light reflected from the eye (as the light source is moved) is observed to help calculate the corrective glasses needed.

ACCOMMODATION TESTS

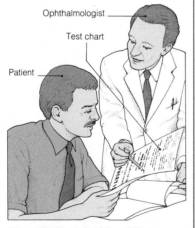

After any distance-focusing ability has been established, the patient's ability to read small print close up is measured to test accommodation.

VISUAL FIELD TESTS

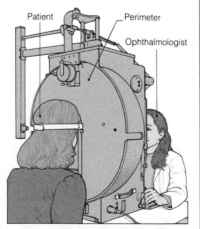

One eye is fixed straight ahead, the other covered, and lights are shone onto a white bowl or screen in front of the patient to find the field of vision of each eye.

V

THE VISUAL FIELDS

Viewed from above, the field of vision of each eye (with the head and eyes immobile) extends through an angle of about 130 degrees and is divided into an area that overlaps with the visual field of the other eye (binocular vision) and an area that can be seen only by one eye.

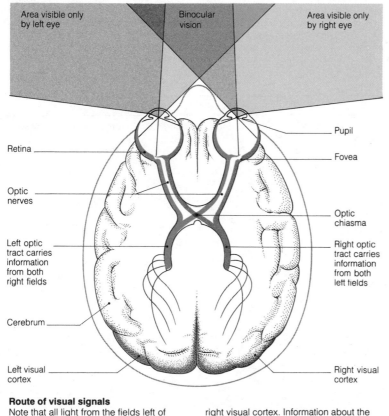

Area visible only by left eye

Binocular vision

Area visible only by right eye

Retina

Optic nerves

Left optic tract carries information from both right fields

Cerebrum

Left visual cortex

Pupil

Fovea

Optic chiasma

Right optic tract carries information from both left fields

Right visual cortex

Route of visual signals
Note that all light from the fields left of center of both eyes (gray) falls on the right sides of the two retinas; information about these fields goes to the right visual cortex. Information about the right fields of vision (pink) goes to the left cortex. Data about the area of binocular vision go to both cortices.

at which one is looking directly. For instance, it is impossible to read fine print as little as 5 degrees to one side of the fixation point. This is especially apparent to people with *macular degeneration*, who have no central vision and must therefore use other parts of the visual field.

Partial loss of visual field is less obvious than loss of central vision; even people with extensive visual field loss, such as from *glaucoma* or *stroke*, may be unaware of it if they still have sharp central visual acuity. (See also *Vision, disorders of; Vision tests*.)

Vital sign

An indication that a person is still alive. Vital signs include chest movements caused by breathing, the presence of a pulse (which indicates that the heart is beating), and the constriction of the pupil of the eye when it is exposed to a bright light. A physician certifies *death* on the basis of the absence of all these signs. Additional tests, such as measurement of brain activity, are sometimes performed.

Vitamin

Any of a group of complex organic substances that are essential in small amounts for the normal functioning of the body. With few exceptions (niacin and vitamin D), the body cannot manufacture these substances itself, making it necessary to obtain them from the diet. There are 13 vitamins—A, C, D, E, K, B_{12}, and the seven vitamins discussed under the heading of *vitamin B complex* (thiamine or B_1, riboflavin or B_2, niacin, pyridoxine or B_6, pantothenic acid, folic acid, and biotin or vitamin H). Each vitamin is present in many different foods. Vitamin D is also produced in the skin when it is exposed to sunlight, and niacin is made by the body from tryptophan (an *amino acid*).

A varied diet is likely to contain adequate amounts of all the vitamins. However, a physician may recommend *vitamin supplements* in certain circumstances, such as for young children, some women who are pregnant or breast-feeding, and for people taking certain *lipid-lowering drugs*, which reduce intestinal absorption of vitamins, or other drugs that interfere with vitamin function.

TYPES

Vitamins can be categorized as fat-soluble or water-soluble vitamins.

FAT-SOLUBLE VITAMINS The fat-soluble vitamins (A, D, E, and K) are absorbed with fats from the intestine into the bloodstream and then stored in fatty tissue (mainly in the liver). Body reserves of some may last for several years and a daily intake is therefore not usually essential; in fact, an excessive intake of a fat-soluble vitamin from pharmaceutical preparations may be harmful, especially vitamin D.

Deficiency of a fat-soluble vitamin is usually due to a disorder in which intestinal absorption of fats is impaired (see *Malabsorption*) or to a prolonged poor or restricted diet.

WATER-SOLUBLE VITAMINS The water-soluble vitamins are C, B_{12}, and the members of the B complex. The body can store only a limited amount of these and they are rapidly excreted in the urine if taken in greater amounts than the body requires. A regular intake is therefore essential to prevent a deficiency. Vitamin B_{12} is an exception because it is stored in the liver and these stores last for several years.

Deficiencies of water-soluble vitamins are thus more likely to occur than fat-soluble vitamin deficiencies. Foods that contain water-soluble vitamins should be eaten daily; moreover, prolonged cooking, storage, and processing tend to damage these vitamins, so fresh or lightly cooked foods are the best sources. Frozen fruits and vegetables can also be a good source of water-soluble vitamins. Taking very large amounts of water-soluble vitamins does not usually cause toxic effects although adverse reactions to very large doses of vitamin C and pyridoxine have been reported.

V

FUNCTION

The role of all the vitamins is not fully understood. Most have several important actions on one or more body systems or functions, and many are involved in the activities of *enzymes* (substances that promote chemical reactions in the body).

Vitamin A

A fat-soluble *vitamin* essential for normal growth, for the formation of bones and teeth, for cell structure, for night vision, and for protecting the linings of the respiratory, digestive, and urinary tracts against infection.

Vitamin A is absorbed by the body in the form of retinol. This is found in animal foods, such as liver, fish-liver oils, egg yolk, and dairy products, and is also added to margarines. *Carotene*, which is converted into retinol in the body, also provides a good source of vitamin A. Carotene is present in carrots, green vegetables, tomatoes, and various fruits.

DEFICIENCY

Vitamin A deficiency is rare in developed countries. In most cases it is due to failure of the intestine to absorb sufficient quantities of the vitamin as a result of *malabsorption*, which may be due to damage, *cystic fibrosis*, or obstruction of the bile duct. Vitamin A deficiency may also occur as an adverse effect of long-term treatment with certain *lipid-lowering drugs*. Deficiency is common in some developing countries.

RECOMMENDED DAILY INTAKES (RDIs) OF SELECTED VITAMINS

Age	Weight (kg)		Protein (g)	Vitamin A (mcg)	Vitamin D (mcg)	Vitamin E (mg)	Vitamin C (mg)	Folate (mcg)	Vitamin B₁₂ (mcg)	Thiamin (mg)	Riboflavin (mg)	Niacin (mg)
0–4 months		6.0	12	400	10[a]	3	20	50	0.3	0.3	0.3	4
5–12 months		9.0	12	400	10[a]	3	20	50	0.3	0.4	0.5	7
1 year		11	19	400	10[a]	3	20	65	0.3	0.5	0.6	8
2–3 years		14	22	400	5	4	20	80	0.4	0.6	0.7	9
4–6 years		18	26	500	5	5	25	90	0.5	0.7	0.9	13
7–9 years	M	25	30	700	2.5	7	25	125	0.8	0.9	1.1	16
	F	25	30	700	2.5	6	25	125	0.8	0.8	1.0	14
10–12 years	M	34	38	800	2.5	8	25	170	1.0	1.0	1.3	18
	F	36	40	800	5	7	25	180	1.0	0.9	1.1	16
13–15 years	M	50	50	900	5	9	30	150	1.5	1.1	1.4	20
	F	48	42	800	5	7	30	145	1.5	0.9	1.1	16
16–18 years	M	62	55	1000	5	10	40[b]	185	1.9	1.3	1.6	23
	F	53	43	800	2.5	7	30[b]	160	1.9	0.8	1.1	15
19–24 years	M	71	58	1000	2.5	10	40[b]	210	2.0	1.2	1.5	22
	F	58	43	800	2.5	7	30[b]	175	2.0	0.8	1.1	15
25–49 years	M	74	61	1000	2.5	9	40[b]	220	2.0	1.1	1.4	19
	F	59	44	800	2.5	6	30[b]	175	2.0	0.8	1.0	14
50–74 years	M	73	60	1000	5	7	40[b]	220	2.0	0.9	1.3	16
	F	63	47	800	5	6	30[b]	190	2.0	0.8	1.0	14
75+ years	M	69	57	1000	5	6	40[b]	205	2.0	0.8	1.0	14
	F	64	47	800	5	5	30[b]	190	2.0	0.8	1.0	14
Pregnancy (extra) 1st Trimester			5	100	2.5	2	0	300	1.0	0.1	0.1	0.1
2nd Trimester			20	100	2.5	2	10	300	1.0	0.1	0.3	0.2
3rd Trimester			24	100	2.5	2	10	300	1.0	0.1	0.3	0.2
Lactation (extra)			20	400	2.5	2	25	100	0.5	0.2	0.4	0.3

[a] Should be doubled in arctic regions.
[b] Smokers should increase vitamin C by 50%.

Vitamin requirements

The table above gives the recommended daily intakes (RDIs) of vitamins for which amounts have been established; when different, the RDIs for males and females are denoted by M and F.

Units

mg = milligrams (thousandths of a gram)

mcg = micrograms (millionths of a gram)

V

The first symptom of deficiency is night blindness (inability to see in dim light), followed by dryness and inflammation of the eyes, *keratomalacia* (damage to the cornea), and eventually blindness. Deficiency also causes reduced resistance to infection, dry rough skin, and, in children, stunted growth.

Worldwide, there are half a million new cases of *xerophthalmia* (dry eye caused by vitamin A deficiency) each year; half of these result in blindness.

EXCESS

Prolonged, excessive intake of vitamin A can result in a condition called hypervitaminosis A. This condition most commonly occurs as a result of taking large quantities of self-prescribed vitamin supplements. (To avoid the risk of overdose, manufacturers of the vitamin limit the potency of their preparations.)

Symptoms of hypervitaminosis A include headache, nausea, loss of appetite, peeling of the skin, hair loss, and, in women, irregular menstruation. In extreme cases, the liver and spleen become enlarged. Excessive intake during pregnancy may cause birth defects. In infants, the condition may cause skull deformities, which disappear if the diet is corrected.

Excessive intake of carrots can give rise to a harmless orange coloration of the skin; this is known as carotenemia and vanishes when the diet is corrected.

MEDICAL USES

Several compounds, known as retinoids, which are chemically related to retinol have recently been under investigation for inhibiting the growth of certain types of tumors; the results so far are conflicting.

The drug *tretinoin* (a derivative of vitamin A) is effective in the treatment of severe *acne*.

Vitamin B

See *Vitamin B₁₂*; *Vitamin B complex*.

Vitamin B₁₂

Also known as cyanocobalamin, vitamin B₁₂ plays a vital role in the activities of several *enzymes* (substances that promote chemical reactions in the body). Vitamin B₁₂ is important in the production of the genetic material of cells (and thus in growth and development), in the production of red blood cells in bone marrow, in the utilization of folic acid (a constituent of the *vitamin B complex*) and carbohydrates in the diet, and in the functioning of the nervous system.

Foods rich in vitamin B₁₂ include liver, kidney, chicken, beef, pork, fish, eggs, and dairy products.

DEFICIENCY AND EXCESS

A balanced diet contains sufficient amounts of vitamin B₁₂ for the body's needs. Deficiency of vitamin B₁₂ is almost always due to an inability of the intestine to absorb the vitamin, most commonly as a result of pernicious anemia (see *Anemia, megaloblastic*). Less commonly, deficiency of vitamin B₁₂ may be an effect of *gastrectomy*, result from *malabsorption* due to an intestinal disorder, or be a consequence of following a vegan diet (one that excludes all kinds of animal products).

VITAMINS AND MAIN FOOD SOURCES

Fat-soluble	Good sources
Vitamin A	Liver; fish-liver oils; egg yolk; milk and dairy products; margarine; various fruits and vegetables (such as apricots and carrots)
Vitamin D	Cod-liver oil; oily fish (such as sardines, herring, salmon, and tuna); liver; egg yolk; margarine
Vitamin E	Vegetable oils (such as corn, soybean, olive, and sunflower oils); nuts; meat; green, leafy vegetables; cereals; wheat germ; egg yolk
Vitamin K	Green, leafy vegetables (especially cabbage, broccoli, spinach, and turnip greens); vegetable oils; egg yolk; cheese; pork liver
Water-soluble	
Thiamine (vitamin B₁)	Wheat germ; bran; whole-grain or enriched cereals; whole wheat bread; brown rice; pasta; liver; kidney; pork; fish; beans; nuts; eggs
Riboflavin (vitamin B₂)	Brewer's yeast; liver; kidney; milk; cheese; eggs; whole grains; enriched cereals; wheat germ
Niacin	Liver; lean meat; poultry; fish; nuts; dried beans; enriched cereals; bread; wheat germ; potatoes
Pantothenic acid	Liver; heart; kidney; fish; egg yolk; wheat germ; most vegetables; most cereals
Pyridoxine (vitamin B₆)	Liver; chicken; pork; fish; whole grains; wheat germ; bananas; potatoes; dried beans
Biotin (vitamin H)	Liver; peanuts; dried beans; egg yolk
Folic acid	Green, leafy vegetables; mushrooms; liver; nuts; dried beans; peas; egg yolk; whole wheat bread; whole grain cereals
Vitamin B₁₂ (cyanocobalamin)	Liver; kidney; chicken; beef; pork; fish; eggs; milk; cheese
Vitamin C	Citrus fruits; tomatoes; green, leafy vegetables; potatoes; green peppers; strawberries; blackcurrants

Vitamin needs

A varied diet usually provides all vitamin needs. For vegans (who eat no animal products), vitamins B₁₂ and D may be lacking; these vitamins can be obtained from supplements or, in the case of vitamin D, through adequate exposure to sunlight.

V

The principal effects of vitamin B_{12} deficiency are megaloblastic anemia, a sore mouth and tongue, and symptoms caused by damage to the spinal cord, such as numbness and tingling in the limbs. There may also be depression and loss of memory.

No harmful effects are known to occur as a result of a high intake of vitamin B_{12}.

Vitamin B complex

A group of *vitamins* that consists of thiamine (vitamin B_1), riboflavin (vitamin B_2), niacin, pantothenic acid, pyridoxine (vitamin B_6), biotin (vitamin H), and folic acid. *Vitamin B_{12}* is discussed separately.

THIAMINE

This vitamin plays a vital role in the activities of various *enzymes* (substances that promote chemical reactions in the body) involved in the utilization of *carbohydrates* and consequently in the functioning of the nerves, muscles, and heart. Wheat germ, bran, whole-grain or enriched cereals, whole wheat breads, brown rice, pasta, liver, kidney, pork, fish, beans, nuts, and eggs are good sources of thiamine.

Those susceptible to deficiency include elderly people on a poor diet relatively rich in sugar and white flour products, those suffering from *hyperthyroidism*, those with disorders of *malabsorption*, and those with severe *alcohol dependence*. Deficiency may also occur as a result of severe illness, major surgery, or serious injury.

Mild thiamine deficiency may cause tiredness, irritability, loss of appetite, and sleep disturbances. Severe deficiency may cause abdominal pain, constipation, depression, memory impairment, and *beriberi* (which may be fatal); in sufferers of chronic alcohol dependence, it may cause *Wernicke-Korsakoff syndrome*.

Excessive intake of thiamine is not known to cause harmful effects.

RIBOFLAVIN

Riboflavin is essential for the activities of various enzymes involved in the breakdown and utilization of carbohydrates, fats, and proteins, the production of energy in cells, the utilization of other B vitamins, and the production of hormones by the adrenal glands.

Particularly good sources of riboflavin are liver and milk, also eggs, whole grains, and brewer's yeast.

People susceptible to deficiency include those taking phenothiazine *antipsychotic drugs*, tricyclic *antidepres-*

sant drugs, or estrogen-containing *oral contraceptives*, those with malabsorption disorders, or those with severe alcohol dependence. Riboflavin deficiency may also occur as a result of serious illness, major surgery, or severe injury.

Prolonged deficiency of riboflavin may cause chapped lips, soreness of the tongue and corners of the mouth, and certain eye disorders, such as *amblyopia* (poor visual acuity) and *photophobia* (abnormal sensitivity to bright light). Excessive intake is not known to cause harmful effects.

NIACIN

This consists of nicotinic acid and nicotinamide, and does not have a designated vitamin number. Niacin plays an essential role in the activities of various enzymes involved in the metabolism of carbohydrates and fats, the functioning of the nervous and digestive systems, the manufacture of sex hormones, and the maintenance of healthy skin.

The principal dietary sources of niacin include liver, lean meat, poultry, fish, nuts, and dried beans. Niacin is present in cereals in a chemically bound form that is not absorbed by the body; part is liberated and becomes available when the cereal is baked. Niacin can be made in the body from tryptophan (an *amino acid* present in proteins).

Most cases of deficiency are due to malabsorption disorders or to severe alcohol dependence. Prolonged niacin deficiency causes *pellagra*, the principal symptoms of which include soreness and cracking of the skin, inflammation of the mouth and tongue, and mental disturbances; pellagra can be fatal.

Excessive intake of niacin is not known to cause harmful effects.

PANTOTHENIC ACID

Pantothenic acid is essential for the activities of various enzymes involved in the metabolism of carbohydrates and fats, the manufacture of corticosteroids and sex hormones, the utilization of other vitamins, the functioning of the nervous system and adrenal glands, and normal growth and development.

Pantothenic acid is present in almost all vegetables, cereals, and animal foods. Particularly rich sources of this vitamin include liver, heart, kidney, fish, egg yolk, and wheat germ.

A dietary shortage is almost never seen; deficiency usually occurs as a result of malabsorption disorders or severe alcohol dependence. Defi-

ciency may also sometimes occur as a result of severe illness, major surgery, or serious injury. The principal effects of deficiency include fatigue, headache, nausea, abdominal pain, numbness and tingling, muscle cramps, and susceptibility to respiratory infections. In severe cases, a *peptic ulcer* may develop.

Excessive intake of pantothenic acid is not known to have harmful effects.

PYRIDOXINE

This vitamin plays a vital role in the activities of various enzymes and hormones involved in the breakdown and utilization of carbohydrates, fats, and proteins, in the manufacture of red blood cells and antibodies, in the functioning of the digestive and nervous systems, and in the maintenance of healthy skin.

Good dietary sources of pyridoxine include liver, chicken, pork, fish, whole grains, wheat germ, bananas, potatoes, and dried beans. Pyridoxine is also manufactured in small amounts by intestinal bacteria. Groups susceptible to deficiency include elderly people on a poor diet, people with a malabsorption disorder, people with severe alcohol dependence, and people who are being treated with certain drugs (including *penicillamine* and *isoniazid*).

Deficiency of pyridoxine may cause weakness, irritability, depression, skin disorders, inflammation of the mouth and tongue, cracked lips, anemia, and, in infants, seizures.

Excessive intake—100 times or more above the normal daily intake—has been reported to cause *neuritis*. Doses of 50 to 100 mg per day are said to be helpful in relieving symptoms of premenstrual syndrome.

BIOTIN

Biotin is essential for the activities of various enzymes involved in the breakdown of fatty acids and carbohydrates and for the excretion of the waste products of protein breakdown.

Biotin is present in many foods. Particularly rich sources of this vitamin include liver, peanuts, dried beans, egg yolk, mushrooms, bananas, grapefruit, and watermelon. Biotin is also manufactured by bacteria present in the intestines.

Deficiency may occur during prolonged treatment with *antibiotic drugs* or *sulfonamide drugs*. It may also result from long-term high consumption of raw egg whites, which contain a substance that interferes with the intestinal absorption of biotin. Otherwise, no dietary shortage has been ob-

V

served. The principal symptoms of biotin deficiency include weakness, tiredness, poor appetite, hair loss, depression, inflammation of the tongue, and eczema.

Excessive intake of biotin is not known to cause harmful effects.

FOLIC ACID

This vitamin plays a vital role in the activities of various enzymes involved in the manufacture of *nucleic acids* (the genetic material of cells) and therefore in growth and reproduction, in the production of red blood cells, and in the healthy functioning of the nervous system. The principal dietary sources of folic acid include green leafy vegetables, mushrooms, liver, nuts, dried beans, peas, egg yolk, and whole wheat bread.

A varied diet that includes fresh vegetables and fruit generally provides enough folic acid for the body's needs. Mild deficiency is relatively common, but can usually be corrected by increasing the daily consumption of foods containing folic acid. More severe deficiency may occur during pregnancy or breast-feeding, in premature or low-birthweight infants, in people undergoing *dialysis*, in people with certain blood disorders, *psoriasis*, malabsorption disorders, or severe alcohol dependence, and in people taking certain drugs, including *anticonvulsant drugs*, antimalarial drugs, estrogen-containing oral contraceptive drugs, and some *analgesic drugs* (painkillers), *corticosteroid drugs*, and sulfonamide drugs.

The principal effects of folic acid deficiency include anemia, sores around the mouth, a sore tongue, and, in children, poor growth.

High intakes of folic acid are discouraged because they can mask vitamin B_{12} deficiency.

Vitamin C

Also known by its chemical name, ascorbic acid, a vitamin that plays an essential role in the activities of various *enzymes* (substances that promote chemical reactions in the body). Vitamin C is important for the growth and maintenance of healthy bones, teeth, gums, ligaments, and blood vessels; in the production of certain *neurotransmitters* (chemicals responsible for the transmission of nerve impulses between nerve cells) and of adrenal gland hormones; in the response of the *immune system* to infection; in wound healing; and in the absorption of *iron*.

The principal dietary sources of vitamin C are fruits and vegetables. Citrus fruits, tomatoes, green leafy vegetables, potatoes, green peppers, strawberries, and blackcurrants are particularly rich sources. Considerable amounts of vitamin C are lost during the processing, cooking, or keeping warm of foods.

DEFICIENCY

Dietary deficiency of vitamin C is rare. Slight deficiency may occur as a result of a serious injury or burn, major surgery, use of *oral contraceptives*, fever, or continual inhalation of carbon monoxide (a constituent of tobacco smoke and traffic fumes). More pronounced deficiency is usually caused by a very restricted diet.

Mild deficiency may cause weakness, general aches and pains, swollen gums, and *nosebleeds*. Severe deficiency leads to *scurvy* and *anemia*.

EXCESS

Large doses of vitamin C are taken by some people who believe this prevents the common cold, but there is no convincing evidence to support this belief. Excessive intake is not usually harmful unless the daily dose exceeds 1 g, when it may cause nausea, stomach cramps, diarrhea, and, rarely, kidney stones.

Vitamin D

The collective term for a group of related substances—including ergocalciferol (vitamin D_2), and cholecalciferol (vitamin D_3)—that play several vital roles in the body. Vitamin D helps regulate the balance of *calcium* and *phosphate*, aids the absorption of calcium from the intestine, and is essential for strong bones and teeth.

Good sources of vitamin D include oily fish (such as sardines, herring, salmon, and tuna), liver, and egg yolk; vitamin D is also added to margarines. In the body, vitamin D is formed by the action of ultraviolet rays in sunlight on a specific chemical in the skin.

DEFICIENCY

Deficiency may occur in people on a poor diet; in premature infants; in those deprived of sunlight, such as night workers; and in dark-skinned people, particularly those living in foggy urban areas, who do not absorb enough ultraviolet rays. It also occurs in certain disorders, most commonly those in which intestinal absorption of the vitamin is impaired (see *Malabsorption*). Other causes include liver disorders, kidney disorders, some genetic defects, and prolonged use of certain drugs, such as *phenytoin* (an anticonvulsant drug). Deficiency in young children causes *rickets* (a condition in which there is poor bone formation). Long-term deficiency in adults leads to *osteomalacia* (the adult equivalent of rickets, in which the bones lose calcium and become very fragile).

EXCESS

Excessive intake of vitamin D disrupts the balance of calcium and phosphate in the body and leads to *hypercalcemia* (an abnormally high level of calcium in the blood). Symptoms of an excessive vitamin D intake include weakness, abnormal thirst, increased urination, gastrointestinal disturbances, and depression. An excess of vitamin D may also lead to abnormal calcium deposits in the soft tissues, kidneys, and blood vessel walls. In children, vitamin D excess may cause growth retardation.

Vitamin E

The collective term for a group of substances—of which alpha-tocopherol is the most important—that play several vital roles in the body, principally concerned with protecting fats from oxidation.

Vitamin E is essential for normal cell structure, for maintaining the activities of certain *enzymes* (substances that promote chemical reactions in the body), and for the formation of red blood cells. This vitamin also protects the lungs and other tissues from damage by pollutants, helps prevent red blood cells from being destroyed by poisons in the blood, and is believed to slow aging of cells.

The principal dietary sources of vitamin E are vegetable oils, nuts, meat, green leafy vegetables, cereals, wheat germ, and egg yolk.

DEFICIENCY

Dietary shortages rarely occur; deficiency usually occurs only through impaired intestinal absorption (see *Malabsorption*), in certain liver disorders, and in premature infants.

Vitamin E deficiency leads to the destruction of red blood cells, which eventually results in *anemia*. In infants, deficiency causes irritability and edema (accumulation of fluid in body tissues).

EXCESS

Prolonged, excessive intake of vitamin E may cause abdominal pain, nausea and vomiting, and diarrhea. It may also reduce intestinal absorption of vitamins A, D, and K, which, in severe cases, may produce symptoms of deficiency of these vitamins.

V

Vitamin K

A *vitamin* that is essential for the formation in the liver of substances that promote blood clotting. Its principal dietary sources are green leafy vegetables (especially spinach, cabbage, broccoli, and turnip greens), vegetable oils, egg yolk, cheese, and pork liver. Vitamin K is also manufactured by bacteria that live in the intestine.

DEFICIENCY AND EXCESS

Dietary deficiency rarely occurs. Deficiency may develop in people suffering from *malabsorption* disorders, from certain liver disorders, and from chronic diarrhea, and it may also develop as a result of prolonged treatment with *antibiotic drugs*. Newborns lack the intestinal bacteria that produce vitamin K and are therefore routinely given supplements.

Deficiency of vitamin K reduces the ability of the blood to clot. This may cause nosebleeds, seeping of blood from wounds, and bleeding from the gums, intestine, and urinary tract. In rare, very severe cases, brain hemorrhage may result.

Excessive intake of vitamin K is not known to cause harmful effects.

Vitamin supplements

A group of dietary preparations containing one or more *vitamins*.

Most people do not usually need vitamin supplements (see *Nutrition*). Eating a variety of foods provides adequate amounts of all vitamins. Excessive amounts of some vitamins (especially A and D) may be harmful.

MEDICAL USES

Vitamin supplements are used to treat diagnosed vitamin deficiency, to prevent vitamin deficiency in susceptible people, and to treat certain medical disorders.

In developed countries, deficiency most commonly occurs in people on a poor diet, such as those with severe *alcohol dependence* or *drug dependence*, those on a low income, and elderly people who are not eating properly. A vegan diet (one that excludes all animal products) may sometimes result in vitamin deficiency. Deficiency may also result from *malabsorption*, *liver disorders*, and *kidney disorders*.

Vitamin supplements are also used to prevent deficiency during periods of increased requirements, such as pregnancy, breast-feeding, and infancy. They are also given to people who are taking certain drugs that may impair the absorption of vitamins, to those suffering from serious illness or injury, or to people who have had major surgery. People who are being fed intravenously are also likely to need vitamin supplements.

Certain vitamins are used to treat some conditions that are not specific deficiency disorders. Vitamin D, for example, is used in the treatment of *osteoporosis* and vitamin A derivatives are prescribed for severe *acne*.

There is no clear medical evidence that vitamin C helps to prevent or cure the common cold, that vitamin B_6 relieves premenstrual syndrome, or that vitamin E improves well-being.

Vitiligo

A common disorder of *skin* pigmentation in which patches of skin lose their color. Depigmented white patches are particularly obvious in dark-skinned people, occurring most commonly on the face, hands, armpits, and groin. Affected skin is particularly sensitive to sunlight.

Vitiligo is thought to be an *autoimmune disorder* that causes an absence of melanocytes, the specialized cells responsible for secreting the skin pigment *melanin*. The condition may occur at any age but usually develops in early adulthood. It affects about one in 200 people. Spontaneous repigmentation occurs in about 30 percent of cases.

TREATMENT

Makeup may be used to disguise areas of vitiligo; in mild cases, no further treatment may be necessary. *Phototherapy* using *PUVA* induces significant repigmentation in more than 50 percent of cases, but many treatments are required. Creams containing *corticosteroid drugs* may also help. If areas of vitiligo are extensive, chemicals may be used to remove pigment from remaining areas of normal skin.

Vitreous hemorrhage

Bleeding into the *vitreous humor*, the gellike substance that fills the main cavity of the *eye* between the crystalline lens and the retina. A common cause of vitreous hemorrhage is diabetic *retinopathy*, in which new, fragile blood capillaries that bleed readily form on the retina.

Any bleeding into the vitreous humor is likely to affect vision; a major hemorrhage into the center of the gel causes very poor vision for as long as the blood remains. Blood released into the periphery of the vitreous humor may be reabsorbed and the transparency of the gel restored, but a large hemorrhage may persist for months or never clear.

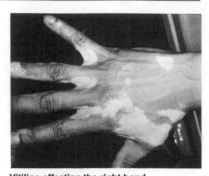

Vitiligo affecting the right hand
Loss of pigment is the only skin change that occurs. The usual remedy is to mask the white patches with cosmetics.

Vitreous humor

The transparent, gellike body that fills the large rear compartment of the *eye* between the crystalline lens and the retina. The vitreous humor consists almost entirely of water. Under certain conditions, it can exert sufficient pull on the retina to cause *retinal tears* and *retinal detachment*.

Vivisection

The performance of a surgical operation on a live animal, particularly for research purposes. However, the term vivisection is popularly used to refer to *animal experimentation* of any kind, even when surgery is not involved in such research activity.

Vocal cords

Two fibrous sheets of tissue in the *larynx* (voice box) that are responsible for voice production. The cords are attached at the front to the inner surface of the thyroid cartilage (Adam's apple) and at the rear to the arytenoid cartilages.

The so-called true vocal cords are the cords that vibrate and make sound; the false vocal cords are merely folds in the larynx, just above the true vocal cords, that have nothing to do with sound production.

Most of the time the vocal cords lie apart, forming a V-shaped opening called the glottis through which air is breathed. Vocal sounds are produced when the cords tighten, close, and vibrate as air expelled from the lungs passes between them. Alterations in the tension of the cords produce sounds of different pitch, which are modified by the tongue, palate, and lips to produce *speech*. (See also *Larynx, disorders of*.)

Voice box

See *Larynx*.

V

Voice, loss of

Inability to speak normally due to a disorder affecting the *vocal cords* or, rarely, to a psychological problem. Loss of voice may be partial or total, temporary or permanent.

Partial loss of voice, also known as *dysphonia*, may be caused by any condition that interferes with the normal working of the vocal cords.

Temporary loss of voice commonly results from straining of the muscles of the *larynx* through overuse of the voice. Temporary dysphonia also often results from inflammation of the vocal cords in *laryngitis*.

Persistent or recurrent dysphonia may be due to *polyps* on the vocal cords, thickening of the vocal cords as a result of *hypothyroidism*, or, less commonly, to interference with the nerve supply to the muscles of the larynx as a result of cancer of the larynx (see *Larynx, cancer of*), thyroid gland (see *Thyroid cancer*), or esophagus (see *Esophagus, cancer of*). In rare cases, the vocal cords themselves or the nerves supplying them may be accidentally damaged during a surgical operation performed to treat thyroid cancer, resulting in permanent dysphonia.

Total loss of the voice, known as *aphonia*, is rare and is usually of psychological origin. (See also *Hoarseness; Larynx, disorders of*.)

Volkmann's contracture

A disorder in which the wrist and fingers become permanently fixed in a bent position. Volkmann's contracture occurs as a result of ischemia (inadequate blood supply) in the forearm muscles that control the wrist and fingers.

CAUSES

Ischemia in the forearm muscles may be caused by damage to the brachial artery as a result of a displaced fracture of the humerus (see *Humerus, fracture of*) or of dislocation of the *elbow*. Ischemia may also follow any forearm injury that leads to *edema* (retention of fluid within tissues), with consequent swelling of tissues and compression of blood vessels.

SYMPTOMS

Initially, the fingers become cold, numb, and white or blue. Finger movements are weak and painful, and no pulse can be felt at the wrist. Unless treatment is started within a few hours, the characteristic wrist and finger deformity develops.

TREATMENT

Any displaced bones are first manipulated back into position under

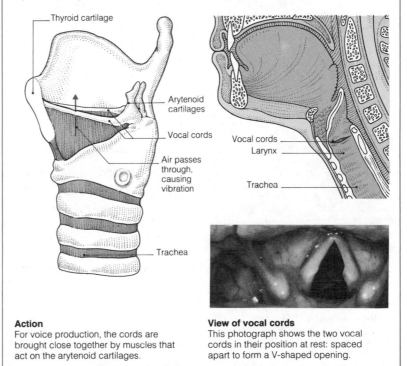

LOCATION OF THE VOCAL CORDS

The vocal cords are located at the top of the larynx (voice box). Their top edges stretch between the thyroid cartilage at the front and the arytenoid cartilages at the back. If brought close together, the cords vibrate and emit sounds as air passes between them.

Thyroid cartilage
Arytenoid cartilages
Vocal cords
Air passes through, causing vibration
Trachea
Vocal cords
Larynx
Trachea

Action
For voice production, the cords are brought close together by muscles that act on the arytenoid cartilages.

View of vocal cords
This photograph shows the two vocal cords in their position at rest: spaced apart to form a V-shaped opening.

general anesthetic. If blood flow to the affected hand fails to improve, an operation is performed in which the tissues in the forearm are cut open to relieve pressure on the underlying muscles. Blockage of the artery may be relieved by injecting a *vasodilator drug* or by cutting open the artery and removing part of the lining. Occasionally, a section of damaged artery is replaced by a graft taken from a vein.

If there is permanent deformity, *physiotherapy* may restore function to an acceptable level. In severe cases, surgery may be required to shorten the bones in the forearm, to cut away damaged muscle, and to transplant healthy muscle from another part of the forearm.

Volvulus

Twisting of a loop of *intestine* or, in rare cases, of the *stomach*. Volvulus is a serious condition that causes obstruction of the passage of intestinal contents (see *Intestine, obstruction of*) and a risk of *strangulation*. If strangulation occurs, blockage of the blood flow to

the affected area leads to potentially fatal *gangrene*. The symptoms of volvulus are severe *colic* followed by vomiting.

Volvulus may be present from birth or may be a result of *adhesions* (bands of scar tissue). It is more common in Africa and Asia than in North America or Europe, possibly because of an association between volvulus and a very high-fiber diet.

Vomiting

Involuntary forcible expulsion of stomach contents through the mouth. Vomiting is usually preceded by nausea, pallor, sweating, excessive salivation, and slowing of the heart rate.

MECHANISM

Vomiting occurs when the vomiting center in the *brain stem* is activated. Activation of the vomiting center may occur as the result of information passing directly to it from the frontal lobes of the brain, the digestive tract, or the balancing mechanism in the inner ear when these mechanisms are either damaged or disturbed. The

V

center may also be activated by the chemoreceptor trigger zone, also in the brain stem, which is itself stimulated by the presence in the blood of poisons or certain other substances.

Once activated, the vomiting center sends messages to the diaphragm (the sheet of muscle separating the chest from the abdomen), which presses sharply downward on the stomach, and to the wall of the abdomen, which presses inward. Simultaneously, the pyloric sphincter between the base of the stomach and the intestine closes and the region between the top of the stomach and the esophagus relaxes. As a result, the stomach contents are expelled upward through the esophagus. As this happens, the larynx (voice box) is tightly closed by the epiglottis (the flap of cartilage at its entrance) to prevent vomit from entering the trachea (windpipe).

CAUSES
Vomiting commonly happens after overindulgence in food or alcohol. It is also a common adverse effect of many drugs and often follows general anesthesia (see *Anesthesia, general*).

Vomiting may also result from disorders of the stomach or intestine that result in inflammation, irritation, or distention (swelling) of either organ. Such disorders include *peptic ulcer*, acute *appendicitis*, *gastroenteritis*, and *food poisoning*. Less commonly, vomiting is a symptom of intestinal obstruction due to *pyloric stenosis*, *intussusception*, or a tumor.

Vomiting may also be caused by inflammation of organs associated with the digestive tract, such as the liver (see *Hepatitis*), the pancreas (see *Pancreatitis*), and the gallbladder (see *Cholecystitis*).

Another possible cause of vomiting is raised pressure within the skull, which may be due to *encephalitis*, *hydrocephalus*, a *brain tumor*, or a *head injury*. When the rise is rapid, it causes sudden, extremely forceful vomiting, often without any prior nausea. Vomiting is a common feature of *migraine*.

Vomiting is also a common feature of disorders affecting the balancing mechanism within the inner ear, such as *Meniere's disease* and acute *labyrinthitis*, or of disturbance of the mechanism by unusual movement, such as that experienced on a boat (see *Motion sickness*).

Disorders of the *endocrine system*, such as *Addison's disease*, may cause vomiting, as do disturbances of hormone production in early pregnancy (see *Vomiting in pregnancy*).

Vomiting may be a symptom of a metabolic disorder, which may be due to poorly controlled *diabetes mellitus*.

Internal bleeding from the esophagus, stomach, or duodenum, or swallowing blood from a nosebleed, can also result in *vomiting blood*.

Vomiting sometimes occurs as a reaction of disgust to a situation or food. It may also be a symptom of a psychological or emotional problem or be part of the psychiatric disorders *anorexia nervosa* or *bulimia*.

Persistent vomiting requires investigation by a physician. Treatment depends on the underlying cause. Do not eat or drink or take any unnecessary medication during the active phase of vomiting.

Vomiting blood
Known medically as hematemesis, vomiting blood is a symptom of bleeding from within the digestive tract. It usually occurs as a result of a serious disorder of the esophagus, stomach, or duodenum.

The cause may be a tear at the lower end of the esophagus (see *Mallory-Weiss syndrome*), bleeding from *esophageal varices* (widened veins in the esophagus and upper stomach), severe erosive *gastritis* (inflammation of the stomach lining), *peptic ulcer*, or, in rare cases, *stomach cancer*. Blood can also be vomited if it is swallowed during a nosebleed.

Vomited blood may be dark red, brown, black, or resemble coffee grounds (as a result of the action of stomach acid). Depending on the extent of internal bleeding and the quantity of stomach contents, the blood may either streak the vomit or constitute a major part of it. Vomiting blood is often accompanied by *melena* (the passing of black, tarry feces).

The underlying cause of vomiting blood is investigated by *endoscopy* (inspection through a viewing instrument) of the esophagus and stomach, or by *barium X-ray examinations*. If blood loss is severe, *blood transfusion* and possibly surgery to stop the bleeding may be needed.

Vomiting in pregnancy
Nausea and vomiting in early *pregnancy* are extremely common. These symptoms are experienced by about half of all pregnant women.

The vomiting usually starts before the sixth week of pregnancy and continues until about the 12th week; in some cases it occurs throughout pregnancy. The probable cause is activation of the vomiting center in the brain due to changed hormone levels during pregnancy. Vomiting occurs most commonly in the morning, often after waking (hence its common name, morning sickness), but can occur at any time. It is sometimes precipitated by emotional stress, traveling, or food. Sufferers may find it helpful to eat small, regular meals.

In rare cases, the vomiting becomes severe and prolonged, a condition known as hyperemesis gravidarum. This can cause dehydration, nutritional deficiency, alteration in blood acidity, liver damage, and weight loss. Immediate hospital admission is required to replace lost fluids and chemicals by *intravenous infusion*, to rule out the possibility of any serious underlying disorder, and to control the vomiting (although *antiemetic drugs* are avoided if possible).

Von Recklinghausen's disease
Another name for *neurofibromatosis*.

Von Willebrand's disease
An inherited lifelong *bleeding disorder* with similarities to *hemophilia*.

CAUSES AND INCIDENCE
Von Willebrand's disease is caused by a defective *gene* and is usually inherited in an autosomal dominant pattern (see *Genetic disorders*). A person needs to inherit only one copy of the defective gene to suffer from the disease. As many as one person in 1,000 is believed to have the gene but its effects are variable. Unlike hemophilia, the disease affects equal numbers of males and females.

The gene defect leads to a reduced concentration in the blood of a substance called von Willebrand factor. This factor plays a dual role in the arrest of bleeding. It helps platelets in the blood to plug injured blood vessel walls, and it forms part of factor VIII (a substance that is vital to blood coagulation). In the absence of von Willebrand factor, neither blood coagulation nor platelet plug formation can proceed normally.

SYMPTOMS
The symptoms may include excessive bleeding from the gums and from cuts and nosebleeds. Women may suffer from *menorrhagia*. In some cases, symptoms are minimal. In the most severe forms, deep bleeding into joints and muscles may be a problem.

DIAGNOSIS
The disease is diagnosed by *blood-clotting tests*, which show a long bleeding

V

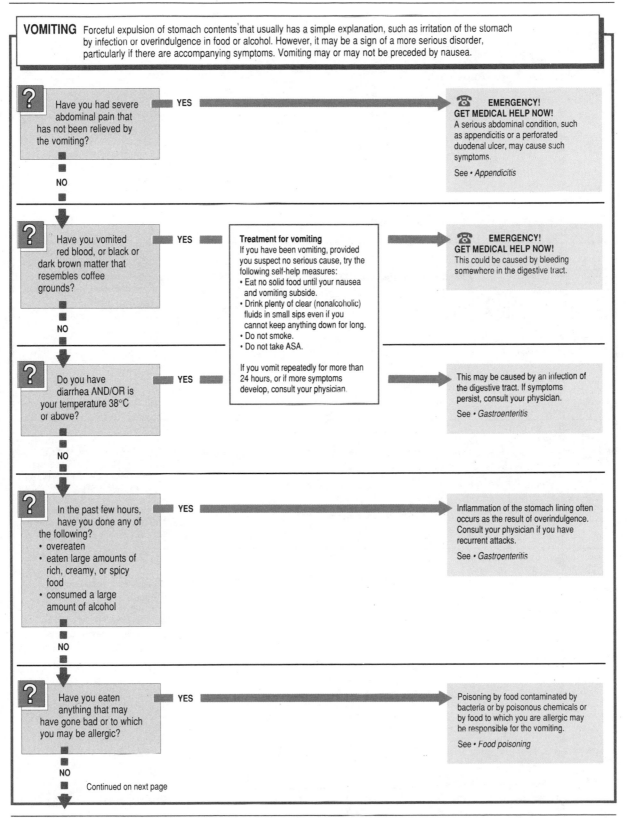

VOMITING Forceful expulsion of stomach contents that usually has a simple explanation, such as irritation of the stomach by infection or overindulgence in food or alcohol. However, it may be a sign of a more serious disorder, particularly if there are accompanying symptoms. Vomiting may or may not be preceded by nausea.

Have you had severe abdominal pain that has not been relieved by the vomiting?

YES

EMERGENCY!
GET MEDICAL HELP NOW!
A serious abdominal condition, such as appendicitis or a perforated duodenal ulcer, may cause such symptoms.

See • *Appendicitis*

NO

Have you vomited red blood, or black or dark brown matter that resembles coffee grounds?

YES

EMERGENCY!
GET MEDICAL HELP NOW!
This could be caused by bleeding somewhere in the digestive tract.

NO

Treatment for vomiting
If you have been vomiting, provided you suspect no serious cause, try the following self-help measures:
• Eat no solid food until your nausea and vomiting subside.
• Drink plenty of clear (nonalcoholic) fluids in small sips even if you cannot keep anything down for long.
• Do not smoke.
• Do not take ASA.

If you vomit repeatedly for more than 24 hours, or if more symptoms develop, consult your physician.

Do you have diarrhea AND/OR is your temperature 38°C or above?

YES

This may be caused by an infection of the digestive tract. If symptoms persist, consult your physician.

See • *Gastroenteritis*

NO

In the past few hours, have you done any of the following?
• overeaten
• eaten large amounts of rich, creamy, or spicy food
• consumed a large amount of alcohol

YES

Inflammation of the stomach lining often occurs as the result of overindulgence. Consult your physician if you have recurrent attacks.

See • *Gastroenteritis*

NO

Have you eaten anything that may have gone bad or to which you may be allergic?

YES

Poisoning by food contaminated by bacteria or by poisonous chemicals or by food to which you are allergic may be responsible for the vomiting.

See • *Food poisoning*

NO

Continued on next page

V

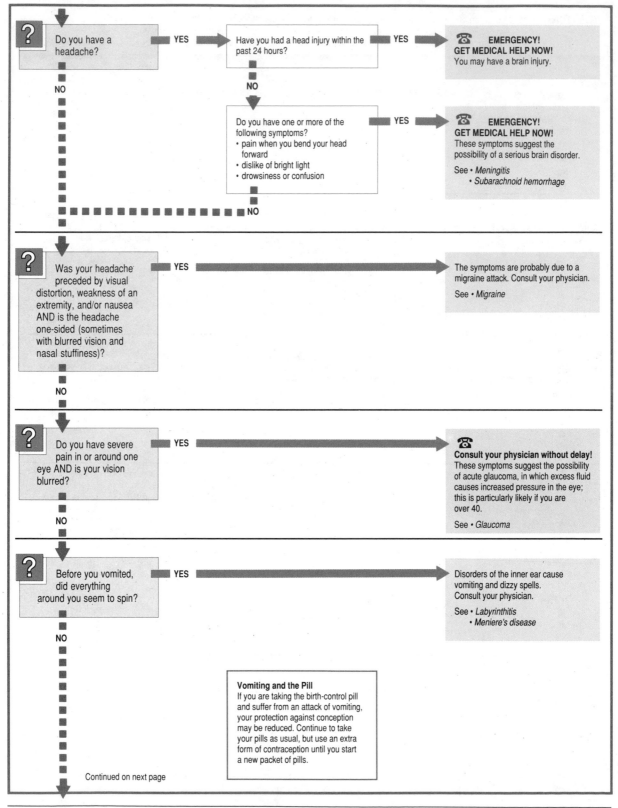

? Do you have a headache?

YES → Have you had a head injury within the past 24 hours?

YES → ☎ **EMERGENCY!**
GET MEDICAL HELP NOW!
You may have a brain injury.

NO ↓

Do you have one or more of the following symptoms?
• pain when you bend your head forward
• dislike of bright light
• drowsiness or confusion

YES → ☎ **EMERGENCY!**
GET MEDICAL HELP NOW!
These symptoms suggest the possibility of a serious brain disorder.

See • *Meningitis*
     • *Subarachnoid hemorrhage*

NO

NO

? Was your headache preceded by visual distortion, weakness of an extremity, and/or nausea AND is the headache one-sided (sometimes with blurred vision and nasal stuffiness)?

YES → The symptoms are probably due to a migraine attack. Consult your physician.

See • *Migraine*

NO

? Do you have severe pain in or around one eye AND is your vision blurred?

YES → ☎
Consult your physician without delay!
These symptoms suggest the possibility of acute glaucoma, in which excess fluid causes increased pressure in the eye; this is particularly likely if you are over 40.

See • *Glaucoma*

NO

? Before you vomited, did everything around you seem to spin?

YES → Disorders of the inner ear cause vomiting and dizzy spells. Consult your physician.

See • *Labyrinthitis*
     • *Meniere's disease*

NO

Vomiting and the Pill
If you are taking the birth-control pill and suffer from an attack of vomiting, your protection against conception may be reduced. Continue to take your pills as usual, but use an extra form of contraception until you start a new packet of pills.

Continued on next page

V

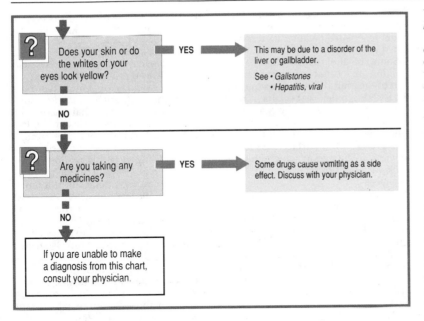

? Does your skin or do the whites of your eyes look yellow?	**YES**	This may be due to a disorder of the liver or gallbladder. See • *Gallstones* • *Hepatitis, viral*

NO

? Are you taking any medicines?	**YES**	Some drugs cause vomiting as a side effect. Discuss with your physician.

NO

If you are unable to make a diagnosis from this chart, consult your physician.

time, and by measurements that reveal reduced levels of von Willebrand factor in the blood.

TREATMENT

Bleeding episodes can be prevented or controlled by the giving of desmopressin (a substance resembling *ADH*), which raises the body's natural production of von Willebrand factor. Another possible treatment is the administration of cryoprecipitate (a preparation obtained from normal blood plasma), which is a rich source of von Willebrand factor.

Voyeurism

The repeated observation of unsuspecting people who are naked, in the act of undressing, or engaging in sexual activity. Commonly called Peeping Toms, voyeurs become sexually aroused through the act of looking and have no wish to engage in sexual activity themselves. Orgasm is achieved (usually by masturbation) while watching or remembering the witnessed events.

Vulva

The external, visible part of the female genitalia. The vulva comprises the *clitoris* and two pairs of skin folds called *labia*.

The most common symptom of a disorder affecting the vulva is *vulval itching*, known medically as pruritus vulvae. Specific vulval conditions include genital warts (see *Warts, genital*), *vulvitis, vulvovaginitis*, and cancer (see *Vulva, cancer of*).

Vulva, cancer of

A rare disorder that most commonly affects postmenopausal women. Cancer of the vulva may be preceded by vulval itching, but in many cases the first symptom is a lump or painful ulcer on the vulva.

A diagnosis of vulval cancer is made by *biopsy*. Treatment is by surgical removal of the affected area. The outlook depends on how soon the cancer is diagnosed and treated.

Vulval itching

A term for irritation of the *vulva* (the female external genitalia), also known as pruritus vulvae.

Most commonly, vulval itching is due to an allergic reaction to chemicals in deodorants, spermicides, creams, and douches. Itching is also very common after the *menopause*, when it is due to low levels of *estrogen hormone*. Vulval itching may also be caused by a vaginal discharge due to an infection of the vagina (see *Vaginitis*). A group of vulval skin changes, collectively called vulval dystrophies (see *Vulvitis*), can cause itching of the vulva.

Treatment of vulval itching may be in the form of *antibiotic drugs* or hormones, sometimes taken orally and sometimes applied in cream form.

Vulvitis

Inflammation of the *vulva*, which may have a variety of different causes.

Infections that may cause vulvitis include *candidiasis*, genital herpes (see *Herpes, genital*), and warts (see

Warts, genital). Infestations with *pubic lice* or *scabies* are other possible causes.

Vulvitis may also occur as a result of changes in the vulval skin. These changes tend to affect women after the menopause, although there is no apparent cause. They may take the form of red or white patches and/or thickened or thinned areas that may be inflamed. Formerly called a variety of names, such as kraurosis vulvae and lichen sclerosus et atrophicus, these conditions are now generally known as vulval dystrophy.

Other possible causes of vulvitis are allergic reactions to soap, cream, or detergent, excessive vaginal discharge, or urinary *incontinence*.

TREATMENT

Treatment depends on the cause. A combination of drugs applied to the vulva along with good hygiene is the usual remedy. In some cases of vulval dystrophy, a *biopsy* may be carried out to exclude the slight possibility of cancer. (See also *Vaginitis; Vulvovaginitis*.)

Vulvovaginitis

Inflammation of the *vulva* and *vagina*. Vulvovaginitis is usually due to the infections *candidiasis* or *trichomoniasis*, which cause a profuse vaginal discharge that also affects the vulva. In children, nonspecific infection may occur. (See also *Vaginitis; Vulvitis*.)

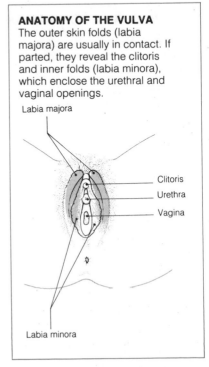

ANATOMY OF THE VULVA
The outer skin folds (labia majora) are usually in contact. If parted, they reveal the clitoris and inner folds (labia minora), which enclose the urethral and vaginal openings.

Labia majora

Clitoris

Urethra

Vagina

Labia minora

V

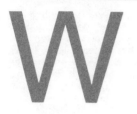

Walking

Movement of the body in one direction by lifting the feet alternately and bringing one foot into contact with the ground before the other starts to leave it. The manner of walking, known as gait, is determined by body shape, size, and posture, and often reflects the individual's personality. A normal pattern of walking is shown in the illustrated box.

Walking is controlled by nerve signals from the motor cortex (part of the *cerebrum* of the brain) and by signals from the *basal ganglia* and the *cerebellum*, located at the back of the brain. The signals are sent via the spinal cord to nerve cells and from there are carried by nerve fibers to the muscles. In response to changes in position, the cerebellum also receives information from the muscles, joints, eyes, and the balance organ in the inner ear. This information is used to adjust new signals sent to the muscles by the brain to ensure balance and coordinated movement.

Some of the nerves that control walking are located in a very primitive part of the brain. This may account for the walking reflex that occurs in newborn babies in which the legs move automatically in a walking motion when the child is held upright and the sole presses on a surface (see *Reflex, primitive*). The age at which children walk varies enormously.

DISORDERS
Abnormal gait may be caused by muscle weakness, by abnormalities of the skeleton, or by joint stiffness, causing immobility in the lower limbs or spine. Abnormal gait may also be the result of neurological disorders that affect the central control of locomotion and the balance and input of information to the nervous system from muscles and joints.

Different disorders affect walking in a variety of ways; the physician can often gain clues to the underlying cause of a disorder by observing the way in which a person walks.

MUSCULAR CAUSES Any condition that causes wasting or loss of any of the muscles connected to the legs or feet may cause abnormal walking. In *muscular dystrophy*, the legs are held wide apart and the person waddles because of weakness of the buttock muscles. In *poliomyelitis* or after severe muscle injury, weakness of individual groups of muscles may cause limping because of unbalanced muscle action.

SKELETAL CAUSES Congenital deformities of the foot, such as *talipes* (clubfoot), may prevent normal walking. In talipes equinovarus, for example, the heel cannot be brought to the ground and a characteristic limping gait results. Congenital dislocation of the hip (see *Hip, congenital dislocation of*) that has not been detected in infancy may be noticed only when the child starts to walk—the foot on the affected side is placed flat on the ground while the opposite knee is flexed. *Scoliosis* (deformity of the spine) can also result in abnormal gait.

During a stage in their growth, children often develop *knock-knee* or *bow-leg*. These conditions may produce a strange walk, but both usually disappear within several years.

Synovitis of the hip is a common cause of limping in children, most often in boys between the ages of 2 and 12 years. The limp, which is accompanied by pain of varying severity, starts suddenly and lasts for only a few days or weeks. Another common cause of limping in boys, usually between the ages of 5 and

---

THE MECHANICS OF WALKING

Many different muscles take part in the walking process. They contract in a complex, rhythmic sequence in response to programs of signals sent from the motor cortex in the brain. Feedback of information from the muscles and joints to the brain helps to ensure that the gait is smooth, steady, and coordinated.

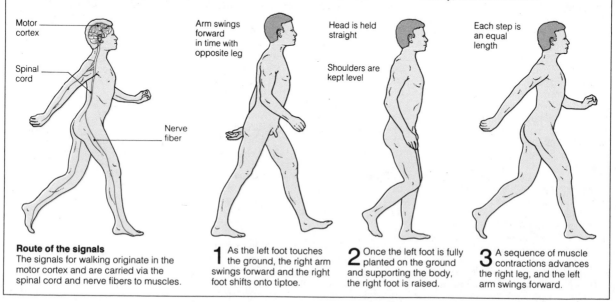

Route of the signals
The signals for walking originate in the motor cortex and are carried via the spinal cord and nerve fibers to muscles.

Motor cortex

Spinal cord

Nerve fiber

Arm swings forward in time with opposite leg

1 As the left foot touches the ground, the right arm swings forward and the right foot shifts onto tiptoe.

Head is held straight

Shoulders are kept level

2 Once the left foot is fully planted on the ground and supporting the body, the right foot is raised.

Each step is an equal length

3 A sequence of muscle contractions advances the right leg, and the left arm swings forward.

10, is *Perthes' disease*. The limp may or may not be painful. Young adolescents may develop a painful limp as a result of a slipped epiphysis (see *Femoral epiphysis, slipped*).

Other causes of limp include a painful *bone tumor* and *arthritis*.

Bone shortening may follow fracture or disease of one of the long bones of the leg (the *tibia, fibula,* or *femur*). This condition always causes an abnormal gait, usually with a dip of the body to the shortened side.

NEUROLOGICAL CAUSES Among the most common of the neurological causes is *stroke*, which commonly results in *hemiplegia* (paralysis or weakness of one side of the body). Because the affected leg is held stiffly extended, it must be swung outward and forward in walking. When both legs are affected by weakness (a condition known as paraparesis), they are held extended and pressed together at the thighs so that only short steps are possible and the toes scrape along the ground. In some people with paraparesis, the legs cross with each step, which produces a characteristic scissor movement.

In *parkinsonism* there is difficulty in starting to walk; the body is bent forward at the waist and hips, with bending at the knees and ankles. The steps are short and shuffling with the feet barely clearing the ground. As progress continues, the steps become more and more rapid, and the person may eventually fall unless assisted.

Other disorders, including severe peripheral *neuritis, multiple sclerosis,* tertiary *syphilis,* and various forms of *myelitis,* may damage the sensory nerves or the spinal cord. The damage causes loss of information to the brain about the position of the joints, resulting in a characteristic gait. The body is bent forward and the eyes are fixed on the ground, the legs are held wide apart, and the feet are carried much higher than normal and thrown forward with sudden movements. People affected in this way are critically dependent on vision for walking; the gait becomes even worse if vision is defective.

Disease of the cerebellum or of the balancing mechanisms in the inner ears, such as *Meniere's disease,* may cause severe loss of balance and instability so that the affected person walks cautiously, with the legs apart, sometimes lurching to one side as though intoxicated (see *Ataxia*). In *chorea,* the gait may be bizarre and dancelike, with sudden thrusting

WALKING AIDS

Various types of walking aids are available for different forms and degrees of disability. The choice depends on such factors as whether the person is usually healthy or chronically disabled and whether the disability affects one or both of the person's legs.

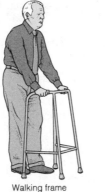
Walking frame

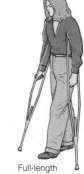
Walking stick

Elbow crutches

Full-length crutches

Walking frame and walking stick
Frames are useful for people affected by weakness on both sides, sticks for those who have one-sided weakness or pain.

Elbow and full-length crutches
Elbow crutches are often useful for people recovering from strokes, full-length crutches for those with leg injuries.

HOW TO USE CRUTCHES
Crutches are suitable only for people who are able to support their weight on at least one leg.

There are various ways of using crutches, as shown in the illustrations below.

FOUR-POINT WALKING

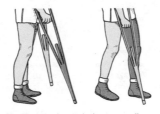

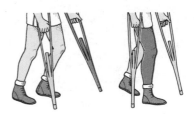

The feet and crutch tips are well separated, and one point is moved at a time. There are two possible sequences—right crutch, left foot, left crutch, right foot (above) or right then left crutch, right then left foot.

THREE-POINT WALKING

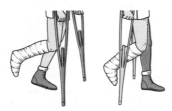

The crutches are advanced together while the person balances on one or both feet; the weight is then borne by the crutches while the feet are moved.

TWO-POINT WALKING

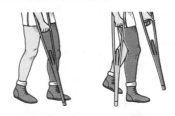

In two-point walking with crutches, the person moves the left foot and right crutch forward together, followed by the right foot and left crutch.

W

movements of the hips and twisting of the trunk and limbs. The steps are irregular and of varying length.

Walking aids

Equipment for increasing the mobility of people who have a disorder that affects *walking*. Support from a walking aid may be required by people with *arthritis* or other diseases affecting mobility, by those recovering from an injury (such as a *fracture* or *sprain*), or by those who are waiting to be fitted with a prosthesis (artificial limb) after an amputation.

WALKING FRAMES

Walking frames provide a very stable form of support and may be useful for people with severe balancing problems or for those who are affected by weakness, pain, or stiffness on both sides. However, walking frames tend to get in the way of the feet, allowing only slow progress.

Walking frames are usually made of a light, strong alloy and have four rubber-tipped legs in order to prevent sliding. They can be supplied with wheels on the front legs to make maneuvering easier.

CRUTCHES

Crutches provide greater mobility than a walking frame, but they are suitable only for people who are able to support their own weight. Crutches are often used by people who need to avoid placing weight on an injured leg or foot while healing takes place. Body weight should be taken by the hands through the crossbar of each crutch.

Full-length crutches are usually used by otherwise healthy people who have suffered a bone fracture or a severe strain or sprain of a joint, ligament, or tendon of a lower extremity. Body weight should not be taken through the armpits with full-length crutches, because this can cause radial nerve palsy.

Elbow crutches are sometimes useful because they allow gradual progression from a high degree of support to almost natural walking. People with arthritis in their upper limbs should not use elbow crutches because the additional strain on the joints may make the arthritis worse.

Crutches are usually made of a light alloy and are rubber-tipped. There are various ways of using crutches (see illustrated box on previous page).

WALKING STICKS

Walking sticks are most commonly used by people who have weakness, pain, or stiffness on one side. They are usually made of wood and have various types of handles to suit different grips. Lightweight aluminum sticks, whose length can easily be adjusted, are also available. A walking stick should have a rubber tip (or ferrule) to prevent slipping. For extra stability, walking sticks with three or four small feet on the end of the shaft can be used; such sticks are called tripods or quadropods.

A walking stick of the correct length should always be used, permitting an upright posture with the elbow slightly bent. It is generally best to walk with the stick on the strong side so that the stick is forward when the foot on the weak side comes forward. However, if one side is very weak, the stick may be held on the weak side, close to the leg, and moved with it, acting as a type of splint.

ELECTROMUSCULAR STIMULATION

Computer-controlled electromuscular stimulation of the leg muscles to facilitate walking in quadriplegics and paraplegics is being investigated.

Walking, delayed

Most children walk by around 15 months of age. Delayed walking may be suspected if the child is unable to walk unassisted by 18 months. (See *Developmental delay*.)

Warfarin

> **WARNING**
> Always check with your physician before taking any other drug with warfarin since many drugs interfere with its anticlotting action.

An *anticoagulant drug* used to treat and prevent abnormal *blood clotting*. Warfarin is used to treat *thrombosis*, to prevent *stroke* and to treat *transient ischemic attack*. It is also prescribed to prevent blood clotting after heart valve replacement (see *Heart valve surgery*), in some *heart valve* disorders, or in persistent *atrial fibrillation*.

Warfarin works by inhibiting the formation of *vitamin K*-dependent clotting factors in the liver. Because warfarin is fully effective only after several days, a faster-acting anticoagulant, such as *heparin*, is usually also prescribed during the first few days.

POSSIBLE ADVERSE EFFECTS

Warfarin may cause abnormal bleeding in different parts of the body; regular blood-clotting (prothrombin time) tests are therefore carried out to allow careful regulation of dosage. Warfarin may also cause nausea, loss of appetite, abdominal pain, and rash.

Wart

A very common, contagious, harmless growth on skin or mucous membranes. Warts affect only the topmost layer of skin. They do not have roots, seeds, or branches. The black dots that are sometimes evident are capillaries that have become clotted due to the rapid skin growth caused by the wart virus.

TYPES

Warts are caused by the human papillomavirus, HPV, of which at least 30 different types are known. These cause different types of warts at various sites, such as the hands or genitals; HPV 16, for example, causes changes in the uterine cervix.

COMMON WARTS These are firm, sharply defined, round or irregular, flesh-colored to brown growths, up to about 6 mm in diameter. They often have a rough surface.

Common warts usually appear on sites subject to injury (such as the hands, face, knees, and scalp), particularly in young children.

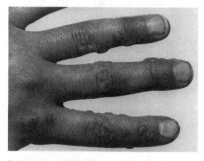

Common warts on hand
Warts often grow in crops. In time, they disappear spontaneously but they can be removed by freezing.

FLAT WARTS Flat-topped, flesh-colored lumps that occur mainly on the wrists, the backs of the hands, and the face. These warts may itch.

DIGITATE WARTS Growths, sometimes dark in color, that have fingerlike projections.

FILIFORM WARTS Long, slender growths that may occur on the eyelids, armpits, or neck.

PLANTAR WARTS These are flat warts on the sole of the foot (see *Wart, plantar*). They are flattened simply as a result of the pressure placed on them; otherwise, they are just like other warts.

GENITAL WARTS These extensive, pink, cauliflowerlike areas may occur on the genitals of men or women (see *Warts, genital*). Genital warts should be treated promptly. There is some evidence that warts infecting a woman's cervix may predispose her to cervical cancer. It is important that both sexual partners be checked and rechecked since the infection can pass back and forth between them. Condoms can sometimes prevent transmission of the causative virus. Warts in the genital region of young children may be a sign of sexual abuse.

TREATMENT
About 50 percent of warts disappear in six to 12 months without any treatment; warts other than genital and painful plantar warts are often left to disappear naturally.

Common, flat, and plantar warts can be treated in various ways. They can sometimes be destroyed by the application of a wart-removing liquid or special plaster. Several treatments may be needed and sometimes a wart returns. Warts are also commonly treated by *cryosurgery*, in which liquid nitrogen is used to freeze the wart solid. As it thaws, a blister forms, lifting the wart off. Alternatively, *electrocautery*, *curettage*, or *laser treatment* may be used.

Wart, plantar
A hard, horny, rough-surfaced area on the sole of the foot caused by a virus called a papillomavirus. Plantar warts, also commonly known as verrucas, may occur singly or in mosaic-like clusters.

Infection is usually acquired from contaminated floors in swimming pools and communal showers. Because of pressure from the weight of the body, the wart is flattened and forced into the skin of the sole, sometimes causing discomfort or pain when walking.

TREATMENT
Many plantar warts disappear without treatment, but some persist for

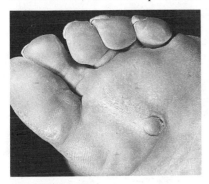

Typical plantar wart
This type of wart may need treatment—a physician may pare it down with a scalpel and apply a corrosive paint.

years or may recur. To relieve discomfort, a foam pad may be worn in the shoe. Plantar warts can be removed by *cryosurgery, electrocautery, curettage, laser treatment*, or by applying salicylic acid plasters.

Warts, genital
Soft warts that grow in and around the entrance of the vagina and the anus and on the penis. Genital warts are transmitted by sexual contact and are caused by a papillomavirus (see *Carcinogen*). There may be an interval of up to 18 months between infection and the appearance of the warts.

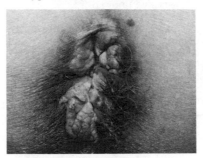

Genital warts around the anus
These growths are painless but need treatment—usually by the application of podophyllin or by surgical removal.

Genital warts have been linked with cases of cervical cancer (see *Cervix, cancer of*). A woman who has had genital warts—or whose partner has had genital warts—should have annual *cervical smear tests*.

Genital warts may be removed by surgery or by the application of *podophyllin*. However, there is a tendency for the warts to recur.

Wasp stings
See *Insect stings*.

Water
Although only a simple chemical (molecularly, two atoms of hydrogen bonded to one of oxygen—H_2O), water is essential to all forms of life. Some simple life-forms, such as certain microorganisms, can survive in a state of suspended animation for years or decades without water. However, even they require water to carry out functions such as growth and reproduction.

Water is the most common chemical in the human body (and also one of the most abundant substances on earth). Water accounts for about 99 percent of all the molecules in the body, but for a comparatively smaller

percentage of the total body weight (about 60 percent in an average man). Thus, a man weighing 70 kg contains about 42 litres of water, of which about 28 litres are within the body cells themselves and 14 litres are extracellular. Of the extracellular water, about 3 to 4 litres are in the blood plasma, lymph, and cerebrospinal fluid; the remaining 10 to 11 litres are in *tissue fluid*.

ROLE IN THE BODY
Water is essential to life because it provides the medium in which all metabolic reactions take place (see *Metabolism*). It also provides the medium for the transportation of chemical substances, such as *ions*, in the body. The blood plasma carries water to all body tissues; it also carries excess water from tissues for elimination from the body by the *liver, kidneys, lungs*, and *skin*. The interchange of water between the blood and tissue cells occurs via the tissue fluid, which bathes all the individual cells. The passage of water in the tissue fluid into and out of cells takes place by a process called *osmosis*.

WATER BALANCE
Water is taken into the body not only by drinking, but also in food. A

WATER BALANCE IN THE BODY

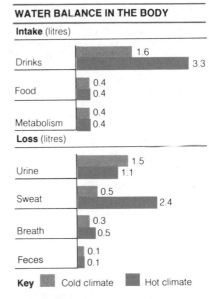

Intake (litres)

	Cold climate	Hot climate
Drinks	1.6	3.3
Food	0.4	0.4
Metabolism	0.4	0.4

Loss (litres)

	Cold climate	Hot climate
Urine	1.5	1.1
Sweat	0.5	2.4
Breath	0.3	0.5
Feces	0.1	0.1

Key ▪ Cold climate ▪ Hot climate

W

Water intake and loss
The charts show average intake of water from various sources and losses in urine, sweat, and so on. In cool climates, people tend to drink more than the amount required to satisfy thirst; the excess water is lost in urine. In hot climates, large amounts of water are lost in sweat, and an increase in fluid intake is essential to avoid dehydration.

small amount of water is actually formed within the body by the metabolism of food.

Water is lost from the body in the *urine* and *feces*, as water vapor breathed out, and by *sweating*. The amount passed out of the body in the urine depends largely on the amount of fluid drunk; the amount lost as sweat depends on physical activity and the external temperature.

The amount of water in the body must remain within relatively narrow limits for the proper functioning of metabolic processes; this balance is achieved by the activities of the kidneys, which control the balance between fluid intake and output by regulating the amount of water excreted from the body in the urine. The minimum daily urinary output necessary to remove waste products is about 0.5 litre, although most healthy adults usually produce about 1.5 litres of urine a day. The amount produced in excess of the minimum is controlled mainly by *ADH* (antidiuretic hormone), which is produced by the posterior portion of the pituitary gland and acts on the kidneys to reduce water excretion.

The body's water balance is also regulated in another way. If there is an excessive amount of any substance (such as sugar or salt) dissolved in the blood that must be excreted by the kidneys, extra water is needed to accomplish this function. This may lead to *dehydration* despite increased production of ADH, but is usually compensated for by increased water intake as a response to *thirst*.

In some disorders, such as *kidney failure* or *heart failure*, insufficient water is excreted in the urine, resulting in *edema* (abnormal accumulation of water in body tissues).

Waterborne infection

Any disease caused by infective or parasitic organisms transmitted via water. Infections can be contracted if infected water is drunk, if it contaminates food, or if individuals swim or wade in it.

DRINKING WATER
Throughout the world, contamination of water used for drinking is an important mode of transmission for various diseases, including viral *hepatitis A*, many viral and bacterial causes of *diarrhea*, *typhoid fever*, *cholera*, *amebiasis*, and some types of *worm infestation*.

Contamination results from the discharge of human or animal excretory products containing infective organ-

isms into rivers, lakes, reservoirs, or wells used as a source of water supply. The discharge may be direct or in the form of untreated sewage. It can also occur through leakage between sewage and water supply systems. This could happen, for example, in a city affected by a major earthquake.

In developed countries, the risks of waterborne infection are minimized through measures such as adequate sanitary facilities, sewage treatment and disposal, and the sterilization and testing of water before it is supplied to homes. Tap water is usually safe to drink therefore (unless there is a specific warning not to drink it).

In developing countries, sanitary facilities, sewage disposal, and water treatment may be inadequate. As a consequence, members of the population are more likely to carry the types of disease organisms spread by water. It is therefore best not to drink tap water in such countries and always to regard with suspicion any water taken directly from rivers, lakes, and wells.

AVOIDANCE OF INFECTION The accompanying table summarizes safe and suspect sources of drinking water in developed and developing countries. If safe tap water is unavailable, bottled or canned water or drinks of well-known brand names are usually safe; do not put ice made from suspect water into drinks. Rainwater is usually free of infective organisms provided it is not allowed to stand for a long period before drinking.

Water that may be infected should be sterilized before drinking. The most reliable method is to boil it for five minutes. Boiling kills any infective organisms present. If boiling is impractical, the alternative is to filter the water and then to sterilize it chem-

ically. Filtering is necessary to remove suspended particles, which can harbor disease organisms and interfere with sterilization. Various types of filters are available; some remove bacteria and other infective organisms as well as inanimate particles. The manufacturer's instructions should be followed carefully. For chemical sterilization, purifying tablets that contain chlorine or iodine are used. Water should be left for 20 to 30 minutes after treatment before being used.

Vegetables or other foods that have been washed in suspect water should not be eaten unless they have been thoroughly cooked or peeled. (See also *Food-borne infection*.)

IMMERSION IN WATER
Swimming in polluted water is liable to cause an ear infection (see *Otitis externa*). The risk can be minimized by shaking the head from side to side after swimming to clear water out of the outer ear canals.

Most swimmers inadvertently swallow some water. If the water is contaminated, there is a risk of contracting any of the diseases transmitted in polluted drinking water. It is therefore advisable to avoid swimming in rivers that may be polluted with sewage (for example, downstream of towns) or in the sea near large coastal resorts.

A form of *leptospirosis* is caused by contact with water contaminated by rat's urine; sewage workers, canal workers, and more recently, trout farmers are most at risk.

In tropical countries, swimming or wading in rivers, lakes, and ponds is very inadvisable due to the risk of contracting *schistosomiasis* (also known as bilharziasis), a serious disease caused by a fluke that can burrow through the swimmer's skin. Swim-

SAFETY OF WATER AND OTHER DRINKS FOR CONSUMPTION

	Developed countries	Developing countries
Usually safe	Tap water from public supply; rainwater; canned or bottled drinks; springwater	Canned or bottled drinks of well-known brands; rainwater
Suspect	Water direct from rivers, streams, lakes, ponds, canals, and wells	Tap water (cities); springwater
Very suspect	Obviously polluted water (i.e., cloudy in appearance or with an unpleasant smell)	Tap water (rural areas); water direct from rivers, streams, lakes, ponds, and canals

Safe and suspect water
Water from any source that falls into the suspect or very suspect categories should be sterilized. Techniques include boiling, filtering, and chemical treatment.

mer's itch is caused by a similar type of fluke, which burrows into the skin and causes an itchy rash.

OTHER MECHANISMS OF WATERBORNE INFECTION

Fish (particularly shellfish) that live in polluted water may collect infective organisms in their bodies. Such fish must be expertly cleaned and prepared and then promptly and thoroughly cooked to avoid possible hepatitis, choleralike illnesses, *food poisoning*, or a *tapeworm infestation*.

Legionnaires' disease is a type of pneumonia caused by a bacterium that can contaminate the water systems of large buildings. It is not apparently contracted from actually drinking contaminated water; the route of infection seems to occur via inhalation of water from showers or from the water used in some air-conditioning systems.

Water brash

Sudden filling of the mouth with tasteless saliva. It is not to be confused with *acid reflux* (the regurgitation of gastric juices), which has an unpleasant, sour taste. Water brash is usually accompanied by other symptoms, such as abdominal pain before a meal. It usually indicates a disorder of the upper gastrointestinal tract.

Waterhouse-Friderichsen syndrome

A serious, but very rare, condition that is caused by infection of the bloodstream by bacteria of the meningococcus group. The main feature is bleeding into the adrenal glands, which leads to acute *adrenal failure* and to *shock*. Waterhouse-Friderichsen syndrome is often associated with *meningitis*.

Watering eye

An increase in the volume of the tear film, usually producing epiphora (overflow of *tears*). Watering may be caused by excess tear production due to emotion or to conjunctival or corneal irritation. It may also be caused by an obstruction to the channel that drains tears from the eye. (See also *Lacrimal apparatus*.)

Water intoxication

A condition caused by excessive water retention in the *brain*. The principal symptoms are headaches, dizziness, nausea, confusion, and, in severe cases, seizures and unconsciousness.

Various disorders can disrupt the body's water balance, leading to accumulation of water in body tissues, including the brain. Such disorders include *kidney failure*, liver *cirrhosis*, severe *heart failure*, diseases of the *adrenal glands*, and certain lung or ovarian tumors that produce a substance with a similar action to *ADH* (antidiuretic hormone).

There is also a risk of water intoxication for about 48 hours after surgery, because the stress of an operation leads to increased ADH production. Water intoxication may also occur during induction of labor with *oxytocin*, which has an action similar to that of ADH.

Water on the brain

A nonmedical term for *hydrocephalus*.

Water on the knee

A popular term for accumulation of fluid within or around the knee joint. The most common cause is *bursitis* (inflammation of a bursa, one of the fluid-filled sacs that cover and cushion pressure points in the body). Another possible cause is fluid within the knee joint (see *Effusion, joint*).

Water tablets

See *Diuretic drugs*.

Wax bath

A type of *heat treatment* in which hot, liquid wax is applied to part of the body to relieve pain and stiffness in inflamed or injured joints. Wax baths are most commonly used to treat sufferers from *rheumatoid arthritis*.

A wax bath is given by dipping the body part into wax kept at a temperature of 50 to 55°C. The limb is held in the wax for a few seconds and then withdrawn; the wax solidifies, forming a thin layer. The procedure may be repeated until the wax coating is about 10 mm thick. The treated area is wrapped in a plastic sheet and blanket to retain the heat. After 20 minutes, the wax is peeled off and exercises are performed to encourage movement in the treated joints.

Weakness

A term used to describe a general lack of vigor or strength, which is a common symptom of a wide range of conditions, including *anemia, emotional problems*, and various disorders affecting the heart, nervous system, bones, joints, and muscles. When associated with emotional disorders (such as depression), weakness may represent a lack of desire or ambition rather than a lack of muscle strength.

More specifically, the term weakness is used to describe loss of power in certain muscle groups, which may or may not be accompanied by muscle wasting and loss of sensation. (See also *Paralysis*.)

Weaning

The gradual substitution of solid foods for milk or milk formula in an infant's diet (see *Feeding, infant*).

Webbing

A flap of skin, as between adjacent fingers or toes. Webbing is a common congenital abnormality that often runs in families and which may affect two or more digits. Although mild webbing is completely harmless, surgical correction may be performed for cosmetic reasons. In severe cases of webbing, adjacent digits may be completely fused (see *Syndactyly*). Webbing of the neck may be a feature of *Turner's syndrome*.

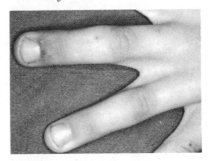

Webbing of the fingers
This curious feature is often an inherited trait, appearing in each of several generations of a family. Most cases are completely harmless and do not require treatment.

Wegener's granulomatosis

A rare disorder in which *granulomas* (nodular collections of abnormal cells) associated with areas of chronic tissue inflammation due to *vasculitis* (inflammation of the blood vessels) develop in the nasal passages, lungs, and kidneys.

CAUSES AND SYMPTOMS

The cause of the condition is unknown, but it is thought to be an *autoimmune disorder* (a disorder in which the body's natural defenses attack its own tissues).

The principal symptoms include a bloody discharge from the nose, coughing (sometimes with the production of bloodstained sputum), breathing difficulty, chest pain, and blood in the urine. There may also be loss of appetite, weight loss, weakness, fatigue, and joint pains.

W

DIAGNOSIS AND TREATMENT

A diagnosis usually requires the microscopic examination of a *biopsy* sample of abnormal tissue, which may be taken from inside the nose, from a lung, or from a kidney.

Treatment is with a combination of *immunosuppressant drugs*, such as *cyclophosphamide* or *azathioprine*, and *corticosteroid drugs* to alleviate the symptoms and, in some cases, to help bring about a *remission* in the disease process.

OUTLOOK

With prompt treatment, most people recover completely within about a year, although *kidney failure* develops in some sufferers.

Without treatment, various complications may occur, including perforation of the nasal septum, causing deformity of the nose; inflammation of the eyes; a rash, nodules, or ulcers on the skin; and damage to the heart muscle, which may be fatal.

Weight

The heaviness (mass) of an object or person. The ideal time to weigh oneself is before breakfast, either naked or wearing light clothing.

In children, weight is one of the indexes of *growth*. At all ages, body weights greater or less than expected for a person's height may have medical implications. In healthy adults, weight remains more or less stable because energy intake from the diet matches energy expenditure used to fuel all body activities (see *Metabolism*).

In the past, a variety of tables of "ideal weights" have been developed, mostly based on data from insurance companies. These are being replaced by a calculated index called the Body Mass Index (BMI).

This index is more useful than ideal body weights because it is always calculated in the same way, and has been shown to be related more closely to health than ideal weight tables. The BMI is calculated by dividing the weight in kilograms by the height in metres squared. For example, a person 1.73 m (5 feet 8 inches) tall weighing 75 kg (165 pounds) would have a BMI of 25.

Another advantage of the BMI is that the same scale can be used for both men and women. Body masses of men and women remain proportional to their heights because, although men have less fatty tissue, they have greater muscle mass. A BMI of less than 20 may be associated with

health problems, such as malnutrition or chronic disease. BMIs between 20 and 25 are considered normal for most people. BMIs between 25 and 27 may be associated with health problems in some people, but may be normal in people with heavy builds (see *Somatotype*). BMIs above 27 indicate an increasing risk of health problems.

Obesity is usually defined as a BMI over 27, but allowance should be made for body type. Another measure, waist/hip ratio, can enter into the definition of obesity.

For men, under the latest calculations, obesity is said to occur when the waist circumference is greater than the hip circumference; for women, when the waist circumference is greater than 80 percent of the hip circumference.

Weight loss

Loss of body weight occurs any time there is a decrease in the net balance of energy intake compared with energy expenditure. This decrease may be due to deliberate *weight reduction*, to a change in diet, or to a change in activity level. Weight loss is also a symptom of many disorders.

CAUSES

Many diseases disrupt the appetite and may lead to weight loss by reducing the intake of energy. *Depression* reduces the motivation to eat, *peptic ulcer* causes pain and may lead to food avoidance, and some kidney disorders cause loss of appetite due to the effect of *uremia* (raised levels of urea in the blood). In *anorexia nervosa* and *bulimia*, complex psychological factors affect the individual's eating pattern.

Energy intake may also be affected by digestive disorders. Persistent *vomiting* due to *gastroenteritis*, for example, leads to weight loss. Cancer of the esophagus (see *Esophagus, cancer of*) or *stomach cancer* causes loss of weight, as does the *malabsorption* of nutrients that occurs in certain disorders of the intestine or pancreas.

Disorders that increase the rate of metabolic activity in cells cause weight loss by increasing the expenditure of energy. These disorders include any type of *cancer*, chronic infection such as *tuberculosis*, and *hyperthyroidism* (overactivity of the thyroid gland). Untreated *diabetes mellitus* also causes weight loss, initially due to a greater fluid loss from the increase in urine

ADULT WEIGHTS

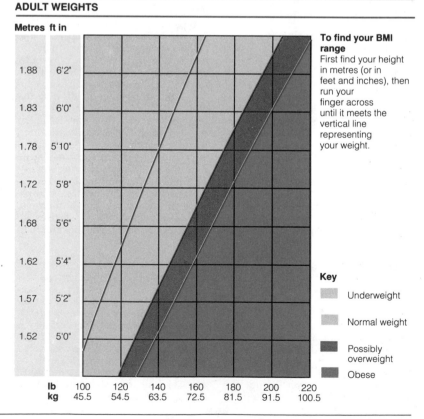

To find your BMI range
First find your height in metres (or in feet and inches), then run your finger across until it meets the vertical line representing your weight.

Metres	ft in
1.88	6'2"
1.83	6'0"
1.78	5'10"
1.72	5'8"
1.68	5'6"
1.62	5'4"
1.57	5'2"
1.52	5'0"

lb	100	120	140	160	180	200	220
kg	45.5	54.5	63.5	72.5	81.5	91.5	100.5

Key

Underweight

Normal weight

Possibly overweight

Obese

W

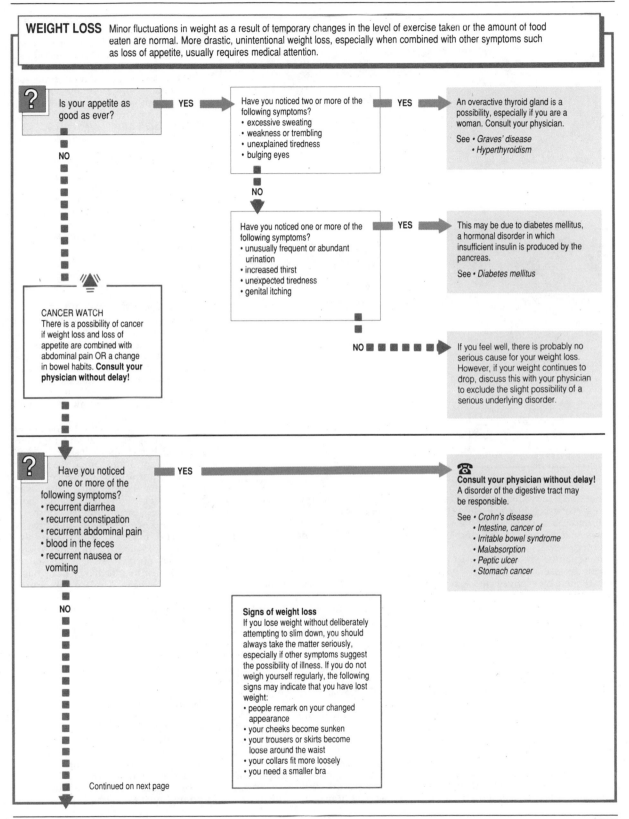

WEIGHT LOSS Minor fluctuations in weight as a result of temporary changes in the level of exercise taken or the amount of food eaten are normal. More drastic, unintentional weight loss, especially when combined with other symptoms such as loss of appetite, usually requires medical attention.

Is your appetite as good as ever?

YES →

Have you noticed two or more of the following symptoms?
• excessive sweating
• weakness or trembling
• unexplained tiredness
• bulging eyes

YES →

An overactive thyroid gland is a possibility, especially if you are a woman. Consult your physician.

See • *Graves' disease*
     • *Hyperthyroidism*

NO ↓

Have you noticed one or more of the following symptoms?
• unusually frequent or abundant urination
• increased thirst
• unexpected tiredness
• genital itching

YES →

This may be due to diabetes mellitus, a hormonal disorder in which insufficient insulin is produced by the pancreas.

See • *Diabetes mellitus*

NO →

If you feel well, there is probably no serious cause for your weight loss. However, if your weight continues to drop, discuss this with your physician to exclude the slight possibility of a serious underlying disorder.

NO ↓

CANCER WATCH
There is a possibility of cancer if weight loss and loss of appetite are combined with abdominal pain OR a change in bowel habits. **Consult your physician without delay!**

Have you noticed one or more of the following symptoms?
• recurrent diarrhea
• recurrent constipation
• recurrent abdominal pain
• blood in the feces
• recurrent nausea or vomiting

YES →

☎
Consult your physician without delay!
A disorder of the digestive tract may be responsible.

See • *Crohn's disease*
     • *Intestine, cancer of*
     • *Irritable bowel syndrome*
     • *Malabsorption*
     • *Peptic ulcer*
     • *Stomach cancer*

NO ↓

Signs of weight loss
If you lose weight without deliberately attempting to slim down, you should always take the matter seriously, especially if other symptoms suggest the possibility of illness. If you do not weigh yourself regularly, the following signs may indicate that you have lost weight:
• people remark on your changed appearance
• your cheeks become sunken
• your trousers or skirts become loose around the waist
• your collars fit more loosely
• you need a smaller bra

Continued on next page

W

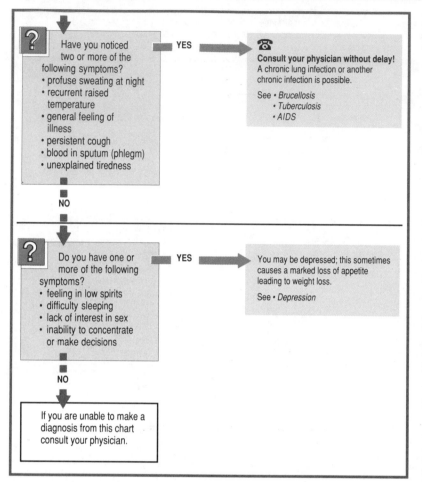

Have you noticed two or more of the following symptoms?
- profuse sweating at night
- recurrent raised temperature
- general feeling of illness
- persistent cough
- blood in sputum (phlegm)
- unexplained tiredness

YES →

☎ **Consult your physician without delay!**
A chronic lung infection or another chronic infection is possible.

See • Brucellosis
      • Tuberculosis
      • AIDS

NO ↓

Do you have one or more of the following symptoms?
- feeling in low spirits
- difficulty sleeping
- lack of interest in sex
- inability to concentrate or make decisions

YES →

You may be depressed; this sometimes causes a marked loss of appetite leading to weight loss.

See • Depression

NO ↓

If you are unable to make a diagnosis from this chart consult your physician.

output and as a result of loss of energy from glycosuria (glucose in the urine); eventually, a wasting of tissue mass causes weight loss as fat stores are broken down.

Unexplained weight loss may be a sign of disease and should always be investigated by a physician. A working diagnosis may be established by means of a careful patient history and a physical examination. Symptoms and signs usually suggest a specific cause, which permits the physician to select appropriate tests.

Weight reduction

The process of losing excess body fat. A person who is severely overweight (see *Obesity*) is more at risk of suffering from various illnesses, such as *diabetes mellitus*, *hypertension* (high blood pressure), and heart disease.

HOW IT IS DONE
The most efficient way to lose weight is to eat less. To lose weight, people should eat 500 to 1,000 calories a day

less than their energy requirements. This reduction in food consumption should result in a weight loss of between 0.5 and 1 kg per week until a desirable weight is achieved. The rate of weight loss may be faster during the first one to two weeks of a weight reduction diet because of the loss of water that occurs during this period.

Exercise forms an important part of a reducing regime, burning excess energy and improving muscle tone. Some people believe *aerobics* speed up the metabolism after exercising, but this is probably true only for regular and strenuous exercise like that undertaken by an athlete in training.

FAD DIETS
Many people who are trying to lose weight want to do so quickly; they may follow fad diets that provide severely restricted energy intakes. Although there may be a rapid weight loss in the beginning, most of these diets do not work in the long term and the lost weight usually returns.

A number of liquid diets providing about 330 calories per day have been developed. Some physicians are concerned about the effects of these liquid diets. Any diet that provides less than 1,000 calories per day should be undertaken only under medical supervision.

Weil's disease
Another name for *leptospirosis*.

Welder's eye
Acute *conjunctivitis* and *keratopathy* (corneal damage) caused by the intense *ultraviolet light* radiation that is emitted by the electric welding arc. Welder's eye results from failure to wear adequate eye protection while welding.

Wen
A name for a *sebaceous cyst*.

Werdnig-Hoffmann disease
A very rare inherited disorder of the *nervous system* that affects infants. Also known as infantile spinal muscular atrophy, Werdnig-Hoffmann disease is a type of *motor neuron disease*. Werdnig-Hoffmann disease affects the nerve cells in the spinal cord that control muscle movement. Its underlying cause is unknown.

Marked floppiness and paralysis occur during the first few months. Affected babies move less than normal babies and sometimes the mother recalls being aware of reduced fetal movements before the baby was born. Severely affected infants tend to lie still in a froglike position with the knees bent up and turned out. The muscles of the face are unaffected, with the result that the child has an alert expression that is in sharp contrast to his or her physical helplessness. The baby becomes increasingly floppy and deformed over the following few months. The muscles that control breathing and feeding are also affected, and this usually causes death before the child is 3 years old.

There is no cure for Werdnig-Hoffmann disease. Treatment aims to keep the affected infant as comfortable as possible.

Wernicke-Korsakoff syndrome
An uncommon *brain* disorder almost always due to the malnutrition·that occurs in chronic *alcohol dependence*. The disorder also occurs in other conditions, such as *cancer*.

RECOMMENDATIONS FOR WEIGHT REDUCTION

Cut down drastically on all visible fats, such as butter, margarine, cream, and cooking oils, as well as the invisible	fats present in pastries, cookies, and cakes. Choose low fat milk, cheeses, and yogurts
Choose lean cuts of meat and avoid processed meat such as salami. Broil or	roast meat without adding fat instead of frying.
Eat more boiled legumes (e.g., lentils and beans), which provide protein but	contain very little fat.
Avoid refined carbohydrates such as sugar (sucrose) as well as refined	grain products such as white flour and white rice.
Increase your consumption of unrefined carbohydrates. Eat whole wheat bread,	whole grain rice and cereals, fresh fruit, and plenty of vegetables.
Reduce your intake of alcoholic drinks,	all of which are high in calories.

Dietary recommendations for weight loss
Careful choice of the right types of food—and, in particular, the avoidance of items with a high calorie content per unit of weight (mainly fats)—makes it easier to achieve a low-calorie diet without necessarily having to reduce the bulk of the food you eat.

Wernicke-Korsakoff syndrome is caused by deficiency of thiamine (vitamin B$_1$, see *Vitamin B complex*), which affects the brain and nervous system. The thiamine deficiency is probably caused by the combined effects of poor eating habits and an inherited defect in thiamine metabolism.

The disease consists of two stages—Wernicke's encephalopathy and Korsakoff's psychosis—each characterized by particular symptoms.

Wernicke's encephalopathy usually develops suddenly and produces *nystagmus* (abnormal jerky eye movements) and other abnormal eye movements), *ataxia* (difficulty in coordinating body movements, especially walking), slowness, and confusion. Sufferers also usually have signs of *neuropathy*, such as loss of sensation, a pins and needles sensation, or impaired reflexes. The level of consciousness progressively falls and may lead to coma and death unless treated.

Korsakoff's psychosis may follow Wernicke's encephalopathy if treatment is not begun soon enough. Symptoms consist of severe *amnesia* (memory loss), apathy, and disorientation. Recent memory is affected more than distant memory, sufferers often not being able to remember what they did even a few minutes previously. Confabulation (invention of stories) may occur to make up for gaps in memory.

TREATMENT AND OUTLOOK
Wernicke's encephalopathy is a medical emergency. If the diagnosis is even suspected, high doses of intravenous thiamine are given to the patient immediately. This treatment reverses most of the symptoms, often within a few hours.

In the absence of prompt treatment, Korsakoff's psychosis is usually irreversible, leaving the sufferer permanently handicapped by memory loss and in need of continual supervision.

Wernicke's encephalopathy
See *Wernicke-Korsakoff syndrome.*

Wheelchair
A chair mounted on wheels used to provide mobility for a person unable to walk. The simplest type of wheelchair is pushed by an attendant or hand-propelled by the disabled person. Manual wheelchairs have small wheels with casters at the front and large, narrow wheels at the back; these wheelchairs are designed so that the hand-rims can be easily gripped by a disabled person.

Powered wheelchairs are battery-operated and controlled electronically by finger pressure or, if necessary, by chin pressure or breath control. The battery provides power for six to eight hours and is recharged overnight by connection to an electrical outlet. Wheels are usually small with wide, low-pressure tires. Several different types of powered chair are available. Those suitable for outdoor use are capable of negotiating raised obstructions but are usually too wide and long for convenient use indoors; conversely, indoor models are lighter and more compact but they cannot mount sidewalks.

Wheelchairs may be made of lightweight metal (such as titanium or an alloy) and are often foldable for easy storage in the trunk of a car.

Wheeze
A high-pitched, whistling sound produced in the chest during breathing; it is caused by narrowing of the airways. A wheeze may be loud enough to be heard by those in the room with the sufferer or just audible with a stethoscope. Wheeze is a feature of *asthma* and also occurs in *bronchitis, bronchiolitis,* and *pulmonary edema* (accumulation of fluid in the lungs). Inhalation of a foreign body, such as a peanut, into the airways may also cause a wheeze. (See also *Breathing difficulty.*)

Whiplash injury
An injury to the soft tissues, *ligaments,* and spinal joints of the neck caused by the neck being bent forcibly and violently forward and then backward or vice versa. Whiplash injury most commonly results from sudden acceleration or deceleration, as in a car collision. However, some degree of whiplash to the neck occurs in all forms of head injury.

Damage to the spine usually involves minor *sprain* of a neck ligament, or *subluxation* (partial dislocation) of a cervical joint. Occasionally, a ligament may rupture or there may be a fracture of a cervical vertebra (see *Spinal injury*). Characteristically, pain and stiffness in the neck are much worse 24 hours after the injury.

Treatment may include immobilization in an orthopedic *collar, analgesic drugs* (painkillers), *muscle-relaxant drugs,* and *physiotherapy.* Recovery is usually complete but it can take several weeks before full pain-free neck movement is possible.

Whipple's disease
A rare disorder that may affect many organs. Also called intestinal lipodystrophy, Whipple's disease causes a variety of symptoms and signs, including malabsorption (impaired absorption of nutrients by the small intestine), diarrhea, abdominal pain, progressive weight loss, joint pains, swollen lymph nodes, abnormal skin

W

CAUSE OF WHIPLASH INJURY

This injury to the neck section of the spine may occur when a car is subjected to a sudden violent force and the occupant's body is restrained in the seat but his or her head is not restrained.

Sudden acceleration
Here, there is a sudden force from behind (usually due to another vehicle striking the rear of the car). As the body accelerates forward, the head jerks violently backward relative to the body, stretching and bending the neck; the head then rebounds forward.

Sudden deceleration
Here, there is a sudden violent force from the front toward the back of the vehicle, due, for example, to a collision with a tree. The seat belt restrains the body, but the head continues to move forward, stretching the neck; the head then rebounds backward.

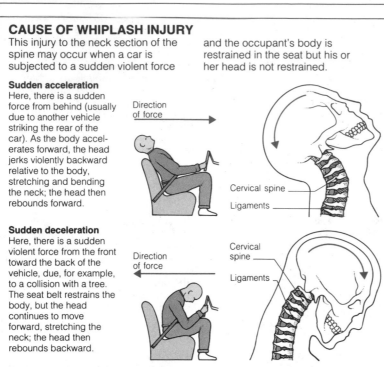

pigmentation, anemia, and fever. The condition most commonly occurs in middle-aged men.

The precise cause of Whipple's disease remains unknown but it is probably due to an unidentified bacterial infection. Diagnosis is by *jejunal biopsy* (removal of a small sample of tissue from the jejunum for microscopic analysis). Affected tissues are found to contain macrophages (a type of scavenging cell) containing rod-shaped bacteria. Treatment is with *antibiotic drugs* for at least one year. Attempts to correct nutritional deficiencies that have arisen from malabsorption are made with dietary supplements.

Whipple's operation

A type of *pancreatectomy* in which the head of the pancreas and the loop of the duodenum are surgically removed. It is named after the US surgeon Allen Whipple (1881-1963).

Whipworm infestation

The whipworm is a small, cylindrical whiplike worm, between 2.5 and 5 cm long, that can live in the human large intestine.

The life cycle of the whipworm is shown in the illustrated box, facing page. A light infestation causes no symptoms. A heavy infestation can cause abdominal pain, diarrhea, and, sometimes, *anemia*, because the worms consume a small amount of the host's blood every day. The condition is diagnosed by finding whipworm eggs during an examination of feces.

Treatment is with *anthelmintic drugs*, such as *mebendazole*, which usually bring about a satisfactory cure; heavy infestations may require more than one course of treatment.

Whitehead

A very common type of skin blemish (see *Milia*).

Whitlow

An abscess on the fingertip or, rarely, on the toe. The most common type is an acute *paronychia*. A whitlow causes the finger to swell and become extremely painful and sensitive to pressure and touch. It may be caused

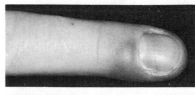

Herpetic whitlow
This extremely painful finger infection, caused by the herpes simplex virus, may be helped by applying an antiviral ointment.

by the virus that causes *herpes simplex* or by a bacterium, which usually enters the body through a cut.

A whitlow caused by bacterial infection may be treated with *antibiotic drugs* or, if the infection is severe, by incision and drainage in a minor surgical procedure under local anesthesia. A whitlow caused by the virus that causes herpes simplex is treated by the application of an *antiviral drug*; such whitlows should not be incised and drained because of the high risk of spreading the infection.

A very rare complication of an untreated whitlow is *osteomyelitis*.

Whooping cough
See *Pertussis*.

Wife beating
See *Spouse abuse*.

Will, living
See *Living will*.

Wilms' tumor
A type of *kidney cancer*, also called nephroblastoma, that occurs mainly in children.

Wilson's disease
A rare, inherited disorder in which copper accumulates in the liver and is slowly released into other parts of the body. Eventually, Wilson's disease causes severe damage to both the liver and the brain.

SYMPTOMS AND SIGNS
Symptoms, which vary in severity from person to person, usually first appear in adolescence but sometimes occur as early as 5 or as late as 50. The toxic effects of copper on the liver can cause various disorders, progressing from *hepatitis* to *cirrhosis*. Accumulation of copper in the brain causes progressive problems ranging from mild intellectual impairment to crippling rigidity, tremor, and dementia.

DIAGNOSIS AND TREATMENT
The diagnosis is based on analysis of blood and urine and a liver *biopsy* (removal of a small sample of tissue for microscopic analysis) to discover the amount of copper in the body.

Wilson's disease requires lifelong treatment with *penicillamine*, a drug that binds with copper and thus enables it to be excreted. If started soon after the onset of symptoms, penicillamine can sometimes improve liver and brain function. If the disease is discovered before toxic effects produce symptoms, the drug may be able to prevent them from developing.

W

LIFE CYCLE OF WHIPWORM

Whipworm infestation (known medically as trichuriasis) occurs worldwide and is particularly common in the tropics, but is very rare in Canada. Adult whipworms are 2.5 to 5 cm long. They may live in a person's intestine for up to 20 years. Most infestations do not cause symptoms.

The female adult worms produce eggs, which are passed in an infested person's faeces.

If personal hygiene is inadequate, worm eggs may contaminate a person's hands and, in turn, food.

The swallowed eggs hatch into larvae. Larvae develop into adults, which live in the infested person's intestines.

Worm eggs may be accidentally ingested in contaminated food, or directly from fingers.

Windpipe
A common name for the *trachea*.

Wiring of the jaws
Immobilization of the jaws by means of metal wires to allow a fracture of the jaw to heal or as part of a treatment for *obesity*. In the most commonly used method, thin, hairpin-shaped wires with a central eyelet (closed loop) are wound around pairs of adjacent teeth; about six wires are fixed to teeth in the upper and lower jawbones. Wires are then threaded through opposing pairs of upper and lower eyelets and twisted together to hold the jaws in a rigid position.

When a fracture is being treated, the jaws are kept wired in a fixed position for about six weeks. For promoting weight loss, the jaws are wired for as long as a year. In both cases, the person is unable to chew and can take

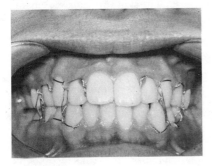

Wired jaws
Eight pairs of teeth have been wired together to immobilize the jaw while a fracture heals.

only a liquid or semiliquid diet. For weight loss purposes, the diet is calorie controlled and the patient is kept under medical supervision. This form of diet treatment, though effective while the jaws are wired, usually fails when the overweight person resumes his or her previous eating habits.

Wisdom tooth
One of the four rearmost *teeth*, also known as third molars. In most people, the wisdom teeth erupt between the ages of 17 and 21. However, in some people, one or more fail to develop or to erupt. In many cases, wisdom teeth are unable to emerge fully from the gum as a result of overcrowding (see *Impaction, dental*).

Witches' milk
A thin, white discharge from the nipple of a newborn infant. Witches' milk occurs quite commonly and is usually accompanied by enlargement of one or both of the baby's breasts. The discharge is caused by maternal hormones that entered the fetus's circulation through the placenta. Witches' milk is harmless and usually disappears within a few weeks.

Withdrawal
The process of retreating from society and from relationships with others. Withdrawal is usually indicated by aloofness, lack of interest in social activities, preoccupation with one's own concerns, and difficulty in communicating with others.

Withdrawal is also a term applied to the psychological and physical symptoms that develop on discontinuing a substance on which a person is dependent (see *Withdrawal syndrome*).

Withdrawal bleeding
Vaginal blood loss that occurs when the body's level of *estrogen hormones*, *progesterone hormone*, or *progestogen drugs* drops suddenly.

Menstruation is a form of withdrawal bleeding because it is preceded in the menstrual cycle by falling levels of both estrogen and progesterone. The withdrawal bleeding that occurs at the end of each month's supply of combined *oral contraceptive* pills mimics menstruation, but is usually shorter and lighter. Discontinuation of an estrogen-only or progestogen-only preparation also produces bleeding.

Withdrawal method
See *Coitus interruptus*.

Withdrawal syndrome
A group of unpleasant mental and physical symptoms that are experienced when a person stops using a drug on which he or she is dependent (see *Drug dependence*).

In general, any drug that causes euphoria or that relieves pain or anxiety can cause dependence and withdrawal symptoms of varying degrees. Withdrawal syndromes most commonly result from *alcohol dependence*, *tobacco smoking*, *narcotic drug* dependence, or regular use of *tranquilizers*. Other drugs that may lead to withdrawal symptoms include *amphetamine drugs*, *cocaine*, *marijuana*, and *caffeine*.

TYPES

ALCOHOL Withdrawal symptoms start six to eight hours after the last drink and may last four to seven days. Common symptoms include trembling of the hands and tongue, sweating, nausea, anxiety, and sometimes cramps and vomiting. More severe symptoms include seizures (see *Delirium tremens*), *confusion*, and *hallucinations*. Withdrawal symptoms may be frightening and frequently result in a resumption of drinking. Many alcohol-dependent people need a drink in the morning to ward off the minor withdrawal syndrome that is experienced on waking.

NARCOTIC DRUGS *Heroin* or *morphine* withdrawal syndrome starts eight to 12 hours after the last dose and may last for seven to 10 days. At first, a craving for the drug is the most promi-

W

nent feature, accompanied by restlessness, sweating, running eyes and nose, and yawning. As the syndrome progresses, a variety of other symptoms appear, including diarrhea, vomiting, abdominal cramps, dilated pupils, loss of appetite, gooseflesh (the origin of the term "cold turkey"), irritability, tremor, weakness, and depression.

Other narcotic drugs, such as *codeine* and some prescription *analgesic drugs*, cause withdrawal symptoms similar to those produced by heroin or morphine. Lower doses may produce withdrawal symptoms that are less intense and that develop more slowly.

TRANQUILIZERS Withdrawal syndrome from *barbiturate drugs* and *meprobamate* begins from 12 to 24 hours after the last dose and has many similarities to alcohol withdrawal. The first symptoms are usually tremor, anxiety, restlessness, and weakness, sometimes followed by delirium, hallucinations, and, in some cases, seizures. A period of prolonged sleep occurs just before the symptoms clear up, which is between three and eight days after onset, depending on the drug.

Withdrawal from *benzodiazepine drugs* may begin much more slowly (up to 14 days after the last dose) and can in some cases be life-threatening.

TOBACCO SMOKING Withdrawal symptoms from *nicotine* (the substance in tobacco responsible for dependence) develop gradually over 24 to 48 hours. In addition to a desperate desire to smoke, the most common symptoms are irritability, difficulty in concentrating, frustration, headaches, and restless anxiety.

OTHER DRUGS Discontinuation of an amphetamine drug or cocaine results in lethargy, extreme tiredness, and dizziness. Cocaine withdrawal may also lead to severe depression, and sometimes to other physical symptoms, such as tremor and sweating.

Chronic marijuana users have reported various withdrawal symptoms, including tremor, sweating, nausea, vomiting, diarrhea, irritability, and sleep disturbances.

Symptoms of caffeine withdrawal, consisting of tiredness, headaches, and irritability, may occur in people accustomed to drinking large quantities of tea, coffee, or caffeine-containing soft drinks.

TREATMENT
Severe withdrawal syndromes require medical treatment. Symptoms may be suppressed by giving the patient small quantities of the drug he or she had been taking. More commonly, however, a substitute drug is given, such as *methadone* for narcotic drugs or *diazepam* for alcohol. The dose of the drug is then gradually reduced. This substitution process requires careful adjustment and can be safely managed only in a medical setting.

Wobble board
A balancing board used during *physiotherapy* to improve muscle strength and coordination in the feet, ankles, and legs. A wobble board is sometimes used after an ankle sprain to reduce the risk of a recurrence.

A wobble board consists of a smooth flat surface with a rocker attached to its underside. The rocker may be cylindrical, so that the board will only rock in one plane, or it may be spherical, allowing movement in all directions.

Womb
See *Uterus.*

Word blindness
See *Alexia; Dyslexia.*

World Health Organization
The World Health Organization (WHO) was established in 1948 as an agency of the United Nations with responsibilities for international health matters and public health. Its headquarters are in Geneva, Switzerland; there are also regional offices for North America, South America, Europe, Africa, Southeast Asia, the Eastern Mediterranean, and the Western Pacific (including Australia).

The WHO has campaigned effectively against certain infectious diseases, notably smallpox (which was declared to have been eradicated throughout the world in 1980), tuberculosis, and malaria. Its other functions include sponsoring medical research programs, organizing a network of collaborating national laboratories, and providing expert advice to its 160 member states on matters such as health service organizations, family health, the use of medicinal drugs, the abuse of drugs, and mental health. The organization's current strategy is described in its campaign "Health for all by the year 2000." The plan gives specific targets for basic measures, such as the provision of piped water supplies and other basic sanitation, the universal provision of immunization of children against infectious diseases, and reductions in the use of tobacco and alcohol.

Worm infestation
Several types of worm, or their larvae, can exist as parasites of humans. These worms range in size from the microscopic to many metres in length and may live in the intestines, blood, lymphatic system, bile ducts, or organs such as the liver. Worms are more common than is realized; in many cases, they cause few or no symptoms, and a person may have an infestation for many years without realizing it. Other worms can cause chronic, sometimes severe and debilitating, illness.

There are two main classes of worm—the *roundworms*, which have long, cylindrical bodies, and the platyhelminths, which have flattened bodies. The platyhelminths are further subdivided into the cestodes (tapeworms) and trematodes (flukes).

Worm diseases found in developed countries include *pinworm infestation, ascariasis, whipworm infestation,* and *toxocariasis* (all caused by different types of roundworm); infestation with *liver flukes;* and some types of *tapeworm infestation.* However, apart from pinworm infestation, these are all very uncommon in Canada. Important types of worm diseases occurring in tropical regions include *hookworm infestation, filariasis,* and *guinea worm disease* (all caused by roundworms); and *schistosomiasis* (caused by a type of fluke).

Worms may be acquired by eating undercooked, infected meat, by contact with soil or water containing worm larvae, or by accidental ingestion of worm eggs (via the fingers or food) from soil contaminated by infected feces. (See box, facing page.)

Wound
Any damage to the skin and/or underlying tissues caused by an accident, act of violence, or surgery. Wounds in which the skin or mucous membrane is broken are called open; those in which they remain intact are termed closed.

Wounds can be divided into the following five broad categories: an incised wound; an abrasion (or graze); a *laceration;* a penetrating wound; and a contusion (see box, p. 1085).

Many penetrating wounds and some contusions are deceptive in appearance, showing little external sign of damage but involving serious internal injury. Low-velocity gunshot injuries cause tissue damage all along the path of the projectile. High-velocity gunshot injuries may also

W

DRUGS USED TO TREAT WORM INFESTATIONS

Infestation	Drug
Pinworm	Mebendazole, piperazine, pyrantel
Common roundworm (ascariasis)	Mebendazole, piperazine, pyrantel
Whipworm	Mebendazole
Hookworm	Bephenium, mebendazole, pyrantel
Strongyloidiasis	Mebendazole, thiabendazole
Toxocariasis	Diethylcarbamazine, thiabendazole
Tapeworms	Niclosamide, praziquantel
Filariasis	Diethylcarbamazine
Schistosomiasis	Praziquantel

Anthelmintic drugs
Drugs such as those listed above are the main treatment for worm infestations. Usually just one or two doses are required but sometimes longer treatment is needed. Laxatives may also be given to aid expulsion of worms living in the intestines.

damage distant structures as a result of shock waves traveling through body tissues. In stab wounds, vital organs may be perforated and major blood vessels may be severed. In contusions, the liver, spleen, or kidney may be ruptured. Many minor wounds can often be treated by first-aid measures (see *Bleeding, treatment of; Dressings;* and *Wounds first aid box*).

More extensive or deeper wounds require professional treatment, which varies according to the type of wound. If the wound contains any foreign material or dead tissue, this is removed; the wound is then cleansed with an antiseptic solution to decrease the risk of *wound infection*.

New, clean, incised wounds may be closed by *suturing* (stitching), and usually heal with minimal scarring. Lacerations may need to have the jagged skin edges cut away before they are stitched. Small incised wounds can be closed by taping the edges together. Contaminated wounds are usually left open in order to prevent abscess formation.

Deep wounds in which there is extensive tissue damage and/or a high risk of infection are usually filled with layers of sterile gauze and covered with a bandage for four or five days. If, after this time, there is no sign of infection and the skin edges can be brought together without tension, the wound may be stitched. Otherwise, the wound may be left open and allowed to heal on its own.

Penetrating wounds or contusions may require an exploratory operation on the abdominal cavity (see *Laparotomy*) or the chest cavity (see *Thoracotomy*). Damage to blood vessels, nerves, or bones often necessitates repair by specialized surgical techniques, such as *microsurgery*.

Wound infection
Any type of *wound* is susceptible to the entry of bacteria; the resultant infection can delay healing, result in disability, or cause death. Infection of a wound is indicated by redness, swelling, warmth, pain, and sometimes the presence of pus and the formation of an *abscess*. Wound infection may sometimes result in complications due to local spread of infection to adjacent organs or tissue, or to distant spread of infection via the blood.

SURGICAL WOUNDS
About 5 to 10 percent of surgical wounds become infected. Primary infection—occurring during the operation itself or while dressing the wound afterward—is a common occurrence despite routine *aseptic technique* (the creation of a germ-free environment). *Antibiotic drugs* are therefore administered as a preventive measure for 24 hours after surgery. Infection is more likely to develop in obese patients or those with reduced natural defenses against infection, such as the elderly and those suffering from cancer.

For surgery in which there is a higher-than-average risk of infection (such as an intestinal operation) or in which infection would have particularly serious consequences, the patient is given antibiotic drugs.

NONSURGICAL WOUNDS
Of nonsurgical wounds, those most likely to become infected are wounds sustained in an agricultural accident or by soldiers in battle. There is a risk of infection by the soilborne bacterium CLOSTRIDIUM TETANI, which causes the serious, sometimes fatal, infection *tetanus*, or of infection by related bacteria, such as CLOSTRIDIUM PERFRINGENS, which cause gas *gangrene*.

In dealing with any serious nonsurgical wound, the physician attempts to prevent infection by removing any foreign material or dead tissue from the wound, thoroughly cleaning it with an antiseptic solution, and giving antibiotic drugs. In addition, if there is a risk that the wound might be contaminated with soil, an anti-tetanus injection is given unless the patient has received one within the previous five years.

TREATMENT
Once infection is discovered, a sample of blood or pus is taken and the patient is given an antibiotic drug. Any abscess that occurs should be drained surgically.

Wrinkle
A furrow in the *skin*. Wrinkling is a natural feature of aging caused by a loss of skin elasticity. Wrinkles are most obvious on the face and other exposed parts of the body but occur all over the skin. Premature deep wrinkling is usually caused by overexposure to the ultraviolet rays in sunlight.

Despite the claims made for various "rejuvenating" skin preparations, no treatment can permanently restore skin elasticity. Nevertheless, treatment with some *vitamin A* derivatives is being evaluated as a means of reducing wrinkling. A *face-lift* smoothes out wrinkles by stretching the skin, but the operation's effects last only about five years.

Wrist
The joint between the *hand* and the arm. The skeleton of the wrist consists of eight bones (known collectively as the carpus) arranged in two rows—the scaphoid, lunate, triquetral, and pisiform bones, which articulate with the radius and ulna (bones of the forearm); and the trapezium, trapezoid, capitate, and hamate, which are

FIRST AID: WOUNDS

DO NOT
- attempt to remove the object from the wound.

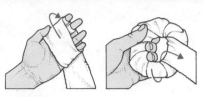

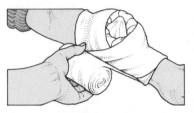

FOREIGN BODY

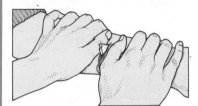

1 Apply direct pressure above and below the object. Lay the victim down and raise and support the limb.

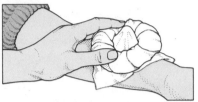

2 Lightly drape a piece of gauze over object and wound and place a ring pad over it. Or use cotton wool to build up a pad around the wound. It should be high enough to prevent pressure on the object.

Ring pad

1 Place a narrow bandage across one hand. Wind one end once or twice around your fingers to make a loop.

2 Bring the other end through the loop, wind it repeatedly around the loop, pulling it tight each time.

3 Secure with a roller bandage. Make two straight turns, overlapping the pad, on either side. Then continue with diagonal turns until the pad is held firmly. Take the victim to hospital.

DEEPER WOUNDS

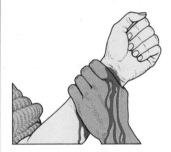

1 Examine the wound for foreign bodies; if there is none, apply direct pressure to control bleeding by pressing on the wound with the fingers or palm. Lay the victim down and raise the injured part higher than the chest and heart.

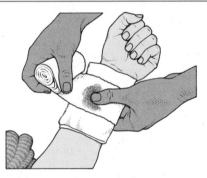

2 Put a sterile, unmedicated dressing over the wound so that it extends well beyond the edges of the wound. Secure the dressing firmly with a bandage.

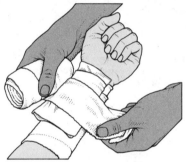

3 If the blood seeps through, do not remove the bandage, but put more dressing and another bandage on top. Watch for *shock* and seek medical help.

CUTS AND SCRAPES

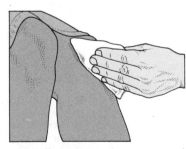

1 Rinse the wound under cold, running water. Then, using cotton wool, gauze or antiseptic wipes, clean around the wound. Work outward, using a clean pad for each stroke.

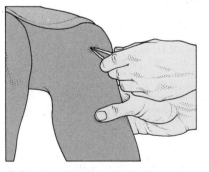

2 Remove any loose foreign bodies, such as metal, glass, or gravel, with the gauze or cotton wool, or with tweezers.

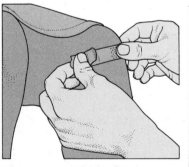

3 Dry the surrounding area and dress the wound. If it is small, use an adhesive dressing. Otherwise, make a dressing with a piece of gauze and cotton wool. Secure with a bandage.

W

TYPES OF WOUNDS

Wounds can be divided into incised wounds, in which the skin is cleanly cut (e.g., surgical incisions); abrasions or grazes, in which surface tissue is scraped away; lacerations, in which the skin is torn (e.g., animal *bites*); contusions, in which the underlying tissues are damaged by a blunt instrument; and penetrating wounds (e.g., stab or gunshot wounds).

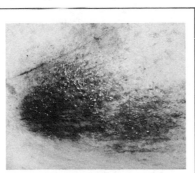

Abrasion on the arm
Abrasions usually result from sliding falls and may contain dirt. They should be carefully cleaned and dressed.

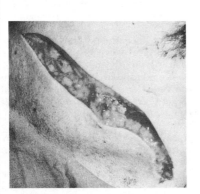

Knife wound down the side of the face
This is a deep incised wound, cleanly cut, and likely to heal with minimal scarring once its edges have been stitched.

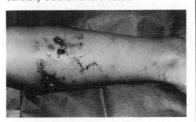

Dog-bite lacerations on the arm
Such wounds are usually cleaned and then left open to heal. Antibiotic and antitetanus treatment may be given.

connected to the bones of the palm. The bones of the carpus articulate with each other. Many tendons, which connect the forearm muscles to the fingers and thumb, run across the wrist. The extensor tendons, which straighten the fingers, are on the back of the wrist; the flexor tendons, which bend the fingers, are on the front.

These tendons pass under ligaments to prevent them from springing away from the wrist. The gap between the ligaments and tendons at the front of the wrist is known as the carpal tunnel.

Also passing across the wrist are the arteries and nerves supplying the muscles, bones, and skin of the hand.

STRUCTURE OF THE WRIST

The wrist is a complex joint that allows the hand to be bent forward and backward relative to the arm (through an angle of almost 180 degrees) and also moved side to side (through about 70 degrees).

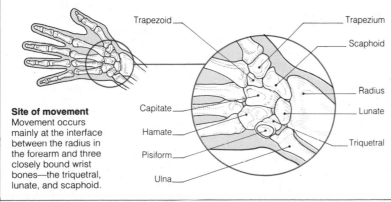

Site of movement
Movement occurs mainly at the interface between the radius in the forearm and three closely bound wrist bones—the triquetral, lunate, and scaphoid.

Trapezoid
Trapezium
Scaphoid
Radius
Lunate
Triquetral
Capitate
Hamate
Pisiform
Ulna

DISORDERS

Wrist injuries may lead to serious disability by limiting hand movement. This is especially likely to occur with fractures of the scaphoid bone, which often fail to heal, and with injuries in which the tendons or nerves in the wrist are severed.

A common wrist injury in adults is *Colles' fracture*, in which the lower end of the radius is fractured and the wrist and hand are displaced backward. In young children, similar displacement results from a fracture through the epiphysis (growing end) of the radius. A *sprain* can affect ligaments at the wrist joint.

Pressure on the median nerve as it passes through the carpal tunnel causes numbness, tingling, and pain in the thumb, index, and middle fingers (see *Carpal tunnel syndrome*). Damage to the radial nerve, which may be caused by fracture of the humerus (upper-arm bone), results in *wristdrop*. Other conditions that may affect the wrist include *tenosynovitis* (inflammation of the inner lining of a tendon sheath) and *osteoarthritis* (degenerative joint disease).

Wristdrop

Inability to straighten the *wrist*, so that the back of the hand cannot be brought into line with the back of the forearm. This causes weakness of grip because the hand muscles can function efficiently only when the wrist is held straight.

Wristdrop is caused by damage to the *radial nerve*, usually at a point where it passes beneath the armpit or where it winds around the *humerus* (upper-arm bone). The radial nerve may be damaged by prolonged pressure in the armpit (see *Crutch palsy*) or by a fracture of the humerus (see *Humerus, fracture of*).

Treatment involves holding the wrist straight. In some cases, this may be achieved by means of a simple splint. However, if damage to the radial nerve is permanent, the usual treatment is *arthrodesis* (surgical fusion) of the wrist bones in a straight position.

Writer's cramp

See *Cramp, writer's*.

Wry neck

Abnormal tilting and twisting of the head. Wry neck may be due to various causes, including injury to, or spasm of, the muscles on one side of the neck (see *Torticollis*).

W

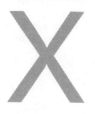

X

Xanthelasma

Yellowish deposits of fatty substance in the eyelids which are sometimes associated with *hyperlipidemias* (a group of disorders in which there are raised levels of fats in the blood). Xanthelasmas may be removed by a simple surgical procedure performed under a local anesthetic. (See also *Xanthomatosis*.)

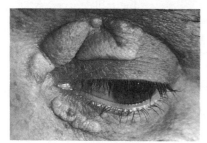

Appearance of xanthelasma
These fatty deposits around the eyes are common in elderly people but are usually of no more than cosmetic importance.

Xanthoma

A yellowish deposit of fatty material in the skin, often on the elbow or buttock. Xanthomas may be associated with *hyperlipidemias* (a group of disorders in which there are raised levels of fats in the blood). (See *Xanthomatosis*.)

Xanthomatosis

A condition in which deposits of yellowish, fatty material occur in various parts of the body, particularly in the skin, internal organs, corneas, brain, and tendons. The deposits may occur only in the eyelids, a condition known as *xanthelasma*. The most important feature of xanthomatosis is the tendency for fatty material to be deposited in the linings of blood vessels, leading to generalized *atherosclerosis*. Xanthomatosis is often associated with *hyperlipidemias* (a group of disorders in which there are raised levels of fats in the blood).

Treatment aims to lower the levels of fats in the blood. This is achieved by means of a diet that is low in *cholesterol* and high in polyunsaturated fat, and by treatment with drugs.

X chromosome

A *sex chromosome*. Every normal female body cell has a pair of X chromosomes; every normal male body cell has one X chromosome and one Y chromosome, whereas each sperm carries either an X or a Y chromosome. Abnormal genes on X chromosomes cause *X-linked disorders*.

Xeroderma pigmentosum

A rare, inherited skin disease. The skin is normal at birth, but *photosensitivity* (extreme sensitivity to sunlight) causes it to become dry, wrinkled, freckled, and prematurely aged by about the age of 5. Benign skin tumors and *skin cancers* also develop. Xeroderma pigmentosum is often accompanied by eye problems, such as *photophobia* and *conjunctivitis*.

Treatment consists of protecting the skin from sunlight by wearing protective clothing and using *sunscreens*. Skin cancers are usually treated surgically or with *anticancer drugs*.

Xerophthalmia

An *eye* disorder in which *vitamin A* deficiency causes the conjunctiva and cornea to become abnormally dry. Without treatment, xerophthalmia may progress to *keratomalacia*, a condition in which there is severe damage to the cornea.

Xerostomia

Abnormal dryness of the mouth (see *Mouth, dry*).

Xiphisternum

An alternative name for the xiphoid process, the small, leaf-shaped projection that forms the lowest of the three parts of the *sternum* (breastbone).

X-linked disorders

Sex-linked *genetic disorders* in which the abnormal gene or genes—the causative factors—are located on the X chromosome, and in which almost all those affected are males; *color vision deficiency* and *hemophilia* are examples. (See also *Fragile X syndrome*.)

X rays

A form of invisible electromagnetic energy of short wavelength that is produced when high-speed electrons strike a heavy metal. X rays were discovered in 1895 by Wilhelm Conrad Roentgen. From the time of their discovery, X rays have been used to an increasingly important degree in medicine both for diagnosis and for treatment. (See box, p. 1008.)

WHY THEY ARE USED
X rays can be used to produce images of bones, organs, and internal tissues. Low doses of X rays are passed through the tissues and cast images—essentially shadows—onto film or onto a fluorescent screen. The X ray image, also known as a radiograph or roentgenogram, shows any structural changes in the area that is being examined.

X rays have the potential to damage living cells, especially those that are dividing rapidly. Because cancer cells divide rapidly, high doses of radiation are used (along with other forms of radiant energy) for treating cancer (see *Radiation therapy*).

HOW THEY WORK
X rays are produced artificially by bombarding a heavy metal tungsten target with electrons in a device known as an X-ray tube (or Coolidge tube). The X rays that are emitted travel in straight lines and radiate outward in all directions from a point on the target. In an X-ray machine, the X-ray tube is surrounded by lead casing, except for a small aperture through which the X-ray beam emerges.

Each of the body's tissues absorbs X rays in a predictable way. Bones, which are dense and contain calcium, absorb X rays well. In contrast soft tissues—skin, fat, blood, and muscle, for example—absorb X rays to a lesser extent. Thus, when an arm, for instance, is placed in the path of an X-ray beam, the X rays pass readily through the soft tissues but penetrate the bones much less easily. As a result, the arm casts a shadow onto film or onto a fluorescent screen, with the bone presenting a clear white image, and the surrounding soft tissues appearing as dark gray.

THE X-RAY EXAMINATION
When a patient arrives for an X-ray examination, the X-ray technician explains the procedure. The patient undresses to expose the area to be X-rayed and must remove any objects that might produce an image on the film, such as jewelry, hair clips, dentures, or a wig.

The position of the patient when the X ray is taken is carefully chosen to provide the clearest view of the part under examination, although this position may require modification if the patient is very ill or in severe pain.

X-RAY EXAMINATION

Probably the best known of all imaging techniques, X rays are also one of the most useful, particularly for imaging the skeleton, the chest, and body conduits such as the blood vessels and digestive tract (after a radiopaque material has been introduced into them). Modern X-ray equipment is designed to produce high-quality images at the lowest possible radiation dose to the patient.

Procedure

The technician makes sure the patient is correctly positioned, checks that the X-ray tube is ready, and then goes to a control panel behind a protective screen and presses a button to take the X ray. The technician can see and talk to the patient from behind the screen.

X-ray machine

X-ray technician

Area of coverage of X rays. This is easily adjusted

Patient

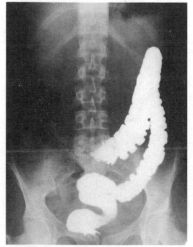

Barium enema
This X ray shows the lower part of the large intestine outlined by a radiopaque contrast medium containing a barium compound.

The X-ray film is usually contained in a flat cassette; the patient lies, sits, or stands with the region to be examined in contact with the cassette. To avoid getting a blurred image, the patient must keep still while the X ray is taken. Every effort is made to keep the patient comfortable and relaxed and to use the shortest possible exposure time—usually just a fraction of a second. If necessary, the region under examination can be supported or immobilized.

When the patient is in the correct position, the film is in place, and the X-ray tube is ready, the technician leaves the room for a few moments and presses the exposure button on the control panel to take the X ray.

Once the X-ray film has been developed, it is interpreted by a radiologist. Some disorders, such as fractures, are immediately recognizable; others, such as some tumors, may take more time to assess.

SPECIAL X-RAY TECHNIQUES

Hollow or fluid-filled parts of the body often do not show up well on X-ray film unless they first have a contrast medium (a substance that is opaque to X rays) introduced into them. Contrast-medium X-ray techniques are used to look at the gallbladder (see *Cholecystography*), the bile ducts (see *Cholangiography*), the urinary tract (see *Urography*), the gastrointestinal tract (see *Barium X-ray examinations*), the blood vessels (see *Angiography; Venography*), the spinal cord (see *Myelography*), and the spaces within joints (see *Arthrography*).

X rays can be used to obtain an image of a "slice" through an organ or part of the body by using a technique known as *tomography*. More detailed and accurate images of a body slice are produced by combining tomography with the capabilities of a computer (see *CT scanning*).

X-RAY SAFETY

Large doses of radiation can be extremely harmful and even small doses carry some risk (see *Radiation hazards*). Modern X-ray film, equipment, and techniques are designed specifically to produce high-quality images with the lowest possible radiation exposure to the patient. The possible hazard of genetic damage can be minimized by using a lead shield to protect the patient's reproductive organs from the X rays. X-ray exam-inations are generally avoided if there is any possibility of pregnancy. X-ray technicians and radiologists wear a *film badge* to monitor their exposure to radiation. (See also *Imaging techniques; Radiography; Radiology*.)

X rays, dental

See *Dental X rays*.

X-ray technician

A person who prepares patients for *X-ray* examinations, takes and develops X-ray pictures, and assists with other imaging techniques.

Xylometazoline

A *decongestant drug* used to relieve nasal congestion caused by a common *cold, sinusitis,* or hay fever (see *Rhinitis, allergic*). Available in nose drops or nasal sprays, xylometazoline works by narrowing the small blood vessels in the lining of the nose. It is also used as an ingredient of eye drops in the treatment of allergic *conjunctivitis*.

Excessive use of xylometazoline may cause headache, palpitations, or drowsiness. Long-term use may cause nasal congestion to become worse when the drug is stopped.

USING X RAYS TO LOOK AT THE BODY

X rays are perhaps the most widely used method of imaging the body. When passed through body tissues onto photographic film, X rays cast images of internal structures, allowing alterations in silhouette to be seen. Soft tissues do not show up as well as bone on X rays, but, by using a contrast medium, they too can be visualized. New computer techniques produce even clearer, more detailed images.

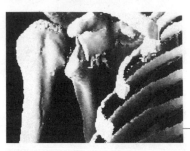

3-D CT scan
A computer can transform X-ray images of body slices into a three-dimensional image of part of the body. This scan shows a badly damaged shoulder-blade.

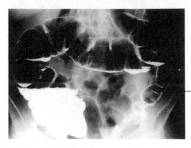

Barium X ray
Introducing barium, which is opaque to X rays, into the large intestine allows it to be visualized.

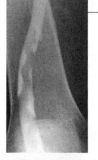

Venography
This technique for examining veins involves injecting them with a contrast medium before they are X-rayed. The femoral vein shown here (in the foreground) is partly blocked by blood clots.

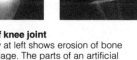

X rays of knee joint
The X ray at left shows erosion of bone and cartilage. The parts of an artificial knee are seen in the X ray at right.

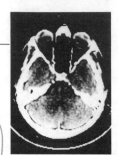

CT scan
Combined use of a computer and X rays produces cross-sectional images. In this brain scan, the eyes and nose are seen at the top; the central light area represents the brain stem.

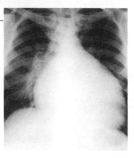

Chest X ray
This heart appears enlarged due to accumulation of fluid around it.

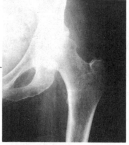

X ray of hip joint
This X ray of an osteo-arthritic hip shows almost complete degeneration of the cartilage.

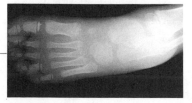

X ray of foot
All the bones can be clearly seen in this X ray of a 4-year-old's foot.

X

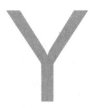

Y

Yawning

An involuntary act, usually associated with drowsiness or boredom, in which the mouth is opened wide and a slow, deep breath taken through it. Yawning is accompanied by a momentary increase in the heart rate, slight narrowing of some tiny blood vessels, and, in many cases, watering of the eyes (possibly because of pressure on the tear glands as a result of the facial movements).

The purpose of yawning is unknown, but one theory suggests it is triggered by raised levels of carbon dioxide in the blood; thus, its purpose could be to reduce the level of carbon dioxide and to increase the level of oxygen in the blood.

Yaws

A disease found throughout poorer subtropical and tropical areas of the world that is caused by a spirochete (spiral-shaped bacterium) very similar to that which causes syphilis. Yaws is not, however, a sexually transmitted disease. The infection is almost always acquired in childhood.

Three or four weeks after infection, a single, highly infectious, itchy, raspberrylike growth appears at the site of infection. Scratching spreads the infection and leads to the development of more growths elsewhere on the skin. Without treatment, the

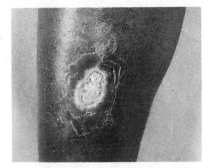

Yaws ulcer on leg
Yaws is an infection that mainly affects the skin and bones. Ulceration and tissue destruction may occur in advanced cases.

growths heal slowly over the course of about six months. Recurrence of the growths is common.

Yaws can be cured by a single large dose of a *penicillin drug*. In about 10 percent of untreated cases, widespread tissue loss eventually occurs. This may lead to gross destruction of the skin, bones, and joints of the legs, nose, palate, and upper jaw.

Y chromosome

A *sex chromosome* that is present in every normal male body cell, paired with an X chromosome.

Yeasts

Types of *fungi*. Certain yeasts can cause infections of the skin or mucous membranes. The most important disease-causing yeast is CANDIDA ALBICANS, which causes *candidiasis*.

Yellow fever

 An infectious disease of short duration and variable severity caused by a virus transmitted by mosquitoes. In severe cases, the skin of the sufferer becomes yellow from *jaundice*—hence the name yellow fever.

CAUSES
Today, yellow fever is contracted only in Central America, parts of South America, and a large area of Africa. In forest areas, various species of mosquitoes may spread the infection from monkeys to humans. In urban areas, it is transmitted between humans by AEDES AEGYPTI mosquitoes.

PREVENTION
Eradication of the causative mosquito from populated areas has greatly reduced the incidence of yellow fever. Vaccination confers long-lasting immunity and should always be obtained before travel to affected areas. A vaccination certificate is required for entry to many countries where the disease is prevalent or when traveling from these areas.

A single injection of the vaccine gives protection for at least 10 years. Children under 1 year old should not be vaccinated. Reactions to the vaccine are rare and usually trivial.

SYMPTOMS AND SIGNS
Three to six days after infection, there is sudden onset of fever and headache, often with nausea and nosebleeds. Characteristically, despite the high fever, the heart rate is very slow. In many cases, the patient recovers in about three days.

In more serious cases, the fever is higher and there is severe headache

and pain in the neck, back, and legs. Damage may occur rapidly to the liver and kidneys, causing jaundice and *kidney failure*. This may be followed by a stage of severe agitation and delirium, leading to coma and death.

DIAGNOSIS AND TREATMENT
During epidemics, diagnosis is easy. A diagnosis can be confirmed by using blood tests to isolate the causative virus or to find *antibodies* to the virus.

No drug is effective against the yellow fever virus; treatment is directed at maintaining the blood volume. Transfusion of fluids is often necessary. In mild and moderate cases, the outlook is excellent and complications are few. Relapses do not occur and one attack confers lifelong immunity. Overall, however, about 10 percent of victims die.

Yin and yang

Fundamental concepts in traditional *Chinese medicine* and philosophy. Yang embodies positive, active, "male" qualities and thus complements yin, which embodies negative, passive, "female" qualities. The concepts of yin and yang are also central to the theoretical basis of *macrobiotics*.

Yoga

A system of Hindu philosophy and physical discipline. The main form of yoga practiced in the West is hatha-yoga, in which the follower adopts a series of poses, known as asanas, and uses a special breathing technique. This maintains flexibility of the body, teaches physical and mental control, and is a useful *relaxation technique*.

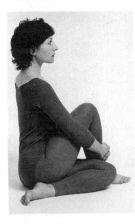

Yoga pose
This photograph shows a stage of the full twist asana, which is excellent for promoting flexibility.

Y

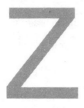

Zidovudine

An *antiviral drug*, formerly known as azidothymidine or AZT. Zidovudine was approved for use in the treatment of *AIDS* in 1987.

WHY IT IS USED

Zidovudine is used to treat serious AIDS-related conditions, such as *pneumocystis pneumonia* and infections of the brain and nervous system caused by *HIV* (the AIDS virus). Zidovudine does not cure these conditions but may improve symptoms or prolong remissions. For example, it may reduce lymph node swelling and promote weight gain. Although zidovudine slows the progress of AIDS, relapse commonly occurs after several months of treatment.

Zidovudine has also proved effective in the treatment of people infected with HIV who have not developed symptoms. In research trials on people infected with HIV, the proportion of people who developed AIDS or AIDS-related complex was lower among those treated with zidovudine than among those who were not given the drug.

HOW IT WORKS

Zidovudine blocks the action of the *enzyme* that stimulates the AIDS virus to grow and multiply. Clinical trials have shown that the resultant reduction in virus activity leads to an increase in the production and number of T-helper lymphocytes (a type of white blood cell). This in turn improves the efficiency of the *immune system*, making the occurrence of *opportunistic infections*, such as candidiasis (thrush), less likely. Zidovudine does not appear to stop the growth of other viruses.

POSSIBLE ADVERSE EFFECTS

By reducing the number of red blood cells produced, zidovudine often causes severe *anemia*, requiring blood transfusion. For this reason, regular blood tests are performed and the drug is withdrawn if the blood count is dangerously low. Too high a dose of zidovudine may cause restlessness, insomnia, and fever.

Zidovudine also impairs the absorption and thus the effectiveness of *trimethoprim* and sulfamethoxazole, the antibiotic drugs used to treat pneumonia in people who have AIDS.

Zinc

A *trace element* that is essential for normal growth, development of the reproductive organs, normal functioning of the prostate gland, healing of wounds, and the manufacture of proteins and nucleic acids (the genetic material of cells). Zinc also controls the activities of more than 100 enzymes and is involved in the functioning of the hormone insulin.

Small amounts of the element are present in a wide variety of foods; particularly rich sources include lean meat, whole wheat breads, whole grain cereals, dried beans, and seafoods.

DEFICIENCY

Zinc deficiency is rare. Most cases occur in people who are generally malnourished. Deficiency may also be caused by any disorder that causes *malabsorption*, by *acrodermatitis enteropathica* (a disorder of zinc absorption), or by increased zinc requirements due to cell damage (for example, as a result of a burn or in *sickle cell anemia*). Symptoms of deficiency include impairment of taste and loss of appetite; in severe cases, there may also be hair loss and inflammation of the skin, mouth, tongue, and eyelids. In children, zinc deficiency impairs physical growth and delays sexual development.

EXCESS

Prolonged, excessive intake of zinc (usually through supplements) may interfere with the intestinal absorption of *iron* and *copper*, leading to a deficiency of these minerals and resultant symptoms of nausea, vomiting, fever, headache, tiredness, and abdominal pain.

MEDICAL USES

Zinc compounds, such as *zinc oxide*, are included in many preparations for treating skin and scalp disorders.

Zinc oxide

An ingredient of many skin preparations that has a mild *astringent* (drying) action and a soothing effect. Zinc oxide is used to treat painful, itchy, or moist skin conditions (such as eczema, bedsores, and diaper rash)

A SELECTION OF ZOONOSES (DISEASES CAUGHT FROM ANIMALS)

Animal	Disease	Animal	Disease
Bat	Histoplasmosis Rabies	Horse	Glanders
Cat	Toxoplasmosis Cat-scratch fever Fungal infections	Pig	Trichinosis Pork tapeworm Brucellosis
Cow	Brucellosis Beef tapeworm Q fever Cowpox	Rabbit	Tularemia
Dog	Rabies Toxocariasis Mite infestations Fungal infections	Rat	Leptospirosis Rat-bite fever
Chicken	Salmonella infection Psittacosis	Sheep	Liver fluke Anthrax

Relative importance
With the exception of fungal infections and mites caught from pets, all the diseases listed above are rare in Canada. Several of the diseases may be caught from animals that are used as food (pigs and cows, for example) but such diseases are prevalent mainly in countries in which food hygiene regulations and/or practices are lax. Rabies, probably the most serious zoonosis, can be caught from various animals in addition to those listed above—foxes, skunks, and mongeese, for example.

and to ease the pain caused by hemorrhoids and insect bites or stings. It also blocks the ultraviolet rays of the sun (see *Sunscreens*).

Zinc oxide is also used to thicken lotions and creams, making them easier to apply.

Zollinger-Ellison syndrome
A rare condition characterized by severe and recurrent *peptic ulcers* in the stomach, duodenum, and upper small intestine. Zollinger-Ellison syndrome is caused by one or several tumors, usually found in the *pancreas*, that secrete the hormone gastrin. This hormone stimulates the stomach and duodenum to produce large quantities of acid, which leads to ulceration. The high levels of acid in the digestive tract also cause diarrhea and steatorrhea (abnormally fatty feces) in almost half the people with Zollinger-Ellison syndrome.

The condition often goes unrecognized until surgery for the peptic ulcers is rapidly followed by a recurrence of the ulceration. Once suspicion is aroused, the physician performs blood tests; high levels of gastrin are usually sufficient to confirm the diagnosis.

The tumors are most often cancerous, although of a slow-growing type. If possible, the tumor or tumors are removed surgically; otherwise, total *gastrectomy* (surgical removal of the stomach) is necessary.

Zoonosis
Any infectious or parasitic disease of animals that can be transmitted to humans. Many disease organisms can infect only humans or particular animals, but zoonotic organisms are more flexible and can adapt themselves to many different species.

Zoonoses are usually caught from animals closely associated with humans, either as pets (such as dogs, cats, or parrots), food sources (such as pigs or cattle), or scavenging parasites (such as rats). Examples include *toxocariasis* (from dogs), *cat-scratch fever* and some *fungal infections* (from cats), *psittacosis* (from parrots or other birds), *brucellosis* (from cows, goats, or pigs), *trichinosis* (from pigs), and *leptospirosis* (from rats). *Rabies* can infect virtually any mammal, but dog bites are a common cause of human infection worldwide. (See the box on the previous page.)

Other zoonoses are transmitted from animals less obviously associated with humans, usually by insect

---

TECHNIQUE OF Z-PLASTY
This relatively simple plastic surgery technique is carried out to revise unsightly scars or to relieve skin tension caused by scar contracture.

It can be particularly useful for dealing with facial scars or scars that cross natural skin creases.

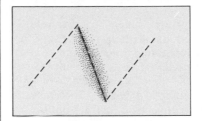

1 Three incisions are made, forming a Z. The central incision is made lengthwise through the scar.

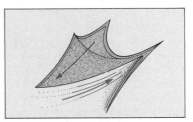

2 Two triangular flaps are developed by cutting skin away from underlying tissue, and the flaps are then transposed.

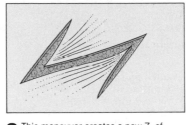

3 This maneuver creates a new Z, of which the central arm is at right angles to the original direction of the scar.

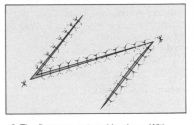

4 The flaps are sutured in place. With careful planning, the suture lines can be hidden in natural skin creases.

---

vectors. For example, some cases of *yellow fever* are transmitted from forest monkeys to humans via the bites of mosquitoes. (See also *Cats, diseases from; Dogs, diseases from; Insects and disease; Rats, diseases from.*)

Z-plasty
A technique that is used in *plastic surgery* to change the direction of a scar so that it can be hidden in natural skin creases or to relieve skin tension caused by *contracture* of a scar. Z-plasty is especially useful for revising unsightly scars on the face and for releasing scarring across joints, such as on the fingers or in the armpits, that may restrict normal movement or cause deformity.

A Z-shaped incision is made with the central arm of the Z along the scar. Two V-shaped flaps are created by cutting the skin away from underlying tissue. The flaps are then transposed and stitched. The procedure has the effect of redistributing tension perpendicular to the original defect.

Zygote
The cell produced when a *sperm* fertilizes an *ovum*. A zygote, measuring about 0.1 mm in diameter in humans,

contains all the genetic material for a new individual—half coming from the sperm, half from the ovum.

The zygote travels down one of the woman's *fallopian tubes* toward the uterus, dividing as it does so. After about a week, the mass of cells (now called a blastocyst) implants into the lining of the uterus, and the next stage of embryological growth begins. (See also *Embryo; Fertilization.*)

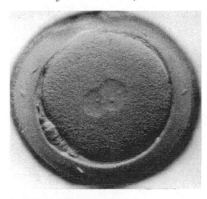

Appearance of a zygote
The photograph shows a human egg just after fertilization by a sperm. The two circular areas at the center are the nuclei of the sperm and egg merging.

SELF - HELP
ORGANIZATIONS

These organizations and support groups—many have provincial and local chapters—exist to help people with particular health problems. Some offer information only; others provide special services, personalized counseling, or referrals. Some have toll-free (800) numbers; a few are equipped with Telecommunication Devices for the Deaf (TDD).

Even if there is no mention of a support group for your specific problem, one of the more broadly based groups, the Canadian Neurological Coalition, for example, may be able to help, or you could check the *Directory of National Health-related Organizations and Associations in Canada*, a publication of the Health Promotion Directorate, Health and Welfare Canada.

ABORTION AND BIRTH CONTROL

Planned Parenthood Federation of Canada
1 Nicholas St., Suite 430
Ottawa, Ont., K1N 7B7
(613) 238-4474

Information and referrals on abortion, birth control, and pregnancy testing.

ACQUIRED IMMUNODEFICIENCY SYNDROME (AIDS) (*See also* SEXUALLY TRANSMITTED DISEASES)

Canadian AIDS Society
170 Laurier Ave. West, Suite 1101
Ottawa, Ont., K1P 5V5
(613) 230-3580

Information and referrals to local support groups.

ADDICTION

Addiction Research Foundation
33 Russell St.
Toronto, Ont., M5S 2S1
(416) 595-6000

Information on alcohol and other drugs, walk-in clinic, community programs throughout Ontario.

Al Anon Family Groups (Canada) National Public Information Canada
P.O. Box 6433, Station J
Ottawa, Ont., K2A 3Y6
(613) 722-1830

Information, family support through group therapy.

Alcoholics Anonymous
Most communities have at least one chapter. Check your local phone book. Information, group support.

Canadian Association for Children of Alcoholics
P.O. Box 159, Station H
Toronto, Ont., M4C 5H9
(416) 533-6293

Information and referrals.

Council on Drug Abuse
698 Weston Rd., Suite 17
Toronto, Ont., M6N 3R3
(416) 763-1491

Preventive drug education, information, referrals.

Parents Against Drugs
70 Maxome Ave.
Willowdale, Ont., M2M 3K1
(416) 225-6601

Information, intervention and other support programs for problems of drug/alcohol abuse.

ALCOHOLISM (*See* ADDICTION)

ALLERGIES

Allergy Foundation of Canada
P.O. Box 1904
Saskatoon, Sask., S7K 3S5
(306) 373-7591

Mutual support groups, newsletter, information.

Allergy Information Association
65 Tromley Dr., Room 10
Etobicoke, Ont., M9B 5Y7
(416) 244-9312

Written information for allergy sufferers.

ALZHEIMER'S DISEASE

Alzheimer Society of Canada
1320 Yonge St., Suite 201
Toronto, Ont., M4T 1X2
(416) 925-3552

Research, education, support services, newsletter.

ARTHRITIS

Arthritis Society
250 Bloor St. East, Suite 401
Toronto, Ont., M4W 3P2
(416) 967-1414

Finances research and patient care.

AUTISM

Autism Society Canada
20 College St., Suite 2
Toronto, Ont., M5G 1K2
(416) 924-4189

Information, newsletter.

BACK PROBLEMS

Back Association of Canada
83 Cottingham St.
Toronto, Ont., M4V 1B9
(416) 967-4670

Information, counseling.

BLOOD-RELATED DISORDERS

Aplastic Anemia Family Association of Canada
14 Lilac Ave.
Thornhill, Ont., L3T 5J9
(416) 731-3499

Family and patient support.

Canadian Hemochromatosis Society
P.O. Box 94303
Richmond, B.C., V6Y 2A6
(604) 271-8001

Information, counseling, referrals to physicians experienced in treating the disease.

Canadian Hemophilia Society
1450 City Councillors St., Suite 840
Montreal, Que., H3A 2E6
(514) 848-0503

Education material, family retreats, workshops.

Canadian Porphyria Foundation Inc.
P.O. Box 1206
Neepawa, Man., R0J 1H0
(204) 476-2800

Education materials and patient support (by phone, correspondence, and group meetings).

CANCER

Canadian Cancer Society
10 Alcorn Ave., Suite 200
Toronto, Ont., M4V 3B1
(416) 961-7223

Information, patient services.

Cancer Information Service
711 Concession St.
Hamilton, Ont., L8V 1C3
(416) 387-1153
1-800-263-6750

Answers questions from patients, family and others.

CELIAC DISEASE

Canadian Celiac Association
6519B Mississauga Rd.
Mississauga, Ont., L5N 1A6
(416) 567-7195

Information and referrals to local self-help groups.

CEREBRAL PALSY

Canadian Cerebral Palsy Association
880 Wellington St., Suite 612
City Centre
Ottawa, Ont., K1R 6K7
(613) 235-2144
1-800-267-6572

Information and referrals. Callers to 800 number get an information kit.

CHARCOT-MARIE-TOOTH DISEASE

Charcot-Marie-Tooth Disease/ Peroneal Muscular Atrophy International Association Inc. CMT International
1 Springbank Dr.
St. Catharines, Ont., L2S 2K1
(416) 687-3630

Information and referrals.

CHILDREN

Canadian Children's Foundation
60 Bloor St. West, Suite 1011
Toronto, Ont., M4W 1A1
(416) 920-5437

Maintains a "Kids Help Phone." Children of all ages may call about any problem they may have.

Canadian Society for the Prevention of Cruelty to Children
356 First Street
P.O. Box 700
Midland, Ont., L4R 4P4
(705) 526-5647

Educational material.

Family Service Canada
55 Parkdale Ave.
Ottawa, Ont., K1Y 4G1
(613) 728-2463

Counseling and various programs for teens and seniors.

CHRONIC FATIGUE

M.E. Association of Canada
246 Queen St., Suite 400
Ottawa, Ont., K1P 5E4
(613) 563-1565

Information on myalgic encephalomyelitis (chronic fatigue syndrome).

COLITIS (See ILEITIS)

CYSTIC FIBROSIS

Canadian Cystic Fibrosis Foundation
2221 Yonge St., Suite 601
Toronto, Ont., M4S 2B4
(416) 485-9149

Provides literature and referrals to local groups.

DIABETES

Canadian Diabetes Association
78 Bond St.
Toronto, Ont., M5B 2J8
(416) 362-4440

Information and referrals to local support groups.

Juvenile Diabetes Foundation Canada
4632 Yonge St., Suite 100
Willowdale, Ont., M2N 5M1
(416) 223-1068
1-800-668-0274

Information on causes, treatment.

DOWN'S SYNDROME

Canadian Down Syndrome Society
501 18th Avenue S.W., Suite 303
Calgary, Alta., T2S 0C7
(403) 228-5239

Information and referrals to local chapters.

DRUG ABUSE (See ADDICTION)

EATING DISORDERS

Bulimia Anorexia Nervosa Association (BANA)
c/o Psychological Services
University of Windsor
Windsor, Ont., N9B 3P4
(519) 253-7421 (hotline)
(519) 253-7545

Information, assessment, referrals.

ENDOMETRIOSIS

Endometriosis International
8585 North 76th Place
Milwaukee, Wis. 53223 USA
(414) 355-2200
1-800-426-2363

Information and referrals in 28 countries.

EPILEPSY

Epilepsy Canada
1470 Pcel St., Suite 745
Montreal, Que., H3A 1T1
(514) 876-7455

Information, client services, and referrals to local associations.

FITNESS

Canadian Fitness and Lifestyle Research Institute
47 Clarence St., Suite 200
Ottawa, Ont., K1N 9K1
(613) 236-0173

Information on fitness.

GENERAL HEALTH

Canadian Centre for Health Information
A division of StatsCan
R H Coats Bldg.
Holland Ave. and Scott St.
Tunney's Pasture
Ottawa, Ont., K1A 0T6
(613) 951-1746

Statistical summaries of incidence and prevalence of diseases.

Canadian Medic-Alert Foundation
250 Ferrand Dr., Suite 301
Toronto, Ont., M3C 3G8
(416) 696-0267
1-800-668-1507

Provides identification for medical conditions that should be known in an emergency.

Canadian Red Cross Society
1800 Alta Vista Dr.
Ottawa, Ont., K1G 4J5
(613) 739-3000

Community-based safety, seniors' and sick-room programs. Contact your local division or branch.

International Association for Medical Assistance to Travellers
40 Regal Rd.
Guelph, Ont., N1K 1B5
(519) 836-0102

Information on immunization requirements, tropical diseases. Provides a list of English-speaking physicians in 500 cities overseas.

HANDICAPS AND DISABILITIES (See also HEARING AND SPEECH and VISION)

Canadian Rehabilitation Council for the Disabled
45 Sheppard Ave. E., Suite 801
Willowdale, Ont., M2N 5W9
(416) 250-7490 (voice/TDD)

Through participating organizations provides coast-to-coast network of services and programs.

Easter Seal Society
250 Ferrand Dr., Suite 200
Don Mills, Ont., M3C 2P2
(416) 421-8377

Physical rehabilitation, summer camps, preschools, and equipment for handicapped children.

Learning Disabilities Association of Canada
323 Chapel St., Suite 200
Ottawa, Ont., K1N 7Z2
(613) 238-5721

Parent support group. Information on dyslexia, referrals to local associations, and services according to location and demand.

War Amputations of Canada
2827 Riverside Dr.
Ottawa, Ont., K1V 0C4
(613) 731-3821

Programs and services for all Canadian amputees.

HEADACHE

Migraine Foundation
390 Brunswick Ave.
Toronto, Ont., M5R 2Z4
(416) 920-4916
(416) 929-5661 (after hours)

Information, counseling, and referral services to people with migraine, cluster headaches, and related pain syndromes, and parents of children who suffer migraine.

HEARING AND SPEECH

Canadian Deaf-Blind and Rubella Association
Box 1625
Meaford, Ont., N0H 1Y0
(519) 538-3431 (voice/TDD)
Fax (519) 538-2812

Services include information, one-on-one intervention, support, consultants.

Canadian Hearing Society
271 Spadina Rd.
Toronto, Ont., M5R 2V3
(416) 964-9595
(416) 964-0023 (TDD)

Services include audiological, interpreter (sign and oral), speech pathology and hearing aid programs, employment, and vocational rehabilitation, seniors' programs, and counseling.

HEART DISEASE

Heart and Stroke Foundation of Canada
160 George St., Suite 200
Ottawa, Ont., K1N 9M2
(613) 237-4361

Referrals, rehabilitation programs.

HOME HEALTH CARE

Saint Elizabeth Visiting Nurses' Association of Ontario
10 Gateway Blvd., Suite 650
Don Mills, Ont., M3C 3A1
(416) 429-0112

Nursing care and counseling in the home on a visiting basis. Specialty programs include palliative care, enterostomal therapy foot care, early obstetrical discharge, gerontology, and psychiatric patient monitoring.

Victorian Order of Nurses for Canada
5 Blackburn Ave.
Ottawa, Ont., K1N 8A2
(613) 233-5694

Visiting nurses help individuals and families cope at home with health problems.

Visiting Homemakers Association
170 Merton St.
Toronto, Ont., M4S 1A1
(416) 489-2500

Under social worker supervision, trained homemakers assist the elderly, handicapped, and others in crisis.

HUNTINGTON'S CHOREA

Huntington Society of Canada
13 Water St. North, Suite 3
P.O. Box 333
Cambridge, Ont., N1R 5T8
(519) 622-1002

Information and referrals to local support groups.

ILEITIS

Canadian Foundation for Ileitis and Colitis
21 St. Clair Ave. E., Suite 301
Toronto, Ont., M4T 1L9
(416) 920-5035
1-800-387-1479

Information and support services.

KIDNEY DISEASES

Kidney Foundation of Canada
5160 Decarie Blvd., Bureau 780
Montreal, Que., H3W 2Z9
(514) 369-4806
1-800-361-7494

Financial assistance to those unable
to pay treatment-related costs.

LEARNING DISORDERS (*See* HANDICAPS AND DISABILITIES)

LIVER DISEASES

Canadian Liver Foundation
1320 Yonge St., Suite 301
Toronto, Ont., M4T 1X2
(416) 964-1953
1-800-563-5483

Information and patient support.

LUNG DISEASE

Canadian Lung Association
75 Albert St., Suite 908
Ottawa, Ont., K1P 5E7
(613) 237-1208

Research and rehabilitation.

LUPUS

Lupus Canada
P.O. Box 3302, Station B
Calgary, Alta., T2M 4L8
1-800-661-1468

Support and information for
patients.

MENTAL HANDICAPS

**The Canadian Association for
Community Living**
Kinsmen Building, York University
4700 Keele St.
North York, Ont., M3J 1P3
(416) 661-9611

Local chapter services include job
training and community living.

MENTAL HEALTH

Canadian Mental Health Association
2160 Yonge St., 3rd Floor
Toronto, Ont., M4S 2Z3
(416) 484-7750

Information and referrals to local
associations.

MULTIPLE SCLEROSIS

Multiple Sclerosis Society of Canada
250 Bloor St. East, Suite 820
Toronto, Ont., M4W 3P9
(416) 922-6065

Information, special services, and
referrals to local branches.

MUSCULAR DYSTROPHY

**Muscular Dystrophy Association of
Canada**
150 Eglinton Ave. East, Suite 400
Toronto, Ont., M4P 1E8
(416) 488-0030
1-800-465-6322

Services (through national network
to registered clients) include
assessment, referrals, education,
medical equipment purchase, and
family research.

NEUROLOGICAL PROBLEMS

Canadian Neurological Coalition
c/o Banting Institute
100 College St., Suite 126
Toronto, Ont., M5G 1L5
(416) 596-7043

An association of voluntary health
agencies concerned with
neurological impairment. The
coalition and member agencies offer
patient education and family
support. Chapters are organized
around specific neurological
conditions such as acoustic neuroma,
Alzheimer's disease, amyotrophic
lateral sclerosis, brain injuries,
craniofacial deformity, dystonia,
epilepsy, Friedreich's ataxia,
geriatrics research, Huntington's
disease, learning disabilities,
muscular dystrophy, narcolepsy,
neurofibromatosis, paraplegia,
Parkinson's disease, schizophrenia,
and Tourette's syndrome.

PAIN

**North American Chronic Pain
Association of Canada**
6 Handel Court
Brampton, Ont., L6S 1Y4
(416) 793-5230

Education, referrals to local self-help
groups.

PARALYSIS AND SPINAL CORD INJURY (*See also* HANDICAPS AND DISABILITIES)

Canadian Paraplegic Association
1500 Don Mills Rd., Suite 201
Don Mills, Ont., M3B 3K4
(416) 391-0203

Help to spinal cord-injured and
mobility-impaired people.

Spinal Cord Society of Canada
120 Newkirk Rd., Unit 32
Richmond Hill, Ont., L4C 9S7
(416) 508-4000

Research, referrals, information.

PARKINSON'S DISEASE

**The Parkinson Foundation of
Canada**
55 Bloor St. West, Suite 230
Toronto, Ont., M4W 1A5
(416) 964-1155

Information and referrals.

PREGNANCY

La Leche League Canada
493 Main St.
Winchester, Ont., K0C 2K0
(613) 774-2850

Information on breast-feeding.

PSORIASIS

Canadian Psoriasis Foundation Inc.
1565 Carling Ave., Suite 400
Ottawa, Ont., K1Z 8R1
(613) 728-4000

Information and referrals.

RARE DISEASES

**National Organization for Rare
Disorders (US)**
P.O. Box 8923
New Fairfield, Conn. 06812 USA
(203) 746-6518

Information and referrals.

SAFETY

Canada Safety Council
2750 Stevenage Dr., Unit 6
Ottawa, Ont., K1G 3N2
(613) 739-1535

Accident prevention information.

Canadian Centre for Occupational Health and Safety
250 Main St. East
Hamilton, Ont., L8N 1H6
(416) 572-4400
1-800-263-8466
On-line 1-800-263-8340
1-800-263-8276 general information and inquiries in French.

Operates a national emporium of information services and products.

SCHIZOPHRENIA

Schizophrenia Society of Canada
75 The Donway West, Suite 814
Don Mills, Ont., M3C 2E9
(416) 445-8204

Family support, information, referrals.

SEXUALLY TRANSMITTED DISEASES

Sexually Transmitted Disease Information Line for Toronto
(416) 392-7400

Information and referrals.
Similar hotlines exist in other major centers. Check your local phone book.

SPINA BIFIDA

Spina Bifida Association of Canada
633 Wellington Cres.
Winnipeg, Man., R3M 0A8
(204) 452-7580

Information and referrals to local organizations.

STROKE VICTIMS

Stroke Recovery Association
170 The Donway West, Suite 122
Don Mills, Ont., M3C 2G3
(416) 441-1421

Support and counseling.

SUDDEN INFANT DEATH SYNDROME

Canadian Foundation for the Study of Infant Deaths
P.O. Box 190, Station R
Toronto, Ont., M4G 3Z9
(416) 488-3260 (24-hour service)

Information for public awareness, emotional support for grieving families, and referrals to local chapters and contacts.

THYROID PROBLEMS

Thyroid Foundation of Canada
P.O. Box 1597
Kingston, Ont., K7L 5C8
(613) 542-8330

Information and referrals.

TRACHEO-ESOPHAGEAL FISTULA

Tracheo-Esophageal Fistula Parent Network
c/o 42 Saskatoon Dr.
Etobicoke, Ont., M9P 2E9
(416) 249-8710

Information and support; provides video.

TUBEROUS SCLEROSIS

National Tuberous Sclerosis Association (US)
4351 Garden City Dr., Suite 660
Landover, Md. 20785
(301) 459-9888
1-800-225-6872

Information, referrals, and support groups.

TURNER'S SYNDROME

Turner's Syndrome Society
York University
Administrative Studies Building
4700 Keele St., Room 006
Downsview, Ont., M3J 1P3
(416) 736-5023

Information and referrals.

VISION (*See also* HANDICAPS AND DISABILITIES)

Canadian National Institute for the Blind
1929 Bayview Ave.
Toronto, Ont., M4G 3E8
(416) 486-2500

Rehabilitation services to blind and visually impaired people, library.

WOMEN

Canadian Pelvic Inflammatory Disease [PID] Society
P.O. Box 33804, Station D
Vancouver, B.C., V6J 4L6
(604) 684-5704

Information on pelvic inflammatory disease.

DRUG
GLOSSARY

This glossary includes the most important generic-name drugs, a broad range of brand-name drugs, and various vitamins and minerals that may be used as drugs. Generic (nonproprietary) names are approved or recommended by such agencies as Health and Welfare Canada and the World Health Organization. Brand (proprietary) names are chosen by drug manufacturers.

If a generic-name drug has a separate entry within the encyclopedia, the entry page number follows the drug's name. If a drug belongs to a group of drugs that has its own encyclopedia entry, the glossary gives the relevant page number. If a generic-name drug belongs to a drug group that does not have an encyclopedia entry, the glossary tells you the disorder, condition, or symptom for which the drug is most commonly used. (Cross-references to encyclopedia non-drug entries—disorders, for example—are in parentheses.)

In the case of brand-name drugs, glossary entries cite equivalent generic-name drugs and page references to encyclopedia entries. If a brand-name drug contains several generic-name drugs, or if its ingredients do not have separate encyclopedia entries, the glossary will direct you to appropriate drug group or disorder entries.

This selection of drugs is designed to reflect the wide diversity of products available. Inclusion of any drug does not imply CMA endorsement, nor does exclusion indicate CMA disapproval.

A

Accutane brand name for isotretinoin 607, the generic name for a drug derived from vitamin A 1060 used to treat acne (63)

Acebutolol 61, generic name of a beta-blocker drug 163

Acet-Am brand name for theophylline 982, the generic name of a bronchodilator drug 213

Acetaminophen 61, generic name of a non-narcotic analgesic drug 96

Acetazolamide 61, generic name of a diuretic drug 363

Acetic acid 61, liquid ingredient of some antiseptics 118

Acetohexamide generic name of a hypoglycemic drug 559

Acetylcholine 61, a neurotransmitter 730

Acetylcysteine 61, generic name of a mucolytic drug 704

Acetylsalicylic acid 61, non-narcotic analgesic drug 736

Achromycin brand-name tetracycline drug 979

Acnomel BP5 brand name for benzoyl peroxide 162

ACTH 65, abbreviation for adrenocorticotropic hormone

Acthar brand name for corticotropin 310, another name for adrenocorticotropic hormone 65

Actifed brand-name decongestant 333 and antihistamine drug 117

Activated charcoal 253, an antidote to poisoning (116)

Acyclovir 66, generic name of an antiviral drug 119

Adalat brand name for nifedipine 732, the generic name of a calcium channel blocker drug 221

Adrenalin brand name for a preparation of epinephrine 410, a hormone (544) whose primary action is vasoconstriction (1045)

Adriamycin brand name for doxorubicin 369, the generic name of an anticancer drug 114

Adrucil brand name for fluorouracil 457, the generic name of an anticancer drug 114

Advil brand name for ibuprofen 565, the generic name of a nonsteroidal anti-inflammatory drug 736

Aerosporin brand-name antibiotic drug 113

Agarol brand-name laxative drug 632

Akineton brand name for biperiden, a drug used to treat parkinsonism (778)

AK-Sulf brand name for sulfacetamide eye drops 957, the generic name of an antibacterial drug 113

AK-Tate brand name for prednisolone eye drops 818, the generic name of a corticosteroid drug 309

Albalon-A brand-name ophthalmic decongestant antihistamine product 117

Albalon Liquifilm brand name for naphazoline eye drops 719, the generic name of a decongestant drug 333

Alcohol, rubbing, liquid preparation used as an antiseptic 118

Alcomicin brand name for gentamicin eye drops 484, the generic name of an antibiotic drug 113

Aldactone brand name for spironolactone 935, the generic name of a potassium-sparing diuretic drug 363

Aldomet brand name for methyldopa 687, the generic name of an antihypertensive drug 117

Aldoril brand-name drug containing hydrochlorothiazide 549, the generic name of a thiazide diuretic drug 363, and methyldopa 687, the generic name of an antihypertensive drug 117

Alfacalcidol another name for vitamin D 1063

Alkeran brand-name anticancer drug 114

Allerdryl brand name for diphenhydramine 358, the generic name of an antihistamine drug 117

Alloprin brand name for allopurinol 87, the generic name of a drug used to treat gout (495)

Allopurinol 87, generic name of a drug used to treat gout (495)

Alpha-tocopherol vitamin E element 1063

Alprazolam 88, generic name of a benzodiazepine antianxiety drug 113

Alprostadil generic name of a prostaglandin drug 830

Altretamine generic name of an anticancer drug 114

Aluminum acetate an astringent 138

Aluminum carbonate an antacid drug 112

Aluminum chloride generic name of an antiperspirant 118

Aluminum hydroxide an antacid drug 112

Alupent brand name for orciprenaline 754, the generic name of a selective bronchodilator drug 213

Alu-Tab brand name for aluminum hydroxide, the generic name of an antacid drug 112

Amantadine 91, generic name of an antiviral drug 119

Ambenonium generic name of a drug used to treat myasthenia gravis (713)

Amcinonide generic name

of a corticosteroid drug 309

Amersol brand name for ibuprofen 565, the generic name of a nonsteroidal anti-inflammatory drug 736

Amikacin generic name of an antibiotic drug 113

Amikin brand-name antibiotic drug 113

Amiloride 92, generic name of a potassium-sparing diuretic drug 363

Aminoglutethimide 92, generic name of an anticancer drug 114

Aminophylline 93, generic name of a bronchodilator drug 213

Aminosalicylate sodium another name for para-aminosalicylic acid 774, the generic name of a drug used to treat tuberculosis (1016)

Amiodarone generic name of an antiarrhythmic drug 113

Amitriptyline 93, generic name of an antidepressant drug 115

Amobarbital generic name of a barbiturate drug 155

Amoxapine generic name of an antidepressant drug 115

Amoxicillin 94, generic name of a penicillin drug 785

Amoxil brand name for amoxicillin 94, the generic name of a penicillin drug 785, an antibiotic drug 113

Amphotericin B 94, generic name of an antifungal drug 117

Ampicillin 95, generic name of a penicillin drug 785, an antibiotic drug 113

Ampicin brand name for ampicillin 94, the generic name of a penicillin drug 785, an antibiotic drug 113

Amrinone generic name of a drug used to treat heart failure (518)

Amyl nitrite 95, generic name of a vasodilator drug 1045

Amytal brand-name barbiturate drug 155

Anacin brand-name non-narcotic analgesic drug 96 containing acetylsalicylic acid 61

Anacin 3 brand name for acetaminophen 61, the generic name of a non-narcotic analgesic drug 96

Anafranil brand name for clomipramine 281, the generic name of an antidepressant drug 115

Anaprox brand name for naproxen 719, the generic name of a nonsteroidal anti-inflammatory drug 736

Anbesol brand-name local anesthetic (105)

Ancef brand-name cephalosporin drug 244, an antibiotic drug 113

Ancotil brand name for an antifungal drug 117

Anectine brand-name muscle-relaxant drug 710 used in anesthesia (103)

Ansaid brand name for flurbiprofen, the generic name of a nonsteroidal anti-inflammatory drug 736

Antabuse brand name for disulfiram 362, the generic name of a drug used to treat alcohol dependence (81)

Anthralin 112, generic name of a drug (also known as dithranol) used to treat psoriasis (835)

Anthranol brand name for anthralin 112, the generic name of a drug used for psoriasis (835)

Anturan brand-name drug used to treat gout (495)

APL brand name for human chorionic gonadotropin 494

Apo-Carbamazepine brand name for carbamazepine 228, generic name of an anticonvulsant drug 115

Apo-Chlordiazepoxide brand name for chlordiazepoxide 267, a benzodiazepine 162 antianxiety drug 113

Apo-Chlorpropamide brand name for chlorpropamide 268, the generic name of a drug used to treat diabetes mellitus (346)

Apo-Chlorthalidone brand name for chlorthalidone 268, the generic name of a thiazide diuretic drug 363, and an antihypertensive drug 117

Apo-Cimetidine brand name for cimetidine 277, the generic name of a drug used to treat ulcers (1021)

Apo-Diazepam brand name for diazepam 354, the generic name of a benzodiazepine 162 antianxiety drug 113

Apo-Diltiaz brand name for diltiazem 358, the generic name of a calcium channel blocker drug 221

Apo-Dimenhydrinate brand name for dimenhydrinate 358, the generic name of an antiemetic drug 116

Apo-Dipyridamole brand name for dipyridamole 359, the generic name of a drug used to treat abnormal blood clotting (182)

Apo-Erythro brand name for erythromycin 414, the generic name of an antibiotic drug 113

Apo-Ferrous Sulfate brand name for ferrous sulfate, an iron supplement 605

Apo-Fluphenazine brand name for fluphenazine 457, the generic name of an antipsychotic drug 118

Apo-Flurazepam brand name for flurazepam 457, a benzodiazepine 162 sleeping drug 920

Apo-Furosemide brand name for furosemide 469, the generic name of a loop diuretic drug 363

Apo-Guanethidine brand name for guanethidine 500, the generic name of an antihypertensive drug 117

Apo-Haloperidol brand name for haloperidol 504, the generic name of an antipsychotic drug 118

Apo-Hydro brand name for hydrochlorothiazide 549, the generic name of a thiazide diuretic drug 363

Apo-Hydroxyzine brand name for hydroxyzine 550, the generic name of an antihistamine drug 117

Apo-Ibuprofen brand name for ibuprofen 565, the generic name of a nonsteroidal anti-inflammatory drug 736

Apo-Imipramine brand name for imipramine 569, the generic name of an antidepressant drug 115

Apo-Indomethacin brand name for indomethacin 580, the generic name of a nonsteroidal anti-inflammatory drug 736

Apo-ISDN brand name for isosorbide dinitrate 607, the generic name of a vasodilator drug 1045

Apo-K brand name for potassium chloride, the generic name of a potassium supplement used with some antihypertensive drugs 117

Apo-Lorazepam brand name for lorazepam 650, the generic name of a benzodiazepine 162 sleeping drug 920

Apo-Meprobamate brand name for meprobamate 683, the generic name of an antianxiety drug 113

Apo-Methazide brand-name antihypertensive drug 117

Apo-Methyldopa brand name for methyldopa 687, the generic name of an antihypertensive drug 117

Apo-Metoprolol brand name for metoprolol, the generic name of a beta-blocker drug 163

Apo-Metronidazole brand name for metronidazole 687, the generic name of an antibiotic drug 113

Apo-Nadol brand name for nadolol 719, the generic name of a beta-blocker drug 163

Apo-Nifed brand name for nifedipine 732, the generic name of a calcium channel blocker drug (221)

Apo-Nitrofurantoin brand name for nitrofurantoin 734, the generic name of an antibiotic drug 113

Apo-Oxazepam brand name for oxazepam 766, the generic name of a benzodiazepine 162 antianxiety drug 113

Apo-Oxtriphylline brand name for oxtriphylline 766, the generic name of a bronchodilator drug 213

Apo-Pen-VK brand name for penicillin V, the generic name of a penicillin drug 785, an antibiotic drug 113

Apo-Perphenazine brand name for perphenazine 791, the generic name of a phenothiazine-type drug 796, an antipsychotic 118 and antiemetic drug 116

Apo-Phenylbutazone brand name for phenylbutazone 796, the generic name of a nonsteroidal anti-inflammatory drug 736

Apo-Pindol brand name for pindolol 800, the generic name of a beta-blocker drug 163

Apo-Prednisone brand name for prednisone 818, the generic name of a corticosteroid drug 309

Apo-Primidone brand name for primidone 827, the generic name of an anticonvulsant drug 115

Apo-Procainamide brand name for procainamide 827, the generic name of an antiarrhythmic drug 113

Apo-Propranolol brand name for propranolol 829, the generic name of a beta-blocker drug 163

Apo-Ranitidine brand name for ranitidine 855, the generic name of a drug used to treat ulcers (1021)

Apo-Salvent brand name for salbutamol 883, the generic name of a bronchodilator drug 213

Apo-Sulfamethoxazole brand name for sulfamethoxazole 957, the generic name of an antibiotic drug 113

Apo-Sulfatrim brand-name drug containing sulfamethoxazole 957, the generic name of an antibiotic drug 113, and trimethoprim, the generic name of an antibiotic drug 113

Apo-Sulfinpyrazone brand name for sulfinpyrazone 957, the generic name of a drug used to treat gout (495)

Apo-Sulin brand name for sulindac 957, the generic name of a nonsteroidal anti-inflammatory drug 736

Apo-Tetra brand name for tetracycline, the generic name of an antibiotic drug 113

Apo-Thioridazine brand name for thioridazine 982, the generic name of an antipsychotic drug 118

Apo-Timol brand name for timolol 992, the generic name of a beta-blocker drug 163

Apo-Tolbutamide brand name for tolbutamide 998, the generic name of a hypoglycemic drug 559

Apo-Triazide brand-name antihypertensive drug 117

Apo-Triazo brand name for triazolam 1012, the generic name of a benzodiazepine sleeping drug 162

Apo-Trifluoperazine brand name for trifluoperazine 1013, the generic name of an antipsychotic drug 118

Apo-Trihex brand name for trihexyphenidyl, the generic name of an anticholinergic drug 114

Apresoline brand name for hydralazine 549, the generic name of an antihypertensive drug 117

Aquasol A brand name for vitamin A 1060

Arachis oil liquid preparation used to treat scaly skin (913)

Aralen brand name for chloroquine 267, the generic name of a drug used to treat malaria (660)

Aristocort brand name for triamcinolone 1012, the generic name of a corticosteroid drug 309

Arlidin brand name for a vasodilator drug 1045

Arnica herbal preparation used to treat bruises (214)

Artane brand name for trihexyphenidyl, the generic name of an anticholinergic drug 114

ASA abbreviation for acetylsalicylic acid 61, a non-narcotic analgesic drug 96

Ascorbic acid 135, another name for vitamin C 1063

Asendin brand name for amoxapine, the generic name of an antidepressant drug 115

Asparaginase generic name of an anticancer drug 114

Aspergum brand-name drug containing acetylsalicylic acid 61, a non-narcotic analgesic drug 96

Aspirin 136, brand name for acetylsalicylic acid 62, a non-narcotic analgesic drug 96

Astemizole generic name of an antihistamine drug 117

Atabrine brand name for quinacrine 847, the generic name of a drug primarily used to treat giardiasis (485)

Atarax brand name for hydroxyzine 550, the generic name of an antihistamine drug 117

Atasol brand name for acetaminophen 61, the generic name of a non-narcotic analgesic drug 96

Atenolol 139, generic name of a beta-blocker drug 163

Ativan brand name for lorazepam 650, the generic name of a benzodiazepine 162 antianxiety drug 113

Atracurium generic name of a muscle-relaxant drug 701 used in general anesthesia 103

Atromid-S brand name for clofibrate 281, the generic name of a lipid-lowering drug 642

Atropine 142, generic name of an anticholinergic drug 114

Atrovent brand name for ipratropium 605, generic name of an anticholinergic drug 114 used as a bronchodilator drug 213

Auralgan brand-name analgesic drug 96 in ear-drop form

Auranofin generic name of an antirheumatic drug 117

Aureomycin brand-name antibiotic drug 113

Aurothioglucose generic name of a gold-based drug 493

Aventyl brand name for nortriptyline 736, the generic name of an antidepressant drug 115

Avlosulfon brand name for dapsone 330, the generic name of an antibacterial drug 113

Axid brand name for nizatidine 734, the generic name of a drug used to treat ulcers (1021)

Ayercillin brand name for penicillin G, the generic name of a penicillin drug 785, an antibiotic drug 113

Azatadine 188, generic name of an antihistamine drug 117

Azathioprine 148, generic name of an immunosuppressant drug 575

Azidothymidine former name for zidovudine 1090, the generic name of an antiviral drug 119 used to treat AIDS (76)

Azo Gantrisin brand-name drug containing a urinary analgesic drug 96 and an antibiotic drug 113

AZT 148, abbreviation of azidothymidine, the former name for zidovudine 1090, the generic name of an antiviral drug 119 used to treat AIDS (76)

B

Bacampicillin generic name for a penicillin drug 785, an antibiotic drug 113

Baciguent brand name for bacitracin 149, the generic name of an antibacterial drug 113

Bacitin brand name for bacitracin 149, the generic name for an antibacterial drug 113

Bacitracin 149, generic name for an antibacterial drug 113

Baclofen 151, generic name for a muscle-relaxant drug 710

Bactopen brand name for cloxacillin 281, the generic name for a penicillin drug 785, an antibiotic drug 113

Bactrim brand-name drug containing sulfamethoxazole 957, the generic name of an antibiotic drug 113, and trimethoprim, the generic name of an antibiotic drug 113

Balminil DM Syrup brand name for dextromethorphan 346, the generic name of a cough suppressant 314

Balminil Expectorant brand name for guaifenesin 500, the generic name of an expectorant 424

Beclomethasone 159, generic name of a corticosteroid drug 307

Beclovent brand name for beclomethasone 159, the generic name of a corticosteroid drug 307

Beconase brand name for beclomethasone 159, the generic name of a corticosteroid drug 307

Belladonna 162, generic name of an anticholinergic drug 114

Bellergal brand-name drug used to treat migraines (690)

Benadryl brand name for diphenhydramine 358, the generic name of an antihistamine drug 117

Bendroflumethiazide generic name of a thiazide diuretic drug 363

Benemid brand name for probenecid 827, the generic name of a drug used to treat recurrent attacks of gout (495)

Benoquin brand-name drug used to treat vitiligo (1064)

Benoxyl brand name for benzoyl peroxide 162, the generic name of a drug used topically to treat acne (63)

Bentylol brand name for dicyclomine 354, an antispasmodic drug 119

Benuryl brand name for probenecid 827, generic name of a drug used to treat recurrent attacks of gout (495)

Benylin-DM brand name for dextromethorphan, the generic name of a cough suppressant 314

Benzagel brand name for benzoyl peroxide 162, the generic name of a drug used topically to treat acne (63)

Benzalkonium chloride generic name of a skin antiseptic 118

Benzathine penicillin G generic name of a penicillin drug 785, an antibiotic drug 113

Benzocaine generic name of a local anesthetic 105

Benzoic acid an antifungal drug 117

Benzoin aromatic resin added to inhalations (588)

Benzonatate generic name of a cough suppressant 314

Benzoyl peroxide 162, generic name of a drug used topically to treat acne (63)

Benztropine generic name of a drug used to treat parkinsonism (778)

Benzydamine generic name of a local anesthetic (105) used to treat acute sore throat (927)

Benzyl benzoate generic name of a drug used to treat scabies (886)

Benzylpenicillin generic name of a penicillin drug 785, an antibiotic drug 113

Berotec brand name for fenoterol, the generic name of a bronchodilator drug 213

Beta-carotene another name for vitamin A 1060

Betaloc brand name for metoprolol, the generic name of a beta-blocker drug 163

Betamethasone 164, generic name of a corticosteroid drug 309

Betaxolol generic name of beta-blocker eye drops 163 used to treat glaucoma (487)

Bethanechol generic name of a drug used to treat urinary retention (1032)

Betnesol brand name for betamethasone 164, the generic name of a corticosteroid drug 309

Betnovate brand name for betamethasone 164, the generic name of a corticosteroid drug 309

Betoptic brand-name beta-blocker eye drops 163 used to treat glaucoma (487)

Bicillin brand-name penicillin drug, an antibiotic drug 113

BiCNU brand-name anticancer drug 114

Biotin part of the vitamin B complex 1062

Biperiden generic name of a drug used to treat parkinsonism (778)

Biquin brand name for quinidine 847, the generic name of an antiarrhythmic drug 113

Bisacodyl generic name of a stimulant laxative drug 632

Bismuth 172, generic name of an antacid 112, and an antidiarrheal drug 116

Blenoxane brand-name anticancer drug 114

Bleomycin generic name of an anticancer drug 114

Blephamide brand-name eye drops used to treat eye infection and inflammation (430)

Blocadren brand name for timolol 992, the generic name of a beta-blocker drug 163

Bonamine brand name for meclizine 670, the generic name of an antiemetic drug 116

Bricanyl brand name for terbutaline 974, a bronchodilator drug 213

Bromazepam generic name of a benzodiazepine 162 antianxiety drug 113

Bromocriptine 211, generic name of a drug used to treat parkinsonism (778)

Brompheniramine generic name of an antihistamine drug 117

Bronkaid Mistometer brand-name bronchodilator 213

Budesonide generic corticosteroid drug 309

Bupivacaine generic name of a local anesthetic 105

Busulfan generic name of an anticancer drug 114

Butabarbital generic name of a barbiturate drug 155, a sleeping drug 920

Butazolidin brand name for phenylbutazone 796, the generic name of a nonsteroidal anti-inflammatory drug 736

Butisol brand-name barbiturate drug 155, a sleeping drug 920

C

Cafergot brand-name drug used to treat migraine (690)

Caffeine 219, generic name of a stimulant (945) used with other drugs to treat headache (506)

Caladryl brand-name drug containing diphenhydramine 358, the generic name of an antihistamine drug 117, and calamine 220, the generic name of drug used to treat skin irritation (917)

Calamine 220, generic name of a drug used to treat skin irritation (917)

Calciferol another name for vitamin D 1063

Calcilean brand name for heparin 531, the generic name of an anticoagulant drug 115

Calcimar brand name for a drug used to treat bone disorders (192)

Calcitonin 220, generic name of a drug used to treat bone disorders (192)

Calcitriol another name for vitamin D 1063

Calcium carbonate antacid drug 112

Camphor drug used to relieve skin itching (607)

Canesten brand-name antifungal drug 117

Cannabis 227, central nervous system depressant 341 (see Marijuana 665)

Cantharidin generic name of a drug used to treat warts (1072)

Cantharone brand-name drug used to treat warts (1072)

Capoten brand name for captopril 228, a generic name of an ACE inhibitor drug 61

Captopril 228, generic name of an ACE inhibitor drug 61

Carbachol 228, generic name of a drug used to treat glaucoma (487)

Carbamazepine generic name of an anticonvulsant drug 115

Carbamide peroxide generic name of a drug used to soften earwax (384)

Carbenicillin generic name of a penicillin drug 785, an antibiotic drug 113

Carbenoxolone 228, generic name of a drug used to treat ulcers (1021)

Carbimide generic name of

a drug used to treat alcohol dependence (81)

Carbocaine brand-name local anesthetic (105)

Carbocysteine generic name of a mucolytic drug 704

Carbolith brand name for lithium 643, the generic name of a drug used to treat manic-depressive illness (664)

Cardilate brand-name nitrate drug 733 used to treat angina pectoris (107)

Cardizem brand name for diltiazem 358, a calcium channel blocker drug 221

Carisoprodol 235, generic name of a muscle-relaxant drug 710

Carmustine generic name of an anticancer drug 114

Casanthranol generic name of a stimulant laxative drug 632

Cascara stimulant laxative drug 632

Castor oil 236, stimulant laxative drug 632

Ceclor brand name for a cephalosporin drug 244, an antibiotic drug 113

Cedocard-SR brand name for isosorbide dinitrate 607, the generic name of a vasodilator drug 1045

CeeNu brand-name anticancer drug 114

Cefaclor 241, generic name of a cephalosporin drug 244, an antibiotic drug 113

Cefadroxil generic name of a cephalosporin drug 244, an antibiotic drug 113

Cefazolin generic name of a cephalosporin drug 244, an antibiotic drug 113

Cefizox brand name for a cephalosporin drug 248, an antibiotic drug 113

Cefobid brand name for cefoperazone, the generic name of a cephalosporin drug 244, an antibiotic drug 113

Cefoperazone generic name of a cephalosporin drug 244, an antibiotic drug 113

Cefotaxime generic name of a cephalosporin drug 244, an antibiotic drug 113

Cefoxitin generic name of a cephalosporin drug 244, an antibiotic drug 113

Ceftazidime generic name of a cephalosporin drug 244, an antibiotic drug 113

Ceftizoxime generic name of a cephalosporin drug 244, an antibiotic drug 113

Ceftriaxone generic name

of a cephalosporin drug 244, an antibiotic drug 113

Cefuroxime generic name of a cephalosporin drug 244, an antibiotic drug 113

Celestone brand name for betamethasone 164, the generic name of a corticosteroid drug 309

Celontin brand-name anticonvulsant drug 115

Centrum brand-name multivitamin and minerals preparation 706

Cephalexin 244, generic name of a cephalosporin drug 244, an antibiotic drug 113

Cephalothin generic name of a cephalosporin drug 244, an antibiotic drug 113

Cephradine generic name of a cephalosporin drug 244, an antibiotic drug 113

Cephulac brand name for lactulose 626, the generic name of a laxative drug 632

Ceporex brand name for cephalexin 244, the generic name of a cephalosporin drug 244, an antibiotic drug 113

Cerubidine brand-name anticancer drug 114

Cerumenex brand-name preparation for softening earwax (384)

Cesamet brand name for an antiemetic drug 116

Cetamide brand name for sulfacetamide eye drops 957, the generic name of an antibacterial drug 113

Cevitamic acid another name for ascorbic acid (vitamin C) 1063

Chloral hydrate 267, generic name of a sleeping drug 920

Chlorambucil 267, generic name of an anticancer drug 114

Chloramphenicol 267, generic name of an antibiotic drug 113

Chloraseptic brand-name preparation used to treat sore mouth (700) or throat (784)

Chlordiazepoxide 267, generic name of a benzodiazepine 162 antianxiety drug 113

Chlorhexidine 267, skin antiseptic 118

Chlormezanone generic name of an antianxiety drug 113

Chloroguanide generic name of a drug used to treat malaria (660)

Chloromycetin brand name for chloramphenicol

267, the generic name of an antibiotic drug 113

Chlorophenothane another name for DDT 330

Chloroptic brand name for chloramphenicol eye drops, the generic name of an antibiotic drug 113

Chloroquine 267, generic name of a drug used to treat malaria (660)

Chlorothiazide generic name of a thiazide diuretic drug 363

Chlorotrianisene generic name of an estrogen drug used to treat cancer 115

Chlorphenesin generic name of an antifungal drug 117

Chlorpheniramine 267, generic name of an antihistamine drug 117

Chlorpromanyl brand name for chlorpromazine 267, the generic name of an antipsychotic drug 118

Chlorpromazine 267, generic name of an antipsychotic drug 118

Chlorpropamide 268, generic name of a drug used to treat diabetes mellitus (346)

Chlorprothixene generic name of an antipsychotic drug 118

Chlortetracycline generic name of a tetracycline drug 979, an antibiotic drug 113

Chlorthalidone 268, generic name of a thiazide diuretic drug 363, an antihypertensive drug 117

Chlor-Tripolon brand name for chlorpheniramine 267, the generic name of an antihistamine drug 117

Cholecalciferol 269, another name for vitamin D 1063

Choledyl brand name for oxtriphylline 766, the generic name of a bronchodilator drug 213

Cholestyramine 271, generic name of a lipid-lowering drug 642

Choline magnesium trisalicylate generic name of a drug used to treat arthritis (130)

Choline salicylate topical anesthetic (105) used in the mouth (700)

Choloxin brand-name lipid-lowering drug 642

Chophylline brand name for oxtriphylline 766, the generic name of a bronchodilator drug 213

Chymopapain enzyme (406)

for chemonucleolysis (255)

Chymotrypsin enzyme (406) used in the treatment of cataracts (237)

Ciclopirox generic name of an antifungal drug 117

Cimetidine 277, generic name of a drug used to treat ulcers (102)

Cisplatin 279, generic name of an anticancer drug 114

Claforan brand name for cefotaxime, the generic name of a cephalosporin drug 244, an antibiotic drug 113

Claripex brand name for clofibrate 281, the generic name of a lipid-lowering drug 642

Claritin brand-name antihistamine drug 117

Clavulin brand-name antibiotic compound 113

Clemastine generic name of an antihistamine drug 117

Clidinium bromide generic name of an antispasmodic drug 119 used to treat irritable bowel syndrome (606)

Clindamycin 280, generic name of an antibiotic drug 113

Clinoril brand-name nonsteroidal anti-inflammatory drug 736

Clioquinol generic name of an antibacterial 113 and an antifungal drug 117

Clobetasol generic name of a corticosteroid drug 309

Clofibrate 281, generic name of a lipid-lowering drug 642

Clomid brand name for clomiphene 281, the generic name of an antifertility drug (582)

Clomiphene 281, generic name of an antifertility drug (582)

Clomipramine 281, generic name of an antidepressant drug 115

Clonazepam 281, generic name of a benzodiazepine drug 162 primarily used to treat epilepsy (409)

Clonidine 281, generic name of an antihypertensive drug 117

Clorazepate 281, generic name of a benzodiazepine antianxiety drug 113

Clotrimazole 281, generic name of an antifungal drug 117

Cloxacillin 281, generic name of a penicillin drug 785 antibiotic drug 113

Coal tar 282, ingredient in some preparations for skin disorders (917)

Cocaine 282, generic name of a central nervous system stimulant 945

Codeine 283, generic name of a narcotic drug 720

Cod liver oil 283, dietary supplement containing vitamin A 1060

Cogentin brand name for benztropine, the generic name of a drug used to treat parkinsonism (778)

Colchicine 284, generic name of a drug used for centuries to treat gout (495)

Colestid brand name for a lipid-lowering drug 642

Colestipol generic name of a lipid-lowering drug 642

Colistin 285, generic name of an antibiotic drug 113 primarily used to treat infections of the external ear (381)

Colprone brand-name progestogen drug 828

Coly-Mycin Otic brand-name ear drops used to treat infections of the external ear (381)

Combantrin brand name for a drug used to treat helminth infestation 525, (see worm infestation 1082)

Conjugated estrogens generic name of estrogen drug 418

Contac C brand-name cold remedy 284

Coptin brand-name antibacterial drug 113

Cordarone brand-name antiarrhythmic drug 113

Corgard brand-name for nadolol 719, the generic name of a beta-blocker drug 163

Coricidin brand-name cold remedy 284

Corium brand-name antispasmodic (119) and antianxiety compound (113)

Coronex brand name for isosorbide dinitrate 607, a nitrate drug 733, the generic name of a vasodilator drug 1045

Corophyllin brand name for aminophylline 93, the generic name of a bronchodilator drug 213

Cortacet brand name for hydrocortisone 549, the generic name of a corticosteroid drug 309

Cortamed brand name for hydrocortisone 549, the generic name of a corticosteroid drug 309

Cortate brand name for hydrocortisone 549, the generic name of a corticosteroid drug 309

Cortef brand name for hydrocortisone 549, the generic name of a corticosteroid drug 309

Corticotropin 310, another name for adrenocorticotropic hormone 65

Cortifoam brand name for hydrocortisone 549, the generic name of a corticosteroid drug 309

Cortisol another name for hydrocortisone 549, the generic name of a corticosteroid drug 309

Cortisone 310, generic name of a corticosteroid drug 309

Cortisporin brand-name preparation containing a corticosteroid drug 309 and antibiotics 113

Cortone brand name for cortisone 310, the generic name of a corticosteroid drug 309

Cosmegen brand-name anticancer drug 114

Co-trimazine generic name for a combination of sulfadiazine, the generic name of an antibacterial drug 113 and trimethoprim, the generic name of an antibiotic drug 113

Cotrimoxazole generic name for an antibacterial drug 113, a combination of sulfamethoxazole 957, the generic name of an antibacterial drug 113 and trimethoprim, the generic name of an antibiotic drug 113

Coumadin brand name for warfarin 1072, the generic name of an anticoagulant drug 115

Cromolyn sodium generic name of a drug used to prevent asthma attacks (136)

Cuprimine brand name for penicillamine 784, the generic name of an antirheumatic drug 119 and chelating agent 253

Curare 322, generic name of a muscle-relaxant drug 710

Cyclamate generic name of an artificial sweetener 134

Cyanocobalamin 323, another name for vitamin B_{12} 1061

Cyclandelate generic name of a vasodilator drug 1045

Cyclizine generic name of an antiemetic drug 116

Cyclobenzaprine 323, generic name of a muscle-relaxant drug 710

Cyclocort brand-name topical corticosteroid drug 309

Cyclomen brand name for danazol 329, the generic name of a drug used to treat endometriosis (401)

Cyclophosphamide 323, generic name of an anticancer drug 114

Cyclospasmol brand name for a vasodilator drug 1045

Cyclosporine 323, generic name of an immunosuppressant drug 575

Cylert brand name for a stimulant drug 945

Cyproheptadine generic name of an appetite stimulant drug 127

Cytadren brand name for aminoglutethimide 92, the generic name of an anticancer drug 114

Cytarabine generic name of an anticancer drug 114

Cytomel brand name for liothyronine, the generic name of a synthetic thyroid hormone 544

Cytosar brand-name anticancer drug 114

Cytosine Arabinoside generic name of an anticancer drug 114

Cytotec brand name for misoprostol 694, the generic name of a prostaglandin drug 829

Cytoxan brand-name anticancer drug 114

D

Dacarbazine generic name of an anticancer drug 114

Dactinomycin generic name of an anticancer drug 114

Dalacin C brand name for clindamycin 280, the generic name of an antibiotic drug 113

Dalmane brand name for flurazepam 457, a benzodiazepine drug 162 used to treat insomnia

Danazol 329, generic name of a drug used to treat endometriosis (401)

Dantrium brand name for dantrolene 330, the generic name of a muscle-relaxant drug 710

Dantrolene 330, generic

name of a muscle-relaxant drug 710

Dapsone 330, generic name of an antibacterial drug 113

Daraprim brand name for pyrimethamine 846, the generic name of a drug used to treat malaria (660) and toxoplasmosis (1004)

Darbid brand-name antispasmodic drug 119

Darvon-N brand name for propoxyphene 829, the generic name of a weak narcotic drug 720, an analgesic drug 96

Daunorubicin generic name of an anticancer drug 114

Decadron brand name for dexamethasone 345, the generic name of a corticosteroid drug 309

Deca-Durabolin brand name for nandrolone 719, an anabolic steroid 95

Declomycin brand-name tetracycline antibiotic 979

Deferoxamine generic name of a drug used to treat iron poisoning (810)

Dehydrocholic acid generic name of a drug used to increase the flow of bile (165)

Delsym brand name for dextromethorphan 346, the generic name of a cough suppressant 314

Deltasone brand name for prednisone 818, the generic name of a corticosteroid drug 309

Demeclocycline generic name of a tetracycline drug 979

Demerol brand name for meperidine 683, also known as pethidine 793, the generic name of a narcotic analgesic drug 720

Depakene brand name for valproic acid 1041, the generic name of an anticonvulsant drug 115

Depo-Medrol brand name for methylprednisolone 687, the generic name of a corticosteroid drug 309

Depo-Provera brand name for medroxyprogesterone 673, a progestogen drug 828

Depo-Testosterone brand-name drug containing testosterone 977, an androgen hormone 98

Deprenyl brand name for selegiline 894, the generic name of a drug used to treat parkinsonism (778)

Dermovate brand name for

clobetasol, the generic name of a corticosteroid drug 309

Desenex brand-name topical antifungal drug 117

Desferal brand-name drug used to treat iron poisoning (810)

Desipramine 343, generic name of a tricyclic antidepressant drug 115

Desonide generic name of a corticosteroid drug 309

Desoximetasone generic name of a corticosteroid drug 309

Desyrel brand name for trazodone 1010, the generic name of an antidepressant drug 115

Detensol brand name for propranolol 829, a generic beta-blocker drug 163

Dexamethasone 345, generic name of a corticosteroid drug 309

Dexasone brand name for dexamethasone 345, the generic name of a corticosteroid drug 309

Dexbrompheniramine generic name of an antihistamine drug 117

Dexchlorpheniramine generic name of an antihistamine drug 117

Dexedrine brand-name central nervous system (244) stimulant 945

Dextroamphetamine 345, generic name of a central nervous system (244) stimulant 945

Dextromethorphan generic name of a cough suppressant 314

Dextrothyroxine generic name of a lipid-lowering drug 642

DHT vitamin D 1063

DiaBeta brand name for glyburide 492, the generic name of a hypoglycemic drug 559

Diabinese brand name for chlorpropamide 268, the generic name of a drug used to treat diabetes mellitus (346)

Diamicron brand name for a hypoglycemic drug 559

Diamorphine generic name of a narcotic analgesic drug 96

Diamox brand name for acetazolamide 61, the generic name of a diuretic drug 362

Diazepam 354, generic name of a benzodiazepine 162 antianxiety drug 113

Diazoxide generic name of an antihypertensive drug 117

Dibucaine generic name of a local anesthetic 105

Diclofenac 354, generic name of a nonsteroidal anti-inflammatory drug 736

Dicloxacillin generic name of a penicillin drug 785, an antibiotic drug 113

Dicumarol 353, generic name of an anticoagulant drug 115

Dicyclomine 354, generic name of an antispasmodic drug 119

Didronel brand name for a drug used to treat Paget's disease 768

Dienestrol 354, generic name of an estrogen drug 418

Diethylcarbamazine generic name of an anthelmintic drug used to treat helminth infestation (525) (see worm infestation 1082)

Diethylpropion generic name of an appetite suppressant drug 127

Diethylstilbestrol 355, generic name of an estrogen drug 418

Diflorasone generic name of a corticosteroid drug 309

Diflunisal 355, generic name of a nonsteroidal anti-inflammatory drug 736

Digitoxin 357, generic name of a digitalis drug 357

Digoxin 357, generic name of a digitalis drug 357

Dihydroergotamine generic name of a drug used to treat migraine (690)

Dihydrotachysterol another name for vitamin D 1063

Dilantin brand name for phenytoin 796, the generic name of a drug used to treat epilepsy (409)

Dilaudid brand name for hydromorphone, the generic name of a narcotic drug 720, an analgesic drug 96

Diltiazem 358, generic name of a calcium channel blocker drug 221

Dimelor brand name for acetohexamide, the generic name of a hypoglycemic drug 559

Dimenhydrinate 358, generic name of an antiemetic drug 116

Dimercaprol generic name of a drug used to treat lead poisoning (632)

Dimetane brand-name antihistamine drug 117

Dimethyl sulfoxide generic name of a drug used to treat cystitis (325)

Dimethyl tubocurarine generic name of a muscle-relaxant drug 710 used in general anesthesia (103)

Dinoprostone generic name of a prostaglandin drug 829 used to stimulate uterine contractions in childbirth (260)

Diodoquin brand-name drug used to treat amebiasis 91

Diphenhydramine 358, generic name of an antihistamine drug 117

Diphenidol generic name of an antiemetic drug 116

Diphenoxylate 358, generic name of an antidiarrheal drug 116

Diphenylpyraline generic name of an antihistamine drug 117

Dipivefrin generic name of a drug used to treat glaucoma (487)

Diprolene brand name for betamethasone 164, the generic name of a corticosteroid drug 309

Dipyridamole 359, generic name of a drug used to treat abnormal blood clotting (182)

Disopyramide 362, generic name of an antiarrhythmic drug 113

Disulfiram 362, generic name of a drug used to treat alcohol dependence (81)

Dithranol 362, also called anthralin 112, generic name of a drug used for psoriasis (835)

Ditropan brand name for oxybutynin 766, the generic name of an anticholinergic drug 114 used to treat urinary incontinence (578)

Dixarit brand-name drug used to treat menopausal flashes (679)

Dobutamine generic name of a drug used to treat heart failure (518)

Dobutrex brand-name drug used to treat heart failure (518)

Docusate generic name of a laxative drug 632

Dolobid brand name for diflunisal 355, a nonsteroidal anti-inflammatory drug 736

Domperidone generic name of an antiemetic drug 116

Dopamine generic name for a natural neurotransmitter 730 used to treat heart failure (518) and shock (905)

Dopram brand-name drug used to stimulate respiration (867)

Doxapram generic name of a drug used to stimulate respiration (867)

Doxepin 369, generic name of a tricyclic antidepressant drug 115

Doxorubicin 369, generic name of an anticancer drug 114

Doxycycline 369, generic name of a tetracycline drug 979

Doxylamine generic name of an antihistamine drug 117, also used to treat nausea (721)

Drenison brand-name corticosteroid drug 309

Drisdol brand name for ergocalciferol 412, another name for vitamin D 1063

Droperidol generic name of an antiemetic drug 116

DTIC brand-name anticancer drug 114

Dulcolax brand-name stimulant laxative drug 632

Duolube brand-name drug used to relieve dry eyes (see keratoconjunctivitis sicca 614)

Durabolin brand name for nandrolone 719, the generic name of an anabolic steroid drug 95

Duralith brand name for lithium 643, the generic name of a drug used to treat manic-depressive illness (664)

Duratears brand name for artificial tear preparation (969)

Duretic brand name for a thiazide diuretic drug 363

Duricef brand name for cephalosporin 244, an antibiotic drug 113

Dyazide brand-name antihypertensive drug 119

Dycholium brand-name drug used to increase the flow of bile (165)

Dynapen brand-name penicillin drug 785, an antibiotic drug 113

Dyrenium brand name for triamterene 1012, the generic name of a potassium-sparing diuretic 363

Dysne-Inhal brand-name bronchodilator aerosol 213

E

Econazole 386, generic name of an antifungal drug 117

Ecostatin brand name for econazole 386, the generic name of an antifungal drug 117

Ecotrin brand-name nonsteroidal anti-inflammatory drug 736

Edecrin brand-name loop diuretic drug 363

EES brand name for erythromycin 414, the generic name of an antibiotic drug 113

Efudex brand name for fluorouracil 457

Elavil brand name for amitriptyline 93, the generic name of an antidepressant drug 115

Eldopaque brand-name preparation used to lighten the skin in disorders of pigmentation (800)

Eldoquin brand-name preparation used to lighten the skin in disorders of pigmentation (800)

Elixophyllin brand name for theophylline 981, the generic name of a bronchodilator 213

Eltroxin brand name for levothyroxine 638, the generic name of a thyroid hormone 544

Emcyt brand name for an anticancer drug 114

Emex brand name for metoclopramide 687, the generic name of an antiemetic drug 116

E-Mycin brand name for erythromycin 414, the generic name of an antibiotic drug 113

Enalapril 397, generic name of an ACE inhibitor drug 61

Enflurane generic name of a general anesthetic (103)

Entacyl brand name for a drug used to treat helminth infestation (525) (see worm infestation 1082)

Entrophen brand-name nonsteroidal anti-inflammatory drug 736

E-Pam brand name for diazepam 354, the generic name of a benzodiazepine 162 antianxiety drug 113

Ephedrine 407, generic name of a bronchodilator drug 213

Epifrin brand-name ophthalmic drug containing epinephrine 410

Epimorph brand name for morphine 698, the generic name of a narcotic analgesic drug 96

Epinephrine 410, hormone (544) which effects vasoconstriction (1045)

EpiPen brand-name injection containing epinephrine 410 for allergy therapy

Equanil brand name for meprobamate 683, the generic name of an antianxiety drug 113

Ergocalciferol another name for vitamin D 1063

Ergomar brand name for ergotamine 412, the generic name of a drug used to treat migraine (690)

Ergometrine 412, another name for ergonovine 412, the generic name of a drug used to stop bleeding after childbirth (260)

Ergonovine 412, generic name of a drug used to stop bleeding after childbirth (260)

Ergotamine 412, generic name of a drug used to treat migraine (690)

Eryc brand name for erythromycin 414, the generic name of an antibiotic drug 113

Erythrityl tetranitrate generic name of a nitrate drug 733 to treat angina pectoris (107)

Erythrocin brand name for erythromycin 414, the generic name of an antibiotic drug 113

Erythromid brand name for erythromycin 414, the generic name of an antibiotic drug 113

Erythromycin 414, generic name of an antibiotic drug 113

Estar brand name for coal tar 282, the generic name of an ingredient in some preparations for skin disorders (917)

Estinyl brand name for ethinyl estradiol 418

Estrace brand name for estradiol 418, the generic name of an estrogen drug 418 used to treat symptoms of menopause (679)

Estradiol 418, generic name of an estrogen drug 418 used to treat

symptoms of menopause (679)

Estramustine generic name of an anticancer drug 114

Estropipate generic name of an estrogen drug 418 used to treat symptoms of menopause (679)

Ethacrynic acid generic name of a loop diuretic drug 363

Ethambutol 418, generic name of a drug used to treat tuberculosis (1016)

Ethchlorvynol generic name of a sleeping drug 920

Ethinyl estradiol generic name of an estrogen drug 418

Ethopropazine generic name of a phenothiazine drug 796 used to treat parkinsonism (778)

Ethosuximide 419, generic name of an anticonvulsant drug 115

Ethrane brand-name general anesthetic (103)

Ethyl alcohol 419, another name for ethanol 419, a chemical name for alcohol in alcoholic drinks, produces intoxication (601), vomiting (1065) and coma (291)

Etidronate generic name of a drug used to treat Paget's disease (768)

Etoposide generic name of an anticancer drug 114

Etretinate 419, generic name of a drug used to treat psoriasis (835)

Euglucon brand name for glyburide 492, the generic name of a hypoglycemic drug 559

Eurax brand-name drug used to treat scabies (886)

F

Famotidine 437, generic name of a drug used to treat ulcers (1021)

Fansidar brand-name drug used to treat malaria (660)

Feldene brand name for piroxicam 801, the generic name of a nonsteroidal anti-inflammatory drug 736

Fenfluramine generic name of an appetite suppressant drug 127

Fenicol brand name for chloramphenicol eye ointment 267

Fenoprofen 442, generic name of a nonsteroidal

anti-inflammatory drug 736

Fenoterol generic name of a bronchodilator drug 213

Fentanyl generic name of an analgesic drug (96) used in general anesthesia (103)

Fer-In-Sol brand name for ferrous sulfate 442, an iron supplement 605

Ferrous sulfate 442, an iron supplement 605

Fibrinolysin generic name of a drug used to treat skin ulcers (1021)

Flagyl brand name for metronidazole 687, the generic name of an antibiotic drug 113

Flamazine brand name for an antibacterial drug 113

Flavoxate generic name of a urinary tract antispasmodic drug 119

Flaxedil brand name for a muscle-relaxant drug 710

Flecainide generic name of an antiarrhythmic drug 113

Flexeril brand name for cyclobenzaprine 323, the generic name of a muscle-relaxant drug 710

Florinef brand-name corticosteroid drug 309

Florone brand-name corticosteroid drug 309

Fluclox brand-name penicillin antibiotic 785

Flucloxacillin 456, generic name of a penicillin drug 785, an antibotic drug 113

Flucytosine generic name of an antifungal drug 117

Fludrocortisone generic name of a corticosteroid drug 309

Flunisolide generic name of a corticosteroid drug 309

Fluocinolone 456, generic name of a corticosteroid drug 309

Fluocinonide generic name of a corticosteroid drug 309

Fluonide brand name for fluocinolone 456, the generic name of a corticosteroid drug 309

Fluorouracil 457, generic name of an anticancer drug 114

Fluothane brand name for halothane 504, the generic name of a general anesthetic (103)

Fluoxetine generic name of an antidepressant drug 115

Fluphenazine 457, generic name of an antipsychotic drug 118

Flurandrenolide generic name of a corticosteroid drug 309

Flurazepam 457, generic name of a benzodiazepine 162 sleeping drug 920

Flurbiprofen generic name of a nonsteroidal anti-inflammatory drug 736

Folic acid 457, a vitamin 1059

Folvite brand name for folic acid 457, a vitamin 1059

Forane brand name for a general anesthetic (103)

Formulex brand name for dicyclomine 354, the generic name of an antispasmodic drug 119

Fortaz brand name for a cephalosporin drug 244, an antibiotic drug 113

Froben brand name for flurbiprofen, the generic name of a nonsteroidal anti-inflammatory drug 736

Frusemide 467, another name for furosemide 469, the generic name of a loop diuretic drug 363

Fulvicin U/F brand name for griseofulvin 497, the generic name of an antifungal drug 117

Fungizone brand name for amphotericin B 94, the generic name of an antifungal drug 117

Furosemide 469, generic name of a loop diuretic drug 363

G

Gallamine generic name of a muscle-relaxant drug 710

Gamma benzene hexachloride another name for lindane 641, the generic name of a drug used to treat scabies (886)

Gantanol brand name for sulfamethoxazole 957, the generic name of an antibacterial drug 113

Garamycin brand name for gentamicin 484, the generic name of an aminoglycoside 93, an antibiotic drug 113

Gastrozepin brand name for a drug used to treat peptic ulcers (1021)

Gemfibrozil 476, generic name of a lipid-lowering drug 642

Gentamicin 484, generic name of an aminoglycoside 93, an antibiotic drug 113

Gliclazide generic name of a hypoglycemic drug 559

Glucophage brand-name hypoglycemic agent 559

Glyburide 492, generic name of a hypoglycemic drug 559

Glyceryl trinitrate 492, vasodilator drug 1045 used to treat angina pectoris (107)

Glycopyrrolate generic name of an anticholinergic 114 and antispasmodic drug 119

Gold sodium thiomalate generic name of an antirheumatic drug 117 containing gold 493, an antirheumatic drug 117 used to treat rheumatoid arthritis (873)

Gramicidin 496, generic name of an antibiotic drug 113

Gravol brand name for dimenhydrinate 358, the generic name of an antiemetic drug 116

Green soap an antiseptic 118 in liquid soap form

Griseofulvin 497, generic name of an antifungal drug 117

Guaifenesin 500, generic name of an expectorant 424

Guanethidine 500, generic name of an antihypertensive drug 117

Gynergen brand name for ergotamine 412, the generic name of a drug used to treat migraine (690)

H

Halcion brand name for triazolam 1012, the generic name of a benzodiazepine sleeping drug 162

Haldol brand name for haloperidol 504, the generic name of an antipsychotic drug 118

Haloperidol 504, generic name of an antipsychotic drug 118

Haloprogin generic name of an antifungal drug 117

Halotex brand-name antifungal drug 117

Halothane 504, generic name of a general anesthetic (103)

HCG abbreviation for human chorionic gonadotropin 494

Heparin 531, generic name

of an anticoagulant drug 115

Herplex brand name for idoxuridine 565, the generic name of an antiviral drug 119

Hexachlorophene an antiseptic 118

Hexadrol brand name for dexamethasone 345, the generic name of a corticosteroid drug 309

Hismanal brand name for astemizole, the generic name of an antihistamine drug 117

Histantil brand name for promethazine 829, the generic name of an antihistamine drug 117

HMS brand-name corticosteroid drug 309 used to treat eye inflammation (425)

Homatropine generic name of an anticholinergic drug 114

Human chorionic gonadotropin generic name of a drug used to treat infertility (582)

Humulin brand name for insulin 593, a hormone (544) that regulates blood sugar levels

Hyaluronidase enzyme that aids in the dispersion of injected drugs 373

Hycort brand name for hydrocortisone 549, the generic name of a corticosteroid drug 309

Hydralazine 549, generic name of an antihypertensive drug 117

Hydrea brand-name anticancer drug 114

Hydrochlorothiazide 549, generic name of a thiazide diuretic drug 363

Hydrocodone generic name of a narcotic drug 720 used mainly in cough remedies 314

Hydrocortisone 549, generic name of a corticosteroid drug 309

HydroDiuril brand name for hydrochlorothiazide 549, the generic name of a thiazide diuretic drug 363

Hydrogen peroxide 549, type of antiseptic 118

Hydromorphone generic name of a narcotic drug 720, an analgesic drug 96

Hydropres brand-name antihypertensive drug 117

Hydroquinone generic name of a drug used to lighten the skin in disorders of skin pigmentation (800)

Hydroxocobalamin 550, synthetic form of vitamin B_{12} 1061

Hydroxychloroquine generic name of a drug used to treat malaria (660)

Hydroxyurea generic name of an anticancer drug 114

Hydroxyzine generic name of an antihistamine drug 117

Hygroton brand name for chlorthalidone 268, the generic name of a thiazide diuretic 363 and antihypertensive drug 117

Hyoscine another name for scopolamine 891, the generic name of an antispasmodic drug 119

Hyoscyamine 551, generic name of an anticholinergic drug 114

Hytrin brand-name antihypertensive drug 117

I

Ibuprofen 565, generic name of a nonsteroidal anti-inflammatory drug 736

Idoxuridine 565, generic name of an antiviral drug 119

Iletin brand name for insulin 593, a hormone (544) that regulates blood sugar levels

Ilosone brand name for erythromycin 414, the generic name of an antibiotic drug 113

Ilotycin brand name for erythromycin 414, the generic name of an antibiotic drug 113

Imipramine 569, generic name of an antidepressant drug 115

Immune serum globulin 569, preparation of antibodies also known as immune globulin and gamma globulin

Imodium brand name for loperamide 650, the generic name of an antidiarrheal drug 116

Impril brand name for imipramine 569, the generic name of an antidepressant drug 115

Imuran brand name for azathioprine 148, the generic name of an immunosuppressant drug 575

Inapsine brand-name antiemetic drug 116

Indapamide generic name

of a thiazidelike diuretic drug 363

Inderal brand name for propranolol 829, the generic name of a beta-blocker drug 163

Inderide brand-name drug containing hydrochlorothiazide 549, the generic name of a thiazide diuretic drug 363, and propranolol 829, the generic name of a beta-blocker drug 163

Indocid brand name for indomethacin 580, the generic name of a nonsteroidal anti-inflammatory drug 736

Indomethacin 580, generic name of a nonsteroidal anti-inflammatory drug 736

Inflamase brand name for prednisolone 818, the generic name of a corticosteroid drug (309) in eye drop form

INH another name for isoniazid 607, the generic name of a drug used to treat tuberculosis (1016)

Inocor brand-name drug used to treat heart failure (518)

Inositol niacinate generic name of a drug used to treat peripheral vascular disease (789)

Insulin 593, a hormone (544) that regulates blood sugar levels

Insulin Toronto brand name for insulin 593, a hormone (544) that regulates blood sugar levels

Intal brand name for cromolyn sodium, the generic name of a drug used for the prevention of asthma (136)

Interferon 598, generic name of an antiviral 119 and anticancer drug 114

Intrabutazone brand name for phenylbutazone 796, the generic name of a nonsteroidal anti-inflammatory drug 736

Intron A brand name for interferon 598, the generic name of an antiviral 119 and anticancer drug 114

Intropin brand name for dopamine, a natural neurotransmitter 730 used to treat heart failure (518) and shock (905)

Iodine 604, an element, compounds of which are used as antiseptics 118

Iodoquinol generic name of a drug used to treat

amebiasis 91

Ionamin brand name for phentermine 796, the generic name of an appetite suppressant drug 127

Iopanoic acid compound used in diagnostic imaging (567)

Ipecac 605, generic name of a drug used to induce vomiting

Ipodate generic name of a drug used in diagnostic imaging (567)

Ipratropium 605, generic name of an anticholinergic drug 114 used as a bronchodilator drug 213

Iron 605, an essential mineral

Ismelin brand name for guanethidine 500, the generic name of an antihypertensive drug 117

Isocarboxazid 607, generic name of an antidepressant drug 115

Isoflurane generic name of a general anesthetic (103)

Isoniazid 607, generic name of a drug used to treat tuberculosis (1016)

Isopropamide generic name of an antispasmodic drug 119

Isoproterenol 607, generic name of a bronchodilator drug 213

Isoptin brand name for verapamil 1050, the generic name of a calcium-channel blocker 221

Isopto Carbachol brand name for carbachol eye drops 228, the generic name of a drug used to treat glaucoma (487)

Isopto Carpine brand name for pilocarpine eye drops 800, the generic name of a drug used to treat glaucoma (487)

Isopto Cetamide brand name for sulfacetamide eye drops 957, the generic name of an antibacterial drug 113

Isordil brand name for isosorbide dinitrate 607, a nitrate drug 733, the generic name of a vasodilator drug 1045

Isosorbide dinitrate 607, generic name of a vasodilator drug 1045

Isotamine brand name for isoniazid 607, the generic name of a drug used to treat tuberculosis (1016)

Isotretinoin 607, generic name of a drug derived from vitamin A 1060 used to treat acne (63)

Isoxsuprine 607, generic name of a vasodilator drug 1045

Isuprel brand name for isoproterenol 607, the generic name of a bronchodilator drug 213

K

Kaochlor brand-name potassium supplement 817

Kaolin 613, generic name of an ingredient of some antidiarrheal drugs 116

Kaon brand-name potassium supplement 817

Kay Ciel brand-name potassium supplement 817

Keflin brand-name cephalosporin drug 244, an antibiotic drug 113

Kefzol brand-name cephalosporin drug 244, an antibiotic drug 113

Kemadrin brand name for procyclidine 827, the generic name of an anticholinergic drug 114 used to treat parkinsonism (778)

Kenalog brand-name corticosteroid drug 309

Ketalar brand name for a general anesthetic (103)

Ketamine generic name of a general anesthetic (103)

Ketoconazole 615, generic name of an antifungal drug 117

Ketoprofen 615, generic name of a nonsteroidal anti-inflammatory drug 736

Kidrolase brand-name anticancer drug 114

Konakion brand name for phytomenadione 799, the generic name of a drug that controls bleeding

Kwellada brand name for lindane 641, the generic name of a drug used to treat scabies (886) and lice (638)

L

Labetalol 625, generic name of a beta-blocker drug 163

Lacrisert brand-name artificial tear preparation (969)

Lactulax brand name for lactulose 626, the generic name of a laxative drug 632

Lactulose 626, generic name of a laxative drug 632

Lanoxin brand name for digoxin 357, the generic name of a digitalis drug 357

Largactil brand name for chlorpromazine 267, the generic name of an antipsychotic drug 118

Larodopa brand name for levodopa 638, the generic name of a drug used to treat parkinsonism (778)

Lasix brand name for furosemide 469, the generic name of a loop diuretic drug 363

Lectopam brand name for bromazepam, the generic name of a benzodiazepine 162 antianxiety drug 113

Leukeran brand-name anticancer drug 114

Leuprolide generic name of an anticancer drug 114

Levate brand name for amitriptyline 93, the generic name of an antidepressant drug 115

Levobunolol generic name of a beta-blocker drug 163 used to treat glaucoma (487)

Levodopa 638, generic name of a drug used to treat parkinsonism (778)

Levo-Dromoran brand name for a narcotic drug 720, an analgesic drug 96

Levonorgestrel 638, generic name of a progestogen drug 828 used in oral contraceptives 751

Levorphan generic name of a narcotic drug 720, an analgesic drug 96

Levothyroxine 638, generic name of a thyroid hormone (544)

Librax brand-name antispasmodic (119) and antianxiety compound (113)

Librium brand name for chlordiazepoxide 267, the generic name of a benzodiazepine 162 antianxiety drug 113

Lidex brand-name topical corticosteroid drug 309

Lidocaine 639, generic name of a local anesthetic (105)

Lincocin brand name for lincomycin 641, the generic name of an antibiotic drug 113

Lincomycin 641, generic name of an antibiotic drug 113

Lindane 641, generic name of a drug used to treat scabies (886) and lice (638)

Linodil brand name for a drug used to treat peripheral vascular disease (789)

Lioresal brand name for baclofen 151, the generic name of a muscle-relaxant drug 710

Liothyronine generic name of a synthetic thyroid hormone (544)

Lithane brand name for lithium 643, the generic name of a drug used to treat manic-depressive illness (664)

Lithium 643, generic name of a drug used to treat manic-depressive illness (664)

Lomine brand name for dicyclomine 354, the generic name of an antispasmodic drug 119

Lomotil brand-name drug containing diphenoxylate 358, the generic name of an antidiarrheal drug 116

Lomustine generic name of an anticancer drug 114

Loniten brand name for minoxidil, the generic name of a vasodilator drug 1045

Loperamide 650, generic name of an antidiarrheal drug 116

Lopid brand name for gemfibrozil 476, the generic name of a lipid-lowering drug 642

Lopresor brand name for metoprolol, the generic name of a beta-blocker drug 163

Loprox brand-name antifungal drug 117

Loratadine 650, generic name of an antihistamine drug 117

Lorazepam 650, generic name of a benzodiazepine 162 sleeping drug 920

Lorelco brand name for probucol 827, the generic name of a lipid-lowering drug 642

Loroxide brand name for benzoyl peroxide 162, the generic name of a drug used topically to treat acne (63)

Losec brand name for a drug used to treat peptic ulcers (1021)

Lovastatin 650, generic name of a lipid-lowering drug 642

Loxapac brand-name antidepressant drug 115

Loxapine generic name of an antidepressant drug 115

Lozide brand name for indapamide, the generic name of a thiazidelike diuretic drug 363

Ludiomil brand name for maprotiline 665, the generic name of an antidepressant drug 115

Lugol's Solution preparation of iodine 604 used to treat hyperthyroidism (563)

Lysergic acid diethylamide another name for LSD 650, a synthetic hallucinogenic drug 503

Lysodren brand-name anticancer drug 114

M

Macrodantin brand name for nitrofurantoin 734, the generic name of an antibiotic drug 113

Mafenide generic name of a topical antibacterial drug 113

Magnesium 659, mineral 692, compounds of which are used in antacid (112) and laxative drugs (632)

Magnesium citrate laxative drug 632

Magnesium gluconate magnesium supplement 659

Magnesium hydroxide antacid drug 112

Magnesium salicylate antirheumatic drug 117

Magnesium sulfate magnesium supplement 659

Malathion generic name of a drug used to treat lice (638)

Mandelamine brand-name drug used to treat urinary tract infections (1030)

Mandol brand-name cephalosporin drug 244

Mannitol 664, generic name of an osmotic diuretic drug 363

Maprotiline 665, generic name of an antidepressant drug 115

Marcaine brand-name local anesthetic 105

Marijuana 665, generic name of a central nervous system depressant 341

Marplan brand name for isocarboxazid 607, the generic name of an antidepressant drug 115

Marzine brand-name antiemetic drug 116

Maxeran brand name for metoclopramide 687, the generic name of an antiemetic drug 116

Maxidex brand name for dexamethasone eye preparations 345, the generic name of a corticosteroid drug 309

Mazepine brand name for carbamazepine 228, the generic name of an anticonvulsant drug 115

Mazindol generic name of an appetite suppressant drug 127

Mebaral brand-name anticonvulsant drug 115

Mebendazole 670, generic name of a drug used to treat helminth infestation (525) (see worm infestation 1082)

Mechlorethamine generic name of an anticancer drug 114

Meclizine 670, generic name of an antiemetic drug 116

Medihaler-Epi brand-name epinephrine bronchodilator aerosol 213

Medihaler-Ergotamine brand name for ergotamine aerosol used to treat migraine (690)

Medihaler-Iso brand-name isoproterenol bronchodilator aerosol 213

Medilium brand name for chlordiazepoxide 267, the generic name of a benzodiazepine antianxiety drug 113

Medrogestone generic name of a progestogen drug 828

Medrol brand name for methylprednisolone 687, the generic name of a synthetic corticosteroid drug 309

Medroxyprogesterone 673, generic name of a progestogen drug 828

Medrysone generic name of a corticosteroid drug 309 used to treat eye inflammation (425)

Mefenamic acid 674, generic name of a nonsteroidal anti-inflammatory drug 118

Mefoxin brand name for cefoxitin, the generic name of a cephalosporin drug 244, an antibiotic drug 113

Megace brand-name progestogen drug (828), an anticancer drug 114

Megacillin brand name for penicillin G, the generic name of a penicillin drug 785, an antibiotic drug 113

Megestrol 675, generic name of a progestogen drug 828, an anticancer drug 114

Mellaril brand name for thioridazine 982, the generic name of an antipsychotic drug 118

Melphalan 676, generic name of an anticancer drug 114

Menadiol another name for vitamin K 1064

Menadione another name for vitamin K 1064

Menotropins 680, generic name of a drug used to treat infertility (582)

Menthol 683, an extract from mint used in inhalations and to treat some skin irritations (917)

Meperidine 683, generic name of a narcotic drug 720, an analgesic drug 96

Mephenytoin generic name of an anticonvulsant drug 115

Mephobarbital generic name of an anticonvulsant drug 115

Mepivacaine generic name of a local anesthetic (105)

Meprobamate 683, generic name of an antianxiety drug 113

Mercaptopurine 683, generic name of an anticancer drug 114

Mesalamine 684, generic name of a drug used to treat inflammatory bowel disease (587)

Mesantoin brand-name anticonvulsant drug 115

Mescaline 684, generic name of a hallucinogenic drug 503

Mesoridazine generic name of an antipsychotic drug 118

Mestinon 684, brand name for pyridostigmine 846, the generic name of a drug used to treat myasthenia gravis (713)

Mestranol 684, generic name of an estrogen drug 418

Metamucil brand-name laxative drug 632

Metandren brand-name androgen drug 98

Metaproterenol 685, another name for orciprenaline 754, the generic name of a bronchodilator drug 213

Metformin 686, generic name of a hypoglycemic drug 559 used to treat non-insulin-dependent diabetes mellitus (346)

Methadone 686, generic

name of a narcotic 720 analgesic drug 96

Methenamine mandelate generic name of a drug used to treat urinary tract infections (1030)

Methimazole 686, generic name of a drug used to treat hyperthyroidism (557)

Methocarbamol 686, generic name of a muscle-relaxant drug 710

Methotrexate 686, generic name of an anticancer drug 114

Methotrimeprazine 686, generic name of an antipsychotic drug 118

Methoxsalen 686, generic name of a drug used to treat psoriasis (835)

Methsuximide generic name of an anticonvulsant drug 115

Methyclothiazide 686, generic name of a thiazide diuretic drug 363

Methylcellulose 687, generic name of a laxative 632 and antidiarrheal drug 116

Methyldopa 687, generic name of an antihypertensive drug 117

Methylphenidate generic name of a central nervous system stimulant (945)

Methylprednisolone 687, generic name of a corticosteroid drug 309

Methyltestosterone generic name of an androgen drug 98

Methyprylon generic name of a sleeping drug 920

Methysergide generic name of a drug used to prevent migraine (690)

Meticorten brand name for prednisone 818, the generic name of a corticosteroid drug 309

Metoclopramide 687, generic name of an antiemetic drug 116

Metocurine generic name of a muscle-relaxant drug 710 used in general anesthesia (103)

Metolazone 687, generic name of a thiazidelike diuretic drug 363

Metopirone brand name for a drug used to treat Cushing's syndrome 322

Metoprolol generic name of a beta-blocker drug 163

Metronidazole 687, generic name of an antibiotic drug 113

Metubine Iodide brand name for a muscle-relaxant drug 710 used in general anesthesia (103)

Metyrapone generic name of a drug used to treat Cushing's syndrome 322

Mevacor brand name for lovastatin 650, the generic name of a lipid-lowering drug 642

Mexiletine 687, generic name of an antiarrhythmic drug 113

Mexitil brand name for an antiarrhythmic drug 113

Micatin brand name for an antifungal drug 117

Miconazole 687, generic name of an antifungal drug 117

Micro-K brand-name potassium supplement used with antihypertensive drugs (117)

Micronor brand name for norethindrone 736, the generic name of a progestogen drug 828 used in oral contraceptives 751

Midamor brand name for amiloride 92, the generic name of a potassium-sparing diuretic drug 363

Midazolam generic name of a benzodiazepine drug 162 used for premedication (822)

Milk of Magnesia brand-name antacid drug 112

Mineral oil 692, lubricant laxative drug 632

Minestrin brand-name oral contraceptive 751

Minipress brand name for prazosin 818, the generic name of a vasodilator drug 1045

Minocin brand name for minocycline, the generic name of a tetracycline drug 979, an antibiotic drug 113

Minocycline generic name of a tetracycline drug 979, an antibiotic drug 113

Minoxidil generic name of a vasodilator drug 1045, also applied topically to stimulate hair growth (502)

Miocarpine brand name for pilocarpine eye drops 800, the generic name of a drug used to treat glaucoma (487)

Miostat brand name for carbachol eye drops 228, the generic name of a drug used to treat glaucoma (487)

Misoprostol 694, generic name of a prostaglandin drug 829

Mitotane generic name of an anticancer drug 114

Mixtard brand name for insulin 593, a hormone (544) that regulates blood sugar levels

Moditen brand name for fluphenazine 457, the generic name of an antipsychotic drug 118

Moduret brand-name drug containing amiloride 92, the generic name of a potassium-sparing diuretic drug 363, and hydrochlorothiazide 549, the generic name of a thiazide diuretic drug 363

Mogadon brand-name benzodiazepine drug 162 used to treat sleep disorders (919) and epilepsy (409)

Monobenzone generic name of a drug used to treat vitiligo (1064)

Monosodium glutamate 697, a food additive 458

Morphine 698, generic name of a narcotic 720 analgesic drug 96

Motilium brand name for domperidone 367, the generic name of an antiemetic drug 116

Motrin brand name for ibuprofen 565, the generic name of a nonsteroidal anti-inflammatory drug 736

Mucomyst brand-name mucolytic drug 704

Muromonab CD3 generic name of an immunosuppressant drug 575

Mustargen brand-name anticancer drug 114

Myambutol brand name for a drug used to treat tuberculosis (1016)

Mycifradin brand name for neomycin 723, the generic name of an antibiotic drug 113

Myciguent brand name for neomycin 723, the generic name of an antibiotic drug 113

Myclo brand name for clotrimazole 281, the generic name of an antifungal drug 117

Mycostatin brand name for nystatin 743, the generic name of an antifungal drug 117

Mydfrin brand name for phenylephrine eye drops 796, the generic name of a decongestant drug 333

Mydriacyl brand name for tropicamide eye drops 1016, the generic name of a drug used to dilate the pupil (844)

Myleran brand-name anticancer drug 114

Myochrisine brand name for a gold compound used to treat rheumatoid arthritis (813)

Mysoline brand name for primidone 827, the generic name of an anticonvulsant drug 115

Mytelase brand-name drug used to treat myasthenia gravis (713)

N

Nabilone generic name of an antiemetic drug 116

Nadolol 719, generic name of a beta-blocker drug 163

Nadopen-V brand name for penicillin V, the generic name of a penicillin drug 785

Nafcillin generic name of a penicillin drug 785, an antibiotic drug 113

Nalbuphine generic name of an analgesic drug 96

Nalcrom brand name for a drug taken orally for gastrointestinal food allergy (459)

Nalfon brand-name nonsteroidal anti-inflammatory drug 736

Nalidixic acid 719, generic name of an antibiotic drug 113

Naloxone 719, generic name of a drug that blocks the action of narcotic drugs 720

Nandrolone 719, generic name of an anabolic steroid drug 944

Naphazoline 719, generic name of a decongestant drug 333

Naprosyn brand name for naproxen 719, the generic name of a nonsteroidal anti-inflammatory drug 736

Naproxen 719, generic name of a nonsteroidal anti-inflammatory drug 736

Narcan brand name for naloxone 719, the generic name of a drug that blocks the action of narcotic drugs 720

Nardil brand name for phenelzine 796, the generic name of a monoamine oxidase inhibitor, an antidepressant drug 115

Natulan brand name for an anticancer drug 114

Naturetin brand name for bendroflumethiazide, the generic name of a thiazidelike diuretic drug 363

Navane brand name for thiothixene 982, the generic name of an antipsychotic drug 118

Naxen brand name for naproxen 719, the generic name of a nonsteroidal anti-inflammatory drug 736

Nebcin brand name for tobramycin 996, the generic name of an antibiotic drug 113

NegGram brand name for nalidixic acid 719, the generic name of an antibiotic drug 113

Nemasol brand name for para-aminosalicylic acid 774, the generic name of a drug used to treat tuberculosis (1016)

Nembutal brand name for pentobarbital 786, the generic name of a barbiturate drug 155

Neo-Bex vitamin B complex preparation containing vitamin C 1063

Neo-Codema brand name for hydrochlorothiazide 549, the generic name of a thiazide diuretic drug 363

Neo-Cortef brand-name drug containing hydrocortisone 549, the generic name of a corticosteroid drug 309, and neomycin 723, the generic name of an antibiotic drug 113

Neo-Medrol brand-name drug containing methylprednisolone 687, a generic name of a corticosteroid drug 309, and neomycin 723, the generic name of an antibiotic drug 113

Neo-Metric brand-name drug containing metronidazole 687, the generic name of an antibiotic drug 113

Neomycin 723, generic name of an antibiotic drug 113

Neosporin brand-name topical antibiotic preparation 113

Neostigmine 723, generic name of a drug used to treat myasthenia gravis (713)

Neo-Synephrine brand name for phenylephrine 796, the generic name of a sympathomimetic drug

Nephronex brand name for nitrofurantoin 734, the generic name of an antibiotic drug 113

Netilmicin 725, generic name of an antibiotic drug 113

Netromycin brand name for netilmicin 725, the generic name of an antibiotic drug 113

Niacin 732, member of the vitamin B complex 1062

Niacinamide 732, a form of niacin, a member of the vitamin B complex 1062

Nicorette brand-name drug used to aid in smoking cessation (996)

Nicotine stimulant drug found in tobacco 995, also used in preparations to aid in smoking cessation (996)

Nicoumalone generic name of an anticoagulant drug 115

Nifedipine 732, generic name of a calcium channel blocker drug 221

Nitrazepam generic name of a benzodiazepine drug 162 used to treat sleep disorders (919) and epilepsy (409)

Nitro-Bid brand name for nitroglycerin 734, the generic name of a vasodilator drug 1045

Nitrofurantoin 734, generic name of an antibiotic drug 113

Nitrogen mustard generic name of an anticancer drug 114

Nitroglycerin 734, generic name of a vasodilator drug 1045

Nitrol brand name for nitroglycerin 734, the generic name of a vasodilator drug 1045

Nitrolingual brand name for nitroglycerin spray 734, the generic name of a vasodilator drug 1045

Nitrostat brand name for nitroglycerin 734, the generic name of a vasodilator drug 1045

Nitrous oxide 734, gas used to induce general anesthesia (103)

Nix brand name for a drug used to treat lice (638)

Nizatidine 734, generic name of a drug used to treat ulcers (1021)

Nizoral brand name for ketoconazole 615, the generic name of an antifungal drug 117

Noctec brand name for chloral hydrate 267, the generic name of a sleeping drug 920

Noludar brand name for methyprylon, the generic name of a sleeping drug 920

Nonoxynol-9 generic name of a spermicide 930

Norcuron brand name for a muscle-relaxant drug 710

Norepinephrine 736, hormone (544)

Norethindrone 736, generic name of a progestogen drug 828 used in oral contraceptives 751

Norflex brand name for orphenadrine 755, the generic name of a muscle-relaxant drug 710

Norfloxacin generic name of an antibiotic drug 113

Norgestrel 736, generic name of a progestogen drug 828

Norinyl brand-name oral contraceptive 751

Norlestrin brand-name oral contraceptive 751

Norlutate brand name for norethindrone 736, the generic name of a progestogen drug 828

Noroxin brand name for an antibiotic drug 113

Norpace brand name for disopyramide 362, the generic name of an antiarrhythmic drug 113

Norpramin brand name for desipramine 343, the generic name of a tricyclic antidepressant drug 115

Nortriptyline 736, generic name of an antidepressant drug 115

Novamoxin brand name for amoxicillin 94, the generic name of a penicillin drug 785

Novo-Ampicillin brand name for ampicillin 95, the generic name of a penicillin drug 785, an antibiotic drug 113

Novobutamide brand name for tolbutamide 998, the generic name of a hypoglycemic drug 559

Novobutazone brand name for phenylbutazone 796, the generic name of a nonsteroidal anti-inflammatory drug 736

Novocain brand name for procaine 827, the generic name of a local anesthetic (105)

Novocarbamaz brand name for carbamazepine 228, the generic name of an anticonvulsant drug 115

Novochlorocap brand name for chloramphenicol 267, the generic name of an antibiotic drug 113

Novochloroquine brand name for chloroquine 267, the generic name of a drug used to treat malaria (660)

Novochlorpromazine brand name for chlorpromazine 267, the generic name of an antipsychotic drug 718

Novocimetine brand name for cimetidine 277, the generic name of a drug used to treat ulcers (1021)

Novoclopate brand name for clorazepate 281, the generic name of a benzodiazepine antianxiety drug 113

Novocloxin brand name for cloxacillin 281, the generic name of a penicillin drug 785, an antibiotic drug 113

Novodigoxin brand name for digoxin 357, the generic name of a digitalis drug 357

Novodipam brand name for diazepam 354, the generic name of a benzodiazepine 162 antianxiety drug 113

Novodoparil brand-name drug containing hydrochlorothiazide 549, the generic name of a thiazide diuretic drug 363, and methyldopa 687, the generic name of an antihypertensive drug 98

Novoferrogluc brand name for ferrous gluconate, the generic name of an iron supplement 605

Novoferrosulfa brand name for ferrous sulfate, the generic name of an iron supplement 605

Novofibrate brand name for clofibrate 281, the generic name of a lipid-lowering drug 642

Novoflupam brand name for flurazepam 457, the generic name of a benzodiazepine 162 sleeping drug 920

Novoflurazine brand name for trifluoperazine 1013, the generic name of an antipsychotic drug 118

Novofuran brand name for nitrofurantoin 734, the generic name of an antibiotic drug 113

Novohydrazide brand name for hydrochlorothiazide 549, the generic name of a thiazide diuretic drug 363

Novohylazin brand name for hydralazine 549, the generic name of an antihypertensive drug 117

Novolexin brand name for cephalexin 244, the generic name of a cephalosporin drug 244, an antibiotic drug 113

Novolin brand-name preparation of insulin 593, a hormone (544) that regulates blood sugar levels

Novolorazem brand name for lorazepam 650, the generic name of a benzodiazepine 162 sleeping drug 920

Novomedopa brand name for methyldopa 687, the generic name of an antihypertensive drug 117

Novomethacin brand name for indomethacin 580, the generic name of a nonsteroidal anti-inflammatory drug 736

Novometoprol brand name for metoprolol, the generic name of a beta-blocker drug 163

Novonaprox brand name for naproxen 719, the generic name of a nonsteroidal anti-inflammatory drug 736

Novonidazol brand name for metronidazole 687, the generic name of an antibiotic drug 113

Novonifedin brand name for nifedipine 732, the generic name of a calcium channel blocker drug 221

Novopen G brand name for penicillin G, the generic name of a penicillin drug 785, an antibiotic drug 113

Novopen-VK-500 brand name for penicillin V, the generic name of a penicillin drug 785, an antibiotic drug 113

Novoperidol brand name for haloperidol 504, the generic name of an antipsychotic drug 118

Novopheniram brand name for chlorpheniramine 267, the generic name of an antihistamine drug 117

Novopirocam brand name for piroxicam 801, the generic name of a nonsteroidal anti-inflammatory drug 736

Novopoxide brand name for chlordiazepoxide 267, the generic name of a benzodiazepine 162

antianxiety drug 113

Novopramine brand name for imipramine 569, the generic name of an antidepressant drug 115

Novopranol brand name for propranolol 829, the generic name of a beta-blocker drug 163

Novoprednisolone brand name for prednisolone 818, the generic name of a corticosteroid drug 309

Novoprednisone brand name for prednisone 818, the generic name of a corticosteroid drug 309

Novoprofen brand name for ibuprofen 565, the generic name of a nonsteroidal anti-inflammatory drug 736

Novopropamide brand name for chlorpropamide 268, the generic name of a drug used to treat diabetes mellitus (346)

Novopurol brand name for allopurinol 87, the generic name of a drug used to treat gout (495)

Novopyrazone brand name for sulfinpyrazone 957, the generic name of a drug used to treat gout (495)

Novoquinidin brand name for quinidine 847, the generic name of an antiarrhythmic drug 113

Novoquinine brand name for quinine 847, the generic name of a drug used to treat malaria (660)

Novoridazine brand name for thioridazine 982, the generic name of a phenothiazine antipsychotic drug 118

Novorythro brand name for erythromycin 414, the generic name of an antibiotic drug 113

Novosalmol brand name for salbutamol 883, the generic name of a bronchodilator drug 213

Novosecobarb brand name for secobarbital, the generic name of a barbiturate drug 155

Novosemide brand name for furosemide 469, the generic name of a loop diuretic drug 363

Novosorbide brand name for isosorbide dinitrate 607, a nitrate drug 733, the generic name of a vasodilator drug 1045

Novosoxazole brand name for sulfisoxazole 957, the generic name of an antibacterial drug 113

Novospiroton brand name for spironolactone 935, the generic name of a potassium-sparing diuretic drug 363

Novospirozine brand-name drug containing spironolactone 935, the generic name of a potassium-sparing diuretic drug 363, and hydrochlorothiazide 549, the generic name of a thiazide diuretic drug 363

Novosundac brand name for sulindac 957, the generic name of a nonsteroidal anti-inflammatory drug 736

Novotetra brand name for tetracycline, the generic name of an antibiotic drug 113

Novothalidone brand name for chlorthalidone 268, the generic name of a thiazide diuretic drug 363, an antihypertensive drug 117

Novotriphyl brand name for oxtriphylline 766, the generic name of a bronchodilator drug 213

Novotriptyn brand name for amitriptyline 93, the generic name of an antidepressant drug 115

Nozinan brand name for methotrimeprazine 686, the generic name of an antipsychotic drug 118

NPH insulin brand-name preparation of insulin 593, a hormone (544) that regulates blood sugar levels

Nubain brand name analgesic drug 96

Numorphan generic name of a narcotic drug 720, an analgesic drug 96

Nupercainal brand-name local anesthetic (105)

Nylidrin generic name of a vasodilator drug 1045

Nystatin 743, generic name of an antifungal drug 117

O

Occlusal brand name for salicylic acid 883, the generic name of a keratolytic drug 614

Ocuclear brand name for oxymetazoline eye drops 767, the generic name of a topical decongestant drug 333

Ocufen brand name for flurbiprofen eye drops,

the generic name of a nonsteroidal anti-inflammatory drug 736

Ocusert brand name for pilocarpine 800, the generic name of a drug used to treat glaucoma (487)

Ogen brand-name estrogen drug 418

Olive oil 747, oil used to treat cradle cap (315)

Omeprazole generic name of a drug used to treat peptic ulcers (1021)

Oncovin brand-name anticancer drug 114

Opcon brand name for naphazoline eye drops 719, the generic name of a decongestant drug 333

Opium 750, a naturally occurring narcotic drug 720, an analgesic drug 96

Optimine brand name for azatadine 148, the generic name of an antihistamine drug 117

Oradexon brand name for dexamethasone 345, the generic name of a corticosteroid drug 309

Oragrafin brand-name drug used in diagnostic imaging (567)

Orajel brand name for benzocaine, the generic name of a local anesthetic (105)

Orap brand name for pimozide 800, the generic name of a drug used to treat Gilles de la Tourette's syndrome (485)

Orbenin brand name for cloxacillin 281, the generic name of a penicillin drug 785, an antibiotic drug 113

Orciprenaline 754, generic name of a bronchodilator drug 213

Orinase brand name for tolbutamide 998, the generic name of a hypoglycemic drug 559

Ornex Cold brand name for pseudoephedrine 834, the generic name of a decongestant drug 333

Ornex-DM brand name for dextromethorphan 346, the generic name of a cough suppressant 314

Orphenadrine 755, generic name of a muscle-relaxant drug 710 used to treat parkinsonism (778)

Orthoclone OKT3 brand-name immunosuppressant drug 575

Ortho-Novum 1/35 brand-name oral contraceptive 751

Orudis brand name for

ketoprofen 615, the generic name of a nonsteroidal anti-inflammatory drug 736

Os-Cal-D brand-name drug containing calcium and vitamin D 1063

Otrivin brand name for xylometazoline 1087, the generic name of a nasal decongestant drug 333

Ovol brand name for a drug used to relieve flatulence (455)

Ovral brand-name oral contraceptive 751

Ovulen brand-name oral contraceptive 751

Oxazepam 766, generic name of a benzodiazepine 162 antianxiety drug 113

Oxprenolol 766, generic name of a beta-blocker drug 163

Oxsoralen brand name for methoxsalen 686, the generic name of a drug used to treat psoriasis (835)

Oxtriphylline 766, generic name of a bronchodilator drug 213

Oxybenzone generic name of a drug used in sunscreen preparations (955)

Oxybutynin 766, generic name of an anticholinergic drug 114 used to treat urinary incontinence (578)

Oxycodone 766, generic name of a narcotic drug 720, an analgesic drug 96

Oxymetazoline 767, generic name of a nasal and ophthalmic decongestant drug 333

Oxymorphone generic name of a narcotic drug 720, an analgesic drug 96

Oxyphenbutazone generic name of a nonsteroidal anti-inflammatory drug 736

Oxytocin 767, a pituitary hormone (544) used to induce labor (580)

P

Paludrine brand-name drug used to treat malaria (660)

Pancrease brand name for preparation of pancreatic hormones 544

Pancrelipase preparation of pancreatic hormones 544

Pancuronium generic name of a muscle-relaxant drug 710

Panectyl brand-name antihistamine drug 117

Panthenol form of pantothenic acid, a member of the vitamin B complex 1062

Pantopon brand-name narcotic drug 720 containing morphine and opium 698, the generic name of an analgesic drug 96

Pantothenic acid member of the vitamin B complex 1062

Papaverine generic name of a vasodilator drug 1045

Para-aminobenzoic acid 774, generic name of a drug used in many sunscreens (958)

Para-aminosalicylic acid 774, generic name of a drug used to treat tuberculosis (1016)

Paradione brand name for an anticonvulsant drug 115

Paraldehyde 774, generic name of an anticonvulsant drug 115

Paramethadione generic name of an anticonvulsant drug 115

Parlodel brand name for bromocriptine 211, the generic name of a drug used to treat parkinsonism (778)

Parnate brand name for a monoamine oxidase inhibitor antidepressant 115

Parsitan brand name for a drug used to treat parkinsonism (778)

Paveral brand name for codeine 283, the generic name of a narcotic drug 720

Pavulon brand-name muscle-relaxant drug 710

Pemoline 774, generic name of a stimulant drug 945

Penglobe brand-name antibiotic drug 113

Penicillamine 784, generic name of an antirheumatic drug 117 and chelating agent 253

Penicillin G generic name of a penicillin drug 785, an antibiotic drug 113

Penicillin V generic name of a penicillin drug 785, an antibiotic drug 113

Pentaerythritol tetranitrate generic name of a nitrate drug 733

Pentamidine generic name of a drug used to treat trypanosomiasis (1016), and leishmaniasis (634)

Pentazocine 786, generic name of a narcotic drug 720, an analgesic drug 96

Pentobarbital 786, generic name of a barbiturate drug 155

Pentothal brand name for thiopental 982, a fast-acting barbiturate 155 used to induce general anesthesia (103)

Pentoxifylline generic name of a drug used to treat peripheral vascular disease (789)

Pen-Vee brand-name penicillin drug 785, an antibiotic drug 113

Pepcid brand name for famotidine 437, the generic name of a drug used to treat ulcers (1021)

Peppermint oil 786, flavoring used in some drug preparations

Peptol brand name for cimetidine 277, the generic name of a drug used to treat ulcers (1021)

Percocet brand-name drug containing acetaminophen 61, the generic name of a non-narcotic analgesic drug 96, and oxycodone 766, the generic name of a narcotic drug 720, an analgesic drug 96

Percodan brand-name drug containing acetylsalicylic acid 61, a non-narcotic analgesic drug 96, and oxycodone 766, the generic name of a narcotic drug 720

Pergonal brand name for menotropins 680, the generic name of a drug used to treat infertility (582)

Periactin brand name for an appetite stimulant drug 127

Peridol brand name for haloperidol 504, the generic name of an antipsychotic drug 118

Peritrate brand-name nitrate drug 733

Permethrin generic name of a drug used to treat lice (638)

Permitil brand name for fluphenazine 457, the generic name of an antipsychotic drug 118

Perphenazine 791, generic name of a phenothiazine drug 796, an antipsychotic 118 and antiemetic drug 116

Persantine brand name for dipyridamole 359, the generic name of a drug used to treat abnormal blood clotting (182)

Pertofrane brand name for desipramine 343, the generic name of a tricyclic antidepressant drug 115

Peruvian balsam ingredient of some preparations used to treat hemorrhoids (530)

Pethidine 793, generic name of a narcotic analgesic drug 96

Petrolatum another name for petroleum jelly 793, a greasy substance used as an emollient (396)

Petroleum jelly 793, greasy substance used as an emollient (396)

Phenazopyridine 796, generic name of an analgesic drug 96 used to treat urinary tract infections (1030)

Phenelzine 796, generic name of a monoamine oxidase inhibitor, an antidepressant drug 115

Phenergan brand name for promethazine 829, the generic name of an antihistamine drug 117

Pheniramine generic name of an antihistamine drug 117

Phenobarbital 796, generic name of a barbiturate drug 155

Phenol antiseptic 118

Phenolphthalein generic name of a laxative 632

Phenoxymethyl penicillin 796, synthetic penicillin drug 785, an antibiotic drug 113

Phentermine 796, generic name of an appetite suppressant drug 127

Phentolamine generic name of an antihypertensive drug 117

Phenylbutazone 796, generic name of a nonsteroidal anti-inflammatory drug 736

Phenylephrine 796, generic name of a decongestant drug 333

Phenylpropanolamine 796, generic name of a decongestant drug 333

Phenyltoloxamine generic name of an antihistamine drug 117

Phenytoin 796, generic name of an anticonvulsant drug 115

pHisoHex brand-name antiseptic 118

Phyllocontin brand name for aminophylline 93, the generic name of a bronchodilator drug 213

Physostigmine 799, generic name of a drug used for glaucoma (487)

Phytomenadione 799, generic name of a drug that controls bleeding (175)

Pilocarpine 800, generic name of a drug used for glaucoma (487)

Pimozide generic name of a drug used to treat Gilles de la Tourette's syndrome (485)

Pindolol 800, generic name of a beta-blocker drug 163

Piperacillin generic name of a penicillin drug 785, an antibiotic drug 113

Piperazine 801, generic name of a drug used to treat helminth infestation (525) (see worm infestation 1082)

Pipracil brand-name penicillin drug 785, an antibiotic drug 113

Pirenzepine generic name of a drug used to treat peptic ulcers (1021)

Piroxicam 801, generic name of a nonsteroidal anti-inflammatory drug 736

Pitressin brand name for ADH (antidiuretic hormone) 68

Pivampicillin 803, generic name of a penicillin drug 785, an antibiotic drug 113

Pivmecillinam 803, generic name of a penicillin drug 785, an antibiotic drug 113

Pizotyline 803, generic name of a drug used to prevent migraine (690)

Placebo 803, substance containing no medically active ingredient given in place of a drug

Placidyl brand-name sleeping drug 920

Plaquenil brand-name drug used to treat malaria (660) and rheumatoid arthritis (130)

Platinol brand name for an anticancer drug 114

PMS Benztropine brand name for benztropine, the generic name of a drug used to treat parkinsonism (778)

PMS Carbamazepine brand name for carbamazepine 228, the generic name of an anticonvulsant drug 115

PMS Docusate Calcium brand name for docusate, the generic name of a laxative drug 632

PMS Flurazepam brand name for flurazepam 457, the generic name of a benzodiazepine 162

sleeping drug 920

PMS Isoniazid brand name for isoniazid 607, the generic name of a drug used to treat tuberculosis (1016)

PMS Lindane brand name for lindane 641, the generic name of a drug used to treat scabies (886) and lice (638)

PMS Nylidrin brand name for nylidrin, the generic name of a vasodilator drug 1045

PMS Procyclidine brand name for procyclidine 827, the generic name of an anticholinergic drug 114 used to treat parkinsonism (778)

PMS Promethazine Syrup brand name for promethazine 829, the generic name of an antihistamine drug 117

PMS Pyrazinamide brand name for pyrazinamide 846, the generic name of a drug used to treat tuberculosis (1016)

PMS Theophylline brand name for theophylline 981, the generic name of a bronchodilator drug 213

PMS Thioridazine brand name for thioridazine 982, the generic name of an antipsychotic drug 118

PMS Trihexyphenidyl brand name for trihexyphenidyl, the generic name of an anticholinergic drug 114

Podophyllin 810, generic name of a drug used to treat warts (1073)

Polaramine brand-name antihistamine drug 117

Polyvinyl alcohol ingredient in some artificial tear preparations 969

Ponderal brand name for an appetite suppressant drug 127

Pondicillin generic name of a penicillin (785) antibiotic drug 113

Ponstan brand name for mefenamic acid 674, the generic name of a nonsteroidal anti-inflammatory drug 118

Pontocaine brand name for tetracaine 979, the generic name of a local anesthetic (105)

Potassium 817, a mineral 692

Potassium chloride potassium supplement sometimes used with antihypertensive drugs 117

Potassium clavulanate generic name of a drug used to enhance the activity of some antibiotic drugs 113

Potassium gluconate potassium supplement 817

Potassium iodide any expectorant agent (424); also used to treat thyrotoxicosis (563)

Potassium permanganate 817, substance formerly used as an antiseptic 118

Pralidoxime generic name of a drug used to treat poisoning with parathion (777) and certain other pesticides (793)

Pramoxine generic name of a local anesthetic (105)

Praziquantel 818, generic name of a drug used to treat helminth infestation (525) (see worm infestation 1082)

Prazosin 818, generic name of a vasodilator drug 1045

Prednisolone 818, generic name of a corticosteroid drug 309

Prednisone 818, generic name of a corticosteroid drug 309

Prefrin Liquifilm brand name for phenylephrine eye drops 796, the generic name of a decongestant drug 333

Premarin brand-name estrogen drug 418

Primaquine 826, generic name of a drug used to treat malaria (660)

Primidone 827, generic name of an anticonvulsant drug 115

Prioderm brand-name drug used to treat lice (638)

Privine brand name for naphazoline 719, the generic name of a decongestant drug 333

Pro-Banthine brand name for propantheline 829, the generic name of an antispasmodic drug 119

Probenecid 827, generic name of a drug used to treat recurrent attacks of gout (495) and to enhance the effect of some antibiotics 113

Probucol 827, generic name of a lipid-lowering drug 642

Procainamide 827, generic name of an antiarrhythmic drug 113

Procaine 827, generic name of a local anesthetic (105)

Procarbazine 827, generic

name of an anticancer drug 114

Prochlorperazine 827, generic name of a phenothiazine drug 796, an antiemetic drug 116

Procyclid brand name for procyclidine 827, the generic name of an anticholinergic drug 114 used to treat parkinsonism (778)

Procyclidine 827, generic name of an anticholinergic drug 114 used to treat parkinsonism (778)

Progestasert brand-name progestogen drug 828

Progestin another name for a progestogen drug 828 or hormone 544

Proglycem brand-name antihypertensive drug 117

Proguanil 828, generic name of a drug used in treating and preventing malaria (660)

Proloprim brand-name antibiotic drug 113

Promazine 829, generic name of a phenothiazine drug 796, an antipsychotic drug 118

Promethazine 829, generic name of an antihistamine drug 117

Pronestyl brand name for procainamide 827, the generic name of an antiarrhythmic drug 113

Propafenone generic name of an antiarrhythmic drug 113

Propantheline 829, generic name of an antispasmodic drug 119

Propine brand-name eye drops used to treat glaucoma (488)

Propoxyphene 829, generic name of a weak narcotic drug 720, an analgesic drug 96

Propranolol 829, generic name of a beta-blocker drug 163

Propylene glycol substance used as an emollient (396)

Propylthiouracil 829, generic name of a drug used to treat hyperthyroidism (557)

Prostigmin brand name for neostigmine 723, the generic name of a drug used to treat myasthenia gravis (713)

Prostin VR brand name for alprostadil, a prostaglandin drug 830

Protopam brand name for a drug used to treat poisoning with parathion

and certain other pesticides (793)

Protriptyline 833, generic name of an antidepressant drug 115

Protropin brand name for growth hormone 500

Protylol brand name for dicyclomine 354, the generic name of an antispasmodic drug 119

Provera brand name for medroxyprogesterone 673, the generic name of a progestogen drug 828

Prozac brand name for fluoxetine, the generic name of an antidepressant drug 115

Pseudoephedrine 834, generic name of a decongestant drug 333

Psilocybin 834, a hallucinogenic drug 503

Psyllium 839, generic name of a laxative drug 632

Pulmicort brand-name drug used to treat bronchial asthma (136)

Purinethol brand name for an anticancer drug 114

Pyopen brand-name penicillin antibiotic 113

Pyrantel 846, generic name of a drug used to treat helminth infestation (525) (see worm infestation 1082)

Pyrazinamide 846, generic name of a drug used to treat tuberculosis (1016)

Pyribenzamine brand-name antihistamine drug 117

Pyridium brand name for phenazopyridine 796, the generic name of an analgesic drug 96 used in the treatment of urinary tract infections (1030)

Pyridostigmine 846, generic name of a drug used to treat myasthenia gravis (713)

Pyridoxine 846, another name for vitamin B_6 complex 1062

Pyrimethamine 846, generic name of a drug used to treat malaria (660) and toxoplasmosis (1004)

Pyrvinium generic name of a drug used to treat helminth infestation (525) (see worm infestation 1082)

Q

Questran brand name for

cholestyramine 271, the generic name of a lipid-lowering drug 642

Quibron-T brand name for theophylline 981, the generic name of a bronchodilator drug 213

Quinacrine 847, generic name of a drug primarily used to treat giardiasis (485)

Quinaglute brand name for quinidine 847, the generic name of an antiarrhythmic drug 113

Quinate brand name for quinidine 847, the generic name of an antiarrhythmic drug 113

Quinidine 847, generic name of an antiarrhythmic drug 113

Quinine 847, generic name of a drug used to treat malaria (660) and leg cramps (315)

R

Ranitidine 855, generic name of a drug used to treat ulcers (1021)

Reglan brand name for metoclopramide 687, the generic name of an antiemetic drug 116

Regonol brand name for pyridostigmine 846, the generic name of a drug used to treat myasthenia gravis (713)

Reserpine 866, generic name of an antihypertensive drug 117

Resorcinol generic name of a chemical used to treat acne (63) and dermatitis (342)

Restoril brand name for temazepam 971, the generic name of a benzodiazepine sleeping drug 162

Retin-A brand-name drug used to treat acne (63)

Retinoic acid derivative of vitamin A 1060

Retinol 872, principal form of vitamin A 1060

Retrovir brand name for zidovudine 1090, the generic name of an antiviral drug 119 used to treat AIDS (76)

Rhinalar brand-name corticosteroid nasal spray 309

Rhodis brand name for ketoprofen 615, the generic name of a nonsteroidal anti-

inflammatory drug 736

Ribavirin generic name of an antiviral drug 119

Riboflavin 878, another name for vitamin B₂ 1061

Ridaura brand name for auranofin 142, the generic name of an antirheumatic drug 117

Rifampin 878, generic name of an antibacterial drug 113

Rimactane brand name for rifampin 878, the generic name of an antibacterial drug 113

Rimso-50 brand-name drug used to treat cystitis (325)

Ritalin brand-name central nervous system stimulant (945)

Ritodrine 879, generic name of a drug used to delay premature labor (260)

Rivotril brand name for clonazepam 281, a benzodiazepine drug (162) primarily used to treat epilepsy (409)

Robaxin brand name for methocarbamol 686, the generic name of a muscle-relaxant drug 710

Robidone brand name for hydrocodone, the generic name of a narcotic drug 720 used mainly in cough remedies 314

Robidrine brand name for pseudoephedrine 834, the generic name of a decongestant drug 333

Robinul brand-name anticholinergic 114 and antispasmodic drug 119

Robitussin brand name for guaifenesin 500, the generic name of an expectorant 424

Rocephin brand-name cephalosporin 244, an antibiotic drug 113

Rogaine brand name for a vasodilator drug 1045, used topically to stimulate hair growth (502)

Rogitine brand-name antihypertensive drug 117

Rouphylline brand name for oxtriphylline 766, the generic name of a bronchodilator drug 213

Rythmodan brand name for disopyramide 362, the generic name of an antiarrhythmic drug 113

Rythmol brand name for propafenone, the generic name of an antiarrhythmic drug 113

S

Saccharin 882, an artificial sweetener (134)

Salazopyrin brand name for a drug used to treat inflammatory bowel disease (587)

Salbutamol 883, generic name of a bronchodilator drug 213

Salicylic acid 883, a keratolytic drug 614

Salofalk brand-name drug used to treat inflammatory bowel disease (587)

Sandimmune brand-name immunosuppressant drug 575

Sandomigran brand name for a drug used to prevent migraine (690)

Sanorex brand name for an appetite suppressant drug 127

Sansert brand name for methysergide, the generic name of a drug used to prevent migraine (690)

SAS-500 brand name for a drug used to treat inflammatory bowel disease (587)

Scopolamine 889, generic name of an antispasmodic drug 119

Sebulex brand-name preparation containing salicylic acid 883, the generic name of a keratolytic drug 614, and sulfur 957, a mineral 692

Sebulon brand-name shampoo used to treat dandruff (329)

Secobarbital 894, generic name of a barbiturate drug 155

Seconal brand-name for secobarbital 894, the generic name of a barbiturate drug 155

Sectral brand name for acebutolol 61, the generic name of a beta-blocker drug 163

Seldane brand name for terfenadine 975, the generic name of an antihistamine drug 117

Selegiline 894, generic name of a drug used to treat parkinsonism (778)

Selenium sulfide agent used to treat dandruff (329) and tinea versicolor (992)

Selexid brand-name penicillin 785 antibiotic drug 113

Selsun brand-name preparation used to treat

dandruff (329) and tinea versicolor (992)

Senna 895, generic name of a stimulant laxative drug 632

Septra brand name for an antibacterial 113 compound of sulfamethoxazole 957, and trimethoprim 113

Serax brand name for oxazepam 766, the generic name of a benzodiazepine 162 antianxiety drug 113

Serentil brand-name antipsychotic drug 118

Serpasil brand name for reserpine 866, the generic name of an antihypertensive drug 117

Sertan brand name for primidone 827, the generic name of an anticonvulsant drug 115

Silver nitrate 910, an astringent 138

Silver sulfadiazine 910, generic name of an antibacterial drug 113

Simethicone 910, generic name of a drug used to relieve flatulence (455)

Sinemet brand-name drug used to treat parkinsonism (778)

Sinequan brand name for doxepin 369, a tricyclic antidepressant drug 115

Sintrom brand name for an anticoagulant drug 115

Slo-Bid brand name for theophylline 981, the generic name of a bronchodilator drug 213

Slow-Trasicor brand name for oxprenolol 766, the generic name of a beta-blocker drug 163

Slow-Fe brand name for ferrous sulfate 442, an iron supplement 605

Slow-K brand name for potassium chloride 817

Sodium bicarbonate 925, an antacid drug 112

Sodium cromoglycate 925, generic name of a drug primarily used to prevent asthma (136)

Sodium fluoride form of fluoride 457

Sodium iodide form of iodine 604 used to treat hyperthyroidism (557) and thyroid cancer (987)

Sodium salicylate 925, generic name of a nonsteroidal anti-inflammatory drug 736

Solganal brand-name antirheumatic drug 117

Solium brand name for chlordiazepoxide 267, the generic name of a benzodiazepine 162 antianxiety drug 113

Solu-Cortef brand name for hydrocortisone 549, the generic name of a corticosteroid drug 309

Solu-Medrol brand name for methylprednisolone 687, the generic name of a corticosteroid drug 309

Soma brand name for carisoprodol 235, the generic name of a muscle-relaxant drug 710

Somnol brand name for flurazepam 457, the generic name of a benzodiazepine 162 sleeping drug 920

Somophyllin brand name for aminophylline 93, the generic name of a bronchodilator drug 213

Sotacor brand name for a beta-blocker drug 163

Sotalol generic name of a beta-blocker drug 163

Spasmoban brand name for dicyclomine 354, the generic name of an antispasmodic drug 119

Spectinomycin generic name of an antibiotic drug 113

Spironolactone 935, generic name of a potassium-sparing diuretic drug 363

Stanozolol 941, generic name of an anabolic steroid drug 944

Stelazine brand name for trifluoperazine 1013, the generic name of an antipsychotic drug 118

Stemetil brand name for prochlorperazine 827, the generic name of a phenothiazine 796, an antiemetic drug 116

Stilbestrol 945, see diethylstilbestrol 335, the generic name of an estrogen drug 418

Stoxil brand name for idoxuridine eye ointment 565, the generic name of an antiviral drug 119

Streptase brand name for streptokinase 948, the generic name of a thrombolytic drug 984

Streptokinase 948, generic name of a thrombolytic drug 984

Streptomycin 948, generic name of an antibiotic drug 113

Streptozocine generic name of an anticancer drug 114

Succinylcholine generic name of a muscle-relaxant drug 710

Sucralfate 955, drug used to treat peptic ulcers (786)

Sudafed brand name for pseudoephedrine 834, the generic name of a decongestant drug 333

Sulcrate brand name for a drug used to treat peptic ulcers (786)

Sulfacetamide 957, generic name of an antibacterial drug 113

Sulfadiazine generic name of an antibacterial drug 113

Sulfamethoxazole 957, generic name of an antibacterial drug 113

Sulfamylon brand name for a topical antibacterial drug 113

Sulfasalazine 957, generic name of a drug used to treat inflammatory bowel disease (587)

Sulfinpyrazone 957, generic name of a drug used to treat gout (495)

Sulfisoxazole 957, generic name of an antibacterial drug 113

Sulfur 957, a mineral 692

Sulindac 957, generic name of a nonsteroidal anti-inflammatory drug 736

Supeudol brand name for oxycodone 766, the generic name of a narcotic drug 720, an analgesic drug 96

Supres brand-name antihypertensive drug 117, containing chlorothiazide, the generic name of a thiazide diuretic drug 363, and methyldopa 687, the generic name of an antihypertensive drug 117

Surgam brand name for a nonsteroidal anti-inflammatory drug 736

Surmontil brand name for trimipramine, the generic name of an antidepressant drug 115

Symmetrel brand name for amantadine 91, the generic name of an antiviral drug 119

Synalar brand name for fluocinolone 456, the generic name of a corticosteroid drug 309

Synkavite brand name for vitamin K 1064

Synthroid brand name for levothyroxine 638, the generic name of a thyroid hormone (989)

Syntocinon brand name for oxytocin 767, a pituitary hormone (544) used to induce labor (580)

T

TACE brand-name estrogen drug used to treat cancer 115

Tagamet brand name for cimetidine 277, the generic name of a drug used to treat ulcers 1021

Talwin brand name for pentazocine 786, the generic name of a narcotic drug 720, an analgesic drug 96

Tambocor brand name for flecainide, the generic name of an antiarrhythmic drug 113

Tamoxifen 966, generic name of an anticancer drug 114

Tantum brand-name drug used to treat acute sore throat (927)

Tapazole brand name for methimazole 686, the generic name of a drug used to treat hyperthyroidism 557

Tarasan brand name for an antipsychotic drug 118

Tebrazid brand name for pyrazinamide 846, the generic name of a drug used to treat tuberculosis (1016)

Teejel brand-name topical anesthetic used in the mouth (700)

Tegison brand-name drug used to treat psoriasis (835)

Tegopen brand name for cloxacillin 281, the generic name of a penicillin drug 785 antibiotic drug 113

Tegretol brand name for carbamazepine 228, the generic name of an anticonvulsant drug 115

Telepaque brand-name compound used in diagnostic imaging (567)

Temazepam 971, generic name of a benzodiazepine sleeping drug 162

Temposil brand-name drug used to treat alcohol dependence (81)

Teniposide generic name of an anticancer drug 114

Tenoretic brand-name drug containing atenolol 139, the generic name of a beta-blocker drug 163, and chlorthalidone 268, the generic name of a thiazide diuretic drug 363, an antihypertensive drug 117

Tenormin brand name for atenolol 139, the generic name of a beta-blocker drug 163

Tenuate brand name for phentermine 796, the generic name of an appetite suppressant drug 127

Terazosin generic name of an antihypertensive drug 117

Terbutaline 974, generic name of a bronchodilator drug 213

Terfenadine 975, generic name of an antihistamine drug 117

Tessalon brand-name cough suppressant 314

Testosterone 997, androgen hormone 98

Tetracaine 979, generic name of a local anesthetic (105)

Tetracycline generic name of an antibiotic drug 113

Tetracyn brand-name tetracycline drug 979, an antibiotic drug 113

Tetrahydroaminoacridine 979, generic name of a drug used to treat Alzheimer's disease (90)

Theo-Dur brand name for theophylline 981, the generic name of a bronchodilator drug 213

Theophylline 981, generic name of a bronchodilator drug 213

Thiabendazole 982, generic name of a drug used to treat helminth infestation (525) (see worm infestation 1082)

Thiamine 982, another name for vitamin B$_1$

Thiethylperazine generic name of an antiemetic drug 116

Thioguanine generic name of an anticancer drug 114

Thiopental 982, generic name of a barbiturate drug 155

Thioridazine 982, generic name of an antipsychotic drug 118

Thiotepa generic name of an anticancer drug 114

Thiothixene 982, generic name of an antipsychotic drug 118

Tiaprofenic acid 991, generic name of a nonsteroidal anti-inflammatory drug 736

Ticar brand-name penicillin 785 antibiotic drug 113

Ticarcillin generic name of a penicillin drug 785, an antibiotic drug 113

Ticlopidine generic name of a drug used to prevent blood clotting (182)

Timolide brand-name

drug containing hydrochlorothiazide 549, the generic name of a thiazide diuretic drug 363, and timolol 992, the generic name of a beta-blocker drug 163

Timolol 992, generic name of a beta-blocker drug 163

Timoptic brand name for timolol eye drops 992, the generic name of a beta-blocker drug 163

Tinactin brand name for tolnaftate 998, the generic name of an antifungal drug 117

Tioconazole generic name of an antifungal drug 117

Tissue-plasminogen activator 994, generic name of a thrombolytic drug 984

Tobramycin 996, generic name of an antibiotic drug 113

Tobrex brand name for tobramycin eye drops 996, the generic name of an antibiotic drug 113

Tocainide 997, generic name of an antiarrhythmic drug 113

Tofranil brand name for imipramine 569, the generic name of an antidepressant drug 115

Tolbutamide 998, generic name of a hypoglycemic drug 559

Tolectin brand name for tolmetin 998, the generic name of a nonsteroidal anti-inflammatory drug 736

Tolmetin 998, generic name of a nonsteroidal anti-inflammatory drug 736

Tolnaftate 998, generic name of an antifungal drug 117

Tonocard brand name for tocainide 997, the generic name of an antiarrhythmic drug 113

Topicort brand-name corticosteroid drug 309

Torecan brand-name antiemetic drug 116

TPA 1004, abbreviation for tissue-plasminogen activator 994, the generic name of a thrombolytic drug 984

Trancopal brand-name antianxiety drug 113

Trandate brand name for labetalol 625, the generic name of a beta-blocker drug 163

Transderm-Nitro brand name for nitroglycerin 734, the generic name of a

vasodilator drug 1045

Transderm-V brand name for scopolamine 891, the generic name of an antispasmodic drug 119

Tranxene brand name for clorazepate 981, the generic name of an antianxiety drug 113

Tranylcypromine 1009, generic name of a monoamine-oxidase inhibitor antidepressant drug 115

Trasicor brand name for oxprenolol 766, the generic name of a beta-blocker drug 163

Trazodone 1010, generic name of an antidepressant drug 115

Trental brand name for pentoxifylline, the generic name of a drug used to treat peripheral vascular disease 789

Tretinoin 1011, generic name of a drug used to treat acne (63)

Triadapin brand name for doxepin 369, a tricyclic antidepressant drug 115

Triamcinolone 1012, generic name of a corticosteroid drug 309

Triamterene 1012, generic name of a potassium-sparing diuretic 363

Triavil brand-name drug containing amitriptyline 93, the generic name of an antidepressant drug 115, and perphenazine 791, the generic name of a phenothiazine drug 796

Triazolam 1012, generic name of a benzodiazepine sleeping drug 162

Trichloroacetic acid liquid used to treat warts (1072)

Triclosan antiseptic 118

Tridesilon brand-name corticosteroid drug 309

Triethylenetetramine generic name of a chelating agent (253) used to treat Wilson's disease (1080)

Trifluoperazine 1013, generic name of an antipsychotic drug 118

Trifluridine 1013, generic name of an ophthalmic antiviral drug 119

Trihexyphenidyl generic name of an anticholinergic drug 114

Trilafon brand name for perphenazine 791, the generic name of a phenothiazine drug 796, an antipsychotic 118 and antiemetic drug 116

Trilisate brand-name drug used to treat arthritis (130)

Trimeprazine generic name of an antihistamine drug 117

Trimethoprim generic name of an antibiotic drug 113

Trimipramine generic name of an antidepressant drug 115

Tripelennamine generic name of an antihistamine drug 117

Triphasil brand-name oral contraceptive 751

Triprolidine generic name of an antihistamine drug 117

Triptil brand-name antidepressant drug 115

Trisoralen brand-name psoralen drug 835 used to treat PUVA (845)

Trobicin brand-name antibiotic drug 113

Tronothane brand name for a local anesthetic (105)

Tropicacyl brand name for tropicamide 1016, the generic name of a drug used to dilate the pupil (844)

Tropicamide 1016, generic name of a drug used to dilate the pupil (844)

Trosyd brand-name antifungal drug 112

Tryptan brand-name antidepressant drug 115

Tryptophan 1016, generic name of an antidepressant drug 115

Tubocurarine generic name of a muscle-relaxant drug 710 used in general anesthesia (103)

Tuinal brand-name barbiturate 155 sleeping drug 920

Tylenol brand name for acetaminophen 61, the generic name of a non-narcotic analgesic drug 96

U

Undecylenic acid generic name of a topical antifungal drug 117

Unipen brand-name penicillin drug 785, an antibiotic drug 113

Uniphyl brand name for theophylline 981, the generic name of a bronchodilator drug 213

Urecholine brand-name drug used to treat urinary retention (1029)

Urispas brand name for urinary tract antispasmodic drug 119

Uritol brand name for furosemide 469, the generic name of a loop diuretic drug 363

Urokinase 1033, generic name of a thrombolytic drug 984

V

Valisone brand name for betamethasone 164, the generic name of a corticosteroid drug 309

Valium brand name for diazepam 354, the generic name of a benzodiazepine 162 antianxiety drug 113

Valproic acid 1041, generic name of an anticonvulsant drug 115

Vancocin brand name for vancomycin 1042, the generic name of an antibiotic drug 113

Vancomycin 1042, generic name of an antibiotic drug 113

Vanquin brand name for a drug used to treat helminth infestation (525) (see worm infestation 1082)

Vasodilan brand name for isoxsuprine 607, the generic name of a vasodilator drug 1045

Vasopressin 1045, generic name of a drug used to treat diabetes insipidus (346)

Vasotec brand name for enalapril 397, the generic name of an ACE inhibitor drug 61

V-Cillin K brand-name penicillin drug 785, an antibiotic drug 113

Vecuronium generic name of a muscle-relaxant drug 710

Velosef brand-name cephalosporin 244, an antibiotic drug 113

Ventolin brand name for salbutamol 883, the generic name of a bronchodilator drug 213

Vepesid brand name for an anticancer drug 114

Verapamil 1050, generic name of a calcium-channel blocker 221

Vermox brand name for mebendazole 670, the generic name of a drug to treat helminth infestation (525) (see worm infestation 1082)

Versed   brand name for a benzodiazepine drug 162 used for premedication (822)

Vibramycin   brand name for doxycycline 369, the generic name of a tetracycline drug 979, an antibiotic drug 113

Vibra-Tabs   brand name for doxycycline 369, the generic name of a tetracycline drug 979, an antibiotic drug 113

Vidarabine   generic name of an antiviral drug 119

Vincristine   generic name of an anticancer drug 114

Vioform   brand-name antibacterial 113 and antifungal drug 117

Vira-A   brand-name antiviral drug 119

Virazole   brand name for an antiviral drug 119

Viroptic   brand name for trifluridine eye drops 1013, the generic name of an antiviral drug 119

Viscorex   brand-name mucolytic drug 704

Visken   brand name for pindolol 800, the generic name of a beta-blocker drug 63

Vistacrom   brand name for anti-allergic eye drops 426

Vivol   brand name for diazepam 354, the generic name of a benzodiazepine

162 antianxiety drug 113

Voltaren   brand name for diclofenac 354, a nonsteroidal anti-inflammatory drug 736

Vontrol   brand-name antiemetic drug 116

Vumon   brand name for an anticancer drug 114

W

Warfarin   1072, generic name of an anticoagulant drug 115

Winpred   brand name for prednisone 818, the generic name of a corticosteroid drug 309

WinRh$_0$ brand name for anti-D(Rh$_0$) immunoglobulin 574

Winstrol   brand name for stanozolol 941, the generic name of an anabolic steroid drug 944

Witch hazel   mild astringent 138

Wycillin   brand-name penicillin drug 785, an antibiotic drug 113

Wydase   brand-name enzyme used to enhance the absorption and dispersion of injected drugs 373

X

Xanax   brand name for alprazolam 88, the generic name of a benzodiazepine antianxiety drug 113

Xylocaine   brand name for lidocaine 639, the generic name of a local anesthetic (105)

Xylocard   brand name for lidocaine 639, the generic name of a local anesthetic (105)

Xylometazoline   1087, generic name of a decongestant drug 333

Y

Yocon   brand-name antihypertensive drug 117

Yohimbine   generic name of an antihypertensive drug 117

Yutopar   brand name for a drug used to delay premature labor (260)

Z

Zanosar   brand-name

anticancer drug 114

Zantac   brand name for ranitidine 855, the generic name of a drug used to treat ulcers (1021)

Zapex   brand name for oxazepam 766, the generic name of a benzodiazepine 162 antianxiety drug 113

Zarontin   brand name for ethosuximide 419, the generic name of an anticonvulsant drug 115

Zaroxolyn   brand name for metolazone 687, the generic name of a thiazidelike diuretic drug 363

Zephiran   brand-name antiseptic 118

Zetar   brand name for coal tar 282, the generic name of an ingredient in some preparations for skin disorders (917)

Zidovudine   1090, generic name of an antiviral drug 119 used to treat AIDS (76)

Zinacef   brand-name cephalosporin antibiotic 113

Zinc gluconate   compound of zinc 1090

Zinc sulfate   astringent 138

Zovirax   brand-name antiviral drug 119

Zyloprim   brand name for allopurinol 87, the generic name of a drug used to treat gout (495)

INDEX

This index covers the encyclopedia sections: **Medicine Today**, **A to Z of Medicine**, and **Drug Glossary**. **Self-help Organizations** (pages 1092-1096) are not included. Most index entries with an initial capital correspond to titles of entries in **Medicine Today** or **A to Z of Medicine**. Other index entries with an initial capital refer you to a **Drug Glossary** entry. Except for a few capitalized abbreviations or eponyms, all other index entries have a lower-case first letter. *Italic* type refers you to illustrations.

1118

1121

C

E

1146

1157

1171

Legionnaires' disease 633;

S

1181

PHOTOGRAPHIC CREDITS

American Society of Plastic and Reconstructive Surgeons, Inc. *177, 431, 763*; AMI Portland Hospital (Ultrasound Dept.) *821*; Argentum *465, 941, 954, 981, 1073, 1085*

Mr. John Browett *539, 623, 1088*; BUPA Medical Centre *203, 663*

Cemax Inc. *1088*; Dr. M. Curling *249, 328*

Dr. Richard Dawood *157, 191, 1087, 1088*; Prof. P. Dieppe and Gower Medical Publishing *495*; Dorling Kindersley (DK)/Steve Bartholomew *21, 40*; DK/Paul Fletcher *1092*; DK/ Stephan Oliver *21, 36, 39*; DK/ Susanna Price *24, 30, 31, 38*; DK/ Clive Streeter *17, 18, 19*; Dr. R. Doshi, Brook Green Hospital *200, 489*; Dr. Andrew Duncombe, St. Thomas's Hospital Medical School *184, 637*

Edwards Laboratories, Orange County, California *523*

Dr. T. Fowler *90, 197*

Gibbs Dental Division *360, 806*; Glaxo *387, 877*; Mr. Brian Glenville *307*

Health Education Authority *22*

The Image Bank *17, 42*; Institute of Orthopaedics, London *75, 738,758, 759, 761, 874, 1088*

Mr. P.H. Jacobson, Dental School, Cardiff *211*; Dr. J.R. Jenner *361*; Mr. R.P. Juniper *1081*

KeyMed Ltd. *36, 214, 327, 586, 787, 910*

Sue Lloyd *486, 789*; London School of Hygiene and Tropical Medicine *634, 661, 921*

Dr. Francis Matthey *102, 181, 930*; Nancy Durrell McKenna *190, 195, 205, 254, 261, 570*; Penny Miller/ Down's Syndrome Association *369*; Lorraine Miller, Hammersmith Hospital *191*

National Medical Slide Bank *194, 250, 430, 446, 468, 493, 504, 514, 520, 555, 629, 631, 633, 634, 651, 653, 657, 691, 697, 706, 720, 764, 784, 823, 845, 878, 907, 931, 941, 951, 953, 963, 981, 992, 1001, 1025, 1033, 1043, 1080, 1085*

Vincent Oliver *160*

Philips Medical Systems *32*

Queen Elizabeth Military Hospital, Woolwich (Histopathology Dept., Jogn Boyd Laboratories) *243, 379*; Queen Square Imaging Centre/ BUPA *703*

Dr. I.R. Reynolds, Eastman Dental Hospital *662, 756, 765*; Adrian Roberts *48*

Saga Holidays Ltd. *17*; Science Photo Library (SPL) *25, 32, 34, 465, 586, 739, 766, 1017*; SPL/Michael Abbey *23*; SPL/Argentum *1086*; SPL/ Dr. Tony Brain *502, 689*; SPL/ Dr. Goran Bredberg *513*; SPL/CDC *48*; SPL/CEA-Orsay/ CNRI *35, 793*; SPL/CNRI *33, 35, 46, 134, 806, 1047*; SPL/Dr. R. Damadian *34*; SPL/ Division of Computer Research and Technology, National Institutes of Health *37*; SPL/Martin Dohrn *45*; SPL/Don Fawcett *572*; SPL/Fawcett/ Hirokawa/ Heuser *1052*; SPL/Prof. C..Ferlaud/ CNRI *1065*; SPL/Malcolm Fielding, The BOC Group PLC *44*; SPL/Grave *1002*; SPL/Jan Hinsch *275, 276*; SPL/Manfred Kage *36, 182*; SPL/David Leah *579*; SPL/Francis Leroy *444*; SPL/R. Litchfield *86*; SPL/London School of Hygiene and Tropical Medicine *582*; SPL/Andrew McClenaghan *42*; SPL/Astrid and Hans-Frieder Michler *23, 728*; SPL/Mark Morgan *621*; SPL/Ohio-Nuclear Corporation *33*; SPL/ Omikron *968*; SPL/David Parker *43, 298*; SPL/Nestlé *394*; SPL/Philippe Plailly *853*; SPL/John Radcliffe Hospital *1021*; SPL/David Scharf *689*; SPL/Dr. Karol Sikora *226,940*; SPL/Dr. Howard Smedley *852*; SPL/St. Bartholomew's Hospital *388*; SPL/St. Mary's Hospital *244*; SPL/Dr. Rob Stepney *46*; SPL/James Stevenson *46, 495, 691, 966*; SPL/Alexander Tsiaras *35, 47, 132*; SPL/USDA *460*; SPL/US National Cancer Institute *78*; SPL/John Walsh *689, 929*; SPL/Don Wong *427*; SPL/J.F. Wilson *1064*; Prof. Crispian Scully, Dental School, University of Bristol *235, 339, 970*; Squibb Surgicare Ltd. *290, 566*; St. Bartholomew's Hospital *160, 167, 216, 241, 243, 270, 315, 393, 401, 576, 613, 623, 676, 809, 811, 919, 1014, 1023, 1072, 1073, 1088*; St. John's Institute of Dermatology *64, 80, 172, 342, 962*; St. Mary's Hospital Medical School (Audio Visual Services) *140, 233, 343, 364, 520, 624, 654, 655, 835, 893, 915, 950, 971, 986, 991, 1005, 1088, 1089, 1091*; Tony Stone/Chris Harvey *16*; Tony Stone/David Joel *39*; Ron Sutherland *25*; Dr. Paul Sweny *174, 222, 321, 350, 568, 620, 644, 1031*

University of Washington School of Medicine/The Lancet *81*; John Watney *80, 278*; C. James Webb *545, 1012, 1029*; Dr. David Wheeler *350*; Dr. A.R. Williams, Charing Cross and Westminster Medical School *549*; Dr. I. Williams *64, 108, 131, 141, 217, 286, 377, 388, 414, 423, 462, 472, 536, 624, 718, 748, 759, 774, 812, 839, 914, 916, 1021,1075*; Woman's Health Concern *660*

Col. Robert M. Youngson *127, 238, 253, 318, 387, 426, 665, 839*

ADDITIONAL CREDITS

Table on page 60 from *Health reports*, Table 12, Catalogue No. 820003, 1989, Vol. 1, No. 1, Statistics Canada. Reproduced with permission.

RESEARCH ACKNOWLEDGMENTS

Reader's Digest acknowledges with thanks the assistance of the following: Acupuncture Foundation of Canada; Addiction Research Foundation; Agriculture Canada (Pesticide Directorate); American Cancer Society; ASTRA Pharmatex; Jack Bernstein, B.Sc, D.D.S.; Pierre Biron, M.D., M.Sc; Canadian Cancer Society; Canadian Centre for Occupational Health and Safety; Canadian Heart Foundation; Canadian Labour Congress; Canadian National Institute for the Blind; Canadian Red Cross; N. L. Cassar M.D.; John P. Collins, M.D.; Henry Goldenberg, D.PH., L.PH.; George Harpur, M.D.; Tobi Louise Harpur; Health and Welfare Canada (Bureau of Biologics, Bureau of Chemical Safety, Bureau of Human Prescription Drugs, Bureau of Non-Prescription Drugs, Chemical Evaluation Division, Communicable Diseases, Epidemiology, Communications Directorate, Emergency Drugs Section, Federal Centre for AIDS, Food Directorate, Health Protection Branch, Laboratory Centre for Disease Control, Nutrition Research Division, Occupational Toxicology Research Section, Youth Protection Bureau); Healthco (Canada); Heart and Stroke Foundation of Canada; Hôpital Notre Dame, Montreal (Département d'audiologie et orthophonie); House of Commons Information Service; Journal Branch of the Senate; Labour Canada (Industrial Statistics Division; Occupational Safety and Health); Prof. Elizabeth Lambie, School of Nursing, Dalhousie University; Royal Victoria Hospital, Montreal (Department of Dietetics); Montreal General Hospital (Judy Tremblay, Department of Nuclear Medicine); National Cancer Institute (US); National Institute of Nutrition; McCain Foods Ltd.; Louis O'Dea, M.B., B.A.O., B.CH., F.R.C.P.(C); Ontario Department of Health; Ottawa Civic Hospital; Pointe Claire CPR Program; Senate Information Service; Statistical Reference Centre; Statistics Canada; US Library of the Census Bureau (International Population Reference Bureau); Vitamin Information Centre; Wyeth Pharmaceuticals.

Dorling Kindersley would like to thank the following organizations, departments, and companies for their help: Alcoholics Anonymous; ASH; British Association of Electrolysists; British Dental Association; British Nutrition Foundation; BUPA; Department of Health; Institute of Chiropodists; IPPF; Office of Population Censuses and Surveys; Olympus Optical Co.; Royal National Institute for the Blind; Thorn EMI; Women against Rape.